THE PHYSIOLOGIC

BASIS OF

SURGERY

Second Edition

THE PHYSIOLOGIC
BASIS OF
SURGERY

Second Edition

EDITED BY

J. Patrick O'Leary, M.D., F.A.C.S.

The Isidore Cohn Jr. Professor and Chairman of Surgery
Louisiana State University School of Medicine
New Orleans, Louisiana

ASSOCIATE EDITOR

Lea Rhea Capote, B.G.S.

Coordinator, Surgical Education
Louisiana State University School of Medicine
New Orleans, Louisiana

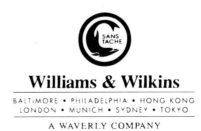

Williams & Wilkins

BALTIMORE • PHILADELPHIA • HONG KONG
LONDON • MUNICH • SYDNEY • TOKYO

A WAVERLY COMPANY

Editor: Carroll C. Cann
Managing Editor: Susan Hunsberger
Production Coordinator: Peter J. Carley
Copy Editor: Kathy Gilbert
Illustration Planner: Peter J. Carley
Typesetter: Maryland Composition
Printer: Maple Press
Digitized Illustrations: Maryland Composition
Binder: Maple Press

Copyright © 1996 Williams & Wilkins

351 West Camden Street
Baltimore, Maryland 21201-2436 USA

Rose Tree Corporate Center
1400 North Providence Road
Building II, Suite 5025
Media, Pennsylvania 19063-2043 USA

Accurate indications, adverse reactions and dosage schedules for drugs are provided in this book, but it is possible that they may change. The reader is urged to review the package information data of the manufacturers of the medications mentioned.

Printed in the United States of America

Second Edition,

Library of Congress Cataloging-in-Publication Data

The physiologic basis of surgery / edited by J. Patrick O'Leary ;
    assistant editor, Lea Rhea Capote.
        p.   cm.
        Includes bibliographical references and index.
        ISBN 0-683-06634-X
        1. Physiology, Pathological.   2. Surgery—Physiological aspects.
    3. Human physiology.   I. O'Leary, J. Patrick, 1941–
    II. Capote, Lea Rhea.
        [DNLM: 1. Surgery.   2. Physiology.   WO 102 P5782   1993]
    RB113.P473   1996
    617—dc20
    DNLKM/DLC   93-17306
    for Library of Congress   CIP

The publishers have made every effort to trace the copyright holders for borrowed material. If they have inadvertently overlooked any, they will be pleased to make the necessary arrangements at the first opportunity.

To purchase additional copies of this book, call our customer service department at **(800) 638-0672** or fax orders to **(800) 447-8438**. For other book services, including chapter reprints and large quantity sales, ask for the Special Sales department.

Canadian customers should call **(800) 268-4178** or **(905) 470-6780**. For all other calls originating outside the United States, please call **(410) 528-4223** or fax us at **(410) 528-8550**.

Visit Williams & Wilkins on the Internet: **http://www.wwilkins.com** or contact our customer service department at **custserv@ wwilkins.com**. Williams & Wilkins customer service representatives are available from 8:30 am to 6:00 pm, EST, Monday through Friday, for telephone access.

95 96 97 98 99
1 2 3 4 5 6 7 8 9 10

To all surgery residents
past, present, and future

Preface for Second Edition

Gratification comes to each individual in slightly different ways. For the teacher there can be no greater sense of achievement than to watch the awakening of understanding in a student as they grasp a new concept or, more importantly, the relationship between two previously known facts. For the editor or the author, the production of the tome is clearly the end product of the work. This product is tangible, has form, substance, occupies space, and has a certain attractiveness to it that is magnified by a sense of ownership or achievement. It is not the tangible product that produces the ultimate long lasting gratification, rather it is seeing the product picked up, read, and incorporated into a life long learning pattern. It is seeing the resident who has spent time delving into the book emerge from the encounter with a fresh understanding and perhaps new knowledge. Nothing in *The Physiologic Basis of Surgery (PBS)* is new. In fact, most every resident in surgery during their medical school experience probably heard these concepts and this rhetoric any number of times. The real purpose of the project was to collapse mountains of information into a reasonable volume that was structured by surgeons in such a way that surgeons-in-training would be able to assimilate those important basic science concepts inherent in the treatment of patients with disease. It was not the purpose of this book to present knowledge for knowledge's sake, but to present salient information that provides the underpinning for an understanding of the patient's disease process. It is only when an understanding of such basic principles reaches a certain critical level that true understanding of disease processes can be attained.

I have heard it said by many residents that spending time on basic science studies is a waste of effort. I contend, however, that it is only when a resident is substantially grounded in basic science that he begins to have a true understanding of disease and is not memorizing a certain litany of arcane signs and symptoms signifying disease.

As discussed in the preface of the first edition, this project was sponsored by the Association of Program Directors in Surgery (APDS) and was in response to a movement in the American Board of Surgery which had hoped to emphasize the basic science curriculum in residency training programs. Although implementation of some of the suggestions by the American Board of Surgery did not occur, the American Board of Surgery In Training Examination (ABSITE) was modified so that basic science topics were emphasized. Because there was no standardized text on the market to serve as a benchmark for residents in training or for the individuals making up the examination, there was a great deal of variability among items in the test, as to how well residents performed on the examination. It would now appear that the *PBS* has demonstrated a substantial penetration into the market with almost as many volumes sold as there are residents currently in categorical positions in the country.

The second edition responds to several criticisms that were couched in a very constructive way by Dr. Francis Moore in his review of the first volume in *The New England Journal of Medicine,* and by Dr. George Higgins, now deceased, in a personal letter. Topics such as shock, fluid and electrolytes, and reproductive physiology have been added. Some chapters have been modified slightly, while other chapters have undergone a near complete revision.

Whenever someone does something for the first time they always silently marvel at their accomplishments. As time passes and experience grows, the individual often begins to realize that although the first foray was a worthy effort, with practice comes refinement and often improvement. So it is with *PBS.* The second edition is an improvement over the first edition in many ways. The most important difference is probably in the computer program that will be a part of the overall package. The multiple choice questions that were included in the first packet have been expanded to include a discussion of each distractor and why the correct answer was chosen by the author. The questions and text are now available together on CD ROM allowing a complete interactive interface for the resident. This will allow a full description of the circumstances surrounding each question. Although this is still a fledgling attempt to use the power of computers to enhance self learning, it is a step in the proper direction.

Acknowledgment

In the acknowledgments that preceded the first edition, a number of people were identified. Each of those individuals has continued to be supportive and each has continued to be integral to the process. As is frequently the case, several individuals were not named in the acknowledgment that should have been mentioned. Probably the most serious omission was the contributions of Dr. Robert Berry of Roanoke, Virginia. Dr. Berry has served as both president and member of the executive committee of the APDS.

The real power behind the production of this edition is the authors who have spent long and arduous hours delving into their collective understanding of disease so that the basic science curriculum could be collated and consolidated. It is also true that without the diligent efforts, compulsive nature, and organizational skills of Mrs. Lea Rhea Capote this project would have failed. Again, to all these individuals I am extremely grateful.

Contributors

Wayne L. Backes, Ph.D
Professor
Department of Pharmacology and Experimental
    Therapeutics
Louisiana State University Medical Center
New Orleans, LA

Lorne H. Blackbourne, M.D., F.A.C.S.
Senior Resident in General Surgery
Department of Surgery
University of Virginia Health Sciences Center
Charlottesville, VA

Kirby I. Bland, M.D.
The J. Murray Beardsley Professor and Chairman
Surgeon-in-Chief
Department of Surgery
Brown University School of Medicine
Rhode Island Hospital
Providence, RI

Mary Brandt, M.D., F.A.C.S.
Department of Pediatric Surgery
Baylor College of Medicine
Houston, TX

L. Michael Brunt, M.D., F.A.C.S.
Assistant Professor of Surgery
Department of Surgery
Washington University School of Medicine
St. Louis, MO

Kennan J. Buechter, M.D., F.A.C.S.
Associate Professor of Surgery
Department of Surgery
Louisiana State University School of Medicine
New Orleans, LA

Patricia M. Byers, M.D., F.A.C.S.
Nutrition and Metabolic Support Services
University of Miami School of Medicine
Miami, FL

Gilbert A. Castro, Ph.D.
Professor
Department of Integrative Biology
University of Texas—Houston Medical School
Houston, TX

Kevin C. Chung, M.D.
Department of Plastic and Reconstructive Surgery
University of Michigan
Ann Arbor, MI

Jeffrey T. Cope, M.D.
Senior Resident in General Surgery
Department of Surgery
University of Virginian Health Sciences Center
Charlottesville, VA

Verne E. Cowles, Ph.D
Associate Professor of Surgery and Physiology,
Medical College of Wisconsin
Research Physiologist
Zablocki Veterans Administration Medical Center
Milwaukee, WI

Alan T. Davis, M.D.
Assistant Professor of Surgery
Butterworth Hospital
Nutritional Research Lab
Grand Rapids, MI

Haile T. Debas, M.D., F.A.C.S.
Professor and Chairman
Department of Surgery
University of California
San Francisco, CA

Frederick J. Doherty, M.D.
Chief of Ultrasound
New England Medical Center
Boston, MA

Keith Donatto, M.D.
Department of Othopedics
Louisiana State University Medical Center
New Orleans, LA

Stanley J. Dudrick, M.D., F.A.C.S.
Surgeon-in-Chief and Clinical Professor of Surgery
Hermann Hospital and University of Texas Medical
    School
Houston, TX

James A. Edney, M.D., F.A.C.S.
Associate Professor of Surgery
Chief of Surgical Oncology
Department of Surgery
University of Nebraska Medical Center
Omaha, NE

Michael Emmett, M.D., F.A.C.P.
Tompsett Professor of Medicine
Chief of Internal Medicine
Baylor University Medical Center
Dallas, TX

Greg R. Eure, M.D.
Assistant Professor of Urology
East Virginia Medical School
Norfolk, VA

Scott Fabozzi, M.D.
Associate Instructor of Surgery
East Virginia Medical School
Norfolk, VA

Andrew Fenves, M.D., F.A.C.P.
Associate Director
Nephrology/Metabolism Division
Baylor University Medical Center
Dallas, TX

Donald E. Fry, M.D., F.A.C.S.
Chairman
Department of Surgery
University of New Mexico
Albuquerque, NM

Jared Gilmore, M.D.
Department of Surgery
Louisiana State University School of Medicine
New Orleans, LA

George Gittes, M.D.
Fellow in Pediatric Surgery
Children's Mercy Hospital
Overland Park, KS

A. Gerson Greenberg, M.D.
Department of Surgery
Brown University Program of Medicine
The Miriam Hospital
Providence, RI

John Halverson, M.D., F.A.C.S.
Department of Surgery
State University of New York
Syracuse, NY

Keith Hansen, M.D., F.A.C.O.G.
Assistant Professor
Section of Reproductive Endocrinology, Infertility,
  and Genetics
Department of Obstetrics and Gynecology
Division of Reproductive Endocrinology
Medical College of Georgia
Augusta, GA

Walter D. Holder, Jr., M.D.
Associate Clinical Professor of Surgery
Chief, Surgical Oncology Division
Director, General Surgery Research
Department of General Surgery
Carolinas Medical Center
Charlotte, NC

William G. Horstman, M.D.
Assistant Professor of Radiology
East Virginia Medical School
Norfolk, VA

Bernard Jaffe, M.D., F.A.C.S.
Department of Surgery
Tulane University Medical Center
New Orleans, LA

Devika N. Jajoo, M.D.
Resident
Hospital of St. Raphael
West Haven, CT

Robert J. Johnson, M.D.
Neurosurgeon
Baptist Medical Center
Birmingham, AL

Gerald Jordan, M.D., F.A.C.S.
Professor of Urology
East Virginia Medical School
Norfolk, VA

Daniel J. Jurusz, M.D.
Assistant Professor of Surgery
Department of Surgery
Louisiana State University School of Medicine
New Orleans, LA

Peter J. Kahrilas, M.D.
Associate Professor of Medicine
Departments of Medicine and Communication
  Sciences and Disorders
Northwestern University
Chicago, IL

Andrew S. Klein, M.D., F.A.C.S.
Associate Professor of Surgery
The Johns Hopkins University School of Medicine
  Baltimore
Chief, Division of Transplantation
Department of Surgery
The Johns Hopkins Hospital
Baltimore, MD

Timothy Koch, M.D.
Associate Professor of Medicine
Assistant Professor of Physiology
Division of Gastroenterology
Medical College of Wisconsin
Froedtert Memorial Lutheran Hospital
Milwaukee, WI

Ivan M. Lang, Ph.D.
Adjunct Associate Professor of Medicine
Director of Dysphagia Research Laboratory
Dysphagia Research Laboratory
Medical College of Wisconsin
Milwaukee, WI

Rafat Latifi, M.D.
Research Associate in Surgery
Hermann Hospital and University of Texas Medical
  School
Houston, TX

W. Thomas Lawrence, M.D., F.A.C.S.
Professor and Chief
Division of Plastic Surgery
University of Massachusetts Medical Center
Worcester, MA

Keith D. Lillemoe, M.D., F.A.C.S.
Associate Professor of Surgery
Department of Surgery
Johns Hopkins Medical Institutions
Baltimore, MD

Donald F. Lynch, M.D., F.A.C.S.
Associate Professor of Urology
East Virginia Medical School
Norfolk, VA

Anne T. Mancino, M.D.
Assistant Professor of Surgery
University of Mississippi Medical Center
Jackson, MS

James M. McGreevy, M.D., F.A.C.S.
Associate Professor of Surgery
Department of Surgery
University of Utah
Salt Lake City, UT

Frank M. Mele, M.D.
Department of Radiology
Hospital of Saint Raphael
New Haven, CT

Joseph M. Moerschbaecher III, Ph.D.
Professor and Head of Pharmacology and
    Experimental Therapeutics
Department of Pharmacology
Louisiana State University Medical Center
New Orleans, LA

Anthony L. Moulton, M.D., F.A.C.S.
Chief of Cardiothoracic Surgery and Professor of
    Surgery
Brown University School of Medicine
The Miriam Hospital
Providence, RI

Mary Pat Moyer, Ph.D.
Professor of Surgery
Department of Surgery
University of Texas Health Science Center
San Antonio, TX

Thomas E. Nolan, M.D., F.A.C.O.G.
Associate Professor of Obstetrics and Gynecology
    and Internal Medicine
 Chief, Section of General Obstetrics and Gynecology
    Department OB/GYN
Louisiana State University School of Medicine
New Orleans, LA

Mary F. Otterson, M.D., F.A.C.S.
Assistant Professor of Surgery and Physiology
Digestive Disease Research Center
Medical College of Wisconsin and Milwaukee
    Veterans Administration Medical Center
Milwaukee, WI

Henry A. Pitt, M.D., F.A.C.S.
Professor and Vice-Chairman
Department of Surgery
The Johns Hopkins Hospital
Baltimore, MD

William J. Pokorny, M.D.
DECEASED
Chief, Pediatric Surgery
Professor of Surgery
Professor of Pediatrics
Baylor College of Medicine
Houston, TX

Riley S. Rees, M.D., F.A.C.S.
Professor of Surgery
Section of Plastic Surgery
Plastic and Reconstructive Surgery
University of Michigan Medical Center
Taubman Health Care Center
Ann Arbor, MI

Randolph Reinhold, M.D., F.A.C.S.
Chairman
Department of Surgery
Hospital of St. Raphael
New Haven, CT

Edward E. Rigdon, M.D., F.A.C.S.
Associate Professor of Surgery
Department of Surgery
University of Mississippi Medical Center
Jackson, MS

James M. Riopelle, M.D.
Professor of Anesthesiology
Louisiana State University Medical Center
Director, Chronic Pain Clinic
Department of Anesthesiology
Charity Hospital
New Orleans, LA

Edwin L. Robey, M.D., F.A.C.S.
Associate Professor of Urology
East Virginia Medical School
Norfolk, VA

Martin C. Robson, M.D., F.A.C.S.
Professor of Surgery and Director of The Division of
    Surgical Research
University of South Florida
Chief of Surgery, Bay Pines Veterans Affairs Medical
    Center
Director, Institute of Tissue Regeneration, Repair,
    Rehabilitation
Tampa, FL

William A. Rock, Jr., M.D.
Professor of Pathology, Division of Clinical
    Pathology
Department of Pathology
University of Mississippi Medical Center
Jackson, MS

Richard Rohrer, M.D., F.A.C.S.
Chief, Division of Transplant Surgery
Associate Professor of Surgery
Tufts University School of Medicine
New England Medical Center
Boston, MA

Steven S. Rothenberg, M.D., F.A.C.S.
Director of Pediatric Surgery
Presbyterian-St. Luke's Medical Center
Assistant Clinical Professor of Surgery,
University of Colorado Health Sciences Center
Denver, CO

Sushil K. Sarna, Ph.D.
Department of Surgery
Medical College of Wisconsin
Clinics at Froedtert
Milwaukee, WI

Paul F. Schellhammer, M.D., F.A.C.S.
Professor and Chairman
Department of Urology of Virginia Prostate Center
Eastern Virginia Medical School
Sentara Cancer Institute
Norfolk, VA

Wayne H. Schwesinger, M.D., F.A.C.S.
Professor of Surgery
University of Texas Health Science Center San
    Antonio
Director of Surgical Endoscopy
University of Texas Health Science Center San
    Antonio and Audie L. Murphy
    Memorial Veterans Hospital
The University of Texas Health Science Center at
    San Antonio

Carol Scott-Conner, M.D., F.A.C.S.
Professor and Head of Surgery
The University of Iowa Hospitals and Clinics
Iowa City, IA

Brett C. Sheppard, M.D., F.A.C.S.
Physician and Surgeon
Assistant Professor of Surgery
Division of General Surgery
Oregon Health Sciences University
Portland, OR

David J. Smith, Jr., M.D., F.A.C.S.
Professor of Surgery
Section Head of Plastic and Reconstructive Surgery
Associate Chairman for the Department of Surgery
Department of Surgery
University of Michigan Medical Center
Ann Arbor, MI

Roger Smith, M.D.
Department of Neurosurgery
Louisiana State University School of Medicine
New Orleans, LA

John F. Stecker, M.D., F.A.C.S.
Associate Professor of Urology
East Virginia Medical School
Norfolk, VA

Gordon L. Telford, M.D., F.A.C.S.
Professor of Surgery
Department of Surgery
Medical College of Wisconsin
Froedtert Memorial Lutheran Hospital
Milwaukee, WI

Susan W. Telford, Ph.D.
Assistant Clinical Professor of Anesthesiology and
   Physiology
Medical College of Wisconsin
Research Physiologist
Zablocki Veterans Administration Medical Center
Milwaukee, WI

Mack A. Thomas, M.D., F.A.C.S.
Professor of Anesthesiology and Surgery
Louisiana State University School of Medicine
Chief, Anesthesiology
Veterans Administration Medical Center
New Orleans, LA

Robert Tiel, M.D.
Assistant Professor of Neurosurgery
Louisiana State University School of Medicine
New Orleans, LA

Curtis Tribble, M.D., F.A.C.S.
Department of Surgery
University of Virginia Health Science Center
Charlottesville, VA

Reid W. Tribble, M.D.
Clinical Assistant Professor of Surgery
University of South Carolina, School of Medicine
Columbia, SC

William V. Tynes II, M.D., F.A.C.S.
Associate Professor of Urology
East Virginia Medical School
Norfolk, VA

Thomas V. Whelan, M.D.
Assistant Professor of Nephrology
East Virginia Medical School
Norfolk, VA

Edwin G. Wilkins, M.D.
Department of Plastic and Reconstructive Surgery
University of Michigan
Ann Arbor, MI

Boyd H. Winslow, M.D., F.A.C.S.
Professor of Urology
East Virginia Medical School
Norfolk, VA

Eugene A. Woltering, M.D., F.A.C.S.
Rives Professor of Surgery
Department of Surgery
Louisiana State University School of Medicine
New Orleans, LA

Charles J. Yeo, M.D.
Associate Professor of Surgery and Oncology
The Johns Hopkins University School of Medicine
Attending Surgeon
The Johns Hopkins Hospital
Baltimore, MD

Contents

1

Cell Biology

Wayne H. Schwesinger | Mary Pat Moyer

There is grandeur in this view of life, with its several powers having been originally breathed into a few forms or into one; and that, whilst this planet has gone cycling on according to the fixed law of gravity, from so simple a beginning endless forms most beautiful and most wonderful have been, and are being, evolved.

—Charles Darwin
The Origin of Species, 1859

Introduction

Our world, with its "endless forms," is populated by an enormous variety of cells; all have evolved from a common ancestor over a span of nearly 4 billion years. This evolution was punctuated by the relatively late appearance of animals 600 million years ago, presumably coincident with an abrupt increase in atmospheric oxygen (1). In spite of the ensuing diversity in size, shape, and function, cells—because of their common origins—can still be shown at a subcellular level to share many features, especially when grouped according to their complexity.

The simplest cells are classified as *prokaryotes* and contain few intracellular membranes and no specialized compartments. Members of this class include all bacteria, certain algae, and the pleuropneumonia-like organisms. Their name is derived from the fact that their nuclear material, or karyon, lacks a discrete membrane, leaving the solitary molecule of double-stranded DNA condensed but not enclosed (Fig. 1.1). Prokaryotes tend to be extremely small, usually measuring between 0.1 and 2.0 mm. From an evolutionary viewpoint, they are distinctively primitive; some microorganisms have been discovered in Proterozoic rock formations that are at least 2.7 billion years old.

By contrast, *eukaryotic* cells have a more developed and complex intracellular organization that allows most of their specialized functions to be performed within unique, membrane-bound compartments or organelles.

This compartmentation is accommodated easily by the larger size of eukaryotic cells; their dimensions range from 5 to 20 mm and beyond. Cells of this class include unicellular protozoa, most algae, and all plant and animal cells (Fig. 1.2). There are more than 250 cell types in the human body, and these cells have grown and differentiated into a highly integrated and complex system of tissues and organs. This relationship between individual cells and their collective environment is critically important, but only partially understood.

In this chapter, we will focus on the relationship between structure and function in the cells of the human body and elucidate known mechanisms that contribute to their control. Because major advances in molecular and cellular biology during the past decade have resulted in explosive progress in this area, this review cannot be comprehensive; rather, it will highlight important aspects of this topic.

Plasma Membrane

General Features

A plasma membrane defines the surface of each cell and effectively separates its internal aqueous environment from the outside world. The most basic function of this barrier is to maintain transmembrane gradients by controlling the passage of small and large molecules. An even more elegant role, however, is to provide a substrate for the various enzyme systems and receptors that, when stimulated, produce appropriate and timely cellular responses. Structurally, biological membranes can appear as a deceptively simple bilayer on electron microscopy, but they are actually remarkably complex and dynamic. They are composed of approximately equal weights of lipids and proteins; carbohydrates account for a small but extremely important fraction of the total.

Lipids

The lipids in the membrane are typically amphipathic molecules composed of a hydrophilic polar head and one or two hydrophobic and nonpolar hydrocarbon tails (Fig. 1.3). The three main lipid classes found in membranes are phospholipids, cholesterol, and glycolipids.

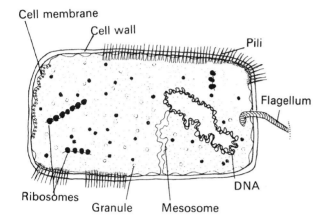

Figure 1.1. The generalized prokaryote, represented by a bacterium. Almost all bacteria are surrounded by a cell wall, which is attached to the cell membrane at relatively few points. Either flagella or pili or both may extend from the cytoplasm through the wall. Ribosomes, granules of various kinds, and DNA are found in the cytoplasm. From Dyson RD. Essentials of cell biology, 2nd ed:1978;12. Reprinted by permission of Prentice Hall, Englewood Cliffs, NJ.

Figure 1.2. The generalized eukaryotic cell. The diagram shows organelles of eukaryotic animal and plant cells as revealed by electron microscopy. From Gennis RB. Biomembranes: molecular structure, and function. New York: Springer-Verlag, 1989. Reprinted by permission.

The most common of these, the phospholipids, are arranged as a stable, bilayer matrix with their hydrocarbon tails juxtaposed to form a hydrophobic interior domain, whereas their hydrophilic polar head groups face the aqueous environment on either side. The phospholipids of most membranes show striking heterogeneity with considerable variation in both their hydrocarbon length and bond saturation. In addition, the different phospholipid molecules exhibit a remarkable degree of lateral and rotational movement. This important phenomena, called *membrane fluidity,* indirectly influences many of the cellular functions specific to the membrane (2).

Large amounts of cholesterol are also present in most eukaryotic membranes, often reaching a molecular ratio as high as 1:1 with phospholipids. Because the smaller cholesterol molecule tends to become packed between adjacent phospholipid molecules, it provides mechanical stability and thus limits membrane fluidity. Glycosphingolipids, however, generally account for only a small fraction of the total lipids in the membrane. Their general structure is similar to the glycerol-based phospholipids, with a polar head group attached to two nonpolar hydrocarbon chains. Although their function is still uncertain, accumulating evidence points to their importance in cell-cell recognition and in the modulation of transmembrane signaling.

The basic function of membrane lipids is to provide

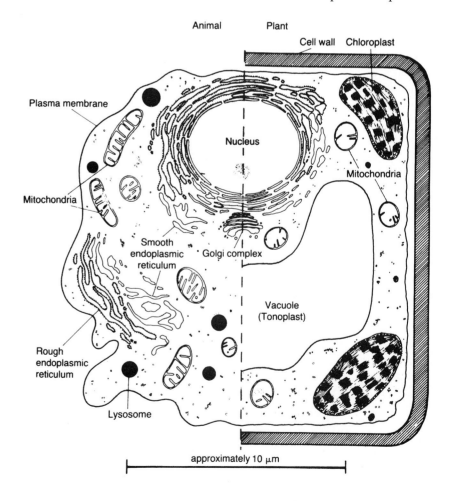

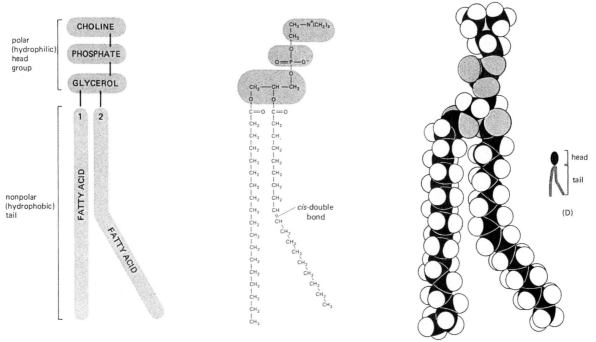

Figure 1.3. The parts of a phospholipid molecule, phosphatidylcholine, represented (far left) schematically, (middle left) in formula, (middle right) as a space-filling model, and (far right) as a symbol. From Alberts B, Bray D, Lewis J, et al. Molecular biology of the cell. 2nd ed. New York: Garland, 1989. Reprinted by permission.

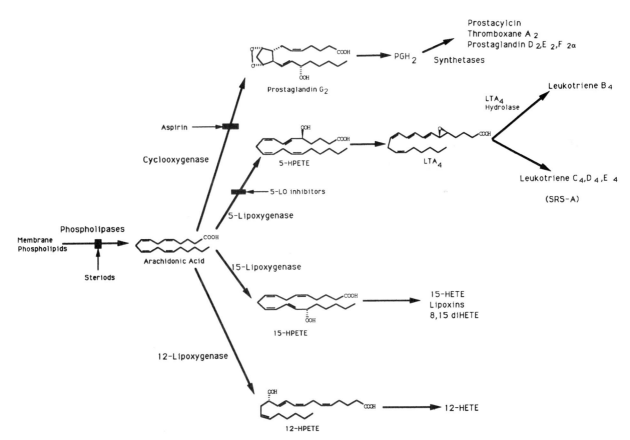

Figure 1.4. Arachidonic acid metabolism via cyclooxygenase and lipoxygenase (LO) pathways. Putative sites of action for steroids, aspirin, and 5-LO inhibitors are indicated by shaded boxes. From Sigal E. The molecular biology of mammalian arachidonic acid metabolism. Am J Physiol 1991;260 (Lung Cell Mol Physiol 4):L13–L28. Reprinted by permission.

a permeability barrier for the cell. However, lipids are not necessarily inert. They may also function as mediators and anchors. Arachidonic acid, a common constituent of membrane phospholipids, is released in response to the local action of phospholipases activated by specific receptors (3). Once released, arachidonate can be oxidized through either cyclooxygenase or lipoxygenase pathways. The active metabolites, leukotrienes, prostaglandins, and thromboxanes have been implicated as critical mediators in a variety of inflammatory disorders (Fig. 1.4).

Another novel class of membrane lipids, the phosphatidylinositols, serve as the sole anchors for a diverse group of cell-surface proteins, including alkaline phosphatase, carcinoembryonic antigen, and acetylcholinesterase. This superficial arrangement apparently provides lateral mobility to the bound proteins and allows their rapid release under appropriate circumstances.

The fact that cells organize to form tissues means that adjacent cells must be attached to each other. The specialized zones within the membrane that form attachments are termed junctions. At *tight junctions*, the external lamella of bordering plasma membranes appear to be fused together, totally sealing the intercellular space. This arrangement forms a continuous belt-like attachment that limits movement and maintains the polarity of individual cells by preventing mixing of their different membrane regions. In this manner, for example, the mucosal enzymes of intestinal epithelia remain segregated to their apical surface.

In highly stressed tissues, *anchoring junctions* bolster the normal mechanical support by linking the interior cytoskeletons of individual cells and distributing their tensile strength across many cells. One form, the adherence junction, is characterized by dense bands of amorphous protein that occupy a portion of the intercellular space and connect through transmembrane links to the actin filamentous network within the cell. Similarly, desmosomes are localized patches of linker glycoprotein that rivet cells together and then anchor them by attachment proteins connected to their intracellular intermediate filaments. Hemidesmosomes, present in epithelial tissues, rivet cells to their underlying basement membrane.

Gap junctions are another area of fixation between cells and represent the most direct form of communication between them. These specialized pores, called connexons, are each formed by a hexagonal arrangement of transmembrane subunits (Fig. 1.5). When the connexons from two cells are coupled, ions and small water-soluble molecules can pass from one cell to the other, whereas larger macromolecules, such as proteins and nucleotides, are excluded. This avenue of rapid and direct solute transfer apparently ensures a high level of cooperative activity among closely related cells. To avoid catastrophe, the pores can also be sealed by such stimuli as changing pH as individual cells approach death.

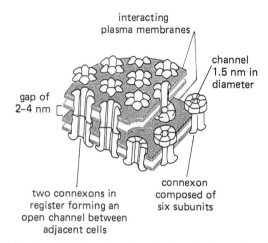

Figure 1.5. A model of gap junction showing the interacting plasma membranes of two adjacent cells. The apposed lipid bilayers are penetrated by protein assemblies called connexons, each of which is thought to be formed by six identical protein subunits. Two connexons join across the intercellular gap to form a continuous aqueous channel connecting the two cells. From Alberts B, Bray D, Lewis J, Raff M, et al. Molecular biology of the cell. 2nd ed. New York: Garland, 1989. Reprinted by permission.

Proteins

General Structure

It is estimated that a typical human cell synthesizes 3000 to 6000 different proteins. They range in complexity from simple to elaborate, yet the entire spectrum is synthesized from a limited set of 20 amino acids. Peptide bonds (Fig. 1.6) link the individual amino acids by joining the α-carboxyl group of one to the α-amino group of the other. In the polypeptide chain that is formed, a series of regularly repeating units forms a molecular backbone that always has an amino and a carboxyl terminus and may have numerous distinctive side chains as well. Each different protein has a unique amino acid sequence, called its *primary structure*, which is genetically determined (Fig. 1.7). The three-dimensional arrangement of amino acids in a specific segment of the protein molecule is referred to as its *secondary structure*. Two common configurations at this structural level are the α-helix and the β-pleated sheet. The α-helix (see Fig. 1.7) is a tightly coiled and stable rod-like structure with hydrogen bonds on the inside and amino acid side chains on the outside. By contrast, the β-pleated sheet is formed when hydrogen bonds join adjacent parallel or antiparallel arrays of polypeptide chains.

On an even larger scale, polypeptide chains often develop complex patterns of folding, and the resulting configurations are referred to as the *tertiary structure* of the protein. Moreover, when spatial relationships develop between multiple polypeptide chains, their schematic representations are referred to as *quaternary structure*. In total, these various configurations occur as the result of rapid self-assembly, i.e., the form that is finally taken is determined by the specific amino acid sequences of the

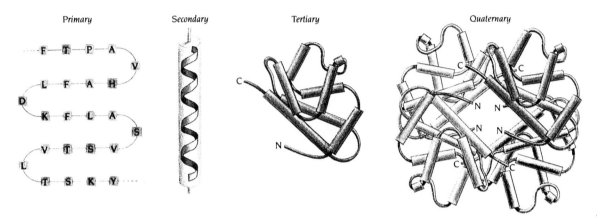

Figure 1.6. Formation of a peptide bond. From Stryer L. Molecular design of life. New York: WH Freeman, 1988: 22. Reprinted by permission.

Primary	Secondary	Tertiary	Quaternary

Figure 1.7. The amino acid sequence of a protein's polypeptide chain is called its primary structure. Different regions of the sequence form local regular secondary structure, such as α- or β-strands. The tertiary structure is formed by packing such structural elements into one or several compact globular units, called domains. The final protein may contain several polypeptide chains arranged in a quaternary structure. By formation of such tertiary and quaternary structures, amino acids far apart in the sequence are brought close together in three dimensions to form a functional region, or an active site. From Branden C, Tooze J. Introduction to protein structure. New York: Garland, 1991. Reprinted by permission.

polypeptides involved and the nature of the surrounding environment. It is precisely the three-dimensional structural features that confer on proteins their unique functions and their ability to recognize and interact with the enormously diverse range of molecules to which they are exposed.

Most functions specific to the membrane depend on the presence of proteins arranged between adjacent lipids, an association that has been depicted as a fluid mosaic pattern (Fig. 1.8). Some of the proteins in this mosaic are attached superficially by loose bonds and can be removed easily. These are termed *peripheral proteins.* Others, known as *integral proteins,* are anchored tightly to the membrane either by covalent bonding with the surface lipids or by incorporation into its hydrophobic core (4).

Transmembrane Proteins. Transmembrane proteins are those amphipathic integral proteins that span the entire membrane in single or multiple passes; their membrane-spanning domains are configured as hydrophobic α-helices. It is important that the extracellular domains of nearly all integral proteins are bound to one or more oligosaccharide chains. This glycosylation results in considerable structural diversity, because of the tremendous potential for branching exhibited by oligosaccharides. Thus these sugars provide unique identities to the proteins on which they are attached.

Membrane proteins play many roles essential to the normal physiology of the cell. Two major classes of integral proteins are particularly important and widespread: transport and receptor proteins.

Transport Proteins. Because the bilipid cell membrane is such an effective barrier, the transfer of many solutes would be drastically impeded without the action of specialized transport mechanisms. In fact, transmembrane traffic would be limited to shifts of water by osmosis and the movement of gases, lipid-soluble substances, and some small, noncharged molecules by *simple diffusion.* But other protein-based mechanisms fortunately have evolved (Table 1.1). For example, in *facilitated diffusion,* specialized transmembrane proteins serve as downhill carriers or channels through which solutes may pass. In the first instance, membrane-embedded carrier proteins couple with hydrophilic solutes, such as glucose and amino acids and transport them through the hydrophobic membrane barrier. In the second, integral membrane proteins form gated, ion-specific (e.g., Na^+, K^+, and Ca^{2+}) aqueous channels that can open in response to either voltage shifts or neurotransmitter signaling (Fig. 1.9). This allows very rapid ion flow (approximately 106/sec) to occur down the existing gradient. Finally, specialized protein pumps provide energy-dependent active transport for selected ions (e.g., Ca^{2+}, Na^+/K^+, and H^+) by working against the prevailing concentration gradient.

Receptors and Cell Signaling. Multicellular organisms have evolved an elaborate system of cell-cell communication as a means of coordinating behavior. Much

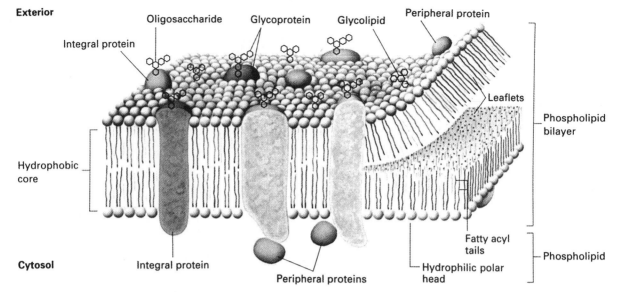

Figure 1.8. The fluid mosaic of cell membranes. A phospholipid bilayer constitutes the basic structure, whereas the hydrophobic fatty acyl tails of the phospholipids form the middle of the bilayer. The polar hydrophilic heads of the phospholipids line both surfaces. Integral proteins have one or more regions embedded in the lipid bilayer. Peripheral proteins are associated primarily with the membrane by specific protein-protein interaction. Oligosaccharides bind mainly to membrane proteins; however, some bind to lipids, forming glycolipids. From Darnell, Lodish, and Baltimore. Molecular cell biology. Copyright ©1990 by Scientific American Books, Inc. Reprinted by permission of W. H. Freeman and Company.

Table 1.1
Classification of Some Transport Proteins Based on Mechanism and Energetics[a]

I. Channels
    A. Voltage-regulated channels (example: Na^+ channel)
    B. Chemically regulated channels (example: nicotine acetylcholine receptor)
    C. Other (unregulated, pressure-sensitive, etc.)
II. Transporters
    A. Passive uniporters (example: erythrocyte glucose transporter)
    B. Active transporters
        1. Primary active transporters
            a. Redox coupled (example: cytochrome c oxidase)
            b. Light coupled (example: bacteriorhodopsin)
            c. ATPases (example: Na^+/K^+-ATPase)
        2. Secondary active transporters
            a. Symporters (example: lactose permease)
            b. Antiporters (example: B and 3)

[a] Adapted from Gennis RB, Biomembranes, structure and function. New York: Springer-Verlag, 1989.

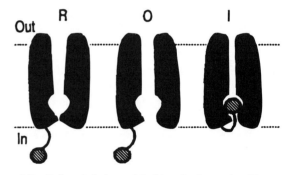

Figure 1.9. Ball-and-chain model of inactivation gating. Three gating states of the channel exist: resting (R), open (O), and inactivated (I). The receptor for the inactivation ball becomes exposed on opening of the channel. From Miller C. 1990: Annus mirabilis of potassium channels. Science 1991;252:1092. Copyright © 1991 by the AAAS. Reprinted by permission.

of this depends on proteins. The extracellular information that cells process is provided in the form of various humoral or contact-mediated signals (see "Extracellular Structure and Function"). These signals (ligands) exert their effects by binding with specific transmembrane receptor proteins, an event that is then transduced into a cytoplasmic signal, which initiates a second messenger cascade within the cell. Thus receptor proteins are able to discriminate between various stimuli and send greatly amplified signals to the interior of the cell.

Large families of receptor proteins have been partially characterized (Table 1.2). The largest of these, the *G protein-linked family,* is a member of the GTPase superfamily, a ubiquitous molecular switch with on and off

Table 1.2.
Some Receptor Families

Receptor	Morphology	Ligands
G protein	Seven-fold Membrane-spanning	Epinephrine Norepinephrine Peptide hormones
Protein tyrosine kinase	Single Membrane-spanning	EGF PDGF Insulin
Integrin	Two membrane-spanning subunits	Fibronectin Vitronectin Fibrinogen
Neurotransmitter	Four-fold membrane spanning	n-acetylcholine GABA

positions triggered by the binding and hydrolysis of guanine nucleotide (5). All of the G protein-coupled receptors have seven membrane-spanning domains, which distinguish them from other receptors (Fig. 1.10). Many ligands, including most peptide hormones, the catecholamines, many drugs, and the protooncogenes, bind to specific receptors, which are coupled to the heterotrimeric G proteins, causing them to interact with GTP. This typically results in the activation of second messengers or the opening of ion channels. In one such system, membrane-bound adenyl cyclase is stimulated,

leading to the generation of cAMP which, together with calcium, controls the activity of various protein kinases. These enzymes, in turn, catalyze the phosphorylation of specific cytoplasmic proteins, thereby inducing changes in their behavior. G protein binding may also cause the degradation of phosphatidylinositol, a membrane phospholipid, to inositol-l,4,5-triphosphate (IP_3) and diacylglycerol (DAG). Cytosolic IP_3 promotes calcium release from intracellular stores, allowing calcium-calmodulin complexes to form, which stimulate further protein phosphorylation. Similarly, increases in DAG stimulate

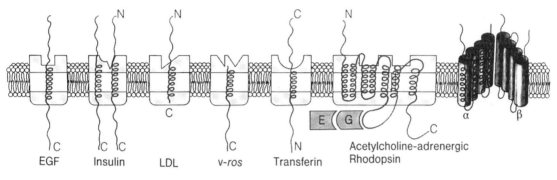

Single membrane-spanning receptors

Sevenfold membrane-spanning receptors

Fourfold membrane-spanning receptor ion channel

Figure 1.10.   Topology of receptor structures in the membrane. E, effector protein; G, G protein; C, C-terminus; *N*, N-terminus; *LDL*, low-density lipoprotein. From Hesch RD. Classification of receptors. Curr Top Pathol 1991;83:13–51. Reprinted by permission of Springer-Verlag.

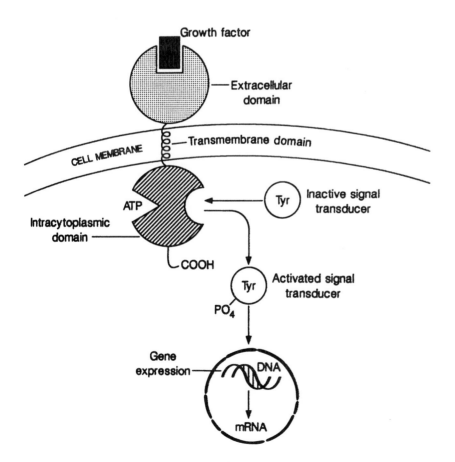

Figure 1.11.   The protein tyrosine kinase receptor and its molecular cascades. *Tyr*, tyrosine. From Arbeit J. Molecules, cancer and the surgeon. Ann Surg 1990;212:3–13. Reprinted by permission.

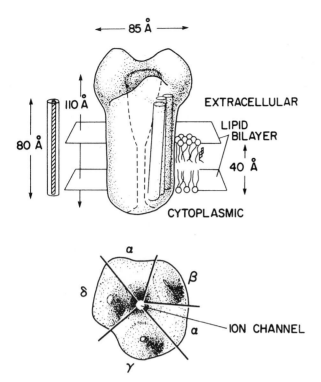

Figure 1.12. Schematic representation of the nicotinic acetylcholine receptor, composed of two a units and separate β, t, and d units around a central ion channel. Reprinted by permission of the publisher, from Williams RC. Molecular biology in clinical medicine. Copyright © 1991 by Elsevier Science Publishing Co., Inc.

protein kinase C activation, which acts to modulate membrane function and activate gene transcription.

G proteins may also be coupled to ion channels, and these pathways open to allow entry of various cations once their receptor is activated. In this way, for example, submembrane and cytoplasmic levels of calcium rapidly increase; such changes, along with phosphorylation, are instrumental in regulating most intracellular processes, including gene transcription, cytoskeletal reorganization, and intracellular mobilization.

Another family of receptors, the *protein tyrosine kinase family*, controls cellular events by phosphorylation of the tyrosine residues located in certain intracellular proteins (6). As noted with G protein systems, this covalent attachment of phosphate groups to proteins at specific sites is catalyzed by protein kinase and induces a conformational change sufficient to initiate a specific intracellular response (Fig. 1.11). This receptor family, which is composed of single membrane-spanning polypeptides, includes such growth factors as epidermal growth factor (EGF), platelet-derived growth factor (PDGF) and transforming growth factor-α (TGFα). Importantly, the insulin receptor is also a member of this family but has a unique dimeric configuration.

A third type of cell membrane receptor is the *nicotinic acetylcholine receptor* (nAchR), which is an archetypical neurotransmitter-gated ionic channel. It is structurally unrelated to the muscarinic acetylcholine receptors,

Figure 1.13. Integrin structure and interactions depicting three binding modes of various integrins. Reproduced from The Journal of Clinical Investigation, 1991, 87:1–5, by copyright permission of the American Society for Clinical Investigation.

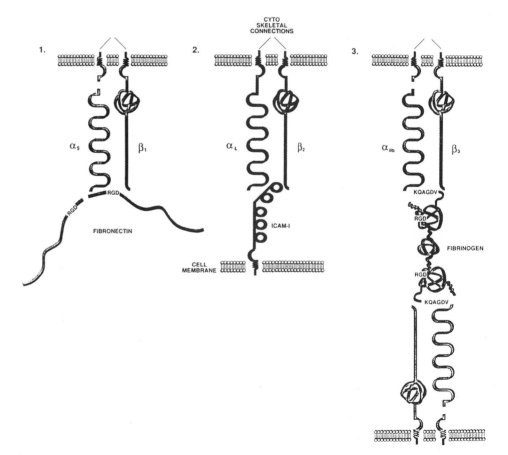

which belong to the G protein superfamily, but acts together with them to regulate the activity of the peripheral cells innervated by the autonomic nervous system and the cholinergic neurons of the central nervous system. The nAchR is composed of four different polypeptide chains located around a single ion channel (Fig. 1.12). Acetylcholine binds to the receptor, thus mediating transmission of nerve impulses to muscle at the motor end plate. This receptor family also includes the GABA and glycine receptor-gated channels, which share considerable structural homology.

Finally, the ubiquitous *integrin receptor family* is composed of receptors that are essential for the adhesion of cells to the extracellular matrix proteins. It is also one of the many families that are active in cell-cell adhesion (7). These properties are of fundamental importance to the cell because they provide anchorage, cues for migration, and signals for growth and migration. Structurally, integrins are composed of two disulfide-linked, membrane-spanning glycoprotein subunits. The external ligand-binding site is formed by sequences from both units, whereas the internal domain forms links with the cytoskeleton. Known ligands include the extracellular matrix proteins; the intercellular adhesion proteins of other cells (ICAM-1, ICAM-2, and VCAM-1); and some components of the coagulation system, including platelets, fibrinogen, and von Willebrand factor (Fig. 1.13).

Nucleus

General Structure

The nucleus is the information center of the eukaryotic cell and contains nearly all of the cell's genetic material. This has been called the *Central Dogma* of molecular biology (Fig. 1.14). Structurally, the nucleus is sur-

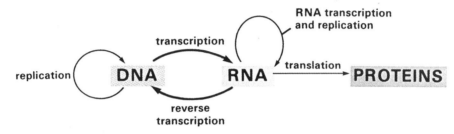

Figure 1.14. Established informational relationships between DNA, RNA, and protein. From Singer M, Berg P. Genes and genomes. Mill Valley, CA: University Science Books, 1991:36. Reprinted by permission.

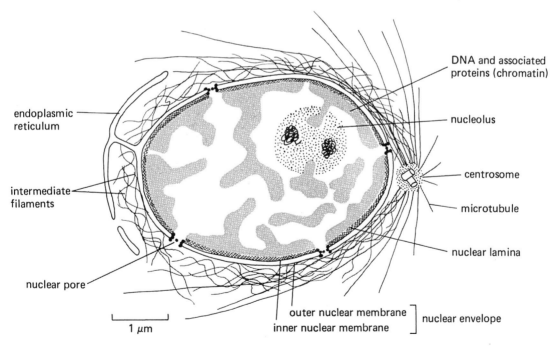

Figure 1.15. Cross-section of a typical cell nucleus. The nuclear envelope consists of two membranes; the outer one is continuous with the endoplasmic reticulum membrane (see bottom). The lipid bilayers of the inner and outer nuclear membranes are fused at the nuclear pores. Two networks of rope-like intermediate filaments (*wavy lines*) provide mechanical support for the nuclear envelope; the filaments inside the nucleus form a sheet-like nuclear lamina. Top, from Alberts B, Bray D, Lewis J, et al. Molecular biology of the cell. 2nd ed. New York: Garland, 1989. Reprinted by permission. Bottom, from Kleinsmith LJ, Kish VM. Principles of cell biology. Copyright ©1988 by Harper & Row, Publishers, Inc. Reprinted by permission of HarperCollins Publishers.

rounded by a nuclear envelope, which consists of two closely approximated bilipid membranes (Fig. 1.15). The outer membrane is continuous with the endoplasmic reticulum and studded with ribosomes, whereas the inner membrane is ribosome-free and supported by a filamentous nuclear lamina. These double membranes are perforated by numerous pores, which serve as conduits for controlled nucleocytoplasmic interchange. Each is filled by a grommet-like arrangement of specialized glycoproteins to form a nuclear pore complex. This complex apparently allows some smaller molecules to diffuse freely through the remaining apertures, although larger proteins require transport by energy-dependent, receptor-mediated processes intrinsic to the glycoproteins.

The interior of the human nucleus contains 23 paired chromosomes carrying at least 30,000 genes, which, taken together, constitute the genome. Each chromosome is composed of nearly equal amounts of deoxyribonucleic acid (DNA) and basic histone proteins, as well as variable quantities of acidic nonhistone proteins and small amounts of ribonucleic acid (RNA). The DNA component is composed of two extremely long deoxyribonucleotide polymers coiled together into the familiar double helix (Fig. 1.16). The basic repeating unit of each

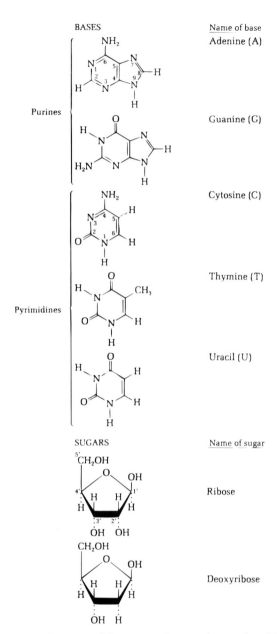

Figure 1.17. Structures of the common bases and sugars found in nucleic acids. From Kleinsmith LJ, Kish VM. Principles of cell biology. Copyright © 1988 by Harper & Row, Publishers, Inc. Reprinted by permission of HarperCollins Publishers.

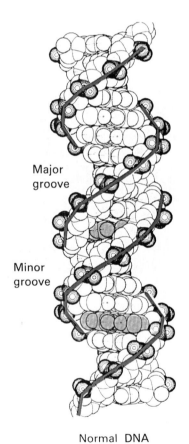

Major groove

Minor groove

Normal DNA

Figure 1.16. Space-filling model of the normal right-handed Watson-Crick DNA. Normal DNA has two grooves (one major and one minor). From Darnell, Lodish, Baltimore. Molecular cell biology. Copyright © 1990 by Scientific American Books, Inc. Reprinted by permission of W. H. Freeman and Company.

polymer is a deoxyribose sugar with a phosphate attached at one end and a nitrogenous base attached to the other (Fig. 1.17). These units are linked by phosphodiester bridges between the 3'-hydroxyl of one sugar and the 5'-hydroxyl of the next sugar to form a polar backbone. In the diploid chromosome, two nucleotide chains so formed are held together by hydrogen bonds, which join the purine bases adenine (A) and guanine (G) with the pyrimidine bases thymine (T) and cytosine (C). Base pairing is invariant; every A on one chain is paired to a T on the other chain and every G is paired to a C. As a consequence, the base sequence on one chain exactly specifies the sequence of bases on the other; two DNA strands attached in this way are complementary.

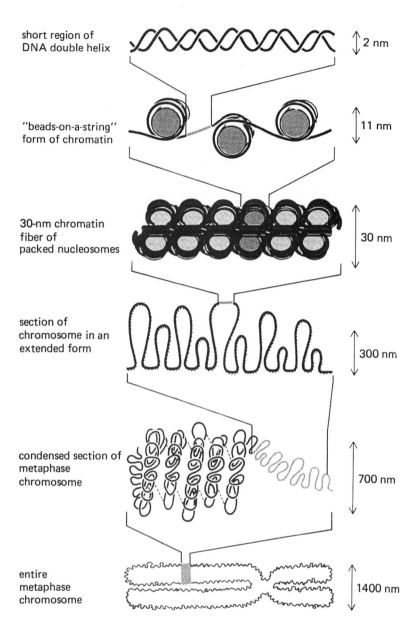

short region of
DNA double helix

‡ 2 nm

"beads-on-a-string"
form of chromatin

‡ 11 nm

30-nm chromatin
fiber of
packed nucleosomes

‡ 30 nm

section of
chromosome in an
extended form

‡ 300 nm

condensed section of
metaphase
chromosome

‡ 700 nm

entire
metaphase
chromosome

‡ 1400 nm

Figure 1.18. Schematic illustration of some of the many orders of chromatin packing that have been postulated to give rise to the highly condensed metaphase chromosome. From Alberts B, Bray D, Lewis J, et al. Molecular biology of the cell. 2nd ed. New York: Garland, 1989. Reprinted by permission.

Each human chromosome contains an average of 50 to 250 million base pairs and, if extended, would measure nearly 40 mm in length. Because all 46 chromosomes need to function within a nucleus that measures approximately 0.006 mm in diameter, the enclosed DNA must be densely packed (8). The hierarchy of organization begins with coils of DNA, called nucleosomes, the basic units of DNA packaging (Fig. 1.18). Each nucleosome is formed by the wrapping of nearly 200 base pairs of DNA twice around an octameric core composed of two copies each of four histones: H2A, H2B, H3, and H4. These small basic proteins bind tightly, but nonspecifically, with the more acidic DNA segments. Another histone, H1, is associated directly with the DNA as it enters and exits the nucleosome and appears to promote the coiling of six or more nucleosomes to form larger complexes, called solenoids. Finally, in an even higher order of packaging, many chromatin loops of varying sizes become permanently attached to a proteinaceous axial scaffold. This genetic material is further attached to a nuclear matrix, which maintains it in position for replication or transcription.

In addition to this necessarily precise structural organization of chromosomes, certain DNA sequence elements are also required for normal chromosomal function. One, the *centromere*, is a specialized area of constriction present in all chromosomes. A *kinetochore* complex assembles at this site and mediates the attachment of the chromosome to the spindle during mitosis. This appears necessary to ensure that the chromosome is divided longitudinally into two equal chromatids. Another element, the *telomere*, is a specialized DNA cap, which is positioned at the end of all chromosomes and consists of simple repeats of nongenomic base se-

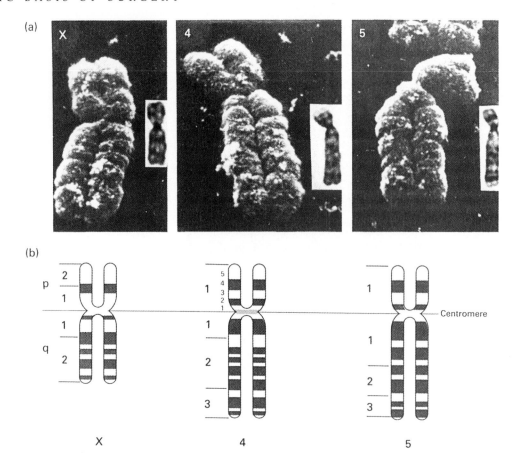

Figure 1.19. Human male chromosomes X, 4, and 5 after G-banding. The chromosomes were subjected to brief proteolytic treatment and then stained with Giemsa reagent, producing distinctive bands at characteristic places. From Harrison CJ et al. Scanning electron miscroscopy of the G-banded human karyotype. Exp Cell Res 1981;134: 141–153. Reprinted by permission of Academic Press.

quences. The major function of the telomere appears to be the prevention of chromosomal shortening during replication. These structural features of chromosomes allow them to be studied best during mitosis, when they are condensed. At that time, they can be stained to yield banding patterns that are sufficiently distinct to individual chromosomes to permit karyotyping (Fig. 1.19).

DNA Replication

DNA Structure and Synthesis

DNA is the chemical basis for inheritance. The double helix structure of DNA allows it to be readily duplicated by the unwinding and use of each chain as a template for copying by complementary base pairing (Fig. 1.20). This results in *semiconservative replication*, in which each new DNA molecule is composed of one old (conserved) and one new strain of DNA. *DNA polymerases* are the enzymes that catalyze the polymerization of deoxynucleoside triphosphates into DNA. There are several types of DNA polymerases, which were numbered in order of their discovery rather than the order of their importance. Thus DNA elongation by nucleotide linkage is promoted by DNA polymerase III, whereas gapfilling and repair functions are accomplished by DNA polymerase I. There are, in fact, many mechanisms by which the fidelity of DNA duplication is scrupulously

preserved, but heritable mutations can occasionally occur, sometimes with drastic consequences (9).

The molecular mechanisms of DNA replication are complex, requiring several additional proteins (Fig. 1.21). These include a *helicase enzyme*, involved in the unwinding step; a *primase*, which catalyzes the formation of RNA primers used to initiate DNA synthesis; and a *ligase*, which joins DNA fragments generated by degradation of the RNA primers. Furthermore, because the DNA polymerase can only function in a 5' to 3' direction, one strand of DNA is copied by discontinuous synthesis of small DNA fragments (Okazaki fragments) initiated by RNA primers, which are later removed and replaced by DNA (see Fig. 1.20).

The DNA polymerase enzyme has other functions in addition to polymerizing DNA. An editing or proofreading function is provided by a 3'-5' exonuclease activity, whereas a 5'-3' exonuclease functions to link Okazaki fragments and repair DNA. Those editing functions are extremely important for maintaining DNA integrity.

Several theories are proposed for the role of the centromeric region in triggering the onset of chromosome separation. Phosphorylation events are known to involve structural proteins of the nuclear lamina. Depolymerization of the lamina, condensation of the chromatin, and breakdown of the nuclear envelope are all temporally related to phosphorylation of the nuclear

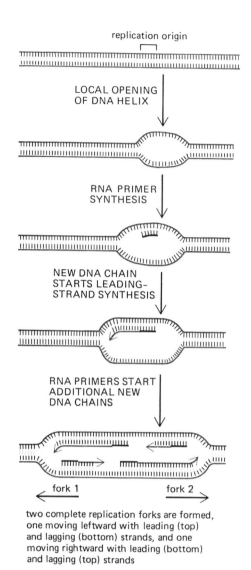

replication origin

LOCAL OPENING
OF DNA HELIX

RNA PRIMER
SYNTHESIS

NEW DNA CHAIN
STARTS LEADING-
STRAND SYNTHESIS

RNA PRIMERS START
ADDITIONAL NEW
DNA CHAINS

fork 1   fork 2

two complete replication forks are formed,
one moving leftward with leading (top)
and lagging (bottom) strands, and one
moving rightward with leading (bottom)
and lagging (top) strands

Figure 1.20. An outline of the processes involved in the initiation of replication forks at replication origins. From Alberts B, Bray D, Lewis J, et al. Molecular biology of the cell. 2nd ed. New York: Garland, 1989. Reprinted by permission.

lamina, as is a significant increase in histone H1 phosphorylation.

Cell Cycle

The cell cycle of eukaryotes has four successive phases (Fig. 1.22). The daughter cells begin *interphase* of a new cycle. The first part of this is the G_1, or first gap, phase when biosynthetic activities of the cells proceed slowly before DNA synthesis, the *S phase*. When the S phase ends, another short gap time occurs, called G_2, which precedes mitosis. Cell cycle times vary, but typically occur as 24-hr cycles. The cell cycle culminates in mitosis (nuclear division) and division of the cells by a process called cytokinesis.

Mitosis is divided into four major stages (Fig. 1.23): *prophase, metaphase, anaphase,* and *telophase.* Distinguishing these phases is based on chromosome features such as appearance and behavior. Mitotic chromosomes are compact, multiple supercoiled structures of chromatin fibers. In prophase, the chromatin fibers begin to condense into the discrete structures that are recognizable as separate chromosomes. A pair of *chromatids*, or the individual parts of the chromosomes, are joined by a *centromere*. Upon condensation of the chromosomes, transcription of the DNA slows down and eventually stops. Nucleoli commonly disperse at this time. Furthermore, the mitotic spindle begins to assemble during this stage of mitosis. Cytoplasmic microtubule-containing structures, called *centrioles,* migrate to opposite sides of the nucleus. Centrioles are self-replicating and are important in stimulating the microtubules to generate the spindle apparatus along which the chromosomes migrate during mitosis. During prophase, the nuclear envelope begins to break down, with final breakdown of the envelope indicating the end of prophase. In metaphase, which is the next step, the nuclear envelope is gone. Spindle microtubules become attached to the centromeres of the chromosomes, and the chromosomes then migrate toward the equator of the spindle, where they line up adjacent to one another. Centromeres of each chromosome are attached to two sets of microtubules, one from each pole of the centriole-associated spindle.

During metaphase, chemical agents can be used to disrupt the mitotic spindle. Because this allows chromosomes to be microscopically examined, karyotypes based on chromosome size, shape, and differential staining patterns can be generated. Thus metaphase is the opportune time for studying individual chromosomes. The next phase of mitosis is anaphase, during which time the two chromatids separate from each other to generate two independent chromosomes. Each of the newly formed chromosomes derived from the chromatid pair migrate to opposite poles of the spindle, thus the two sets of chromosomes are separated from each other. When the chromatids attach to the spindle microtubules, their specialized structures known as *kinetochores* attach to the centromere at opposite sides. Because of this structural arrangement, the kinetochore attachment ensures that the chromosomes are sent to opposite poles of the spindle during anaphase. The second function of the centromere is to hold the two chromatids together until the beginning of anaphase. Several theories have been proposed to explain the mechanisms of chromosome separation, but the exact mechanisms have yet to be defined.

When the chromosomes arrive at opposite poles of the spindle, this is the beginning of the next step of mitosis, called telophase. During this step, the chromosomes unfold and disperse into typical interphase chromatin fibers. Nuclear changes include the reformation of the nuclear envelope and the reappearance of nucleoli, which is followed by *cytokinesis,* or division of the cytoplasm.

Figure 1.21. A simplified outline of the initial steps leading to the formation of replication forks at the *E. coli* and bacteriophage λ replication origins. Discovery of the indicated mechanism required in vitro studies that used a mixture of highly purified proteins. Subsequent steps cause the initiation of three more DNA chains by a pathway that is not yet clear. For *E. coli* DNA replication, the initiator protein is the dnaA protein and the primosome is composed of the dnaB (DNA helicase) and dnaG (RNA primase) proteins. From Alberts B, Bray D, Lewis J, et al. Molecular biology of the cell. 2nd ed. New York: Garland, 1989. Reprinted by permission.

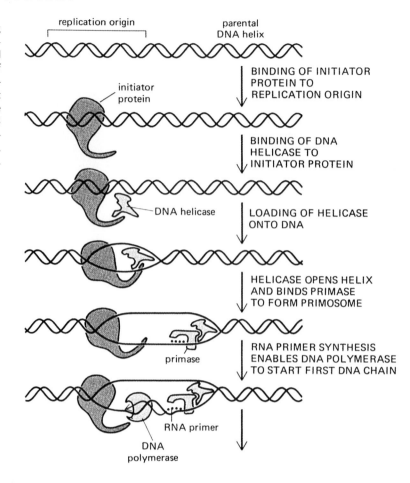

Controls

Many proteins are involved in the control of the cell cycle (Table 1.3). Chromosome condensation and folding involves protein phosphorylation events via certain proteins such as the maturation-promoting factor (MPF). Cyclins play a critical role, partially by their association with a universal eukaryotic cell regulator called p34cdc^2. The mechanisms by which these proceed through the cell cycle are just beginning to be explained, but the cyclin B protein associates with p34 in the transition from G_2 to S phase of the cell cycle, whereas the p34 protein kinase associated with cyclin A may function earlier in the cell cycle than mitosis (Fig. 1.24). Cyclins are known to be involved in cell differentiation and embryogenesis.

Mechanisms associated with cell proliferation have become better defined in recent years. Included among myriad candidate modulators are protooncogenes and growth factors, such as EGF (10). Protooncogenes (also called c-*onc*'s, referring to the cellular "oncogenes") are normal cell growth and regulatory genes that correspond to a variety of aberrant oncogenes isolated from tumor-causing viruses or cancer cells. Viral oncogenes are called collectively v-*onc*'s. Some protooncogene-encoded proteins that have been defined include growth factors, growth factor receptors, GTP-binding proteins,

protein kinases, and nuclear proteins (Table 1.4). Changes in cellular protooncogene sequences or expression can contribute to altered growth control. However, multiple stages are likely to be involved in the carcinogenesis process, not a single gene mutation. The protein products of two of these genes (*fos* and *jun*) are known as members of the AP1 transcription factor family. Because the cell cycle is well-controlled in regard to timing, transcription of genes such as the c-*jun* and c-*fos* oncogene are highly regulated (11).

Various growth factors and agents that are known to be "tumor promoters" (i.e., they enhance DNA synthesis and cell replication), activate *fos* and *jun* mRNAs. Thus normal cellular DNA synthesis is stimulated by a mitogen or tumor promoter. Activation of the cellular protein kinase may in turn phosphorylate cellular proteins involved in the cell cycle, thus enhancing synthesis of transcriptional regulators, including subsets of oncogenes that stimulate synthesis in new mRNAs. Accompanying these actions are changes in lipid metabolism and alterations in the intracellular ionic environment, particularly signaling by calcium and by monovalent cation changes. Changes may persist or may be transient after the initial stimulus. Both constant and intermittent repeated alterations in up-regulation of the cells or down-regulation of cellular regulatory mechanisms are

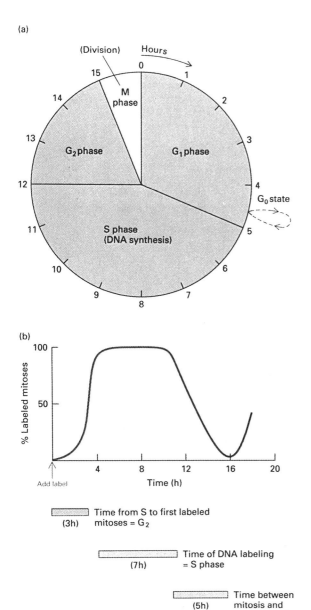

Figure 1.22. The mammalian cell cycle with a generation time of 16 hr. **(a)** The three phases spanning the first 15 hr or so—the G_1 (first gap) phase, the S (synthetic) phase, and the G_2 (second gap) phase—make up interphase, during which DNA and other cellular macromolecules are synthesized. The remaining hour is the M (mitotic) phase, during which the cell actually divides. **(b)** The phases of the cell cycle were determined by exposing a culture briefly to labeled thymidine, which is incorporated into DNA, and then observing the time of appearance of labeled mitotic cells. From Darnell, Lodish, and Baltimore, Molecular Cell Biology. Copyright © 1990 by Scientific American Books, Inc. Reprinted by permission of W. H. Freeman and Company.

involved in the normal changes that accompany cell growth regulation. Structural considerations of a tissue, which are relevant to differences in cell-cell associations, basement membrane, and other features, lead to temporal and positional control of cell division. In addition, certain genes may be overexpressed during the course of conversion of cells into cancer cells.

Transcription

Site of RNA Synthesis

The nucleus has one or more prominent organelles, called nucleoli, which have no membrane but instead consist of densely packed proteins and RNA. The nucleolus is the site where most cellular RNA is produced and organized (Fig. 1.25). Assembly with specific proteins results in the formation of two separate subunits of mature ribosomes (40S and 60S), which are then passed into the cytoplasm through the nuclear pores.

The process of RNA synthesis, or *transcription*, generally resembles DNA synthesis, but there are two major differences: (a) the base uracil (U) is substituted in RNA for thymine (T) such that U pairs with A as its complementary base, and (b) transcription is asymmetric because the polymerase selectively copies only one of the two DNA strands; the choice of strands depends on the gene. All cells synthesize three major types of RNA: ribosomal RNA (rRNA), transfer RNA (tRNA), and messenger RNA (mRNA). Each plays an important role in synthesis of cellular proteins, but only mRNA contains the base sequence that codes for the amino acids of the newly synthesized protein. It obtains this as a result of the action of RNA polymerase, which catalyzes the polymerization of multiple ribonucleoside triphosphates into RNA, using DNA as the template.

In eukaryotes, mRNA synthesis is more complicated than in prokaryotes because larger precursor molecules called *heterogeneous nuclear* RNAs (hnRNAs) must be shortened into mRNA by a process called splicing (Fig. 1.26). This is necessary because the protein-coding sequences of RNA, called *exons*, are separated by intervening, noncoding sequences, called *introns*. Splicing involves *spliceosomes*, which contain small nuclear ribonucleoprotein molecules and specialized cellular enzymes acting on the complex hnRNAs to generate mRNAs, which contain only exons.

Regulatory Mechanisms

Important regulatory features controlling the transcription process also exist. The sites on the DNA molecule where the RNA polymerase begins and ends transcription are determined by the base sequence and by the complex, tertiary, or quaternary structure of the molecule. Regions of the parent DNA that precede and follow the protein-coding structural region of the mRNA are called, respectively, the upstream and downstream *regulatory regions*. The detailed complexities of how these regions govern RNA synthesis are beyond the scope of this chapter, but some general features of its components are important to note (Table 1.5). A common upstream structure in the start-site region for RNA synthesis is the TATA box. Other regulatory regions include binding sites for transcription factors, proteins that play key roles in regulating the initiation of tran-

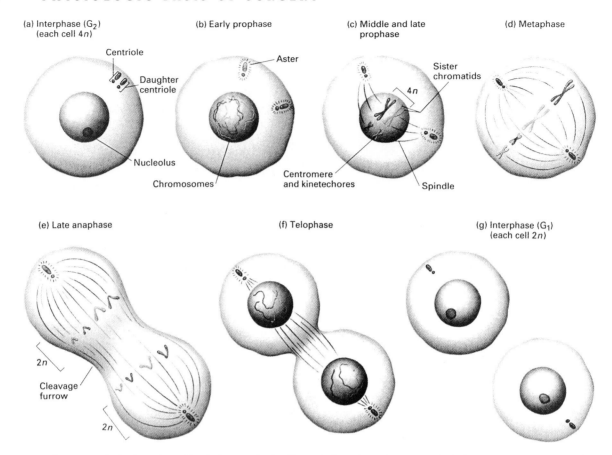

(a) Interphase (G_2)
(each cell 4n)

Centriole

Daughter
centriole

Nucleolus

Chromosomes

(b) Early prophase

Aster

(c) Middle and late
prophase

Sister
chromatids

4n

Centromere
and kinetechores

Spindle

(d) Metaphase

(e) Late anaphase

2n

Cleavage
furrow

2n

(f) Telophase

(g) Interphase (G_1)
(each cell 2n)

Figure 1.23. The stages of mitosis and cytokinesis in an animal cell. (a) Interphase. During the S phase, chromosomal DNA is replicated and bound to protein, but the chromosomes are not seen as distinct structures. The nucleolus is the only nuclear substructure that is visible under the light microscope. (b) Early prophase. The centrioles begin moving toward opposite poles of the cell; the chromosomes can be seen as long threads. The nuclear membrane begins to disaggregate. (c) Middle and late prophase. Chromosome condensation is completed; each visible chromosome structure is composed of two chromatids held together at their centromeres. Each chromatid contains one of the two newly replicated daughter DNA molecules. The microtubular spindle begins to radiate from the regions just adjacent to the centrioles, which are moving closer to their poles. Some spindle fibers reach from pole to pole, but most go to chromatids and attach at kinetochores. (d) Metaphase. The chromosomes move toward the equator of the cell, where they become aligned in the equatorial plane. The sister chromatids have not yet separated. This is the phase in which morphologic studies of chromosomes are usually carried out. (e) Late anaphase. The two sister chromatids separate into independent chromosomes. Each contains a centromere that is linked by a spindle fiber to one pole to which it moves. Thus one copy of each chromosome is donated to each daughter cell. Simultaneously, the cell elongates, as do the pole-to-pole spindles. Cytokinesis begins as the cleavage furrow starts to form. (f) Telophase. New membranes form around the daughter nuclei; the chromosomes uncoil and become less distinct, the nucleolus becomes visible again, and the nuclear membrane forms around each daughter nucleus. Cytokinesis is nearly complete, and the spindle disappears as the microtubules and other fibers depolymerize. Throughout mitosis, the daughter centriole at each pole grows until it is full-length. At telophase, the duplication of each of the original centrioles is completed, and a new daughter centriole will be generated during the next interphase. (g) Interphase. Upon the completion of cytokinesis, the cell enters the G_1 phase of the cell cycle and proceeds again through the system. From Darnell, Lodish, Baltimore. Molecular cell biology. Copyright © 1990 by Scientific American Books, Inc. Reprinted by permission of W. H. Freeman and Company.

scription by associating either directly with the DNA (usually in a complex with other molecules) or indirectly via other mediators. These interactions cause the controlled synthesis of mRNAs and are responsible for the production of specific proteins. The complement of transcription factors expressed by a cell ultimately plays a role in determining the specific cell type and its unique properties (12).

Based on amino acid homologies and protein structures, transcription factors can be categorized into three major families of related molecules. For example, steroid hormone receptors and the glucocorticoid receptor are part of a *zinc finger* family that includes thyroid hor-

mone, retinoic acid, and vitamin D_3 receptors. These receptors have a molecular design with a domain in the protein structure that contains zinc atom(s) which bind to multiple amino acids, generating a three-dimensional structure with looped-out "zinc finger" regions, which bind to the major groove of DNA (Fig. 1.27). In the case of steroid receptors, zinc fingers bind to *hormone-responsive elements* (HREs) in DNA. When a hormone binds to this receptor, the receptor-ligand complex is transported to the nucleus and then binds to DNA, thus activating transcription.

Another type of transcription factor protein has a *helix-turn-helix* structure. The best known example in eu-

Table1.3.
Functions Proposed for Some of the Known Regulatory Factors Involved in Mitosis[a]

Proposed Function	Factor(s)	Biochemical Mechanism(s)
Promotes mitosis and meiosis	MPF	ser/thr protein kinase
Regulartory subunit of MPF	Cyclins	Substrate for kinases
Induces mitotic arrest; stabilizes MPF	CSF	ser/thr protein kinase
	wee-1	ser/thr protein kinase
Regulates timing of MPF activation	per^{cdc2}	ser/thr protein kinase
	mos	ser/thr protein kinase
Catalytic subunit of MPF	Histone H1	DNA binding protein
Activator of MPF in meiosis	MAP-2	Microtubule-associated protein
In vitro substrate of p34^{cdc2}	src	Tyrosine protein kinase
In vivo p34^{cdc2} substrate	Lamins	Nuclear matrix structure

[a] Abbreviations: MPF (maturation promotion factor); CSF (cytostatic factor); MAP (microtubule associated protein).

Table 1.4.
Some General Classes of Protein Products Encoded by Representative Oncogenes

General Class	Representative Oncogene(s)
Protein kinases	
Tyrosine-specific	src, yes, fes, abl, neu, fgr
Tyrosine-specific (EGF receptor fragment)	erb-B
Serine-threonine specific	raf, mil, mos
GTP-binding proteins	ras^H, ras^K, ras^N
Nuclear binding proteins, affecting DNA replication and transcription	fos, jun, myc, ski, myb
Growth factors (analogue, platelet-derived growth factor)	sis
EGF receptor (tyrosine kinase)	erb-B
Macrophage colony-stimulatory factor	fms
Thyroid hormone receptor	erb-A

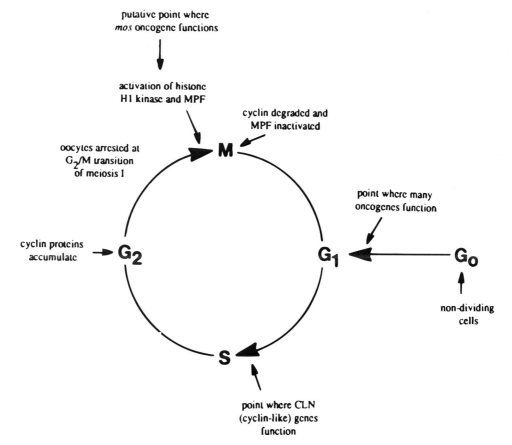

Figure 1.24. Location of regulatory events in the eukaryotic cell cycle. Quiescent somatic cells are arrested in a nongrowth state known as G$_0$. Various mitogenic agents and numerous oncogenes can stimulate cells to enter the cell cycle at G$_1$. In contrast, oocytes are arrested at the G$_2$/M-phase border. Hormones such as progesterone and several oncogenes stimulate oocytes to undergo meiotic maturation, which involves two successive nuclear divisions. Reprinted with permission from Freeman RS, Donoghue DJ. Protein kinases and proto-oncogenes: biochemical regulators of the eukaryotic cell cycle. Biochemistry 1991;30:2294. Copyright © 1991 American Chemical Society.

Figure 1.25. The function of the nucleolus in ribosome synthesis. The 45S rRNA transcript is packaged in a large ribonucleoprotein particle containing many ribosomal proteins imported from the cytoplasm. While this particle remains in the nucleolus, selected pieces are discarded as it is processed into immature large and small ribosomal subunits. The two subunits are thought to attain their final functional form only as they are transported individually through the nuclear pores into the cytoplasm. From Alberts B, Bray D, Lewis J, et al. Molecular biology of the cell. 2nd ed. New York: Garland, 1989. Reprinted by permission.

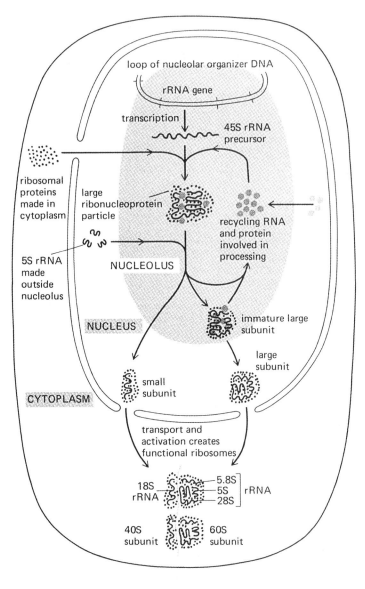

karyotes is the *homeodomain* protein, which is encoded by *homeobox* regions of DNA. It has a region 60 amino acids long that functions as a DNA-binding region and is composed of three a-helixes. These proteins play a critical role in development and thus are expressed characteristically and temporally in subsets of embryonic cells.

Leucine zippers, which are a third motif of transcription factors, are short coils of two parallel a-helices with about eight turns per helix. The zipper motif of the protein characteristically occurs as a Y-shaped "scissor-grip" structure within the DNA molecule (Fig. 1.28). Juxtaposed regions of basic amino acids within the protein cause a bipartite DNA-binding domain from each of the basic regions of the dimer. Leucine zipper motifs are found in some eukaryotic transcription factors and some nuclear oncogenes (e.g., *jun, fos,* and *myc*).) For example, dimers of *c-jun*, with itself or other protooncogene products, may occur via phosphorylation-dephosphorylation events that regulate binding of monomer or multimer structures of regulatory proteins to DNA (13).

Table 1.5.
Components of Transcriptional Regulation in Eukaryotes

Factor(s) or Structure(s)	Description
Transcription factors	Site-specific DNA binding proteins
Structural motifs	
Zinc fingers	Contains intrinsic zinc in protein that forms finger-like projections that bind to DNA
Leucine zippers	
Helix-turn-helix	
Control module	DNA sequence associated with transcription factor(s); over 50 modules are known; thus, large numbers of combinations are possible
Upstream promotor element	Usually 100-200 base pairs in length and close to site of transcription initiation; includes A-T base pair rich region known as TATA box
Enhancer elements	Short DNA sequences that enhance transcription; sometimes close to promoter, but may be far away (e.g., over 20,000 or more base pairs) or not even in the 5' region

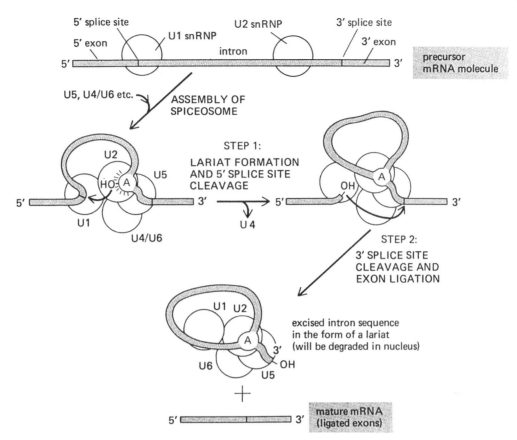

Figure 1.26. RNA splicing catalyzed by a spliceosome formed from the assembly of multiple small nuclear ribonucleoproteins (RNPs) arbitrarily designated U1, U2, etc. After the assembly of the spliceosome, the reaction occurs in two steps. As a result, the two exon sequences are joined to each other, and the intron sequence is released as a lariat. These splicing reactions occur in the nucleus and generate mRNA molecules from mRNA precursor molecules. From Alberts B, Bray D, Lewis J, et al. Molecular biology of the cell. 2nd ed. New York: Garland, 1989. Reprinted by permission.

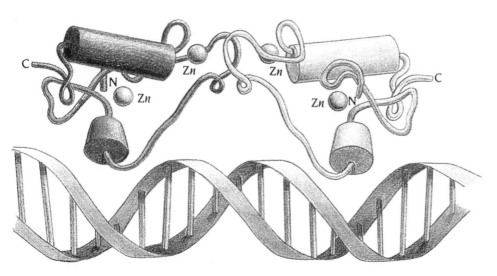

Figure 1.27. A hypothetical model of the DNA-binding domain of the glucocorticoid receptor bound to DNA as a dimer. The α-helices of the first zinc finger of each subunit are positioned in successive major grooves on one face of the DNA double helix, while the second zinc finger of each subunit is involved in dimer formation. From Branden C, Tooze J. Introduction to protein structure. New York: Garland, 1991. Reprinted by permission.

Gene expression can also be regulated by association of the DNA with the nuclear matrix (Fig. 1.29). Nuclear matrix proteins may be involved in binding and localization and positioning of specific DNA sequences so that they are available actively to transcribe genes for specific cell types or tissues. This control of the three-dimensional confirmation of the DNA confers specific-ity for binding of the transcription factors and receptors that regulate *cell differentiation,* with the resultant production of unique cell-type-specific proteins. Thus the nuclear matrix should not be viewed as simply a structural system but also as a functional system that helps to organize and coordinate the function of individual cell types. In addition to this matrix component, soluble, *trans*-acting factors clearly are involved in these processes of organization and gene regulation.

Cytoplasm

General Structure and Organelles

Conventional histology generally depicts the interior of the eukaryotic cell as the relatively amorphous envi-

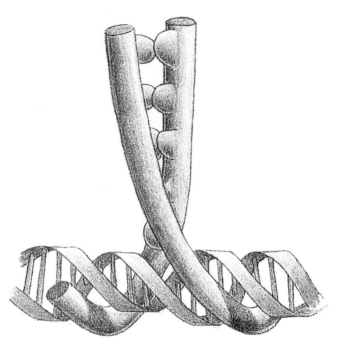

Figure 1.28. The scissors-grip model of DNA recognition by the leucine zipper motif. Two DNA-binding domains dimerize through their α-helical leucine zipper region to form a Y-shaped molecule. The arms of the "Y" each form a single α-helice that contains the DNA recognition region of the domain and is positioned in the major groove of the DNA molecule. Each of these helices is kinked so that it can follow the path of the major groove. From Branden C, Tooze J. Introduction to protein structure. New York: Garland, 1991. Reprinted by permission.

ronment in which subcellular organelles are suspended, but, in fact, the cytoplasm is complex and has many components. In the typical cell, the soluble fraction, or *cytosol*, consists of about 70% water and 20% protein, a combination that produces a viscous gel. The remainder of the cytoplasm is composed of smaller proportions of the various other enzymes, metabolites, and inorganic constituents that are involved in cellular metabolism. In addition, many cells have inclusion bodies to provide storage for metabolic fuels such as glycogen and fat.

The cytoplasm is compartmentalized further by a number of membrane-bound organelles, with each type capable of performing its own unique set of functions. One such compartment, the *endoplasmic reticulum* (ER), consists of an extensive network of interconnected tube-like structures and flattened cisternae all formed by a single membrane. The rough ER is that portion with *ribosomes* attached to it (Fig. 1.30). All nucleated cells contain perhaps as many as 20,000 to 50,000 ribosomes. Those attached to the ER are sites where proteins are synthesized either for incorporation into the cell's various membranes or for export outside the cell. Other ribosomes are free in the cytoplasm, where they participate in the synthesis of most of the remaining proteins destined to stay within the cell. The smooth ER, devoid of ribosomes, serves as the primary site for many other important reactions, including steroid and lipoprotein biosynthesis, xenobiotic detoxification, molecular conjugation, and fatty acid desaturation.

The *Golgi apparatus* is associated closely with the smooth ER but is physically separate from it. It is a complex membranous organelle that consists of multiple flat cisternae arranged in stacks and joined by interconnecting tubules. Three morphologically and functionally distinct units can be identified: the cis, medial, trans subsections. Newly synthesized lipids and proteins are transported and modified within this system before their directed release (14).

Lysosomes are membranous, sac-like organelles hav-

Figure 1.29. Hypothesis depicting DNA organization and gene activity. Tissue-specific nuclear matrix proteins are involved in the binding and localization of specific DNA sequences and determining the position of genes in proper configuration for transcription factors to interact and allow activation of gene expression. By controlling the three-dimensional conformation of DNA, the tissue-specific nuclear matrix proteins confer specificity controlling the three-dimensional conformation of DNA, the tissue-specific nuclear matrix proteins confer specificity to transcription factor/receptor binding. Reprinted with permission from Pienta KJ, Getzenberg RH, Coffey DS. Cell structure and DNA organization. Crit Rev Eukaryotic Gene Expression 1991;1: 355. Copyright CRC Press, Inc., Boca Raton, FL.

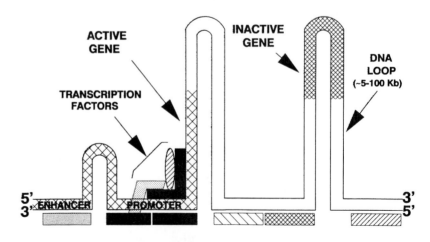

NUCLEAR MATRIX PROTEINS

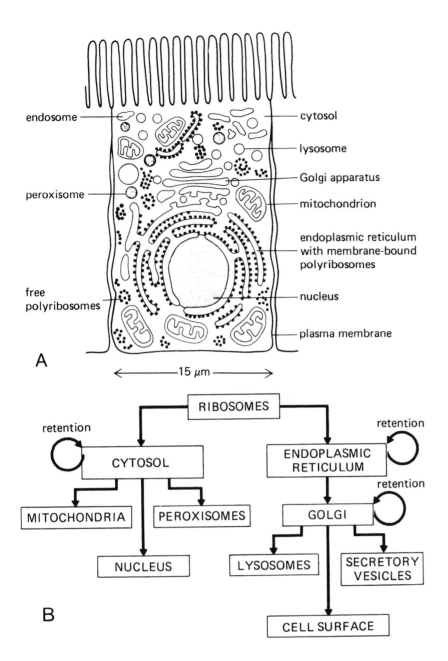

endosome —

— cytosol

— lysosome

— Golgi apparatus

peroxisome —

— mitochondrion

— endoplasmic reticulum with membrane-bound polyribosomes

free polyribosomes —

— nucleus

— plasma membrane

A

←——— 15 μm ———→

RIBOSOMES

retention

CYTOSOL

retention

ENDOPLASMIC RETICULUM

retention

MITOCHONDRIA   PEROXISOMES   GOLGI

NUCLEUS   LYSOSOMES   SECRETORY VESICLES

B

CELL SURFACE

Figure 1.30. (A) A drawing of an animal cell, emphasizing the major intracellular compartments. The cytosol, endoplasmic reticulum, Golgi apparatus, nucleus, mitochondrion, endosome, lysosome, and peroxisome are distinct compartments isolated from the rest of the cell by at least one selectively permeable membrane. [In Alberts 8-1.] (B) A simplified road map of biosynthetic protein traffic. The signals that direct a given protein's movement through the system, and thereby determine its eventual location in the cell, are contained in its amino acid sequence. The journey begins with the synthesis of a protein on a ribosome and terminates when the final destination is reached. At each intermediate station (*boxes*), a decision is made as to whether to retain the protein or to transport it further. In principle, a signal could be required either for retention or for leaving each of the compartments shown, with the alternative fate being the default pathway (one that requires no signal). From Alberts B, Bray D, Lewis J, et al. Molecular biology of the cell. 2nd ed. New York: Garland, 1989. Reprinted by permission.

ing diverse shapes and sizes. Each contains a large variety of acidic hydrolases capable of the controlled enzymatic degradation of many intracellular macromolecules. Lysosomes are important in the autolysis of dead and dying cells and worn-out organelles. Furthermore, they digest the particulate or fluid materials taken into healthy cells by the process of endocytosis.

Another saccular organelle present in the cytoplasm, the *peroxisome*, contains a variety of active enzymes sequestered within a single membrane. Morphologically, it is characterized by its fine granular matrix; frequently, a dense core or nucleoid is also present. The enclosed enzymes are capable of breaking down smaller molecules such as amino acids, xanthine, and fatty acids, often producing toxic hydrogen peroxide. Fortunately, this highly reactive molecule is metabolized by the action of catalase, another peroxisomal enzyme, to yield

water and oxygen. Peroxisomes are thought by some to represent primitive, vestigial organelles whose functions have been replaced largely by the mitochondria.

Mitochondria are motile, sausage-shaped organelles that are formed by a double membrane enclosing a fluid-filled matrix. Numerous infoldings, or cristae, extend from the inner membrane into the central matrix. This results in four specialized compartments: the inner and outer membranes, the intermembrane space, and the matrix; each has specific functions associated with its diverse proteins (Fig. 1.31). Some of these functions are strikingly different among different tissues. However, the one fundamental property common to all mitochondria is the production of ATP, the universal currency of energy in biological systems. ATP is generated by the oxidative phosphorylation of a variety of energy-rich metabolic substrates, which are stored in the cytoplasm

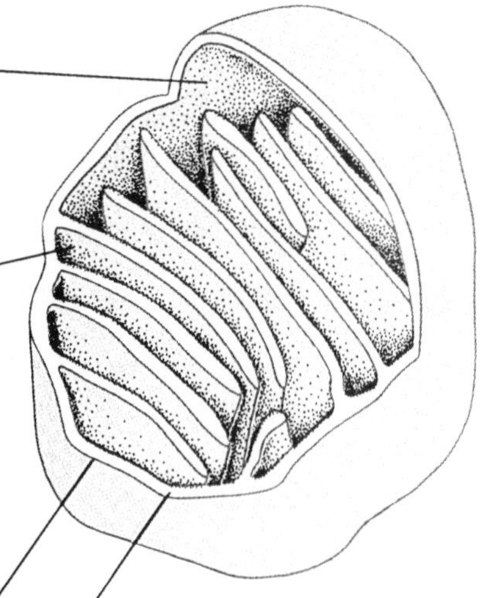

Matrix. The matrix contains a highly concentrated mixture of hundreds of enzymes, including those required for the oxidation of pyruvate and fatty acids and for the citric acid cycle. The matrix also contains several identical copies of the mitochondrial DNA genome, special mitochondrial ribosomes, tRNAs, and various enzymes required for expression of the mitochondrial genes.

Inner Membrane. The inner membrane is folded into numerous cristae, which greatly increase its total surface area. It contains proteins with three types of functions: (1) those that carry out the oxidation reactions of the respiratory chain, (2) an enzyme complex called *ATP synthetase* that makes ATP in the matrix, and (3) specific transport proteins that regulate the passage of metabolites into and out of the matrix. Since an electrochemical gradient that drives the ATP synthetase is established across this membrane by the respiratory chain, it is important that the membrane be impermeable to most small ions.

Outer membrane. Because it contains a large channel-forming protein (called porin), the outer membrane is permeable to all molecules of 10,000 daltons or less. Other proteins in this membrane include enzymes involved in mitochondrial lipid synthesis and enzymes that convert lipid substrates into forms that are subsequently metabolized in the matrix.

Intermembrane Space. This space contains several enzymes that use the ATP passing out of the matrix to phosphorylate other nucleotides.

Figure 1.31. Structural and functional components of the mitochondrion are depicted in this diagram. From Alberts B, Bray D, Lewis J, et al. Molecular biology of the cell. 2nd ed. New York: Garland, 1989. Reprinted by permission.

as fats, proteins, and glycogen (Fig. 1.32). When needed, these substrates are transported across the double membrane of the mitochondria as fatty acids and pyruvate (Fig. 1.33). Once in the matrix, both molecules are converted enzymatically to acetyl-CoA and then metabolized by the citric acid (Krebs) cycle to produce NADH and FADH$_2$. These are the reducing equivalents that fuel oxidative phosphorylation by chemiosmotic mechanisms. High-energy electrons from these fuels are passed along the electron transport chain, a series of three enzyme complexes embedded in the inner mitochondrial membrane (Fig. 1.34). Protons are pumped out of the matrix at these sites, thus creating a proton electrochemical gradient across the inner membrane. In response to the gradient, protons move passively back into the matrix through another trans-membrane complex, ATP-synthase, where the energy of their flow is coupled to the synthesis of ATP from ADP and P$_i$. Thus ATP becomes available for movement into the cytoplasm, where its potential energy can be used to perform work. Some of the remaining electrons ultimately are transferred to cytochrome c oxidase, inducing this enzyme complex to catalyze the reduction of molecular oxygen to two molecules of water.

Considering how important energy and the mitochondrial powerhouse are to the normal function of the eukaryotic cell, it is interesting that these organelles are now recognized to be symbiotic descendants of primitive bacteria. The evidence is compelling: the inner mitochondrial membrane is structurally typical for bacteria.

In addition, mitochondria possess and use some of their own genetic material; from 2 to 10 circular DNA molecules are present per organelle. Mitochondrial DNA (mtDNA) is transmitted only by the mother because sperm cells contain few mitochondria. Mutations or deletions in mtDNA have been observed and can be associated with rare, maternally transmitted diseases, particularly defects of the electron transfer chain and oxidative phosphorylation (15).

Cytoskeleton

In addition to the separation of different functions into organelles, internal cellular architecture is further organized by a fibrous scaffolding. As characterized by ultrastructural and biochemical studies, the *cytoskeleton* is a complex structural framework composed of three major types of protein polymers: actin filaments, microtubules, and intermediate filaments. These systems can be dynamic; evidence exists of both active and ongoing polymerization and depolymerization. Each is assembled from repeating subunits, which are held in a linear array by noncovalent bonds and are modified by numerous regulatory proteins. Cytoskeletal polymers can also interact with at least four families of motor proteins: myosin, kinesin, dynein, and dynamin. These motors serve as mechanochemical enzymes, producing unidirectional movement along polymers by using ATP or GTP as their immediate energy source. Together, the structural, accessory, and motor components of the cyto-

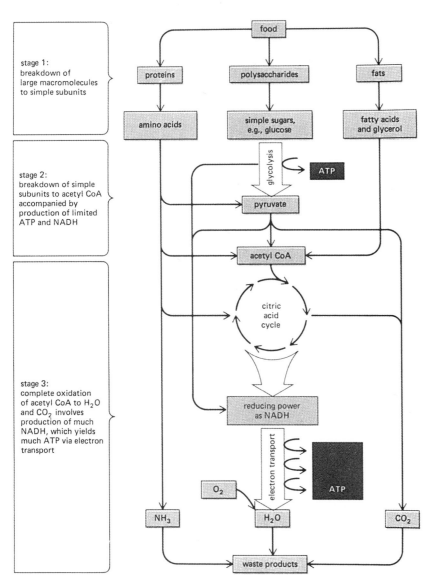

Figure 1.32. Simplified diagram of the three stages of catabolism that lead from food to waste products. This series of reactions produces ATP, which is then used to drive biosynthetic reactions and other energy-requiring processes in the cell. From Alberts B, Bray D, Lewis J, et al. Molecular biology of the cell. 2nd ed. New York: Garland, 1989. Reprinted by permission.

skeleton act to maintain cellular shape, produce movement inside and outside the cell, and provide anchorage for the subcellular organelles.

Actin filaments are rigid linear polymers of globular actin, a contractile protein found in nearly all cells. They are formed by self-assembly from the available pool of actin, a process in which the speed of elongation is more rapid at one end of the filament than at the other. The precise three-dimensional arrangement that filamentous actin assumes in each cell is tailored to the functional demands of that specific cell type and is controlled largely by the diverse group of actin-binding proteins, which can stabilize, alter, or bundle actin filaments. One common structural form, an orthogonal meshwork, is found in the cortex of all animal cells just beneath the plasma membrane. It is responsible for providing peripheral rigidity and preventing contact between the membrane and intracellular granules and organelles. The cortex is produced by specialized actin-binding proteins, which serve as flexible cross-linkages with the actin filaments. When major changes occur in the contour of the plasma membrane, such as seen with formation of pseudopods or blebs, localized disassembly of this diffuse network is required (16).

Actin filaments may also be organized into tight or loose bundles. In one such system, large bundles, or stress fibers, are attached to the adhesion plaques situated immediately adjacent to the plasma membrane. These contacts are then linked with the extracellular matrix through integrin-type membrane receptors; this provides a sensitive mechanism for the interaction of cytoskeletal polymers with a variety of signal transduction systems sensitive to extracellular changes.

Actin filaments may be highly specialized. The intestinal epithelial cells provide one example (Fig. 1.35). In the core of each brush-border microvillus, tightly aligned bundles of actin extend from the tip of the microvillus to the cell cortex where they are then anchored in a terminal web. The specialized binding proteins—villin, fimbrin, and tropomyosin—are essential to maintain the

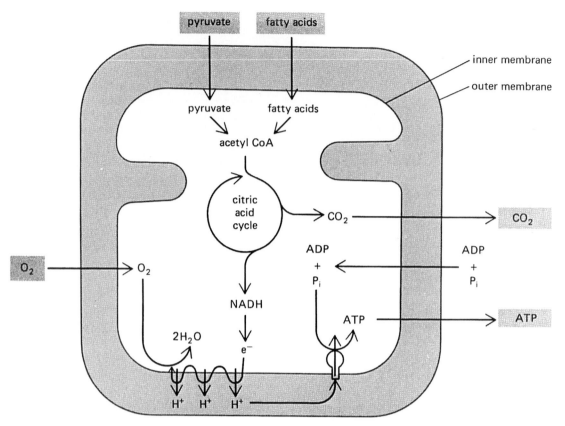

Figure 1.33. A summary of the flow of major reactants into and out of the mitochondrion. Pyruvate and fatty acids enter the mitochondrion and are metabolized by the citric acid cycle, which produces NADH. In the process of oxidative phosphorylation, high-energy electrons from NADH are then passed to oxygen by means of the respiratory chain in the inner membrane, producing ATP by a chemiosmotic mechanism. NADH generated by glycolysis in the cytosol also passes electrons to the respiratory chain (not shown). Because NADH cannot cross the mitochondrial inner membrane, the electron transfer from systolic NADH must be accomplished indirectly by means of one of several shuttle systems that transport another reduced compound into the mitochondrion; after being oxidized, this compound is returned to the cytosol, where it is reduced by NADH again. From Alberts B, Bray D, Lewis J, et al. Molecular biology of the cell. 2nd ed. New York: Garland, 1989. Reprinted by permission.

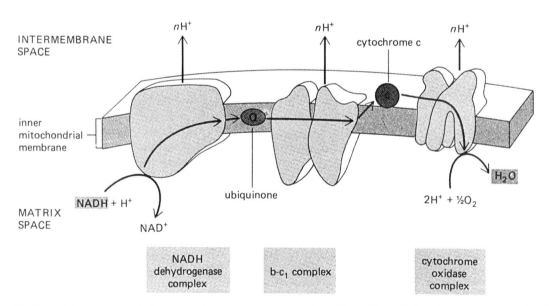

Figure 1.34. The flow of electrons through the three major respiratory enzyme complexes during the transfer of two electrons from NADH to oxygen. Ubiquinone and cytochrome c serve as carriers between the complexes. From Alberts B, Bray D, Lewis J, et al. Molecular biology of the cell. 2nd ed. New York: Garland, 1989. Reprinted by permission.

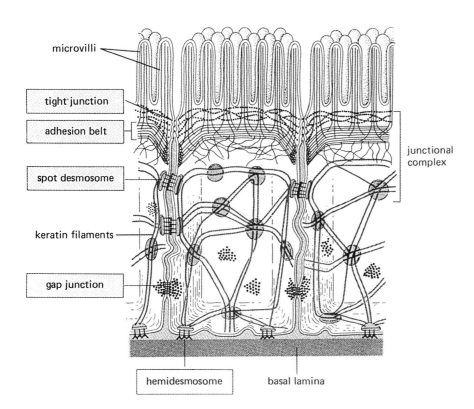

microvilli

tight junction

adhesion belt

spot desmosome

keratin filaments

gap junction

junctional complex

hemidesmosome   basal lamina

Figure 1.35. Distribution of the various cell junctions formed by epithelial cells of the small intestine. Bundles of actin microfilaments run down the centers of the microvilli of the intestinal epithelial cell and intersect with a layer of filaments called the terminal web. From Alberts B, Bray D, Lewis J, et al. Molecular biology of the cell. 2nd ed. New York: Garland, 1989. Reprinted by permission.

microvilli in their most efficient, erect position and provide the structural framework that allows efficient cell function. In addition, they are integral to maintaining cell-cell associations through specialized structures, such as desmosomes.

Skeletal and cardiac muscle are other examples of specialization and are the most extensively studied filamentous systems in the human body. Each muscle cell contains numerous cylindrical fibrils, packed in parallel alignment. The individual myofibrils have multiple repeating contractile subunits called sarcomeres, which are, in turn, composed of parallel thick filaments of myosin alternating with thin filaments of actin. Muscle contraction occurs when the thick filaments are stimulated to slide inside of the thin filaments as a result of calcium-dependent molecular interactions occurring between them (Fig. 1.36).

Another component of the cytoskeleton, the *microtubule,* is a cylindrical linear polymer formed by the aggregation of heterodimeric proteins called tubulins, which are themselves formed from two different protein molecules, α- and β-tubulin. Polymerization of tubulins is initiated in the centrosome, the cell's microtubule-organizing center. This small organelle is positioned adjacent to the nucleus and contains two centrioles and γ-tubulin. Microtubular assembly originating from this site is intrinsically polar with a slow-growing end embedded in the pericentriolar area and a fast-growing end directed toward the plasma membrane. Microtubules are not inherently static; they switch rapidly between phases of assembly and disassembly, a unique property referred to as *dynamic instability.* However,

once they have reached their optimal intracellular configuration, they generally are stabilized by the binding of specialized proteins called microtubule-associated proteins (MAPs). In most interphase cells, microtubules play a supportive role and, as such, are oriented along the long axis of the cell between the centrosome and the plasma membrane. They also serve as tracks on which intracellular membrane traffic travels, carried by the unidirectional motor proteins dynein (centrifugal) and kinesin (centripetal). In this manner, lysosomes, vesicles, the endoplasmic reticulum, and the Golgi apparatus are moved along microtubules by the motor proteins to which they are attached.

Specialized microtubules also participate in the motility of cilia and flagella. These motile cylinders share a similar structural arrangement, consisting of nine microtubule doublets surrounding two central tubules and enclosed by a membrane. Their characteristic movements occur when adjacent doublets slide longitudinally over one another, apparently as a result of conformational changes in the dynein bridges (motors) that link them (Fig. 1.37).

Similarly, normal cell division requires microtubular participation. During mitosis, centrosomes are replicated, initiating the growth of a unique array of microtubules that interdigitate to form the mitotic spindle. By attaching to chromosomes at their kinetochores, spindle microtubules precisely segregate and then parcel the DNA of the dividing cell into two equal parts. These sliding movements of spindle components, once again, appear to be mediated by the action of motor proteins (17).

Figure 1.36. Structure of myocardial cells at the level of light and electron microscopy is portrayed. (top) The drawing shows a portion of ventricular myocardium with branching muscle cells enmeshed in collagen. Nuclei are placed centrally, and intercalated discs contain sites for end-to-end attachment of cells. (middle) The drawing shows ultrastructure of portions of two cells in a cutaway view; the arrangement of myofibrils is evident. A network of intermediate filaments, which surrounds the myofibrils like a cage, is periodically anchored to cell membrane plaques at the Z bands and at transverse regions of the intercalated discs. Within the sarcomeres, the contractile units of the muscle delimited at each end by a Z band consist of three sets of filaments. Thick filaments containing primarily myosin are located in the A band; thin filaments containing actin, tropomyosin, troponin, and thin elastic filaments of titin extend from each Z band toward the middle of the sarcomere. (bottom) The thick and thin filaments interdigitate regularly to form a hexagonal array seen in cross-section. The exact placement of the titin filaments is not known, but they are thought to attach periodically along the thick filament. The Z band is a lattice of axial and cross-connecting Z filaments. The ends of the thin filaments from adjacent sarcomeres overlap and interdigitate in a centered tetragonal array and are held together periodically by cross-connecting filaments (four sets are shown here). From Goldstein MA, Schroetter JP, Michael LH. Role of the Z band in the mechanical properties of the heart. FASEB J 1991;5:2167–2174. Reprinted by permission.

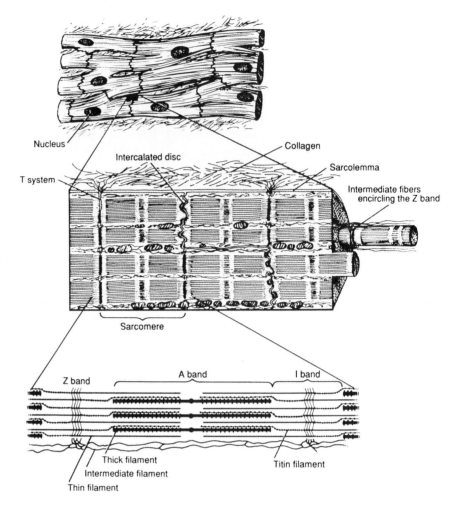

The third major component of the cytoskeleton, the *intermediate filament* protein family, is a heterogenous group of long, rope-like fibrous proteins (Fig. 1.38) with high tensile strength. All share a common central region of approximately 300 amino acids formed into an α-helix; however, the terminal segments may vary greatly. There are at least six types of intermediate filaments; five are relatively tissue specific. The cytokeratins type I (acidic) and type II (basic), are found in epithelial cells; vimentin, in mesenchymal tissues; desmin, in muscle; glial fibrillary acidic protein, in glial cells; and neurofilaments, in neurons. Intermediate filaments extend from the nucleus to the cell surface and interact with a variety of binding proteins and with other cytoskeletal filaments to produce their effects. By contrast, the nuclear lamins are present in all cells. As highly organized, dynamic sheets of filaments, they form the nuclear lamina that lines the inside surface of the nuclear envelope. During mitosis, the nuclear envelope and lamina rapidly disassemble, then reassemble as daughter cells begin to develop.

Proteins—From Translation to Sorting

All proteins are synthesized in the cell cytoplasm where the ribosomes serve as the sites for *translation* of the mRNA. This is the second stage of the process by which genes encoded in the DNA are synthesized into proteins. The reactions are complex; there are many steps in the transcription/translation process. Critical to understanding the process of translation is the *genetic code* by which triplets of bases encode a single amino acid (Fig. 1.39). The mRNA triplets, called *codons*, are always written in the 5' to 3' direction. There are 64 triplet codes for only 20 different amino acids, with 3 of the triplets coding for termination codons or stop signals. Because more than one codon may specify the same amino acid (in a pattern in which the first two bases are the same and the third base may vary), the genetic code has been termed *degenerate.*

Transfer RNA is involved intimately in translation (Fig. 1.40). Multiple forms of tRNA exist, with a separate tRNA population for each amino acid. Each tRNA has a triplet base sequence, an *anticodon,* which is complementary to the codon sequence and acts as an acceptor site for its specific amino acid. Structurally, tRNA molecules are folded into a cloverleaf-like pattern to make the bound amino acid and the anticodon loop more readily available for the translation sequence involved in synthesis.

Newly synthesized proteins require sorting, and the

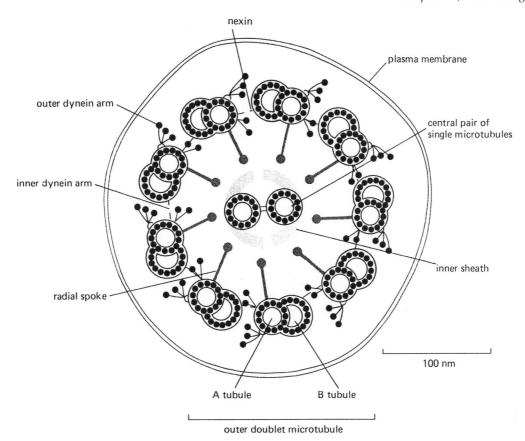

nexin

plasma membrane

outer dynein arm

central pair of single microtubules

inner dynein arm

inner sheath

radial spoke

100 nm

A tubule   B tubule

outer doublet microtubule

Figure 1.37. A cilium shown in cross-section. The various structural projections from the microtubules that occur at regular intervals along the cilium are responsible for ciliary function. Dynein arms, which project from microtubule doublets, interact with adjacent doublets to produce bending upon ATP hydrolysis and removal of cross-links by proteolysis. Nexin links hold adjacent microtubule doublets together. Radial spokes extend from each of the nine outer doublets inward to the central pair. Sheath projections that occur as a series of side arms from the central pair of microtubules regulate the form of the ciliary beat in concert with the radial spokes. From Alberts B, Bray D, Lewis J, et al. Molecular biology of the cell. 2nd ed. New York: Garland, 1989. Reprinted by permission.

regulation of their intracellular traffic is a function of the membranous organelles, which act together as a central vacuolar system. The ER acts as the initial assembly point for most of those proteins destined for extracellular secretion or residence within membranes. Protein synthesis begins in the cytoplasm on free ribosomes, but is quickly targeted to the ER by a signal peptide present on the leading portion of the new peptide chain. This leads the ribosomal complex to dock over a protein-conducting channel, stimulating synthesis to continue and ensuring that the nascent polypeptide chain translocates into the lumen of the ER. The signal peptide is subsequently cleaved, and the new proteins are *processed* and *sorted* according to specific targeting signals contained within them. Some proteins are retained within the ER. Others are enclosed within vesicles that bud from the smooth ER and fuse to the cis-Golgi network. Here posttranslational modification is sequentially completed through a series of steps that may include proteolytic cleavage, glycosylation, phosphorylation, and sulfation. The resulting product is released from the trans-Golgi subsection after being targeted to its final destination (18). Secretory proteins are either released continuously (constitutive) or stored in granules until an appropriate stimulus is received (regulated). Integral membrane proteins are delivered selectively to specific plasma membrane domains by a final transport vesicle that fuses to the inner membrane surface (Fig. 1.41).

Endocytosis

Cellular traffic is not one way. Substances on the surface of the cell can be enclosed in membrane-bound vesicles and taken into the cell by the process of endocytosis. Three kinds of *endocytosis* can be observed. In *pinocytosis*, solutions are internalized; in *phagocytosis*, particles are ingested. The contents of the early endosomes so formed generally are degraded by fusing with lysosomes, which contain autolytic enzymes. *Receptor-mediated endocytosis* occurs when certain ligands (nutrients, hormones, proteins, and viruses) migrate with their receptor to clathrin-coated pits and are then internalized as coated vesicles. Ligands and receptors commonly are dissociated in the endosome, allowing recycling of the receptors to the plasma membrane and routing of the ligands to lysosomes for disposal.

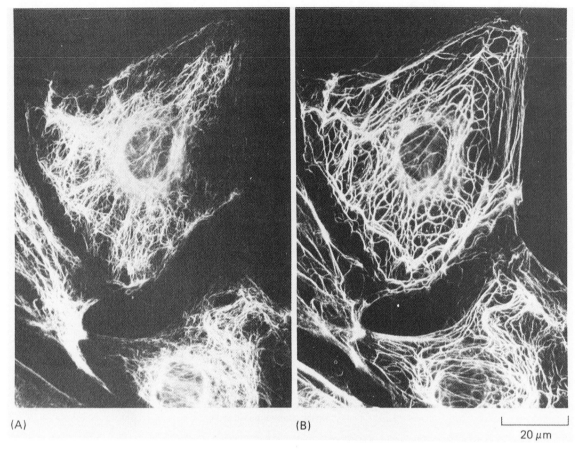

(A)   (B)

20 μm

Figure 1.38. Immunofluorescence micrographs of rat kangaroo epithelial cells (PtK2 cells) in interphase. The cells have been labeled with antibodies to vimentin (A) and to keratin (B). The cells contain separate arrays of vimentin filaments and keratin filaments, although the two arrays have a similar distribution. From Alberts B, Bray D, Lewis J, et al. Molecular biology of the cell. 2nd ed. New York: Garland, 1989. Reprinted by permission.

Figure 1.39. The genetic code. Sets of three nucleotides (codons) in an mRNA molecule are translated into amino acids in the course of protein synthesis, according to the rules shown. For example, the codons GUG and GAG are translated into valine and glutamic acid, respectively. Note that those codons with U or C as the second nucleotide tend to specify the more hydrophobic amino acids. From Alberts B, Bray D, Lewis J, et al. Molecular biology of the cell. 2nd ed. New York: Garland, 1989. Reprinted by permission.

1st position (5' end)	\	2nd position			3rd position (3' end)
	U	**C**	**A**	**G**	
U	Phe Phe Leu Leu	Ser Ser Ser Ser	Tyr Tyr STOP STOP	Cys Cys STOP Trp	U C A G
C	Leu Leu Leu Leu	Pro Pro Pro Pro	His His Gln Gln	Arg Arg Arg Arg	U C A G
A	Ile Ile Ile Met	Thr Thr Thr Thr	Asn Asn Lys Lys	Ser Ser Arg Arg	U C A G
G	Val Val Val Val	Ala Ala Ala Ala	Asp Asp Glu Glu	Gly Gly Gly Gly	U C A G

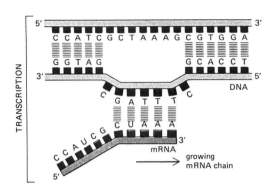

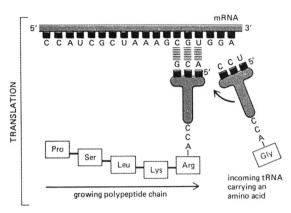

Figure 1.40. Information flow in protein synthesis. The nucleotides in an mRNA molecule are joined together to form a complementary copy of a segment of one strand of DNA. They are then matched three at a time to complementary sets of three nucleotides in the anticodon regions of tRNA molecules. At the other end of each type of tRNA molecule, a specific amino acid is held in a high-energy linkage, and when matching occurs, this amino acid is added to the end of the growing polypeptide chain. Thus translation of the mRNA nucleotide sequence into an amino acid sequence depends on complementary base pairing between codons in the mRNA and corresponding tRNA anticodons. In fact, the molecular basis of information transfer in translation is similar to that in DNA replication and transcription. The mRNA is both synthesized and translated starting from its 5' end. From Alberts B, Bray D, Lewis J, et al. Molecular biology of the cell. 2nd ed. New York: Garland, 1989. Reprinted by permission.

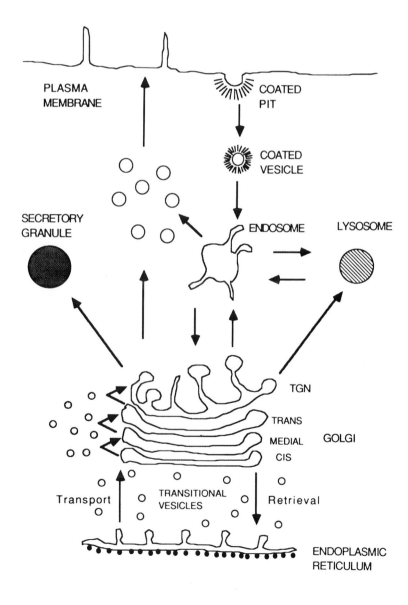

Figure 1.41. Sorting and traffic in the central vacuolar system. The organelles within this system include the rough and smooth ER; the cis-, medial-, and trans-Golgi; the trans-Golgi network (TGN), secretory vesicles, secretory granules, the endosomal system, lysosomes, and the plasma membrane. In addition, an unknown variety of transitional and/or transport organelles mediate the communication between these multiple compartments. Each of these organelles possesses characteristic resident membrane proteins that define the unique and differentiated structure and function of that compartment. From Klausner RD. Sorting and traffic in the central vacuolar system. Cell 1989;57:703. Copyright Cell Press. Reprinted by permission.

Figure 1.42. Pathways for MHC proteins. MHC proteins, which regulate the immune system, must be linked to antigens to reach the cell surface. The class I proteins, unlike the class II proteins, rely on transporter molecules to bring them antigens. A new theory suggests that defective transporters and MHC class I deficiencies could cause autoimmune disorders. From Renie J. First-class culprit. Copyright © 1992 by Scientific American, Inc. All rights reserved. Reprinted by permission.

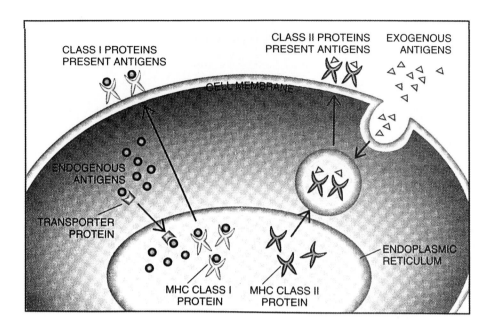

Antigen Processing

A specialized form of protein sorting occurs when foreign proteins are processed as antigens by certain immune cells, including B cells and macrophages, and presented to the other immune component, the helper T cell. Processing begins after a virus or other endogenous antigen is transferred into the ER by specialized transport proteins and binds to the proteins of the class I major histocompatibility complex (MHC). The MHC-peptide complex is carried to the cell's membrane where it is inserted with its peptide moiety pointing outward. Here it can be detected by specific receptors on the T cells, which then initiate immune-response cascades that involve cytokine production and cell stimulation (19). Exogenous antigents are processed differently. They interact with class II MHC proteins and then are taken into the cell and degraded before presentation on the cell surface (Fig. 1.42).

Extracellular Structures and Function

Extracellular Matrix

Most eukaryotic cells are surrounded by, or are in contact with, a complex scaffolding of insoluble structural macromolecules collectively termed the extracellular matrix (ECM). The form taken by this matrix (Fig. 1.43) varies from that of the basement membrane in epithelial tissues to the ground substance of mesenchymal tissues (20). The ECM must not only provide requisite structural support for cells, but also help to regulate cell behavior. In complex tissues, connective tissues may have large amounts of ECM and mesenchymal cells, which provide an important substrate for attachment and growth of the parenchymal cells of the tissue. An example of this is the epithelium lining the gut (Fig. 1.44).

The ECM is composed of at least four types of macromolecules: collagens, noncollagenous glycoproteins, proteoglycans, and elastin. The *collagens* are its major constituents and are the most abundant proteins in the human body; current nomenclature identifies at least 15 distinct types. Collagens are glycoproteins, and each is characterized by the presence of one or more triple-helical regions in its tertiary structure. This motif requires that glycine be present in every third amino acid position in the three polypeptide a-chains; frequently, proline and hydroxyproline are also present. The fibrillar collagens (Types I, II, III, V, XI) are mainly found in connective tissue where they are secreted in their inactive procollagen form with long nonhelical extensions at both ends. Once the terminal propeptides are cleaved enzymatically, the collagen molecules self-assemble into fibrils and assume their typical striated appearance, a result of the incomplete overlapping of adjacent molecules (Fig. 1.45). The prototypical Type I collagen is the most common type in mammals and forms the large bundles of collagen fibers present in many stromal matrices. Its specific architecture is adapted to the needs of the surrounding tissue: from a loose weave in skin to a highly oriented, nearly complete alignment in tendons to a tight orthogonal network in bone. Type II collagen is distributed in cartilage and corneal tissue, whereas the nonfibrillar Type IV collagen is present exclusively as a sheet-like mesh in the basement membrane. Many of the remaining types influence tissue properties by combining with Types I and II to form heterotypic fibrils.

The *noncollagenous glycoproteins* are adhesive macromolecules that interact with cells and with other ECM

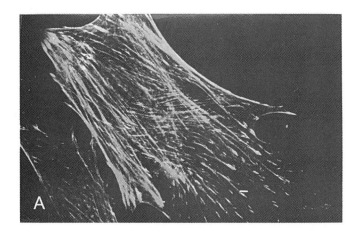

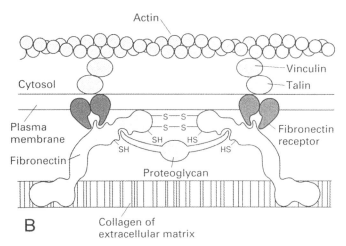

Figure 1.43. (A) Immunofluorescence of a fixed, stationary cultured fibroblast showing co-localization of the fibronectin receptor and actin-containing stress fibers. At the ends of the stress fibers, where the cells contact the substratum, there is coincidence of actin and the fibronectin receptor. Reproduced from The Journal of Cell Biology, 1988;107:1385, by copyright permission of the Rockefeller University Press. (B) Model of the connections between actin, fibronectin, and the extracellular matrix at the regions of contact between stationary fibroblasts and the substratum. The two-subunit transmembrane fibronectin receptor binds to fibronectin on its exoplasmic side and talin on its cytoplasmic side. Vinculin binds to talin and probably directly to an actin filament; fibronectin binds to fibrous collagen and to many proteoglycans. From Darnell, Lodish, Baltimore. Molecular cell biology. Copyright ©1990 by Scientific American Books, Inc. Reprinted by permission of W. H. Freeman and Company.

components to promote adhesion, migration, and proliferation and to influence gene expression (Fig. 1.46). The best characterized of these, fibronectin, is a large dimeric protein in which each polypeptide arm contains separate domains for binding to collagen, heparin, and fibrin and to specific cell-surface receptors. Binding can also occur to the glycoprotein envelope of viruses, to *Candida*, and to various bacteria. Fibronectin is produced by fibroblasts and by several other cells in both a soluble form (serum) and an insoluble form (cellular). Its cell-attachment domain contains a specific tripeptide recognition sequence, Arg-Gly-Asp (RGD), which is the segment recognized by the integrin-type receptors of many

cells. Because fibronectin is widely distributed and multifunctional, it is able to play an important role in such diverse biologic activities as cell-to-cell attachment, clot stabilization, wound healing, nerve regeneration, and phagocytosis.

Laminin is a large multidomain glycoprotein that has three polypeptide chains bonded into a cruciform shape. It is located primarily in the basement membrane, where it interacts with many cells and with other ECM molecules. Some of its newly discovered properties include the promotion of differentiation in muscle and epithelium and the stimulation of neurons to extend new processes. Other adhesive glycoproteins, such as entactin and tenascin, appear to have a much more restricted distribution; much remains to be discovered about their function.

The *proteoglycans* are large molecules composed of protein cores to which are attached side chains of glycosaminoglycans (GAGs); these polysaccharide chains are formed from repeating disaccharide units in which one of the two residues in each pair is always an amino sugar. The classification of proteoglycan aggregates is based on their dominant disaccharide unit and includes hyaluronate, chondroitin, dermatan, keratan, heparan, and heparin. Because they form bulky hydrated gels, they fill most of the extracellular space, providing a milieu in which water-soluble molecules can readily diffuse and cells can easily migrate. In addition, they interact with other ECM components to help determine the biomechanical properties of the surrounding tissue, such as the compressibility of cartilage. Their glycosaminoglycan side chains may bind and modulate various growth factors, thus acting as a reservoir for these and other soluble bioactive molecules.

Elastin is an unfolded hydrophobic protein that provides resiliency to tissue; its highly cross-linked, random-coiled structure allows it to stretch and relax. Not surprisingly, it is most prominent in the tissues of skin, blood vessels, and lungs.

Soluble and Insoluble Messengers

Cells are surrounded by a constantly changing environment and, through signal transduction, can respond to it with programmed multilevel intracellular actions. Some actions are rapid and do not require protein or RNA synthesis; others can only occur as a result of the induction of nuclear transcription. The signals themselves are derived from a wide variety of sources, but individual cells are able to be selective in their choices because the expression of their receptors is not uniform.

Insoluble or *contact-mediated signals* are provided by the ECM glycoproteins and proteoglycans that, when linked to the interior of the cell through integrin-like receptors, can promote adhesion and de-adhesion and stimulate cell migration, morphologic changes, and cytoskeletal reorganization. Insoluble matrix proteins may

Figure 1.44. Cell interactions and cell function. The connective tissue underlying an epithelial cell sheet. From Alberts B, Bray D, Lewis J, et al. Molecular biology of the cell. 2nd ed. New York: Garland, 1989. Reprinted by permission.

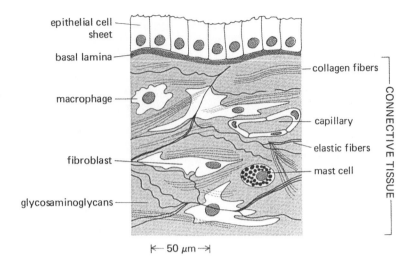

Figure 1.45. Fibroblast assembly of collagen fibrils. (A) Intracellular posttranslational modifications of precursor chains. (B) Enzymic cleavage of procollagen to collagen, self-assembly of collagen monomers into fibrils, and crosslinking of fibrils. Reprinted, by permission of The New England Journal of Medicine (311;377,1984).

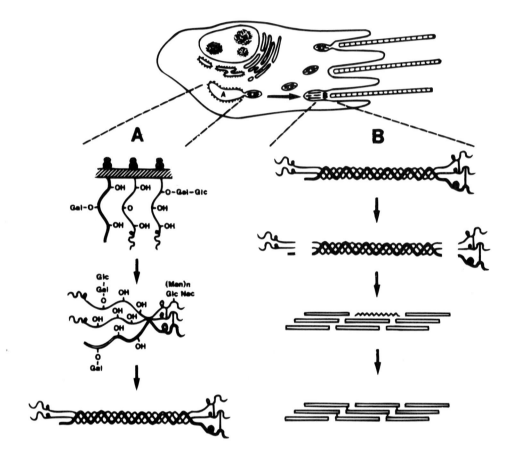

also interact with many local soluble factors to initiate inflammatory responses and to promote healing when wounding has occurred. Cell-cell contact similarly induces extracellular and intracellular changes by the transduction of signals across specific transmembrane receptors. In specialized cells, such as leukocytes, membrane-bound adhesive proteins serve to maintain cell contact and optimize cell-cell interaction.

The *soluble signals* include the cytokines, peptide hormones, and neuropeptides. Because of the hydrophobicity of cell membranes, these hydrophilic signals can-

not pass to the inside of the cell but instead communicate by binding to receptors on the cell surface. There they initiate various intracellular biochemical cascades. They may have only a local effect (paracrine and autocrine) or may act at multiple distant sites to which they are transported by blood (Table 1.6).

Cytokines are nonenzymatic, extracellular signaling proteins that generally act locally to both modify cell-specific behavior and to remodel the extracellular architecture. Interactions are complex, and single agents may exhibit a plethora of activities with different cell types

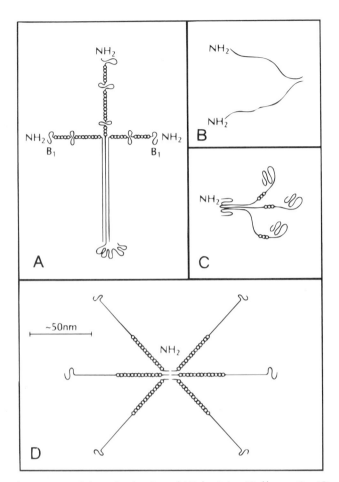

Figure 1.46. Schematic drawing of (A) laminin, (B) fibronectin, (C) thrombospondin, and (D) tenascin with epidermal growth-factor-like domains indicated by circles. The molecules are drawn approximately to scale. From Engel J. Common structural motifs in proteins of the extracellular matrix. Curr Opin Cell Biol 1991;3:782. Reprinted by permission of Current Science.

Table 1.6.
Delivery Pathways of Vertebrate Hormones and Growth Factors

Pathways	Transport of Bioactive Molecules
Endocrine	Hormone-producing cells synthesize and release into circulation
Paracrine	Nonneural cells synthesize factors that are released locally and affect neighboring target cells
Autocrine	Molecules reenter and affect (e.g., stimulation, inhibition) the cells synthesizing the bioactive factors
Neuroendocrine	Neural origin cells synthesize and release molecules into the circulation
Neurocrine	Local release of neurotransmitter or other neural cell molecules into the intercellular space adjacent to a target cell

and matrix proteins. Specific classes of cytokines include, but are not limited to, the growth factors, tumor necrosis factors, interleukins, and interferons (21). One important example of cytokine function is depicted in the response of the immune system to foreign antigens (Fig. 1.47).

The peptide hormones are synthesized in specialized cells of the endocrine glands, the central nervous system, and the gastrointestinal tract and either remain in the local environment or are transported in serum to relatively remote target sites where they bind to specific receptors. Many hormones are synthesized initially as inactive precursors and must be modified by proteolytic cleavage and/or chemical binding to become active before their secretion (Fig. 1.48). As with other biological systems, a variety of negative- and positive-feedback mechanisms are available to fine-tune the final effects.

Various neurotransmitters are released by exocytosis from cells within the central nervous system and from the synapses of peripheral neurons. These chemical signals mediate their effect focally by binding to cell membrane receptors of two different types. The channel-linked receptors provoke abrupt changes in channel conformation that allow specific ions to cross the membrane rapidly, thus producing short-lived voltage changes in the cell. These excitatory cationic channels in the periphery are primarily linked to acetylcholine (Ach) receptors and glutamate receptors in the brain. They are counterbalanced by inhibitory, mainly chloride, channels that are linked to receptors for γ-aminobutyric acid (GABA) and glycine.

By contrast, binding of non-channel neuroreceptors activates either G protein or protein tyrosine kinase pathways, which are slower, more sustained and relatively diffuse. Included in this group are the monoamines (e.g., epinephrine, norepinephrine, dopamine, and secretonin) and certain neuropeptides (e.g., vasoactive intestinal peptide, somatostatin, substance P, enkephalin, and β-endorphin). Complex interactions of multiple factors are often present; regulation of gastric parietal cell secretion is a prototype (Fig. 1.49).

Another signaling molecule, as yet incompletely characterized, is nitric oxide (NO). This potentially toxic gas is freely permeable through membranes and, therefore, able to diffuse from its original cell into nearby cells. It was previously known as the endothelium-derived relaxing factor because it causes blood vessels to relax when released from endothelium after stimulation by Ach. It is synthesized enzymatically from α-arginine and acts predominantly as a nonadrenergic, noncholinergic inhibitory neurotransmitter. Its enzyme, nitric oxide synthase, has been identified not only in neurons and endothelial cells but also in mast cells, the myenteric plexus, and the pancreatic β-cells. It has also been implicated as a cause of irreversible shock in endotoxemia (22). Another candidate for neurotransmitter gas is carbon monoxide, also normally found in brain tissue. Investigation of both these agents is proceeding rapidly.

Steroid hormones are synthesized from cholesterol and are thus lipophilic and able to cross cell membranes easily. Together with several other molecular signals such as thyroid hormone, vitamin D_3, and retinoic acid, glucocorticoids form complexes with cytoplasmic receptors

Figure 1.47. Proliferation of T cells is controlled by interleukin-2 (IL-2) after an antigen, ingested and presented by a macrophage, activates individual T cells. The antigen stimulates the T cells to secrete IL-2 and to make IL-2 receptors. Subsequently, the binding of IL-2 with its receptors signals the T cells to divide, thereby producing pairs of daughter cells that can also be activated by the antigen. In this way, a clone of identical antigen-specific T cells grows until the immune system eliminates the antigen from the body. From Smith KA. Interleukin-2. Copyright © 1990 by Scientific American, Inc. All rights reserved. Reprinted by permission.

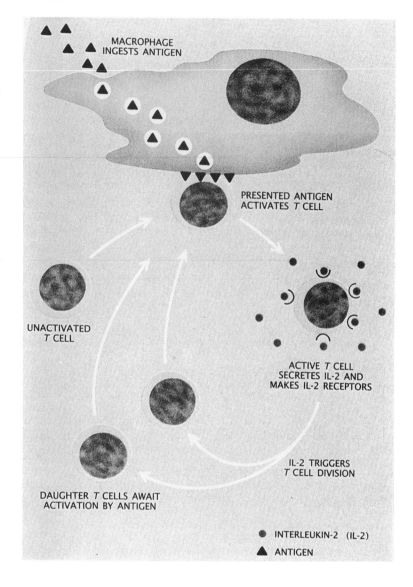

MACROPHAGE INGESTS ANTIGEN

PRESENTED ANTIGEN ACTIVATES *T* CELL

UNACTIVATED *T* CELL

ACTIVE *T* CELL SECRETES IL-2 AND MAKES IL-2 RECEPTORS

IL-2 TRIGGERS *T* CELL DIVISION

DAUGHTER *T* CELLS AWAIT ACTIVATION BY ANTIGEN

● INTERLEUKIN-2 (IL-2)

▲ ANTIGEN

that become activated and rapidly move into the nucleus to bind to regulatory units on the DNA. In this way, the hormones activate the transcription of certain genes and increase the production of the proteins that they encode (Fig. 1.50).

Applications

Molecular Technology

As with surgery, technical advances in methodology have had a major impact on cellular and molecular investigations. This new technology has its own nomenclature, as exemplified in Table 1.7. Sophisticated biochemical techniques for nucleic acid purification and analysis include a variety of nucleic acid hybridization methods for which the relatedness of two nucleic acid chains are compared by testing the ability of their bases to form complementary hybrids with one another. Con-

ditions have been defined to generate hydrogen-bonded DNA-DNA, DNA-RNA, or RNA-RNA hybrids. The method of nucleic acid hybridization, combined with the discovery of restriction-modification endonucleases (*restriction enzymes*), has led to an unprecedented explosion of knowledge on gene organization and expression. Restriction enzymes normally function to protect bacteria and other microbes from foreign DNAs such as viruses. Because they recognize specific mirror-image, 4- to 8-pair base sequences, called *palindromes*, they can be used as ''molecular scalpels'' to dissect DNA into reproducible sets of fragments according to specific base sequences.

When DNA is cut into fragments by restriction enzymes, the restriction fragments that result can be used to generate recombinant molecules, for structural analyses and other studies (Fig. 1.51). When locations of enzyme cleavage sites relative to one another in a long strand of DNA are compared, a DNA structural map can be created. The exact sequence of each base in the map can also be determined with relative ease by ana-

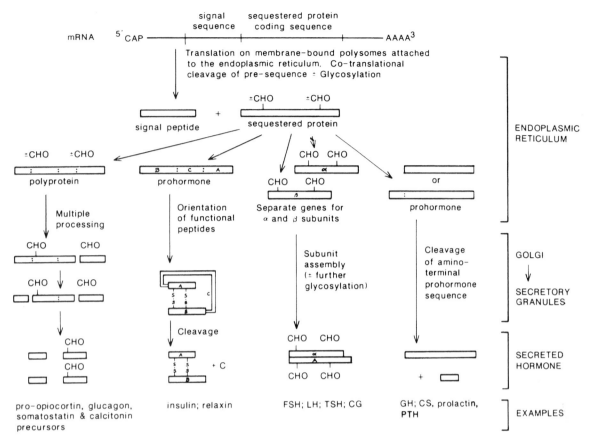

Figure 1.48. Several schemes whereby various groups of hormones are assembled from signal and subsequent prohormone products. Reprinted by permission of the publisher, from Williams RC. Molecular biology in clinical medicine. Copyright © 1991 by Elsevier Science Publishing Co., Inc.

lyzing restriction enzyme-generated fragments using automated DNA sequencing methods. The ability to sequence DNA is an extremely powerful tool, as it also permits predictions of the amino acid sequences of large proteins by using the genetic code and selecting the appropriate reading frame (i.e., the one that proceeds for long stretches without interruption by termination codons). Because these predictions of amino acid sequences do not require that the protein be isolated and purified, proteins that are difficult to obtain because of a short half-life or limited synthesis can now be studied more readily. This information can lead to production of clinically important proteins; examples include vaccine production to prevent disease, immunoassays for diagnostic use, and therapeutic products for injection or local application.

Another important technique is the generation of complementary DNA (cDNA) from mRNA molecules using the enzyme reverse transcriptase (Fig. 1.52). These cDNAs can then be used to prepare genetic *libraries,* which are recombinants between the cDNA molecules and vector DNAs, such as plasmids. Thus each library will contain the relevant information about mRNAs expressed by specific cells or tissues.

The *polymerase chain reaction* (PCR) technique has revolutionized molecular medicine, and it is responsible for

a number of applications, including detection of pathogens, gene cloning, forensics studies, paternity testing, and assessments of genetic mutations or rearrangements (Fig. 1.53). In the PCR technique, unique oligonucleotide primers, which are complementary to flanking regions of opposite DNA strands, are used to amplify a specific DNA segment. This yields PCR product, which is usually a single band of DNA detected by gel electrophoresis assay. Sequence specificity and integrity depend on the choice of primers, the quality of reagents, and the conditions used for amplification. Choice of oligonucleotides is based on knowing the base sequence of the opposite strand flanking regions, each of which must be unique. Verification by nucleic acid hybridization and sequence analyses are done when necessary, and where appropriate other procedures (e.g., immunoassays for diagnoses of pathogens) may be used in conjunction with PCR. The power of this procedure is that it can amplify a specific sequence of DNA by millions so that even rare molecular events, limited starting material, and partially degraded DNA can be studied (23).

Disease

Important to the overall changes in cells as they progress toward malignancy are the alterations of cell-

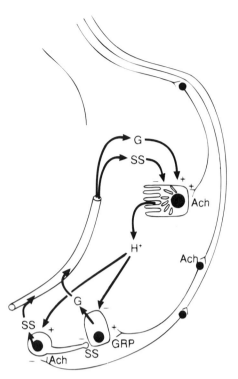

Figure 1.49. Regulation of acid secretion is a complex interplay of hormonal, neurocrine, and paracrine influences. Vagal cholinergic stimulation directly causes H^+ secretion from the parietal cell and indirectly via release of gastrin from antral G-cells. The latter effect is mediated via gastric GRP-containing neurons. The released gastrin acts hormonally to further stimulate acid secretion. Luminal acidification stimulates somatostatin release from d cells. Somatostatin acts in a paracrine manner to inhibit further gastrin release and in both paracrine and endocrine fashion to inhibit H^+ secretion. H^+, hydrogen ion; *G*, gastrin; *SS*, somatostatin; *GRP*, gastrin-releasing peptide. From Debas HT. Neuroendocrine design of the gut. Am J Surg 1991;161:246. Reprinted by permission.

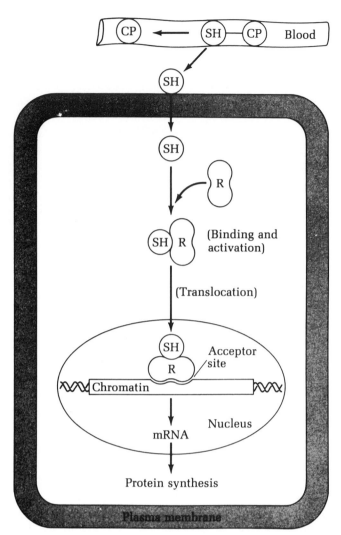

Figure 1.50. A general model for the mechanism of action of steroid hormones. The steroid hormone (SH) is transported in the blood bound to a carrier protein (CP). This complex dissociates and the hormone moves into the cytoplasm, where it binds to a receptor (R). This results in activation and translocation of the steroid hormone-receptor complex into the nucleus, where it binds to a specific acceptor site in chromatin, leading to transcription of a specific gene. The resulting mRNA is translated in the cytoplasm into a polypeptide molecule. This model applies to the action of estradiol as well as to that of other steroid hormones. From Kleinsmith LJ, Kish VM. Principles of cell biology. Copyright © 1988 by Harper & Row, Publishers, Inc. Reprinted by permission of HarperCollins Publishers.

signaling pathways, frequently combined with changes in responsiveness to various types of factors, and the not uncommon production of autocrine growth-stimulation factors by malignant cells. Collectively, these changes in the cells provide a growth advantage to the cells as they advance toward the malignant phenotype or acquire new abilities, particularly the ability to grow in different sites from the site of tumor initiation. A challenge exists to find new and more effective diagnostic strategies and therapeutic agents to manage patients, particularly those for whom long-term survival has generally been poor. The ability to diagnose disease earlier, based on deletion of certain tumor factors or cells, by new methods strongly suggests that a better knowledge of tumor biology gained through basic research efforts may be a prelude to developing more organ- or cell-specific treatment to control or eradicate tumors. Recent applications of growth factors, introduction of modified tumor-infiltrating lymphocytes, and modulation of tumor cell surfaces followed by reinjection are all approaches that have shown promising results in cancer treatment. As an example, knowledge of estrogen and progesterone receptor status impacts the treatment and prognosis in

patients with breast cancer. Nevertheless, the complex interactive networks involved at the cellular level are just beginning to be understood (Fig. 1.54). Care must be taken in the use of these new tools because there are still many things that are yet to be understood.

One perplexing problem in the effort to develop new therapeutic agents is that cells themselves have protective mechanisms, such as the ability to induce drug-resistant genes (e.g., the multiple drug-resistant gene, *mdr*). Some organs constitutively express *mdr* genes and are thus naturally refractory (24). On the positive side, de novo expression or amplification of specific genes

Table 1.7.
Glossary of Terms Used in Recombinant DNA Studies

Term	Definition
DNA Types	
Genomic	All chromosomal sequences of organisms
Plasmid	Extrachromosomal, independently replicating circular DNA molecules
Phage	Bacterial virus-derived DNA, commonly used as vector
cDNA	"Complementary" DNA copied from an mRNA molecule
Recombinant	Pieces of DNAs from two or more sources ligated into a single vector
General Terms	
Vector	Plasmid or virus DNA molecule containing inserted gene or DNA fragment of interest (prokaryotic or eukaryotic)
Host cell	Cell (prokaryotic or eukaryotic) in which vectors are propagated
Clone	Genetically identical molecule, cell, or organism
Library	Complete set of genomic or cDNA clones from one cell or microbe type; maintained in plasmids or phage
Restriction endonuclease	Enzyme that site-specifically recognizes and cuts in DNA regions with mirror-image sequences (i.e., palindromes of usually four to eight bases)
Cleavage maps	Structural "maps" generated by use of multiple restriction endonucleases to determine arrangements of genomic regions in DNA
DNA probe	DNA labeled radioactively or with chromogen, then hybridized with other nucleic acid to determine sequence relationships
Methods:	
Blot or Blotting	Methods used to study macromolecules separated by gel electrophoresis, then transferred onto membrane filters, can be visualized by specific probes and/or staining methods
Southern	Transfer and binding of DNAs; allows probing for presence of specific genes
Northern	Transfer and binding of RNAs; allows probing for DNA expression of specific genes
Western	Transfer and binding of proteins; allows comparative protein analyses, augmented with use of protein-specific antibodies to establish identity
RNA Terms	
Splicing	Process by which RNA transcript is cleaved, and religated to generate a functional mRNA
Intron	Regions of RNA removed during splicing
Exon	Regions of RNA that are part of protein-coding sequences
Untranslated regions	Regions at the 5' and 3' ends of mRNA that do not code for protein but have regulatory functions
PolyA	Polyadenylated regions at 3' end of mRNA; important for nuclear transport and mRNA longevity
Cap	Modified bases at 5' terminus of mRNA
Reverse transcriptase	Enzyme that copies RNA into cDNA
Methods, General	
Gel electrophoresis	Biochemical separation of macromolecules based on size and charge
Polymerease chain reaction	Method to enzymatically amplify a specific segment of DNA many millionfold
Mutagenesis	Induction of mutation; can be random but certain methods can yield site-specific mutagenesis
Nucleic acid hybridization	Denaturation of two sources nucleic acids followed by reassociation and base pairing to assess genetic identity or relatedness
DNA sequencing	Determining the series of bases comprising a sequence
Immunoassays	Immunological methods in which antibodies are used as tools to measure very low concentrations of biological agents

may herald a new strategy that can capitalize on those changes. Thus biotechnology-derived products combined with a working knowledge of each type of tumor and normal cell types can lead to new approaches based on changes of what are normal homeostatic mechanisms. Ultimately, this will lead to rational drug design, with biologically based approaches to cancer diagnosis, therapy, and prevention.

Human and other mammalian cells are also used to produce various biologicals, which collectively include vaccines and released products (such as peptides or growth factors). These biologicals cannot be produced by lower organisms, such as bacteria, because those microbes lack the secretory functions of mammalian cells and many proteins must be modified, by glycosylation or tight association with lipids, for example, to be func-

tional. In addition, biologicals from human sources are more likely to lack the immunogenic properties that could cause them to be rejected by the patient. The latter issues are also relevant when nonhuman mammalian cells are used to produce new diagnostic and therapeutic tools; problems may be encountered with immunological rejection.

In addition, technological advances made in cellular and molecular biology have increased the ability to introduce functional genes into a variety of cell types. This has enhanced the probability of successful gene therapy and stimulated numerous other clinical applications. Many types of recombinant vectors have been constructed and used to transfect human and other mammalian cells. Multiple factors are involved in expression, persistence, and recombination of the introduced genes.

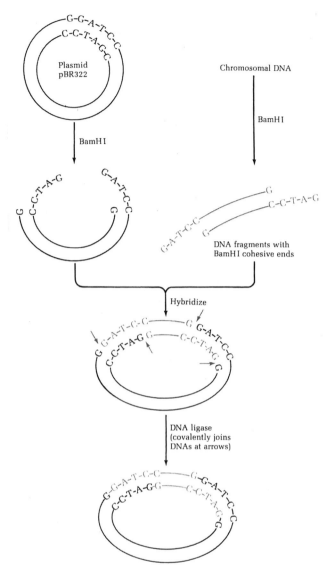

Figure 1.51. One way in which restriction enzymes can be used to generate recombinant DNA molecules. This general approach can be used with restriction enzymes that cut the cloning vector in a single location and that also generate suitable fragments of the DNA sample being cloned. From Kleinsmith LJ, Kish VM. Principles of cell biology. Copyright © 1988 by Harper & Row, Publishers, Inc. Reprinted by permission of HarperCollins Publishers.

Although progress is being made, technology still needs to be advanced in several areas: (a) development of an injectable, "targetable" vector that may not require that the target cells be dividing; (b) improved site-specific integration into the host DNA; (c) regulation of physiologic signals; and (d) propagation and characterization of specific types of human cells. Through continued research and a better understanding of pathophysiology at the cellular and molecular levels comes the logical next step of adding genetically engineered human cells to the repertoire of acceptable biomedical technologies. Indeed, some clinical trials are already under way.

The Human Genome Project is a worldwide endeavor to sequence the entire human genome and to identify specific human genes. It has stimulated ever-advancing molecular technologies and promoted a keen understanding of gene expression in various cell types (25). Critical to this goal will be the dramatic increase in automation of molecular biology, combined with the development of human cell culture models and tissue banks from multiple organ sites with representation from various ages of donors. These strides will continue to impact the feasibility of genetically engineering human cells and the associated clinical applications of treating diseases, producing biologicals, and providing gene therapy.

Current thought is that genes that normally function to suppress tumorigenicity are somehow inactivated by deletions, methylations, point mutations, or other changes as a prelude to malignant transformation of cells. Such models propose that this lost genetic material is important during the progressive stages of tumorigenesis, with a variety of studies pointing to specific regions of chromosomes involved in certain types of cancers (26). One example of the concept of tumor suppressor genes involves retinoblastoma (Rb), an uncommon childhood cancer that forms in neural precursor cells of the immature retina. When mutations and deletions occur in both alleles of chromosome 13, where the retinoblastoma gene is located, retinoblastoma will develop in 100% of the individuals. The *Rb* gene is involved in binding to nuclear DNA and commonly is associated with the variety of protooncogenes in the cell. Mutation of this particular gene has a known end point, retinoblastoma, and is the best understood example of a tumor-suppressor gene.

In another example, colon cancer, chromosomes 5, 17, and 18 have been identified as candidate regions for tumor-suppressor genes. The *p53* gene, which is involved intimately in the formation of many types of cancers, may have a deletion in one allele and another change in the second allele, such as a point mutation. Thus the *p53* gene is one of those genes implicated in the series of stages of colon carcinogenesis. Other genes are involved in colon cancer, including the *DCC* gene located on chromosome 18. Collectively, these putative tumor-suppressor genes play some role, which is yet to be clearly defined.

Because cancer development is made up of various stages, including initiation, promotion, and progression, there are many opportunities for mutations to occur. In various models using either cell cultures or animal subjects, a single event is usually inadequate to convert cells that are normal into cells that are malignant. Thus several preneoplastic stages commonly precede the development of particular types of cancer. An example of this is the formation of polyps during the progression of colon cancer or other types of premalignant lesions, such as hyperplasia, seen in the prostate as a prelude to potential formation of a tumor at that organ site. The formation of the tumor and its complete conversion to

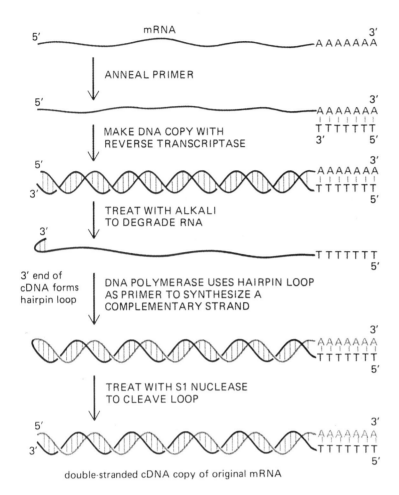

Figure 1.52. Recombinant DNA from mRNA; the synthesis of cDNA. A DNA copy of an mRNA molecule is produced by the enzyme reverse transcriptase, thereby forming a DNA/RNA hybrid helix. Treating the DNA/RNA hybrid with alkali selectively degrades the RNA strand into nucleotides. The remaining single-stranded cDNA is then copied into double-stranded cDNA by the enzyme DNA polymerase. As indicated, both reverse transcriptase and DNA polymerase require a primer to begin their synthesis. For reverse transcriptase, a small oligonucleotide is used; in this example, oligo(dT) has been annealed with the long poly A tract at the 3' end of most mRNAs. Note that the double-stranded cDNA molecule produced here lacks cohesive ends. From Alberts B, Bray D, Lewis J, et al. Molecular biology of the cell. 2nd ed. New York: Garland, 1989. Reprinted by permission.

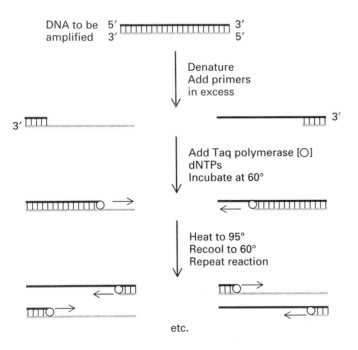

Figure 1.53. The polymerase chain reaction. Taq polymerase, a heat-resistant DNA polymerase from *Thermus aquaticus* is used to extend primers between two fixed points on a DNA molecule. All the components for chain elongation (primers, deoxynucleotides, and polymerase) are heat stable. Thus multiple heating and cooling cycles cause alternating DNA melting and synthesis. DNA between the recognition sites of the two oligonucleotide primers accumulates exponentially. Overnight, it may be amplified as much as a millionfold. From Darnell, Lodish, Baltimore. Molecular cell biology. Copyright ©1990 by Scientific American Books, Inc. Reprinted by permission of W. H. Freeman and Company.

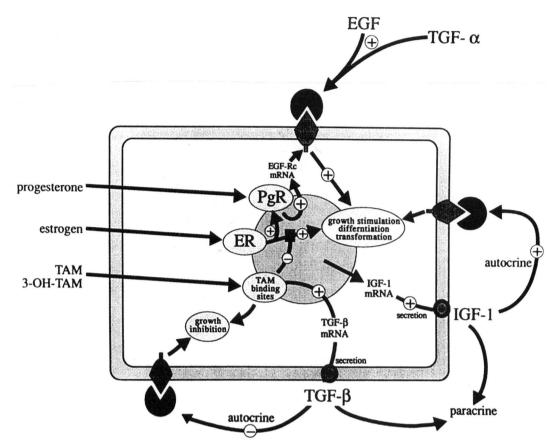

Figure 1.54. Complex interactive network between steroid and peptide hormones and related receptors exemplified for the mammary carcinoma cell line MCF-7. Estrogen binding to EGF stimulates PgR synthesis, which, after activation, enhances EGF receptor synthesis. Overexpressed EGF receptors are stimulated by EGF and TGF-a, inducing cellular growth, differentiation, and/or transformation. During this process, IGF-I synthesis, secretion, and receptor expression are elevated. TAM and 3-OH- TAM inhibit estrogen-induced growth and stimulate production and secretion of the negative growth factor TGF-*β*. *PgR*, progesterone receptor; *ER*, estrogen receptor; *IGF*, insulin-like growth factor; *TAM*, tamoxifen; *+*, stimulation; *−*, inhibition. From Dietel M. Morphological characterization of cell receptors. Curr Top Pathol 1991;83:108. Reprinted by permission of Springer-Verlag.

malignancy may then be followed by metastases. Additional genetic changes may accompany metastases as the tumor cells acquire the ability to leave the primary site of tumor formation and migrate to other sites in the body. Some of the genetic changes appear to be caused by carcinogens in the environment or by specific types of viruses that have been implicated in various human cancers. These viruses contain either DNA or RNA. For example, DNA viruses in the herpesvirus, papovavirus, poxvirus, adenovirus, and other groups have been implicated in the formation of cancers. In the RNA viruses, only the retrovirus group has been implicated as potential tumor-causing viruses. This group includes the human T cell leukemia virus, which causes adult T cell leukemia and lymphoma, and the human immunodeficiency virus (HIV), which is the causative agent of acquired immunodeficiency syndrome (AIDS) and has been implicated in the formation of lymphomas and Kaposi's sarcomas.

Combined understanding of many features of cell biology and cell regulation and identification of the specific genes associated with tumor-causing viruses have

led to an interface of fields and a greater understanding of how these factors have coevolved and of how changes in these factors can lead to malignant phenotypes. Thus tumor-causing viruses have specific genes that are involved in the process of converting cells from a normal to a malignant state. Their effects may include changes in the regulation of RNA synthesis, modification of membranes, the binding of growth-factor receptors, and complexing with tumor-suppressor genes such as cellular *p53*. In addition, these collections of factors may interact with other types of proteins important for the regulation of mitosis or the response to growth factors.

Mechanisms are now being elucidated for many of these proteins, but much more remains to be learned. By understanding the changes associated with the conversion of a cell from normal to malignant, a better understanding has come of not only abnormal cell growth regulatory processes, but normal processes as well. New targets for cancer chemotherapeutics, diagnosis, and prevention can be gleaned from a better understanding of the mechanisms involved at the cellular and genetic level in these models. Indeed, newly targeted approaches in clinical trials are using knowledge gained from these types of studies.

Cell Death

Cells are not immortal. In multicellular organisms they may die either as the result of an accident (necrosis) or in response to an internally-coded suicide program (apoptosis). These two terminal processes appear to be morphologically and functionally distinct, although areas of overlap can sometimes be observed.

The first, necrosis, represents the cell's response to such injuries as ischemia or irradiation. By contrast, apoptosis is a natural process that begins under the precise control of diverse intra-and extracellular signals, which act as either enhancers or inhibitors. These signals are highly dependent on the cell type and its microenvironment. The progression of apoptosis is then regulated by a variety of different genes, including p53 and members of the *bcl*-2 related gene family. It is characterized by a fixed sequence of events that begin when the cell shrinks and loses its normal membrane contacts. Cellular budding and fragmentation follow; the resultant apoptotic bodies are then phagocytosed rapidly by macrophages and other neighboring cells (Fig. 1.55).

Early studies of apoptosis have already yielded numerous intriguing discoveries, and enormous potential exists for further progress. In particular, the characterization of genes that are uniquely responsible for regulating or modifying cell death promises to have broad applications to such areas as cancer research, cardiovascular disease, developmental biology and immunology (27).

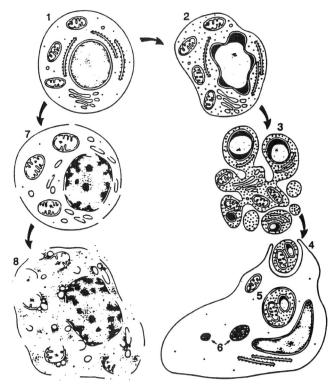

Figure 1.55. The sequence of ultrastructural events that takes place in apoptosis (right) and necrosis (left). A normal cell is represented at 1. In the early stages of apoptosis (2), the chromatin compacts to form sharply delineated masses on the nuclear envelope, the cytoplasm begins to condense, and the nuclear and cellular outlines become mildly convoluted (3). Marked convolution of the cell surface occurs with breaking-up of the nucleus into discrete, membrane-enclosed fragments, and budding of the cell as a whole to produce membrane-bound apoptotic bodies containing well-preserved organelles. In tissues, these are phagocytosed by adjacent cells (4) and degraded within lysosomal vacuoles (5), and reduced to compact debris within telolysosomes (6). There is no inflammation, and unaffected cells close ranks as the apoptotic bodies are phagocytosed. Cell deletion is effected without disruption of overall tissue architecture. The onset of necrosis in irreversibly injured cells (7) is characterized by condensation of chromatin, without radical change in its distribution, producing irregular clumps with ill-defined edges. Simultaneously, all cytoplasmic compartments undergo marked swelling, and membranes begin to break down. At a later stage (8), the nuclei and organelles disintegrate, but the cells tend to retain their overall configuration until removed by mononuclear phagocytes. From Kerr JFR. Neglected opportunities in apoptosis research. Trends in Cell Biology 1995; 5:55–57. Reprinted by permission.

Summary

The proteins within a cell determine its character. The identity of these proteins as specified by their amino acid sequence is a direct function of the genetic code. In this way, the code programs the range of properties that can be exhibited by a given cell. Even cell death appears to be encoded by a genetic clock, a phenomena called apoptosis.

Ultimately, the survival of a cell depends on its ability to relate to its environment and to respond appropriately to the myriad stimuli surrounding it. The pathways of these responses can be enormously complex and are largely uncharted; they occur in several time frames and at multiple levels of function. Metabolic, muscular, or neurobiologic responses may occur within seconds to minutes, whereas new protein synthesis requires minutes to hours. None of these responses occur in isolation; rather, each is integrated closely with the functions of many other cells, tissues, and organs.

The fundamental processes of cell differentiation and growth basically are controlled by the regulation of gene transcription, but in each instance, numerous environmental cues play a major role. Other functions that require much more rapid execution may depend on cytoplasmic metabolic mechanisms, but they are still modulated by the information contained within the genetic code. Any abnormalities within the genetic code or an inability of the cell to respond appropriately to the variety of internal and external stresses to which it is exposed will lead to cell death, placing the entire organism at risk. Fortunately, these complex and interactive relationships will continue to become more comprehensible as a result of the many interdisciplinary efforts that are now under way. Moreover, the diagnosis and treatment of medical and surgical disease will be increasingly predicated on a knowledge of the intricacies of cell biology. It is thus imperative that the disciplines of molecular biology become integrated into our knowledge base, and, by inference, into our daily practice.

REFERENCES

1. Knoll AH. End of the Proterozoic eon. Sci Am 1991;259:64–73.
2. Schacter, O. Fluidity and function of hepatocyte plasma membranes. Hepatology 1984;4:140–151.
3. Sigal E. The molecular biology of mammalian arachidonic acid metabolism. Am J Physiol 1991;260(Lung Cell Mol Physiol 4):L13–L28.
4. Singer SJ. The structure and insertion of integral proteins in membranes. Annu Rev Cell Biol 1990;6:247–296.
5. Bourne HR, Sanders DA, McCormick F. The GTPase superfamily: a conserved switch for diverse cell functions. Nature 1990;348:125–132.
6. Hunter T. Protein modification: phosphorylation on tyrosine residues. Curr Opin Cell Biol 1989;1:1168–1181.
7. Ruoslahti R, Pierschbacher MD. New perspectives in cell adhesion: RGD and integrins. Science 1987;283:491–497.
8. Getzenberg RH, Pienta KJ, Ward WS, Coffey D. Nuclear structure and the three-dimensional organization of DNA. J Cell Biochem 1991;47:289–299.
9. Radman M, Wagner R. The high fidelity of DNA duplication. Sci Am 1988;259:40–46.
10. Freeman RS, Donoghue DJ. Protein kinases and protooncogenes: biochemical regulators of the eukaryotic cell cycle. Biochemistry 1991;30:2293–2302.
11. Angel P, Karin M. The role of Jun, Fos and the AP-1 complex in cell-proliferation and transformation. Biochim Biophys Acta 1991;1072:129–157.
12. Ptashne M. How eukaryotic transcriptional activators work. Nature 1988;334:683–689.
13. McKnight SL. Molecular zippers in gene regulation. Sci Am 1991;264:54–64.
14. Mellman I, Simons K. The Golgi complex; in vitro veritas? Cell 1992;68:829–840.
15. Harding AE. The other genome. Br Med J 1991;303:377–378.
16. Bray D, White JG. Cortical flow in animal cells. Science 1988;239:883–888.
17. McIntosh JR, McDonald KL. The mitotic spindle. Sci Am 1989;261:48–56.
18. Rothman JE, Orci L. Molecular dissection of the secretory pathway. Nature 1992;355:409–415.
19. Rudensky AV, Preston-Hurlburt P, Hong SC, Barlow A, Janeway CA Jr. Sequence analysis of peptides bound to MHC class II molecules. Nature 1991;353:622–627.
20. Hay ED. Extracellular matrix, cell skeletons, and embryonic development. Am J Med Genet 1989;34:14–29.
21. Nathan C, Sporn M. Cytokines in context. J Cell Biol 1991;113:981–986.
22. Snyder SH, Bredt DS. Biological roles of nitric oxide. Sci Am 1992;266:68–77.
23. Mullis KB. The unusual origin of the polymerase chain reaction. Sci Am 1990;262:56–60.
24. Fairchild CR, Cowan KH. Multi-drug resistance: a pleiotropic response to cytotoxic drugs. Int J Radiat Oncol Biol Phys 1991;20:361–379.
25. Green ED, Waterson, RH. The human genome project. Prospects and implications for clinical medicine. JAMA 1991;266:1966–1975.
26. William CL, Fenoglio-Preiser CM. Oncogenes, suppression genes, and carcinogenesis. Hum Pathol 1987;18:896–902.
27. Monti D, Grassilli E, Troiano L, Cossarizzi A, et al. Senescence, immortalization, and apoptosis: An intriguing relationship. Ann N Y Acad Sci 1992;673:70-82.

SUGGESTED READINGS

Alberts B, Bray D, Lewis J, et al. Molecular biology of the cell. 3rd ed. New York: Garland, 1994.

Branden C, Tooze J. Introduction to protein structure. New York: Garland, 1991.

Darnell JE, Lodish H, Baltimore D. Molecular cell biology. New York: WH Freeman, Scientific American Books, 1990.

Gennis RB. Biomembranes: molecular structure, and function. New York: Springer-Verlag, 1989.

Hay ED. Cell biology of extracellular matrix. 2nd ed. New York: Plenum Press, 1991.

Kleinsmith LJ, Kish VM. Principles of cell biology. New York: Harper & Row, 1988.

Sambrook J, Fritsch EF, Maniatis T. Molecular cloning. A laboratory manual. 2nd ed. Cold Spring Harbor, NY: Cold Spring Harbor Laboratory Press, 1989.

Leder P, Clayton DA, Rubenstein E. Introduction to molecular biology. New York: Scientific American, Inc., 1994.

2 Growth and Development

William J. Pokorny | Steven S. Rothenberg | Mary L. Brandt

Introduction

The DNA messages that are brought to an individual and the intrauterine environmental factors met by the fertilized egg and developing embryo are critical to the eventual outcome of the pregnancy and the fetus. Although the etiology of human malformations is often difficult to ascertain, it has been estimated that 15% are primarily of genetic origin, 10% result from chromosomal aberrations, 10% are of viral or teratogenic origin, and 65% are of unknown origin (1,2). Only 30% of fertilized eggs result in normal babies (Fig. 2.1) (3). As many as 58% of fertilized eggs fail to implant or are lost before the next menstrual period so that a clinical pregnancy is not established (3,4). Nearly 50% of these losses are due to chromosomal abnormalities. Pregnancy outcome based on fetal loss and infant death for 92 weeks after conception is shown graphically in Figure 2.2 (5,6). By the forty-second week of gestation, and before birth, there are an estimated 295 deaths per 1000 conceptions with implantation. Of the 705 live births, approximately 13 will have died by 92 weeks from conception (6). The majority of these deaths are caused by fetal maldevelopment, usually as a result of environmental factors during or after the pregnancy.

About 66% of malformations occur in the first month of gestation, and almost 25% occur during the second month (7). Only an estimated 9% occur after the second month of gestation, emphasizing the critical role early prenatal care can play in a successful outcome. In Figure 2.3, the probable age at which developmental errors arise is shown for 203 different congenital anomalies of concern to the surgeon (1).

Genetics

Understanding genetics and embryology provides a guide to the events in development as well as in many disease processes. As our understanding of the genetic events of a human lifetime evolve, it is apparent that this "map" of our existence has a direct bearing on surgical intervention. Surgery is no longer limited to dissection with the scalpel and scissors but has now entered the realm of molecular "dissection" as well.

To understand the new frontier of molecular surgery, it is important to understand the building blocks of the genome, beginning with DNA. Deoxyribonucleic acid (DNA) is a polymer composed of a sugar (deoxyribose), nitrogen-containing bases (purines and pyrimidines), and a phosphate. The sequencing of the purine (adenine and guanine) and pyrimidine (thymine and cytosine) bases provides the code for subsequent protein synthesis.

The translation of the DNA code is carried out by messenger RNA (mRNA). Transcription of the DNA into RNA is carried out in the nucleus. The mRNA is then extruded into the cytoplasm where transfer RNA (tRNA) transfers amino acids onto the mRNA template, creating a protein.

DNA sequences containing codes for proteins (exons) and noncoding sequences (introns) are found in certain locations on the chromosomes called genes. In addition to the exons and introns, a gene will also have segments that regulate gene expression, i.e., protein synthesis. Each gene is matched with an identical gene on the second chromosome in each chromosome pair. The different gene forms for a specific site are called alleles. In each pair of alleles, one was inherited from the mother and one from the father.

There are 46 chromosomes in the human, 22 pairs of autosomes, and one pair of sex chromosomes, XX in the female and XY in the male. All of the genetic information required for the maintenance of life and expression of individuality is contained within these chromosomes. Certain disease states are transmitted from the parents with specific patterns of inheritance.

Patterns in Human Genetics

Single Gene Disorders

Nearly 4000 disorders in humans have been attributed to single genes. These single-gene disorders

Figure 2.1. Graph of postovulatory survival and development in humans. Baselines give age and developmental periods. Under assumed favorable conditions, 30% of eggs develop to normal babies (**Good Eggs**); 1% become live-born infants with cognitive defects (*hatched*), of which about 1 in 25 have chromosome anomalies; 69% perish (*reabsorbed or aborted*), this class (**Malformations**) may be chromosomally normal (*white*) or anomalous (*black*). Cl., cleavage; Impl., implantation; Neur., neurula. From Witschi 1970.

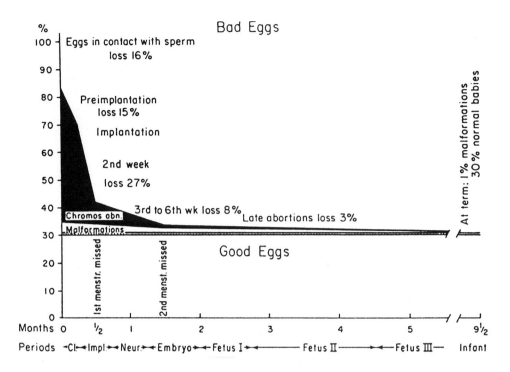

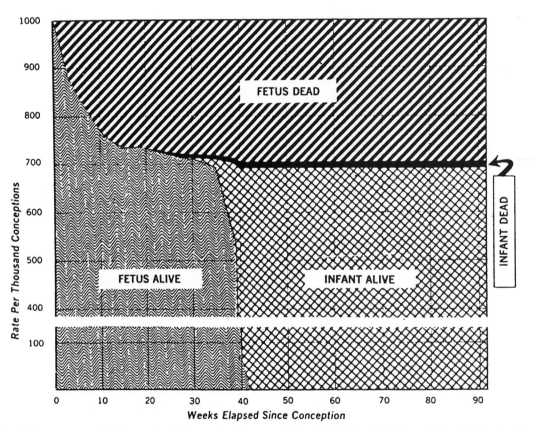

Figure 2.2. Cumulative outcome of 1000 pregnancies by weeks after conception. By week 44 there will have been 705 live births of which 13 infants have died after having been born alive. The remaining 295 will have died before birth. From Stickle G. Defective development and reproductive wastage in the United States. Am J Obstet Gynecol 1968; 100:442–447. Reprinted by permission.

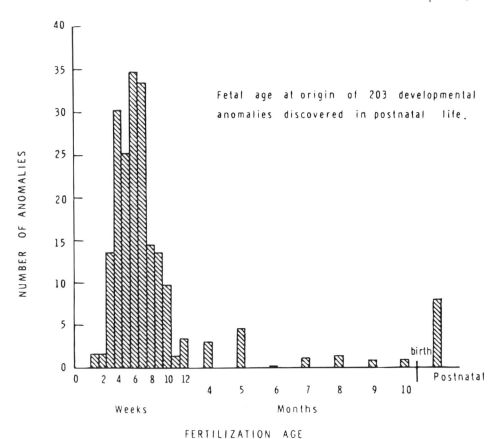

Fetal age at origin of 203 developmental anomalies discovered in postnatal life.

Figure 2.3. The probable age at which developmental errors arise to produce 203 of the congenital anomalies discussed in this volume. Only anomalies that may be present in postnatal life are included. From Gray SW, Skandalakis JE. Embryology for surgeons. Philadelphia: WB Saunders, 1972. Reprinted by permission.

follow the classic Mendelian pattern of inheritance (8).

Autosomal Dominant Disorders. An autosomal dominant disorder implies that only one of the two genes in a pair needs to be abnormal for the individual to exhibit characteristics of a disease (9). Because the abnormality is carried on an autosomal chromosome, the sexes are equally affected and the risk of an affected individual having an affected child is one out of two.

Unlike autosomal recessive diseases, a carrier state does not commonly occur in autosomal dominant diseases. That is, a person with the gene for an autosomal dominant disease has the disease, and a person with no evidence of the disease can be assumed not to be a carrier of the gene. These simple Mendelian rules are complicated by incomplete penetrance, variable expressivity, and mutation. Incomplete penetrance describes the unusual situation in which a person may carry the gene but show no signs of the disease and yet can still pass the gene and disease to the offspring. Variable expressivity refers to the variability of manifestations among individuals with the same genetic disorder. A mutation describes the appearance of the disease in the offspring of normal parents with no family history of affected members. Examples of autosomal dominant disorders include Ehlers-Danlos syndrome, osteogenesis imperfecta, Marfan's syndrome, neurofibromatosis, and achondroplasia (10).

Autosomal Recessive Disorders. Autosomal recessive disorders are manifested only when both genes are abnormal. Males and females are equally affected. Unlike autosomal dominant disorders, which show vertical transmission (affected parent to affected child), autosomal recessive disorders are horizontal, with multiple affected members within the same generation born to normal parents. The normal parents are carriers of the disorder. When two carriers mate, the risk is one in four that the pregnancy will result in an affected child, two in four that the child will be a carrier of the abnormal gene, and one in four that the child will have no abnormal gene and not be a carrier. Examples of autosomal recessive diseases include sickle cell anemia, cystic fibrosis, β-thalassemia, and Tay-Sachs disease.

X-Linked Recessive Disorders. Males are affected almost exclusively by X-linked recessive disorders. This is because females with a mutant gene on one X chromosome will usually have a normal gene on the other X chromosome. Males have no genes on the Y chromosome to match those on the X chromosome. The abnormal gene is transmitted to the male child by a carrier mother. The risk of a male child being affected is one in two, and the risk of a female child being a carrier is one in two. Hemophilia A and B, Duchenne's dystrophy, and hemolytic anemia related to glucose-6-phosphate dehydrogenase (G6PD) deficiency are well-known examples of X-linked recessive disorders. Screening tests are available for the detection of the carriers of these disorders.

X-Linked Dominant Disorders. X-linked dominant disorders are very rare. Because an affected male cannot pass an X chromosome to his son, these disorders do not have male to male transmission, and because the affected father can pass only an abnormal gene to his daughter, all of his female offspring will be affected. Vitamin-D resistant rickets and telecanthus-hypospadias syndrome are two examples of an X-linked dominant disorder.

Multifactorial Disorders. Multifactorial refers to familial disorders that cannot be explained by a single mutant gene; such disorders are attributed to the additive effects of multiple genes and environmental factors. Within an affected family, these disorders tend to have an occurrence of 3% to 7%. Parents, siblings, and offspring are all equally likely to be affected. However, the risk increases if more than one family member is affected. Examples of multifactorial disorders include pyloric stenosis, neural tube defects, cleft lip and palate, club foot, and congenital hip dislocation.

Chromosomal Abnormalities

The normal number of human chromosomes, 46, is referred to as the diploid number. Each gamete has a haploid number, 23. The addition of an extra complete set of chromosomes within a cell is referred to as polyploidy. The presence or absence of a single or several chromosomes is referred to as aneuploidy. A trisomy, the presence of three chromosomes, is a common example of aneuploidy. Trisomies result from an accident in meiosis during the formation of the gametes—eggs and sperms. The chromosome pair fails to segregate appropriately during meiosis so that one gamete gets both chromosomes. This is referred to as nondisjunction. This gamete then joins with the normal gamete (now a zygote), which is trisomic for the involved chromosome. Because nondisjunction occurs during formation of a single gamete only, future gametes and, therefore, offspring are not likely to be affected. Nondisjunction is more likely to occur in older women. Down syndrome can occur as either nondisjunction (95%) or translocation (5%). In about 33% of individuals with Down syndrome as a result of translocation, one of the parents will have 45 chromosomes with a balanced translocation between a chromosome 21 and one of the D or G group chromosomes. That parent is at substantial risk of having another child with Down syndrome. The most common example of an internal structural abnormality is a translocation. A translocation refers to a chromosomal abnormality in which part or all of a chromosome becomes attached to another chromosome. Translocations occur as the result of chromosome breakage and recombination.

Although most trisomies result in spontaneous abortion, trisomies 21, 18, and 13 frequently result in live births. Trisomy 21 results in Down syndrome. Trisomies 18 and 13 both have a very poor prognosis with severe mental retardation and only 10% to 20% survive to 1 year of age.

Sex chromosome abnormalities include Turner's syndrome (XO) and Klinefelter's syndrome (XXY). Turner's syndrome is the result of loss of a sex chromosome during early meiotic division in the zygote after fertilization. This results in complex forms of mosaicism in which the individual has two or more populations of cells, each with a different chromosome complement (XO, XX). However, Klinefelter's syndrome is thought to be the result of meiotic nondisjunction in one of the parents.

Recombinant DNA

Bacteria have no immune system yet can be infected by foreign DNA from a virus. The method of defense used by bacteria against these attacking viruses is an enzyme called restriction endonuclease. This enzyme "cuts" DNA into segments at a specific site (restriction site). More than 200 of these restriction endonucleases have been discovered, and their discovery was the first step in developing the concept of recombinant DNA. DNA fragments, cut by the restriction endonuclease, can be sequenced and, therefore, the protein for which they code can also be sequenced.

Recombinant DNA means, simply, combining DNA from two different organisms. The foreign DNA is attached to a vector and inserted into the genome of the host. In other words, and most commonly, a human gene can be introduced into a bacteria. The two vectors used are bacterial plasmids and viral phages. This allows, at least conceptually, the introduction of a "missing gene" into a genome, for example, the gene for α-1-antitrypsin could be introduced into a patient with α-1-antitrypsin deficiency.

Embryology

An overview of the early stages of development is helpful in understanding the malformations that are of surgical importance. The first 2 weeks, or the time from fertilization to completion of implantation in the uterine wall, is known as the period of the ovum. The third to eighth week following conception is considered the embryonic period, and the eighth to the fortieth week of gestation is known as the fetal period. During the embryonic period, nearly 90% of congenital anomalies occur. Unfortunately, it is difficult to obtain exact dates of conception and it is very difficult to measure the embryo accurately. Although embryologists use more precise and complex methods to estimate embryonic and fetal age, for the interested surgeon embryonic size may be most simply and adequately given as crown-rump length and age from conception, which is estimated as

Table 2.1.
Age and Size of Embryos

Crown-Rump Length in mm	No. of Somites	Estimated Age (Days)
0.05		7–8
0.10		7–9
0.15		11–15
0.30		14–17
0.7		19
1.5		20
2.0		21
2.8	1–4	24
3.3	5–12	27
3.5	13–20	28
4.0	21–24	30
4.3	28–29	31
5.4	30–32	35
6.0	38	35–37
8.0		35–38
10.0		40
12.0		42
14.0		44
17.0		49
22–250		56

14 days after the onset of the last menstrual period. Table 2.1 compares the crown-rump length with the number of somites and estimated age from fertilization (1,11–13).

The period of the ovum extends from fertilization until implantation in the wall of the uterus. During this period, fertilization occurs with restoration of the diploid number of chromosomes, determination of chromosomal sex, and the initiation of cleavage. The cells of the zygote arrange in an outer mass to form the trophoblast and an inner mass to form the embryo proper. By the end of the second week the zygote, now known as the blastocyst, has become embedded in the endometrial stroma, and a primitive uteroplacental circulation develops. During the second week, the embryo formed from the inner cell mass is known as the embryoblast, which differentiates into a bilaminar germ disc. The ectoderm cells surround the amnion cavity and the endoderm cells surround the primitive yolk sac (Fig. 2.4) (14).

During the third week of gestation, the three germ layers of the embryo are established. The primitive streak appears at the beginning of this week. At the cephalic end of the primitive streak, the primitive node invaginates to form the endoderm and the mesoderm (Fig. 2.5) (14). Cells of the mesoderm migrate between the ectoderm lining the amnion and endoderm lining the yolk sac. Cells of the ectoderm invaginate in the primitive pit and move forward in a tube-like process forming the notochordal or head process (Fig. 2.6) (14).

During the embryonic period, which extends from the third week through the eighth week of development, each of the three germ layers gives rise to specific tissues and organs. The ectodermal germ layer forms the central and peripheral nervous system, including the sensory epithelium of the ear, nose, and eye. It also forms the epidermis, nails, hair, subcutaneous glands, mammary glands, pituitary gland, adrenal medulla, and the enamel of the teeth. Tissues and organs of mesodermal origin include supporting tissues (connective tissue, cartilage, bone, and muscle); blood and lymph cells; heart, blood, and lymph vessels; kidneys, gonads, and their ducts; cortical portion of the adrenal gland; and the spleen. The endoderm forms the epithelial lining of the gastrointestinal, respiratory, and urinary tracts. It also forms the thyroid, parathyroid, liver, and pancreas. The

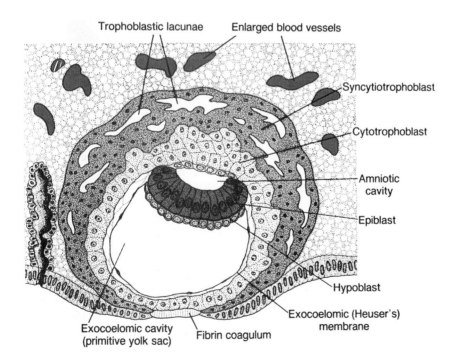

Figure 2.4. Drawing of a 9-day human blastocyst. The syncytiotrophoblast shows a large number of lacunae. Note the flat cells that form the exocoelomic membrane. The bilaminar germ disc consists of a layer of columnar epiblast cells and a layer of bucoidal hypoblast cells. The original surface defect is closed by a fibrin coagulum. From Sadler TW. Langman's medical embryology. 6th ed. Baltimore: Williams & Wilkins, 1990. Reprinted by permission.

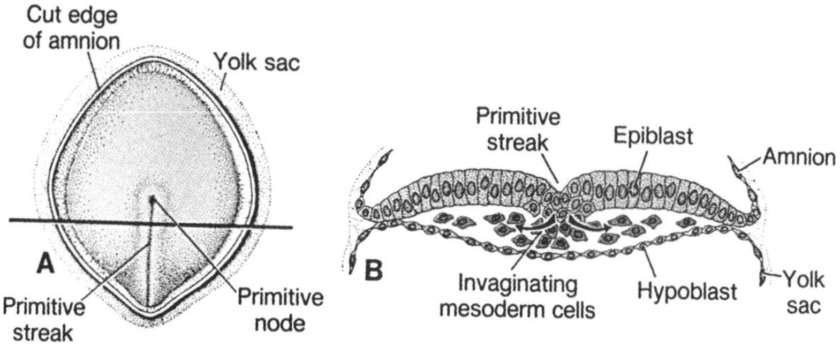

Figure 2.5. **A,** Schematic drawing of the dorsal side of a 16-day presomite embryo. The primitive streak and node are clearly visible. Modified after Streeter. **B,** Transverse section through the region of the primitive streak (as indicated in **A**), showing the invagination and subsequent lateral migration of the epiblast cells that will form the embryonic mesoderm and endoderm. From Sadler TW. Langman's medical embryology. 6th ed. Baltimore: Williams & Wilkins, 1990. Reprinted by permission.

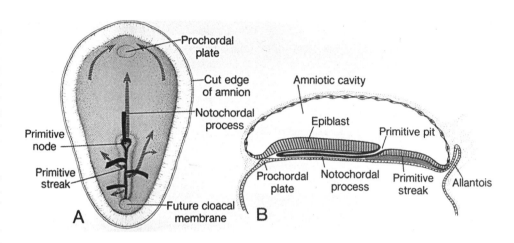

Figure 2.6. **A,** Schematic representation of the dorsal side of the germ disc, indicating the movement of surface cells (solid black lines) toward the primitive streak and node and the subsequent migration of cells between the hypoblast and epiblast germ layers (broken lines). **B,** Cephalocaudal midline section through a 16-day embryo. The notochordal process occupies the midline region extending from the prochordal plate to the primitive node. Note the notochordal or central canal in the center of the notochordal process. From Sadler TW. Langman's medical embryology. 6th ed. Baltimore: Williams & Wilkins, 1990. Reprinted by permission.

epithelial lining of the tympanic cavity and eustachian tubes are also of endodermal origin.

The fetal period extends from the ninth week until birth, usually at 38 weeks after fertilization or 40 weeks after the onset of the last menstruation. Although the embryonic period is characterized by differentiation of tissues and development of organs, the fetal period is characterized by rapid growth and maturation of tissues and organs. Growth in length is most striking during the third through the fifth months. Weight gain is most prominent during the last 2 months of gestation, when the fetal weight nearly doubles. The proportion of the head to the body also changes rapidly during fetal development (Fig. 2.7) (15). During the fetal period, perinatologists can assess growth and development of the fetus by ultrasound, amniocentesis, and chorionic villus biopsy. Intrauterine growth retardation (IUGR) applies to an infant who is at or below the tenth percentile for the expected weight at a given gestational age. This is thought to occur in approximately 1 in 10 babies. Individuals with IUGR will be at increased risk of neurologic deficiencies, congenital malformations, meconium aspiration, hypoglycemia, hypocalcemia, and respiratory distress syndrome. Factors responsible for IUGR babies include chromosomal abnormalities, congenital infections, drug abuse, and poor maternal nutrition and health (16,17).

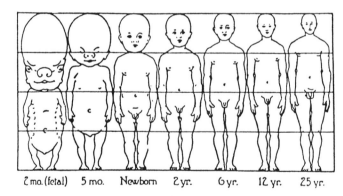

Figure 2.7. Illustration of the change in body proportions during the fetal period.

Congenital malformations are recognized in 2% to 3% of all live births (7,14,18). This number doubles by 1 year of age as other anomalies manifest symptoms and are recognized (19). The factors responsible for these congenital malformations include environmental, chromosomal, and genetic. Environmental factors are now estimated to account for 10% of human malformations (14). These factors include infectious agents, radiation, chemical agents, hormones, nutritional deficiencies, and hypoxia (20–23). Chromosomal and genetic factors also account for an estimated 10% of human malformations. These factors include chromosomal numerical abnormalities, structural chromosomal abnormalities, and gene abnormalities.

Immune System

The immune system in the fetus develops from stem cells, which originate in the extraembryonic yolk sac. These cells, after migrating to different sites in the developing fetus, are stimulated to develop into the neutrophils and lymphoid cells of the immune system. The initial lymphoid cells appear in the thymus and elsewhere in the fetus such as the bone marrow and fetal liver. The T cells responsible for the cellular immune response develop under the influence of the thymus. B cells, which are primarily responsible for the humoral immune response, develop chiefly in the bone marrow (24).

At birth, the term infant is essentially immunologically competent but suffers from several problems that may increase the risk of sepsis. First, the barriers that prevent entry of bacteria may be compromised. The newborn has very thin, permeable skin, which is easily injured. The newborn ileum may absorb macromolecules, even entire bacteria (25). This may be accentuated even more in the presence of compromised intestine, such as necrotizing enterocolitis. At birth, infants have a high level of maternal IgG and quickly develop their own IgM and IgA immunoglobulins. The premature infant, however, has a delayed ability to manufacture immunoglobulins, with an increased risk of sepsis as a result (25).

Deficiencies in any of the components of the immune system may lead to dramatic clinical presentations with multiple or unusual infections. B cell deficiencies, or an inability to produce normal immunoglobulins, results in recurrent, invasive infection from pyogenic bacteria. T cell deficiencies result in both a decreased cellular response and, because the T cells are important in regulating the function of the B cells, may also result in defective immunoglobulin production as well. Examples of these syndromes include severe combined immunodeficiency syndrome (SCIDS), immunodeficiency with ataxia and telangiectasia, Wiskott-Aldrich syndrome (eczema, thrombocytopenia, multiple infections), and DiGeorge syndrome (congenital thymic aplasia, hypoparathyroidism) (26).

Cardiovascular System

Development of the fetal heart begins at approximately the third week of gestation. The mesoderm splits into a somatic dorsal and splanchnic ventral portion.

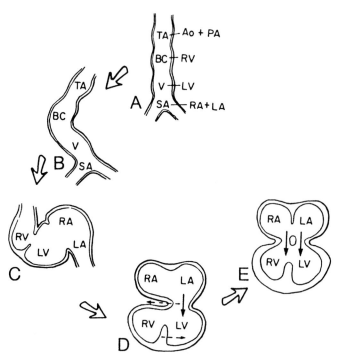

Figure 2.8. Transition from straight cardiac tube to four-chamber heart. **A,** Straight cardiac tube stage with four segments in series. The sinoatrium (SA) is destined to become the right atrium (RA) and left atrium (LA), the primitive ventricle (V) is precursor to the left ventricle (LV), the bulbus cordis (BC) becomes the right ventricle (RV), and the truncus arteriosus (TA) divides into the aorta (Ao) and main pulmonary artery (PA). The proximal and distal ends of the tube are fixed. **B,** Differential growth causes the tube to bend toward the right. **C,** The bulboventricular portion of the tube doubles over on itself, so that the right and left ventricles lie side by side. **D,** The right and left atria still connect to the left ventricle by the atrioventricular canal. The atrioventricular canal migrates toward the right, so that it lies over both ventricles. **E,** The anterior and posterior endocardial cushions meet and divide the atrioventricular canal into tricuspid and mitral orifices. From Kramer TC. The partitioning of the truncus and conus and the formation of the membranous portion of the interventricular septum in the human heart. Am J Anat 1942;71; 343–370. Copyright © 1942 Kramer; reprinted by permission of Wiley-Liss, a division of John Wiley and Sons, Inc.

This results in the development of a column that later divides into a series of vesicles. The cranial and medial portions evolve into the pericardial cavity. The ventral portion of the mesoderm contains the neomyocardium or the cardiogenic plate and this then becomes lined with an angioblastic layer, which forms the cardiac tube or endocardium (Fig. 2.8) (27). During the fourth gestational week the epimyocardium becomes enfolded at a number of sites, developing sulci that will eventually define the chambers of the heart. These include the infundibulotruncal sulcus, the interventricular sulcus, and the atrioventricular sulcus. These give rise to the truncus arteriosus, the right infundibulum and the right and left ventricles, and the left and right aorta, respectively. During the fifth week of gestation, the heart tube undergoes a rotation forward and to the right with demarcation of the sinus venosus, atrium, ventricles, and truncus arteriosus (1). During the fourth to sixth weeks, the atrioventricular canal divides into two channels. The anterior and posterior edges become thickened and fuse to form the endocardial cushions. This results in division of the A-V canal into right and left orifices. Failure of the fusion may result in septal defects or malformation of the atrioventricular valves. During this time, the atrial septum (septum primum) also forms and migrates toward the fused endocardial cushion, thereby dividing the atria and closing the foramen primum. Concurrently, the foramen secundum develops in the cranial portion of the septum thus maintaining communication between the left and right atria. Following this, a second septum develops to the right of the septum primum. This second septum never becomes complete and the opening in it becomes the foramen ovale. The septa and their foramina form a one-way valve allowing flow from right to left but not from left to right. This correlates with fetal circulation in which right atrial pressures are greater than left atrial pressures. This difference is due to umbilical vein flow from the placenta and a lack of pulmonary venous flow secondary to a patent ductus arteriosus and relative pulmonary arterial constriction. At birth the lungs expand, pulmonary artery constriction decreases, and systemic pressure increases, resulting in a preferential flow to the pulmonary bed. This causes an increase in pulmonary return and left atrial pressure relative to the low systemic venous pressure of the right atrium, which functionally closes the one-way valve (1,28,29). Following functional closure a fibroplastic hypertrophy of the septum primum occurs, and it adheres to the septum secundum, resulting in an anatomical closure of the flap. Anatomic defects as well as various causes of pulmonary hypertension can result in persistence of the right-to-left shunt through the atria (30). These will be discussed later.

The ventricles also form during this period of fetal growth. Two areas of trabeculation and rapid growth occur proximally and distally in the endocardial tube. The proximal area is ventral and eventually develops into the left ventricle; distally, the trabeculation occurs dorsolaterally and develops into the right ventricle. These two plates grow toward each other to develop into the muscular portion of the interventricular septum. The membranous portion of the septum develops as connective tissue outgrowths from the valvular and truncus ridges as well as the endocardial cushions. Fusion of the membrane and muscular portions results in closure of the interventricular canal. Failure of this process results in the majority of ventriculoseptal defects.

The pulmonary and aortic trunks develop from ridges that develop in the truncus arteriosus and eventually divide into two separate tubes (1,31). This process starts at approximately the fifth week of gestation. These ridges eventually fuse proximally with the developing interventricular septum. Thickening of endocardial tissue at this site eventually develops into the semilunar valves (Fig. 2.9) (32). Distally, the ridges develop between the fourth and sixth aortic arches, eventually separating these into the systemic and pulmonary outflow, respectively. Appropriate orientation of the truncal separation to the ventricular septum is essential for normal development between the right ventricle and pulmo-

Figure 2.9. The developing heart from the cardiac loop.

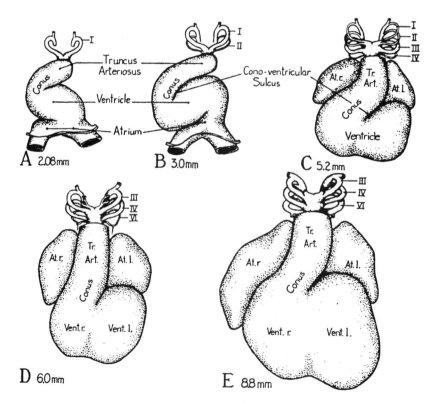

nary artery and the left ventricle and the aorta. Failure of proper orientation results in various types of transposition of the great vessels (31,33).

Fetal Circulation

During fetal development, the pulmonary bed is almost entirely excluded from fetal circulation (Fig. 2.10) (29,34). Studies by Fox et al. suggest the pulmonary circulation receives only 7% of the cardiac output (34,35). Instead, most of the blood is shunted in a right-to-left fashion via the patent foramen ovale or patent ductus arteriosus. In general, blood returns to the fetus from the placenta via the umbilical vein. This flows into the right atrium with the majority of flow crossing the foramen ovale and entering the left atrium. The remainder flows into the right ventricle and then to the pulmonary artery. However, because of the high resistance in the pulmonary vascular bed and the low pressure in the systemic bed, the blood bypasses the lung via the patent ductus arteriosus. Premature closure of the foramen ovale in utero is usually fatal. The defect results in a marked increase in right ventricular work and a decrease in flow to the left ventricle, causing it to become hypoplastic. The patent ductus arteriosus may provide enough systemic flow to maintain the fetus in utero, but at birth cyanosis and left heart failure usually result in death.

Transitional Circulation

With the infant's initial breaths, the lungs expand, resulting in a marked decrease in the pulmonary vascular resistance. This allows for increased flow from the right ventricle into the pulmonary artery and into the pulmonary vascular bed. Concurrently, there is an increase in the systemic vascular pressure, which causes an increase in the left atrial and ventricular pressures. These changes result in decreased flow across the foramen ovale and ductus arteriosus, essentially obliterating the right-to-left shunt. In the initial postnatal period, these changes are not irreversible and alterations in oxygenation, acid-base status, and pulmonary artery pressures can result in a shift back toward fetal circulation. This period is known as the transitional phase between fetal and newborn circulation. The hallmarks of this phase are right and left ventricles that are relatively equal in size and musculature. The foramen ovale and

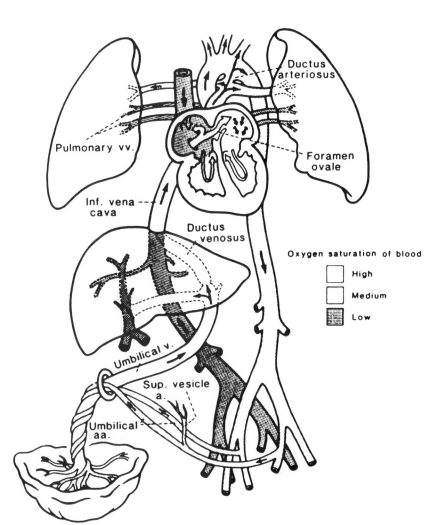

Figure 2.10. Normal fetal circulatory pattern. From Krummel TM, Greenfield LJ, Kirkpatrick BV, et al. Alveolar-arterial oxygen gradients vs neonatal pulmonary insufficiency index for prediction of mortality in ECMO candidates. J Pediatr Surg 1984; 19:380–384. Reprinted by permission.

ductus arteriosus have not yet fibrosed and remain anatomically patent. Furthermore, the smooth muscle in the pulmonary arterioles is relatively hypertrophied, is reactive, and is very sensitive to changes in blood pH and Pa_{O_2} (28).

Therefore, changes during the first weeks of life that result in hypoxia and acidosis can cause an increase in pulmonary arterial pressures. This is known as persistent pulmonary hypertension of the newborn (PPHN). The pulmonary hypertension causes an increase in right-sided heart pressures and can result in right-to-left shunting across the foramen ovale and patent ductus arteriosus, a phenomenon known as persistent fetal circulation. Besides hypoxia and acid-base status, the pulmonary vasculature is also affected by prostaglandins. Briefly, PGE_1, PGE_2, and prostacyclin (PGI_2) act as pulmonary vasodilators, whereas the F-series prostaglandins are vasoconstrictors. It is likely that thromboxane also acts as a pulmonary vasoconstrictor. Therefore, in the normal newborn, an increased Pa_{O_2}, increased pH, PGE_2, and PGI_2 all work together to decrease pulmonary vascular pressures and functionally close the right-to-left shunt (29,36,37). Then over a period of days to weeks the foramen ovale and ductus arteriosus become fibrosed and anatomically closed.

Another issue is primary failure of the ductus to close (patent ductus arteriosus), which can result in a large left-to-right shunt with congestion of the pulmonary bed and evidence of congestive heart failure. This is especially common in the premature infant whose immature lungs, coupled with some degree of persistent pulmonary hypertension, prevent normal closure of the ductus (38). This can be a progressive problem as hypoxia and acidosis can cause increased pulmonary arterial spasm and increased pulmonary hypertension. Clinically, the patent ductus results in a holosystolic murmur, bounding pulses with a widened pulse pressure, and evidence of congestive heart failure. Treatment is either with Indomethacin, which blocks the synthesis of certain prostaglandins that inhibit duct closure, or with direct surgical ligation (30). The merits of the various techniques are beyond the scope of this discussion.

Neonatal and Infant Circulation

Once the transition has been made from fetal circulation to neonatal circulation, the cardiovascular physiology is in general similar to that of children and adults (Fig. 2.11) (34). Initially, the newborn is relatively hyperdynamic with increased cardiac output. This primarily presents itself as an increased pulse rate, decreased blood pressure, and an increased respiratory rate. Table 2.2 shows normal blood pressures for various age groups (39–41). It should be noted that the differences are even more extreme in the severely premature infant.

Cyanotic Congenital Heart Disease

Cyanotic congenital heart disease consists of lesions that result in a right-to-left shunt, the bypass of the pul-

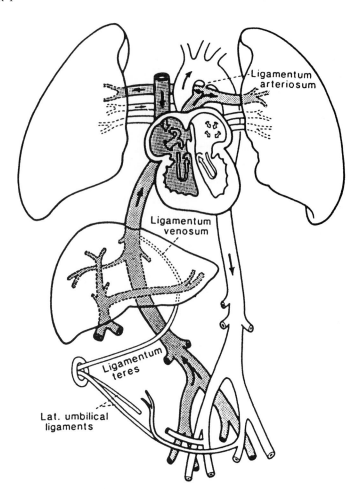

Figure 2.11. Normal newborn circulatory pattern. From Krummel TM, Greenfield LJ, Kirkpatrick BV, et al. Alveolar-arterial oxygen gradients vs neonatal pulmonary insufficiency index for prediction of mortality in ECMO candidates. J Pediatr Surg 1984;19:380–384. Reprinted by permission.

monary bed, a relative peripheral hypoxia, and varying degrees of cyanosis. These lesions include (a) defects in the development of the truncus arteriosus; (b) transposition of the great vessels; (c) persistent truncus arteriosus; (d) total anomalous pulmonary venous return; (e) a combination of lesions also affecting the endocardial cushion; and (f) maldevelopment of the atrioventricular and/or similar valves, i.e., tricuspid atresia, pulmonary atresia with associated hypoplastic right heart, and Fallot's tetralogy (right ventricular outflow stenosis; ventriculoseptal defect, VSD; right ventricular hypertrophy; and dextroposition of the aorta) (30,36). There are a number of surgical procedures that attempt to provide adequate flow to the pulmonary bed for oxygenation and of oxygenated blood to the systemic circulation. These include the Blalock-Taussig operation (subclavian artery to pulmonary artery), Waterson shunt (ascending aorta to right pulmonary artery), Fontan procedure (right atrium to pulmonary artery), Potts's operation (descending aorta to left pulmonary artery), Glenn's operation (superior vena cava to right pulmonary artery),

Table 2.2.
Percentiles of Blood Pressure[a]

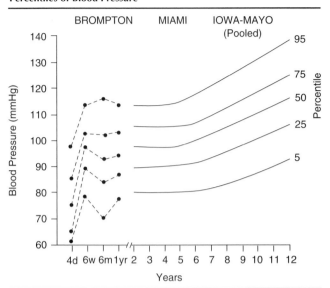

[a]Infants 4 days to 1 year: percentiles of blood pressure (BP) in infants awake, both sexes pooled (Brompton study). At age 6 weeks the percentile values were calculated from the 594 boys and 538 girls who were awake at the time of BP measurement. At ages 6 months and 1 year all infants were awake. At age 4 days there were only 174 infants awake at the time of BP measurement, and the percentile values were, therefore, taken from these measurements plus the measurements made on the sleeping infants after correction for wakefulness. Children ages 2 to 14 years: percentiles from the values for 29 to 45 boys from the Miami study and 453 to 592 boys from the Muscatine and Rochester studies (Iowa-Mayo pool) as summarized by the Task Force for Blood Pressure Control in Children.

Blalock-Hanlon operation (creation of atrial septal defect), balloon septostomy (creation of atrial septal defect with a catheter and balloon), and total correction of a transposition.

Congestive or Noncyanotic Lesions

Congestive lesions result in a left-to-right shunt and include atrioseptal defects (ASDs), VSDs, and atrioventricular canal defects. As previously mentioned, these defects arise from abnormal development of the septa or the endocardial cushion. Surgical correction usually requires simple closure or patching of the defects.

Associated Thoracic Vascular Anomalies

Most of the other major thoracic vascular defects arise from abnormal development of the aortic arch. This includes two primary categories that are of significance in the neonate: coarctation and vascular ring.

The thoracic aorta arises from pairs of arteries (aortic arches) that migrate from the primitive heart forming laterally around the gut and moving posteriorly and caudad (Fig. 2.12) (31). The vessels fuse on the fetus's dorsal surface to form a common aorta. During development there are six pairs of arches that develop and re-

gress at various stages. Initially, there are two dorsal aortae, but eventually they fuse to form a single posterior aorta. The first and second aortic arches regress and become small local arteries. The third arch develops into the internal carotid artery. The right fourth arch usually regresses and the left fourth arch becomes the proper aortic arch, occurring at approximately the eighth week of gestation. The sixth arch fuses with primordial vessels developing off the truncus to form the pulmonary artery. Persistence of the right aortic arch, or various elements, can lead to *vascular rings*, which can encircle the trachea, esophagus, or both, causing partial airway or gastrointestinal obstruction at birth (1,36,42,43).

Coarctation of the aorta has been classified into two types: (*a*) infantile, a long, narrow segment proximal to the ductus arteriosus, and (*b*) adult, a short, constricted segment either preductal or postductal (33). Development of a coarctation is thought to be secondary to an imbalance of aortic and pulmonary artery blood flow in the fetus. This may be secondary to an inadequate foramen ovale, aortic stenosis, or mitral valve deficiency. Lack of adequate blood flow following birth results in a failure of dilatation of the aortic isthmus and a persistence of fetal narrowing or coarctation. Other short-segment coarctations may simply be secondary to local atresias and lack of adequate development in utero. Treatment consists of either resection with end-to-end anastomosis or graft, or using the subclavian artery as a patch. Spontaneous or surgical closure of a significant ductus arteriosus in a patient with a preductal stenosis can result in substantial distal ischemia.

Pulmonary System

Embryology

During the fourth week of gestation, a groove begins to develop in the ventral surface of the primitive foregut (Fig. 2.13) (43). This groove (the laryngotracheal groove) develops from the formation of a thickened epithelial ridge that encroaches on the lumen of the foregut. As the groove develops, it also grows caudad and will eventually become the neotrachea. During this stage, cells of primitive mesenchyma from the mediastinal mesentery start to proliferate. These cells will eventually grow into the cartilage, muscle, and connective tissue of the lungs. During the cranial and caudal growth of the laryngotracheal groove, the epithelial ridges continue to grow, thereby separating the respiratory and alimentary tracts. Failure of complete separation can result in numerous congenital anomalies, including tracheoesophageal fistula, which may have dire consequences after birth (44–46).

As the neotrachea grows caudally it bifurcates to form the right and left main stem bronchus and two

Figure 2.12. **Left,** Diagram of the aortic arches and dorsal aorta during early fetal stage. **Right,** The aorta after transformation into the definitive vascular pattern. The obliterated components are indicated by broken lines. *RECA,* right external carotid artery; *RICA,* right internal carotid artery; *LICA,* left internal carotid artery; *LECA,* left external carotid artery; *RPA,* right pulmonary artery; *MPA,* main pulmonary artery; *LPA,* left pulmonary artery; *RSA,* right subclavian artery; *LSA,* left subclavian artery; *TA,* truncus arteriosis; *Ao,* aorta. From Congdon ED. Transformation of the aortic-arch system during the development of the human embryo. Contrib Embryol 1922;14:47–110. Reproduced by permission of the Carnegie Institution of Washington.

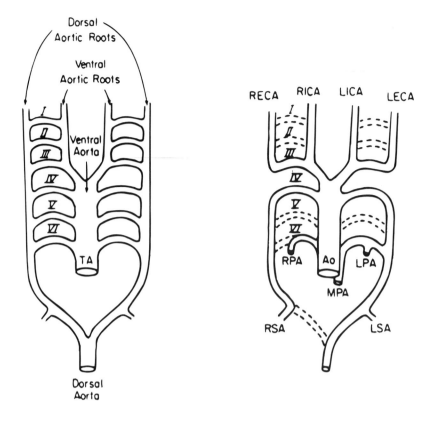

Figure 2.13. Development of trachea and bronchia. **A,** Four anterior views and lateral view of lung buds at the end of the 5th week (Horizon SIII). **B,** Lateral view at the middle of the 6th week (Horizon XV). **C,** Lateral view near the end of the 6th week (Horizon XVI). From Streeter GL. Development horizons in human embryos. Contrib Embryol 1948; 32:133–203. Reproduced by permission of the Carnegie Institution of Washington.

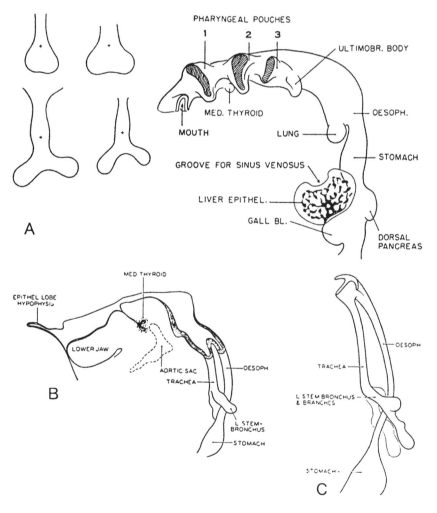

discrete lung buds. Initially, the level of the bifurcation is high in the cervical region, but by the sixth week it is descended to the level of the first thoracic vertebra, and at birth, it has reached T4 or T5. The primitive lung begins its true growth at approximately the fourth week of gestation and continues its critical glandular development until the sixteenth week. During this period, the lung bud is extremely susceptible to environmental influences and any disruptions can result in hypoplasia or even agenesis of the lung (see "Diaphragm," below). The development of the lung can be divided into four stages (Fig. 2.14) (47–52). The first stage, or pseudoglandular, lasts from 5 to 17 weeks' gestation. During this period the major airways develop and the lung has a glandular appearance. Budding and branching occurs only if the surrounding mediastinal mesenchyma is present, suggesting that this tissue is the stimulus for growth. The next stage is the canalicular stage (17–26 weeks). By this time, all the airways from the trachea to the terminal bronchioles are laid down. During this period there is proliferation of the mesenchyma into cartilage, connective tissue, muscle, and blood vessels.

The airways also begin to differentiate with evidence of increased size of endobronchial lumens and decreased epithelial lining. The terminal sac, or saccular stage, goes from 24 weeks to birth. This period is marked by further differentiation of the respiratory portion of the lung with transformation of some terminal bronchioles into respiratory bronchioles. These are immature alveoli or sacculi and contain alveolar epithelial type II cells, which secrete surfactant. The sacculi are capable of gas exchange; however, they are larger and have thicker epithelial linings than true alveoli and are incapable of efficient gas exchange. The development and maturation of the surfactant system occurs during this stage. The fourth stage of growth actually occurs postnatally. This period is marked by formation of alveoli, maturation of airways, and the production and secretion of numerous substances, including surfactant within the lung. The larger immature sacculi are divided by septa into alveolar sacs and ducts. Nearly 90% of alveoli form after birth. It is generally accepted that alveolar development continues until 8 years of age (49,51).

Pulmonary Anomalies

Anomalies of the respiratory tract are closely related to the stage of development when the abnormality occurs. However, no matter how severe the anomaly, it will usually not interfere with intrauterine life even if the defect is lethal in the immediate postnatal period.

Tracheal Atresia. The most severe defect, tracheal atresia is extremely rare and is incompatible with life. The tracheal primordium develops normally both proximally (larynx) and distally (lungs), but the mid-portion of the foregut fails to divide and develops into the esophagus only. The origin of this defect is likely to occur by the fourth week of gestation. Tracheal stenosis is a defect of variable severity and can run the spectrum of disease between tracheal agenesis and lung agenesis.

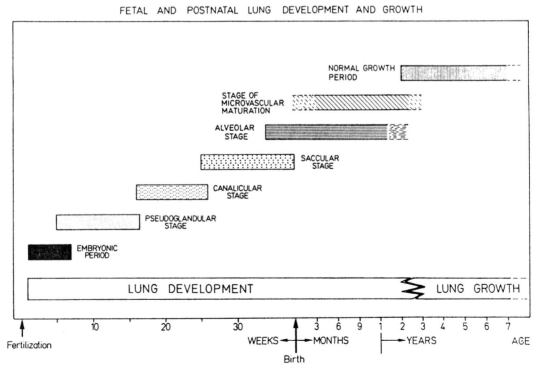

Figure 2.14. Diagram of the stages of fetal and postnatal lung development and growth. From Burri PH. Fetal and postnatal development of the lung. Ann Rev Physiol 1984;46:617–628. Reproduced with permission from the Annual Review of Physiology, Volume 46, copyright 1984 by Annual Reviews Inc.

Bilateral Agenesis of the Lungs. Bilateral agenesis is a rare disorder that is incompatible with life. It results from a failure of the progression of development of the distal or caudal tracheolaryngeal groove. This results in an absence of lung bud development and eventual pulmonary agenesis. In general, these defects are secondary to an abnormal division of the foregut endoderm and variable growth of the lung buds.

Unilateral Agenesis of the Lung. Unilateral agenesis is likely to be secondary to a failure to maintain normal development rather than a simple arrest of normal development. It seems likely that some environmental force acts to inhibit or slow normal growth on one side.

Pulmonary Hypoplasia. Pulmonary hypoplasia is an example of one model of environmental forces causing abnormal development and a congenital diaphragmatic hernia. A large number (>50%) of patients with unilateral agenesis also have associated anomalies, including esophageal atresia, tracheoesophageal fistula, spina bifida, fused ribs, laryngeal and palate malformations, imperforate anus, and cardiac defects (45,46,50). There is no clear underlying or common factor that has been discovered to date.

In addition to various degrees of hypoplasia and agenesis, there are a number of other congenital pulmonary defects that may develop as a result of abnormal foregut differentiation (53–55).

Bronchogenic Cysts. Bronchogenic cysts, also called lung buds, are buds of developing embryonic lung that become separated from the developing tracheobronchial tree before the bronchi are formed. Because they arise from ectopic foregut they may be lined with squamous epithelium. Although many of these cysts have ciliated columnar epithelium, they rarely have any connection to the normal bronchial lumens and may be located anywhere along the trachea or bronchi, either extraparenchymal or intraparenchymal, but the majority are in the posterior mediastinum at the level of the carina. Clinically, they present as space-occupying lesions, which may cause obstruction or become infected. During infancy they may partially obstruct one bronchus causing air trapping and may be confused clinically with congenital lobar emphysema or an intrabronchial foreign body. In many ways, they are the respiratory equivalent of foregut duplications. Treatment consists of simple excision.

Congenital Pulmonary Cysts. Congenital pulmonary cysts are similar to bronchogenic cysts as they are a portion of the developing lung bud that becomes entrapped. These cysts, however, communicate with the bronchi and may present as a thin-walled, large pneumatocele. Infants born with large lung cysts may develop acute respiratory distress and tension pneumothoraces, which may require emergency thoracotomy.

Pulmonary Sequestrations. Another type of anomaly in the spectrum of anomalous lung bud development are the pulmonary sequestrations (55,56). In this case the isolated lung bud segment returns or develops a systemic vascular circuit. It is not clear whether this happens because the initial separation of the sequestered segment occurs before the division of the pulmonary and aortic circulation or if persistence of the early embryonic splanchnic systems results in traction on a part of the lung bud, causing this tissue to break away. In either case the result is the development of accessory lung tissue that has no connection to the normal tracheobronchial tree and receives its blood supply directly from the systemic (aorta) circulation. There are two types of sequestration: (a) intralobar, in which the venous drainage is into the pulmonary vein, and (b) extralobar, which drains into the azygous system. It is likely that the more ectopic extralobar sequestration is a result of an isolation of the lung bud segment at an earlier stage of development.

Adenomatoid Malformations. Adenomatoid malformation appears to be the result of an arrest in bronchial development while there is a persistence and, perhaps, overgrowth of mesenchymal elements. Histologically, this defect is characterized by the absence of cartilage in the bronchi and proliferation of terminal bronchioles, which gives the lung a cystic and glandular appearance. These lesions have been classified into three types based on the histological and clinical presentation (1,54). Type I lesions are composed of a large single cyst or multiple cysts in which mucous-secreting cells and cartilage are rarely seen. Relatively normal alveoli are usually adjacent to these cysts. This type of lesion often causes marked mediastinal shift. Type II lesions are composed of multiple small cysts (<1 cm), again with a paucity of mucous cells or cartilage, and there is a high association with other congenital lesions. Type III lesions are bulky noncystic lesions that often occupy the entire lobe. Bronchial-like structures are separated by masses of cuboidal epithelium-lined, alveolus-like structures. The most commonly affected portion of the lung is the left lower lobe, but multiple lobar involvement is frequent and can often be bilateral. Treatment consists of total excision, but the prognosis may be poor if there is multilobar involvement or there are type II and type III lesions.

Congenital Lobar Emphysema. Congenital lobar emphysema is usually limited to the upper lobes or right middle lobe and is characterized by severe air trapping and overdistention of the lung parenchyma. The dilated lobe causes compression of the adjacent lung parenchyma and can cause a shift of the mediastinum to the unaffected side. The etiology of this lesion may be manifold, but the common factor seems to be some pathologic entity that causes partial obstruction of the bronchi, resulting in a one-way, or ball valve, effect. This causes overexpansion of the lung with destruction of the normal alveolar architecture. Causes may include bronchial kinking, bronchomalacia, mucous plugging, external compression by aberrant vessels or lymph nodes, or intrinsic bronchial obstruction, i.e., stenosis. In the majority of cases no specific etiology can be discovered. Because the degree of lung destruction is irreversible, treatment consists of excision of the affected lobe.

Diaphragm

The diaphragm evolves from four structures: the septum transversum, the pleuroperitoneal membranes, the esophagus and its mesentery, and ingrowth of muscular components from the lateral and dorsal body wall. The septum transversum first appears at the end of the third week as a thick plate of mesodermal tissue between the pericardium and the stalk of the yolk sac. The septum transversum becomes the central tendon of the diaphragm. The pleuroperitoneal folds develop as crescent-shaped folds along the caudal border of the pleural cavity. These folds form membranes that grow mediad to meet the esophageal mesentery in the midline and dorsad and ventrad to fuse with the septum transversum to form the primitive diaphragm; complete partition of the thoracic and peritoneal cavities occurs by the seventh week (57). There is then an ingrowth of cells from the lateral body wall into the pleuroperitoneal membrane to form the muscular portion of the diaphragm so that the membranous portion of the diaphragm in the newborn is very small. The crura of the diaphragm develop from the dorsal mesentery of the esophagus.

During the fourth week the septum transversum begins to develop at the level of the third, fourth, and fifth cervical somites. Ventral folding and rapid growth of the dorsal and cephalic portions of the embryo result in an apparent caudal descent of the diaphragm. Whereas the dorsal part of the diaphragm lies at the level of the first lumbar vertebra, the motor innervation is from the ventral rami of C3, C4, and C5, which lengthen and fuse into the phrenic nerve. Some of the sensory fibers come from the lower intercostal nerves (1). This explains diaphragmatic irritation being manifest as referred pain to the shoulder.

If the pleuroperitoneal membranes fail to develop by the eighth week, a posterior-lateral defect, Bochdalek's hernia, occurs and allows the abdominal viscera to herniate into the chest (Fig. 2.15). This is particularly important because the midgut returns to the abdomen from the umbilical stalk during the eighth to tenth week of gestation. This is an early stage in the lung bud development, and the presence of the space-occupying abdominal viscera in the chest prevents normal lung development, causing the lung to become hypoplastic (58–60). Although the lung on the involved side is most severely affected, the contralateral lung may also be hypoplastic to varying degrees. In 30% to 50% of affected newborns the lungs are so hypoplastic that survival is not possible.

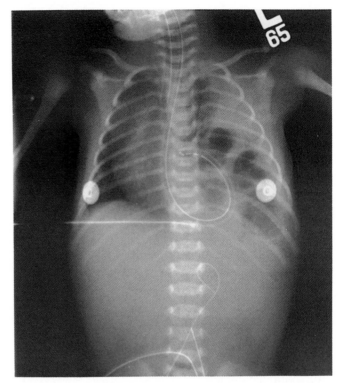

Figure 2.15. Roentgenogram of an infant with a left Bochdalek's diaphragmatic hernia. The heart is shifted to the right, the position of the nasogastric tube indicates the stomach is in the left side of the chest, and the intestinal gas pattern is entirely within the chest.

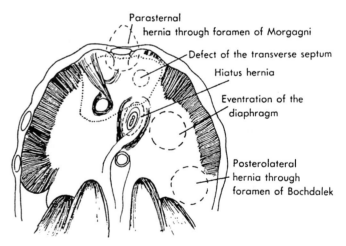

Figure 2.16. Sites of diaphragmatic anomalies. From Gray SW, Skandalakis JE. Embryology for surgeons. Philadelphia: WB Saunders, 1972. Reprinted by permission.

The right diaphragm seems to be protected during final development by the liver, and 90% of these hernias occur on the left.

Abnormal development of the diaphragm may result in hernias at various sites (Fig. 2.16) (1). Hernias may also occur directly behind the sternum through Morgagni's foramen; these account for 2% to 6% of congenital diaphragmatic hernias. Morgagni's hernias result from failure of the septum transversum to join the sternum. Most of these hernias are first recognized in middle-aged individuals, but they may also be symptomatic in the newborn (61). Depending on the size and amount of abdominal viscera herniated into the chest, they can present with respiratory compromise and a clinical picture similar to that of a Bochdalek's hernia (62). They may also be one component of a group of midline anomalies known as pentalogy of Cantrell.

Other uncommon anomalies of the diaphragm include eventration, congenital hiatal hernia, and phrenic nerve paralysis. Eventration may be difficult to differentiate from phrenic nerve paralysis and a small posterior-lateral hernia with a sac (63). In fact, many eventrations may be the result of phrenic nerve injury (64,65). Phrenic nerve injuries occurring during birth trauma are often associated with brachial plexus injuries or Erb's palsy. The paralyzed hemidiaphragm typically rises to the fourth or fifth interspace and is thin and fibrotic and moves paradoxically with respirations on fluoroscopic or ultrasound examination. Because newborn infants rely primarily on their diaphragms for ventilation, many of these infants are ventilator dependent. Many phrenic stretch injuries will recover if given time. Eventration of the diaphragm has also been associated with muscular dystrophy. Hiatal hernias, like Morgagni's hernias, are usually seen later in life and are associated with obesity. When seen during infancy they may be associated with a congenitally short esophagus.

Gastrointestinal System

Foregut Formation

The development of the foregut into the neotrachea and esophagus begins at approximately the third week of gestation. This differentiation involves three major processes (44,46,53). The first is the formation of two separate organ-forming fields from the primitive mesoderm. This causes differentiation of the ventral endoderm into the tracheal mucosa and differentiation of the dorsal endoderm into esophageal mucosa. Second, lateral ridges of proliferative ectoderm grow into the lumen of the foregut to divide into separate esophageal and tracheal tubes. And, last, the third major step is elongation of both the primitive tubes. This division becomes complete by approximately the fifth week, and the submucosa and circular muscle layer are apparent by the end of the sixth week. The outer longitudinal muscle layer is well-formed by the ninth week. At no time during development does the esophagus become completely obliterated by the neoepithelium, so failure of recanalization is not a cause of esophageal atresia, as is the case with duodenal atresia. The majority of defects of the esophagus are a result of abnormal or incomplete separation of the trachea from the esophagus during the fourth and fifth weeks of gestation (1). The extent of malformation ranges from failure of separation of the trachea and esophagus (a persistent foregut) with a common lumen to a fistula or cleft between the trachea and esophagus. An example of the latter defect includes incomplete cranial growth of the septum. This will result in a laryngeal cleft or, in more severe cases, a laryngotracheoesophageal fistula. Local failure of the septum to form will result in a simple tracheoesophageal fistula. In approximately 90% of these cases, this is associated with the section of adjacent esophagus coming under the influence of the tracheal mesoderm, causing a local atresia of the esophagus. Any number of variations are possible based on relatively small alterations in the growth process. Figure 2.17 illustrates the classification of esophageal atresia and tracheoesophageal fistula proposed by Gross (66). Type C is the most common and accounts for nearly 87% of these anomalies (Fig. 2.18) (67). Type A, which is an isolated esophageal atresia, is characterized by a gasless abdomen and esophageal atresia. Type A occurs in approximately 8% of infants in whom the anomaly is diagnosed at birth. Infants with Type E anomalies usually present at an older age with recurrent respiratory tract infections or coughing when

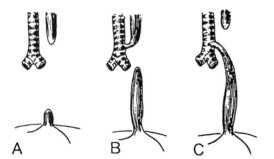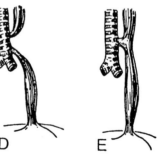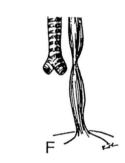

Figure 2.17. Types of congenital abnormalities of the esophagus. **A,** Esophagea atresia. There is no esophageal communication with the trachea; under such circumstances the lower esophageal end is apt to be quite short. **B,** Esophageal atresia. The upper segment communicates with the trachea. **C,** Esophageal atresia. The lower segment communicates with the back of the trachea; more than 90% of all esophageal malformations fall into this group. **D,** Esophageal atresia. Both segments communicate with the trachea. **E,** Esophagus has no disruption of its continuity but has a tracheoesophageal fistula. **F,** Esophageal stenosis. From Gross RE. The surgery of infancy and childhood. Philadelphia: WB Saunders, 1953. Reprinted by permission.

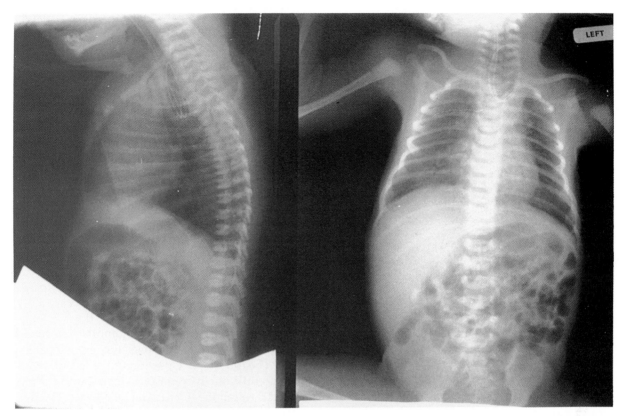

Figure 2.18. Lateral and P-A roentgenograms of a newborn with an esophageal atresia and distal tracheoesophageal fistula (type C). The catheter is curled in the blind upper esophageal pouch. Air has entered the intestine through the fistula.

swallowing liquids. Types B and D are uncommon. Anomalies of the trachea and esophagus have a high frequency (approximately 50%) of association with other defects (68). One constellation of defects has been identified as the VATER or VACTERL syndrome. This classifies the association of tracheoesophageal anomalies with vertebral, cardiac, renal, radial bone, anal, and limb defects (69,70). All patients with tracheoesophageal fistula should be examined closely for other anomalies and a thorough family history should also be obtained (71).

Stomach

The stomach begins to develop during the fifth week as a fusiform dilatation of the lower end of the foregut. The dorsal portion grows faster than the ventral portion and forms the greater curvature. As the stomach grows it undergoes a 90° clockwise rotation on its longitudinal axis so that the posterior wall, the greater curvature, becomes the left wall. The left wall and left vagus nerve are carried anteriorly while the right wall and right vagus nerve move posteriorly. The dorsal mesentery is also carried to the left, forming a cavity to the right of the dorsal mesentery and dorsal to the stomach. This cavity is called the omental bursa or lessor sac of the peritoneum and communicates with the peritoneal cavity through the epiploic foramen or foramen of Wins-

low. Except for congenital pyloric stenosis and heterotrophic pancreatic mucosa, congenital anomalies of the stomach are rare.

Duodenum

The duodenum is formed by the distal foregut and proximal midgut, which are considered to meet just distal to the biliary ampullae. The duodenum is supplied by branches of the celiac artery, which supplies the foregut, and by branches of the superior mesenteric artery, which supplies the midgut. The proximal duodenum is pulled to the right by the bending of the stomach to form a C-shaped loop. The clockwise rotation and bending of the duodenum also draws the common duct behind the duodenum so that the biliary ampulla enters the posterior wall of the duodenum.

During the fifth and sixth weeks, the lumen of the duodenum becomes temporarily obliterated by proliferating epithelial cells from the gut lining. By the eighth week, the lumen is reestablished by a process of recanalization. Atresia and stenosis of the duodenum are thought to be the result of a failure of the recanalization process (72). Atresia or stenosis occur most commonly at or just distal to the papilla of Vater, so that emesis is nearly always bilious (Fig. 2.19*A–C*) (73). The most common type of duodenal atresia is that caused by a diaphragm or web formed of mucosa and submucosa

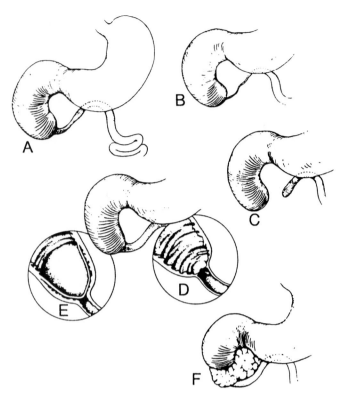

Figure 2.19. Various types of anomalies causing duodenal obstruction. **A,** Type 1 atresia with intact membrane producing marked discrepancy in size between proximal and distal segments. **B,** Blind ends of duodenum connected by a fibrous cord. **C,** Blind ends of duodenum are separated, and the mesentery is absent at the separation. **D,** Intraluminal membrane with a perforation. **E,** Wind-sock anomaly; note that an incision in the distal portion of the dilated segment would still be beyond the obstruction. **F,** Annular pancreas. From Duodenal atresia, stenosis and annular pancreas. In: Welch KJ, Randolph JG, Ravitch MM, et al, eds. Pediatric surgery. 4th ed. Chicago: Year Book Medical Publishers, 1986. Reprinted by permission.

(Fig. 2.19*D*). The membrane may become stretched by the peristaltic action on the swallowed amniotic fluid forming a wind-sock anomaly (Fig. 2.19*E*) (74). The ampullae of Vater frequently is located on or adjacent to the web and great care must be taken when dissecting in this area.

Duodenal atresia is the most frequent location of intestinal atresia and is one of the more common major congenital anomalies requiring surgical correction to allow extrauterine survival (75). Associated anomalies are common and nearly 30% are associated with Down syndrome (73,76). Annular pancreas and malrotation may also present as duodenal obstruction (Fig. 2.19*F*).

Liver and Pancreas

The liver primordium is first seen in the fourth week of development, but is not identified as a separate organ until it grows from the septum transversum when the embryo is 6 to 8 mm in length. The bare area of the liver is the remaining evidence of the liver's intimate association to the septum transversum. The liver paren-

chyma arises from the hepatic bud of the distal foregut. This diverticulum grows into the transverse septum. The fetal liver is primarily an organ of hematopoiesis. At 9 weeks of gestation, the liver represents 10% of the body weight of the fetus. By birth, when it is no longer functioning as a hematopoietic organ, it represents approximately 5% of body weight. The most common anomaly of liver formation is the presence of an abnormal lobe called Riedel's lobe. This is an elongated, tongue-like lobe that extends from the right lobe. The lobe is functional and is only important in that it may be misdiagnosed as an abdominal mass if not recognized.

Conceptually, the most difficult, but also the most important for the surgeon, is the development of the blood vessels of the liver (Fig. 2.20) (77). The vitelline and umbilical veins start as paired structures, which are not associated with the liver parenchyma in the fourth week of gestation. The liver parenchyma envelops the vitelline veins by the end of the fifth week. At the same time, the extrahepatic portion of the vitelline veins undergoes a spontaneous anastomosis. The superior, or dorsal anastomosis, becomes the extrahepatic portal vein. The intrahepatic portion of the left umbilical vein becomes the ductus venosus, which shunts the placental blood through the liver to the fetal heart. The right umbilical vein regresses. In the newborn infant, the ductus venosus may remain patent for several days. This allows for passage of a catheter into the umbilical vein, through the ductus venosus and into a central venous position to sample blood or measure pressures in the newborn. In the adult, the umbilical vein remnant can be seen as a white, cord-like structure in the free edge of the falciform ligament, which extends to the umbilicus in the preperitoneal space. In patients with portal hypertension, the umbilical vein may recanalize and provide a spontaneous portosystemic shunt (caput medusae).

The pancreas is first identifiable as the two pancreatic diverticular buds from the ventral and dorsal side of the foregut in the sixth week of gestation. The dorsal diverticulum grows to form the majority of the body of the pancreas. As the duodenum elongates; the ventral diverticulum rotates inferiorly and mediad. This accomplishes two things: the common bile duct is brought into position to join the pancreatic duct at the sphincter of Oddi and the ventral diverticulum of the pancreas takes up a position inferior to the dorsal anlage, where it becomes the uncinate process (Figs. 2.21 and 2.22) (14). Both diverticular buds contain a pancreatic duct, but the proximal portion of the dorsal duct (Santorini's duct) regresses in 30% of people after it anastomoses with the ventral duct (Wirsung's duct).

There are two important anomalies of pancreatic development: anomalous pancreatic ducts and annular pancreas. Anomalous pancreatic ducts may occur if anastomosis between the two ducts fails (pancreatic divisum) or if both ducts enter the duodenum independently. There is some evidence that pancreas divisum

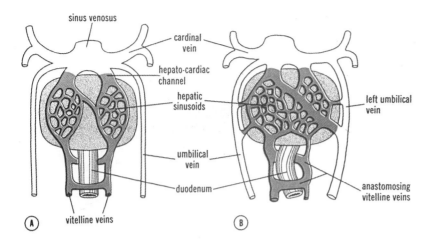

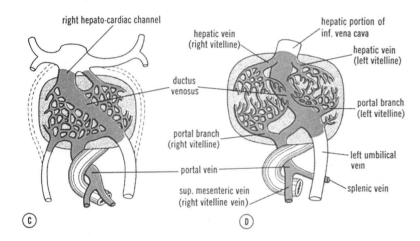

Figure 2.20. Schemes showing the development of the umbilical and vitelline veins. **A,** At the end of the fourth week; **B,** in the fifth week; **C,** in the sixth week; **D,** in the third month. Note the formation of the ductus venosus between the left umbilical vein and the inferior vena cava. From Sadler TW. Langman's medical embryology. 6th ed. Baltimore: Williams & Wilkins, 1990. Reprinted by permission.

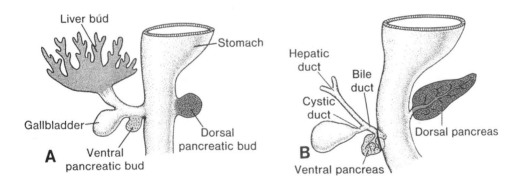

Figure 2.21. Successive stages in the development of the pancreas. **A,** At 30 days (approximately 5 mm). **B,** At 35 days (approximately 7 mm). The ventral pancreatic bud is initially located close to the hepatic diverticulum but later migrates posteriorly around the duodenum in the direction of the dorsal pancreatic bud. From Sadler TW. Langman's medical embryology. 6th ed. Baltimore: Williams & Wilkins, 1990. Reprinted by permission.

may lead to pancreatitis in some patients. Annular pancreas occurs when the ventral anlage of the pancreas fails to rotate. In this condition, it remains anterior to the duodenum. Subsequent joining of the dorsal and ventral anlages leads to a ring of pancreatic tissue around the second portion of the duodenum (78). This may be an incidental finding in a totally asymptomatic patient or may cause complete duodenal obstruction in the newborn. Heterotopic pancreatic tissue has been described throughout the GI tract, although it is most often found in the duodenum or stomach. This too may be found incidentally at a laparotomy, when it may be con-

fused with a neoplastic process. Ectopic pancreatic tissue may also act as a lead point for a small bowel intussusception.

Midgut

Embryologists consider the midgut to be that portion of the gut between the cephalic fold and caudal fold. On the other hand, the surgeon considers the midgut as that portion of the intestine supplied by the superior mesenteric artery, that is, beginning immediately distal to the entrance of the bile duct into the duodenum and

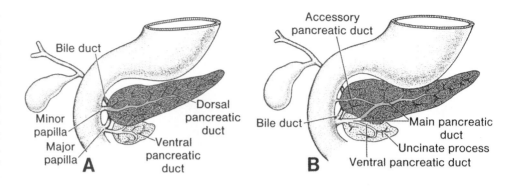

Figure 2.22. **A,** The pancreas during the sixth week of development. The ventral pancreatic bud is in close contact with the dorsal pancreatic bud. **B,** Drawing showing the fusion of the pancreatic ducts. The main pancreatic duct enters the duodenum in combination with the bile duct at the major papilla. The accessory pancreatic duct enters the duodenum at the minor papilla. From Sadler TW. Langman's medical embryology. 6th ed. Baltimore: Williams & Wilkins, 1990. Reprinted by permission.

terminating at the junction of the proximal two-thirds of the transverse colon with the distal one-third.

The primitive gut results from the cephalocaudal and lateral folding of the embryo to incorporate a portion of the endodermal-lined yolk sac (Fig. 2.23) (14). The middle part, or midgut, remains connected to the yolk sac by the vitelline duct. Whereas the epithelial lining of the digestive tract and the liver and the pancreas are derived from the endoderm, the muscular components of the gut form from the splanchnic mesoderm.

The midgut rapidly elongates, forming an intestinal loop that is connected through the vitelline duct at its apex with the yolk sac. Failure of the vitelline duct to obliterate completely results in various anomalies, including Meckel's diverticulum, vitelline cysts, and patent omphalomesenteric sinus or an umbilicoileal fistula (1,79–81). Although nearly 2% of the population have a Meckel's diverticulum only 4% of this group will produce symptoms (80,82). Meckel's diverticulum typically presents with symptoms during early childhood (83). During the 6th week as the gut rapidly elongates, it enters the extraembryonic coelom in the umbilical cord. This process is known as physiologic umbilical herniation. The herniated intestine returns to the abdominal cavity before the twelfth week of development.

The midgut normally undergoes a 270° rotation between the sixth and twelfth week, when it has fully returned to the abdominal cavity (Fig. 2.24) (84). The point of reference of the rotation is the superior mesenteric artery (Fig. 2.25) (74). This rotation can be divided into two portions: the proximal, or duodenal, and the distal, or colonic, segments. The duodenum starts in the right side and rotates counterclockwise 270° below the superior mesenteric artery to become fixed retroperitoneally in the left upper quadrant at Treitz's ligament. The colon is located to the left and also rotates counterclockwise 270° over the superior mesenteric artery and duodenum to become fixed on the right side of the abdomen. Approximately 90° of this rotation occurs while the intestine is herniated out of the peritoneum and 180° occurs as the intestine returns to the abdominal cavity. The cecum is the last portion to return to the abdomen and, initially, is located just below the liver in the right upper quadrant. From this location, it descends into the right iliac fossa. During this time the small intestinal loops continue to elongate and form a number of loops. As the intestine returns to the abdominal cavity the mesenteries shorten and fuse with the posterior parietal peritoneum resulting in fixing the position of the intestinal loops.

Intestinal length nearly doubles during the last trimester from approximately 142 cm at 19 to 27 weeks' gestation to 304 cm at term (Fig. 2.26) (85). Patients with short gut syndrome who have undergone reoperation have been found to double their intestinal length during the 1st year of life (86). This normal growth is important to consider when decisions are made as to whether an infant with massive intestinal loss can survive.

Malrotation

Although the normal rotation can arrest at various stages, the classic malrotation consists of the colon malpositioned on the left of the abdomen, with the cecum in the right upper or mid-abdomen (66,84,87). The duodenum fails to undergo its normal counterclockwise rotation posterior to the superior mesenteric artery but rather descends retroperitoneally to the right of the vena cava. Peritoneal bands, known as Ladd's bands, extend from the cecum and proximal colon across the duodenum to attach to the retroperitoneum on the right side of the duodenum (88). These bands may entrap and obstruct the duodenum. The degree of obstruction is variable as is the age of presentation. In contrast to a duodenal atresia, which presents with a double bubble and no gas beyond the duodenum, an infant with a malrotation typically presents with a double bubble and small amounts of gas scattered beyond the duodenum. The amount of duodenal distention is also less than that seen with duodenal atresia. Although the majority present with signs of obstruction as newborns, 28% present after the neonatal period (89). In older children and adults, malrotation may present in one of three ways: (*a*) Acute intestinal obstruction usually results from obstruction of the duodenum by peritoneal band; (*b*) Abdominal pain with or without vomiting occurs. The pain typically follows meals and is ascribed to peristaltic rushes in a

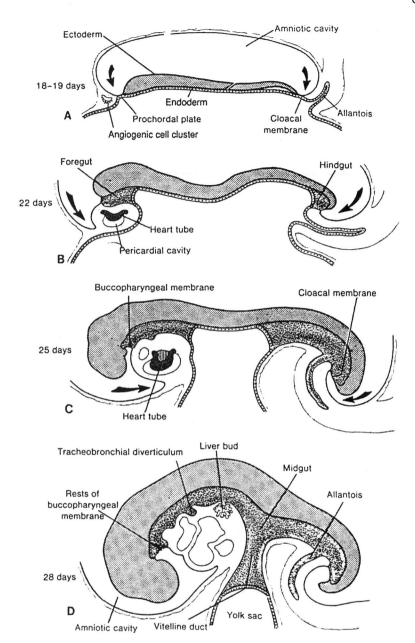

Figure 2.23. Schematic drawings of sagittal sections through embryos at various stages of development to demonstrate the effect of the cephalocaudal and lateral flexion on the position of the endoderm lined cavity. Note the formation of the foregut, midgut, and hindgut. **A,** Presomite embryo; **B,** 7-somite embryo; **C,** 14-somite embryo; **D,** at the end of the first month. From Sadler TW. Langman's medical embryology. 6th ed. Baltimore: Williams & Wilkins, 1990. Reprinted by permission.

dilated partially obstructed duodenum. Patients may get relief from the pain by vomiting the bile-stained meal; *(c)* Chronic diarrhea and malabsorption often with protein losing enteropathy are present. These symptoms are usually associated with twisting and obstruction of the mesentery, which results in chronic lymphatic obstruction and edema of the bowel wall. This is associated with malabsorption and loss of protein into the intestinal lumen (90).

The entire mesentery of the malrotated midgut is very long and fixed to the retroperitoneum by a small pedicle containing the superior mesenteric artery and vein. This single point of fixation allows the entire small bowel and mesentery to twist on this pedicle, resulting in a midgut volvulus with vascular occlusion of the mesenteric vessels (91). In a midgut volvulus, the gut and mesentery uniformly rotate in a clockwise direction, which

is the opposite of normal rotation. The diagnosis and operative correction of a midgut volvulus is a surgical emergency.

Malrotation is associated to a varying degree with a large number of other congenital anomalies (92). However, it is consistently associated with conditions in which the midgut does not return to the peritoneum by the 12th week of gestation and the presence of gastroschisis and omphalocele. In diaphragmatic hernia, as the midgut returns to the peritoneal cavity, it immediately moves into the chest and does not undergo rotation or fixation.

Small Bowel and Colon Atresia

In contrast to duodenal atresia, which results from a failure of the lumen to recanalize, the lumen of the

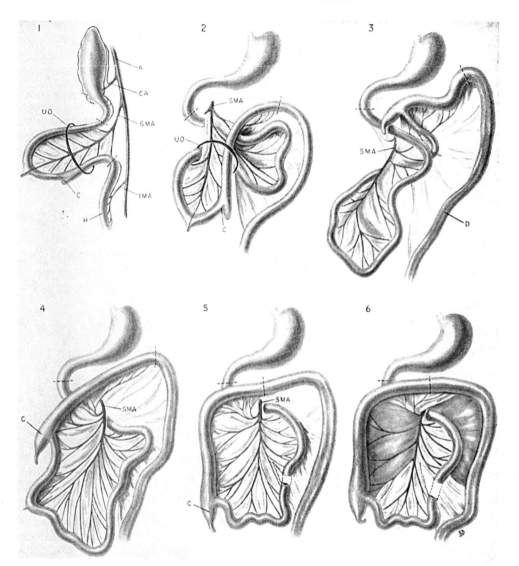

Figure 2.24. Schematic drawing of normal development, rotation, and attachment of the midgut. The midgut in each sketch is that part included between the dotted lines and represents that portion of the alimentary tract from duodenum to midtransverse colon which is supplied by the superior mesenteric artery. **1,** Age: Fifth week of fetal life, lateral view. The foregut, midgut, and hindgut with their respective blood supplies are indicated. Most of the midgut is extruded into the base of the umbilical cord where it normally resides from about the fifth to the tenth week. **2,** Age: Tenth week of fetal life. The intestine is elongating and the hindgut is displaced to the left side of the abdomen. The developing, intraabdominal intestines come to lie behind the superior mesenteric artery. A portion of the midgut still protrudes through the umbilical orifice into the base of the cord. **3,** Age: Eleventh week of fetal life. All of the alimentary tract is withdrawn into the abdomen. The cecum lies in the epigastrium, beneath the stomach. **4,** Age: late in the eleventh week of fetal life. The colon is rotating; the cecum lies in the right upper quadrant of the abdomen. **5,** Rotation of the colon is complete, and the cecum lies in final position. There is a common mesentery; the mesocolon of the ascending colon is continuous with the mesentery of the ileum. There is no posterior attachment of this common mesentery except at the origin of the superior mesenteric artery. **6,** Final stage in attachment of the mesenteries. The ascending and the descending mesocolons become fused to the posterior abdominal wall; thereby the mesentery of the jejunum and ileum gain a posterior attachment from the origin of the superior mesenteric artery obliquely downward to the cecum. *A,* aorta; *C,* cecum; *CA,* celiac axis; *D,* descending colon; *H,* hindgut; *IMA,* inferior mesenteric artery; *SMA,* superior mesenteric artery; *UO,* umbilical orifice. From: Classification of the abnormalities of intestinal rotation. In: Welch KJ, Randolph JG, Ravitch MM, et al, eds. Pediatric surgery. 4th ed. Chicago: Year Book Medical Publishers, 1986:838–848. Reprinted by permission.

remaining small bowel and colon does not become obliterated and hence does not recannulate. Instead, atresia of the small intestine and colon occur as the result of a late intrauterine mesenteric occlusion, which results in varying lengths of intestinal infarction. Mesenteric occlusion may result from volvulus, intussusception, internal hernia, complications of meconium ileus, and herniation of the bowel and mesentery through a small

abdominal wall defect such as a hernia or umbilical ring defect (76). Louw and Barnard (93) demonstrated a spectrum of intestinal atresia, similar to that seen clinically in infants, that could be produced in puppies by intrauterine ligation of the mesenteric Louw (74) classified jejunoileal atresia into three types (Fig. 2.27): type 1, a septum or membrane with an intact bowel wall and mesentery; type 2, two atretic ends connected by a fi-

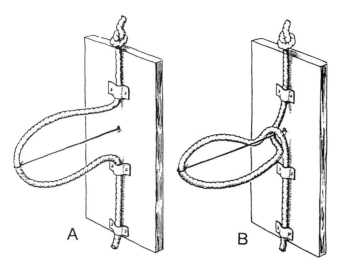

Figure 2.25. Mechanical demonstration of intestinal rotation. A rope is attached to a board at both ends with a wire extending at right angles from the board to the base of the loop. **A,** The top limb of the rope corresponds to the duodenojejunal loop; the wire, to the superior mesenteric artery; and the bottom limb, to the cecocolic segment. **B,** The rope loop has been grasped by the hand and rotated through an arc of 270°, or three-fourths of a complete turn around the wire (the axis), in a counterclockwise direction. Thus in **B** the top limb has become the bottom one, and the bottom limb the top. By following the movements of the two limbs around the wire close to the board, one can visualize the process of rotation of the intestine in the embryo. From Classification of the abnormalities of intestinal rotation. In: Welch KJ, Randolph JG, Ravitch MM, et al, eds. Pediatric surgery. 4th ed. Chicago: Year Book Medical Publishers, 1986:838–848. Reprinted by permission.

brous cord and an intact mesentery; and type 3, two atretic ends with no connection and a gap in the mesentery (75). Other authors have added type 3b and type 4 (74,94). Type 3b is characterized by the loss of the majority of the midgut supplied by the superior mesenteric artery (95–97). A short segment of jejunum remains, which is supplied by collaterals from the celiac artery, and a segment of ileum remains, which is supplied by the ileocolic and right colic arteries via anastomotic arcades from the inferior mesenteric artery. The terminal ileum is wrapped in a spiral fashion about the ileocolic vessel. This unusual appearance gives the anomaly the name "apple-peel" or "Christmas-tree" deformity. Type 4 consists of multiple atresias that have the appearance of a "string of sausages" (98,99). Types 3b and 4 both have a familial pattern (100–102). Unlike duodenal atresia, which most often is type 1, jejunoileal atresias are most often types 2 and 3. In contrast to duodenal atresia, jejunoileal atresias are thought to occur later in fetal development as an intrauterine accident and are not commonly associated with extraperitoneal anomalies. Jejunoileal atresias are multiple in nearly 10% of cases (103).

Hindgut

During the third week, as a result of cephalocaudal and lateral folding of the embryo, a portion of the endoderm-lined yolk sac becomes incorporated into the body of the embryo as the early gut. The tail region of

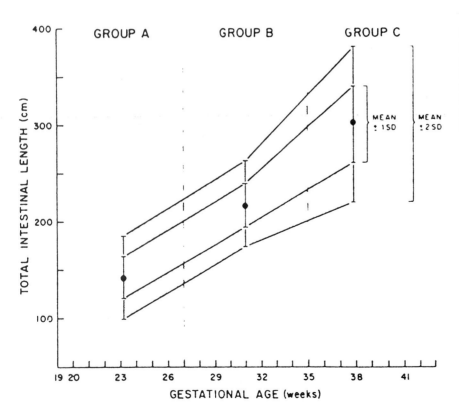

Figure 2.26. Mean total intestinal length [fcplm]1 and 2 standard deviations, calculated by gestational ages from 19 to 27 weeks (**Group A**), 27 to 35 weeks (**Group B**), and older than 35 weeks (**Group C**). From Touloukian RJ, Walker-Smith GJ. Normal intestinal length in preterm infants. J Pediatr Surg 1983;18:720–723. Reprinted by permission.

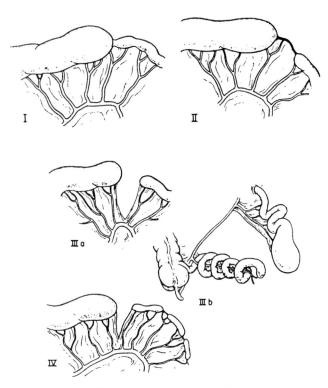

Figure 2.27. Classification of intestinal atresia. Type I, mucosal (membranous) atresia with intact bowel wall and mesentery. Type II, blind ends are separated by a fibrous cord. Type IIIa, blind ends are separated by a V-shaped mesenteric defect (gap). Type IIIb, apple-peel atresia. Type IV, multiple atresias (string of sausages). From Grosfeld JL. Jejunoileal atresia and stenosis. In: Welch KJ, Randolph JG, Ravitch MM, et al, eds. Pediatric surgery. 4th ed. Chicago: Year Book Medical Publishers, 1986: 838–848. Reprinted by permission.

this newly formed canal is the hindgut. Also during this time, the hindgut terminates at the cloacal membrane (Fig. 2.28) (11). The caudal-most portion of the hindgut dilates to become the cloaca, which then is divided by a transverse ridge (the urorectal septum) into the urogenital sinus anteriorly and the anorectal canal posteriorly. This occurs by two processes. First is a downgrowth of Torneaux's septum, which stops its cranial to caudal growth at the level of the verumontanum or Müller's tubercle. Below this point, the urorectal septum consists of an ingrowth from the lateral walls that fuse in the midline (Rathke's fold). The point at which the Torneaux's septum joins Rathke's fold is the site at which rectourethral fistulas occur most often in the male (104). The urorectal septum completely separates the primitive rectum and urogenital sinus by the seventh week. Developmental failure of the urorectal septum results in the various fistulae between the rectum and the genitourinary tracts. At this time the urorectal septum divides the cloacal membrane into an anal membrane and an anterior urogenital membrane. During the ninth week, the anal membrane ruptures at the anal pit to form an opening on to the perineum. Failure of the anal membrane to rupture results in an imperforate anus without a rectogenitourinary fistula. Whereas the proxi-

mal portion of the rectum is of endodermal origin and supplied by the inferior mesenteric artery, the distal third forms from ingrowth of ectodermal tissue of the anal pit and is supplied by branches of the internal iliac artery. The columnar endothelium of endodermal origin meets the squamous epithelium of ectodermal origin at the pectinate line.

Anomalies of the hindgut vary from anal stenosis to cloacal anomalies and are frequently associated with urogenital anomalies (Table 2.3) (105). Imperforate anus is used to describe a large number of hindgut anomalies characterized by an abnormally located and/or nonpatent anus (Fig. 2.29) (105).

Abdominal Wall

Omphalocele

The three embryonic folds that are important in the formation of the developing intestinal tract are also important in the formation of the anterior abdominal wall. Each of these folds is composed of somatic and splanchnic layers (106,107). The somatic layer of the cephalic fold forms the thoracic and epigastric wall and the septum transversum. Developmental failure of this layer results in an epigastric abdominal wall defect referred to as an epigastric omphalocele. This is often associated with features of pentalogy of Cantrell, including lower thoracic wall malformations, anterior diaphragmatic defects (Morgagni's hernia), and cardiac anomalies (108). Developmental failure of the somatic layer of the caudal fold leads to a lower abdominal wall defect, which is referred to as a hypogastric omphalocele. This is usually associated with bladder exstrophy. If the splanchnic layer of the caudal fold is involved, the hindgut will be malformed most commonly as an imperforate anus with an intestinal fistula to the open bladder. Failure of the somatic layer of the lateral folds to develop completely and fuse at the umbilical ring causes the umbilical ring to remain open. This allows the extraembryonic coelom to communicate with the intraembryonic coelom and allows herniation of the midgut and, at times the liver, into the extraembryonic coelom (Fig. 2.30). An anomaly in which the umbilical ring is greater than 4 cm is referred to as an omphalocele; one smaller than 4 cm and containing only small bowel is referred to as a hernia of the cord (109). The herniated viscera is contained in a sac consisting of the avascular amniotic membrane which is an extension of the peritoneum.

As described in the section on the midgut, the midgut normally migrates into the cord or extraembryonic coelom during the fifth week and returns to the abdominal cavity by the eleventh week. The finding of the gut in the cord after the twelfth week by ultrasound is diagnostic of an omphalocele. Between 33% and 50% of infants

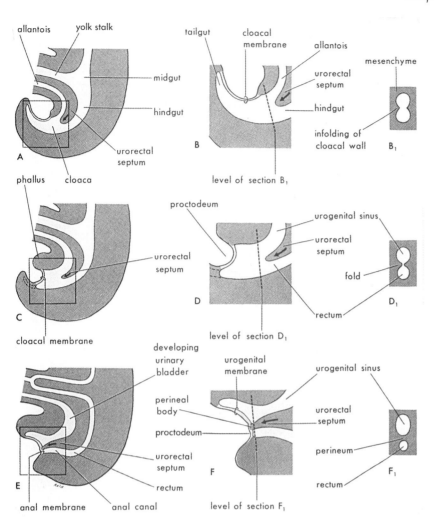

Figure 2.28. Drawings illustrating successive stages in the partitioning of the cloaca into the rectum and urogenital sinus by the urorectal septum. **A, C,** and **E,** Views from the left side at 4, 6, and 7 weeks, respectively. **B, D,** and **F,** are enlargements of the cloacal region. **B₁, D₁,** and **F₁,** are transverse sections through the cloaca at the levels shown in **B, D,** and **F,** respectively. Note that the tailgut (shown in **B**) degenerates and disappears (shown in **C**), as the rectum forms from the dorsal part of the cloaca. From Moore KL. The developing human; clinically oriented embryology. Philadelphia: WB Saunders, 1973. Reprinted by permission.

Table 2.3.
Anatomical Classification of Anorectal Malformations[a]

Female	Male
High	High
Anorectal agenesis	Anorectal agenesis
With rectovaginal fistula	With rectoprostatic urethral fistula[b]
Without fistula	Without fistula
Rectal atresia	Rectal atresia
Intermediate	Intermediate
Rectovestibular fistula	Rectobulbar urethral fistula
Rectovaginal fistula	Anal agenesis without fistula
Anal agenesis without fistula	
Low	Low
Anovestibular fistula[b]	Anocutaneous fistula[b]
Anocutaneous fistula[b,c]	Anal stenosis[b,d]
Anal stenosis[d]	
Cloacal malformations[e]	
Rare malformations	Rare malformations

[a] From Welch. Pediatric surgery. 1986. Reproduced with permission.
[b] Relatively common lesion.
[c] Includes fistulae occurring at the posterior junction of the labia minora often fourchette fistulae or vulvar fistulae.
[d] Previously called covered anus.
[e] Previously called rectocloacal fistulae. Entry of the rectal fistula into the cloaca may be high or intermediate, depending on the length of the cloacal canal.

with omphaloceles have other major anomalies, including cardiac and chromosomal anomalies, and should be evaluated for these. Beckwith-Wiedemann syndrome (omphalocele-macroglossia-gigantism and hypoglycemia) has a high association with hypoglycemia and should be considered in each infant with an omphalocele. While the survival of infants with omphalocele is only 70%, the mortality reflects the serious associated anomalies (110). Infants with isolated omphaloceles are expected to survive and develop normally.

Gastroschisis

Gastroschisis is a full-thickness defect in the anterior abdominal wall through which the stomach and the midgut herniate (Fig. 2.31). The following characteristics differentiate gastroschisis from omphalocele (111): (*a*) the abdominal wall defect is nearly always (97%) to the right of an intact umbilical cord; (*b*) there is no sac; (*c*) the liver and spleen rarely, if ever, herniate through the defect; (*d*) the mesentery of the herniated bowel may be obstructed as it passes through the umbilical ring resulting in intrauterine infarction and small bowel atresia in 15% of the cases; and (*e*) other major congenital malformations are infrequent. Unlike patients with om-

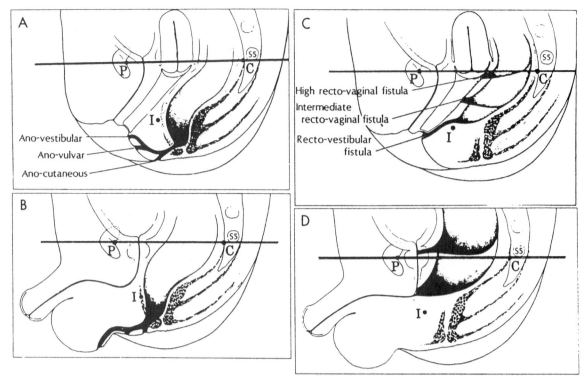

Figure 2.29.   Imperforate anus and kinds of fistulae. **A,** Low imperforate anus anomalies in the female almost always have an external fistulous tract. The tract is named for the point at which it exits: cutaneous (perineal), vulvar (labia majora), or vestibular (just distal to the hymen). A hemostat placed inside all these fistulous tracts will pass posteriorly before turning cephalad to enter the rectum. **B,** Low imperforate anus anomalies in the male usually have an external fistulous tract. The tracts are all anocutaneous, but they vary in how far removed the exit site is from the true anus. When the fistula extends up to and along the scrotal raphe, meconium can often be seen through the thin overlying skin. **C,** Intermediate and high imperforate anus lesions in the female are usually associated with a fistula to the posterior vagina. The passage of stool from above the hymen confirms the presence of an intermediate or high lesion. Patients with a vestibular fistula should be carefully evaluated because the underlying rectal pouch may be intermediate and not low. **D,** Intermediate and high imperforate anus in the male is usually associated with a fistula to the urinary tract. Most of these fistulae involve the prostatic urethra; the rectal pouch is therefore high. A few involve the bulbous urethra. Fistulae at this level are usually larger and enter the urethra more obliquely. From Templeton JM, O'Neill JA. Anorectal malformations. In: Welch KJ, Randolph JG, Ravitch MM, et al, eds. Pediatric surgery. 4th ed. Chicago: Year Book Medical Publishers, 1986:1022–1034. Reprinted by permission.

Figure 2.30.   Omphalocele. This is classified as a hernia of the cord because the defect measures less than 4 cm in diameter. The sac contained nearly all of the small bowel and much of the colon. Note the intact cord coming off the top of the sac.

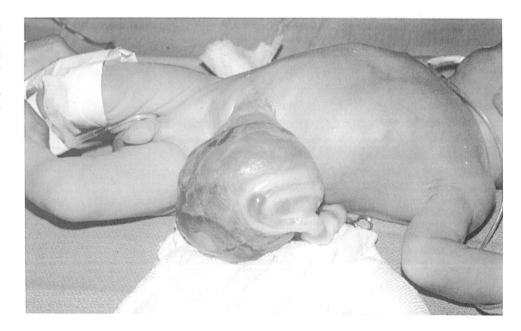

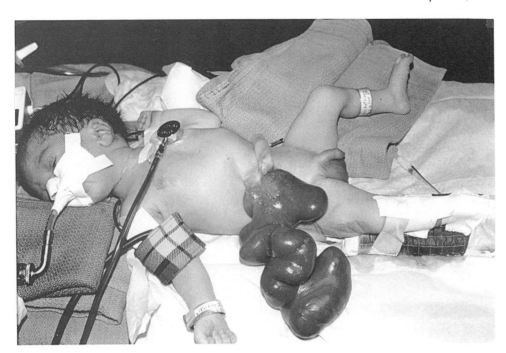

Figure 2.31. Gastroschisis. The intestine prolapses through a defect in the abdominal wall to the right of the umbilical cord. The intestine is edematous and appears short. As the inflammation resolves the intestinal length will be normal.

phaloceles, those with gastroschisis rarely have associated anomalies outside the gastrointestinal tract (110). On the other hand, although malformations of the small bowel are rare in patients with omphalocele, nearly one in five patients with gastroschisis have an associated small bowel atresia (112,113). The jejunoileal atresia is thought to result from mesenteric vascular compromise as the intestine and mesentery herniates through the small umbilical ring (75,113).

Shaw postulated that gastroschisis is a hernia of the umbilical cord in which rupture or tear of the membrane occurred before closure of the umbilical ring and fixation of the bowel in the peritoneal cavity (113). The rupture of the umbilical membrane occurs during a normal embryologic phase rather than the result of a chromosomal or teratologic insult. This would explain the low incidence of associated anomalies. The occurrence to the right of the cord has been postulated to be the result of a weak area of the cord where the right umbilical vein disappears by the seventh week of development. The left vein remains on the left side of the cord and adds support to the left side of the sac in hernias of the cord. Glick and his associates have demonstrated by serial antenatal ultrasound, the transformation of an antenatally ruptured hernia of the cord into a typical gastroschisis (114).

The amniotic fluid is irritating to the exposed viscera and results in varying amounts of serosal edema and thickening (115,116). The bowel may be matted together, appear short, and exhibit poor peristalsis. It was formerly thought that the degree of serosal reaction corresponded to the length of time the bowel was exposed to the amniotic fluid. However, recent clinical studies with serial antenatal ultrasound examinations have shown poor correlation between the length of time the bowel is exposed to the amniotic fluid and the extent of serosal change (117). These serosal changes are reversible after the intestine is returned to the peritoneal cavity and the defect closed immediately after birth (112).

Survival of patients with gastroschisis is nearly 95%. After a period of adaptation—which may last several weeks to allow the intestine to develop normal peristalsis—intestinal function is typically normal. As there are rarely anomalies of other organ systems, patients with gastroschisis can be expected to grow and develop normally.

Urogenital

Both the urinary and genital system arise from the intermediate mesoderm and the mesodermal ridge from the level of the seventh somite caudad. The process of differentiation begins during the fourth and fifth week. The cephalad portions sequentially form the pronephros, then the mesonephros, and finally the metanephros or permanent kidney (Fig. 2.32) (14). The pronephros and mesonephros have degenerated and disappeared by the end of the first and second month, respectively. The permanent kidney develops from the more caudad mesoderm known as the metanephric mesoderm. The collecting ducts form from the ureteric bud, an outgrowth of the mesonephric duct near the cloaca. The ureteric bud forms the major and minor calyces as well as the collecting tubules. The renal tubules continue to form until the end of the fifth month. From the ureteric bud develops the ureter, renal pelvis, calyces, and collecting tubules (Fig. 2.33) (14).

Figure 2.32. **A,** Schematic diagram showing the relation of the intermediate mesoderm of the pronephric, mesonephric, and metanephric systems. In the cervical and upper thoracic regions, the intermediate mesoderm is segmented; in the lower thoracic, lumbar, and sacral regions it forms a solid, unsegmented mass of tissue, the nephrogenic cord. Note the longitudinal collecting duct, initially formed by the pronephros, but later taken over the mesonephros. **B,** Schematic representation of the excretory tubules of the pronephric and mesonephric systems in a 5-week-old embryo. Note the remnant of the pronephric excretory tubules and longitudinal collecting duct. From Sadler TW. Langman's medical embryology. 6th ed. Baltimore: Williams & Wilkins, 1990. Reprinted by permission.

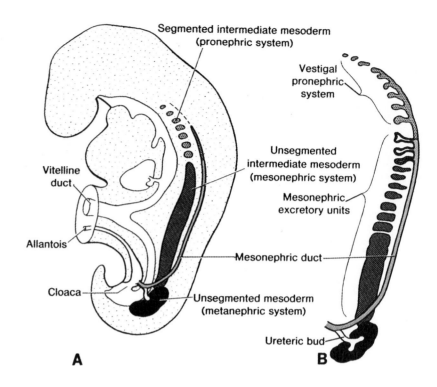

Figure 2.33. Schematic representation of the development of a metanephric excretory unit. *Arrows* indicate the place where the excretory unit establishes an open communication with the collecting system, thus allowing for the flow of urine from the glomerulus into the collecting ducts. From Sadler TW. Langman's medical embryology. 6th ed. Baltimore: Williams & Wilkins, 1990. Reprinted by permission.

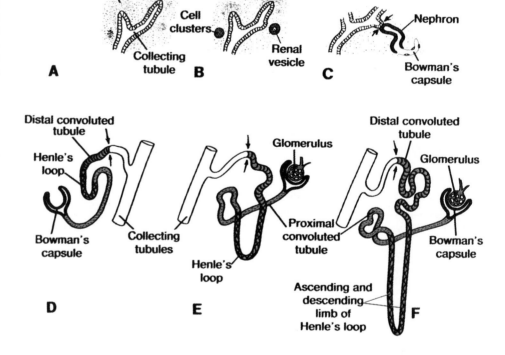

The excretory units develop from a metanephric tissue cap or blastema that forms at the distal end of each collecting tubule. This is known as nephrogenesis. Cells from the metanephric cap form small renal vesicles that form tubules, which, along with glomeruli and tufts of capillaries, make up the nephrons, or excretory units. The proximal end of the nephron forms Bowman's cap-

sule. As the tubule lengthens it forms the proximal convoluted tubule, the loop of Henle, and the distal convoluted tubule before draining into the collecting tubule. Although development of the collecting system is nearly complete by the twentieth week of gestation, nephrogenesis occurs primarily between the twentieth and thirtieth week (Fig. 2.34) (118). Cystic dysplasia appears to

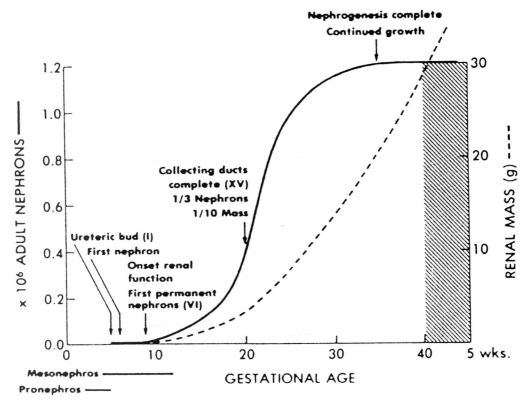

Figure 2.34. Fetal renal development is presented schematically. The branching of the collecting system (15 generations) is complete by 20 weeks, but the majority of nephrons and most of the functional mass form in the cortex after 20 weeks. Obstruction interferes with nephrogen-esis; relief of obstruction may allow further development. From Harrison MR, Golbus MS, Filly RA, et al. Management of the fetus with congenital hydronephrosis. J Pediatr Surg 1982;17:728–741. Reprinted by permission.

Table 2.4.
Normal Values of Renal Function[a]

	Premature Infant	Term Infant			
	First 3 days	First 3 days	2 weeks	8 weeks	1 year
Daily excretion of urine					
mL/kg/24 hour	15–75	20–75	25–120	80–130	40–100
Percent of fluid intake	40–80		50–70	45–65	40–60
Voiding size					
mL/kg per voiding	4–6	4–6	4–7	4–6	3–6
Maximal urine osmolality					
mosm/kg H$_2$O	400–500	600–800	800–900	1000–1200	1200–1400
Glomerular filtration rate					
mL/min per 1.73 m^2	10–15	15–20	35–45	75–80	90–110

[a] From Holiday, Pediatric nephrology. 1987. Reproduced with permission.

be a developmental consequence of obstruction during the development of the excretory units (118).

Initial renal morphogenesis occurs in the area of upper sacral segments, but the kidney undergoes growth in a cranial direction, which is completely in the adult position by the 9th week. As the kidney ascends it rotates 90° so that the renal pelvis and ureter moves from the ventral to a medial position. If one kidney fails to ascend, it remains in the pelvis close to the iliac artery and is known as a pelvic kidney. The kidneys may be pushed together so that the lower poles fuse, resulting

in the formation of a horseshoe kidney. The ascent of a horseshoe kidney is prevented by the root of the inferior mesenteric artery.

During the first year of life, renal function is imma-ture. The glomerular filtration rate is low and the in-fant's ability to concentrate is decreased, which reflects immature tubular function (Table 2.4) (118). During this time, under normal circumstances, the infant takes in only human milk, which provides a small excretory load. This decreased renal function requires a lower rate of energy expenditure at a time when calories are needed for rapid growth (118). However, the system may not adequately handle the increased excretory load associated with operative or other stress. This low urinary concentrating capacity also makes the infant more sensitive to extrarenal water losses and the development of hypertonic dehydration. The newborn is able to dilute the urine so that as much as 165 mL water/kg/day can be given without developing fluid retention. This high volume of water may be necessary to provide adequate urinary volume for the infant to excrete the solid load, which may result from tissue breakdown following stress or increased calories to satisfy the nutritional needs of the infant.

REFERENCES

1. Gray SW, Skandalakis JE. Embryology for surgeons. Philadelphia: WB Saunders, 1972.
2. Fraser FC. Causes of congenital malformations in human beings. J Chron Dis 1959;10:97–110.
3. Witschi E. Teratogenic effects from overripeness of the egg. In: Fraser FC, McKusick VA, eds, Robinson R, co-ed. Congenital malformations, proceedings of the third international conference. Amsterdam: Excerpta Medica, 1969:157–169.
4. Hertig AT. Traumatic abortion and prenatal death of the embryo. In: Holt LE, Ingalls TH, Hellman LB, eds. Prematurity, congenital malformation and birth injury. New York: Association for the Aid of Crippled Children 1953:174–176.
5. Erhardt CL. Pregnancy losses in New York City. Am J Public Health 1963;53:1337–1352.
6. Stickle G. Defective development and reproductive wastage in the United States. Am J Obstet Gynecol 1968;100:442–447.
7. Stevenson SS, Worcester J, Rice RG. 677 congenitally malformed infants and associated gestational characteristics. I. General considerations. Pediatrics 1950;6:37–50.
8. Smith DW. Recognizable patterns of human malformation, genetic, embryologic, and clinical aspects. 2nd ed. Philadelphia: WB Saunders, 1982.
9. Nadler HL, Sacks AJ, Evans MI. Genetics in surgery and prenatal diagnosis. In: Raffensperger JG, ed. Swenson's pediatric surgery. Chicago: Appleton, Century, Crofts, 1980.
10. Baraitser M, Winter R. A colour atlas of clinical genetics. London: Wolf Medical, 1984.
11. Moore KL. The developing human; clinically oriented embryology. Philadelphia: WB Saunders, 1973.
12. Streeter GL. Developmental horizons in human embryos: age group XI, 13–20 somites, and age group XII, 21–29 somites. Contrib Embryol 1942;30:211.
13. Streeter GL. Developmental horizons in human embryos: age group XIII, embryos 4 or 5 mm long, and age group XIV, indentation of lens vesicle. Contrib Embryol 1945;31:26.
14. Sadler TW. Langman's medical embryology. 6th ed. Baltimore: Williams & Wilkins, 1990.
15. Seeds JW. Impaired fetal growth: definition and clinical diagnosis. Obstet Gynecol 1984;64:303–310.
16. Jones M, Battaglia F. Intrauterine growth retardation. Am J Obstet Gynecol 1977;127:540–549.
17. Kennedy WP. Epidemiologic aspects of the problem of congenital malformations. In: Bergsma D, ed. Birth defects original article series. New York: Alan R. Liss, 1967:1.
18. McIntosh R, Merritt KK, Richards MR, et al. Incidence of congenital malformations; a study of 5964 pregnancies. Pediatrics 1954; 14:505–522.
19. Warkany J, Kalter H. Congenital malformations. N Engl J Med 1961;265:993.
20. Kalter H, Warkany J. Experimental production of congenital malformations in mammals by metabolic procedure. Physiol Rev 1959;39:69.
21. Wilson JG. Environment and birth defects. New York: Academic Press, 1973.
22. Wilson JG, Fraser FC. Handbook of teratology. Vols. 1–3. New York: Plenum Press, 1977.
23. Simmons RL, Sutherland DER, Lower RR, et al. Transplantation. In: Schwartz, ed. Principles of surgery. 5th ed. New York: McGraw-Hill, 1989:387–458.
24. Kosloske A, Stone HA. Surgical infections. In: Welch KJ, Randolph JG, Ravitch MM, et al, eds. Pediatric surgery. 4th ed. Chicago: Year Book Medical Publishers, 1986:78–88.
25. Rosen FS. The immunocompromised child. In: Welch KJ, Randolph JG, Ravitch MM, et al, eds. Pediatric surgery. 4th ed. Chicago: Year Book Medical Publishers, 1986:89–95.
26. Hoffman JIE. The circulatory system. In: Rudolph AM, ed. Pediatrics. 18th ed. Norwalk: Appleton & Lange, 1987:1219–1358.
27. Rudolph AM. Fetal and neonatal pulmonary circulation. Ann Rev Physiol 1979;41:383–395.
28. Anderson KD. Congenital diaphragmatic hernia. In: Welch KJ, Randolph JG, Ravitch MM, et al, eds. Pediatric surgery. 4th ed. Chicago: Year Book Medical Publishers, 1986:589–618.
29. Holder TM, Ashcraft KW. Cardiac disease. In: Welch KJ, Randolph JG, Ravitch MM, O'Neill JA, Rowe MI, eds. Pediatric surgery. 4th ed. Chicago: Year Book Medical Publishers, 1986: 1385–1397.
30. Congdon ED. Transformation of the aortic-arch system during the development of the human embryo. Contrib Embryol 1922; 14:47–110.
31. Kramer TC. The partitioning of the truncus and conus and the formation of the membranous portion of the interventricular septum in the human heart. Am J Anat 1942;71;343–370.
32. Waldhausen JA, Pae WE. Thoracic great vessels. In: Welch KJ, Randolph JG, Ravitch MM, et al, eds. Pediatric surgery. 4th ed. Chicago: Year Book Medical Publishers, 1986:1399–1419.
33. Krummel TM, Greenfield LJ, Kirkpatrick BV, et al. Alveolar-arterial oxygen gradients vs neonatal pulmonary insufficiency index for prediction of mortality in ECMO candidates. J Pediatr Surg 1984;19:380–384.
34. Fox WW, Duara S. Persistent pulmonary hypertension in the neonate: diagnosis and management. J Pediatrics 1983;103:505.
35. Colvin E. Cardiac embryology. In: Garson T, Bricker JT, McNamara DG, eds. The science and practice of pediatric cardiology. Philadelphia: Lea & Febiger, 1990:71–108.
36. Van Mierop LHS, Kutsche LM. Anatomy and embryology of the right ventricle. In: Hurst JW, ed. The heart. 6th ed. Chicago: McGraw-Hill, 1986;1:3–16.
37. Pokorny WJ, Adams JM, McGill CW, et al. Ligation of patent ductus arteriosus in the neonatal intensive care unit. Mod Probl Paediatr 1985;23:133–142.
38. Anonymous. Report of the task force on blood pressure control in children. Pediatrics 1977;59(suppl):799.
39. de Sweit M, Fayers P, Shinebourne EA. Systolic blood pressure in a population of infants in the first year of life: the Brompton study. Pediatrics 1980;65:1028–1035.
40. Hennekens CH, Jesse JM, Klein BE, et al. Aggregation of blood pressure in infants and their siblings. Am J Epidemiol 1976;103: 457.
41. Greenwood RD, Rosenthal A. Cardiovascular malformations associated with tracheoesophageal fistula and esophageal atresia. Pediatrics 1976;57:87–91.
42. Streeter GL. Development horizons in human embryos. Contrib Embryol 1948;32:133–203.
43. Smith EI. The early development of the trachea and esophagus in relation to atresia of the esophagus and tracheoesophageal fistula. Embryology 1957;36:41.
44. DeLorimier AA. Congenital malformations and neonatal problems of the respiratory tract. In: Welch KJ, Randolph JG, Ravitch MM, et al, eds. Pediatric surgery. 4th ed. Chicago: Year Book Medical Publishers, 1986:631–644.
45. Randolph JG. Esophageal atresia and congenital stenosis. In: Welch KJ, Randolph JG, Ravitch MM, et al, eds. Pediatric surgery. 4th ed. Chicago: Year Book Medical Publishers, 1986:682–694.
46. Zeltner TB, Burri PH. The postnatal development and growth of the human lung. II. Morphology. Respir Physiol 1987;67:269–282.
47. Tooley WH. The respiratory system. In: Rudolph AM, ed. Pediatrics. 18th ed. Norwalk: Appleton & Lange, 1987:1359–1446.
48. Inselman LS, Mellins RB. Growth and development of the lung. J Pediatr 1981;98:1–15.
49. O'Brodovich HM, Huddad GG. The functional basis of respira-

tory pathology. In: Chernick V, Kendig EL, eds. Kendig's disorders of the respiratory tract in children. 5th ed. Philadelphia: WB Saunders, 1990.

50. Bucher U, Reid L. Development of the intrasegmental bronchial tree: the pattern of branching and development of cartilage of various stages of intrauterine life. Thorax 1961;16:207–218.

51. Burri PH. Fetal and postnatal development of the lung. Ann Rev Physiol 1984;46:617–628.

52. Heithoff KN, Sane SM, Williams HG, et al. Bronchopulmonary foregut malformations. Am J Radiol 1976;126:46–55.

53. Stocker JT, Madewell JE, Drake RM. Congenital cystic adenomatoid malformation of the lung. Hum Pathol 1977;8:155–171.

54. Side RM, Clouse M, Ellis FH. The spectrum of pulmonary sequestration. Ann Thorac Surg 1974;18:644–658.

55. Fowler CL, Pokorny WJ, Wagner ML, et al. Review of bronchopulmonary foregut malformations. J Pediatr Surg 1988;23:793–797.

56. Wells LJ. Development of the human diaphragm and pleural sacs. Contrib Embryol 1954;35:107.

57. DeLorimier AA, Tierney DF, Parker HR. Hypoplastic lungs in fetal lambs with surgically produced congenital diaphragmatic hernia. Surgery 1967;62:12.

58. Ohi R, Suzuki H, Kato T, et al. Development of the lung in fetal rabbits with experimental diaphragmatic hernia. J Pediatr Surg 1976;11:955.

59. Starrett RW, deLorimier AA. Congenital diaphragmatic hernia in lambs: hemodynamic and ventilatory changes with breathing. J Pediatr Surg 1975;10:575.

60. Comer TP, Clagett OT. Surgical treatment of hernia of the foramen of Morgagni. Thorac Cardiovasc Surg 1966;62:461–468.

61. Pokorny WJ, McGill CW, Harberg FJ. Morgagni hernias during infancy: presentation and associated anomalies. J Pediatr Surg 1984;19:394–397.

62. Berdon WE, Baker DH, Amoury RA. The role of pulmonary hyperplasia in the prognosis of infants with diaphragmatic hernia and eventration. Am J Roentgenol 1968;103:413.

63. Haller JA, Rickard LR, Tepas JJ, et al. Management of diaphragmatic paralysis in infants with special emphasis on selection of patients for operative plication. J Pediatr Surg 1979;14:779.

64. McNamara JJ, Paulson DJ, Urschel HC, et al. Eventration of the diaphragm. Surgery 1968;64:1013.

65. Gross RE. The surgery of infancy and childhood. Philadelphia: WB Saunders, 1953.

66. Holder TM, Cloud DT, Lewis JE, et al. Esophageal atresia and tracheoesophageal fistula. A survey of its members by the Surgical Section of the American Academy of Pediatrics. Pediatrics 1961;34:542.

67. Waterson DJ, Bonham Carter RE, Aberdeen E. Oesophageal atresia, tracheoesophageal fistula—a study of survival in 218 infants. Lancet 1962;1:819.

68. Barry JE, Auldist AW. The VATER association: one end of a spectrum of anomalies. Am J Dis Child 1984;128:769.

69. Quan L, Smith DW. The VATER association. J Pediatr 1973; 82:104–107.

70. Andrassy RJ, Mahour H. Gastrointestinal anomalies associated with esophageal atresia or tracheoesophageal fistula. Arch Surg 1979;114:1125–1128.

71. Tandler J. Zur entwicklungsgeschichte des menschlichen duodenums. Morphol Jb 1902;29:187.

72. Harberg FJ, Pokorny WJ, Hahn H. Congenital duodenal obstruction: a review of 65 cases. Am J Surg 1979;138:825–828.

73. Grosfeld JL. Jejunoileal atresia and stenosis. In: Welch KJ, Randolph JG, Ravitch MM, et al, eds. Pediatric surgery. 4th ed. Chicago: Year Book Medical Publishers, 1986:838–848.

74. Louw JH. Resection and end-to-end anastomosis in the management of atresia and stenosis of the small bowel. Surgery 1967;62:940.

75. DeLorimier AA, Fonkalsrud EW, Hays DM. Congenital atresia and stenosis of the jejunum and ileum. Surgery 1969;65:819.

76. Langman J. Medical embryology. 3rd ed. Baltimore: Williams & Wilkins, 1975:245.

77. Lecco TM. Zur morphologie des pankreas annulare. Sitzungsb Akad Wissensch Cl 1910;119:391.

78. Sibley WL. Meckel's diverticulum: dyspepsia Meckeli from heterotopic gastric mucosa. Arch Surg 1944;49:156–166.

79. Soltero MJ, Bill AH. The natural history of Meckel's diverticulum. Ann Surg 1937;105:44–55.

80. Soderland S. Meckel's diverticulum, a clinical and histologic study. Acta Chir Scand Suppl 1959;248:13–233.

81. Benson CD. Surgical implications of Meckel's diverticulum. In: Ravitch MM, Welch KJ, Benson DC, et al, eds. Pediatric surgery. 3rd ed. Chicago: Year Book Medical Publishers 1979:955–960.

82. Amoury RA. Meckels diverticulum. In: Welch KJ, Randolph JG, Ravitch MM, et al, eds. Pediatric surgery. 4th ed. Chicago: Year Book Medical Publishers, 1986:859–867.

83. Snyder WH, Chaffin L. Embryology and pathology of the intestinal tract: presentation of 48 cases of malrotation. Ann Surg 1954;140:368–380.

84. Touloukian RJ, Walker-Smith GJ. Normal intestinal length in preterm infants. J Pediatr Surg 1983;18:720–723.

85. Pokorny WJ, Fowler CL. Isoperistaltic intestinal lengthening for short bowel syndrome. Surg Gynecol Obstet 1991;172:39–43.

86. Mall FP. Development of the human intestine and its position in the adult. Int Abstr Surg 1956;103:417–438.

87. Ladd WE. Surgical diseases of the alimentary tract in infants. N Engl J Med 1936;215:705.

88. Brandt ML, Pokorny WJ, McGill CW, et al. Late presentations of midgut malrotation in children. Am J Surg 1985;150:767–771.

89. Stewart DR, Colodny AL, Daggett WC. Malrotation of the bowel in infants and children: a 15 year review. Surgery 1976;79:716–720.

90. Dott NM. Anomalies of intestinal rotation: their embryology and surgical aspects, with report of 5 cases. Br J Surg 1923;11:251–286.

91. Filston HC, Kirks DR. Malrotation[fcmol]the ubiquitous anomaly. J Pediatr Surg 1981;16:614–620.

92. Louw JH, Barnard CN. Congenital intestinal atresia: observations on its origin. Lancet 1955;2:1065.

93. Martin LW, Zerella JT. Jejunoileal atresia: a proposed classification. J Pediatr Surg 1976;11:399–403.

94. Weitzman JJ, Vanderhoof RS. Jejunal atresia with agenesis of the dorsalmesentery with "Christmas tree" deformity of the small intestine. Am J Surg 1966;111:443.

95. Zerella JT, Martin LW. Jejunal atresia with absent mesentery and a helical ileum. Surgery 1976;80:550.

96. Zwiren GT, Andrews HG, Ahmann P. Jejunal atresia with agenesis of the dorsal mesentery ("apple-peel small bowel"). J Pediatr Surg 1972;7:414.

97. Hays DM. Intestinal atresia and stenosis. Curr Probl Surg 1969;1:3–48.

98. Rittenhouse EA, Beckwith JB, Chappell JS, et al. Multiple septa of the small bowel: description of an unusual case with review of the literature and consideration of etiology. Surgery 1972;71:371.

99. Guttman FN, Braun P, Garance PH, et al. Multiple atresias and a new syndrome of hereditary multiple atresias involving the gastrointestinal tract from stomach to rectum. J Pediatr Surg 1974;8:633.

100. Blyth H, Dickson JAS. Apple peel syndrome (congenital intestinal atresia): a family study of 7 index patients. J Med Genet 1969;6:275.

101. Seashore J, Collins F, Markwitz R, et al. Familial apple peel jejunal atresia: surgical, genetic and radiologic aspects. Pediatrics 1987;80:540.

102. Grosfeld JL. Alimentary tract obstruction in the newborn. Curr Probl Pediatr 1975;5:3–47.

103. Stephens FD, Smith ED. Anorectal malformations in children. Chicago: Year Book Medical Publishers, 1971.

104. Templeton JM, O'Neill JA. Anorectal malformations. In: Welch KJ, Randolph JG, Ravitch MM, et al, eds. Pediatric surgery. 4th ed. Chicago: Year Book Medical Publishers, 1986:1022–1034.

105. Duhamel B. Embryology of exomphalos and allied malformations. Arch Dis Child 1963;38:142–147.

106. Hutchin P. Somatic anomalies of the umbilicus and anterior abdominalwall. Surg Gynecol Obstet 1965;170:1075.

107. Cantrell JR, Haller JA, Ravitch MM. A syndrome of congenital defects involving the abdominal wall, sternum, diaphragm, pericardium and heart. Surg Gynecol Obstet 1958;107:602.

108. Benson CD, Penherthy GC, Hill EJ. Hernia into the umbilical cord and omphalocele (amniocele) in the newborn. Arch Surg 1949;58:833.

109. Schwaitzberg SD, Pokorny WJ, McGill CW, et al. Gastroschisis and omphalocele. Am J Surg 1982;144:650–654.
110. Schuster SR. Omphalocele and gastroschisis. In: Welch KJ, Randolph JG, Ravitch MM, et al, eds. Pediatric surgery. 4th ed. Chicago: Year Book Medical Publishers, 1986:740–763.
111. Pokorny WJ, Harberg FJ, McGill CW. Gastroschisis complicated by intestinal atresia. J Pediatr Surg 1981;16:261–263.
112. Moore TC. Gastroschisis and omphalocele: clinical difference. Surgery 1977;82:561.
113. Shaw A. The myth of gastroschisis. J Pediatr Surg 1975;10:235–244.
114. Glick LG, Harrison MR, Azick NS, et al. The missing link in the pathogenesis of gastroschisis. J Pediatr Surg 1985;20:406–409.
115. Moore TC. Gastroschisis with antenatal evisceration of intestines and urinary bladder. Ann Surg 1963;158:263.
116. Bond SJ, Harrison MR, Filly RA, et al. Severity of intestinal damage in gastroschisis: correlation with prenatal sonographic findings. J Pediatr Surg 1988;23:520–525.
117. Harrison MR, Golbus MS, Filly RA, et al. Management of the fetus with congenital hydronephrosis. J Pediatr Surg 1982;17:728–741.
118. Holliday MA, Barratt TM, Vernier RL, eds. Pediatric nephrology. Baltimore: Williams & Wilkins, 1987.

3 Fluids and Electrolytes

Andrew Z. Fenves | Michael Emmett

Introduction

Fluid and electrolyte management in the surgical patient has become increasingly important over the last several decades. The advance of medical science and improved surgical techniques have allowed us to operate on higher risk patients; close attention to fluid balance constitutes a critical aspect of the care of these patients. This chapter focuses on the changes in fluid homeostasis and electrolyte balance that occur in the peri- and postoperative period. We will also review treatment options.

Normal Fluid Spaces and Dynamics

In critically ill patients, the alteration in fluid balance is a dynamic process characterized by major hemodynamic changes and fluid shifts between body compartments. The extent of these changes is a function of the severity of the underlying disease process. Close monitoring of these fluid shifts helps the clinician to gauge the clinical course of the patient. Knowledge of the body's normal fluid distribution is necessary to understand these changes.

In a normal human, about 60% of the total body weight is water (e.g., 42 L in a 70 kg man and slightly less in women). Approximately two-thirds of this fluid resides inside cells and is called intracellular fluid (ICF). The remaining one-third of the water, called the extracellular fluid (ECF), is outside the cells. The ECF is further separated into two compartments; the vascular compartment (plasma fluid) constitutes about one-third of the ECF, and the fluid present between cells (interstitial fluid) constitutes about two-thirds of the ECF. Within the vascular compartment (e.g., 4.6 L in our 70

kg man), approximately 85% of the fluid resides in the venous side of the circulation and 15% in the arterial side.

A number of forces govern the movement of fluid between, and the relative volumes of, the interstitial space and the vascular compartment. In the capillaries, a balance of forces exists between hydrostatic and oncotic pressure. This concept is expressed mathematically by the Starling equation:

$$Qf = Kf \times (Pv - Pt) - \sigma \times (COP - TOP)$$

where Qf is fluid flux, Kf is capillary filtration coefficient, Pv is vascular hydrostatic pressure, Pt is interstitial hydrostatic pressure, σ is a reflection coefficient (which defines the effectiveness of the membrane in preventing solute flow), COP is colloid osmotic pressure, and TOP is tissue osmotic pressure (1). Fluid leaves the capillary at the arterial end because hydrostatic pressure exceeds oncotic pressure. As blood continues to flow down the capillary, hydrostatic pressure falls and oncotic pressure increases as a result of increasing protein concentration. When the oncotic pressure exceeds the hydrostatic pressure—in the venous end of the capillary—fluid returns from the interstitium to the capillary. Some of the fluid that is not returned to the venous end of the capillaries by virtue of the Starling forces eventually is returned to the vascular compartment by lymphatic drainage. Under some circumstances, lymphatic flow can be massive. For example, in cirrhotic patients, hepatic fibrosis leads to high capillary hydrostatic pressures, which, in conjunction with low capillary oncotic pressures due to hypoalbuminemia, cause a twenty-fold increase in daily lymphatic flow (from 1 liter to 20 liters per day) (2). Serum albumin is the major determinant of capillary colloid osmotic pressure, and hypoalbuminemia can lead to excess transudation of fluid from the vascular to the interstitial compartment. As discussed later, this is one of the more important factors contributing to the development of interstitial edema and expansion of ECF volume in the surgical patient.

Postoperative Changes in Body Fluid Compartments

A number of perioperative events contribute to ECF volume expansion. These nonspecific events also occur with many other pathologic conditions such as sepsis, extensive burns, multiple trauma, pancreatitis, bone marrow transplants, etc. A major stimulus to ECF expansion is a reduced intravascular volume. First, hemorrhage may directly reduce blood volume. Second, a generalized increase in capillary permeability occurs in many patients, especially after major abdominal and chest surgery. This results from a loss of endothelial integrity and the opening of intercellular clefts. The mediators that cause increased capillary permeability are probably identical to those responsible for some elements of the inflammatory response. These include, but may not be limited to, cytokines (interleukin-1, interleukin-6, tumor necrosis factor), β integrins, thrombin, bradykinin, and platelet activating factor (1). As a result of increased capillary permeability, protein-rich fluid escapes from the vascular compartment and expands the interstitial fluid. Third, negative interstitial fluid hydrostatic pressure may develop and *increase* the intravascular to interstitial pressure gradient generating interstitial edema (3).

The above alterations lead to reduced cardiac output and decreased effective blood volume. The sensors for effective blood volume are in the intra-arterial side of the intravascular compartment. In response to these signals, volume is regulated by modulation of renal sodium and water reabsorption. A decrease in cardiac output, decreased peripheral arterial vasodilation, or any combination thereof leads to arterial underfilling, and thus initiates and sustains a sodium and water retaining state (4).

Failure to maintain adequate intravascular volume leads to systemic hypoperfusion, decreased oxygen delivery, lactic acidosis, and ultimately tissue death. Thus, it is imperative to replace intravascular volume with appropriate amounts of colloid and crystalloid. The aim is to maintain a systolic blood pressure above 100 mm Hg, and a urinary output of about 30-50 cc/hr. However, in some patients, aggressive volume expansion markedly increases ECF volume while only producing a limited increase in the intravascular volume. Under these circumstances, avid renal sodium and water retention persists because the effective blood volume remains low. Indeed, increases in body weight of 10% to 30% are common after major surgery, trauma, or sepsis. Bock et al. found a 55% expansion of the interstitial compartment following the resuscitation of severely traumatized patients with isotonic salt solution (5). Generalized pitting

edema indicates an excess of extracellular fluid, but the intravascular volume may be decreased, normal, or increased. Intravascular volume status should be estimated whether generalized edema is present or not.

No known direct treatment can reverse the increased capillary permeability which develops in such patients. As patients recuperate from their underlying illness, the "capillary leak" resolves. Although substances that counteract the pro-inflammatory mediators could theoretically attenuate this pathologic state, none have proven to be effective. As long as clinical parameters suggest low effective intravascular volume, the best approach is the judicious administration of balanced electrolyte solutions and colloid to expand this compartment. Acceptable cardiac output and tissue perfusion remain the paramount concerns, even at the price of a marked increase in ECF and total body weight. In the severely anemic or bleeding patient, blood transfusions are used to expand intravascular volume and improve tissue oxygen delivery. To optimize intravascular volume replacement, pulmonary arterial pressure monitoring can be accomplished via a Swan-Ganz catheter, which measures pulmonary capillary wedge pressure and cardiac output. A pulmonary capillary wedge pressure of 16 to 18 mm Hg and a stable blood pressure is consistent with optimal fluid resuscitation in the patient with normal cardiac function. When the pulmonary capillary wedge pressure rises above 18 mm Hg, the rate of fluid infusion should be decreased to reduce the risk of pulmonary edema.

Adult respiratory distress syndrome (ARDS) may develop as a consequence of major surgical procedures, sepsis, burns, or multiple trauma. ARDS is a state of noncardiogenic pulmonary edema stemming from pulmonary capillary endothelial damage and functional disruption of the capillary-alveolar epithelial permeability barrier (6). Endothelial injury favors the exudation of the protein-rich fluid into the lung's interstitial spaces and fluid accumulated in the alveoli. Patients with ARDS may require lower pulmonary capillary wedge pressures, in the 10 to 12 mm Hg range, to reduce pulmonary congestion and facilitate hemoglobin oxygenation.

Another indirect measure of intravascular volume status is the fractional excretion of sodium calculated from measurements of sodium and creatinine in urine and blood

$$\frac{U_{Na} \times P_{cr}}{U_{cr} \times P_{Na}} \times 100 = FeNa$$

where U_{Na} = urinary sodium; U_{cr} = urinary creatinine; P_{cr} = plasma creatinine; P_{Na} = plasma sodium.

When patients develop oliguria, usually defined as a urine output of less than 600 cc of urine per 24 hours, distinguishing between intrinsic acute renal failure and intravascular volume depletion or prerenal renal dysfunction is critical. A fractional excretion of sodium lower than 1% in this setting suggests intravascular (absolute or relative—i.e., effective) volume contraction and renal hypoperfusion. As long as renal function is normal, the kidneys will retain salt and water until intravascular volume is optimized.

Resuscitation fluids are divided into two groups: colloid and crystalloid. Colloid refers to albumin or protein solutions (i.e., plasmanate) or synthetic hydroxy ethyl starch (hetastarch). Crystalloid refers to salt solutions such as normal saline or Ringer's lactate solution. A larger volume of crystalloid than colloid is required to produce an equal expansion of the ECF. Albumin is much more expensive, and probably offers little advantage over synthetic colloid solutions. Among the crystalloid solutions, one could use normal saline or Ringer's lactate. Table 3.1 depicts the electrolyte composition and osmolality of various intravenous solutions.

While it is tempting to use diuretics during the early phase of resuscitation of oliguric critically ill patients, oliguria in this early phase may be appropriate and may simply reflect decreased intravascular volume and cardiac output. If this is the case, diuretics should not be used because they could further reduce circulatory volume, peripheral perfusion, and thereby contribute to the development of lactic acidosis and acute renal failure.

Diuretics are appropriate when cardiogenic pulmonary edema develops following aggressive fluid resuscitation or when progressive ARDS occurs. Also, during the recovery phase, a large amount of interstitial fluid may reenter the intravascular compartment leading to pulmonary edema. Diuretics may then be required. Generally, loop diuretics are selected because they are most potent. Loop diuretics have several important effects: 1) they inhibit active sodium absorption in the thick ascending limb of Henle; 2) they increase blood flow to the kidney by stimulating vasodilatory prostaglandins; and 3) they increase venous capacitance, which can quickly relieve pulmonary edema, even before diuresis and natriuresis have occurred. Loop diuretics, such as furosemide or bumetanide, are extensively protein-bound and must reach their intratubular site of action via active proximal tubular secretion. Usually they are administered as intermittent intravenous boluses every 4 to 12 hours. When patients are found to be resistant to bolus doses of loop diuretics, continuous intravenous infusion may be used; for example, bumetanide may be infused at a dose of 0.5 to 1.0 mg per hour. This method of administration can produce as much as a 30% increase in urine volume compared to conventional intermittent intravenous doses. A schematic representation of the human nephron is depicted in Figure 3.1 showing the primary site of action of various diuretics.

The role of low dose intravenous dopamine in postoperative fluid management remains controversial. Some advocate the continuous infusion of dopamine at a dose of 2 to 3 μ/kg/min to cause an increase in the cortical perfusion of the kidney and thereby an increased urinary output (i.e., "renal dose dopamine"). This effect occurs by both increased cardiac output and renal vasodilation. It also directly inhibits renal tubular sodium reabsorption. The major potential side effect of dopamine is tachycardia, and occasionally tachyarrhythmias. It may be used when diuresis is needed and diuretics alone are not producing an adequate effect.

Hemodialysis or peritoneal dialysis should be considered if pulmonary edema exists and the above described maneuvers are ineffective. Peritoneal dialysis removes volume much slower than hemodialysis, and the initial instillation of fluid into the abdomen may further compromise respiratory status as the diaphragm is forced upward. In addition, peritoneal dialysis may not be feasible after major abdominal procedures. Hemodialysis, on the other hand, may be less well tolerated hemodynamically and can produce hypotension and cardiac arrhythmias. Continuous arteriovenous hemofiltration (CAVH) is another means to rapidly remove excess fluid and electrolytes. In general, it is better tolerated than hemodialysis. However, it requires placement of vascular catheters and systemic anticoagulation.

In summary, appropriate peri- and postoperative fluid management is critically important. Effective arterial blood volume must be maintained as close to normal as possible, even at the price of an expanded ECF volume and increased total body weight. Close monitoring of the intravascular compartment permits the physician to adjust to the various stages of recovery and the dynamic fluid shifts between compartments.

Table 3.1.
Intravenous Solutions

	Na (mEq/L)	Cl (mEq/L)	Glucose (gm/L)	Osmolality (mOsm/kg)
Ringer's lactate[a]	130	109	*	272
0.9% NaCl (normal saline)	154	154	*	308
0.45% NaCl ($^1/_2$ normal saline)	77	77	*	154
5% D/W	—	—	50	252
10% D/W	—	—	100	505
50% D/W	—	—	500	2520
3% NaCl (hypertonic saline)	513	513	—	1026

[a] Also coantains K^+ (4 mEq/L), Ca^{++} (3 mEq/L), and lactate (28 mEq/L)

Electrolyte Disturbances

Electrolyte disturbances occur commonly in the postoperative patient and may produce significant morbidity and mortality. This section focuses on hypo- and hypernatremia, hypo- and hyperkalemia, hypomagnesemia, and hypocalcemia. Metabolic alkalosis will also be discussed.

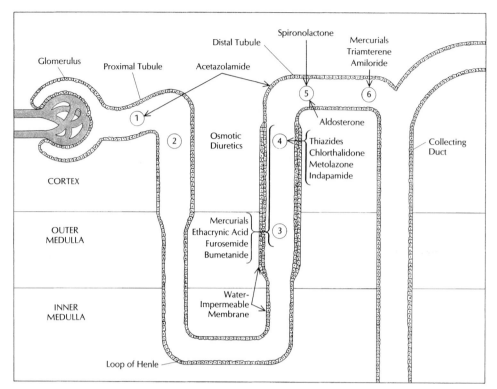

Figure 3.1. Diuretics primarily inhibit tubular reabsorption of sodium to increase excretion. However, other tubular functions are also affected at the discrete sites along the nephron where diuretics act. Thus, the proximal tubule is sensitive to diuretics inhibiting carbonic anhydrase and hydrogen ion section (1). Proximal-acting diuretics increase delivery of sodium and water to the ascending limb of Henle and more distal nephron and ultimately increase free water reabsorption or production, depending on ADH activity or its absence. An osmotic diuretic (e.g., mannitol) acting in the proximal tubule (2) also would enhance free water reabsorption or production. If a diuretic works in the medullary diluting segment of the ascending limb (3), it inhibits sodium chloride reabsorp- tion at a site where major free water generation would also be inhibited. At the same time, such an agent impedes delivery of osmotically active material into the medullary interstitium, impairing its ability to reabsorb free water. A diuretic acting solely in the cortical diluting segment (4) affects free water production but not reabsorption. Diuretics that enhance sodium passage proximal to the distal nephron will enhance potassium secretion, thereby increasing potassium loss. Diuretics acting in the distal tubule conserve potassium either by inhibiting aldosterone's action (5) or independently of aldosterone (6). From Thier SO. Diuretic mechanism as a guide to therapy. Hospital Practice 1987; 7:69.

Hyponatremia

Hyponatremia is one of the most frequent electrolyte abnormalities that occur in hospitalized patients. Hyponatremia usually is equated with hypoosmolality with two exceptions. Pseudohyponatremia results when some unusual biochemical abnormality interferes with correct measurement of the sodium concentration. For example, marked hyperlipidemia or hyperproteinemia displace water and generate measured hyponatremia with flame photometry. Introduction of newer instruments using direct ion selective electrodes have eliminated many of these problems. Hyponatremia can also be produced by very high concentrations of glucose, mannitol, glycine, or the presence of other impermeant solutes which can shift water from the intracellular to the extracellular space and thereby dilute other ECF solutes.

If these problems are excluded, hyponatremia usually indicates hypoosmolality. Plasma osmolality can be measured directly by an osmometer or estimated using the following equation:

$$P_{osm} = 2 \times Na(mEq/L) + \frac{glucose(mg\%)}{18} + \frac{BUN(mg\%)}{2.8}$$

Usually, simply doubling the serum sodium concentration gives a good approximation of the plasma osmolality.

Hypoosmolality indicates excess water relative to solute in the extracellular fluid. Water moves freely across most cell membranes so the ICF and ECF will have the same osmolality. Therefore, hypoosmolality in the plasma equals hypoosmolality in the ICF. In general, intracellular hypoosmolality is caused by increased intracellular water, i.e., cell swelling, rather than reduced intracellular solute.

Hyponatremia develops in 4 to 5% of all postoperative patients (conversely about 25% of all episodes of hospital acquired hyponatremia affect postoperative patients) (7). In most cases, the serum sodium concentration falls between 125 to 140 mEq/L, and these patients are generally asymptomatic. When the serum sodium falls below 125 mEq/L, clinical signs and symptoms may occur. These include headache, nausea, lethargy, hallucinations, seizures, hypothermia, bradycardia, hypoventilation, and occasionally coma.

One of the most important factors contributing to the development of hyponatremia in the perioperative period is persistent secretion of antidiuretic hormone (ADH). Usually the osmolality of the ECF is the major factor controlling ADH secretion. Hyperosmolality stimulates ADH, whereas hypoosmolality is a potent inhibitor. However, some non-osmotic stimuli can override the inhibition produced by hypoosmolality. Potent non-osmotic stimuli to ADH include intravascular volume depletion, nausea, anxiety, pain, and potent narcotics. All of these factors contribute to postoperative "inappropriate" (for osmolality) ADH secretion. Postoperative ADH levels are 5 to 50-fold higher than preoperative values (8). ADH levels generally decline to control values by the third to fifth postoperative day. A second important factor contributing to postoperative hyponatremia is decreased renal function. Postoperative hypotension decreases the glomerular filtration rate, which in turn reduces fluid delivery to the distal nephron. This limits the renal capacity to excrete free water and sets the stage for hyponatremia. The functional processes for regulation of salt and water transport are illustrated schematically in Figure 3.2.

A third factor contributing to postoperative hyponatremia is the administration of excessive free water in the form of hypotonic intravenous fluids. The perioperative patient with elevated ADH levels and decreased renal perfusion is likely to retain hypotonic intravenous fluids and thereby develop hyponatremia. Women in their reproductive years seem to be unusually susceptible to the neurologic complications of hyponatremia. As little as 3 liters of intravenous water over 36 hours can lead to devastating symptoms of hyponatremia, severe neurologic morbidity, and death (9,10). Although the exact mechanism responsible for this unusual syndrome has not been fully elucidated, the administration of hypotonic fluid perioperatively has clearly played a major role. In high risk patients, only isotonic fluids should be used, and the serum sodium should be evaluated frequently.

Another important, often overlooked hyponatremic syndrome occurs in patients undergoing a transurethral prostate resection (11). During this procedure, the prostatic bed is irrigated with large volumes of hypotonic glycine solutions. Absorption of this fluid into the intravascular space can generate hyponatremia, whereas the plasma osmolality may only be reduced slightly (as a result of the glycine). When the syndrome is severe, these men become hypertensive, confused, dyspneic, and nauseated. Hypotension, seizures, coma, and even death can follow. The altered mental and hemodynamic status may be caused by hyponatremia, ammonia generated from the glycine, or a direct toxic effect of the glycine itself (11). The full-blown syndrome occurs in 1% to 7% of patients undergoing a transurethral resection of the prostate.

Diuretic administration is the most common cause of hypovolemic hyponatremia in hospitalized patients. Thiazide diuretics are more likely than loop diuretics to cause hyponatremia because of their site of action in the distal convoluted tubule where urinary diluting capacity is blunted. Although hyponatremia secondary to thiazide diuretics is usually mild and asymptomatic, on occasion it can be acute, develop over 48 hours, and be severe. Furthermore, many diuretics will also produce significant urinary potassium and magnesium losses, further complicating the postoperative care of patients. It is often best to limit diuretic use in the postoperative patient and allow spontaneous diuresis to occur as interstitial fluid floods the intravascular compartment.

The treatment of hyponatremia in the postoperative patient is guided by identifying the cause of the hypoosmolality. Administration of excess free water should be discontinued. If diuretics have generated volume depletion, infusion of normal saline to expand the ECF will cause a brisk water diuresis and correction of the hyponatremia. In severely hyponatremic patients who are symptomatic, especially when the hyponatremia develops acutely, hypertonic saline may be used. The therapeutic goal in these patients with profound hyponatremia is not to restore the sodium concentration to normal; rather, it is to aim for a sodium concentration of about 120 mEq/L and improvement of the neurologic symptoms. The serum sodium level should be monitored closely during the correction phase.

Hypernatremia

Hypernatremia occurs much less commonly than hyponatremia in the perioperative patient. A high serum sodium concentration is always associated with a high serum osmolality and hypertonicity, and water is needed to restore isotonicity. Hypernatremia is normally a potent stimulus to thirst. Therefore, for a patient to develop hypernatremia, some impairment of water intake must exist, such as an inappropriate lack of thirst or no access to water. Excessive water loss or salt intake may contribute as well. The ECF volume status of hypernatremic patients is high when they have excess total body solute; normal when total body solutes are normal but water is inadequate, or low when total body solutes are low and water is reduced even more. For example, excessive sweating and large evaporative losses from the skin and lungs, especially with fever or high environmental temperatures, may cause a disproportionate loss of water compared to the loss of salt from the body. This can generate severe hypernatremia. In such instances, both solute and water are depleted, but water loss exceeds solute loss. Initial therapy with isotonic sa-

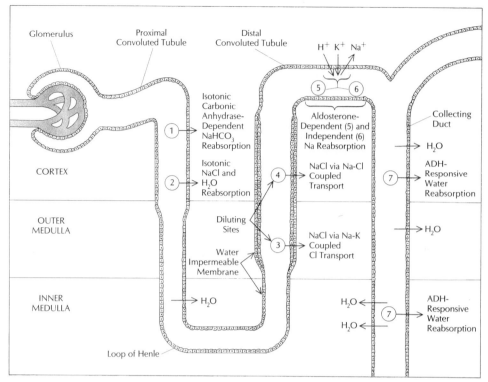

Figure 3.2. Functional processes for regulation of salt and water transport are illustrated schematically. Fluid formed by glomerular filtration of plasma is modified by transtubular reabsorption of sodium in the proximal tubule. Solute reabsorption in the proximal tubule is isotonic, being accompanied by reabsorption of water. In the first portion, the principal anion accompanying sodium reabsorption is bicarbonate (1); farther along, sodium is reabsorbed mainly with chloride (2). Differing permeability properties in Henle's loop provide for water reabsorption in the descending thin limb and some sodium chloride reabsorption in the ascending thin portion. The thick ascending limb, impermeable to water, is a major site for reabsorption of sodium chloride (3, 4). Two mechanisms are operative in the ascending limb: The first is a sodium-potassium transport coupled to chloride transport; the second is a coupled sodium-chloride transport in the cortical diluting segment. Sodium reabsorption in the distal tubule is related to potassium and hydrogen ion secretion (5, 6). Last, in the presence of antidiuretic hormone, the cortical and medullary collecting ducts become permeable to water; this produces further water reabsorption and concentrates the urine (7). From Thier SO. Diuretic mechanism as a guide to therapy. Hospital Practice 1987; 7:69.

line usually is indicated to restore normal intravascular volume before addressing the free water deficit.

Similarly, when diarrhea is induced by osmotic cathartics such as lactulose, sorbitol, or by carbohydrate malabsorption, large quantities of hypotonic fluid will be lost in the stool and can cause severe hypernatremia. However, this occurs only when patients have no access to water or lack appropriate thirst mechanisms.

An often overlooked and relatively common cause of an elevated serum sodium is osmotic diuresis, such as that produced by prolonged glycosuria. The glucose acts as an osmotic agent and generates large losses of electrolyte-free water into the urine. Osmotic diuresis can also occur in catabolic postoperative patients who develop severe prerenal azotemia. Later, as renal function improves and urea is excreted, it generates an osmotic diuresis leading to hypernatremia.

Whenever hypernatremia develops, a relative free water deficit exists and must be replaced. The water deficit can be approximated using the formula:

$$\text{water deficit} = \text{total body water} \times (1 - 140 \div \text{serum sodium})$$

Usually, the rate of correction of hypernatremia should not exceed about 12 mEq/L/day (12). The aim should be to correct about half the deficit over the first 24 hours. Too rapid a correction of hypernatremia may lead to cerebral edema and seizures.

Hypokalemia

Hypokalemia is an important and common electrolyte abnormality in the surgical patient. It is defined as a plasma potassium concentration below 3.5 mEq/L. Most of the body's potassium stores are intracellular, and the degree of hypokalemia correlates poorly with total body potassium deficit.

Hypokalemia can have profound physiologic consequences. Of greatest clinical concern are cardiac arrhythmias and exacerbation of digitalis toxicity. Muscle weakness, cramps, myalgias, paralysis, and when severe, rhabdomyolysis can result. Hypokalemia also enhances renal acid excretion, which can generate and maintain metabolic alkalosis.

Potassium may be lost via the gastrointestinal tract, primarily in patients with diarrhea, and via the kidneys.

Table 3.2.
Electrolyte Content of Sweat and Gastrointestinal Secretions

Sweat or Gastrointestinal Secretion	Electrolyte Concentration (mEq/liter)					Replacement Amount for Each Liter Lost			
	Na+	K+	H+	Cl⁻	HCO₃⁻	Isotonic Saline (ml)	5% D/W (ml)	KCl (mEq)	NaHCO₃ (mEq)
Sweat	30–50	5		45–55		300	700	5	
Gastric secretions	40–65	10	90	100–140		300	700	20	
Pancreatic fistula	135–155	5		55–75	70–90	250	750	5	90
Biliary fistula	135–155	5		80–110	35–50	750	250	5	45
Ileostomy fluid	120–130	10		50–60	50–70	300	700	10	67.6
Diarrhea fluid	25–50	35–60		20–40	30–45		1000	35	45

The most important causes of renal potassium loss are diuretics. Metabolic alkalosis also contributes to renal potassium wasting. Whenever large quantities of NaHCO₃ transit the distal parts of the nephron, potassium secretion is stimulated. High levels of aldosterone, whether due to volume depletion or autonomous secretion, also stimulate potassium secretion. When hypokalemia develops in patients with vomiting or nasogastric suction, it is primarily caused by renal potassium losses, rather than the small amount of potassium lost in the vomitus. The high aldosterone levels and metabolic alkalosis associated with the gastric losses combine to stimulate renal potassium excretion. The electrolyte content of sweat and gastrointestinal secretions is shown in Table 3.2.

The treatment of hypokalemia should be guided by the severity of the disorder and by the presence of complications such as cardiac arrhythmias or musculoskeletal symptoms. If no medical indication exists to rapidly correct the potassium deficit, oral or slow intravenous replacement (i.e., 40 mEq/L over 8 to 12 hours) is adequate. When rapid replacement becomes necessary and the hypokalemia is severe, a central venous access should be used to correct the deficit. This avoids discomfort, venous irritation or sclerosis, and potential severe tissue damage if the fluid extravasates (10–20 mEq KCl can be dissolved in 50–100 cc of fluid). The rate of intravenous potassium repletion should not exceed 20 mEq/ hour.

Hyperkalemia

Hyperkalemia is defined as a plasma potassium concentration above 5.4 mEq/L, and it is considered severe if the concentration exceeds 7.0 mEq/L. Hyperkalemia developing in the perioperative patient may be the result of excessive intake, decreased excretion, redistribution of potassium from the intracellular to the extracellular fluid compartment, or any combination of these derangements. Excessive intake is usually the result of overzealous intravenous potassium administration. Sometimes, excessive oral intake occurs when potassium-containing salt substitutes are used. Decreased excretion is usually caused by acute, chronic, or acute superimposed on chronic renal failure. Addison's disease,

mineralocorticoid deficiency, potassium-sparing diuretics, angiotensin converting enzyme inhibitors, nonsteroidal anti-inflammatory drugs, and cyclosporine are other conditions and drugs that reduce renal potassium excretion.

Several circumstances may cause a shift of potassium out of cells into the extracellular fluid compartment. The cells may be damaged or destroyed, with hemolysis or rhabdomyolysis, for example. Alternatively, potassium can shift out of intact cells in exchange for hydrogen ions when metabolic acidosis develops. Hyperosmolality (i.e., hyperglycemia) will also produce a shift of potassium into the ECF. Certain drugs, such as beta adrenergic antagonists, digitalis, or succinylcholine, can also produce such potassium shifts. The most important clinical consequences of hyperkalemia are cardiac in nature. Typical electrocardiographic changes include peaked T waves, prolonged PR interval, widening of the QRS complex, and eventually loss of P waves. Wide complex ventricular tachycardia, ventricular fibrillation, and asystole may result. Severe hyperkalemia can also produce profound neuromuscular dysfunction, including flaccid paralysis and respiratory failure.

Severe hyperkalemia is a medical emergency because of potential life-threatening cardiac arrhythmias. Sodium bicarbonate can be given intravenously to promote cellular entry of potassium. This is especially important when metabolic acidosis exists. Potassium can also be shifted into cells by the administration of glucose and insulin. Inhaled beta adrenergic agents such as albuterol may also be useful in shifting potassium back into cells. When severe hyperkalemia results in dangerous cardiac arrhythmias, calcium salts (chloride or gluconate) may be injected intravenously. This will quickly suppress cardiac excitability by altering the cell membrane threshold potential. However, it is often necessary not only to shift potassium into cells, but to remove it from the body. If kidney function is adequate, this can be accomplished by inducing a brisk diuresis with diuretics. In addition, the cation exchange resin, sodium polystyrene, can be given by mouth or enema to bind potassium in the GI tract and remove it via the stool. When a large load of plasma potassium needs to be removed, hemodialysis may be necessary.

Hypomagnesemia

Hypomagnesemia is a less common and frequently overlooked electrolyte abnormality. It should be suspected in patients on an insufficient diet, especially alcoholics, or in patients chronically using diuretics. Both alcohol and most diuretics increase renal magnesium excretion. Hypomagnesemia is clinically important not just because it has direct effects, but also because it can produce hypocalcemia and contribute to the persistence of hypokalemia. Magnesium deficiency will cause renal potassium wasting. When hypokalemia and hypomagnesemia coexist, magnesium should be aggressively replaced to restore potassium balance. The same is true for hypocalcemia. The level of plasma magnesium is a poor indicator of the degree of total body magnesium stores. Magnesium should be replaced until the plasma level returns to the upper normal range. Magnesium can be replaced either intravenously or, in less acute circumstances, via oral supplements. Gastrointestinal absorption of this cation, which occurs with greatest facility in the duodenum, is variable. In addition, all magnesium salts have a laxative effect when taken by mouth.

Hypocalcemia

The majority of the body's calcium is contained within the bone matrix; only about 0.1% of body calcium is in the ECF. Normally, the serum calcium concentration is maintained at a level between 9.0 and 10.4 mg/dL or 2.25 and 2.6 mmol/L. Calcium in the serum is found in three forms: about 40% is protein-bound, 10% is complexed to phosphate and other anions, and 50% exists in the ionized form. Normally, the concentration of ionized calcium is remarkably constant despite marked variations in the level of total calcium concentration. A fall in serum albumin of 1 gm/dL usually is associated with a 0.8 mg/dL fall in total calcium concentration, yet the ionized calcium may remain normal. Alterations in systemic pH will affect albumin binding of calcium. Metabolic acidosis decreases protein binding and increases the ionized calcium concentration, whereas metabolic alkalosis has the opposite effect. Direct measurement of the ionized calcium can be done with special electrodes and is often helpful.

Hypocalcemia is defined as a reduction in the ionized component of serum calcium. Patients with hypoalbuminemia and a low total serum calcium concentration may or may not have a reduction in ionized calcium. Consequently, the clinical presentation of the patient with hypocalcemia is crucial when deciding whether therapy is indicated.

The principal clinical manifestations of hypocalcemia are neurologic and include, in order of increasing severity: perioral paresthesias, carpal pedal spasm, tetany, and generalized seizures. Chvostek's sign (twitching of the corner of the mouth produced by tapping over the facial nerve) and Trousseau's sign (spasm of the fingers produced by inflating a blood pressure cuff above systolic) are also manifestations of neuromuscular irritability. Electrocardiographic changes include prolonged corrected QT and ST intervals and peaked T waves. Rarely, heart block may develop.

Perioperative hypocalcemia may be the result of hypomagnesemia, acute renal failure, septic shock, rhabdomyolysis, or acute pancreatitis. Hypocalcemia associated with acute renal failure usually is not severe and rarely requires specific therapy. When rhabdomyolysis occurs, it produces extensive skeletal muscle necrosis and results in calcium deposition in the injured tissue and subsequent hypocalcemia. Similarly, when acute pancreatitis results in the local release of pancreatic enzymes, retroperitoneal and omental fat digestion releases fatty acids which bind calcium. Though severe hypocalcemia may develop, only clinically symptomatic hypocalcemia should be treated with calcium supplementation. Aggressive calcium infusion will often cause a period of hypercalcemia in patients who recover from the acute insult and in whom deposited calcium is released.

Metabolic Alkalosis

Metabolic alkalosis in the postoperative patient is associated with increased morbidity and mortality (13). The pathogenesis of this acid-base disorder may be divided into two distinct phases: the generation of excessive bicarbonate, and the maintenance of the metabolic alkalosis (14). The generation of excess bicarbonate results either from renal or extrarenal acid loss or the addition of base to the extracellular fluid. In the perioperative patient, metabolic alkalosis is most often due to vomiting or gastric drainage. When hydrochloric acid is secreted by the gastric mucosa, an equal amount of bicarbonate is added to the extracellular fluid compartment. Normally, the HCl is neutralized by bicarbonate in the duodenum and small bowel, resulting in no net acid-base imbalance. However, if the HCl is removed via vomiting or nasogastric suction, then net bicarbonate addition to the ECF results. Diuretics also contribute to the metabolic alkalosis in many patients. Bicarbonate may be infused via intravenous solutions, TPN, or blood products that contain sodium citrate, a bicarbonate precursor.

The kidneys have an enormous capacity to rapidly excrete large quantities of bicarbonate. Consequently, for metabolic alkalosis to persist, impaired renal corrective mechanisms, or strong signals to the kidney to retain bicarbonate, must exist. If renal function is impaired markedly, the kidney cannot excrete the generated bicarbonate load. This represents the most common situation. If renal function is preserved, then three major stimuli act to enhance bicarbonate reabsorption: 1) effective arterial volume depletion; 2) mineralocorticoid excess; and 3) hypokalemia. Decreased effective arterial volume increases proximal tubular bicarbonate reabsorption. Hypokalemia also increases proximal reabsorption of bicarbonate and stimulates distal acid excretion. Mineralocorticoid increases distal acid excretion and contributes to the development of hypokalemia.

The therapy of metabolic alkalosis is focused on reversal of those factors generating bicarbonate (i.e., stopping diuretics, decreasing gastric acid secretions), and also reversing those factors which act to maintain the alkalosis. To the extent possible, renal function should be normalized, normal effective intra-arterial volume should be restored, and hypokalemia should be corrected. Thus, if renal function is reasonable, the simple infusion of isotonic saline will quickly produce bicarbonaturia and correct the metabolic alkalosis.

Metabolic Acidosis

Metabolic acidosis is characterized by a fall in the serum bicarbonate concentration, which results in a fall in pH (or a rise in the hydrogen ion concentration). This acid-base disorder can develop in several ways: 1) bicarbonate may be lost from the body via the gastrointestinal tract or the kidney; 2) the kidney may fail to regenerate bicarbonate due to inadequate acid excretion; or 3) bicarbonate may be consumed in the titration of excessive endogenously produced acid (e.g., lactic acidosis/ketoacidosis), or by the ingestion of exogenous acid producing compounds, such as methanol or ethylene glycol.

The kidney plays a pivotal role in maintaining acid-base balance in the human body. The metabolism of an average western protein-containing diet will generate approximately 1 mEq/kg body weight of acid. This daily acid is titrated in the ECF, primarily by the bicarbonate anion. The kidney's role is twofold: 1) it must reclaim all of the bicarbonate which is filtered; and 2) it must excrete the acid anion produced and regenerate the bicarbonate that was consumed by the titration outlined above.

Bicarbonate is regenerated by tubular pumping of hydrogen ions, which are buffered as titratable acid (mainly phosphate), and by ammonia. When the kidney is unable to excrete an adequate quantity of acid (such as NH_4), a variety of distal renal tubular acidoses may result. When the kidney's ability to reabsorb all of the filtered bicarbonate is impaired, then bicarbonate wastage results in proximal renal tubular acidosis.

Patients with chronic renal insufficiency (a decreased GFR) also have reduced acid excretory capacity. Chronic metabolic acidosis must be recognized in such patients preoperatively because worsening renal function and more severe metabolic acidosis may ensue in the postoperative period. The development of postoperative severe metabolic acidosis can adversely affect cardiac function, vascular resistance and the response to catecholamines. Metabolic acidosis must be addressed appropriately and treated according to the clinical circumstances.

Acknowledgement

The authors wish to express their appreciation to Ann Drew for her assistance in preparation of this manuscript.

REFERENCES

1. Weissman C. Ensuring perioperative fluid homeostasis in critically ill patients. Journal of Critical Illness 1994;9:1077–1093.
2. Schrier RW. The edematous patient: cardiac failure, cirrhosis and nephrotic syndrome. In: Schrier RW, ed. Manual of nephrology. 4th ed. Boston: Little, Brown and Company, 1995;1–19.
3. Lund T, Wiig H, Reed RK. Acute postburn edema: Role of strongly negative interstitial fluid pressure. Am J Physiol 1988;255: H1069–H1074.
4. Schrier RW. A unifying hypothesis of body fluid volume regulation. J R Coll Physicians Lond 1992;26:297.
5. Bock JC, Barker BC, Clinton AG, et al. Post-traumatic changes in, and effect of colloid osmotic pressure on the distribution of body water. Ann Surg 1989;210:395–405.
6. Raffin TA. ARDS: Mechanisms and management. Hosp Pract (Off Ed) 1987;15:65-80.
7. Chung, HM, Kluge R, Schrier RW, et al. Postoperative hyponatremia: A prospective stud. Arch Intern Med 1986;146:333–336.
8. Carlos AJ, Arieff AI. Symptomatic hyponatremia: Making the diagnosis rapidly. Journal of Critical Illness 1990;5:846–856.
9. Arieff AI. Hyponatremia, convulsions, respiratory arrest, and permanent brain damage after elective surgery in healthy women. N Engl J Med 1986; 314:1529–1535.
10. Fraser CL, Arieff AI. Fatal central diabetes mellitus and insipidus resulting from untreated hyponatremia: A new syndrome. Ann Intern Med 1990; 112:113–119.
11. Agarwal R, Emmett M. The post-transurethral resection of prostate syndrome: therapeutic proposals. Am J Kidney Dis 1994;24: 108–111.
12. Sterus R. Hypernatremia. In: Greenberg A, ed. Primer on kidney diseases. New York; Academic Press, 1994:370–371.
13. Jones ER. Metabolic alkalosis. In: Greenberg A, ed. Primer on kidney diseases. New York; Academic Press, 1994:382–387.
14. Emmett M, Seldin DW. Metabolic acidosis and metabolic alkalosis. In: Seldin DW, Giebish G, ed. The Kidney: Physiology and Pathophysiology. New York: Raven Press, 1985:1567–1639.

4 Shock and Hypoperfusion States

Daniel J. Jurusz / Jared Y. Gilmore

Introduction and History

Since the 16th century, the condition of shock has mystified and stimulated physicians. Even today, the condition occupies a seminal position in the research efforts of many scientists. Although much has been learned, a great deal remains to be understood.

One of the first classic descriptions of the symptomatology occurring after traumatic shock was written by Ambroise Paré in 1575 (1). While Paré described the symptoms of shock, the first use of the word was credited to the French surgeon, H. LeDran in 1743 (2). Soon thereafter, the term shock began to evolve and its definition became more varied. Frequent monographs on shock were published by such writers as T. Woolcomb (1770), John Hunter (1776), and J. P. Latta (1795) (3)(4)(5). In 1815, G. J. Guthrie cautioned surgeons to delay operations "until the alarm and shock have subsided." (6) It was discovered that situations other than trauma could be associated with shock. L. O'Shaughnessey, in 1831, described the presence of circulatory collapse in patients suffering from cholera (7). In 1876, A. Blum described shock as it was associated with burns and strangulated hernias (8).

As the 19th century came to a close, most interested investigators continued to focus on circulatory failure as the most important feature of shock. Crile, in numerous monographs published at the turn of the century, continued this trend. Moreover, he was one of the first researchers who could consistently reproduce the shock state in various experimental models (9)(10). His investigative work established his reputation as one of the leading investigators in the understanding of the shock state.

The horrors of World War I allowed for numerous studies and experiments to be carried out on victims of traumatic shock. Joint projects were conducted between American, British, and French teams. It was during this time period that Macleod (1921) postulated that following a reduction in oxygen to the tissues, a liberation of metabolic acids occurred (11). This led him to discover the presence of lactic acid in the advanced hypovolemic state.

Before the beginning of World War II, the definitions of shock were becoming more precise and formed the basis of its current definition. Freeman, in 1940, defined shock as, "The clinical condition characterized by progressive loss of the circulating blood volume, brought about by the tissue anoxia which results from inadequate circulation." (12) However, in 1941, Harkins demonstrated his depth of perception when he wrote: "The question of shock is not yet settled and while transfusion therapy is helpful, it is not the entire solution of the problem." (13) This statement is as true now as it was then.

In the aftermath of World War II, further hemodynamic data of shock was collected by Cournand through the application of cardiac catheterization. Since most of the human data were the result of battle injuries, almost all the observations were on patients who were hypovolemic secondary to blood loss. Research continued aggressively as the United States entered the Korean War. During this time, most emphasis was placed on the renal failure resulting from severe shock. Following this period, the era of the Vietnam War saw the research emphasis change towards adequate crystalloid resuscitation and the development of pulmonary failure.

With the development of the Swan-Ganz catheter in 1970, further knowledge was gained. The relationships of preload, afterload, and myocardial contractility to the shock state were investigated. Emphasis also shifted to the septic state, resultant shock, and the respiratory distress syndrome. More recently, researchers are now enthralled with the pathophysiology of multisystem organ failure (MSOF).

Definition

Evolving knowledge has shaped the modern definition of shock. Early definitions were based on a clinical description of injured soldiers in whom hypovolemia was associated with collapse of the cardiovascular system. Weakness, apathy, pallor, and poor circulatory function were considered the hallmarks. More recent definitions have focused on etiologic factors which cause dysfunction and ultimately result in tissue hypoperfusion. In essence, shock is a disturbance of circulatory and metabolic homeostasis. From a physiologic perspective, it is a failure to maintain the pressure/flow relationships necessary for adequate tissue perfusion. Semantic variations aside, all modern definitions of shock have, at their core, the concept of inadequate delivery or decreased utilization of fuels at the cellular level.

Basic Mechanisms

The cellular and molecular events that result from tissue hypoperfusion have similarity regardless of the etiology of shock. Decreased oxygen delivery to peripheral tissues occurs at reduced levels of perfusion. The result is a mandatory conversion from aerobic to anaerobic metabolism. Energy made available from glucose oxidation is decreased considerably in the anaerobic state. Instead of producing carbon dioxide, the normal end product of aerobic metabolism, cells produce lactic acid. Lactic acid, once produced, cannot be removed from the local milieu as could carbon dioxide. As lactic acid accumulates, metabolic acidosis ensues. Although many acid-base derangements can occur with different types of shock, the cellular events are primarily acid producing. In many shock states, the acidosis at the cellular level is more profound than that measured in the blood. As end organs become impaired, their loss of function exacerbates the shock state. The heart, for example, is less able to pump blood to deprived tissues when its metabolic needs are not being met. Thus shock is a self perpetuating disorder, particularly when therapy is either inadequate or delayed. Eventually, the cellular machinery becomes unhinged to an irreversible point. Adenosine triphosphate (ATP), the energy molecule of the cell, becomes so depleted that the transmembrane potential is lost. Sodium leaks into the cell while potassium leaks out. Energy is no longer available for cell respiration, protein synthesis, and the enzymes necessary to maintain cell life. When this occurs, cellular death ensues.

Hemodynamics

The pathogenesis of shock can be appreciated by applying the principles of hemodynamic physiology. The relationship of pressure, flow, and resistance is described by Ohm's law:

$$\text{Pressure} = \text{Flow} \times \text{Resistance}$$

When translated into clinically useful terminology, the following relationship can be constructed:

$$\text{MAP} = \text{CO} \times \text{SVR}$$

where MAP is mean arterial pressure, CO is cardiac output, and SVR is systemic vascular resistance. Therefore, the perfusion necessary to provide adequate tissue oxygenation is determined by cardiac output (CO) and systemic vascular resistance (SVR). Cardiac output, the key variable, is determined by preload, afterload, heart rate, and contractility. These factors will be considered individually.

Preload, described by Starling in 1915, is the stretch on myocardial fibers (14). In clinical terms, it refers to the left ventricular end diastolic volume (LVEDV). The force of contraction of ventricular fibers increases as LVEDV increases. Many factors can affect LVEDV, but blood volume and distribution are the most critical. Beyond a certain level, further increases in LVEDV (preload) no longer increase cardiac output (CO). This was demonstrated by the Starling curve and occurs on the flat, upper part of the curve (Fig. 4.1). At this part of the curve, cardiac failure and pulmonary edema occur. The most common clinical tool for estimating LVEDV is a pulmonary artery catheter passed through the right heart as described by Swan (15). Pulmonary capillary wedge pressure (PCWP) estimates left atrial pressure (LAP), which in turn estimates left ventricular end diastolic pressure (LVEDP). This, in turn, (in most circumstances) parallels LVEDV and therefore correlates with preload. Many factors and disease processes impact these measurements and can confound attempts to measure preload (Fig. 4.2). Of special note are mitral valve disease and intrinsic pulmonary disease, both of which alter pressure relationships between the pulmonary capillaries and the left ventricle. Contractility of the heart

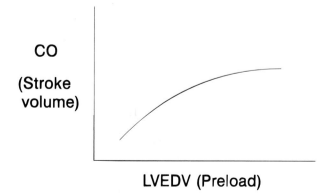

Figure 4.1. The Frank-Starling curve. This curve relates left ventricular end diastolic volume (LVEDV) to cardiac output (CO). Beyond a certain level, further increases in LVEDV (preload) no longer increases cardiac output. This occurs on the flat, upper part of the curve.

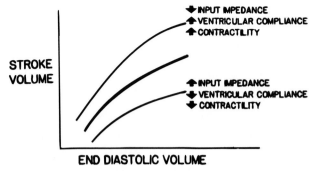

Figure 4.2. The Frank-Starling mechanism. As end-diastolic volume increases, stroke volume also increases (*middle line*). An increase in contractility, an increase in ventricular compliance, or a decrease in input impedance (vascular resistance), all cause an increase in stroke volume for a given end-diastolic volume (*top line*). Stroke volume decreases when the various cardiac factors are reversed (*bottom line*). Reprinted with permission from Sabiston DC, ed. Textbook of surgery. 13th ed. Philadelphia: WB Saunders Company, 1986: 41.

relates to the force of contraction of the myocardial musculature independent of preload or afterload. This so called inotropic state describes the heart's ability to squeeze at a constant preload (LVEDP) and afterload (SVR). The most important factor governing contractility is perfusion of the myocardium. Without adequate perfusion, the heart muscle cannot work optimally. Since coronary perfusion occurs during diastole, coronary perfusion pressure (CPP) dictates the amount of coronary perfusion. CPP is the pressure differential between the mean diastole pressure (DPmean) and LVEDP and can be described by the following equation:

$$CPP = DPmean - LVEDP$$

As will be discussed in more detail, the type of shock most often equated with contractility problems is cardiogenic shock. Also, any shock state that significantly decreases coronary perfusion has a tendency to adversely affect cardiac contractility and therefore cardiac function, further exacerbating the problem. In addition to its relationship to coronary perfusion, contractility is also governed by endogenous hormonal mediators (catecholamines) and external mediators (pharmacologic agents).

Afterload is the resistance against which the heart muscle contracts. It is physiologically equivalent to ventricular wall tension during systole. Clinically, the systemic vascular resistance (SVR) is the measurable entity that estimates afterload. It can be calculated from the MAP, CO, and central venous pressure (CVP) using the following equation:

$$SVR = \frac{MAP - CVP}{CO} \times 80$$

The normal value is 900–1,400 dynes/sec/cm^{-5}. Types of shock that typically have a direct affect on SVR are septic shock and neurogenic shock.

The last component of CO to be considered is heart rate (HR). In general, increases in HR will increase CO up to a rate of 150 beats/min. This value may be age and "general conditioning" dependent. Increases beyond this defined maximum usually impair diastolic filling and increase O_2 demand. Both of these factors negatively impact CO. Bradycardia can also have detrimental influences on CO for obvious reasons. Of all parameters affecting CO, HR is the easiest to measure with standard continuous electrocardiography (EKG).

Categorization

Shock is a clinical state with many etiologies and many manifestations. It is useful to group shock into four major categories that are related to etiology. The categories are: 1) hypovolemic, 2) cardiogenic, 3) septic, and 4) neurogenic.

This system was proposed by Blalock (1934) and has remained the basis for all modern classifications. Several subcategories and considerable overlap in clinical expression exist among the categories. This classification is nonetheless extremely useful because it forms a framework that allows organization of clinical patterns and guides therapeutic strategy and intervention. Each category will be discussed separately, although the considerable overlap between categories will be obvious.

Hypovolemic Shock

Hypovolemic shock is the most common cause of shock encountered by surgeons and is most often related to hemorrhage. Numerous causes of hypovolemic shock exist, but all of the causes lead to the determining principle of reducing both preload and the filling pressures of the heart. This, in turn, is associated with a reduction in cardiac output and, therefore, a decrease in peripheral perfusion. If allowed to continue without intervention, the decrease in peripheral perfusion pressure may lead to severe biochemical changes at the cellular level, which leads to cellular dysfunction and cell death.

The decrease in the preload may be effected by anything that depletes intravascular volume. The loss of volume may occur after blood loss (external or internal) or with the loss of plasma into burned or injured tissue. It may also be secondary to a decrease in intravascular volume associated with pancreatitis, peritonitis, or bowel obstruction. Long bouts of vomiting or diarrhea, or the presence of an enterocutaneous fistula may lead to water and electrolyte abnormalities and also cause hypovolemic shock.

Clinical Manifestations of Hypovolemic Shock

The clinical manifestations of hypovolemic shock depend on several factors. First, the degree of hypovolemia or the amount of intravascular volume loss is the principle factor in determining hemodynamic instability. Whether a patient has lost 15% or 40% of his or her intravascular volume will determine the symptoms expressed. The second factor involved is the rate at which the blood volume is lost. A slower rate of volume depletion is better tolerated since compensatory mechanisms have more time to adjust. Finally, the third factor involved is the ability of an individual's body to compensate. Older, frailer patients will not have the same degree of compensatory mechanisms as younger, more vigorous individuals.

Some of the more common signs associated with hypovolemic shock are hypotension, cold clammy skin, tachycardia, oliguria, and mental status changes. EKG changes consistent with myocardial ischemia occur at an advanced stage. The various organ systems are affected sequentially with the integument being impacted first, followed by various other systems with the heart and brain being affected last.

In acute blood loss (hemorrhagic shock), use of the hematocrit level as a reliable indicator of the amount of blood loss is inappropriate and unreliable. Large amounts of blood loss may produce only a minimal decrease of the hematocrit in the acute setting. Therefore, the physician must be aware that a normal hematocrit does not rule out substantial blood loss.

Classification of Hypovolemic Shock

Based on the signs, symptoms, involved organ systems, and the volume of acute blood loss, hypovolemic shock may be classified as either mild, moderate, or severe (Table 4.1). However, the distinction between classes does not necessarily clearly exist in the clinical situation. These classifications are used to emphasize the evolutionary processes and the pathophysiology of the hypovolemic shock state (16).

Mild hypovolemia is defined as an intracellular volume loss of less than 20% of the circulating blood volume. This reduction in volume will cause a decrease in perfusion to those organs designed to tolerate some ischemia without profound consequences. These organs include the integument, skeletal muscle, and bone. The

clinical symptoms found in this degree of shock are minimal. Adrenergic discharge to the skin is the most subtle sign. The constriction of blood vessels in the skin causes collapse of the veins and a decrease in capillary filling pressure which is associated with pale, cool extremities. The lower extremities are especially prone to these early signs of shock. No measurable changes occur in blood pressure, pulse pressure, or respiratory rate. Urinary output would be expected to show only minimal change. The patient with mild hypovolemia may feel cold and may also report feeling thirsty.

A 20–40% loss of blood volume constitutes moderate shock. In this subgroup, the poor perfusion is extended to those visceral organs (kidneys) that have a low tolerance to ischemia. The adrenergic discharge intensifies and continues to affect the integument and the musculoskeletal system. The kidneys experience vasoconstriction, retain sodium, and urine output falls. Blood pressure may remain normal but only a slight increase in the patient's heart rate may result. The patient may appear anxious and combative. The respiratory rate increases and the resulting tachypnea causes a compensatory respiratory alkalosis.

Severe hypovolemia is categorized by a deficit of greater than 40% of the patient's total blood volume. This degree of volume loss places a patient in eminent danger as decreased perfusion to the heart and brain occurs. The "classic" signs of severe hypovolemia include: cold, clammy skin, oliguria, tachycardia, hypotension, and a severely narrowed pulse pressure. Respirations may become deep, rapid and agonal. The patient shows a markedly depressed mental status. At this stage in the progression of shock, every cell in the body is rendered ischemic. If immediate resuscitative measures are not undertaken, the patient's heart and brain may suffer severe injury leading to loss of consciousness, severe hypotension, myocardial cell loss, and eventually, the death of the patient.

Physiologic Mechanisms

In dealing with the physiology of hypovolemic shock, it is important to realize that the primary initiating mechanism involved is a reduction in intravascular vol-

Table 4.1.
Classification of Hypovolemic Shock

	Blood Volume Loss (%)	Blood Loss (ml)	Blood Pressure	Heart Rate	Respiratory Rate	Skin	Urine Output	Mental Status Changes
Mild	<20	<1000	Normal	Normal	Normal	Pale, cool	Normal to Slightly Decreased	Minimal
Moderate	20–40	1000–2000	Normal	Slightly Increased	Increased	Pale, cool	Decreased	Anxious
Severe	>40	>2000	Decreased	Increased	Increased	Cold, clammy	Decreased	Confused, Lethargic

ume. This lack of volume primarily affects the cardio-vascular system. In decreasing the intravascular volume, the preload will be decreased substantially. This decrease negatively influences the cardiac output. Other factors that influence cardiac output (myocardial contractility, afterload, and heart rate) will be affected by the loss of volume and also by the resulting compensatory mechanisms.

A reduction in intravascular volume causes a reduction in mean arterial pressure and diminishes the stimulation of baroreceptors. These baroreceptors are located in the aortic arch, atria, and carotid bodies. Lowering the stimulation of the receptors inhibits parasympathetic activity and activates sympathetic outflow. Norepinephrine is released from the sympathetic nerve endings, and both norepinephrine and epinephrine are released from the adrenal medulla. Through this reflex, heart rate and myocardial contractility are augmented, and the vascular smooth muscle of the arterioles and venules are constricted. Constriction of these vessels allows for an increase in total peripheral vascular resistance which helps offset the decrease in both preload and myocardial contractility. All of these mechanisms are the body's attempt to maintain an adequate perfusion pressure at the cellular level.

Along with the baroreceptors, chemoreceptors are also stimulated. A decrease in oxygen content and an increase in carbon dioxide production (acidosis) are the primary stimulants for these receptors. The resulting activation accounts for the respiratory changes and also adds a further generalized vasoconstricting effect.

The vasoconstriction causes selective reductions in blood flow to the skin, muscle beds, and splanchnic circulation. However, highly oxygen-dependent tissues such as the brain, heart, and kidneys are spared from this vasoconstricting effect. Maintenance of blood flow and oxygen delivery to these organs preserves function. Thus, in the early phases of hypovolemic shock, there is minimal or no impairment of blood pressure, urine output, or consciousness.

In summary, adrenergic discharge is the main compensatory mechanism involved in early hypovolemic shock. The selective vasoconstriction restores blood pressure and cardiac output, increases myocardial contractility and heart rate, increases venous return, and finally diverts blood away from less essential organs towards the more essential organ systems of the body. The adrenergic response can counterbalance, to a considerable degree, acute volume loss (up to 30%) and maintain the integrity of the vital organs while volume resuscitation is occurring.

As the shock state progresses, there is a shift of fluid from the extracellular compartment into the intravascular space. This fluid shift helps to restore blood volume. The hematocrit level will fall as this fluid shift takes place. The mechanism for this shift is based on a reduction of hydrostatic pressure in the capillary beds (Fig.

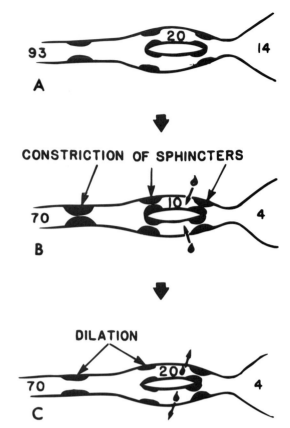

Figure 4.3. Mechanism of fluid shifts in hypovolemic shock. **A,** In a normal arteriole, the mean arterial, capillary, and venular pressures are 93, 20, and 14 mm. Hg, respectively. **B,** In hypovolemic shock, a reduction of hydrostatic pressure occurs in the capillary beds. This pressure decrease is a consequence of the arteriolar vasoconstriction of the pre-capillary sphincters that is greater than the vasoconstriction of the post-capillary sphincters in the venule. This mechanism allows redistribution of water and electrolytes into the vascular space. **C,** In late shock, the arterioles and precapillary sphincters lose their constriction, while the postcapillary sphincters maintain their constriction. Capillary hydrostatic pressure increases, and water and electrolytes extravasate out of the vascular space and back into the interstitial space. Reprinted with permission from Sabiston DC. Textbook of surgery. 13th ed. Philadelphia: WB Saunders Company, 1986:42.

4.3). This pressure decrease is a consequence of the arteriolar vasoconstriction of the precapillary sphincters, which is greater than the vasoconstriction of the post-capillary sphincters in the venule. Thus the fall in the capillary hydrostatic pressure results from a combination of the precapillary vasoconstriction plus the already present systemic arterial hypotension and a decreased resistance to outflow on the venule end. The low hydrostatic pressure that results allows redistribution of water and electrolytes into the vascular space with the expectation of replacing the intravascular volume and therefore improving cardiac output.

These compensatory mechanisms are eventually slowed when the interstitial oncotic pressure becomes greater than the plasma oncotic pressure. A reversal occurs in moderate to severe shock because the capillary permeability becomes altered and proteins extravasate out of the plasma and into the interstitial space. As the amount of protein increases in the interstitial space, more water and osmotically active particles are drawn away from the vascular space into the interstitium. Also, as the shock state progresses, the precapillary sphincters no longer constrict, leading to an increase in capillary hydrostatic pressure. This too results in a shifting of water and electrolytes away from the vascular space back into the interstitium. When this process becomes fully established, shock may become irreversible.

At the same time, other compensatory mechanisms also become active. As previously mentioned, the kidneys are also affected by the adrenergic response, and blood flow is diverted away from the cortex of the kidneys and towards the heart and brain. The sympathetic discharge lowers kidney perfusion as a result of renal artery constriction. This action reduces the glomerular filtration rate (GFR) and is manifested by a decreased urine output. Oliguria in turn stimulates the posterior pituitary gland to release vasopressin (ADH) which acts to potentiate the reabsorption of water from the kidney tubules. Vasopressin also has a powerful vasoconstricting action.

Additionally, renin is released by the kidney in response to the decrease in renal artery perfusion (Fig. 4.4). Renin acts as a catalyst for the formation of Angiotensin II from Angiotensin I. This hormone has a dual

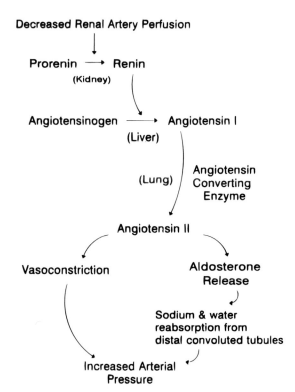

Figure 4.4. Renin-angiotensin system. Renin is released by the kidney in response to a decrease in renal artery perfusion. It acts as a catalyst for the formation of Angiotensin II from angiotensinogen. This system results in an increase in arterial pressure by causing vasoconstriction and reabsorption of sodium and water from the distal convoluted tubules of the kidney via aldosterone.

role in the compensatory process. First, it is another powerful systemic vasoconstrictor, and secondly, it stimulates the release of aldosterone. Aldosterone is a potent stimulant for sodium reabsorption in the distal convoluted tubules of the kidney. As sodium is reabsorbed, it is accompanied by free water retention, therefore helping to replenish vascular volume.

The complex compensatory mechanisms continue to respond as the shock state progresses. The massive adrenergic discharge remains in effect as the patient's symptomatology becomes more prevalent. The patient becomes more tachycardic, more tachypneic, and more oliguric. The extremities become cooler, and mental status changes ensue as cerebral circulation diminishes. Eventually, the patient's compensatory mechanisms become overwhelmed. The severe vasoconstriction leads to even further reduction in tissue perfusion, and cell injury occurs. Blood flow to the heart and brain continues to substantially decrease. The continuing adrenergic response increases afterload of the right ventricle via an increase in pulmonary vascular resistance. The afterload of the left ventricle also increases through a rise in systemic vascular resistance. Increasing the resistance to outflow for both ventricles eventually results in lowered cardiac output. A decrease in coronary perfusion pressures occurs, resulting in myocardial ischemia. A similar fall in perfusion pressure to the cerebrum eventually occurs. Clinical manifestations of cerebral ischemia results in a wide range of mental status changes and, if severe enough, leads to complete loss of consciousness.

The shunting of blood away from muscle and the splanchnic organs leads to irreversible ischemia. The patient's metabolism shifts from aerobic to anaerobic as tissues continue to be underperfused with oxygen. Serum lactic acid levels rise as anaerobic metabolism continues, leading to a fall in the blood pH and in the generation of a metabolic acidosis. Acidosis promotes arteriolar vasodilation, which is a more potent stimulus than the sympathetic discharge. The acidosis is also responsible for a negative cardiac inotropic effect.

As cell death continues, a myriad of vasoactive substances, potassium ions, oxygen-free radicals, and lysosomal enzymes are released through the disrupted cell membrane, into the interstitial space, then into the circulation. All of these substances have a profound adverse effect on the remaining viable organs. This eventually leads to multisystem organ failure (MSOF) with concomitant pulmonary, hepatic and renal failure (17). Failure of these organs results in an extremely high mortality rate.

Treatment

Progressive hypovolemic shock eventually results in death. Thus, the ultimate goal in treating the shock state is to identify the condition and the etiology and adequately treat the patient before permanent damage to cells and organs has occurred. Obviously, preexisting medical conditions, such as coronary artery disease, chronic pulmonary disease, kidney disease or liver disease, make the treatment of shock even more challenging.

The main goal of therapy is to restore adequate oxygen delivery to all the tissues of the body. The early effort should be directed toward replacing the blood volume as rapidly as possible. The amount of fluid to be replaced and the rate of infusion should be guided by the patient's history (if obtainable), a physical examination, hemodynamic parameters, and the response to infusion of intravascular fluids. A crystalloid solution should be used for initial resuscitation. If the etiology of the shock is thought to be hemorrhage, then blood and blood products may be needed in combination with the crystalloid solutions (18). Venous access should be obtained at a peripheral site. At least two large-bore catheters should be used in patients with severe hypovolemia. A central venous catheter should not be used early in the resuscitative phase. Fluid can more effectively be infused through a shorter, large caliber peripheral line rather than a longer central line with a smaller diameter. Also, the central veins may be difficult to access secondary to the hypovolemic state. When the patient is in a more stable condition, a central venous catheter can be placed more safely for central venous pressure (CVP) monitoring and for infusion purposes.

The successful response to volume replacement can be monitored by the improvement in a number of parameters. A rise in blood pressure and a falling pulse are good indicators of repletion of the intravascular volume. As the vascular volume is restored, cardiac output increases and systemic vasoconstriction falls. This leads to improvement in mental status and to increased hourly urine output. With adequate fluid resuscitation, metabolic acidosis should improve. The persistence of acidosis should be treated with larger volumes of fluid infusion.

Electrolyte imbalance may occur during resuscitation. A change in the choice of fluid infusion may be needed to correct imbalances. Because of the role of the kidneys during shock, great attention should be given to shifts in serum levels of sodium, potassium, and calcium. Uncorrected electrolyte imbalances can precipitate organ systems failure, especially the heart.

Early attention should also be directed toward the pulmonary and renal systems. Ischemia to these organ systems leads to immediate dysfunction and adds to the instability of the patient. Impairment of gas exchange secondary to leaking pulmonary capillaries and pulmonary edema causes a decrease in pulmonary compliance and a decrease in the functional residual capacity. These physiologic changes lead to the development of acute respiratory distress syndrome (ARDS). Azotemia may result from progressive oliguria, and acute tubular necrosis (ATN) may result from the prolonged hypoperfu-

sion. The patient may then develop chronic renal insufficiency. Methods should be instituted promptly that promote adequate oxygenation and maximize continued kidney perfusion. The treating physician should also be aware that some patients can develop high output renal failure. Early recognition and treatment of both pulmonary and renal dysfunction may help prevent deleterious systemic effects and chronic organ failure.

Cardiovascular Monitoring

A central venous catheter is a good tool in helping to assess the circulatory status of the resuscitated patient. The CVP can be used to determine right ventricular preload and therefore, indirectly, the adequacy of intravascular volume. Observing the CVP in response to a fluid challenge is of substantial benefit if the catheter is positioned correctly. If a fluid bolus is given and the CVP does not change, this could indicate continued hypovolemia. However, if the fluid bolus results in a rise in the CVP, this suggests normovolemia or hypervolemia. This last scenario can be seen in pump failure. If the CVP continues to rise in response to fluid challenges, and the patient manifests continuing hypotension and persistent evidence of shock, pump failure should be suspected.

A Swan-Ganz catheter is the most accurate means of assessing central pressures for both the left and right sides of the heart. The catheter can be used to measure CVP, pulmonary capillary wedge pressure (PCWP), cardiac output, pulmonary artery pressures, systemic vascular resistance, pulmonary vascular resistance, and mixed venous oxygen saturation. Wedge pressure gives a reasonable estimate of left-sided heart pressures.

The "typical" patient with moderate to severe hypovolemic shock would demonstrate decreases in the CVP, PCWP, cardiac output, and mixed venous oxygen saturation. As expected, there would be increases in both the pulmonary vascular resistance (PVR) and the systemic vascular resistance (SVR).

Cardiovascular Drugs

The first line of treatment for hypovolemic shock is fluid resuscitation. However, in some situations, cardiotonic drugs may be necessary to improve cardiac output. During resuscitation, there may come a point when the heart is no longer able to meet the demands placed on it. This may be secondary to preexistent cardiac disease or from acute damage to the myocardium. At this point, pump failure occurs. This may be manifested as congestive heart failure, pulmonary edema, or both.

At this junction, a positive inotrope (i.e., dobutamine) may be necessary to maintain adequate perfusion pressures and cardiac output. However, cardiovascular drugs are not a substitute for volume replacement. Various drugs have been used at this juncture with each having its own particular indications. A more detailed discussion of the various cardiovascular drugs can be found elsewhere in this chapter.

Cardiogenic Shock

The syndrome of cardiogenic shock occurs as the result of a primary disturbance of the heart. In a mechanical sense, it can be thought of as pump failure. As a result of impairment of the pumping function of the heart, there is inadequate blood flow to meet the metabolic needs of the body's tissues. From a clinical standpoint, it is characterized by poor cardiac output with evidence of tissue hypoxia in the presence of adequate intravascular volume. When hemodynamic parameters are measured, a more precise definition would include: 1) low systolic blood pressure (<90 mmHg or 30 mmHg below basal levels for 30 minutes); 2) an elevated arteriovenous oxygen difference (> 5.5ml/dl); 3) depressed cardiac index (< 2.2 1/min/m^2); and 4) an elevated or at least adequate wedge pressure (>15 mmHg).

Prior to diagnosing cardiogenic shock, it is critical to correct or exclude non-myocardial factors contributing to hypoperfusion, most commonly hypovolemia. Cardiogenic shock has several etiologies and can be classified accordingly as shown in Table 4.2.

Clearly, this categorization creates arbitrary boundaries. For instance, caval obstruction may be thought of as a volume distribution problem. Arrhythmias may be a manifestation rather than a cause of shock. Despite this, distinguishing primary myocardial dysfunction from secondary dysfunction is still useful.

Myocardial Infarction

The form of cardiogenic shock most familiar to clinicians is secondary to acute myocardial infarction. Autopsy studies have revealed that a loss of 40% or more of the left ventricular myocardium generally is associated with cardiogenic shock (19). The cumulative nature of myocardial damage must be recognized in patients who have had previous myocardial damage. Such patients are less able to tolerate future cardiac insults and are more likely to exhibit pump failure. Equally as important as the volume of impaired myocardium is the location of ventricular damage. Injury to critical areas, such as valvular support structures (papillary muscles) or the septal wall, may predispose to hemodynamic decompensation with lesser amounts of damage.

The pathophysiology of myocardial infarction is a continuum from the onset of ischemia through the healing fibrotic phase. Evidence suggests that the underlying defect is a reduction in myocardial strength. A predictable decrease in stroke volume and minute output of the ventricle occur. This produces hypotension and hypoperfusion. Reflex responses via the baroreceptor mechanism and sympathetic output serve to increase peripheral vascular resistance. The extent and location of the cumulative myocardial damage will determine whether these compensatory mechanisms are able to achieve hemodynamic stability. In a favorable situation, the uninvolved myocardium is able to compensate, peripheral perfusion is maintained, and the patient usually has an uncomplicated convalescence. When compensatory mechanisms cannot offset the degree of myocardial damage, cardiac output continues to fall, and shock ultimately ensues. Adequate intravascular volume must be established to differentiate between these two scenarios. The unfortunate subset of patients who progress to cardiogenic shock after infarction have a poor prognosis. Depending on underlying factors and the level of intervention, mortality ranges from 30% to 90% (20, 21).

Experimental and clinical investigations have clearly indicated that after coronary occlusion with resultant infarction, an area of reversibly injured myocardium exists that surrounds the infarct zone. This area is referred to as "stunned" myocardium. The recovery of this area is related to the extent and duration of blood flow deprivation. Prompt reperfusion of the infarct related vessel can limit the size of the infarcted zone and accelerate the recovery of reversibly injured myocardium. The benefits of reperfusion of severely injured myocardium are limited to 1–2 hours after the infarct. Less severely injured myocardium may be benefited by reperfusion up to 3–6 hours. Reperfusion beyond 12 hours is unlikely to have substantial beneficial effects on injured myocardium, but it may prevent further progression in that region of the heart. These findings form the basis for the administration of thrombolytic agents after acute myocardial infarction.

The grim prognosis of cardiogenic shock after myocardial infarction raises serious questions about diagnostic and therapeutic intervention. Aggressive pharmacologic therapy and mechanical support devices have increased survival in a subset of patients with post infarct cardiogenic shock. Since we cannot differentiate this subset, almost all patients should be treated aggressively initially. The advent of cardiac transplant has further complicated this difficult issue.

Table 4.2.
Etiologies of Cardiogenic Shock

Primary Myocardial Dysfunction	Secondary Myocardial Dysfunction
Myocardial Infarction	Tension Pneumothorax
Cardiac Arrhythmias	Vena Caval Obstruction
Myocardial depression from other causes (cardiomyopathy, etc)	Cardiac Tamponade
	Pulmonary Embolus

Post Open Heart Surgery and Miscellaneous Causes

Another type of cardiogenic shock frequently seen by surgeons occurs after open heart operations. This is referred to as the "low output syndrome" and is manifested by ventricular dysfunction, low CO, and raised LVEDP following surgical procedures using cardiopulmonary bypass (CPB). Almost all of these intracardiac procedures are associated with some evidence of myocardial damage despite modern methods of myocardial preservation. Advances in postoperative care have allowed the manipulation of hemodynamic parameters, which have also reduced the mortality of left ventricular dysfunction. When these factors are considered, it follows that the patients most susceptible to postoperative cardiogenic shock are those that have extensive myocardial damage preoperatively. Patients in this category are those with long standing valvular defects, severe congestive failure, severe coronary artery disease with depressed ventricular function, and patients with complex congenital anomalies who evidence ventricular depression.

There are various miscellaneous causes of cardiogenic shock that are beyond the scope of this text. It is most important to distinguish between primary and secondary causes. If the cause is secondary (tension pneumothorax, cardiac tamponade, pulmonary embolism), then treatment of the underlying problem will correct the shock state. If the cause is primary, supportive treatment should be instituted in a sequential fashion.

Treatment

Once secondary causes of cardiogenic shock are excluded or treated, one should approach primary cardiogenic shock systematically. Although there are different approaches depending on the underlying cause (i.e. post infarct vs post intracardiac valve repair), certain tenets remain. The first concern should be the establishment of an optimal cardiac rate and rhythm and the maintenance of optimal ventricular filling pressures. Left-sided filling pressures should be maximized with the infusion of crystalloid, colloid, or blood until left atrial pressure is at least 15 mmHg. Adequate oxygenation and ventilation must be assured. If the cardiac index remains low (< 2.0 L/min/m^2) despite these measures, pharmacologic intervention is indicated. Augmentation of cardiac output with inotropic support or afterload reduction therapy will depend on the patient's SVR. If the SVR is low or normal, inotropic agents are initiated. The choice of inotropic drug will depend on hemodynamic parameters and the clinical situation. Dobutamine is often a first line choice because of its selectivity for cardiac receptors and its vasodilatory properties. Amrinone, a phosphodiesterase inhibitor, has inotropic and vasodilatory properties similar to dobutamine. If the situation warrants a drug that will increase peripheral resistance and provide inotropic support, several choices are available. Most often dopamine, epinephrine, or norepinephrine are used. Patients with a low cardiac output and elevated peripheral resistance are treated with an afterload reducing agent, usually nitroprusside or nitroglycerin. Often, combinations of all of these agents are used.

Failure to respond to pharmacologic support warrants consideration of mechanical support of the heart. Numerous devices are available, and the choice is tailored to the clinical situation. Initially, intraaortic balloon pump (IABP) counterpulsation usually is employed. The IABP, which is positioned in the descending aorta, inflates during diastole and deflates during systole. The physiologic effect is to increase coronary perfusion pressure during diastole and decrease afterload during systole. The net effect is an increase in myocardial oxygen supply and a decrease in demand, thus improving ischemia. IABP appears most useful if myocardial dysfunction is expected to be transient.

Numerous ventricular assist devices exist, both external and implantable. They can provide support for the left, right, or both ventricles, and the power source may be pneumatic or electrical. The far end of this spectrum is the total artificial heart, which requires removal of the native heart. These have been used clinically primarily as a bridge to transplant for patients who meet appropriate criteria. The National Heart, Blood, and Lung Institute is currently sponsoring the development of mechanical circulatory support devices for permanent use (22). The use of these various devices depends on the clinical situation but, in general, is restricted to patients with post infarct refractory shock, post cardiotomy shock, and as a bridge to transplant in select patients. At present, their use is intended to buy time until myocardial recovery occurs or until a new heart can be found. Eventually, these devices may be used as a permanent replacement for the heart. It should be noted that while most of the assist devices mentioned are designed for intermediate to prolonged support (weeks to months), short term support (hours to days) can be provided and is useful as a resuscitative measure. Either standard cardiopulmonary bypass or extracorporeal membrane oxygenation (ECMO) are used when only transient support is anticipated. For example, when a patient who has just undergone coronary bypass fails to wean from the pump. Often, a limited reinstitution of CPB while volume resuscitation and pharmacologic support are maximized is sufficient so that the patient can be weaned without further mechanical support.

A variety of other invasive and noninvasive options exist in the treatment of cardiogenic shock, including heparinization, thrombolytic therapy, percutaneous transluminal coronary angioplasty (PTCA), and emergent coronary bypass. A detailed discussion of these modalities is beyond the scope of this text.

Septic Shock

Because sepsis is an even more elusive and ambiguous term than shock, defining septic shock is a formidable challenge. Most connotations of the word sepsis equate it with severe infection. Historically, it was most commonly related to gram negative bacterial infection, although any infectious agent could be implicated. Today, many patients have all the findings of sepsis, but no clear identifiable infectious etiologic agent. In this context, it is appropriate to view sepsis as a systemic response of the body to overwhelming infection or other severe insult. Septic shock, by extension, would be defined as inadequate tissue perfusion as a result of this systemic response.

Although any infectious agent (including viruses and fungi) may cause septic shock, the most important etiologic agents are gram negative bacteria. The rising incidence of gram negative sepsis has been attributed to several factors, including: 1) the use of broad spectrum antibiotics that "select" out gram negative organisms; 2) the concentration in hospitals of large reservoirs of patients with established infections; and 3) a greater percentage of elderly and immunocompromised patients. Host defense mechanisms against microbial infection play a key role in the development of septic shock. Factors that depress the host defense system include malignancy, severe trauma, burns, immunologic diseases, and chronic inflammatory diseases.

During septicemia, the most common organism isolated in blood cultures is Escherichia coli, with species of Klebsiella, Proteus, Pseudomonas, and Bacteroides frequently found. Common gram positive offenders include species of streptococcus and staphylococcus. The portal of entry varies with the organism but the site is almost always the patient him or herself with the genitourinary, gastrointestinal, biliary tracts, and the tracheobronchial tree seen most common. Often these sites have been subjected to trauma or mechanical manipulation predisposing to infection. Frequently, the infection will be with multiple organisms, often crossing the boundary between gram negative and gram positive and often including both aerobic and anaerobic organisms.

Pathophysiology

The hypoperfusion state in gram negative septic shock is thought to result from the release of a bacterial wall component, also called endotoxin. This compound is a phospholipopolysaccharide protein complex which is present in the cell wall of all gram negative bacteria. The polysaccharide component of the endotoxin is the so-called "O antigen." This moiety probably provides a carrier function, whereas the true toxicity of endotoxin

derives from the lipid component. Even without bacteria, introduction of endotoxin into the bloodstream can result in "septic shock." The quantity of endotoxin and host defense factors largely determine the extent of the septic response.

A growing body of evidence suggests that the body's response to endotoxemia causes septic shock. That is, various inflammatory mediators become activated and result in the hemodynamic derangements that characterize septic shock. These mediators are the subject of intense investigation and will be discussed separately. For the purposes of this discussion, it is sufficient to understand that endotoxin activates several mediators of the inflammatory response which result in septic shock.

The hemodynamic abnormalities that ensue are varied and can follow several patterns. It is convenient to think of two different categories of hemodynamic patterns in septic shock (Table 4.3). The first pattern is referred to as hypodynamic septic shock, also called "uncompensated" septic shock. Circulatory blood volume is decreased, while the CVP and PCWP are usually low. Oxygen consumption is normal or slightly raised, and the arterial-venous oxygen differential or (a-v)d O_2 is widened. Peripherally, anaerobic metabolism results in lactic acidemia. The physiologic effect appears to be an altered venous capacitance with peripheral pooling of blood and depressed myocardial function.

The second pattern is found in patients presenting with a hyperdynamic presentation of septic shock known as the "compensated" form. Alterations in vascular tone with resultant decreased peripheral resistance are profound. Unlike the first form, cardiac output usually increases dramatically while CVP and PCWP are normal or elevated. This results in a markedly narrowed (a-v)d O_2. The primary physiologic event appears to be metabolic with a failure of oxygen utilization by the cells of vital organs. Considerable overlap exists between these two groups, and volume resuscitation probably plays a pivotal role. Unfortunately, almost all peripheral organs potentially can be affected directly in septic shock. It is theorized that the activated mediators have direct toxic effects on the heart, lungs, liver, brain, and kidneys. The result is progressive failure of these organ

Table 4.3.
Hemodynamic Patterns in Septic Shock

Hypodynamic Septic Shock	Hyperdynamic Septic Shock
Altered venous capacitance	Failure of oxygen utilization by cells of vital organs
Hypotension	Hypotension
Decreased peripheral resistance	Decreased peripheral resistance
Decreased cardiac output	Increased cardiac output
Decreased CVP	Normal or Elevated CVP
Decreased PCWP	Normal or Elevated PCWP
Widened (a-v)d O_2	Narrowed (a-v)d O_2

Table 4.4.
Prognosis in Multisystem Organ Failure

Number of Failing Systems	Mortality (%)
0	3
1	30
2	50–60
3	85–100
4	72–100
5	100

systems, called multisystem organ failure (MSOF). The extent and severity of dysfunction in these organs directly impacts on prognosis (Table 4.4). When three or more fail, the mortality is as high as 95%. Thus MSOF syndrome is a form of end-stage septic shock. The pathophysiologic events that have been described as a result of endotoxemia can be extrapolated to any agent or insult which activates the mediators of sepsis or the "septic shock syndrome."

Mediators

A great deal of emphasis has recently been focused on describing the endogenous mediators of the septic response. They fall into two main categories: 1) the mediators of the inflammatory response, and 2) neuroendocrine mediators. Mediators of the inflammatory response can have either local or systemic effects. Activation of the complement cascade is one of the initial events during injury or infection (Fig. 4.5). Specifically, the anaphylotoxins (C3a and C5a) are the components that have immediate hemodynamic effects. These effects include increased vascular permeability, vasodilatation, and chemotaxis.

The metabolites of arachidonic acid are also an important inflammatory mediator of the septic response. Arachidonic acid can be metabolized by either cyclooxygenase or lipoxygenase producing prostaglandins or leukotrienes respectively (Fig. 4.6). Prostaglandin H_2 (PGH_2) is the precursor of the main prostaglandins, the most important of which are thromboxane A_2 (TxA_2) and prostacyclin (PGI_2). These prostaglandins are metabolized quickly and therefore have a primarily local effect (Table 4.5). TxA_2 is a potent vasoconstrictor and bronchoconstrictor. It promotes platelet aggregation, and has membrane destabilizing properties. Prostacyclin has essentially opposite effects. It is a vasodilator, bronchodilator, membrane stabilizer, and platelet aggregation antagonist. The primary source of prostacyclin is vascular endothelium, whereas thromboxane A_2 is produced by platelets. The relative amounts of these prostaglandins will determine the predominant hemodynamic effect. The cyclooxygenase pathway of arachidonic acid metabolism can be blocked by salicylate and nonsteroidal anti-inflammatory drugs. Arachidonic acid can also be metabolized by lipoxygenase, pro-

Classical Pathway

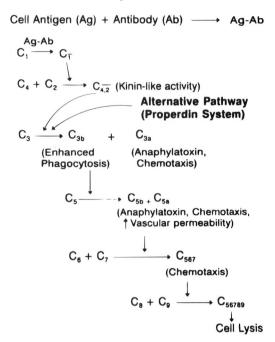

Figure 4.5. The complement cascade. The classical pathway begins with a specific antigen-antibody reaction. This pathway consists of nine separate components (numbered C_1 through C_9) that, when activated, interact sequentially with one another in a "cascade-like" fashion. Many of the activated components of the complement system, (bars above the numbers are used to indicate activated complement components exhibiting enzymatic activity), have profound hemodynamic effects. The alternative pathway (properdin system) is initiated by certain cell surfaces and antibodies. Both pathways converge at the C_3 step where the biologic activity of the complement system begins. The activity of the complement system eventually results in cell lysis.

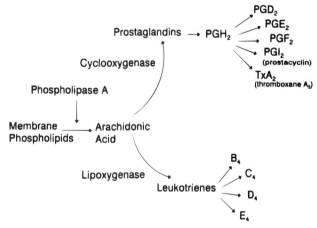

Figure 4.6. Synthesis of prostaglandins and leukotrienes. Arachidonic acid can be metabolized by either cyclooxygenase or lipoxygenase, producing prostaglandins or leukotrienes respectively.

ducing the leukotrienes. These substances are slower acting and cause bronchoconstriction, chemotaxis, and increased vascular permeability.

The plasma kinins are another group of inflammatory mediators that have a role in septic shock (Fig. 4.7).

Table 4.5.
Comparison of Prostacyclin and Thromboxane A₂

Prostacyclin (PGI₂)	Thromboxane A₂ (Tx A₂)
Derived from vascular endothelium	Produced by platelets
Vasodilator	Vasoconstrictor
Bronchodilator	Bronchoconstrictor
Platelet aggregation antagonist	Platelet aggregation
Membrane stabilizer	Membrane destabilizer

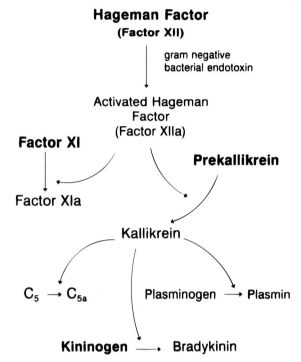

Figure 4.7. The kinin-generating system. Four plasma proteins make up the kinin-generating system: Hageman factor (Factor XII), Factor XI, Prekallikrein, and Kininogen. Activated Hageman factor can interact with factor XI to activate factor XI to factor XIa (activated factor XI). It is this factor that can activate the intrinsic coagulation cascade. Activated Hageman factor also initiates the conversion of prekallikrein to kallikrein. Kallikrein activates plasminogen and also acts directly on the complement pathway by cleaving activated C₅ₐ from C₅. The conversion of kininogen to bradykinin is also initiated by kallikrein. Bradykinin is the major final product of the kinin-generating system. The effects of bradykinin are varied and include: vasodilatation, increased vascular permeability, hypotension, contraction of smooth muscle, activation of phospholipase A₂, and edema production.

These substances are synthesized when the coagulation system is activated in response to inflammation or injury. Bradykinin is the most widely studied, and its effects include vasodilatation, increased vascular permeability, and edema production. Endogenous opioids are mediators that come under the neuroendocrine category. They are produced in the pituitary gland and other neurologic tissues. These substances cause respiratory depressant effects, hypotension, and bradycardia. The role of these substances in sepsis is still being investigated.

The most prominent mediators of the septic response

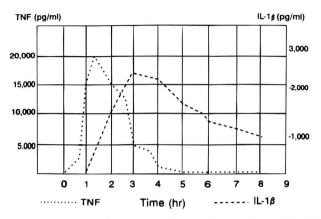

Figure 4.8. Patterns of appearance of TNF and IL-1. Infusion of E coli into baboons results in a rapid rise in TNF and IL-1 in the circulation. Similar patterns of appearance of TNF and IL-1 have been documented in humans after an endotoxin challenge.

are lymphocyte and monocyte derived peptide hormones called lymphokines and monokines respectively (Table 4.6). Interleukin-1 (IL-1) is derived from mononuclear cells and is released during infection or inflammation. It is known to promote fever, stimulate neutrophilia, and initiate the production of hepatic phase proteins. Cachectin or tumor necrosis factor (TNF) is also produced from monocytes and has biologic properties similar to IL-1 (Fig. 4.8). Infusion of TNF into experimental animals results in altered perfusion, lactic acidosis, intravascular coagulation, and increased capillary permeability. In fact, the response is almost identical to that of endotoxin infusion, suggesting that TNF may be a key mediator. TNF can also cause organ dysfunction directly, most profoundly seen in the lungs, kidneys, and liver.

Many other inflammatory mediators probably play a role in septic shock, including corticosteroids, growth hormone, somatomedin, glucagon, insulin, and catecholamines. The complex interaction of these substances is just beginning to be understood.

Metabolic Derangements

The characteristics of hypermetabolism in septicemia include increased energy expenditure, oxygen consumption, and carbon dioxide production. The resting energy expenditure is increased, using a mixed fuel source comprised of carbohydrate (40%), fat (30%), and protein (up to 30%). The protein depletion is mandatory, regardless of intake, and results in increased nitrogen loss in the urine (negative nitrogen balance). Inflammatory mediators probably govern this phenomenon, although the mechanism is not completely understood.

Progressive abnormalities exist in the substrate levels of the fuel sources during septic shock. Hyperglycemia is considered an early indicator of the septic response. This state is often refractory to the administration of exogenous insulin. Serum triglyceride levels also rise

Table 4.6.
Cytokines

Cytokine	Source	Activity
IL-1	Monocytes, macrophages, dendritic cells, NK cells, astrocytes, keratinocytes	Induces lymphokine release from T cells, growth of fibroblasts and synovial cells, PGE release, fever
IL-2	Activated T cells	Induces cytotoxic activity; growth of activated T, NK, B, and LAK cells; lymphokine production
IL-3	Activated T cells, lectin-stimulated PBL[a]	Stimulates the growth of multipotential stem cells
IL-4	Activated T cells	B cell stimulating-factor (BSF), also stimulates T and B lymphocytes and macrophages
IL-5	T cells	Induces differentiation of eosinophils
IL-6	Monocytes, fibroblasts, some tumors	Induces class I HLA expression on fibroblasts and production of acute phase proteins by hepatocytes
IL-7	T cells	Stimulates T cell proliferation, promotes expansion of B cell populations
IL-8	Activated T cells	Activation of granulocytes, induction of chemotactic response
IL-9	T helper cells	Mitogen for T_H subpopulations, promotes growth of mast cells
IL-10	T helper cells	Suppresses cytokine production in other T_H populations producing IL-2 and IFN
Interferon gamma (γ-IFN)	T cells	Activates macrophages T_c, T_{DH}, and NK cells; increases MHC expression
GM-CSF	Activated T cells	Mitogenic for many cells, activates macrophages and granulocytes promotes T cell proliferation
Tumor-necrosis factor (TNF)	Macrophages, T cells	Antitumor activity, mitogenic for many lymphoid cells

[a] Peripheral blood leukocyte.
Reprinted from Pellis N, Balch C. Basic concepts in immunology. In: O'Leary JP, ed. The physiologic basis of surgery, 1st ed. Williams & Wilkins, 1993.

progressively, and evidence of increased hepatic lipogenesis exists. Free fatty acid and ketone levels are elevated. The catabolism of muscle protein to amino acids and then the metabolism of these building blocks contribute to the negative nitrogen balance. Normally, body metabolism is moderated by the neurohumoral system. In sepsis, impairment of normal modulation and eventual failure of the metabolic machinery occur.

Current evidence suggests that there is a primary defect in mitochondrial function which underlies the changes in substrate metabolism. The inability to regenerate nicotinamide-adenine dinucleotide (NAD) probably plays a role, as does inhibition of the enzyme pyruvate dehydrogenase. The result is a failure of substrate to enter mitochondria for high energy phosphate production. When the mitochondria are unable to produce ATP and its derivatives, energy is not available for cell function.

Clinical Characteristics

Septic shock is characterized by fever, tachycardia, and hypotension. Patients usually have warm, moist skin with bounding pulses and, often, mental status changes. Oliguria may or may not occur. Vomiting and diarrhea are nonspecific symptoms that occur frequently, and clinical jaundice occasionally is seen. Laboratory evaluation reveals evidence of infection with leukocytosis and a left shifted differential. Blood cultures are usually positive. A marked respiratory alkalosis often occurs initially caused by hyperventilation, but

this usually progresses to a compensated metabolic acidosis.

As the hypoperfusion state persists, various target organs become dysfunctional. Humans appear to be particularly susceptible to pulmonary dysfunction, while in canines, the gut is an early target organ. The reasons underlying this difference are unknown; however, in humans, pulmonary manifestations tend to predominate the early picture of septic shock. The spectrum of pulmonary insufficiency ranges from mild transient hypoxemia to moderate atelectasis and on to pneumonia and then severe acute respiratory distress syndrome (ARDS) or "shock lung." ARDS is an acute deterioration of pulmonary function manifested by progressive hypoxia despite increasing oxygen administration. Pulmonary compliance falls and inspiratory pressures increase accordingly. The physiologic basis appears to be a disruption of the pulmonary capillary endothelium and basement membrane with the resultant extravasation of fluid into the interstitial space, producing a physiologic diffusion gradient. Alveolar disruption also occurs. A decrease in functional residual capacity (FRC) is usually present. What causes the full blown spectrum in some patients while others are spared is unknown. Proposed etiologic factors include aspiration, recumbency, fluid overload, pulmonary infection, fat embolization, prolonged mechanical ventilation, and oxygen toxicity. The increasing frequency of ARDS in intensive care settings is probably partially due to the fact that many patients survive insults that formerly would not have been compatible with life.

Other susceptible target organs include the kidney, brain, liver and gut. There has been renewed interest recently in the role of the gut as a source of bacteria and bacterial by-products after insult or infection. These theories suggest that in addition to being a target organ, the gut may be a part of the problem. Further studies in this area are ongoing and should help to elucidate the precise and undoubtedly major role of the gut in septic shock. When the cascade of multiple organ failure progresses, the cycle is difficult to break, and patients often succumb to the septic insult.

Treatment

The most important factor in treating septic shock is prompt recognition. The unexplained presence of hyperventilation, tachycardia, fever, or mental status changes must be investigated with a high index of suspicion. Early recognition can help attenuate the high mortality of this disease. Many causes of septic shock are iatrogenic and preventative measures can certainly influence its incidence. This includes judicious use of antibiotics, attention to nutrition, meticulous care of indwelling lines and catheters, strict adherence to sterile technique during invasive procedures, and avoidance of indiscriminant use of steroids and other immunosuppressive drugs.

If septicemia is suspected, broad spectrum antibiotics should be instituted. Combinations of newer synthetic penicillins, aminoglycosides, and clindamycin are often used. The empiric choice should be guided by clinical impression and local experience. Cultures of blood, urine, sputum, wounds, and any other potential source of infection should be obtained. The presence of an abscess or other surgical source of infection is an indication for urgent drainage.

From a hemodynamic standpoint, the patient's volume status must be evaluated and maximized. Most often this involves placement of a Swan-Ganz catheter, and intravascular volume should be expanded to the limits dictated by Starling's mechanism. What constitutes an adequate cardiac output is often debated, but in general it should be increased until further increases no longer augment the oxygen consumption index:

$$[(a - v)dO_2 \times cardiac\ output]$$

Expressed differently, the CO should be increased to such a point that a further increase is not associated with improved oxygen delivery and extraction. After all, it is the oxygen used at the cellular level that is most important. Afterload reduction is rarely indicated in septic shock, but inotropic support is often useful. The sympathomimetic drugs including dopamine, dobutamine, epinephrine, isoproterenol, and norepinephrine are used either alone or in combination The unique benefit of increased renal perfusion with dopamine makes it particularly attractive.

Oxygen administration is invariably indicated, and often mechanical ventilatory support becomes necessary. Frequent analysis of blood gases and arterial pH are used to guide ventilatory support. Hemoglobin levels should be maintained at 13 mg/dl or greater to assure adequate oxygen carrying capacity. The development of ARDS should be treated aggressively with positive end-expiratory pressure (PEEP) and other supportive measures discussed elsewhere.

Nutritional and metabolic support are extremely important in treating septic shock. When possible, the gastrointestinal tract is the preferable route of nutritional support. Early enteral feeding has been reported to improve dysfunction in the MSOF syndrome (23). When enteral feedings are not possible, parenteral support is used. Regardless of the modality, 30 to 40 nonprotein cal/kg/day provides adequate substrate in most patients with sepsis. Protein demands are great, and 2 to 3 gm/kg/day of amino acids are often necessary to support nitrogen balance. In patients with ongoing sepsis, the attainment of neutral or positive nitrogen balance is rarely possible until the septic state is controlled. The ratio of nonprotein calories to grams of nitrogen should be in the 100 to 1 range. The details of nutritional support are discussed elsewhere in this book.

One of the newest areas of investigation in the treatment of septic shock is directed toward counteracting the mediators of the inflammatory response. A monoclonal antibody to TNF has been shown in experimental animals to block the response to lethal doses of endotoxin and bacteria (24). Monoclonal antibodies against the lipid component of endotoxin have also shown promise. The limiting factor with these treatment modalities is timing; they generally have to be administered before or during the septic insult to be beneficial. This severely limits their practicality. Other manipulations of the immune response, including the use of nonsteroidal anti-inflammatory agents, have been used successfully to counteract sepsis in animal models but have limited clinical application at this time. Nonetheless, investigation in these areas continues to be one of the most exciting forefronts in the realm of critical care.

Neurogenic Shock

The basic fundamental mechanism involved in neurogenic shock is an increase in the circulatory capacity of the body. However, unlike hypovolemic shock, the blood volume in neurogenic shock is relatively normal. The unique feature of this type of shock is a massive vasodilatation throughout the entire body which allows for an increase in the circulatory capacity and a "pooling" of blood.

Etiologies of neurogenic shock vary, but the most

common is from a traumatic cervical spinal cord transection (spinal shock). With this injury, there is an interruption in the connection between the brainstem and spinal cord. Other etiologies include high spinal anesthesia and the overdosing of vasodilator drugs. Acute gastric dilatation may also lead to this type of shock (vasovagal effect). Sudden exposure to unpleasant events, such as the sight of blood, an unexpected encountering of severe pain, or an episode of grief may also be possible etiologies.

The treating physician must be aware that the symptomatology of neurogenic shock is different than that found in other types of shock. The diagnosis must be based on sound clinical suspicion. This requires an early recognition of spinal cord trauma, knowledge of previous spinal anesthesia, or the elicitation in the patient's history of other problems. The "typical" presentation is that of hypotension without tachycardia and without vasoconstriction of the skin. Cold, clammy extremities are *not* a part of this presentation. The pulse pressure is not narrowed as in other types of shock, and urine output is not decreased. Thus, a patient who develops neurogenic shock will indeed be hypotensive but will manifest bradycardia and possess warm extremities. The quantity of hourly urine output will range from normal to high.

Physiologic Mechanisms

The pathophysiology of neurogenic shock begins with an etiology that causes a reduction in sympathetic discharge. The lack of sympathetic nervous system outflow will result in vasodilation of the systemic and visceral vasculature. Such vasodilation produces a large decrease in systemic vascular resistance. Venous dilation will allow blood to pool in the capillary beds, and hypotension will result.

The massive vascular dilatation causes a significant reduction in preload. Using the Frank-Starling mechanism, a subsequent reduction in cardiac output may occur. In a patient not suffering from neurogenic shock, a fall in the preload and cardiac output is compensated for by an outpouring of sympathetic discharge. The resulting adrenergic discharge gives rise to tachycardia, augmentation of myocardial contractility, an increase in total peripheral resistance, and a decrease in renal perfusion. In addition, blood flow to the integument, muscles, and splanchnic circulation will be diverted to more essential organ systems. However, these reflexes are lost in the patient suffering from neurogenic shock. Since these reflexes will not be activated, the results are the "typical" neurogenic shock signs of bradycardia, polyuria, and warm extremities.

The lack of sympathetic tone to the heart is also responsible for the absence of a reflex tachycardia. Cardiac output decreases due to a loss of adrenergic stimulation of heart rate, a decrease in peripheral vascular resistance, and the pooling of blood, especially if the patient is hypovolemic. However, the cardiac output may remain normal or slightly increased in a hypervolemic patient because the already increased blood volume helps to stabilize filling pressures of the heart. Also, the decrease in sympathetic outflow will result in a decrease in the afterload. This may allow for less resistance to left ventricular emptying and allow maintenance of the cardiac output.

Treatment of Neurogenic Shock

With many of its etiologies, neurogenic shock usually is a benign and short-lived state. However, without immediate recognition and treatment, severe consequences similar to other types of shock may be the result. Traumatic spinal shock, on the other hand, is a more severe form and can be longer lasting. Even this more severe type of neurogenic shock may only last a few days, and it may resolve when the severed spinal cord begins to independently function and restore adrenergic discharge. Therapy should be directed towards correction of the underlying etiology. This will allow the adrenergic system to return to its normal stimulation of the systemic and visceral vasculature. Until the underlying etiology can be corrected, expansion of the "lost" intravascular compartment with an intravenous fluid infusion should be instituted. This will aid in increasing the preload and augmenting cardiac output. Since a "true" hypovolemia generally does not occur in neurogenic shock, massive fluid infusion may more readily lead to volume overload.

In some instances, fluid resuscitation alone will not substantially improve the hypotension. In this type of situation, a vasoconstrictor should be administered to improve the low peripheral vascular resistance and help increase venous capacitance. The increase in compliance of the veins will allow for an additional increase in preload and optimize cardiac output. Before a vasopressor is instituted, the patient should receive adequate fluid resuscitation. This will help to avert further decreased perfusion caused by the vasoconstrictor. Atropine may be necessary to treat the bradycardia if present.

Conclusion

Shock is a complex array of clinical entities with multiple expressions. Tremendous strides have been made in our understanding of this difficult subject, yet there is still a great deal to learn. Despite extensive investigation, it is unclear whether shock represents a pathologic state, the body's response to a pathologic state, or a combination of the two. Perhaps it was best summed up by John Collins Warren many years ago with his description of shock as "a momentary pause in the act of death."

REFERENCES

1. Paré A. Les Oeuvres d' Ambroise Paré. Paris: Dupuye, 1582.
2. Le Dran HF. A treatise or reflections drawn from practice on gunshot wounds (translated). London: Clarke, 1743.
3. Woolcomb, T. The philosophical transaction of the Royal Society of London, 1770; 13:21.
4. Hunter J. A treatise on the blood, inflammation, and gun-shot wounds. London: Sherwood, Gilbert and Piper, 1828.
5. Latta J. A practical system of surgery. Mudie: London, 1795.
6. Guthrie GJ. On gunshot wounds of the extremities. London: Longman, 1815.
7. Wiggers CJ. Physiology of shock. New York: The Commonwealth Fund, 1950: 1–25.
8. Blum A. Arch gén de méd 1876;1:5.
9. Crile GW. An experimental research into surgical shock. Philadelphia: Lippincott, 1899.
10. Crile GW, and Lower WE. Surgical shock and the shockless operation through anoci-association. Philadelphia: WB Saunders Company, 1920: 17–24.
11. MacCleod JJ. The concentration of lactic acid in the blood in anoxemia and shock. Am J Physiol 1991;55:184.
12. Freeman NE. Cortin and traumatic shock. Science 1933;77: 211–212.
13. Harkins, HN. Recent advances in the study and management of traumatic shock. Surgery 1941;9:231,447,607.
14. Starling EH. The Linacre lecture on the law of the heart. London: Longmans, Green, 1918.
15. Swan HJC, Ganz W, Forrester J, et al. Cardiac catheterization with a flow directed balloon tipped catheter. N Engl J Med 1970;283: 447–451.
16. Holcroft JW. Surgical intensive care: Shock and adult respiratory distress syndrome. In: Way LW. ed. Current surgical diagnosis and treatment. Norwalk: Appleton & Lange, 1988:174–186.
17. Carrico CJ, Meakins JL, et al. Multiple organ system failure syndrome. Arch Surg 1986;121:196–208.
18. Gann DS, et al. The role of solute in the early restitution of blood volume after hemorrhage. Surgery 1983;94:439.
19. Alonso DR, Scheidt S, Post M, Killip T. Pathophysiology of cardiogenic shock: quantification of myocardial necrosis, clinical, pathologic, and electrocardiographic correlations. Circulation 1973;48: 588–596.
20. Goldberg RT, Gore JM, Alpert JS, et al. Cardiogenic shock after acute myocardial infarction: incidence and mortality from a community wide perspective, 1975 to 1988. N Engl J Med 1991; 325: 1117–1122.
21. Bengston JR, Kaplan AJ, Pieper KS, et al. Prognosis in cardiogenic shock after acute myocardial infarction in the interventional era. J Am Coll Cardiol 1992;20:1482–1489.
22. Pennington DG, Swartz MT. Clinical use of assisted circulation. Ann Surg 1994; 26:169–191.
23. Cerra FB, Shronts EP, Konstantinides NN. Enteral feeding in sepsis: A prospective randomized double-blind trial. Surgery 1985; 98:632.
24. Tracey KJ, Fong Y, Hesse DG, et al. Anticachectin/TNF monoclonal antibodies prevent septic shock during lethal bacteremia. Nature 1987;330:662.

SUGGESTED READINGS

Anderson RW, Visner MS. Shock and circulatory collapse. In: Sabiston & Spencer, eds. Surgery of the chest. 5th ed. Philadelphia: WB Saunders, 1990:151–188.
Barrett J, and Nyhus LM. Treatment of shock: Principles and practice, 2nd. ed. Philadelphia: Lea & Febiger, 1986.
Califf RM, Bengston JR. Cardiogenic shock. N Engl J Med 1994; 330(24): 1724–1730.
Davis HA. Shock and allied forms of failure of the circulation. New York: Grune & Stratton, 1949:1–12.
Deitch, EA. Multiple organ failure: Pathophysiology and potential future therapy. Ann Surg 1992;216:117–130.
Gann DS. Shock. In: Cameron, ed. Current Surgical Therapy. 4th ed. St. Louis: Mosby Year Book, 1992:819–822.
Guyton AC. Textbook of medical physiology. Philadelphia: WB Saunders Company, 1985:332–344.
Hardaway RM. Clinical management of shock. Springfield: Thomas, Publ, 1968.
Lucas CE. The renal response to acute injury and sepsis. Surg Clin North Am 1976;56:953.
Mouchawar A, Rosenthal M. A pathophysiologic approach to the patient in shock. Int Anesthesiol Clin 1993;31(2):1–20.
Shires TG (III), Canizaro PC, Carrico CJ, et al. Shock. In: Schwartz, Shires, & Spencer, eds. Principles of surgery. 5th ed. New York: McGraw-Hill, 1989:115–165.
Shires GT, Carrico CJ, and Canizaro PC. Shock. Philadelphia: WB Saunders Company, 1983.
Shires GT, Cunningham JN, Baker CR, et al. Alterations in cellular membrane function during hemorrhagic shock in primates. Ann Surg 1972;176:288–295.

5 Nutrition and Metabolism

Kennan J. Buechter | Patricia M. Byers

Overview of Intermediary Metabolism

Basal energy expenditure in a healthy adult male is approximately 20 kcal/kg/day. With normal activity, this caloric requirement increases to 30 to 40 kcal/kg/day. During the fed and exercised state, this caloric requirement is met by the use of the three main foodstuffs—carbohydrates, fats, and proteins. With fasting, available bodily stores of glucose and glycogen are insufficient for basal energy expenditure, and an increase in fat and protein metabolism occurs. Basic requirements of living cells include protein synthesis for repair and replication and a readily available energy source to drive these reactions. The ultimate goal of adaptation to starvation is the continual generation of adenosine triphosphate (ATP) to fuel required metabolic activities and cellular reactions. In humans, cells use or store energy by hydrolysis or condensation of high-energy bonds. The majority of usable energy in the body is found in the form of ATP, which consists of the purine adenosine (6-amino purine), a pentose sugar, and three high-energy phosphate bonds. Hydrolysis or condensation of these bonds releases or stores energy.

Carbohydrate Metabolism

Gut digestion of sugars yields glucose, fructose, and galactose, with minor amounts of mannose, xylose, and arabinose. These sugars are absorbed readily in the gut and transported to the liver, where fructose and galactose are rapidly converted to glucose. Most glucose in the liver is phosphorylated to glucose 6-phosphate (G6P); the remainder passes into the systemic circulation to maintain serum glucose homeostasis. G6P is split to form pyruvate (glycolysis). Pyruvate formed in glycolysis is transported into the mitochondria and coupled with coenzyme A (CoA) to form acetyl-CoA. The acetyl moiety of acetyl-CoA subsequently is degraded to hy-

drogen and carbon dioxide via the tricarboxylic acid cycle (TCA) (Fig. 5.1). In the presence of oxygen, hydrogen atoms are oxidatively phosphorylated to form ATP and water. Glycolysis and the TCA will be inhibited by the buildup of pyruvate and/or hydrogen atoms. With inadequate oxygenation, oxidative phosphorylation cannot proceed. The end result is the formation of lactic acid and subsequent lactic acidosis, which, in turn, impedes glycolysis.

Lipid Metabolism

Approximately 40% of calories in the average American diet is derived from fat. For biochemical accuracy, lipids are compounds that are insoluble in water, soluble in one or more organic solvents, and have a relation to fatty acids as esters. Fats and oils are triesters of glycerol and various fatty acids. The ability of lipids to be stored as body fat and thus provide a source for continuous energy production on demand is essential. Glucose and hepatic stores of glycogen are metabolized within 12 hours. Because humans do not continuously eat, fat stores are essential for energy homeostasis.

Lipid absorption and digestion is a complex process. In brief, bile salts interact with free fatty acids and monoglycerides to form micelles. These are subsequently absorbed through the small bowel mucosa. Once absorbed, the long-chain fatty acids are esterified to triglycerides and transported via the lymphatic system, whereas short- and medium-chain fatty acids enter the portal venous system directly. The ultimate fate of absorbed fatty acids is to provide a source of lipids for energy storage as fat and to provide constituents of cell membranes in the form of phospholipids.

A decrease in carbohydrate intake causes an increase in hydrolysis of triglycerides into glycerol and free fatty acids. These products are then transported directly to tissues for oxidation. Virtually all tissues, except the brain, can use lipids as an energy source. Tissues oxidize lipids by a process called β-oxidation. This involves multiple cleavages of two carbon fragments from the fatty acid (i.e., at the β-carbon).

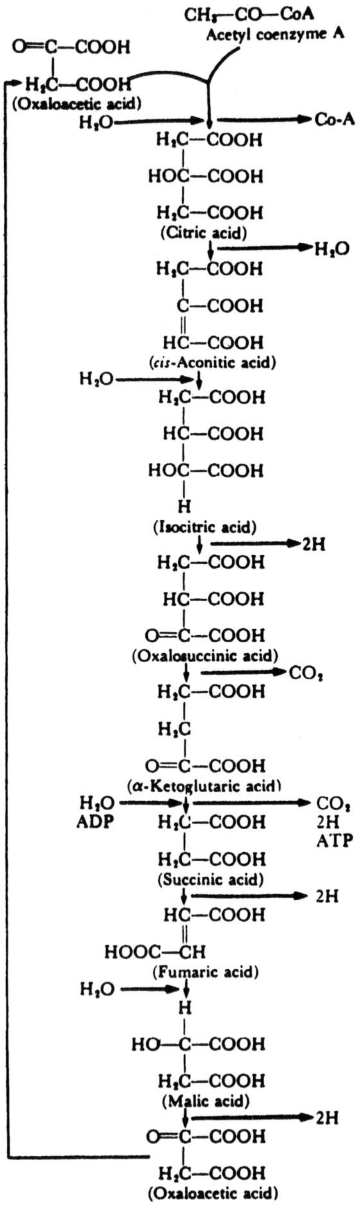

Figure 5.1. The tricarboxylic acid cycle. Note the continuing reentry of oxoacids into the pathway and the generation of hydrogen. Reprinted with permission from Guyton AC. Textbook of medical physiology. 7th ed. Philadelphia: WB Saunders, 1986:813.

Multiple systems regulate the activity of the TCA, including NAD-NADH, ATP-ADP, and feedback inhibition by stoichiometric reactions. Although these systems typically regulate oxidation of glucose, the absence of or inability to use glucose has a substantial effect on metabolic homeostasis. When excessive amounts of lipid are used for energy (e.g., diabetes), two molecules of acetyl-CoA condense to form acetoacetic acid. Acetoacetic acid normally is converted to β-hydroxybutyric acid and minute quantities of acetone. With excessive production of acetoacetic acid however, acetoacetic acid, β-hydroxybutyric acid, and acetone accumulate in large quantities and freely diffuse into the circulation. This results in the clinical condition of ketosis or ketoacidosis.

Protein Metabolism

The goal of clinical nutritional support is to provide nonprotein fuel sources so that protein can be used for anabolic cellular processes. Although protein can and is used as a fuel source via gluconeogenesis, thus offering a readily available reserve fuel source in times of stress and/or fasting, this catabolic process can be detrimental when protein availability is diminished. This would also be true at times of increased need for protein synthesis.

Ingested protein is hydrolyzed to dipeptides and amino acids, absorbed rapidly across the small bowel mucosa, and subsequently transported to the liver via the portal circulation. Although the serum levels of amino acids are low and relatively constant, there is a tremendous continuous turnover of bodily protein with many grams of protein carried throughout the body per hour. Most intracellular amino acids are linked quickly into cellular proteins and stored as protein or used in the cellular system. However, with the exception of certain specific protein stores (e.g., muscle contractile proteins), this linkage is readily reversible and thus liberation of free amino acids to replenish the amino acid pool readily occurs. Any particular cell has a limit to protein storage. Once that limit is reached, unused excess amino acids are either transaminated or deaminated. Transamination is the reaction whereby amino groups are transferred in reverse between amino acids and ketoacids. Thus an amino acid becomes a ketoacid and vice versa. Transamination serves two principal purposes: 1) it allows inter conversion of amino acids to replenish one in short supply; and 2) it serves to transport amino groups to form glutamate and aspartate. Glutamate, with the addition of a second amino group, becomes glutamine, an amino acid whose importance has become increasingly recognized. Deamination is the process of removing amino groups, either oxidatively or nonoxidatively, to yield ammonia. Because ammonia is a highly toxic metabolite, an efficient mechanism is available for its detoxification and removal. Therefore, blood ammonia concentration remains low (Fig. 5.2). Glutamine and glutamate play major roles in ammonia elimination.

Nucleic Acid Synthesis

Deoxyribose nucleic acid (DNA) and ribose nucleic acid (RNA) are nucleic acids. Nucleic acids are formed of phosphoric acid, a sugar, and a base. DNA consists of phosphoric acid, deoxyribose, and one of the four bases: adenine, guanine, cytosine, and thymine. RNA consists of phosphoric acid, ribose, and one of the bases adenine, guanine, cytosine, or uracil. The difference between DNA and RNA is slight, with the principal difference being the substitution of uracil for thymine in RNA. DNA is a nuclear-based molecule, whereas 90% of RNA is found in cell cytoplasm and only 10% is found in the nucleolus. Any unit of a base, sugar, and phosphoric acid is termed a nucleotide. Sequential bonding of nu-

Figure 5.2. Urea formation.

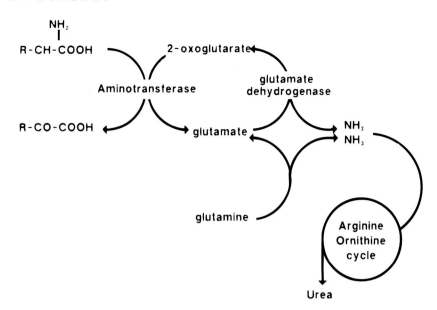

cleotides form the nucleic acids. The purines (adenine and guanine) and pyrimidines (cytosine, thymine, and uracil) are formed of simple precursors: amino acids; carbon monoxide; ammonia; phosphate; and sugar. The amino acid moiety for all three pyrimidines is aspartic acid, whereas the purines use nitrogen contributions from aspartic acid, glycine, and glutamine. The biosynthesis of the nucleotides is a complex process involving several intermediates.

A key point concerning nucleotide synthesis is that the reaction is phosphate dependent and inhibited by nucleotide buildup. Accelerated catabolism of these compounds will liberate phosphate and drive the reaction forward. Conversely, hypophosphatemia results in a deficiency of ATP, with resultant global effects on metabolism.

Although the amino acids involved as direct nitrogen donors for purine and pyrimidine synthesis are considered nonessential, the essential amino acid methionine has a crucial role in the synthesis of nucleic acids. Methionine has the unique property of being the methyl donor in the formation of various compounds (including RNA), a process called transmethylation. Adequate diets that are deficient in methionine have been reported to induce nucleolar RNA alterations, including enlargement and alteration of the molecule and increased activity of RNA polymerase. Diets without any amino acid supplementation cause the same findings, suggesting a key role for methionine in the scheme of nucleotide and ultimately RNA synthesis (1).

Nutritional Requirements

Nutritional requirements vary with age, sex, and body size and can be influenced by drugs, hormones, and disease states. Macronutrients support growth, cellular maintenance, repair, host defenses, and motility through the provision of energy and building blocks. Micronutrients, in contrast, are not used for energy or structure, but are required in small amounts to maintain the physiologic processes essential for life.

Carbohydrates provide approximately 45% of the human energy requirement. They may be ingested as simple monosaccharides and disaccharides or as the more complex polysaccharides, which subsequently undergo intestinal hydrolysis to simpler forms. Certain tissues such as brain, erythrocytes, and renal medulla have an obligate fuel requirement for glucose. Exogenous carbohydrate is not essential for normal growth and metabolism as long as gluconeogenic precursors, such as glycerol or amino acids, are available to satisfy tissue needs (2,3).

Lipids are another important fuel source and, as triglycerides, are the primary storage fuel in the human body. They also play an important role in structure and function. The obligatory nutrient function of lipids is to serve as a source of the essential fatty acids linoleic and α-linolenic acid, which are required for normal growth and function. These unsaturated fatty acids contain double bonds at the number 6 and the number 3 carbon positions. Because humans lack the enzymatic capability to insert double bonds at these locations, these fatty acids must be supplied by the diet. They are needed both for cellular structure and as precursors for prostaglandins, prostacyclins, thromboxanes, and leukotrienes. During periods of starvation, individuals with very low body stores of fat are most susceptible to essential fatty acid deficiencies. However, during periods of carbohydrate intake, with increased insulin levels and inhibition of lipolysis, essential fatty acid deficiency can be manifested rapidly in the absence of fat supplementation (2,4–7).

Table 5.1.
The Aminio Acids

Essential	Semiessential	Nonessential
Leucine		Glycine
Isoleucine		Arginine
Valine		Proline
Lysine		Glutamic acid
Threonine		Aspartic acid
Methionine <------>	Cystine	Serine
Phenylalanine<--->	Tyrosine	Alanine
Tryptophan		
Histidine		

Adapted with permission from Solomons NW Young VR. The major nutrient. In: Paige DM. Clinical nutrition, 2nd ed. St. Louis: CV Mosby Company, 1988:22.

Protein comprises approximately 20% of the lean body mass, but unlike carbohydrate and lipids, it is not stored. Thus any decrease in the body's supply results in a decreased functional capacity or loss of structural integrity. A portion of the protein mass is dynamic and in a continual state of flux. This allows for metabolic control via regulatory enzymes and enables priority use of a limited amino acid pool. Proteins are ingested and hydrolyzed into amino acids, which then enter the amino acid pool. These amino acids are then either synthesized into new protein, catabolized via transamination and oxidative reactions, or converted into other physiologically active compounds such as nucleic acids, porphyrins, glutathione, and creatine. Thus one nutritional protein requirement is to provide a source of usable nitrogen (8–10).

The other nutritional protein requirement is to provide an exogenous source of essential amino acids, because the enzymatic capacity for their synthesis is lacking in the human (Table 5.1). Essential amino acids are defined as those that are needed for normal body function but cannot be produced by the body. The amino acids cystine and tyrosine are considered semiessential because when methionine and phenylalanine are supplied in adequate amounts, their requirement is satisfied. Nonessential amino acids can be synthesized endogenously if sufficient nitrogen is provided. The usual daily protein requirement is 0.8 g/kg/day; however, this does not account for conditions of growth, repletion, or stress. Dietary proteins contain essential amino acids in varying concentrations. Animal sources yield higher concentrations of essential amino acids than vegetable sources. Requirements of essential amino acids change with age and physiologic state. During early growth and development, requirements are high and subsequently decline with age (2,10).

Vitamins are essential nutrients that are required in small amounts to maintain the physiologic processes necessary for life. In addition, deficiencies cause well-defined diseases that are prevented or cured by the appropriate vitamin supplementation. A total of 13 vita-

mins have been identified as essential in human nutrition: 5 are fat soluble and 9 are water soluble. The B-complex vitamins, which include thiamine, biotin, niacin, pantothenic acid, and B₆, serve as precursors of coenzymes. Another group of vitamins (A, K, and D) function in the expression of genetic information either during transcription, translation, posttranslational modification, or cell-surface regulation. Vitamins E and C have electron transport functions and are antioxidants. Finally, a number of vitamins perform specialized yet miscellaneous functions that cannot be grouped into one of the other categories. Requirements are defined by the recommended daily allowances (RDAs) for nutrients and are reevaluated every 5 years by the Food and Nutrition Board of the National Research Council. This is done by first determining the mean requirement and degree of variability for the U.S. population. The average is then increased sufficiently so that the needs of all group members are met. Occasionally, data must be extrapolated carefully. In the case of certain vitamins and trace minerals, insufficient data exists to establish RDAs, so safe and adequate daily dietary intakes (SADDIs) are used (Table 5.2).

There are 19 minerals and trace minerals that are essential to humans, and they may be grouped into four categories based on function. Calcium, phosphorous, magnesium, and zinc are structural components of bone. A second group—sodium, potassium, and chloride—functions as the major charged ions. Calcium and magnesium are both structural components of bone and function as charged ions. Trace minerals are components of metalloproteins and metalloenzymes. These include iron, zinc, copper, selenium, manganese, molybdenum, cobalt, iodine, and chromium.

Nutritional Assessment

The purpose of performing a nutritional assessment is not only to evaluate the nutritional status of a given patient but also to identify those patients at risk for developing malnutrition. Although there is controversy regarding the identification of clinically significant malnutrition, the following is a useful definition: a state of caloric, protein, or micronutrient deficiency that is acute or chronic and adversely affects prognosis.

History and Physical Examination

The many new and sophisticated techniques available to assess nutritional status are not helpful without a thorough, problem-oriented history and physical examination. The history should elicit dietary information, social background, and medical information regarding chronic diseases or malabsorptive states. The patient's

Table 5.2.
A Summary of Essential Daily Nutrient Requirements

Nutrient	RDA or SADDI[1]	Deficiency Function	Deficiency Syndrome
Energy	1400–3300 Kcal	Growth, maintenance, repair, motility	Marasmic malnutrition
Protein	44–56 g	Structure, enzymatic function	Kwashiorkor malnutrition
Essential Fatty Acids	2–4% dietary calories	Precursors of prostaglandins	Dermatitis, impaired water balance, organ degeneration
Vitamins			
Biotin	100–200 μg	Precursor of coenzyme	Dermatitis, atrophy of lingual papillae
Niacin	13–19 mg	Precursor of coenzyme	Pellagra
Pantothenic acid	4– mg	Precursor of coenzyme	Paresthesias, heel tenderness
Pyridoxine (B6)	2.0–2.2 mg	Precursor of coenzyme	Anemia, weakness, cheilosis, glossitis
Vitamin A	800–1000 μg	Transmission of genetic information	Night blindness, keratomalacia
Vitamin K	70–140 μg	Transmission of genetic information	Bleeding
Vitamin D	5–7.5 μg	Transmission of genetic information	Rickets, osteomalacia
Folic Acid	400 μg	Carbon transfer of DNA synthesis	Megaloblastic anemia
Vitamin E	8–10 mg	Antioxidant & electron transport	Ataxia, areflexia, anonal degeneration
Vitamin C	60 mg	Antioxidant & electron transport	Gingivitis, scurvy, psychological disturbances
Riboflavin	1.2–1.7 mg	Flavoprotein enzymes	Cheilosis, glossitis
Thiamin (B1)	1.0–1.5 mg	Neutral transmission	Warniche-Korsakoff Syndrome, wet beriberi
Cobalamin (B12)		Coenzyme for demthylation	Megaloblastic anemia
Minerals			
Sodium	90–3300 mg	Major charged soluble element involved in electrochemical neutrality	Nausea, central nervous system depression, exhaustion
Potassium	1875–5625 mg	Major charged soluble element involved in electrochemical neutrality	EKG changes, lethargy, respiratory failure, muscle weakness
Chloride	1700–5100 mg	Major charged soluble element involved in electrochemical neutrality	Metabolic alkalosis
Calcium	800 mg	Bone structure, charged ion, neuromuscular conduction	Tetany, cardiac arrhythmias
Magnesium	300–350 mg	Bone structure, charged ion, neuromuscular conduction	Seizures, cardiac arrhythmias, muscular irritability, delirium
Phosphorous	800 mg	Bone structure, high energy compounds	Tissue hypoxia, neurologic and psychiatric disturbances
Iron	10–18 mg	Oxygen and electron transport	Anemia
Zinc	15 mg	Enzymes in energy metabolism and transmission of genetic information	Bullous skin lesions, hypogeusia
Iodine	150 mg	Thyroid hormones	Goiter
Copper	2.0–3.0 mg	Oxidative enzymes, interaction with iron, cross-linking of elastin	Anemia, ossification changes
Manganese	2.5–5.0 mg	Mucopolysaccharide metabolism, superoxide dismutase	Unknown
Fluoride	1.5–4.0 mg	Bone, tooth structure	Increased incidence of caries
Chromium	0.05–0.2 mg	Potentiation of insulin	Glucose intolerance, hyperlipidemia
Selenium	0.05–0.2 mg	Glutathione peroxidase, interactions with heavy metals	Keshan disease (cardiomyopathy)
Molybdenum	0.15–0.5 mg	Xanthine and Aldehyde oxidases	Unknown

[1] Recommended dietary allowance and safe and adequate daily dietary intake.

usual weight and recent weight should be recorded with reference to the period of time elapsed.

The physical examination needs to focus on specific signs of protein-calorie malnutrition, signs of micronutrient deficiencies, and evidence of obesity. The patient's height and weight should be measured and compared with the premorbid weight and standard weight tables. Genetic factors, sex, dietary habits, and exercise all influence body weight. In ill patients, well weight may be underestimated and the measured weight may include an increase in intracellular water. A weight loss of greater than 20% of usual weight may be associated with an increase in morbidity and mortality. This is typical of severe catabolic illness for which weight loss may be as high as 500 g/day of lean tissue (11–16).

In addition to weight loss, obesity must be identified. Body mass indices such as Quetelet's index (weight/height in m^2) have been developed to provide an accurate measure of obesity. Life insurance companies have noted that there is an excessive death rate at both ends of the Quetelet's index. Obese individuals are especially prone to death secondary to accidents. A Quetelet's index of 20 to 25 is associated with a minimal risk of mortality. Another measurement that is used to evaluate obesity is the waist-to-hip circumference ratio. Cardiovascular risk increases sharply when this exceeds 1.0 in men and 0.8 in women (17,18).

All portions of the physical examination must be interpreted as they relate to nutritional status. The vital signs may indicate that increased nutritional risk or altered nutritional requirements exist. The texture and color of the hair, skin, lips, tongue, and nails may reveal signs of micronutrient deficiencies. The thyroid should always be checked for signs of enlargement. The lungs are examined for chronic respiratory changes that may affect metabolic rate and the heart for size and rhythm. On palpation of the abdomen, liver size is specifically noted. The extremities are evaluated for skeletal deformities, tenderness, or edema. Finally, the examination is concluded with a detailed neurologic examination that evaluates orientation, memory, calculation, cranial nerves, motor performance, deep tendon reflexes, and sensation.

For a more sophisticated evaluation, further examination and specific tests can be done to estimate the different compartments that comprise body weight. In the stable patient, these measurements are relatively static and thus most accurate (Fig. 5.3).

Anthropometric

Numerous methods have been developed to estimate the amount of adipose tissue in the human body. The simplest is by the anthropometric technique of skinfold thickness. The triceps skinfold (TSF) is most commonly used, but the subscapular, suprailiac, thigh, abdominal, chest, and axillary skinfolds can also be measured. These values can then be compared with measured standards. When using these values, it is assumed that the ratio of subcutaneous fat to total body fat is reasonably constant for a given sex and age group (19).

Skeletal muscle or somatic protein stores can be estimated using the anthropometric technique of mid-arm muscle circumference (MAMC). This is a measurement of lean arm tissue, which is then compared with standards. At the midpoint of the arm, the circumference is measured to the nearest 0.1 cm. The mid-arm muscle circumference is then calculated by subtracting the mid-arm fat circumference from the mid-arm circumference (MAC), using the TSF measurement:

$$MAMC = MAC - (TSK \cdot \pi)$$

These values are obtained easily but are clearly invalid in patients with upper-extremity edema or injury.

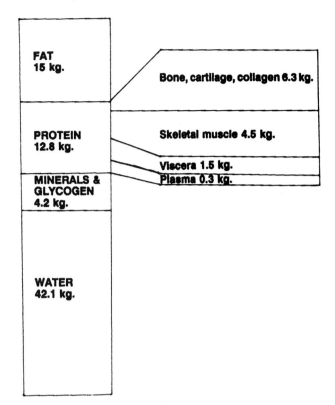

Figure 5.3. The components of body weight in a healthy male subject. Adapted with permission from Hill GL, Beddo AH. Dimensions of the human body and its compartments. In: Kinney JM, Jeejeebhoy KN, Hill GL, Owen OE, eds. Nutrition and metabolism in patient care. Philadelphia: WB Saunders, 1988:90; and Byers PM, Trauma and nutritional support. In: Kreis DJ Jr, Gomez GA, eds. Trauma management. Boston: Little, Brown, & Co., 1989:494.

Other Measurements of Body Composition

Another method that has been developed to measure body fat is densitometry. The patient is submerged in water and his or her body density is determined from a weight measurement. This method is based on the assumptions that: 1) variations in body density are the result of variations in fat content; 2) the density of the fat-free body is constant; and 3) body fat is much less dense than the fat-free body. The following equation is used:

$$M_f/M - 1/D$$

where M_f is fat mass, M is body mass, and D is the density of the fat-free body (1.1 g/nml). Although this method is considered to be the gold standard for the estimation of body fat, it is limited by logistical difficulties and the fact that the fat-free body mass does vary with illness.

Imaging techniques used to estimate body fat include radiometry of plain films, computerized tomography, and ultrasound. Computerized tomography is useful in evaluating both subcutaneous and intra-abdominal fat and in determining changes that may occur in fat distribution with aging. Limitations of computerized tomography include cost and radiation exposure.

Electrical conductivity or impedance measurements can be used to estimate body fat and are based on the differential conductivity of lean and fat tissue. Lean tissue has a far greater conductivity as a result of its electrolyte content. Variance is then believed to be related to the fat mass with the assumption of consistency of the fat-free mass. This is a rapid, reproducible, and safe technique (17,20).

Evaluation of the protein compartment is more complicated because it may be defined and delineated in different ways. For example, *lean body mass* consists of all body tissue other than adipose tissue. *Fat-free mass* differs in that it considers body fat to be ether-extractable tissue. Another differentiation occurs between the dynamic protein mass, which is responsible for daily protein turnover, and the inert protein mass, consisting of bone, cartilage, and collagen. The body cell mass is considered to be the sum of all body cellular components.

One method to define muscle mass was described in the section of anthropometric measures. Another method that may be used to assess skeletal muscle mass is the Creatinine Height Index (CHI). This is based on the assumption that in patients younger than age 55 with normal renal function, urinary creatinine excretion reflects skeletal muscle mass. The CHI is the ratio of the 24-hr urinary creatinine excretion divided by the standard value for that gender, height, and ideal body weight. The rate of protein accretion versus breakdown can be measured with nitrogen balance studies. Urinary urea nitrogen or total urinary nitrogen values are measured in 24-hour urine samples and compared with nitrogen intake. Measurement of the visceral and plasma compartments is more difficult, and an estimation of the adequacy of these is based on laboratory tests. Circulating transport protein levels, such as albumin, transferrin, prealbumin, and retinol-binding protein, can be measured by most chemistry laboratories. In the absence of confounding factors, the rate of change in the level of these markers in response to nutritional status is proportional to their half-lives (Table 5.3) (21).

In markedly catabolic patients, the measurement of acute phase reactants may be useful. Because the immune system is adversely affected by malnutrition, markers of immune function may represent visceral protein stores in the absence of other complicating factors. The total lymphocyte count and delayed hyper-sensitivity testing are used for this purpose.

Table 5.3.
Measurement of the Visceral Protein Compartment

Protein Marker	Half-life days
Albumin	20
Transferrin	8.5
Prealbumin	1.3
Retinol-binding protein	0.4

The fat-free mass can be estimated by in vivo neutron activation analysis in which total body nitrogen is measured and multiplied by 6.25 to achieve an estimate of total body protein. Another technique is cadaver analysis, but this is cumbersome and not frequently done (18).

Several methods have been developed that are able to estimate the body cell mass (22,23). Two methods use a measurement of potassium (K^+) to accomplish this determination. Potassium is the primary intracellular cation and has been shown to be related closely to metabolic expenditure and body cell mass. A dilution technique can be done using ^{42}K. The tagged radioisotope is placed into a known volume of solute (V_1). The concentration of radioisotope in this volume is known (c_i), and then the solution is injected into the patient where it is then distributed within the compartment to be estimated. The new concentration of the isotope is then measured (c_m) and the size of the compartment (V) calculated using the following equation:

$$V = c_i/c_m \cdot V_2$$

For this technique to be valid, the tracer must not redistribute to any other compartment during the equilibration period. To eliminate problems arising from lengthy equilibration periods, the whole-body counter technique using ^{40}K, a naturally occurring radioisotope, was developed. This form has a fixed ratio of 0.01% to the more stable forms ^{39}K and ^{41}K and has a half-life of 109 years. This method has the advantage of being rapid and independent of ongoing fluid shifts (18).

Phosphorous magnetic resonance spectroscopy is a new method being developed to quantitate cellular metabolism and to assess the delivery of substrate for oxidative metabolism. At the cellular level, nutrition is considered to be the process by which electrons are delivered to the respiratory chain within the mitochondria such that the synthesis of ATP can occur. Using this technique, the phosphorylation potential can be quantified (see refs. 24 and 25 for calculation and definition). This value is related to the oxidation-reduction state of cellular cofactors, plasma membrane gradients, intracellular pH, and amino acid synthesis. Phosphorous magnetic resonance can be used to diagnose the cellular defect and monitor the effectiveness of therapy. The phosphorylation potential of cells may be manipulated by controlling the redox state of the permeant, monoanionic nutrients supplied to the patient. This tool may prove useful in that it can measure the steady state of the cell as the phosphorylation potential and can determine the relative velocity of intracellular metabolism.

The evaluation of total body water (TBW) can also be determined using the dilution technique and one of several radioisotopes (tritium, deuterium, ^{18}O, or ^{3}H). To delineate extracellular water (EW), ^{82}Br dilution is commonly used and has an accuracy within $\pm 4\%$. Intracellular water may then be calculated as the difference between TBW and EW (18).

Other Useful Tests

Separate from the determination of the various body compartments, other various laboratory tests exist that may be done to clarify a patient's nutritional status. For example, electrolytes and trace minerals should always be checked when malabsorption or chronic malnutrition is a consideration. Iron levels, iron transport proteins, hemoglobin, and hematocrit with indices may delineate an anemia of nutritional origin. Red blood cell folate levels and vitamin B_{12} levels can be obtained to clarify the deficiency. Glucose levels or a glucose tolerance test may lead to the diagnosis of diabetes. In addition, creatinine, blood urea nitrogen levels, and hepatic function tests are important so that organ dysfunction can be identified and an appropriate nutritional plan developed. Cholesterol and triglyceride profiles should also be checked.

Many vitamin levels, such as those for A, D, E, C, and B-complex, can be measured directly. To assess vitamin K deficiency, prothrombin time and proteins C and S can be checked as indirect measurements. To evaluate pyridoxine, the serum glutamic oxaloacetic transaminase level may be checked. Malabsorption may be assessed by measuring carotene levels in serum, the carotene tolerance test, or the vitamin A absorption test. Related tests that are done with urine samples include the D-xylose test for malabsorption and the Schilling test, which evaluates cobalamin absorption.

Specific Consideration in Nutrition and Metabolism

The Acute Phase Response

For any organism to survive during times of stress, infection, or injury, an appropriate and timely defensive response must be initiated. The constellation of clinical findings and the underlying cellular and metabolic changes in the human response to tissue injury has been termed the acute phase response. Inflammation has long been recognized as a clinical manifestation of this response. Recently, attention has focused on defining the cellular and metabolic initiators and mediators of the acute phase response. It appears there is a characteristic and consistent response regardless of the instigating event. In addition, although the response to an acute injury is characteristic, there are similarities between this response and the body's response to chronic illness.

Trauma, burns, tissue infarction, neoplasia, and pregnancy have all been shown to elicit a predictable metabolic and physiologic response. Classic hallmarks in the diagnosis of the response have been fever and leukocytosis. The diversity of the response at the cellular and metabolic levels, and the influence of nutritional sub-

Table 5.4.
The Acute Phase Response Results in Increases in Serum Levels of the Following Endocrine Hormones:

Glucagon	Growth hormone
Insulin	TSH
ACTH	Hyroxin
Cortisol	Aldosterone
Catecholamine	Vasopressin

Table 5.5.
Metabolic Consequences of the Acute Phase Response

Increased protein synthesis
Increased protein catabolism
Increase gluconeogenesis
Negative nitrogen balance

strate availability on that response, have only recently been appreciated.

Tissue injury generates an endocrine response (Table 5.4). It is unknown whether the hormonal milieu changes as a direct result of tissue injury (manifestation of that injury) or if the observed hormonal changes via various endocrine mediators contribute to the propagation of the response. Regardless of the various interactions, the end result is an increase in net protein catabolism, an increase in protein synthesis, an increase in gluconeogenesis, and the development of a negative nitrogen balance (Table 5.5). Interestingly, while protein catabolism is increased, protein synthesis is also increased. Enzyme systems such as hydroxymethyl-glutaryl-CoA and NADH cytochrome reductase are activated. Activation and increased activity of glutaminolysis has also been reported (26–29).

Fever is a common feature of the acute phase response. In the normal animal, body temperature is regulated via nervous feedback mechanisms through the hypothalamus. There is an abundant supply of cold and warm receptors in the skin, and core body temperature is regulated through receptors in the spinal cord, abdominal viscera, and major veins. Because there are many more cold receptors than warm receptors, it appears the main function of temperature regulation is the prevention of hypothermia. There are multiple factors that affect body temperature besides ambient temperature. Exercise, protein digestion, thyroid hormone, growth hormone, male sex hormone, sleep, and malnutrition all affect metabolic rate and thus body temperature. Sympathetic stimulation and circulating catecholamines cause an immediate increase in the rate of cellular metabolism and body temperature, probably due to uncoupling of oxidative phosphorylation and the subsequent generation of heat. Fever as a manifestation of the acute phase response is a direct effect of interleukin-1

Table 5.6.
Acute Phase Proteins

Ceruloplasmin
C_3 - third component of complement
α_1 - acid glycoprotein
α_1 - antitrypsin
α_1 - antichymotrypsin
Fibrinogen
Hepatoglobin
C-reactive protein
Serum amyloid-A-protein

(IL-1) (alteration in thermal regulation). IL-1 causes an increase in synthesis of prostaglandin E_2 (PGE_2), which has a direct effect on the hypothalamic temperature center. PGE_2 increases the hypothalamic set point and activates the bodily responses of vasoconstriction and shivering, which results in raising the core temperature (30,31).

A variety of hepatic-synthesized plasma proteins are altered in the acute phase response and are thus referred to as the acute phase proteins (Table 5.6). While it is clear that these proteins originate via hepatic synthesis, the instigators and modulators of these synthetic processes remain unclear.

One aspect of protein metabolism in the acute phase response is reprioritization of hepatic protein synthesis. Mobilization of amino acids occurs in concert with increased production of C-reactive protein, alpha-1-acid glycoprotein, alpha-1-Antitrypsin, and other acute phase reactants. Concurrently, there is a decrease in production of constitutive proteins such as albumin, prealbumin, and transferrin. In the absence of any other ongoing insult, this adaptation returns to normal within several days.

The magnitude of response of these proteins is widely varied. As an example, serum levels of C-reactive protein increase dramatically whereas complement 3 increases only slightly. This implies that C-reactive protein may have a distinct role in the pathogenesis of adaptation to the acute phase response and also that its role during nonstressed periods is minimal. At the present time, how this diverse group of proteins interacts during the acute phase response is unknown.

The cytokines, a group of proteins from diverse origins, act as hormones with direct cell-to-cell interactions. Although a multitude of cytokines exist, the principal ones studied for their role in the acute phase response are interleukin-1 (IL-1) and tumor necrosis factor (TNF). IL-1 may actually represent a group of proteins released from macrophages after a variety of stimuli. Because IL-1 infusion in the experimental animal generates the classic response of endotoxemia, it may be part of the mechanism by which endotoxin has its effect.

While the clinical relevancy of many of the actions of cytokines is unknown, some cytokines do have pro-

found clinical significance. IL-1 may be the underlying instigator of the acute phase response. Infusion of IL-1 causes fever, leukocytosis, and accelerated synthesis of acute phase proteins. TNF has many similar properties with IL-1 and may either cause the release of IL-1 or may act synergistically with IL-1. Besides its interactions with IL-1, TNF, may have a role in the development and/or propagation of the cachectic state. Figure 5.4 shows the multitude of effects currently ascribed to IL-1. IL-1 induces skeletal muscle proteolysis, probably through the increased synthesis of PGE_2 which stimulates protein degradation. In addition, a 33-amino acid peptide termed proteolysis-inducing factor (PIF) has been described in the serum of septic patients with increased muscle catabolism (32,33). Certain cells have been demonstrated to have the ability to develop cytokine-specific receptors, which has led to clinical attempts to block the effects of cytokines by receptor blockade. In the future, this may offer a promising area for clinical intervention (34–36).

Interleukin-2 (IL-2) is a more recently discovered cytokine and probably is secreted from T cells after activation by IL-1. The main effect of IL-2 appears to be the stimulation and proliferation of T cells. A specific IL-2 receptor (IL-2-R) appears to be necessary for this action (34,37).

The importance of an adequate acute phase response to the integrity of the immune system, specifically, the end result of that response being immunocompetence, is vitally important for successful recovery from infection and/or injury. Nutritional modulation and interaction in the acute phase response is, therefore, of paramount importance. Several specific nutritional substrates have been investigated for their roles in the acute phase response. Glutamine, with its central role in various aspects of intermediary metabolism, has received the most attention.

Glutamine

It is becoming clear that the acute phase response can be modulated by early enteral nutrition. Enteral nutrition has been shown to maintain higher levels of constitutive proteins with respect to acute phase reactants. In contrast, parenteral nutrition alone results in an exaggerated acute phase and febrile response and an increase in TNF and C-reactive protein levels. Clinical studies have collaborated basic science studies of the protective effect of early enteral feeding in patients with the shock/trauma response (38–43).

The acidic amino acid glutamic acid occurs in protein largely as its corresponding acid-amide, glutamine. Recent evidence has demonstrated unique and specific metabolic properties of glutamine. Glutamine is an important nutrient for replicating cells, and cellular proliferation bears a close relationship to glutaminase activity. Different hypotheses have been proposed to account for

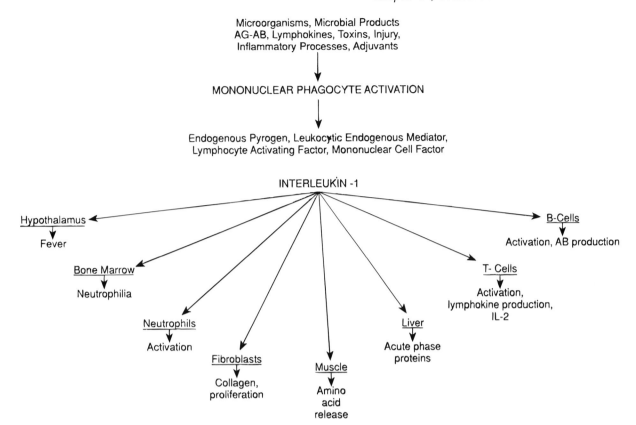

Figure 5.4. Effects of interleukin-1. Reprinted with permission from Dinarello CA. Interleukin-1 and the pathogenesis of the acute-phase response. New Engl J Med 1984;311 (32). *AG,* antigen complex; *AB,* antibody complex.

these findings. One is that high glutamine use may indicate a high rate of usage of glutamine as a nitrogen donor for nucleotide and/or other essential protein synthesis. A second is that glutamine may, via glutaminolysis, provide a source of energy and that during this process, glutamine offers a pathway for the transfer of carbon and nitrogen to other specific metabolites. Most likely, glutamine functions at several points in various pathways in replicating cells. Regardless of its specific activities, it is an important amino acid for these proliferating cells (28,29,38,39, 44–45).

A high rate of use of glutamine is characteristic of macrophages and lymphocytes and other cells. These cells show only partial oxidation of glutamine (glutaminolysis) with less than 10% of glutamine entering the citric acid cycle as acetyl-CoA and undergoing complete oxidation. Because these cells are capable of complete oxidation of fatty acids, excess glutaminolysis is probably not required as an energy source. It has been suggested that high rates of glutaminolysis are maintained in cells even when metabolically quiescent (for example, nonactivated lymphocytes) to furnish substrate for purine and pyrimidine synthesis in various cells of the immune system (28).

As a response to injury, sepsis, or burns, branched-chain amino acid (BCAA) metabolism in muscle preferentially increases. Although it was initially thought that increases in the use of branched-chain amino acids were

a mechanism to provide energy through gluconeogenesis, recent investigators have reported that this increase in BCAA use enables carbon and nitrogen donation in transamination for the formation of glutamine and alanine. Oxoacids from BCAA deamination are released by muscle and subsequently metabolized by other tissues. The net result is an increase in the amount of glutamine and alanine released from muscles, a change in the glutamine flux favoring that release, and therefore an increased availability of glutamine for rapidly replicating cells. This mechanism would thus provide a large and available pool to meet the increased need for glutamine (39,40).

Glutamine also has an established role in the renal response to acidosis and the subsequent generation of ammonia. The renal flux of glutamine increases substantially in acidosis. Glutamine is a principal substrate for proton disposal in the form of ammonia. The primary source of glutamine for the kidney appears to be via increased metabolism of branched-chain amino acids in the skeletal muscle.

In the nonstressed state, the principal organ of glutamine use is the gut. While glutamine is probably a major fuel source for gut mucosa, its role in providing purine and pyrimidine precursors and thus maintaining healthy gut mucosa is also predominant. The entero cycle can transport glutamine into the cell either from its luminal surface or from its interface with its vascular supply.

After surgical stress, intestinal glutamine metabolism is increased, and this increase appears to be mediated via glucagon and glucocorticoid hormones. This hormonal axis is also key in the metabolic demands during stress, including the increased requirements for synthesis of acute phase protein and antibodies. A component of this increased nitrogen turnover is autocannibalism of protein stores. While increased muscle proteolysis in stressed septic patients has been known for some time, only recently have cellular factors driving this proteolysis been elucidated. Interleukin-1 appears specifically to increase muscle proteolysis in vivo and in this regard has a synergistic effect with TNF. Thus one of the many manifestations of mediators of the acute phase response may account for the cachexia and muscle wasting apparent in the critically ill patient (33,36).

Amino acids liberated from skeletal muscle stores under the influence of these mediators are not necessarily used in the synthesis of required protein. Stressed patients preferentially metabolize skeletal muscle reserves of branched-chain amino acids. Multiple studies have demonstrated hyperglycemia, insulin resistance, and increased nitrogen excretion in these patients. Thus part of the manifestations of the "septic state" is a lack of ability to use glucose and fat as a fuel source. Ketogenesis is virtually completely suppressed in sepsis. This differs markedly from the fasting non-stressed individual in whom oxidation of fats becomes the primary fuel source. In the face of adequate glucose but an ineffectual metabolic machine for its oxidation, amino acids are metabolized for energy. Alanine, which is the major nitrogen transporter from skeletal muscle amino acid metabolism, is increased consistently in septic patients, whereas serum levels of the branched-chain amino acids (leucine, isoleucine, and valine) are decreased consistently. This lends strong support to the conclusion that branched-chain amino acids are being metabolized as fuel.

Glucose infusions, even in modest amounts, will decrease nitrogen losses in fasting patients. Although glucose and fat infusions in septic patients also lower nitrogen losses, this effect is much less dramatic. The addition of amino acids to carbohydrate and fat emulsions promotes a more rapid activation of the stress response and thus an increase in glutamine activity in gut mucosa. This may be protective of the integrity of the gut mucosa during nonseptic stress. Of prime importance is the maintenance of the integrity of the gut immune system (gut-associated lymphatic tissue—GALT). Gut glutamine flux is decreased during catabolic stress, and the lack of glutamine supplementation results in a decrease in IgA and an increase in bacterial translocation. These findings are reversed with adequate glutamine supplementation either parentally or via the gut lumen.

Stress associated with sepsis, however, has an opposite effect in gut glutamine activity. Gut glutamine uptake and glutaminase activity are decreased. Endotoxin infusion results in a loss of the gut mucosal barrier and subsequent septicemia. Although increases in cortisol increase proteolysis and glutamine availability, the gut use of glutamine becomes impaired despite increases in serum glutamine. Addition of glutamine to parenteral solutions has shown a reversal of the impaired immune responses, again demonstrating substrate-specific immune deficiencies. This lack of a specific substrate for gut mucosa has a direct effect on subsequent septicemia and, ultimately, mortality (39).

Arginine

Arginine is another amino acid that has been shown to have specific effects on the immune system, in particular tumor growth. Arginine promotes protein synthesis, and augments T cell mitogenesis and delayed hypersensitivity. Supplemental arginine impedes growth of immunogenic tumors in experimental animals and this may be secondary to augmentation of host antitumor responses (44). This effect was differentiated as a specific effect of arginine, as the effect was not apparent in glycine or low-protein-diet fed animals. Arginine augments thymic lymphocyte reactivity to a mitogen and increases production of interleukin-2. Thus arginine may enhance T cell proliferation with the development of specific cytotoxicity to tumor-associated antigens. Protein malnutrition should favor the growth of antigenic tumors because of the associated depression of the immune response. However, protein malnutrition has been shown to retard the growth of many experimental tumors, possibly because of the lack of substrate availability (37,45). Thus the enhancement of the immune response, in particular T cell responses in an immunosuppressive state by specific nutritional substrates, may have important clinical implications.

Arginine, in its L-form, is a precursor for the generation of nitrates, nitrites, and nitric oxide. These substances, which are vasodilatory, complement macrophage killing of tumor and bacteria, and thus are immunoenhancing.

Arginine is metabolized actively by the enterocyte. One pathway of arginine metabolism produces ornithine, which is a precursor for the polyamines putrescine, spermidine, and spermine. These polyamines are thought to be essential for cell growth and protein synthesis and have been shown to modulate hypo- and hyperplasia of the gut. Enteral fasting with parenteral nutritional support results in a decreased content of polyamines in the gut, which is reversed with resumption of enteral feeds. It is yet unknown how much arginine is required to maintain polyamine synthesis in the gut, and what quantities of polyamines are necessary for immunocompetence (46–48).

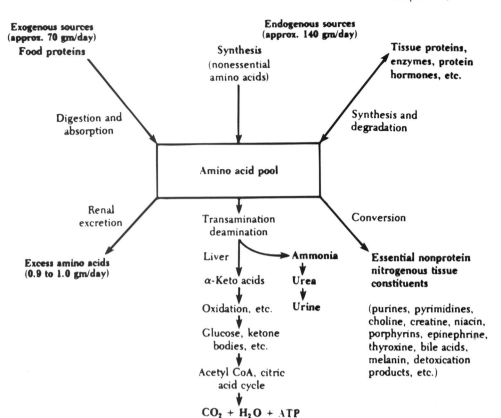

Figure 5.5. General paths of amino acids in metabolism in an average adult male. Reprinted with permission from Orten J, Neuhaus O. Human biochemistry. 10th ed. St. Louis: CV Mosby, 1968:327.

Amino Acid Metabolism and Protein-Sparing Therapy

Amino Acid Metabolism

Various sources contribute amino acids to aid metabolic function. Proteins from foodstuffs are broken down to free amino acids and allow transport to the liver. The exogenous source of protein approximates 70 g/day. In addition, there is an ongoing catabolism of body tissues, and a large proportion of these endogenous amino acids are derived from tissue recycling. This mechanism may provide up to 140 g of protein per day. A third source of amino acids is synthesis of nonessential amino acids, i.e., those that can be synthesized from other amino acid precursors, either through transamination or deamination reactions. As shown in Figure 5.5, these sources form the *amino acid pool*. There are essentially three pathways out of the pool. The first is through various conversion reactions to form essential nonprotein but nitrogen-containing compounds. Examples are purines and pyrimidines for DNA and RNA synthesis. A second major use of the pool is through transamination and deamination reactions with conversion to α-keto acids and eventually oxidation as an energy source. The remaining pathway is by product excretion, usually via the kidneys, in the form of urea.

The Concept of Protein Sparing

There is a continual turnover of amino acid nitrogen in the body. In healthy adult males on a protein-free diet, the average obligatory nitrogen loss is approximately 0.05 g/kg/day. Thus a 70-kg man has an obligatory nitrogen loss of approximately 3.5 g/day. This nitrogen is lost mostly in the urine, primarily as urea. Secondary losses occur through the feces, saliva, and wounds. In stressed patients, nitrogen loss has been reported as high as 15 to 20 g/day. While most of this nitrogen is a reflection of increased negative nitrogen balance, it is also the result of stimulated protein synthesis and decreased protein usage. In particular, solutions with high concentrations of branched-chain amino acids have been shown to be superior to those without such high concentrations with regard to protein sparing. Hence, the working hypothesis is that protein can be spared and thus be made available for required metabolic functions (wound healing, immunoglobulin synthesis, etc.) by infusions of specific substrates that can be used as preferred fuel sources. Unfortunately, although measurements of protein metabolism and synthesis (e.g., 3-methylhistidine excretion and nitrogen balance) can become normalized, it has not been documented that the return of these values toward normal significantly decreases morbidity or improves patient outcome (27,32,49–55).

The recent recognition of glutamine as a key amino acid in proliferating cells, and in particular its role in the competency of the immune system, has led to an alternate hypothesis as to the preferential oxidation of branched-chain amino acids. Muscle takes up branched-chain amino acids and releases alanine and glutamine.

Rodent experiments have documented that in the septic state, the increase in branched-chain amino acid metabolism in skeletal muscle may not be to provide a fuel source but rather to provide a nitrogen source for the synthesis of glutamine. The oxoacids generated through branched-chain amino acid metabolism are released by muscle and are then further metabolized by other tissues. Thus preferential oxidation of branched-chain amino acids may not signify an inability of glucose use by skeletal muscle in the septic state as much as being an essential adaptation to ensure a continuous source of glutamine in the stressed individual (28).

The goal of clinical nutritional support is to furnish sufficient substrate to maintain an adequate energy source to fuel the metabolic functions of the individual. It is also to provide adequate protein so that body auto-cannibalism of protein stores is minimized. Clinical studies have documented that between 100 to 150 cals per gram of nitrogen is sufficient in the mild to moderately stressed patient to provide enough calories to avoid the use of administered protein as a fuel source. This ratio varies, however, depending on the disease process and the quality of protein given. Continuing measurements of nitrogen balance are most beneficial in assessing the appropriateness of fuel sources and the success of protein-sparing therapy.

Nutrition and Immunity

Protein-calorie malnutrition has a profound effect on the integrity of the immune system. Not only is there a lack of available substrate for energy production and protein synthesis, but there are specific substrates with specific actions on immunoresponsiveness. The converse is that the lack of these nutrients can cause immune deficiencies.

Protein-calorie malnutrition results in a clinical syndrome of anergy, weight loss, and cachexia. There is a decrease in the generation of recall antigens, a decrease in migration of polymorphonucleocytes (PMNs) in response to bacterial chemotactic factors, and a decrease in phagocytosis. These deficiencies are related directly to protein-calorie malnutrition and are evidenced by the fact that all are restored to normal with adequate protein-calorie repletion (56).

Multiple reports have shown that enteral feeding in patients enhances the global immune response. Burn patients have probably been studied more extensively than any other group. Major thermal injury results in decreased levels of complement with impaired opsonic and neutrophil activity. Lack of enteral feeding results in increases in bacterial translocation, macrophage activation by endotoxin, and the accelerated release of interleukins, TNF, thromboxanes, and prostaglandins. Immunosuppression can be decreased by increasing protein content in an enteral diet. In addition, the amount of jejunal mucosa atrophy that occurs after major thermal injury can be decreased with gut feedings (57–60).

Fibronectin is an immune system protein strongly related to nutrition. Decreased serum levels of fibronectin invariably reflect protein malnutrition—so closely, in fact, that fibronectin can be used as a nutritional marker. In addition, fibronectin has parallel relationships with other commonly measured immune proteins such as prealbumin and transferrin. Decreases in fibronectin are seen with short-term starvation. It is a ubiquitous protein with multiple effects. Although its role as an opsonin has been well-documented, it is now known to be a monocyte stimulator and enhances monocyte phagocytosis of complement immunoglobulin-coated cells. In addition, it appears that fibronectin by-products also possess immunoregulatory properties (61, 62). Thus decreases in fibronectin due to malnutrition have considerable implications in immune system competence.

Natural immunity refers to the general processes of immune functions, which are not particularly related to any specific toxin. Examples of this include resistance of the skin to invasion by organisms and destruction of organisms by acid secretions of the stomach. The complement cascade is a system of about 20 different proteins that, through a series of reactions, generates by-products with specific activities in the immune system. Because of the generic by-products produced, the complement system can be considered a component of the innate immune system. Tissue injury, in general, causes complement activation and bradykinin production. This generates inflammatory mediators that cause degranulation of tissue mast cells. The net effect is an increase in vascular permeability, accumulation of acute phase proteins and immune complexes, and chemotaxis of leukocytes. Mobilized neutrophils phagocytose and kill pathogenic organisms. In acute protein depletion, the intensity of this response is decreased, granulocytosis and chemotaxis are decreased, and fever is attenuated. In addition, the intensity of the acute phase response is lessened. Levels of IL-2, the underlying mediator for the effects of malnutrition on innate immunity may be a deficiency of IL-1 (63).

Acquired immunity is a more specific immunity that is developed against individual invading organisms. There are two basic types of acquired immunity: 1) humoral, modulated by B cell activation in which circulating antibodies are directed toward specific antigens; and 2) cell-mediated, which is immunity based on the formation of activated lymphocytes (T cells). In prolonged malnutrition, there is a persistent and constant lymphopenia. Several abnormalities in T lymphocytes have been documented. There is a decrease in the rate and number of rosette-forming E lymphocytes, T helper cell function is decreased, and the relationship of T suppressor (T8) to T helper (T4) cells is altered. While the total population of T cells is reduced with malnutrition, the ratio of T8 to T4 is also reduced, thus resulting in excessive T suppressor cell activity. Although serum levels of immunoglobulins may remain normal, there is a detrimental effect on the production of antibodies. Antibody response to T cell-dependent antigens is inhibited specifically, and IgG is more affected than IgM. Antibodies that show the highest specificity are those that appear to have the most pronounced effects from malnutrition (62–64).

The role of lipids as essential nutrients and their role in immunomodulation has recently been better defined. Particularly, the ω-3 polyunsaturated fatty acids (ω-3 PUFA) have demonstrated immunoenhancing properties. The main immunoenhancing role of ω-3 PUFA may be in decreasing PGE$_2$ production. Polyunsaturated fatty acids have been shown to have effects on immunocompetence. PGE$_2$ in the presence of antigens, and activated complement induces a subset of T suppressor cells and directly inhibits T cell function, most likely by suppressing IL-1. PGE$_2$ may also suppress the production of other cytokines. Whether this response is harmful or beneficial to host immunocompetency is unknown (58).

Metabolic Diseases

All known human diseases have metabolic consequences. However, there are some in which the primary derangement is metabolic in origin. Some of these diseases will be discussed.

Diabetes Mellitus

Diabetes mellitus is the third leading cause of death in the United States and represents a spectrum of inherited and acquired disorders characterized by blood sugar levels greater than 140 mg/dl in the fasting subject. Because insulin is the primary hormone of anabolism and growth and the effector of fuel storage, a lack of insulin function results in catabolism. Glucose uptake and oxidation in muscle is decreased, and glycogenolysis predominates. Gluconeogenic amino acids (primarily alanine) are released from muscle to provide the liver with substrate. In untreated diabetes mellitus, there is a decrease in adipose tissue, fatty acid, and glucose uptake and an increase in lipolysis. The released fatty acids are metabolized to ketones in the liver. The result is an excess of glucose in the circulation secondary to overproduction and underutilization.

The two main types of diabetes are Type I (insulin dependent) and Type II (non-insulin dependent). In Type I, there is an insulin deficiency caused by pancreatic β cell destruction, whereas in Type II, there is an insulin deficit, insulin resistance, and a defect in the intracellular postreceptor response. Type I is controlled by diet and insulin therapy. Type II should be managed by weight control, exercise, and diet combined with either oral hypoglycemic agents or insulin (64–65). Recent studies have shown that in patients with severe obesity and diabetes, weight loss induced by a gastric partition has controlled the diabetes (66–Pories Ann Surg.).

Primary Hyperlipoproteinemias

The primary hyperlipoproteinemias are metabolic disorders characterized by an excess of one or more lipoproteins in the circulation. They have been subdivided into five categories by Fredrickson, a categorization that bears his name. Type 1 is rare; it is characterized by an elevation of exogenous triglycerides in the form of chylomicrons as a result of a genetic defect in the clearance of chylomicrons from the blood. Familial hypercholesterolemia, also known as type 2a, results from a single-gene defect in the cell receptor that binds circulatory low-density lipoprotein (LDL). Normally, the cell-surface receptor delivers cholesterol to the cells, which in turn regulates endogenous cholesterol synthesis and suppress the synthesis of the LDL receptor. In the homozygote, there is a marked increase in LDL synthesis, a decrease in its removal, and minimal regulation of endogenous cholesterol synthesis. These patients have hypercholesterolemia from birth, corneal arcus, and tendon xanthomas. They also have an incidence of coronary artery disease 25 times that of the normal population and an average life expectancy of 21 years. Childhood myocardial infarctions are common in these patients. Type 2b differs in that there is both hypercholesterolemia and hypertriglyceridemia with increases in LDL and very low density lipoprotein (VLDL). Type 3 hyperlipoproteinemia is associated with an increase in intermediate-density lipoprotein (IDL). In Type 4, endogenous triglycerides and VLDL levels are mildly elevated. Severe increases in triglycerides with elevated chylomicrons and VLDL levels characterize the Type 5 defect. Both Type 1 and Type 5 can present as recurrent pancreatitis. The clinical response to dietary therapy primarily depends on the severity of the underlying lipemia and is relatively independent of the clinical type. The goals of therapy are to reduce plasma LDL, maximize high-density lipoprotein (HDL) concentrations, and reduce plasma triglyceride concentrations (65).

Acromegaly

Acromegaly is a disease characterized by excessive growth hormone secretion. Growth hormone stimulates long bone growth, protein synthesis, and fatty acid oxidation. It is associated with a positive calcium balance and suppressed peripheral glucose intake. Characteristically, patients with acromegaly have physical findings that result from increased bone and connective tissue synthesis. In addition, there is an increase in basal metabolic rate, glucose intolerance, and a resultant decrease in total body fat (67).

Hyperthyroidism

The thyroid hormones thyroxine (T_4) and triiodothyronine (T_3) regulate many aspects of cellular metabolism. Through the modulation of cellular functions, they regulate oxygen consumption and determine resting metabolic rate.

Hyperthyroidism is associated with an increase in basal temperature, cellular thermogenesis, caloric requirement, and activity of the sodium-potassium pump. Patients also demonstrate weight loss in spite of hyperphagia and are predisposed to an accelerated rate of starvation. Adipose tissue lipolysis is accelerated with increased blood levels of fatty acids and glycerol, and increased fatty acid oxidation and ketonuria are often present. A mild impairment of glucose tolerance usually occurs because of increased gastrointestinal transport and absorption and accelerated hepatic gluconeogenesis. Glucose use via oxidative phosphorylation is increased in extrahepatic tissues.

Other metabolic derangements have been noted in states of hyperthyroidism. There is an increase in bone turnover and destruction with resultant hypercalcemia and raised urinary clearance of calcium and phosphorus. Patients may develop osteoporosis and osteitis fibrosa. Depression of the vitamin A transport system exists, with resultant decreases in serum levels of vitamin A, retinol-binding protein, and prealbumin. However, intestinal absorption and hepatic stores of vitamin A are increased. Because thyroid hormones directly stimulate the conversion of riboflavin to flavin mononucleotide and flavin adenine dinucleotide, there is an increased requirement for riboflavin. Also, the stimulation of pyridoxine degradation appears to result in decreased tissue levels and increased requirements of pyridoxine (68,69).

Cushing's syndrome

Glucocorticoids are the major secretory products of the adrenal cortex and are responsible for the long-term control of intermediary metabolism. These are counterregulatory hormones to insulin and are responsible for the maintenance of adequate blood glucose levels during periods of decreased intake and stress. They also affect the state of negative nitrogen balance by increased protein catabolism and nitrogen excretion. This is done via the proteolysis of muscle, stimulation of gluconeogenesis, and the inhibition of protein synthesis in peripheral tissues. Lipolysis is stimulated, whereas lipid synthesis is inhibited owing to decreased glucose uptake and glycerol synthesis by adipose cells. Because calcium is transported into the cells, urinary excretion is increased and serum calcium levels are lowered.

Chronic hypercortisolism produces important nutritional and metabolic abnormalities which include impaired glucose tolerance and a net loss of lean body mass. Decreased calcium levels stimulate a secondary rise in parathyroid hormone levels with resultant osteopenia (70).

Addison's Disease

Addison's disease is adrenal insufficiency usually associated with weight loss that is directly proportionate to the severity of the disease. Despite this relationship, it is unclear whether cortisol is required to maintain lean body mass. Weight loss may result from decreased caloric intake secondary to anorexia and other gastrointestinal symptoms. During periods of reduced caloric intake or stress, these patients develop hypoglycemia. The associated mineralocorticoid deficiency promotes sodium loss and volume depletion. This, coupled with abnormalities in calcium metabolism, results in hypercalcemia (67).

Pheochromocytoma

Although the secretion of epinephrine and norepinephrine vary with each individual pheochromocytoma, consistent metabolic alterations exist due to the similar effects of these hormones. Energy expenditure and rates of glucose oxidation may be increased up to 40%. There is impaired insulin secretion and glucose intolerance and substantial weight loss. Episodic hypertension, the hallmark of the pheochromocytoma, usually presents along with symptoms of flushing, headache, anxiety, and, in advanced cases, symptoms of renal insufficiency. The condition will be described in greater detail in another portion of the text.

Inborn Errors of Metabolism

In 1908, Sir Archibald Garrod first described inborn errors of metabolism (71). The modern definition includes any genetically determined biochemical disorder that results in inherited abnormalities of protein molecules. Currently, approximately 4000 disorders have been described, and most are inherited as either autosomal recessive or X-linked recessive traits. Whether a particular trait is dominant or recessive depends on the degree of disruption the mutation has on the gene product and on the capability of homeostatic systems. The variability seen among individuals grouped together having a particular disorder is the result of: 1) variability among mutant alleles at the particular locus; 2) variability in the genetic makeup of all other loci; and 3) environmental differences in habits, customs, and experiences (70). The general mechanism involved in producing a disorder results from either the accumulation of a toxic precursor, the overproduction of a product from an alternate pathway, a deficit of product, or some combination of these factors. If diet is the most important source of the metabolite, accumulated precursors can be reduced through dietary restriction. Nutritional therapy may also be directed at providing a deficient product, but this requires that a biologically usable form of the product can be supplied in the diet. The following disorders are illustrative of these principles.

Phenylketonuria

Phenylketonuria (PKU) is a relatively common disease that results from a deficiency of hepatic phenylalanine hydroxylase (Fig. 5.6). Before current neonatal screening, the diagnosis was not made until 6 to 8 months of age with the appearance of developmental delays, mental retardation, eczematoid dermatitis, and seizures. The accumulation of the precursor, phenylalanine, produced the observed toxicity (70). Nutritional therapy restricts phenylalanine intake sufficient to meet growth requirements and obligatory losses. Adequate amounts of tyrosine are also supplied. Therapy is monitored by studying growth parameters, intellectual development, and plasma amino acid concentrations (72).

Maple Syrup Urine Disease

Maple syrup urine disease is a rare disorder that is associated with a deficiency of the branched-chain keto acid decarboxylase (Fig. 5.7). Infants with this disorder have lethargy, anorexia, vomiting, ketosis, metabolic acidosis, and central nervous system depression, eventually resulting in death. Because the transamination reactions are reversible, both the branched-chain amino acid and keto acid accumulate are responsible for the clinical symptoms. The keto acids are excreted in the urine and are responsible for the characteristic odor. Therapy is aimed primarily at restricting branched-chain amino acid intake to an amount that is just sufficient for normal

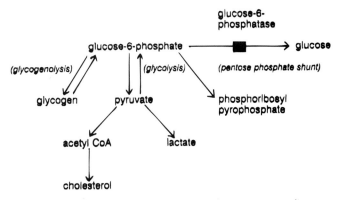

Figure 5.8. The metabolic block in type I glycogen storage disease. Abnormal symptoms are the result of both product deficiency and alternate pathway overproduction.

growth. Because the decarboxylase enzyme is thiamine dependent, occasional cases will respond favorably to thiamine administration. Plasma amino acid concentrations and growth parameters must be monitored carefully (70).

Type I Glycogen Storage Disease

Also known as von Gierke's disease, this disorder is characterized by a deficiency of glucose 6-phosphatase activity. This enzyme is essential for the release of glucose from the liver. Hepatic glucose production is responsible for the maintenance of blood sugar concentrations between meals. In patients with von Gierke's disease, blood glucose levels fall, stimulating the secretion of epinephrine and glucagon, which in turn stimulates hepatic glycogenolysis and gluconeogenesis , a glucose 6-phosphate dependent process (Fig. 5.8). Alternate pathways, such as glycolysis, glycogen synthesis, and the pentose phosphate shunt, are used in excess. Clinical features include neonatal growth failure, hepatomegaly, increased facial fat, xanthomas, and hepatic adenomas. Hypoglycemia and metabolic acidosis are often severe. The pathophysiologic mechanism includes both product deficiency and alternate pathway overproduction. Nutritional therapy requires frequent feeding with glucose or glucose polymers as the sole source of carbohydrate. As the patient grows older, the addition of cornstarch to the diet has been shown to be useful in prolonging intervals between feedings. The long-term outlook is good when treated early and symptomatic hypoglycemia is circumvented (73).

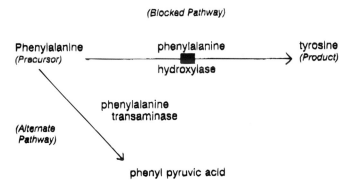

Figure 5.6. Metabolic clock and alternate pathway in phenylketonuria. The diagram includes schematic labels to demonstrate the principles of metabolic derangements in inborn errors.

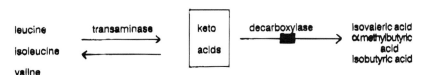

Figure 5.7. The metabolic block in maple syrup urine disease. The deficiency of decarboxylase coupled with the reversibility of transamination cause the accumulation of both branched-chain amino acids and keto acids.

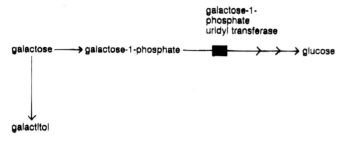

Figure 5.9. The metabolic block in galactosemia. Toxicity is the result of the accumulation of the precursors galactose and galactose 1-phosphate in addition to galactitol, a product of an alternate pathway.

Galactosemia

Galactosemia is an autosomal recessive disorder resulting in the deficient activity of galactosyl-1-phosphate uridyl-transferase (Fig. 5.9). This is one of the enzymes in the pathway by which galactose is converted to glucose. Both precursors accumulate in addition to galactitol, a product of an alternate pathway. Infants with this disease present with poor feeding, vomiting, diarrhea, failure to thrive, jaundice, abnormal liver function, metabolic acidosis, and a mild hemolytic anemia only a few days after the introduction of dietary lactose. After several months, cataracts may be observed. Nutritional therapy is aimed at the elimination of dietary lactose (70).

Summary

Nutritional support in the 1990's is no longer merely ensuring the provision of adequate calories to the surgical patient. Rather, the explosion of scientific research in the field of nutritional support, in particular as it relates to the severely injured or critically ill patient, has defined numerous areas for interventional nutritional therapy. Altering the biological response to disease or enhancing host defense mechanisms by using specific substrates has come out of the basic science laboratory and into the clinical arena. Indeed, the coining of the terms "nutritional pharmacology" and "nutritional immunology" emphasizes not only the complexities of nutritional support, but the importance of its correct application. This chapter has been an attempt to give an overview of the current status of what would be expected for nutritional support as surgery moves into the 21st century.

REFERENCES

1. Aoi S, Wen L, Kuwahata T, et al. Alteration in the ribonucleic acids in rat liver induced by methionine-free total parenteral nutrition. Am J Clin Nutr 1986;117:673–677.
2. Solomons NW, Young VR. The major nutrients. In: Paige DM, ed. Clinical nutrition. 2nd ed. St. Louis: CV Mosby, 1988:16–35.
3. Kirkpatrick JR. Fat and energy metabolism. In: Kirkpatrick JR, ed. Nutrition and metabolism in the surgical patient. Mount Kisco: Futura, 1983:3–28.
4. Cahill GF Jr. Starvation in man. N Engl J Med 1980;282:668–675.
5. Wolfe BM, Ney DM. Lipid metabolism in parenteral nutrition. In: Rombeau JL, Caldwell MD, eds. Clinical nutrition. Vol. 2. Parenteral nutrition. Philadelphia: WB Saunders, 1986:72–99.
6. Burr GO, Burr MM. A new deficiency disease produced by the rigid exclusion of fat from the diet. J Biol Chem 1929;82:345–367.
7. Burr GO, Burr MM. On the nature of the role of the fatty acids essential in nutrition. J Biol Chem 1930;86:587–621.
8. Blackburn GL, Bistrian BR, Homsy FN. Protein metabolism in the surgical patient. In: Kirkpatrick JR, ed. Nutrition and metabolism in the surgical patient. Mount Kisco: Futura, 1983:59–87.
9. Stein TP. Protein metabolism and parenteral nutrition. In: Rombeau JL, Caldwell MD, eds. Clinical nutrition. Vol. 2. Parenteral nutrition. Philadelphia: WB Saunders, 1986:100–134.
10. Stein TP, Buzby GP. Protein metabolism in surgical patients. Surg Clin North Am 1981;61:519–527.
11. Morgan DB, Hill GL, Burkinshaw L. The assessment of weight loss from a single measurement of body weight: the problems and limitations. Am J Clin Nutr 1980;33:2101–2105.
12. Studley HO. Percentage of weight loss. A basic indicator of surgical risk in patients with chronic peptic ulcer. JAMA 1936;106:458–460.
13. Gadisseux P, Ward JD, Young HF, Becker DP. Nutrition and the neurosurgical patient. J Neurosurg 1984;60:219–232.
14. Pettigrew RA, Hill GL. Indicators of surgical risk and clinical judgement. Br J Surg 1986;73:47–51.
15. Moore FD. Energy and the maintenance of the body cell mass. JPEN 1980;4:228–260.
16. Moore FD, Olesen KG, McMurray JD, Parker HV, Ball MR, Boyden CM. The body cell mass and its supporting environment: body composition in health and disease. Philadelphia: WB Saunders, 1963:19–28.
17. Hill GL, Beddoe AH. Dimensions of the human body and its compartments. In: Kinney JM, Jeejeebhoy KN, Hill GL, Owen OE, eds. Nutrition and metabolism in patient care: Philadelphia: WB Saunders, 1988:89–118.
18. Wolfe BM, Ruderman RL, Pollard A. Basic principles of surgical nutrition: metabolic response to starvation, trauma, and sepsis. In: Deitel M, ed. Nutrition in clinical surgery. 2nd ed. Baltimore: Williams & Wilkins, 1985:14–23.
19. Frisancho AR. New standards of weight and body composition by frame size and height for assessment of nutritional status of adults and the elderly. Am J Clin Nutr 1984;40:808–819.
20. Harrison GG, Van Italie TB. Estimation of body composition: A new approach based on electromagnetic principles. Am J Clin Nutr 1982;32:524–526.
21. Byers PM. Trauma and nutritional support. In: Kreis DJ Jr, Gomez GA, eds. Trauma management. Boston: Little, Brown, 1989;491–522.
22. Moore FD, Olesen KH, McMurray JD, Parker HV, Ball MR, Boyden CM. The body cell mass and its supporting environment: Body composition in health and disease. Philadelphia: WB Saunders Company, 1963:19–28.
23. Kinney JM, Lister J, Moore FD. Relationship of energy expenditure to total exchangeable potassium. Ann N Y Acad Sci 1963;110:711–722.
24. Chance B, Veech RL. Phosphorous magnetic spectroscopy as a probe of nutritional state. In: Kinney JM, Jeejeebhoy KN, Hill GL, Owen OE, eds. Nutrition and metabolism in patient care. Philadelphia: WB Saunders, 1988:119–128.
25. Veech RL. The toxic impact of parenteral solutions of the metabolism of cells: a hypothesis for physiological parenteral therapy. Am J Clin Nutr 1986;44:519–551.
26. Kushner I. The phenomenon of the acute phase response. Ann N Y Acad Sci 1982;39–48.
27. Hasselgren O, Jagenburg R, Karlstrom L, et al. Changes of protein metabolism in liver and skeletal muscle following trauma complicated by sepsis. J Trauma 1984;24(3):224–228.
28. Newsholme EA, Newsholme P, Curi R. The role of the citric acid cycle in cells of the immune system and its importance in sepsis, trauma, and burns. Biochem Soc Symp 1987;54:145–161.
29. Newsholme EA, Parry-Billings N. Properties of glutamine release from muscle and its importance for the immune system. J Parent Ent Nutr 1990;14(4):40S–45S, 45S–50S, 63S–67S.

30. Brown JM, Grosso MA, Harken AH. Cytokines, sepsis and the surgeon. Surg Gynecol Obstet 1989;169:568–575.

31. Dinarello CA. Interleukin-1 and the pathogenesis of the acute-phase response. New Engl J Med 1984;311(32):1413–1418.

32. Cerra FB, Mazuski JE, Chute E, et al. Branched chain metabolic support. Ann Surg 1983;199(3):286–291.

33. Clowes GH, George BC, Villee CA, et al. Muscle proteolysis induced by circulating peptide in patients with sepsis or trauma. New Engl J Med 1983;308(10):545–552.

34. Grzelak I, Olszewski WL, Rowinski W. Blood mononuclear cell production of IL-1 and IL-2 following moderate surgical trauma. Eur Surg Res 1989;21:114–122.

35. Beisel WR. Role of nutrition in immune system diseases. Compr Ther 1987;13(1):13–19.

36. Pomposelli JJ, Flores EA, Bistrian BR. Role of biochemical mediators in clinical nutrition and surgical metabolism. JPEN 1988;12(2):212–218.

37. Reynolds JV, Shou J, Sigal R, et al. The influence of protein malnutrition on T-cell, natural killer cell, and lymphokine-activated killer cell function, and on biological responsiveness to high-dose interleukin-2. Cell Immunol 1990;128:569–577.

38. Smith RJ. Glutamine metabolism and its physiologic importance. JPEN 1990;14(4):40S–44S.

39. Souba WW, Herskowitz K, Salloum R, et al. Gut glutamine metabolism. JPEN 1990;14(4):40S–44S, 45S–50S, 63S–67S.

40. Firmansyah A, Penn D, Lebenthal E. Isolated colonocyte metabolism of glucose, glutamine, n-butyrate, and B-hydroxybutyrate in malnutrition. Gastroenterol 1989;97:622–629.

41. Kudsk KA, Minard G, Wojtysiak SL, Croce M, Fabian T, Brown RO. Visceral protein response to enteral versus parenteral nutrition and sepsis in patients with trauma. Surgery 1994;116(3):516–523.

42. Cynober L. Can arginine and ornithine support gut functions. Gut 1994;Supplement 1:S42–S45.

43. Brown RO, Hunt H, Mowatt-Larssen CA, Wojtysiak SL, Henningfield MF, Kudsk KA. Comparison of specialized and standard enteral formulas in trauma patients. Pharmacotherapy 1944;14(3):314–320.

44. Reynolds JV, Thom AK, Zhang SM, et al. Arginine, protein malnutrition, and cancer. J Surg Res 1988;45:513–522.

45. Karpeh MS, Kehne JA, Choi SH, et al. Tumor immunogenicity, nutritional repletion, and cancer. Surgery 1987;102(2):283–290.

46. Cerra FB, Lehmann S, Konstantinides N, Dzik J, Fish J, Konstantinides F, LiCari JJ, Holman RT. Improvement in immune function in ICU patients by enteral nutrition supplemented with arginine, RNA, and menhaden oil is independent of nitrogen balance. Nutrition 1991;7(3):193–199.

47. Alexander JW, Gottschlich MM. Nutritional immunomodulation in burn patients. Crit Care Med 1990;18(2):S149–S153.

48. Alexander JW. Nutrition and translocation. Journal of Parenteral and Enteral Nutrition 1990;Suppl 14(5):170S–174S.

49. von Meyenfeldt MF, Soeters PB, Vente JP, et al. Effect of branched-chain amino acid enrichment of total parenteral nutrition of nitrogen sparing and clinical outcome of sepsis and trauma: a prospective randomized double blind trial. Br J Surg 1982;92(2):192–199.

50. O'Donnell TF, Clowes G, Blackburn GL, et al. Proteolysis associated with deficit of peripheral energy fuel substrates in septic man. Surg 1976;80(2):192–200.

51. Cerra FB, Mazuski J, Teasley K, et al. Nitrogen retention in critically ill patients is proportional to the branched-chain amino acid load. Crit Care Med 1983;11(14):775–778.

52. Cerra FB, Mazuski JE, Chute E, et al. Branched chain metabolic support. Ann Surg 1983;199(3):286–291.

53. Herndon DN, Stein MD, Rutan TC, et al. Failure of TPN supplementation to improve liver function, immunity, and mortality in thermally injured patients. J Trauma 1987;27(2):195–204.

54. Daly JM, Reynolds J, Sigal RK, et al. Effect of dietary protein and amino acids on immune function. CCM 1990;18(2):586–593.

55. Hoyt DB, Ozkan N, Easter D, et al. Isolation of an immunosuppressive trauma peptide and its relationship to fibronectin. J Trauma 1988;28(7):907–913.

56. Garre MA, Boles JM, Youinou PY. Current concepts in immune derangement due to undernutrition. JPEN 1987;11(3):309–313.

57. Waymack JP, Herndon DN. Nutritional support of the burned patient. World J Surg 1992;16:80–86.

58. Peck MD. Omega-3 polyunsaturated fatty acids: Benefit or harm during sepsis? New Horizons 1994;2(2):230–236.

59. Lowry SF. The route of feeding influences injury responses. J Trauma 1990;Supplement 12(30):S10–S15.

60. Alexander JW. Immunoenhancement via enteral nutrition. Arch Surg 1993;128:1242–1245.

61. Wan J, Haw M, Blackburn GL. Proceedings of the nutrition, immune function, and inflammation; an overview. Proc Nutr Soc 1989;48:315–335.

62. Nohr CW, Tchervenkov JI, Meakins JL, et al. Malnutrition and humoral immunity: long-term protein deprivation. J Surg Res 1986;40:432–437.

63. Abbott WC, Tayek JA, Bistian BR, et al. The effect of nutritional support on T-lymphocyte subpopulations in protein calorie malnutrition. J Am Coll Nutr 1986;5:577–584.

64. Shuman CR. Diabetes mellitus. In: Kinney JM, Jeejeebhoy KN, Hill GL, Owen OE, eds. Nutrition and metabolism in patient care. Philadelphia: WB Saunders, 1988:360–385.

65. Katzeff JL, Rivlin RS. Endocrine diseases. In: Kinney JM. Jeejeebhoy KN, Hill GL, Owen OE, eds. Nutrition and metabolism in patient care. Philadelphia: WB Saunders, 1988:342–359.

66. Pories, WJ, Swanson, MS, MacDonald, KJ, et al. Who would have thought it? An operation proves to be the most effective therapy for adult onset diabetes mellitus. Presented at the American Surgical Association, Chicago, Illinois, April, 1995. In press, Annals of Surgery.

67. Kimberg DV, Baerg RD, Gershon E, Graudusius RT. Effect of cortisone treatment on the active transport of calcium by the small intestine. J Clin Invest 50:1309–1321.

68. Mundy GR, Shapiro JL, Bandelin JG, Canalis EM, Raiez LG. Direct stimulation of bone resorption by thyroid hormones. J Clin Invest 1976;58:529–534.

69. Cama HR, Goodwin TW. Studies in vitamin A. The role of the thyroid in carotene and vitamin A metabolism. Biochem J 1949;45:236–241.

70. Valle D, Mitchell GA. Inborn errors of metabolism. In: Paige DM, ed. Clinical nutrition. 2nd ed. St. Louis: CV Mosby, 1988:609–627.

71. Gerrod A. Inborn errors of metabolism [Croonian lectures]. Lancet 1908;2:1–7.

72. Scriver CR, Clow CL. Phenylketonuria: epitome of human biochemical genetics. N Engl J Med 1980;303:1336–1342, 1394–1400.

73. Chen YT, Cornblath M, Sidbury JB. Cornstarch therapy in type I glycogen storage disease. N Engl J Med 1984;310:171–175.

6 Wound Healing Biology and its Application to Wound Management

W. Thomas Lawrence

I dressed the wound; God healed it.

-Ambroise Paré, 16th Century (1)

Introduction

Over the centuries, many medicinal agents have been placed on wounds in hopes of improving healing. To date, nothing has been identified that can accelerate healing in a clinically meaningful manner in a normal individual. Many agents have hindered the healing process more than they have helped it. As Paré's statement suggests, a surgeon's goal in wound management is to create an environment where the healing process can proceed in an optimal fashion. To accomplish this goal, a biologically oriented surgeon must understand the physiologic mechanisms involved in the wound healing process. Paré, himself, was one of the first to use the scientific method to study wound healing. He demonstrated the deleterious effect of applying hot oils to fresh open wounds, a common practice in 16th century Europe.

The capacity for direct scientific measurements has exploded in recent decades. A great deal has been learned about the biochemistry, molecular biology, and cell physiology of the individual events that lead to a healed wound. Although the healing process varies slightly in different tissues, the physiologic mechanisms are similar. In this chapter, healing in skin will be discussed primarily, although the principles outlined are applicable to all mammalian tissues.

The healing process can be broken down into early, intermediate, late, and terminal phases. Each phase is characterized by specific biologic processes. The primary activities involved in the early phase of healing are inflammation and the creation of hemostasis. Mesenchymal cell proliferation and migration, epithelialization, and angiogenesis are the primary events of the intermediate phase. Central events of the late phase of

118

healing include the synthesis of collagen and other matrix proteins and wound contraction. The terminal phase of healing is characterized by wound remodeling. Each of these phases will be discussed as a separate entity even though the phases blend from one to another with no clear boundaries between them (Fig. 6.1).

Phases of Healing

Early Wound Healing Events

In all injuries that penetrate the epidermis, blood vessels are disrupted, resulting in hemorrhage. Hemostasis must be the first event achieved in the healing process. Cellular damage occurs with any injury, and this initiates an inflammatory response. The inflammatory response triggers events that have implications for the entire healing process.

Hemostasis is created primarily by aggregated platelets and fibrin. Platelets aggregate when exposed to extravascular collagen (2,3). Platelets adhere to collagen and release adenosine diphosphate (ADP), which, in the presence of calcium, stimulates further platelet aggregation. Thrombin produced by the coagulation cascade and fatty acids released by injured cells also contribute to continuing platelet aggregation (4). Platelet adhesion to other platelets and to collagen is mediated by four adhesive glycoproteins: fibrinogen, fibronectin, thrombospondin, and von Willebrand factor. These factors derive from both the serum and the alpha granules of platelets (5). Platelet aggregation also leads to the release of cytokines that reside in the alpha granules. These include platelet-derived growth factor (PDGF), transforming growth factor-alpha (TGF-α), and transforming growth factor-β (TGF-β), and they play critical roles in later aspects of healing.

The intrinsic and extrinsic coagulation cascades are triggered by separate events (6). The intrinsic coagula-

Injury

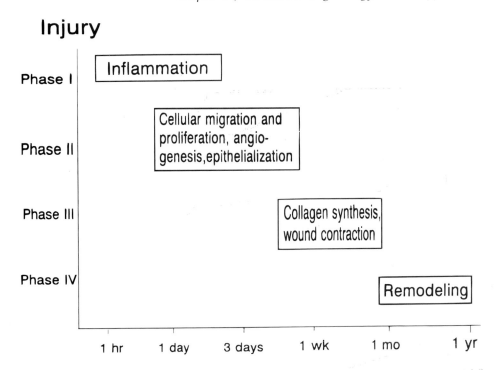

Figure 6.1. Sequence of events in wound healing. Modified from Stevenson TR, Mathes SJ. Wound healing. In: Miller TA, ed. Physiologic basis of modern surgical care. St. Louis: CV Mosby, 1988:1011.

tion pathway is initiated by activation of Factor XII, which occurs when blood is exposed to foreign surfaces. This process is not essential in that individuals deficient in Factor XII clot normally. The alternative extrinsic coagulation pathway is initiated by exposure to tissue factor, which binds Factor VII or VIIa and is essential for normal clotting. Tissue factor is not found in vascular endothelial cells but is found in abundance in extravascular cellular surfaces, particularly in adventitial fibroblasts. Both pathways result in the production of thrombin, which catalyzes the conversion of fibrinogen to fibrin. In addition to contributing to hemostasis, both thrombin and fibrin contribute to other aspects of wound healing. Thrombin contributes to the increased vascular permeability seen after injury and also facilitates the extravascular migration of inflammatory cells (6,7). It may also have a role in both epithelialization and angiogenesis. Fibrin provides a scaffold for the migration of inflammatory and mesenchymal cells. Fibrin also has direct effects on inflammatory cells, and its breakdown products are a stimulus to angiogenesis (8).

The physical signs of inflammation were described initially by Hunter in 1794; they include erythema, edema, pain, and heat. These signs are largely a result of changes that occur in the microcirculation, particularly in the 15–20 micron in diameter micro venules. Immediately after injury, intense local vasoconstriction of arterioles and capillaries occurs, which contributes to hemostasis and produces blanching in the wounded area. This process is mediated by circulating catecholamines (epinephrine) and the sympathetic nervous system (norepinephrine) and prostaglandins released by injured cells. Vasoconstriction reverses after 10 to 15 minutes and is replaced by vasodilation. Vasodilation

generates erythema and heat in the area of injury. Vasodilation is mediated by histamine, kinins, prostaglandins(9), and possibly additional factors such as leukotrienes (10) and endothelial cell products (11,12). Mast cells in connective tissue are the primary source of histamine (13), which directly increases vascular permeability and indirectly causes vasodilation through stimulation of prostaglandin synthesis (14). Mast cells also release heparin, several enzymes, and a tumor necrosis factor-like peptide. The kinins are a family of peptides with nine amino acids that act predominantly as short-term vasodilators. They are released from protein-binding molecules by activation of kallikrein, another by-product of the clotting cascade. PGE_1 and PGE_2 are the prostaglandins that increase capillary permeability. Prostaglandins affect vasodilatation through activation of adenyl cyclase and production of cAMP (15). Prostaglandins accumulate in injured tissue, probably from activation of phospholipases located on injured cell membranes. Phospholipase activity causes arachidonic acid release and the subsequent induction of prostaglandin synthetase.

In addition to stimulating vasodilation, histamine and prostaglandins contribute to gap formation between endothelial cells lining the capillaries. Neutrophil factors may contribute to this gap formation as well (16, 17). These gaps allow plasma to leak from the intravascular space to the extravascular compartment (18–20). Plasma proteins such as fibrin, albumin, and globulin begin to establish a structural matrix in the wound. Fibronectins are a class of glycoproteins that facilitate attachment of migrating fibroblasts to the fibrin latticework, and they contribute to early matrix formation as well (21). Leukocytes migrate into wounded tissues through an active phenomenon known as diapedesis. They initially loosely adhere to endothelial cells lining capillaries in a process mediated by selectins (22). They then roll along the capillary walls before finally becoming firmly adherent to endothelial cells through a process mediated by integrins. The cells then actively migrate between endothelial cells into the wounded tissues. The migration of cells and fluid into the injured area generates edema.

Chemotaxis is the movement of an organism or cell in response to a chemical concentration gradient. A substance that can stimulate a cell to migrate in this fashion is known as a chemotactic agent for that cell type. Chemotactic agents contribute to the migration of leukocytes into the extravascular space. Once in wounded tissue, leukocytes phagocytose injured tissue and bacteria. Alterations in pH resulting from breakdown products of tissue and bacteria, along with swelling and decreased tissue oxygenation from damage to the blood supply, produce the pain noted in areas of injury.

Neutrophils, macrophages, and lymphocytes are leukocytes involved in the inflammatory response to injury. Bacterial products (23), complement factors (24,25), histamine (26), PGE_2, leukotriene (27), and PDGF (28) are chemotactic for leukocytes. Neutrophils, also known as polymorphonuclear leukocytes (PMNs), are the first of the leukocytes to be found in wounded tissue in large numbers. Neutrophils function as defensive units that engulf foreign material and digest it through the action of hydrolytic enzymes. After phagocytosing damaged tissue or bacteria, neutrophils die. They do not appear to have a role in the subsequent events of healing in an uncomplicated wound.

As monocytes migrate from the capillaries into the extravascular space, they transform into macrophages in a process mediated by serum factors (29,30) and fibronectin (31). Chemotactic factors then stimulate the migration of macrophages throughout the wounded area (32–38). Macrophages are tremendously important in normal wound healing (39). Macrophages phagocytose bacteria and dead tissue and also secrete collagenases and elastases that break down damaged matrix (40,41). Macrophages are a primary source of cytokines that stimulate fibroblast proliferation, collagen production, and other healing processes. Macrophages may be the most important cells in the healing process.

Lymphocytes produce factors essential for normal healing (42) in addition to functioning as immunoreactants involved in cellular immunity and antibody production. Heparin-binding epidermal growth factor (EGF) and a form of basic fibroblast growth factor (FGF) may be the critical lymphokines (43,44). Interleukin-2 and other factors have been demonstrated to be chemotactic for lymphocytes (45,46).

In normal healing, changes that occur in tissue over time are extremely reproducible. After hemostasis has been accomplished, inflammatory cells migrate into the wound, with neutrophils initially predominating. At 48–72 hours, macrophages begin to outnumber neutrophils. Large numbers of macrophages remain in the wound for several days. This is critical in that macrophages (47), unlike neutrophils (48), are essential for normal healing. After 5–7 days, few inflammatory cells remain in normal healing wounds (Fig. 6.2).

Foreign material or bacteria can change a scenario of normal healing into one of chronic inflammation. Although the acute phases of inflammation are necessary, the persistence of inflammation can be deleterious to the host (49). Neutrophils release destructive proteolytic enzymes and generate free oxygen radicals which damage tissue. Complement cleavage products, along with metabolic byproducts of peroxide radicals, contribute to the formation of a "cytotoxic membrane attack complex" which perpetuates tissue destruction. An area of foreign material and/or chronic bacterial infection eventually is surrounded by a fibrous capsule isolating the process. These encapsulated areas of chronic inflammation are known as granulomas. In some clinical situations, chronic inflammation can be used by the surgeon for the benefit of the patient. An example is injection of Teflon into a paralyzed vocal cord. This procedure incites a chronic granulomatous reaction that results in fibrous tissue accumulation, allowing apposition of the vocal cords and improved phonation.

Intermediate Wound Healing Events

Intermediate wound healing events include mesenchymal cell chemotaxis, mesenchymal cell proliferation, angiogenesis, and epithelialization. These processes predominate 2–4 days after wounding and are all mediated by cytokines. Cytokines are proteins that mediate cellular function by binding receptors located on cell membranes. Different cytokines have different biologic effects. Some cytokines can stimulate a variety of different cellular activities depending on their concentration and the cells to which they bind. Well described cytokines include platelet-derived growth factor (PDGF), transforming growth factor-β (TGF-β), epidermal growth factor (EGF), acidic and basic fibroblast growth factor (aFGF, bFGF), transforming growth factor-alpha (TGF-α), tumor necrosis factor (TNF), interleukin-1 (IL-1), and insulin-like growth factor (IGF) (see section on Cytokines and Growth Factors.)

Fibroblasts are the primary mesenchymal cell involved in wound healing, though smooth muscle cells are also involved. Fibroblasts normally reside in dermis and are damaged by wounding. Undifferentiated mesenchymal cells in the area may subsequently differentiate into fibroblasts when stimulated by macrophage products secreted into the wound (50). Additional fibroblasts migrate to the wounded area under the influence of chemotactic factors. PDGF has been demonstrated to be chemotactic for both fibroblasts (51) and smooth mus-

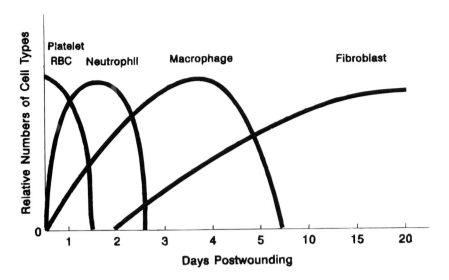

Figure 6.2. Cellular phase of wound healing. Relative concentrations of various cellular components versus time in the healing wound. *RBC* = red blood cell.

cle cells (52). Fibronectin (53–55), EGF (56), and other substances (57,58) have also been demonstrated to be chemotactic for fibroblasts. Fibronectin is a primary component of extracellular matrix, and it facilitates fibroblast migration directly.

The mesenchymal cell population in a wound is augmented further by proliferation of both resident and newly arrived cells. PDGF is a potent mitogenic stimulant for both fibroblasts and smooth muscle cells (59,60). TGF-β is another important stimulant of fibroblast proliferation (61,62). Mesenchymal cell proliferation can also be stimulated by TNF, IL-1, lymphokines (63), insulin, and IGF (64,65).

Angiogenesis reconstructs the vasculature in areas where it has been damaged by wounding and is stimulated by high lactate levels, acidic pH, and decreased oxygen tension in the tissue. Small capillary sprouts initially develop on venules at the periphery of the devascularized area (66). As capillary sprouts grow with endothelial cell proliferation, the cells develop a curvature which results in a lumen. The capillary sprouts continue to grow until they contact other sprouts growing from other directions. The sprouts then interconnect, forming a vascular loop, and the sprouting process begins anew.

Endothelial cell migration and tube formation are facilitated by changes in matrix (67,68). Cytokines directly and indirectly stimulate the endothelial cell migration and proliferation required for angiogenesis. Many of these are derived from macrophages (69–71). Basic fibroblast growth factor is the most potent angiogenic stimulant identified (72); heparin is an important cofactor for this growth factor (73). TGF-alpha, TGF-β (74), vascular endothelial growth factor (75), wound fluids (76,77), prostaglandins, adipocyte lipids (78), and other factors (79–81) also are angiogenic stimulants. Stimulatory cytokines diminish in number when the wounded area is completely revascularized. This flux in angiogenic factors may stimulate maturation of the vascular system (82).

The epidermis provides a barrier between the external environment and internal milieu. It prevents the entry of hostile elements from the environment and the escape of fluid and electrolytes. Epithelial cells in the epidermis must constantly regenerate to survive continuing insults from the external environment. The gastrointestinal, genitourinary, and respiratory systems also have epithelial linings that serve a similar function.

The epidermis is composed of multiple layers of epithelial cells superficial to the dermis. The first layer above the dermis is the basal layer, followed by a prickle cell layer, a granular layer, and finally the most superficial layer, the stratum corneum. The stratum corneum consists primarily of dead cells and keratin. After injury, the process of epithelial renewal is called epithelialization. Epithelialization is particularly important in the healing of partial thickness wounds, such as abrasions or superficial burns, although it plays a role in the healing of all wounds. Partial thickness wounds are those in which the epidermis and a portion of the dermis are damaged while some dermis is preserved. Epithelial cells involved in the closure of partial thickness wounds derive from both the wound edges and epithelial appendages, such as hair follicles, sweat glands, and sebaceous glands in the more central portions of the wound. These appendages extend into the underlying dermis and subcutaneous tissues and persist in partial thickness injuries (83). In contrast, epithelialization in an incisional wound involves cellular migration over a distance of less than a millimeter from one side of the incision to the other. Incisional wounds generally are re-epithelialized completely in 24–48 hours.

The sequence of events that comprise epithelialization include cellular detachment, migration, proliferation, and differentiation (84). In the first 24 hours after injury, thickening of the basal cell layer begins. Marginal basal cells then elongate, detach from the underlying basement membrane, and migrate into the wound. They migrate essentially as a monolayer across the denuded area. Migrating basal cells usually orient themselves along collagen fibers and exhibit what is called contact guidance (85). The cells secrete a provisional matrix including fibronectin if a basement membrane is not present to facilitate migration (86). Laminin and type IV collagen, two normally important basement membrane components, are not seen during this migratory period. Basal cells at the edge of the denuded area begin to divide 48–72 hours after injury. This follows cellular migration of PMN and monocytes (87,88). Epithelial cell proliferation contributes new cells to the advancing epithelial monolayer. Cells migrate until they reach cells migrating from a different direction. At that point, 'contact inhibition' is re-established, and migration ceases. Cells of the monolayer then differentiate into more basal-like cells. Cellular proliferation continues in the new basal cells as a multilayered epidermis is re-established (89). Subsequently, new surface cells begin to keratinize. The migration and proliferation of epithelial cells is stimulated by EGF (90,91). TGF-β stimulates epithelial migration, although it slows epithelial proliferation.

Unfortunately, regenerated epithelium does not retain all of the functional advantages of normal epithelium. There are fewer basal cells in regenerated epidermis, and the interface between epidermis and dermis is abnormal (84). Rete pegs, undulating projections of epidermis that penetrate papillary dermis, are not found on reepithelialized surfaces (92). The epithelium is thicker at the wound edge than in the midportion of a re-epithelialized area.

Late Wound Healing Events

Fibroplasia is the production of fibrous protein in the wound. Collagen makes up 25% of all body proteins and more than 50% of the protein found in scar tissue (93). Collagen is synthesized primarily by fibroblasts in a complex process that begins 3 to 5 days after injury. The rate of collagen synthesis increases rapidly and continues at an accelerated rate for 2 to 4 weeks in most wounds. After 4 weeks, collagen synthesis rates decline, eventually balancing the rate of collagen destruction by collagenase. Age, tension, pressure (94), and stress (95) affect the rate of collagen synthesis. TGF-β stimulates collagen synthesis (96), whereas glucocorticoids inhibit it (97).

At least 11 types of collagen have been described, with slight differences in their component polypeptide chains. Type I is most common. It can be isolated from virtually all tissues. Type I collagen makes up 80–90% of collagen in skin, with the remaining 10–20% being Type III. Increased levels of Type III collagen are seen embryonically and in early phases of wound healing. Type V predominates in smooth muscle. Types II and XI are seen primarily in cartilage, whereas Type IV is seen predominantly in basement membranes. The remaining collagen types are found in small quantities in specific parts of the body.

The molecular inscription for Type I collagen is found on chromosome 17 (98,99). Collagen consists of three polypeptide chains which are individually synthesized in a manner similar to other proteins. Each chain is twisted into a right-hand helix. The alignment of three of these chains into a triple helix is facilitated by nonhelical terminal peptide sequences. The chains align themselves in the characteristic triple helix configuration within the endoplasmic reticulum. The aggregate of three peptide chains is subsequently twisted into a left-hand superhelix (100). Most polypeptide chains used in collagen assembly are alpha-chains. Every third amino acid residue of alpha chains is glycine, and this structure facilitates helix formation. The alpha-chains are further subtyped into alpha$_1$, alpha$_2$, and alpha$_3$ according to variations in other residues.

Another critical component of collagen synthesis is the hydroxylation of lysine and proline moieties within the polypeptide chains. This process occurs in the endoplasmic reticulum. Hydroxylysine is required for covalent crosslink formation. Hydroxyproline is found almost exclusively in collagen and serves as a marker of the quantity of collagen in tissue. This hydroxylation process requires specific enzymes for lysine and proline and, in addition, requires as cofactors oxygen, vitamin C, alpha-ketoglutarate, and ferrous iron. Deficiencies in vitamin C, oxygen, or suppression of enzymatic activity by corticosteroids may lead to under hydroxylated collagen, which is incapable of generating strong cross links and is broken down easily.

After the collagen molecule is synthesized, it is secreted into the extracellular space. Galactosyl-glucose is linked enzymatically to hydroxylysine residues within the molecule and probably contributes to the transport of synthesized collagen across the plasma membrane (101). When collagen is secreted into the extracellular space, it appears in the form of procollagen. Procollagen can be identified by persistent nonhelical extensions of the alpha-chains. This linear extension, or registration peptide, interferes with the subsequent aggregation of collagen molecules into fibrils. Successful cleavage of the registration peptide by specific enzymes yields tropocollagen, which can aggregate into collagen fibrils. A transverse section of a fibril generally demonstrates four to five molecules aligned in a staggered fashion. Fibril formation is facilitated by proteoglycans in the extracellular matrix.

Aggregates of tropocollagen form the quaternary structure of collagen fibrils. Electron microscopy demonstrates a banding pattern in the fibrils with a band width of 640 A (102). This pattern is produced by the overlap of individual molecules in a specific manner determined by electrostatic bonds that form between charged areas of molecules. Approximately 25% of the length of consecutive molecules overlap.

As mentioned, individual polypeptide chains within the collagen molecule are held together by intramolecular cross-links. Intermolecular cross-links form between separate collagen molecules. The initial bonds formed both between individual polypeptide chains and between molecules are electrostatic. These are replaced eventually by covalent bonds, which are formed as a Schiff base reaction (103). Covalent bonding of collagen molecules is initiated by lysyl oxidase, an enzyme that causes deamination of the terminal NH group on the side chain of lysine (104). Oxidation at this site forms an aldehyde group. Neighboring aldehyde groups from parallel peptide chains form a covalent bond through an aldol condensation (105). A Schiff base reaction can occur between residues of lysine to lysine, lysine to hydroxylysine, or hydroxylysine to hydroxylysine. The strongest cross-links are formed between two hydroxylysine residues. Therefore, the strongest collagen molecules are found where the density of hydroxylysine is the greatest (106).

Unaggregated tropocollagen molecules are soluble in cold saline. Fibril formation decreases the solubility of collagen (26) as a result of these intermolecular bonds, and dilute acid is generally required to solubilize aggregated tropocollagen. Strong acid and high temperatures are needed to solubilize maturely cross-linked collagen.

The extracellular connective tissue matrix contains components other than collagen, including proteoglycans, attachment proteins such as fibronectin, and elastin. Proteoglycans consist of a protein core covalently linked to a glycosaminoglycan (GAG) (107). Proteoglycans are synthesized primarily by fibroblasts. Chondroitin sulfate, dermatan sulfate, heparin, heparin sulfate, keratan sulfate, and hyaluronic acid are the more common proteoglycans. The biologic functions of proteoglycans are less well understood than those of collagen. They generally anchor specific proteins in certain locations and affect the biologic activity of target proteins. These processes often involve interactions with cytokines whose function proteoglycans can potentiate. Heparin, for example, is an important cofactor for basic fibroblast growth factor during angiogenesis. It may also directly influence cellular activity including the direct stimulation of cellular proliferation. Hyaluronic acid can stimulate cellular migration for certain cell types.

Attachment proteins, such as fibronectin, are another key component of matrix. Fibronectin is produced by fibroblasts and epithelial cells (108). It is found in plasma and in connective tissue, and it has a variety of functions. Primarily, it aids in cellular attachment and modulates the migration of various cell types into the wound (109–111). It facilitates binding of epithelial cells to matrix and, in so doing, contributes to epithelialization (112). It is chemotactic for fibroblasts (113) and also greatly facilitates fibroblast migration.

Elastin is a third component of the connective tissue matrix; however, it is not synthesized in response to injury. Normal skin has elastic properties that scar lacks due to the lack of elastin in scar.

Wound Contraction

Wound contraction, like collagen synthesis, begins approximately 4 to 5 days after wounding. Wound contraction represents the centripetal movement of the wound edge towards the center of the wound. Maximal wound contraction continues for 12–15 days, though it will continue for longer periods if the wound remains open. The wound edges move towards each other at an average rate of 0.6 to 0.75 mm/day. The rate of contraction depends on tissue laxity with great variability among tissues. A wound in the buttock, where the tissue is loose, will contract much more than a wound on the scalp or pretibial area where the skin is tighter. The relative contribution of wound contraction to the healing process also varies depending on wound type. Wound contraction is a trivial component in the healing of a closed incisional wound, whereas it is a major contributor to the healing of a full thickness open wound.

Wound shape can also affect contraction. Wounds with square edges contract more rapidly than circular wounds. Forces of contraction in a circular wound cancel each other to some degree, preventing effective centripetal movement of the wound edge. It is important to create a circular wound for intestinal stomas to limit stenosis from wound contraction.

Wound contraction occurs to a greater extent in relatively immobile areas, such as the back, abdomen and the midportion of extremities. Contraction of a large wound across a joint surface, however, can lead to a contracture. A contracture is a physical constriction limiting joint motion which results from wound contraction. Contractures are often seen as a result of burn wounds across the neck, axillae, and other joint surfaces that heal secondarily. Some animals have a separate anatomical layer, called the panniculus carnosus, which allows substantial wound contraction without contracture production. Humans do not have a well-defined panniculus carnosus, although the platysma muscle is an analogous structure.

Disagreement exists as to the mechanism by which wounds contract. Large numbers of myofibroblasts are found in wounds during wound contraction, and many feel they mediate the process. Myofibroblasts were first described by Gabbiani in 1971 (114). They can only be differentiated from other fibroblasts by electron microscopy. Their defining characteristics include microfilaments in their cytoplasm, a multi lobulated nucleus, and abundant rough endoplasmic reticulum. They most likely derive from normal fibroblasts in the wound area. They first appear in wounds on the third day after wounding and persist in large numbers until approximately day 21 post-wounding (115). They are primarily found at the periphery of the wound, thus generating the theory that they pull the wound edges together in a "picture frame" fashion. The concept that the "picture frame" is the location of dynamic forces in contraction has been supported by experiments in which the central portion of healing wounds was excised in some wounds and the peripheral area in others (116). No effect on contraction was measured after central tissue excision, whereas wound contraction could be stopped completely by excising a peripheral picture frame strip.

Alternatively, experimental work in contracting collagen matrices has suggested that fibroblasts within the wound are primary contributors to wound contraction through interactions with surrounding matrix (117). Contraction in this model occurs as fibroblasts elongate and migrate through matrix and effectively retract collagen fibrils (118,119) in a serum dependent process (120). Advocates of this theory suggest that myofibroblasts at the wound perimeter are merely fibroblasts with stress fibers in their cytoplasm. The stress fibers are prominent because the cells are in close proximity to each other at the wound edge where contraction has, for the most part, been completed.

Additional work with collagen matrices suggests that fibroblasts exposed to mechanical stress elongate and demonstrate stress fibers in their cytoplasm, making them more myofibroblast-like. This observation may explain why more myofibroblasts or myofibroblast-like cells are seen in actual contracting wounds where there is more stress than in floating contracting lattices (121). As stress is relieved in contracting matrices, these cells differentiate to less active cells.

Contraction is a cell directed process that requires cell division but not collagen synthesis. Radiation and cytolytic drugs delay contraction, adding further evidence that cellular activity is required. Collagen deposition may be involved in fixing the tissues in their final state, however. TGF-β can stimulate collagen lattice contraction and appears to be a mediator of wound contrac-

tion (122). It may also facilitate the transition of fibroblasts into myofibroblasts (123). PDGF can also stimulate contraction of matrices by a TGF-β independent mechanism (124) whereas FGF (125) and interferon-gamma (126) inhibit the process.

Although wound contraction cannot be eliminated, it can be limited. Full thickness skin grafts with a full complement of dermis can limit wound contraction to a greater degree than split thickness skin grafts (127). Myofibroblasts disappear from the wound more quickly after a full thickness skin graft than after a split thickness skin graft. The timing of grafting is also important. Grafting early in the course of wound healing will prevent wound contraction to a greater degree than delayed grafting. Splints can temporarily slow wound contraction, though wound contraction will proceed at an accelerated rate after splint removal. Topical dressings may also delay wound contraction, though they will not prevent it. Pharmacologic manipulations to limit wound contraction have generally been unsuccessful, though in experimental models, smooth muscle antagonists have effectively inhibited wound contraction (128).

Terminal Wound Healing Event

Scar remodeling is the hallmark of the terminal period of healing. Approximately 21 days after injury, net accumulation of wound collagen becomes stable (129). Although collagen content is maximal at this point, bursting strength of the wound is only 15% of that of normal skin. The process of scar remodeling dramatically increases wound bursting strength. The greatest rate of increase occurs between 3 and 6 weeks after wounding. By 6 weeks after wounding, the wound has reached 80–90% of its eventual strength (130) (Fig. 6.3). The bursting strength of scar never reaches that of unwounded skin, however, and it reaches its maximum of approximately 90% of skin breaking strength at 6 months.

Figure 6.3. Graphs demonstrating collagen synthetic activity (specific activity of hydroxyproline) in healing wounds and unwounded skin at different time points and relating collagen synthetic activity to gain in tensile strength in wounds over time. Reproduced with permission from Peacock EE, Jr. Wound repair. 3rd ed. Philadelphia: WB Saunders, 1984:111.

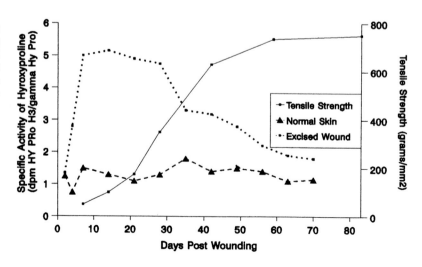

During terminal wound healing, a continual turnover of collagen molecules occurs as old collagen is broken down and new collagen is synthesized in a denser, more organized fashion along stress lines (131). Several metalloproteinases (MMP) have been identified with collagenolytic activity. They are found in scar tissue and in normal connective tissues (132). The activity of collagenolytic enzymes is modulated by several tissue inhibitors of metalloproteinases (TIMP). Other enzymes, such as hyaluronidase, are probably also involved in scar remodeling.

During this period of scar remodeling, the number of intra- and inter-molecular cross-links between collagen fibers increases dramatically. This increase in cross linking is a major contributor to the increase in wound breaking strength. As collagen matures during scar remodeling, the quantity of type III collagen decreases and is replaced by type I collagen. The quantity of water and glycosaminoglycans in matrix decreases as well. Wound remodeling is visible to the surgeon as a change in the texture, thickness, and color of a healing wound. Remodeling continues over a period of nearly 12 months so that decisions regarding operative scar revision should not be made prematurely.

Cytokines and Growth Factors

Normal healing requires the successful completion of multiple coordinated biochemical and cellular functions that occur in a reproducible manner. Cytokines have emerged as primary mediators of most wound healing events. The wound healing process appears to be orchestrated by the carefully regulated release of specific cytokines at appropriate time intervals after injury. The term growth factor is often used interchangeably with cytokines, though technically, growth factors only stimulate cellular proliferation, whereas cytokines can mediate all types of cellular processes.

Cytokines can function in either an endocrine, a paracrine, autocrine or intracrine fashion. A factor functioning in an endocrine fashion is released by a cell and affects a target cell at a distance. Endocrine factors generally are carried to the target cell via the bloodstream. Paracrine factors are released by one cell and affect a different cell in the same locale. Autocrine factors are released by a cell and affect the function of that same cell. Intracrine stimulation differs from the other modes of action in that it does not involve the extracellular release of the cytokine. The cytokine is released intracellularly and mediates function through internal binding (133). A given factor may mediate cellular activity in a variety of locations by acting on some cells in an endocrine fashion and others in a paracrine or autocrine fashion.

Cytokines have often been named for the cell of origin or a characteristic known about the factor when it was first described. Many of the names are misleading because they suggest that a polyfunctional factor has one function or that a factor is derived from only one cell type when many types of cells produce it. PDGF was named after the platelet from which it was originally discovered, although it has since been learned that multiple cell types produce it. TGF-β was named because in vitro studies suggested that the factor was capable of transforming normal cells into malignant ones, although it has since been learned that TGF-β is incapable of inducing malignant transformation.

Several factors determine whether a cytokine is involved in a particular cellular activity. First, it has to be released at the appropriate time and be available at the appropriate site in sufficient concentration. Second, the factor must not be broken down by proteolytic enzymes or bound to matrix. Third, affected cells must have receptors for the cytokine. Bound receptors primarily have direct kinase activity and facilitate the phosphorylation of proteins, which initiates a cascade of intracellular activities, eventually resulting in the stimulation of a cellular function. In some cases, the number of receptors bound is critical with a limited amount of binding producing one function, whereas a greater amount produces a different cellular function.

The functions of many of these cytokines have been discussed in previous sections. Growth factors which have been reasonably well characterized include EGF, PDGF, FGF, and TGF-β. These factors will be discussed individually to clarify their sources, characteristics, and functions. Table 6.1 summarizes information regarding these factors and several additional ones.

Epidermal Growth Factor

Epidermal growth factor (EGF) was the first cytokine described, and it was originally isolated from the salivary glands of mice. It is found in a wide variety of tissues, and most cells have its receptors (134). Epithelial cells have the largest number of receptors, although large numbers are also present in endothelial cells, fibroblasts, and smooth muscle cells. EGF is a potent mitogenic stimulant for epithelial cells, endothelial cells, and fibroblasts, and it is chemotactic for epithelial cells and fibroblasts. It stimulates fibroplasia in wound chambers in addition to increasing collagenase activity (135), stimulating neovascularization (136), and fibronectin synthesis (137).

Fibroblast Growth Factor

Fibroblast Growth Factor (FGF) was originally discovered as a mitogen for mesenchymal cells and secondarily was found to be a primary stimulant of angiogenesis. Both an acidic and basic fibroblast growth factor (aFGF and bFGF) have been identified in addition to a

Table 6.1.
Growth Factors in Wound Healing

Growth Factor	Cell Source	Function
PDGF	Macrophages Platelets Endothelial cells	Stimulates fibroblast & smooth muscle cell chemotaxis and proliferation, collagen synthesis, collagenase activity, fibronectin synthesis
TGF-β	Platelets Macrophages Lymphocytes	Stimulates fibroblast chemotaxis and proliferation, collagen synthesis, proteoglycan synthesis, fibronectin synthesis, angiogenesis, wound contraction
EGF	Multiple	Stimulates epithelial cell chemotaxis and proliferation, fibroblast chemotaxis and proliferation, endothelial cell proliferation
FGF	Macrophages Endothelial cells	Stimulates fibroblast proliferation, epithelial cell proliferation, endothelial cell proliferation, collagen synthesis, proteoglycan synthesis, fibronectin synthesis, angiogenesis, wound contraction
TGF-α	Macrophages Platelets Keratinocytes	Same as EGF.
IL-1	Macrophages	Stimulates inflammatory cell chemotaxis, epithelial cell chemotaxis, fibroblast proliferation, collagen synthesis, collagenase activity
TNF	Macrophages Lymphocytes	Stimulates fibroblast proliferation, collagen synthesis, collagenase activity, angiogenesis
IGF	Fibroblasts Liver cells	Stimulates fibroblast proliferation, collagen synthesis, proteoglycan synthesis

Modified from: Peacock JL, Lawrence WT, Peacock EE Jr. Wound healing. In: O'Leary JP, ed. The physiologic basis of surgery, 1st ed. Baltimore: Williams & Wilkins, 1993.

number of types. Endothelial cells can synthesize and respond to FGF (138). Topical FGF can stimulate wound contraction in experimental wounds (139) though it has no effect in collagen matrix collagen models (125). It has also been shown to stimulate collagen synthesis, proteoglycan synthesis, fibronectin synthesis (140) and epithelialization (141).

Platelet-Derived Growth Factor (PDGF)

The observation that platelet-derived growth factors contribute to the healing process was made in the early 1970s. The initial factor identified was PDGF, which was localized to the alpha-granules of platelets. Tumors, endothelial cells, and macrophages also secrete PDGF-like factors. PDGF exists in AA, BB, and AB isoforms with slightly different activities (142). PDGF stimulates the chemotaxis and proliferation of fibroblasts and smooth muscle cells as well as collagen synthesis and collagenase activity (143). It also stimulates fibronectin and hyaluron synthesis (144,145) and collagen matrix contraction. PDGF may influence the expression of TGF-β and influence cellular activity indirectly by that mechanism as well (146). The concentration of PDGF in an area determines which cells are most attracted because different cells are attracted by different concentrations of PDGF. Somatomedins, or insulin-like growth factors (IGF), are synthesized primarily by hepatocytes and fibroblasts and act as co-factors with PDGF in stimulating fibroblast proliferation. IGF may also contribute to epithelial cell proliferation (147).

Transforming Growth Factor

Transforming growth factor-β (TGFβ) was discovered originally as a stimulant of anchorage-independent cellular proliferation in soft agar, and it has now been isolated from a number of tissues, including platelets, macrophages, lymphocytes, bone, and kidney (148). At least 5 subtypes have been identified, all with similar biologic functions (149). Like PDGF, TGF-β is found in high concentrations in the alpha-granules of platelets and is released during platelet degranulation at the site of injury. TGF-β regulates its own production by macrophages in an autocrine manner. It also stimulates monocytes to secrete other growth factors, including FGF, PDGF, TNF, and IL-1. TGF-β stimulates fibroblast chemotaxis and proliferation. In different concentrations, it can either stimulate or inhibit cellular proliferation, and its effect may be modulated by other cytokines in the milieu. TGF-β may be the most potent stimulant of collagen synthesis, and it further contributes to collagen accumulation by decreasing protease activity. Specific antibodies to TGF-β can limit collagen accumulation in wounds (150). TGF-β has also been demonstrated to stimulate fibronectin synthesis, proteoglycan synthesis, and epithelial cell proliferation. In addition, it stimulates wound contraction, and it indirectly stimulates angiogenesis, although it has no stimulatory effect on endothelial cell proliferation (151).

As is apparent, many cytokines have similar functions. Which factors are the most critical stimulants of the various wound healing functions is not altogether clear. Factors with similar functions may be acting at different time points in the wound healing process.

Disturbances of Wound Healing

Wound healing does not always occur in the undisturbed fashion as described. Both local and systemic factors have the capability of interfering with healing. Local factors include infection, foreign bodies, tissue hypoxia, radiation damage, mechanical trauma, local toxins, venous insufficiency, and cigarette smoking. Systemic factors include malnutrition, cancer, diabetes mellitus, alcoholism, uremia, corticosteroids, chemotherapeutic agents, jaundice, and old age. Several of these local and systemic factors will be discussed in more detail (Table 6.2).

Local Factors

Infection

The body maintains a symbiotic relationship with bacteria. Normal dry skin contains up to 1000 bacteria per gram (152) and saliva contains 100 million bacteria per ml (153). The bacterial population is kept in control by several mechanisms. Bacterial invasion is mechanically limited by an intact stratum corneum in the skin and intact oral mucosa intraorally (154). In addition, sebaceous secretions contain bactericidal and fungicidal fatty acids which modulate bacterial proliferation (155). Edema dilutes these fatty acids rendering edematous areas more infection-prone. Lysozymes in skin hydrolyze bacterial cell membranes and further limit bacterial proliferation (156). The immune system augments the local barriers to infection.

A difference between infection and contamination should be recognized. Contamination is the presence of bacteria from skin or other sources in a wound. Infection occurs when the number or virulence of bacteria has exceeded the ability of local tissue defenses to control them. Generally, infection exists when bacteria have proliferated to levels beyond 10^5 organisms per gram of tissue. At this level, bacteria overwhelm host defenses

and proliferate in an uncontrolled fashion . This number has been arrived at by studies done at the United States Army Institute of Surgical Research and elsewhere (157–160). Group B streptococci are the only bacterial species identified to cause infection at lower bacterial concentrations (161). Several factors can alter the balance point where infection develops, including foreign bodies or necrotic tissue in the wound. Hematomas function like foreign bodies as adjuvants promoting infection (162). Both local and systemic factors can compromise the ability of the host to defend against infection. Local factors such as impaired circulation or radiation injury increase the risk of infection. Systemic diseases such as diabetes, AIDS, uremia, and cancer have all been shown to increase susceptibility to wound infection.

Operative procedures are classified as clean, clean-contaminated, contaminated, and dirty. Table 6.3 lists the characteristics of each classification (163). Classification of wounds allows the surgeon to predict the likelihood of wound infection and alter wound management accordingly. Predicting the chances of wound infection is important because the most cost effective treatment of infection is prevention. Prevention requires meticulous surgical technique, judicious use of perioperative systemic antibiotics, and precise judgment as to which wounds should be closed primarily. Factors that should be considered in choosing to use prophylactic antibiotics are the condition of the patient, the status of the host defense, the degree of wound contamination, and factors increasing the risk to the patient should an infection occur (e.g., prosthetic device). Once the decision for prophylactic antibiotics has been made, they must be administered preoperatively so that serum and tissue levels of antibiotics are maximal at the time of wounding.

Hypoxia and Smoking

Delivery of oxygen to healing tissues is critical for prompt wound repair. Oxygen is necessary for cellular respiration and for hydroxylation of proline and lysine residues. Adequate tissue oxygenation requires an adequate circulating blood volume (164), adequate cardiac function, and adequate local vasculature. Vascular disorders may be systemic because of peripheral vascular disease or they may be localized because of scarring from trauma or prior surgery. Anemia is not associated with impaired healing unless the anemia is severe enough to limit the circulating blood volume.

Smoking can impair tissue oxygenation as it acutely

Table 6.2.
Factors Impairing Wound Healing

Local	Systemic
Infection	Malnutrition
Foreign bodies	Cancer
Ischemia/Hypoxia	Diabetes mellitus
Cigarette smoking	Systemic corticosteroids
Radiation	Uremia
Previous trauma	Alcoholism
Venous insufficiency	Chemotherapeutic agents
Local toxins (e.g. spider venom)	Jaundice
	Old Age

Table 6.3.
Classification and Infection Rates of Wound Contamination

Classification	Infection Rate	Wound Characteristics
Clean	1.5–5.1%	Atraumatic, uninfected; no entry of GU, GI, or respiratory tracts.
Clean-Contaminated	7.7–10.8%	Minor breaks in sterile technique; Entry of GU, GI, or respiratory tracts without significant spillage.
Contaminated	15.2–16.3%	Traumatic wounds; gross spillage from GI tract; entry into infected tissue, bone, urine or bile.
Dirty	28.0–40.0%	Drainage of abscess; debridement of soft tissue infection.

stimulates vasoconstriction (165-167) and contributes to the development of atherosclerosis and vascular disease over time. Three to six percent of cigarette smoke is carbon monoxide, which binds to hemoglobin, producing carboxyhemoglobin. Smokers have carboxyhemoglobin levels between 1% and 20% (168). Carboxyhemoglobin limits the oxygen carrying capacity of the blood and also increases platelet adhesiveness (169) producing endothelial changes (170,171).

Radiation

Radiation damages the DNA of cells in exposed areas. Some cells die, whereas others are rendered incapable of undergoing mitosis. When radiation is administered therapeutically, doses are fractionated and tangential fields are used to limit damage to normal cells and maximize tumor cell damage. In spite of such techniques, normal cells are damaged by radiation.

Radiation therapy initially produces inflammation and desquamation in a dose-dependent fashion (172). After a course of radiation has been completed, healing ensues if surrounding normal tissues have not been irreparably damaged. Additional cells must migrate into the treated area for adequate healing to occur. Fibroblasts that migrate into irradiated tissue are often abnormal because of radiation exposure. These cells are characterized by multiple vacuoles, irregular rough endoplasmic reticulum, degenerating mitochondria, and cytoplasmic crystalline inclusion bodies. Increased levels of inflammatory mediators contribute to the abnormal healing response. Collagen is synthesized to an abnormal degree in irradiated tissue, causing a characteristic fibrosis. The media of dermal blood vessels in irradiated areas thickens and some blood vessels become occluded, resulting in a decrease in the total number of blood vessels. Superficial telangiectasias may be seen. The epidermis becomes thinned, and pigmentation changes often develop. Irradiated skin is dry because of damage to sebaceous and sweat glands, and it has little hair. The epidermal basement membrane is abnormal and nuclear atypia is common in keratinocytes.

In previously irradiated tissue, abnormal healing after wounding is predictable. The decreased vascularity and increased fibrosis limits the ability of platelets and inflammatory cells to gain access to wounds in the area. The quantity of cytokines released is therefore limited. This relative cytokine deficiency causes impairment of essentially all cellular aspects of healing. Damaged fibroblasts and keratinocytes in the area may not respond normally to stimulants. In addition, irradiated tissue is predisposed to infection, which can further slow the healing process.

Clinically, impairment in healing is manifested by a higher rate of complication when an operation is done in irradiated tissue (173). Vitamin A has been used to reverse the healing impairment induced by radiation therapy (174). Difficult wounds in irradiated tissue can often be managed surgically by bringing a new blood supply to the area with flaps from nonirradiated areas.

Systemic Factors

Malnutrition

Adequate amounts of protein, carbohydrates, fatty acids, vitamins, and other nutrients are required for wounds to heal. Malnutrition frequently contributes to suboptimal healing (175). Hypoproteinemia inhibits proper wound healing by limiting the supply of critical amino acids required for the synthesis of collagen and other proteins. Collagen synthesis essentially stops in the absence of protein intake (176), resulting in impaired healing (177,178). Arginine and glutamine appear to be particularly important amino acids. Cystine residues are found along the nonhelical peptide chain associated with procollagen, and in their absence, the proper alignment of peptide chains into a triple helix is inhibited (179).

Carbohydrate and fat provide an energy source for healing. Wound healing slows when carbohydrate or fat stores are limited. Protein is broken down as an alternative energy source instead of contributing primarily to tissue growth (180). Fatty acids are also vital components of cell membranes.

Several vitamins are also essential for normal healing. Vitamin C is a necessary co-factor for hydroxylation of lysine and proline during collagen synthesis. The ability of fibroblasts to produce new, strongly cross-linked collagen is diminished if Vitamin C is deficient. Clinically, existing scars dissolve because collagenolytic activity continues without adequate compensatory collagen synthesis. New wounds do not heal. In addition, Vitamin C deficiency is associated with an impaired resistance to infection (181). Vitamin A is essential for normal epithelialization, proteoglycan synthesis, and normal immune function (181–183). Vitamin A and thiamine deficiencies impair healing (184). Vitamin D is required for normal calcium metabolism and is therefore required for bone healing. Exogenous Vitamin E impairs wound healing in rats, most likely by influencing the inflammatory response in a corticosteroid-like manner (185).

Certain minerals are necessary for normal healing as well. Zinc, a trace element, is a necessary cofactor for DNA polymerase and reverse transcriptase. Zinc deficiency can therefore result in an inhibition of cellular proliferation and deficient granulation tissue formation (186) and healing (187). Pharmacologic overdosing with zinc does not accelerate wound healing and can have detrimental effects (26).

Cancer

A cancer-associated wound healing impairment has been demonstrated experimentally (188) and is often noted clinically. Cancer-bearing hosts may have impaired healing for a variety of reasons. Cancer-induced cachexia, which manifests itself as weight loss, anorexia, and asthenia, significantly limits healing. Cachexia is a result of either decreased caloric intake, increased energy expenditure, or both. Several other causes of cancer cachexia have also been proposed.

Decreased oral intake may be caused by anorexia or mechanical factors. Anorexia is mediated through, as yet, imperfectly defined circulating factors. Changes in taste perception, hypothalamic function, and tryptophan metabolism may contribute to anorexia. Tumors in the gastrointestinal tract can produce obstruction and/or fistulae that limit nutrient absorption. Other cancers generate peptides such as gastrin and vasoactive intestinal polypeptide (VIP) that alter transit times and interfere with absorption of nutrients.

Cancers alter host metabolism in a detrimental fashion as well. First, glucose turnover may be increased, sometimes leading to glucose intolerance. The effect of increased glucose use is higher energy needs (189). Second, protein catabolism may be accelerated. Protein breakdown in muscle is increased as is hepatic utilization of amino acids. Such changes in protein metabolism produce a net loss of plasma protein. Third, cancer patients may be unable to alter their metabolism to conserve energy by relying on fat for most of their energy needs. In tumor-bearing animals, fat has been shown to accumulate, whereas other more vital tissues are broken down for energy. Fourth, Vitamin C may be preferentially taken up by some tumors, limiting the vitamin's availability for hydroxylation of proline and lysine moieties in collagen. All of these metabolic changes contribute to a negative energy balance and inefficient energy use.

Cancer patients may be relatively anergic, most likely because of abnormal inflammatory cell activity. Macrophages do not migrate or function normally in cancer patients. Inflammatory cell dysfunction may limit the availability of cytokines required for healing and may also predispose to infection.

Impaired healing must be anticipated in cancer patients because of the many alterations in metabolism and immune function. It has been suggested that vitamin A can improve healing in tumor-bearing mice (190), but this effect has not yet been demonstrated in cancer patients.

Old Age

The elderly have been shown to heal less efficiently than younger individuals. Dunuoy and Carrell studied patients with war injuries in World War I and demonstrated that wounds in 20 year old patients contracted more rapidly than those in 30 year old patients (191). In a blister epithelialization model, younger patients healed more rapidly than older patients (192). In elderly subjects, wound disruption occurred with less force than in younger individuals (193).

Diabetes

Diabetes mellitus is also associated with impaired healing. The risk of infection in clean incisions was five times greater in diabetics than nondiabetics in a review of 23,649 patients (194). This diabetes-induced healing impairment has been experimentally demonstrated in several models as well (195–197). Diabetes is associated with impaired granulocyte chemotaxis (198) and phagocytic function (199–201). The diabetes-induced healing impairment may be improved by controlling hyperglycemia with insulin (202–204).

Steroids and Immunosuppression

Adrenocortical steroids inhibit all aspects of the healing process. Steroids slow the development of breaking strength in incisional wounds (205). In open wounds healing secondarily, steroids impede wound contraction (206,207) and epithelialization.

This healing impairment is a result of derangements in cellular function induced by steroids. A primary feature of wounds in steroid-treated individuals is a deficiency in inflammatory cell function. Inflammatory cells, particularly macrophages, mediate essentially all aspects of healing through cytokine release. By diminishing the supply of cytokines, steroids and other immunosuppressive agents profoundly impair all aspects of healing. Macrophage migration, fibroblast proliferation, collagen accumulation, and angiogenesis are among the processes diminished by steroid administration. The effects of steroids on healing are most pronounced when the drug is administered within several days before or after wounding (208).

All aspects of steroid-induced healing impairment other than wound contraction can be reversed by supplemental vitamin A. The recommended dose is 25,000 IU per day. Topical vitamin A has also been found to be effective for open wounds (209). Anabolic steroids and growth hormone-releasing factor have reversed steroid-induced healing impairments as well.

Chemotherapeutic Agents

Chemotherapeutic agents impair healing primarily through inhibition of cellular proliferation. Many agents have been examined in experimental models, and virtually all agents impair healing (210). Nitrogen mustard, cyclophosphamide, methotrexate, BCNU (carmustine), and doxorubicin are the most damaging to the healing process. Most chemotherapeutic regimens use a combination of agents compounding their deleterious effects. Clinical trials with chemotherapeutic agents have not been associated with as high an incidence of complications as might be anticipated from experimental evidence. The timing of drug administration and the doses used may explain this apparent contradiction. Doxorubicin, for example, is a more potent inhibitor of wound healing when delivered preoperatively than postoperatively (211).

Hypertrophic Scars and Keloids

In normal healing, the events progress in an orderly, controlled fashion producing flat, unobtrusive scars. Healing is a biologic process, and as in all biologic processes, there are cases where the process may vary. Healing disturbances with diminished healing have already been discussed. Excessive healing can result in a raised, thickened scar with both functional and cosmetic complications. If the scar is confined to the margins of the original wound, it is called a hypertrophic scar (212). In contrast, keloids extend beyond the confines of the original injury such that the original wound can often no longer be distinguished.

Certain patients and certain wounds are at higher risk for abnormal scarring. Dark-skinned individuals and patients between the ages of 2 and 40 are at higher risk for the development of hypertrophic scars or keloids. Wounds in the presternal or deltoid area, wounds that cross skin tension lines, and wounds in thicker skin have a greater tendency to heal with a thickened scar. Some parts of the body almost never develop abnormal scars, such as the genitalia, the eyelids, the palms of the hands, and the soles of the feet.

Certain patient and wound characteristics increase the relative likelihood of developing a hypertrophic scar as opposed to a keloid (213). Keloids are more likely to be familial than hypertrophic scars. Hypertrophic scars are more likely to be seen in light skinned individuals, though both occur more frequently in dark skinned people. Hypertrophic scars generally develop soon after injury, whereas keloids may develop up to a year after an injury. Hypertrophic scars may subside in time whereas keloids rarely do. Hypertrophic scars are more likely to be associated with a contracture across a joint surface.

Keloids and hypertrophic scars result from an overall net increase in the quantity of collagen synthesized by fibroblasts in the wound area. Recent evidence suggests that the fibroblasts within keloids are different than those within normal dermis in terms of their biologic responsiveness. The etiology of keloids and hypertrophic scars is unknown, although many theories as to etiology have been suggested. Treatment of hypertrophic scars and keloids has included surgical excision, steroid injection, pressure garments, topical silastic gel, radiation therapy, and combinations of these modalities. The absence of a uniform treatment program accurately suggests that no modality of treatment is predictably effective for these lesions (214).

Repair of Skin Wounds

The initial step in the management of a wound is a careful history and physical examination. It must first be assured that another more life threatening problem does not require more immediate attention. In relation to the wound itself, it must be determined when and how the wound was created. The presence of coexisting problems that could interfere with wound management or wound healing must be ascertained. It should also be determined whether the patient smokes and if he or she is taking medications. The patient's nutritional status should be evaluated as well as their cardiac and vascular status.

The wound must be examined to assure that the injured tissue is viable and to determine whether foreign bodies are present. Dusky discoloration of tissue implies poor vascular supply. The possibility of injuries to nerves, ducts, muscle, or bones within the wound must be addressed; radiographic evaluation may be required. The patient's tetanus status should be considered. Antirabies treatment must also be considered for patients bitten by wild animals such as skunks, raccoons, foxes, and bats.

The first decision should be whether to primarily close the defect. Primary wound closure refers to closing the wound at the time of presentation and is preferred unless prevented by coexisting factors. Factors that might prevent primary closure include excessive or uncontrollable bleeding, significant quantities of necrotic and foreign material that cannot be removed easily from the wound, and excessive bacterial contamination. Excessive bacterial contamination is determined optimally by quantitative bacteriology, though this service is not always available. The level of bacterial contamination can be suggested by the time elapsed since injury and the mechanism of injury. The initial 6–8 hours after injury has been referred to as the "golden period" in that closure can usually be accomplished without a markedly increased risk of infection. Experimental data suggest that bacteria trapped within the wound exudate cause infections seen in wounds closed after 6–8 hours and that the bacteria require that time period to reach levels of 10^5/gm of tissue (215,216). Some mechanisms of injury are associated with excessive bacterial contamination. Human bites are a prime example in that saliva contains large quantities of bacteria. Human bites should rarely, if ever, be closed. Other mechanisms of injury, such as farm injuries, are associated with intermediate levels of bacterial contamination. The time and mechanism of injury have to also be considered in light of the location of injury and coexisting problems. Because of better vascularization, one can be more lenient in closing slightly older wounds that have a less favorable mechanism of injury in the head and neck than the foot. Malnourished or steroid-treated patients have less competent immune systems and may not be able to tolerate levels of bacteria that may accumulate in less than 6–8 hours. Another variable would be how aggressively the wound can be treated before closure. If a wound can be excised completely back to fresh tissue, one can be more aggressive in pursuing primary closure than in wounds where such aggressive debridement is not possible. Aggressive debridement may be contraindicated because of a lack of excess tissue or because adjacent structures must be preserved.

If primary closure is not feasible, then a period of wound management is initiated. Wounds initially left open may be closed in a tertiary fashion once the original problem preventing primary closure has been corrected.

In some cases, the level of bacterial contamination is unclear, and a technique of wound closure known as delayed primary closure may be implemented (217). When this technique is used, the wound edges are left open at the time of injury or surgery, and the wound is examined 3 to 4 days later. If the wound appears healthy and uninfected at that point, the wound edges may be approximated with sutures or adhesive strips.

Wounds not closed primarily or in a tertiary fashion may be allowed to heal secondarily. Secondary healing is healing through wound contraction and epithelialization. This method of healing may be preferable, not only for heavily contaminated wounds, but also for small or superficial wounds that will heal in a short period of time. The surgeon can estimate the ability of wound contraction to close the majority of wounds simply by physically coapting the skin edges. If a great deal of force and tension is required to coapt the skin edges, then wound contraction itself will not cover the defect in a reasonable period of time. Conversely, if the skin edges coapt easily without a great deal of tension or contraction of surrounding joints, wound contraction will probably be successful in covering the majority of the wound surface.

Wound Closure

If a wound is deemed adequate for closure, a decision must be made regarding the most appropriate method of closure. Options in order of complexity are 1) direct wound approximation; 2) skin grafts; 3) local flaps; and 4) distant flaps (Table 6.4). The least complex method possible generally is used unless a more complex technique offers an advantage that outweighs the disadvantages of the added complexity. For example, it may be preferable to use a flap instead of a graft for a hand injury with damaged tendons, as a flap will better facilitate subsequent tendon reconstruction.

Direct Wound Approximation

The method used most commonly for incisional wounds is direct wound approximation. The steps involved in wound closure include 1) anesthesia, 2) irrigation, 3) shave and prep, 4) debridement, and 5) wound closure. Anesthesia should virtually always be induced first and wound closure always last, although the order of the intermediate three steps sometimes varies. Local, regional, or general anesthesia may be chosen to facilitate wound closure depending on the wound and the patient.

A variety of local anesthetics are available, but for most limited injuries, lidocaine is most commonly used at a concentration of 0.5% or 1.0%. Increased concentrations are not associated with improved anesthesia and have a higher risk of toxicity. Lidocaine's advantages include its rapid onset of action and its 2–3 hour duration of activity. In addition, few individuals are allergic to lidocaine. Epinephrine, in a concentration of 1:100,000 or 1:200,000, can be added in almost all locations. In the fingers and toes, the addition of epinephrine should be avoided as it can induce vasospasm leading to digital loss. Epinephrine aids in hemostasis, prolongs the duration of action of the anesthetic, and increases the volume of local anesthetic that can safely be injected by delaying absorption, thereby spreading out the metabolism of the agent over a longer period of time (218). Maximum safe doses for lidocaine are 4 mg/kg without epinephrine and 7 mg/kg with epinephrine. Lidocaine, like all local anesthetics, causes pain when it is injected, both due to the injection itself and because of the acidity of the agent. Pain induced by the local administration of lidocaine can be minimized by using the smallest needle possible and minimizing the number of skin punctures. It is also helpful to inject the agent slowly. Subcutaneous injections are less painful than intradermal injections because fatty tissue is displaced more easily by the injected drug, though the anesthetic will take effect more slowly with subcutaneous administration (219). Warming the lidocaine and buffering it with sodium bicarbonate to decrease its acidity also decreases the pain associated with its injection (220).

Closure of wounds in hair bearing areas may be complicated by surrounding hair. In such areas, the hair may be clipped. Bacteria that reside within hair follicles are displaced if the area is shaved. This increases the risk of contamination of the wound and therefore wound infection (221). Shaving of the area should be avoided.

The wound should then be irrigated to decrease the number of bacteria and remove foreign material. High-

Table 6.4.
Methods of Wound Closure

Direct Wound Approximation
Skin Graft
Local Flap
Distant Flap

pressure irrigation (>8 psi) is much more effective at diminishing bacterial concentrations than low pressure irrigation or scrubbing with a saline soaked sponge (222–224). Pulsatile irrigation is the best mechanism for cleansing fragments of foreign debris from soft tissue. Pulsatile irrigation can help minimize the amount of sharp excision that is required to convert a contaminated wound into a clean-contaminated wound. Though a pressurized pulsatile irrigation device is optimal, such machines rarely are available in emergency departments. Alternative methods of providing irrigation with some force include the use of a 60 cc syringe and a 19 gauge angiocath or a flexible IV bag surrounded by a blood pressure cuff (222) and then attached to tubing and an angiocath.

Acceptable agents for irrigation include Ringers lactate, 0.9% saline, and fluids containing a surfactant (225–228). One should avoid the use of surgical hand cleaning soaps in irrigation, as all of these agents have been demonstrated to impede healing (229–232). Alcohol is toxic to tissues and should not be placed on a wound (233). Dakin's solution (0.5% sodium hypochlorite) is toxic to fibroblasts, impairs neutrophil function, slows epithelialization, and slows tensile strength development in incisional wounds (234,235). Similarly, 0.5% acetic acid is lethal to cultured fibroblasts, impairs epithelialization, and slows development of tensile strength in experimental models (235). Hydrogen peroxide may be useful for dissolving blood clots in the wound, but it has no antibacterial function. It has also been demonstrated to kill fibroblasts in culture and cause mild histologic damage to tissue (226). Even standard hand soap induces tissue damage (226). A general guideline is that one should not irrigate an open wound with any solution that would not be comfortable in one's own conjunctival sac (236).

The skin around the wound itself should be prepared with an antibacterial solution. Skin preparation is carried out to limit cross contamination of the wound from bacteria residing on surrounding skin. Povidone-iodine is most commonly used; it has a broad spectrum of antibacterial activity and is tolerated by most individuals (237,238).

Wound debridement is carried out to remove foreign material and necrotic tissue which can contribute to wound infection (239). Wounds with perpendicular edges are more likely to heal with a fine scar than those with beveled or irregular wound edges. Unfavorable wound edges should be excised to create a more favorable wound.

The ideal wound closure method has not been identified. An ideal method would support the wound until it had reached near full strength (at least 6 weeks), would not penetrate the epidermis thereby predisposing to additional scars, would not impair any cellular function required for healing, and would not induce inflammation or ischemia. No method accomplishes all of these goals, and therefore all existing methods represent a compromise. Methods for direct wound closure include sutures, staples, tapes, and tissue adhesives.

Sutures of various type are probably used most commonly. One should choose the smallest caliber suture that is able to maintain the sutured tissues in approximation. This philosophy limits the quantity of foreign material placed in the wound. Sutures are classified as absorbable or nonabsorbable. Absorbable sutures include catgut, chromic catgut, and synthetic sutures made primarily from polyglycolic acid derivatives. Catgut is derived from beef and sheep intestine. Chromic catgut is catgut treated with chromium salts to slow its absorption. Catgut generally is absorbed within a week, whereas chromic catgut persists for up to 2 weeks. Both catgut sutures incite a significant inflammatory response and are digested by proteolytic enzymes. Polyglycolic acid polymer sutures are synthetic absorbable sutures synthesized from organometallic compounds. They maintain substantial strength for 2–3 weeks, depending on location. They do not induce a significant inflammatory response. Absorbable sutures are useful for visceral wounds where healing is rapid, suture removal is difficult, and bacterial contamination makes a permanent suture a potential liability.

Nonabsorbable sutures include nylon and a variety of synthetic materials. Silk is also considered permanent, even though it is absorbed slowly over a 2 year period. Nonabsorbable sutures are used in superficial locations where they can be removed and in deeper tissues where wound support is required for a long period of time.

Some sutures are monofilament and some are multifilamentous weaves. Monofilament sutures have the advantage of inducing a limited tissue reaction, although they have the disadvantages of being less easy to tie and manipulate and producing stiff, rigid knots. Multifilament suture are generally more pliable and easy to tie, although bacteria can multiply in the interstices of the multi filamentous weave and may induce a more severe reaction in the surrounding tissues.

Sutures are left in place until healing has created enough wound strength to allow their removal. Removal of sutures too early can result in widening of a scar or even disruption of a wound. However, an epithelialized tract will develop around a suture left in skin for longer than 7–10 days (240). The tract will fill with scar after suture removal, resulting in unsightly suture marks. Sutures should therefore be removed at or before 10 days if possible. The decision as to when to remove sutures from a particular wound necessitates developing a compromise between factors that require prolonged wound support and those that promote early removal. The factors involved include the age, site and type of wound, the general condition of the patient, and whether the wound is further supported by buried sutures. Skin wounds in most anatomic locations generally are not subjected to significant tension and can maintain satisfactory closure with 15% or less of the tensile strength of normal skin. Therefore, skin sutures can often be removed relatively soon after wound closure. Facial wounds are subjected to little stress, and healing in the head and neck is facilitated because of the excellent blood supply. A general rule is to remove sutures in the face at 4 to 5 days. Abdominal skin sutures are generally left in slightly longer and are removed at 7–10 days. Sutures on the lower extremity are left in longer (241). Wounds subjected to excessive tension, such as in skin overlying joints, or wounds in individuals with impaired healing due to diabetes, steroids or other factors, may require longer periods of suture closure to avoid disruption (Fig. 6.3). Any wound must be inspected carefully before sutures are removed. Evidence of undue tension or delayed healing may require that sutures be left in place longer than originally anticipated.

Closure with staples is more rapid than suture closure although tissue approximation may not be as precise (242). This can be improved by additional sutures placed in the dermis. Like sutures, additional scars will result if staples are left in place too long. Tapes such as Steri strips are easy to apply, comfortable for the patient, and leave no marks in the skin (243–245). However, they can be displaced inadvertently and may be less precise than sutures if used alone. In addition, wound edema tends to cause inversion of taped wound edges.

Tissue adhesives that have been used include cyanoacrylate and fibrin. Cyanoacrylate tissue adhesives slow healing by increasing wound inflammation and increasing the likelihood of infection (246). They are not widely used clinically at this time. Fibrin glue has been used to improve the adherence and take of skin grafts (247,248) and for blepharoplasty closure along with the judicious use of sutures (249). Although a useful adjunct, fibrin glue does not produce a strong enough bond to allow its use alone for incisional wounds. Commercially produced fibrin glue is available in Europe, although, as a homologous product, it carries a theoretical risk of virus transmission. In the United States, only autologous fibrin has been utilized.

The old surgical dictum that dead space should be closed or obliterated seems to call for the use of stitches in subcutaneous tissues. However, this is not true; both laboratory and human studies have demonstrated that multiple layers of closure contribute to an increased risk of wound infection (250,251). Stitches in fat convey no additional strength to a wound closure and should be avoided; however, deeper fascial layers should be closed because they contribute to the structural integrity of the wound closure. Closed suction drains are preferable to subcutaneous stitches for the prevention of fluid collections beneath the skin. In addition to limiting the accumulation of blood and serum, suction drains aid in the approximation of tissues. Although most drains are relatively inert, all drains can potentiate infections and

should be removed as soon as drainage is at an acceptable level.

Skin Grafts

Grafts or flaps are used in larger wounds when direct wound approximation cannot be accomplished without unduly distorting normal structures. Grafts are generally simpler to use than flaps. Skin grafts are taken at precise thicknesses that have traditionally been measured in thousandths of an inch. Split-thickness skin grafts (STSG's) consist of epidermis and a portion of the underlying dermis. Thinner STSG's include less dermis, whereas thicker grafts include more dermis. Full-thickness skin grafts (FTSG's) include the full thickness of dermis and epidermis. Full-thickness grafts can only be harvested from areas where skin is thin, or the graft will be too thick to survive. Thin and thick grafts have different characteristics, and the choice between them is based on the nature of the wound to be covered. Thin grafts take more readily and are preferred for less reliable recipient sites. Thicker grafts, especially full-thickness grafts, tend to maintain a more normal appearance than thin grafts. Thicker and full-thickness grafts are therefore commonly used in areas like the face where cosmesis is important. Full-thickness grafts also have the capability of maintaining hair growth when taken from hair-bearing areas.

Primary and secondary graft contracture is directly related to graft thickness. Primary graft contracture is the contraction noted after graft harvest, before placement on the wound bed, and is produced by dermal elastin. Only thicker grafts that include a significant amount of dermis undergo a large degree of primary contraction. Secondary graft contracture refers to the contraction that occurs after the graft is placed on a wound during healing. In secondary contracture, the wound is contracting, not the graft. Thicker grafts limit secondary graft contracture to a greater degree than thinner grafts (127). The critical variable is not the absolute thickness of the skin, but rather the amount of deeper dermis included in the graft. This is important because skin varies considerably in thickness from one part of the body to another, and a full-thickness graft from an area where the skin is thin (i.e., the upper eyelid) may be the same thickness as a split-thickness graft taken from the back where skin is thicker. The eyelid graft will be a more potent inhibitor of wound contraction.

Another consideration is whether to mesh the graft. Meshing involves rolling the graft through a device that places small incisions within it, allowing it to expand like a pantograph. Meshing provides several advantages but also produces some disadvantages. Meshed grafts can expand and cover more area than nonmeshed grafts, limiting the amount of graft required. Meshing provides drain holes that limit the possibility of blood or serum collecting beneath the graft. Meshed grafts may also conform to irregular contours better than nonmeshed grafts. Wounds closed with meshed grafts have a less aesthetic irregular contour than wounds closed with nonmeshed grafts, however. Wounds closed with meshed grafts may also contract more than wounds closed with unmeshed grafts because the interstices of meshed grafts must heal secondarily by wound contraction and epithelialization (252). Meshed grafts should therefore be avoided over joint surfaces.

Any reconstructive method has some cost associated with it. For skin grafts, the primary cost is the second wound at the donor site. The donor sites of split-thickness grafts will heal secondarily by epithelialization, whereas those of full-thickness grafts must be closed. Direct wound approximation is possible if the full-thickness donor site is small, although split-thickness grafting may be required if the donor site is large. Preferred donor sites for all grafts are from places not easily visible. The buttocks and upper thighs, which are often covered by clothes, are the most commonly used donor sites for split-thickness grafts.

Skin harvested from the supraclavicular area and cephalad resembles facial skin more than skin from the back, abdomen, or extremities. For that reason, head and neck donor sites are preferred for grafts to the facial region. Commonly used donor sites include the postauricular area, the supraclavicular area, and the scalp. The postauricular area is commonly used for smaller full-thickness grafts. Larger full- or split-thickness grafts can be harvested from the supraclavicular area. The scalp is an excellent donor site for split-thickness grafts. The donor site is hidden after hair regrowth, and split-thickness scalp grafts generally do not grow hair. The head must be shaved to take the graft, however, and this may not be acceptable to some patients.

Wounds closed with grafts are durable once the graft has healed. Full-thickness grafts grow predictably as the patient grows, although split thickness grafts grow less predictably. Grafted skin, especially thinner grafts, tends to become more darkly pigmented after transfer. Only full-thickness grafts will grow hair. Sebaceous activity generally returns after several months in grafts thick enough to include sebaceous glands. Sensation and sweating return after a variable period of months or even years. Sensation is most like that in the recipient area (253).

Skin Flaps

The decision whether to use a skin graft or a flap for the closure of a large wound is based on the nature of the wound and the desired aesthetic and functional result. Skin grafts will only take on a well-vascularized bed. Skin grafts cannot be used where the wound base includes relatively avascular tissue such as bone, cartilage, nerve, or tendon. Skin grafts also do poorly in areas

rendered relatively avascular by radiation or chronic scarring. Such wounds require the use of a flap for closure.

Flaps may be used in place of skin grafts to provide either an improved aesthetic result or tissue with a specific desired characteristic. In general, local flaps are used if a flap of the appropriate dimension and type is available, and distant or free flaps are used when local tissue of the desired type is not available. The aesthetic and functional cost of any flap must be considered before flap transfer to ensure an appropriate cost/benefit ratio.

Flaps have been characterized in a variety of ways. The most meaningful categorization divides flaps into random-pattern and axial flaps (254) according to their blood supply. Random-pattern flaps are supplied by blood flowing through perforating vessels to the subdermal plexus proximal to the flap base. Generally, a large number of such small, unnamed perforating blood vessels exist. In random-pattern flaps, no single blood vessel is critical to flap survival, and their length is generally limited. Axial pattern flaps are based on a known, major blood vessel that has the capability of nourishing the entire flap. In many anatomic locations, axial vessels enter deep to muscle, allowing the elevation of muscle and skin as a single musculocutaneous flap. In other locations, axial vessels run adjacent to the fascia above the muscle, allowing the elevation of a fasciocutaneous flap. Most axial flaps have been defined by careful anatomic studies of the tissue supplied by a specific blood vessel, and many are large.

Flaps tissue is unchanged in color, texture, thickness, hair-bearing characteristics, and sebaceous activity by the transfer process. Flaps will grow with the patient. Sensation and sweating will be maintained if a nerve supply is transferred intact. When a nerve supply is not maintained, some sensation usually returns to the flap over a matter of months. Flaps can be designed that allow the transfer of viable bone or specialized structures such as jejunum when such tissue is required for complex restorations.

Dressings

Different types of wounds have different needs and therefore require different dressings. Partial thickness injuries where the epidermis and a portion of the dermis are lost heal primarily by epithelialization and are best treated by dressings that maintain a warm moist environment (255,256). A variety of dressings can meet this need, including biologic dressings like allograft (257), amnion (258) or xenografts (259), synthetic biologic dressings (260), hydrogel dressings, and semipermeable or nonpermeable membranes (256). These dressings do not require changing as long as they remain adherent. Other types of dressing require frequent dressing changes (261).

Wet to dry dressings are preferred where the goal of dressing changes is debridement of necrotic tissue, foreign bodies or other debris. Saline soaked wide-meshed gauze dressings are applied, allowed to dry, and then changed every 6–8 hours. Granulation tissue and wound exudate, including necrotic tissue and other debris, become incorporated within the interstices of the meshed gauze as it dries, and thus debridement is accomplished when the dressing is changed (262,263). Enzymatic agents, such as collagenase, may augment the debriding effect of wet to dry dressing changes (264).

The disadvantage of a wet to dry dressing change regimen is that viable cells are damaged by the desiccation and mechanical debridement. Wet to dry dressings should be discontinued when adequate debridement has been accomplished. Wet to wet dressing changes in which the gauze is not allowed to dry minimize tissue damage. Wet dressings can also be used to facilitate heat transfer, which decreases pain and increases capillary perfusion (236). Wet dressings can be harmful if the wounded area becomes overly moist and maceration occurs.

Virtually any type of dressing change regimen will lower the bacterial count in infected wounds (265). Regimens using antibacterial agents that directly effect the offending bacteria generally decrease the bacterial count in wounds more rapidly than other regimens. Silver sulfadiazine is a frequently used broad spectrum antibacterial that has the secondary benefit of maintaining a moist environment and accelerating epithelialization (265–267).

For wounds with exposed tendons or nerves, it is particularly important that a moist environment be maintained to prevent desiccation. Options include biologic and membrane dressings, though they are both difficult to use in deep irregular wounds or if a wound drainage is present. Wet to wet dressings or dressings including creams such as silver sulfadiazine are particularly useful in these settings.

For incisional wounds, dressings optimally include several layers with different functions. The layer immediately adjacent to the wound should be sterile and non-adhering and should not be occlusive. A fine meshed gauze impregnated with a hydrophilic substance is available and meets those needs. The layer over the contact layer should be absorptive and should wick exudate or transudate away from the wound surface. Wide meshed gauze facilitates this capillary action and drainage (268). Such absorptive layers must not become saturated in that exudate will then collect on the wound surface and produce maceration. The outermost layer of the dressing is the binding layer that fixes the dressing in place. Tape is used most commonly, although wraps are useful on extremities. Dressings may generally be discontinued after 48 hours if no drainage occurs; the epithelial layer will have sealed the wound by that time. An alternative method of treating a minimally draining incisional wound is antibacterial ointment. The ointments are occlusive and maintain a sterile moist environment for the 48 hours required for epithelialization. The ointment prevents crusting and scab formation. Ointments, however, are washed away if drainage from the wound is excessive and can easily be inadvertently mechanically removed. This approach is best applied to the face.

For small wounds in difficult areas, it may be easier not to dress the wound and to allow a scab to form. Scabs consist of fibrin, red blood cells, and exudate which protect the wound and limit bacterial invasion and desiccation. Epithelial cells advancing beneath the scab must break down the scab-wound interface as they migrate across the wound (269). Epithelialization is slower under a scab than under an occlusive dressing.

Horizons in Wound Healing

The focus for wound healing in the future will be repair with little or no scarring. At present, scar tissue is the unavoidable result of successful repair. No scar is desirable, and as mentioned, scarring can lead to functional and aesthetic deformities such as wound contractures, anastomotic strictures, and unsightly keloids. In internal organs, liver cirrhosis with secondary portal hypertension, pulmonary fibrosis, and urethral strictures are sequelae of excess scar formation. Complications of scarring might be palliated by pharmacologic agents that restrict collagen synthesis and cross-linking, although exploration of these avenues has produced limited results. The fetal environment is notable for scarless healing (270). A better understanding of how healing occurs in the fetus may help us modulate the healing process in adults. The challenge for investigators in the control of scar tissue is to find agents that accomplish these goals without the debilitating side effects. The ultimate challenge is to stimulate tissue regeneration instead of wound healing through genetic manipulation. Such methodology could allow restoration of even complex damaged structures, such as hands or internal organs, instead of simply sealing the damaged areas with a scar.

Acknowledgements

I acknowledge the contributions of James L. Peacock, MD and Erle E. Peacock, MD which were maintained from the original chapter in the first edition of Physiologic Basis of Surgery.

REFERENCES

1. Singer DW. Selections from the works of Ambroise Paré. New York: William Wood, 1924:38.
2. Meyer FA, Fromjmovic MM, Vic MM. Characteristics of the major platelet membrane site used in binding collagen. Thromb Res 1979;15:755–767.
3. Santaro SA. Identification of a 160,000 Dalton platelet membrane protein that mediates the initial divalent cation-dependent adhesion of platelets to collagen. Cell 1986;913–920.
4. Detwiler TC, Feinman RD. Kinetics of thrombin-induced release of calcium by platelets. Biochemistry 1973;12:282–289.
5. Plow EF, Ginsberg MH, Marguerie GA. Expression and function of adhesive proteins on the platelet surface. in Biochemistry of platelets. Phillips, DR and Shuman, MA, eds. New York: Academic Press, 1986;226–256.
6. Esmon CT. Cell mediated events that control blood coagulation and vascular injury. Annu Rev Cell Biol 1993;9:1–26.
7. Stiernberg J, Redin WR, Warner WS, Carney DH. The role of thrombin and thrombin receptor activating peptide (TRAP-508) in initiation of tissue repair. Thromb Haemost 1993;70:158–162.
8. Tanaka K, Sueishi K. Biology of disease. The coagulation and fibrinolysis systems and atherosclerosis. Lab Invest 1993;69:5–18.
9. Williams TJ, Peck MJ. Role of prostaglandin-mediated vasodilation in inflammation. Nature 1977;270:530.
10. Bisgaard H, Kristensen J, Sondergaared J. The effect of leukotriene C4 and D4 on cutaneous blood flow in humans. Prostaglandins 1982;23:797–801.
11. Cherry PD, Furchgott RF, Zawadzki JV, Jothianadan D. Role of endothelial cells in relaxation of isolated arteries by bradykinin. Proc Natl Acad Sci U S A 1982;72:2106–2110.
12. Griffith TM, Edwards DH, Lewis MJ, Newby AC, Henderson AH. The nature of the endothelium derived vascular relaxant factor. Nature 1984;308:645–647.
13. Lewis T, Grant R. Vascular reactions of the skin to injury. Part II. The liberation of a histamine-like substance in injured skin; the underlying cause of factitious urticaria and of wheals produced by burning, and observations upon the nervous control of certain skin reactions. Heart 1924;11:209–265.
14. Hebda PA, Collins MA, Tharp MA. Mast cell and myofibroblast in wound healing. Derm Clin 1993;11:685–696.
15. Singfelder JR. Prostaglandins: A review. N Engl J Med 1982;307:746–747.
16. Ammeland E, Prasad CM, Raymond RM, Grega GJ. Interactions among inflammatory mediators on edema formation in the canine forelimb. Circ Res 1981;49:298–306.
17. Williamson LM, Sheppard K, Davies JM, Fletcher J. Neutrophils are involved in the increased vascular permeability produced by activated complement in man. Br J Haematol 1986;64:375–384.
18. Majno G, Schoefl GI, Palade G. Studies on inflammation. II. The site of action of histamine and serotonin on the vascular tree; a topographic study. Journal of Biophysics, Biochemistry 1961;11:607–626.
19. Majno G, Shea SM, Leventhal M. Endothelial contraction induced by histamine type mediators. An electron microscopic study. J Cell Biol 1969;42:647–672.
20. McLean AEM, Ahmed K, Judah JD. Cellular permeability and the reaction to injury. Ann N Y Acad Sci 1964;116:986–989.
21. Stevenson TR, Mathes SJ. Wound healing. In: Miller TA, ed. Physiologic basis of modern surgical care. St. Louis: CV Mosby 1988:1010–1018.
22. Ley K. Leukocyte adhesion to vascular endothelium. J Reconstr Microsurg 1992;8:495–503.
23. Marasco WA, Phan SH, Krutzsch et al. Purification and identification of formyl-methionyl-leucyl-phenylalanine as the major peptide neutrophil chemotactic factor produced by Escherichia coli. J Biol Chem 1984;259:5430–5439.
24. Snyderman R, Phillips J, Mergenhagen SE. Polymorphonuclear leukocyte chemotactic activity in rabbit serum and guinea pig serum treated with immune complexes: Evidence for C5a as the major chemotactic factor. Infect Immun 1970;1:521–525.
25. Tonnesen MG, Smedly LA, Henson PM. Neutrophil-endothelial cell interactions: Modulation of neutrophil adhesiveness induced by complement fragments C5a and C5a des arg and formyl-methionyl-leucyl-phenylalanine in vitro. J Clin Invest 1984;745:1581–1592.
26. Peacock EE Jr. Wound repair. 3rd ed. Philadelphia: WB Saunders, 1984.
27. Ford-Hutchinson AW, Bray MA, Doig MV, Shipley ME, Smith MJH. Leukotriene B, a potent chemokinetic and aggregating substance released from polymorphonuclear leukocytes. Nature 1980;286:264–265.
28. Deuel TF, Senior RM, Huang JS, Griffin GL. Chemotaxis of monocytes and neutrophils to platelet-derived growth factor. J Clin Invest 1982;69:1046–1049.
29. Musson RA. Human serum induces maturation of human monocytes in vitro. Am J Pathol 1983;111:331–340.
30. Proveddini DM, Deftos LJ, Manolagas SC. 1,25-dihydroxyvitamin D3 promotes in vitro morphologic and enzymatic changes in normal human monocytes consistent with their differentiation into macrophages. Bone 1986;7:23–28.
31. Wright SD, Meyer BC. Fibronectin receptor of human macrophages recognizes sequence Arg-Gly-Asp-Ser. J Exp Med 1985;162:762–767.
32. Ishida M, Honda M, Heyashi H. In vitro macrophage chemotactic generation from serum immunoglobulin G by neutrophil neutral seryl protease. Immunology 1978;35:167–176.
33. Marder SR, Chenoweth DE, Goldstein IM, Perez HD. Chemotactic responses of human peripheral blood monocytes to the complement-derived peptides C5a and C5a des Arg. J Immunol 1985;134:3325–3331.
34. Norris DA, Clark RAF, Swigart LM, Huff JC, Weston WL, Howell SE. Fibronectin fragment(s) are chemotactic for human peripheral blood monocytes. J Immunol 1982;129:1612–1618.
35. Postlethwaite AE, Kang AH. Collagen- and collagen peptide-induced chemotaxis of human blood monocytes. J Exp Med 1976;143:1299–1307.
36. Senior RM, Griffin GL, Mecham RP, Wrenn DS, Prasad KU, Urry DW. Val-Gly-Val-Ala-Pro-Gly, a repeating peptide in elastin is chemotactic for fibroblasts and monocytes. J Cell Biol 1984;99:870–874.
37. Snyderman R, Fudman EJ. Demonstration of a chemotactic factor receptor on macrophages. J Immunol 1980;124:2754–2757.
38. Wahl SM, Hunt DA, Wakefield LM et al. Transforming growth factor induces monocyte chemotaxis and growth factor production. Proc Natl Acad Sci U S A 1987;84:5788–5792.
39. Diegelmann RF, Cohen IK, Kaplan AM. The role of macrophages in wound repair: A review. Plast Reconstr Surg 1981;68:107–113.
40. Huybrechts-Godin G, Peeters-Joris C, Vaes G. Partial characterization of the macrophage factor that stimulates fibroblasts to produce collagenase and to degrade collagen. Biochim Biophys Acta 1985;846:51–54.
41. Werb Z, Banda MJ, Jones PA. Degradation of connective tissue matrices by macrophages I. Proteolysis of elastin, glycoproteins and collagen by proteinases isolated from macrophages. J Exp Med 1980;152:1340–1357.
42. Peterson JM, Barbul A, Breslin RJ, Wasserkrug HL Efron, G. Significance of T-lymphocytes in wound healing. Surgery 1987;102:300–305.
43. Blotnick S, Peoples GE, Freeman MR, Eberlein TJ, Klagsbrun M. T-lymphocytes synthesize and export heparin-binding epidermal growth factor-like growth factor and basic fibroblast growth factor, mitogens for vascular cells and fibroblasts: Differential production and release by CD4$^+$ and CD8$^+$ T cells. Proc Natl Acad Sci U S A 1994;91:2890–2894.
44. Ross R. The role of T lymphocytes in inflammation. Proc Natl Acad Sci U S A 1994;91:2879.
45. Robbins, RA, Klassen, L, Rasmussen, H, Clayton, MEM, Russ, WD. Interleukin-2-induced chemotaxis of human T-lymphocytes. J Lab Clin Med 1986;108:340–345.
46. Van Epps, D.E. Mediators and modulators of human lymphocyte chemotaxis. Agents Actions Suppl 1983;12:217–233.
47. Leibovich, SJ, Ross, R. The role of the macrophage in wound repair. A study with hydrocortisone and antimacrophage serum. Am J Pathol 1975;78:71–100.
48. Simpson, DM, Ross, R. The neutrophilic leukocyte in wound repair. A study with antineutrophil serum. J Clin Invest 1972;51:2009–2023.
49. Baxter, CR: Immunologic reactions in chronic wounds. Am J Surg 1994;167(Suppl):12S–14S.

50. Ross R, Everett NB, Tyler R. Wound healing and collagen formation. VI. The origin of the wound fibroblast studied in parabiosis. J Cell Biol 1970;44:645–654.

51. Seppä, H, Grotendorst, GR, Seppä, S, Schiffman, E, Martin, GR. Platelet-derived growth factor is chemoattractant for fibroblasts. J Cell Biol 1982;92:584–588.

52. Grotendorst, GR, Chang, T, Seppä HEJ, Kleinman, HK, Martin, GR. Platelet-derived growth factor is a chemoattractant for vascular smooth muscle cells. J Cell Physiol 1982;112:261–266.

53. Gauss-Muller, V, Kleinman, HK, Martin, GR, Schiffman, E. Role of attachment factors and attractants in fibroblast chemotaxis. J Lab Clin Med 1981;96:1071–1080.

54. Postlethwaite, AE, Keski-Oja, J, Ballan, G, Kang, A. Induction of fibroblast chemotaxis by fibronectin. J Exp Med 1981;153:494–499.

55. Tsukamoto, Y, Helsel, WE, Wahl, SE. Macrophage production of fibronectin, a chemoattractant for fibroblasts. J Immunol 1981;127:673–678.

56. Westermark, B and Blomquist, W: Stimulation of fibroblast migration by epidermal growth factor. Cell Biol Int 1980;4:649–654.

57. Postlewhaite, AE, Snyderman R, Kang, AH. The chemotactic attraction of human fibroblasts to a lymphocyte derived factor. J Exp Med 1976;144:188–1203.

58. Postlethwaite, AE, Seyer, JM, Kang, AH. Chemotactic attraction of human fibroblasts to type I, II, and III collagens and collagen derived peptides. Proc Natl Acad Sci U S A 1978;75:871–875.

59. Grotendorst, GR, Pencev, D, Martin, GR, Sodek, J. Molecular mediators of tissue repair. In: Hunt TK, Heppenstall RB, Pines E, Rovee D, eds. Soft and hard tissue repair: biological and clinical aspects. New York: Praeger, 1984;20–41.

60. Rutherford, RB and Ross, R: Platelet factors stimulate fibroblasts and smooth muscle cells quiescent in plasma serum to proliferate. J Cell Biol 1976;69:196–203.

61. Roberts AB, Anzano MA, Wakefield LM, Roche NS, Stern DF, Sporn MB. Type-β transforming growth factor: A bifunctional regulator of cellular growth. Proc Natl Acad Sci U S A 1985;82:119–123.

62. Assoian RK, Grotendorst GR, Miller DM, Sporn MB. Cellular transformation by coordinated action of three peptide growth factors from human platelets. Nature 1984;309:804–806.

63. Wahl SM, Wahl LM, McCarthy JB. Lymphocyte-mediated activation of fibroblast proliferation and collagen production. J Immunol 1978;121:942–946.

64. Clemmons DR. Interaction of circulating cell-derived and plasma growth factors in stimulating cultured smooth muscle cell replication. J Cell Phys 1984;121: 425–430.

65. Ronning OW, Pettersen EO. Effect of different growth factors on cell cycle traverse and protein growth of human cells in culture. Exp Cell Res 1985;157:29–40.

66. Folkman J, Klagsbrun M. Angiogenic factors. Science 1987;235:442–447.

67. Sholley MM, Ferguson GP, Seibel HR, Montour JL, Wilson JD. Mechanisms of neovascularization. Vascular sprouting can occur without proliferation of endothelial cells. Lab Invest 1984;51:624–634.

68. Madri JA, Williams SK. Capillary endothelial cell cultures: Phenotypic modulation by matrix components. J Cell Biol 1983;97:153–165.

69. Polverini PJ, Coltran RS, Gimbrone MA, Unanue ER. Activated macrophages induce vascularization. Nature 1977; 269:804–806.

70. Polverini PJ, Leibovich SJ. Induction of neovascularization in vivo and endothelial cell proliferation in vitro by tumor-associated macrophages. Lab Invest 1984;51:635–642.

71. Koch AE, Polverini PJ, Leibovich SJ. Induction of neovascularization by activated human monocytes. J Leukoc Biol 1986;39:223–238.

72. Gospodarowicz D, Neufeld G, Schweigerer L. Fibroblast growth factor: Structural and biologic properties. J Cell Physiol Suppl 1987;5:15–26.

73. Shing Y, Folkmann J, Sullivan R, Butterfield C, Murray J, Klagsbrun M. Heparin affinity: Purification of a tumor-derived capillary endothelial cell growth factor. Science 1984;223:1296–1299.

74. Roberts AB, Sporn MB, Assoian RK et al. Transforming growth factor type Beta: Rapid induction of fibrosis and angiogenesis in vivo and stimulation of collagen formation in vitro: Proc Natl Acad Sci U S A 1986;83: 4167–4171.

75. Gospodarowicz D, Abraham J, Schilling J. Isolation and characterization of a vascular endothelial cell mitogen produced by pituitary-derived follicular stellate cells. Proc Natl Acad Sci U S A 1989;86:7311–7315.

76. Banda MJ, Dwyer KS Beckman A. Wound fluid angiogenesis factor stimulates the directed migration of capillary endothelial cells. J Cell Biochem 1985;29:183–193.

77. Banda MJ, Knighton DR, Hunt TK, Werb Z. Isolation of a nonmitogenic factor from wound fluid. Proc Natl Acad Sci U S A 1982; 79:7773–7777.

78. Castellot JJ Jr, Karnovsky MJ, Spiegelman BM. Differentiation-dependent stimulation of neovascularization and endothelial cell chemotaxis by 3T3 adipocytes. Proc Natl Acad Sci U S A 1982; 79:5597–5601.

79. Teuscher E, Weidlich V. Adenosine nucleotides, adenosine and adenine as angiogenesis factors. Biomed Biochim Acta 1985;44:493–495.

80. Clemmons DR, Isley WL, Brown MT. Dialyzable factor in human serum of platelet origin stimulates endothelial replication and growth. Proc Natl Acad Sci U S A 1983;80:1641–1645.

81. Schott RJ, Morrow LA. Growth factors and angiogenesis. Cardiovasc Res 1993;27:1155–1161.

82. Ansprunk DH, Falterman K, Folkman J. The sequence of events in the regression of corneal capillaries. Lab Invest 1978;38:284–294.

83. Pang C, Daniels RK, Buck RC. Epidermal migration during the healing of suction blisters in rat skin: A scanning and transmission electron microscopic study. American Journal of Anatomy 1978;153:177–191.

84. Johnson FR, McMinn RM. The cytology of wound healing of body surfaces in mammals. Biol Rev 1962;35:364–412.

85. Odland G, Ross R. Human wound repair. I. Epidermal regeneration. J Cell Biol 1968;39:135–151.

86. Woodley DT, Chen JD, Kim JP et al. Re-epithelialization: Human keratinocyte locomotion. Dermatol Clin 1993;11:641–646.

87. Dunlap MK, Donaldson DJ. Inability of colchicine to inhibit newt epidermal cell migration or prevent concanavalin-A mediated inhibition of migration studies. Exp Cell Res 1978;116:15–19.

88. Sullivan DJ, Epstein WS. Mitotic activity of wounded human epidermis. J Invest Dermatol 1963;41:39–43.

89. Mackenzie IC, Fusenig NE. Regeneration of organized epithelial structure. J Invest Dermatol 1983;81:1895–1945.

90. Niall M Ryan GB, O'Brien BM. The effect of epidermal growth factor on wound healing in mice. J Surg Res 1982;33:164–169.

91. Nanney LB, Magid M, Stoscheck CM, et al. Comparison of epidermal growth factor binding and receptor distribution in normal human epidermis and epidermal appendages. J Invest Dermatol 1984;83:385–393.

92. Gillman T. Healing of cutaneous abrasions and of incisions closed with sutures or plastic adhesive tape. Medical Proceedings 1958; 4:751.

93. Nimmi ME. Collagen: Its structure and function in normal and pathological connective tissues. Semin Arthritis Rheum 1974;4:95–150.

94. Caterson B, Lowther DA. Changes in the metabolism of the proteoglycans from sheep articular cartilage in response to mechanical stress. Biochem Biophys Acta 1978;540:412–422.

95. Weiss PH, Klein L. The quantitative relationship of urinary peptide hydroxyproline excretion to collagen degradation. J Clin Invest 1969;48:1–10.

96. Ignotz RA, Massaugue J. Transforming growth factor-beta stimulates the expression of fibronectin and collagen and their incorporation into the extracellular matrix. J Biol Chem 1986;261:4337–4345.

97. Cutroneo KR, Rokowski R, Counts DF. Glucocorticoids and collagen synthesis: comparison of in vivo and cell culture studies. Collagen and Related Research 1981;1:557–568.

98. Sunder R, Church CV, Klobutcher LA, et al. Genetics of the connective tissue proteins. Assignment of the gene for human type I procollagen to chromosome 17. Proc Natl Acad Sci U S A 1977; 74: 4444–4448.

99. Church RL. Chromosome mapping of connective tissue proteins. International Review of Connective Tissue Research 1981;9:99.

100. Madden JW, Arem AJ. Wound healing: biologic and clinical features. In: Sabiston DC Jr, ed. Textbook of surgery. 13th ed. Philadelphia: WB Saunders, 1986;193–213.

101. Fleischmajer R, Olsen BR, Kuhn K. Biology, chemistry and pathology of collagen. Ann N Y Acad Sci 1985;460:1–13.
102. Chapman JA, Kellgren JH, Steven FS. Assembly of collagen fibrils. Federal Proceedings 1966;25:1811–1812.
103. Petruska JA, Hodge AJ. A subunit model for the tropocollagen macromolecule. Proc Natl Acad Sci U S A 1964;51:871–876.
104. Siegel RC, Pinnel SR, Martin GR. Cross linking of collagen and elastin. Properties of lysyl oxidase. Biochem 1970;9:4486–4492.
105. Tanzer ML. Cross linking of collagen. Science 1973;180:561–566.
106. Veis A, Averey J. Modes of intermolecular cross linking in mature insoluble collagen. J Biol Chem 1965;240:3899–3908.
107. Hassel JR, Kimura JH, Hascall VC. Proteoglycan core protein families. Annual Rev Biochem 1986;55:539–567.
108. Hynes RO. Fibronectins. Sci Am 1986;254:42–51.
109. Oh E, Pierschbacher M, Ruoslahti E. Deposition of plasma fibronectin in tissue. Proc Natl Acad Sci U S A 1981;78:3218–3221.
110. Hynes RO, Yamada KM. Fibronectins: Multifunctional modular glycoproteins. J Cell Biol 1982;95:369–377.
111. Grinnell F. Fibronectin and wound healing. J Cell Biochem 1984;25:107–116.
112. Clark RAF, Folkvord JM, Wertz RL. Fibronectin as well as other extracellular matrix proteins mediate human keratinocyte adherence. J Invest Dermatol 1985;84:378–383.
113. Postlethwaite A, Keski-Oja J, Balian G, et al. Induction of fibroblast chemotaxis by fibronectin. Localization of the chemotactic region of a 140,000 molecular weight non-gelatin-binding fragment. J Exp Med 1981;153:494–499.
114. Gabbianni G, Ryan GB, Majno G. Presence of modified fibroblasts in granulation tissue and their possible role in wound contraction. Experientia 1971;27:549–550.
115. McGrath MH, Hundahl SA. The spatial and temporal quantification of myofibroblasts. Plast Reconstr Surg 1982;69:975–983.
116. Rudolph R. Location of the force of wound contraction. Surg Gynecol Obstet 1979;148:547–551.
117. Ehrlich HP. The role of connective tissue matrix in wound healing. In: Growth factors and other aspects of wound healing: biological and clinical implications. New York: Alan R Liss, Inc, 1988;243–258.
118. Harris AK, Stopak D, Wild P. Fibroblast traction as a mechanism for collagen morphogenesis. Nature 1981;290:249–251.
119. Grinnell F, Lamke DR. Reorganization of hydrated collagen lattices by human skin fibroblasts. J Cell Sci 1984;66:51–63.
120. Guidry C, Grinnell F. Studies on the mechanism of hydrated collagen gel reorganization by fibroblasts. J Cell Sci 1985;79:67–81.
121. Farsi JMA, Aubin JE. Microfilament rearrangements during fibroblast-induced contraction of three-dimensional hydrated collagen gels. Cell Motil Cytoskeleton 1984;4:29–40.
122. Montesano R, Orci L. Transforming growth factor Beta stimulates collagen-matrix contraction by fibroblasts: Implications for wound healing. Proc Natl Acad Sci U S A 1988;85:4894–4897.
123. Ronnov-Jensen L, Peterson OW. Induction of alpha-smooth muscle actin by transforming growth factor-1 in quiescent human breast gland fibroblasts. Lab Invest 1993;68:696–707.
124. Clark RAF, Folkvord JM, Hart CE, et al. Platelet isoforms of platelet-derived growth factor stimulate fibroblasts to contract collagen matrices. J Clin Invest 1989;84:1036–1040.
125. Dubretet LF, Brunner-Ferber F, Misiti J, et al. Activities of human acidic fibroblast growth factor in an in vitro dermal equivalent model. J Invest Dermatol 1991;97:793–798.
126. Gillery P, Serpier H, Polette M, et al. Gamma-interferon inhibits extracellular matrix synthesis and remodeling in collagen lattice cultures of normal and scleroderma skin fibroblasts. Eur J Cell Biol 1992;57:244–253.
127. Rudolph R. The effect of skin graft preparation on wound contraction. Surg Gynecol Obstet 1976;142:49–56.
128. Madden JW, Morton D Jr, Peacock EE Jr. Contraction of experimental wounds. I. Inhibiting wound contraction by using a topical smooth muscle antagonist. Surgery 1974;76:1–8.
129. Madden JW, Peacock EE Jr. Studies on the biology of collagen during wound healing. I. Rate of collagen synthesis and deposition in cutaneous wounds of the rat. Surgery 1968;64:288–294.
130. Levenson SM, Geever EF, Crowley LV, et al. The healing of rat skin wounds. Ann Surg 1965;161:293–308.
131. Forrester JC, Zederfeldt BH, Hayes TL, et al. Wolff's law in relation to the healing skin wound. J Trauma 1970;10:770–779.
132. Riley WB Jr, Peacock EE Jr. Identification, distribution and significance of a collagenolytic enzyme in human tissue. Proc Soc Biol Med 1967;214:207–210.
133. Clark RAF. Growth factors and wound repair. J Cell Biochem 1991;46:1–2.
134. Cohen S. Epidermal growth factor. Biosci Rep 1986;6:1017–1028.
135. Laato M, Niinikoski J, Lebel L, et al. Stimulation of wound healing by epidermal growth factor. Ann Surg 1986;203:379–381.
136. Schreiber AB, Winkler ME, Derynck R. Transforming growth factor alpha: A more potent angiogenic mediator than epidermal growth factor. Science 1986;232:1250–1253.
137. Nishida T, Tanaka H, Nakagawa S, et al. Fibronectin synthesis by the rabbit cornea: Effects of mouse epidermal growth factor and cyclic AMP analogs. Jpn J Ophthalmol 1984;196:196–202.
138. Gospodarowicz D, Neufeld G, Schweigerer L. Fibroblast growth factor: structural and biologic properties. J Cell Physiol Suppl 1987;5:15–26.
139. Klingbeil CK, Cesar LB, Fiddes JC. Basic fibroblast growth factor accelerates tissue repair in models of impaired healing. In: Barbul A, Caldwell MC, Eaglestein WH et al., eds. Clinical and experimental approaches to dermal and epidermal repair: normal and chronic wounds. New York: John Wiley and Sons, 1991;443–458.
140. McGee GS, Davidson JM, Buckley A, et al. Recombinant basic fibroblast growth factor accelerates wound healing. J Surg Res 1988;45:145–153.
141. Hebda PA, Klingbeil CK, Abraham JA, et al. Basic fibroblast growth factor stimulation of epidermal wound healing in pigs. J Invest Derm 1990;95:626–631.
142. Heldin C-H, Westermark B. Platelet-derived growth factors: A family of isoforms that bind to two distinct receptors. Br Med Bull 1989;45:453–464.
143. Ross R. Platelet-derived growth factor. Annu Rev Med 1987;38:71–79.
144. Blatti SP, Foster DN, Ranganathan G, et al. Induction of fibronectin gene transcription and mRNA is a primary response to growth-factor stimulation of AKR-2B cells. Proc Natl Acad Sci U S A 1988;85:1119–1123.
145. Heldin P, Laurent TC, Heldin C-H. Effect of growth factors on hyaluronan synthesis in cultured human fibroblasts. Biochem J 1989;258:919–922.
146. Pierce GF, Mustoe TA, Lingelbach J, et al. Platelet-derived growth factor and transforming growth factor enhance tissue repair activities by unique mechanisms. J Cell Biol 1989;109:429–440.
147. Maciag T, Nemore R, Weinstein R, et al. An endocrine approach to the control of epidermal growth: serum-free cultivation of human keratinocytes. Science 1981;211:1452–1454.
148. Assoian RK, Komoriya A, Meyers CA, et al. Transforming growth factor-B in human platelets. J Biol Chem 1983;258:7155–7160.
149. Masssague J. The TGF-β family of growth and differentiation factors. Cell 1987;49:437–438.
150. Shah M, Foreman DM, Ferguson MWJ. Neutralizing antibody to TGF-$\beta_{1,2}$ reduces cutaneous scarring in adult rodents. J Cell Science 1994;107:1137–1157.
151. Ignotz RA, Endo T, Massague J. Regulation of fibronectin and type I collagen mRNA levels by transforming growth factor. J Biol Chem 1987;262:6443–6446.
152. Peebles K, Boswick JA Jr, Scott FA. Wounds of the hand contaminated by human or animal saliva. J Trauma 1980;20:383–389.
153. Kligman AM. The bacteriology of normal skin. In Wolcott BW, Rund DA, eds. Skin bacteria and their role in infection. New York: McGraw-Hill Book Co., 1965;13–21.
154. Edlich RF, Rodeheaver GT, Morgan RF, et al. Principles of emergency wound management. Ann Emerg Med 1988;17:1284–1302.
155. Ricketts CR, Squire JR, Topley E. Human skin lipids with particular reference to the self sterilizing power of the skin. Clinical Science 1951;10:89–110.
156. Heggers JP. Natural host defense mechanisms. Clin Plast Surg 1979;6:505–513.
157. Lindberg RB, Moncrief JA, Switzer WE, et al. The successful control of burn wound sepsis. J Trauma 1965;5:601–616.
158. Teplitz C, Davis D, Mason AD, et al. Pseudomonas burn wound sepsis. I. Pathogenesis of experimental pseudomonas burn wound sepsis. J Surg Res 1964;4:200–216.
159. Kass EH. Asymptomatic infections of the urinary tract. Trans Assoc Am Physicians 1956;69:56–64.
160. Bendy RH, Nuccio PA, Wolfe E, et al. Relationship of quantitative

bacterial counts to healing of decubiti: effect of gentamycin. Antimicrobial Agents and Chemotherapy 1964;147–153.

161. Robson MC, Heggers JP. Surgical infection. II. The B-hemolytic streptococcus. J Surg Res 1969;9:289–292.
162. Krizek TH, Davis JH. The role of the red cell in subcutaneous infection. J Trauma 1965;5:85–95.
163. Cruse PJE. Wound infection. In: Howard RJ, Simmons RL, eds. Surgical infectious disease. East Norwalk, CT: Appleton & Lange, 1988:319.
164. Hunt TK, Zederfeldt BH, Goldstick TK, et al. Tissue oxygen tensions during controlled hemorrhage. Surgical Forum 1967;18:3–4.
165. Roth GJ, McDonald JB, Sheard C. The effect of cigarettes and of intravenous injections of nicotine on the electrocardiogram, basal metabolic rate, cutaneous temperature, blood pressure, and pulse rate of normal persons. JAMA 1944;125:761–767.
166. Bruce JW, Miller JR, Hooker DR. The effect of smoking upon the blood pressures and upon the volume of the hand. Am J Physiol 1909;24:104–116.
167. Wright IS, Moffat D. The effects of tobacco on the peripheral vascular system. JAMA 1934;103:315–323.
168. Sackett DL, Gibson RW, Bross IDJ, et al. Relation between aortic atherosclerosis and the use of cigarettes and alcohol: An autopsy study. N Engl J Med 1968;279:1413–1420.
169. Birnstingl MA, Brinson K, Chakrabarti. The effect of short-term exposure to carbon monoxide on platelet stickiness. Br J Surg 1971;58:837–839.
170. Astrup P, Kjeldsen K. Carbon monoxide, smoking and atherosclerosis. Med Clin North Am 1973;58:323–350.
171. Kjeldsen K, Astrup P, Wanstrup J. Ultra-structural intimal changes in the rabbit aorta after a moderate carbon monoxide exposure. Atherosclerosis 1972;16:67–82.
172. Fajardo LF, Berthong M. Radiation injury in surgical pathology: Part III salivary glands, pancreas and skin. Am J Surg Pathol 1981;5:279–296.
173. Rudolph R. Complications of surgery for radiotherapy skin damage. Plast Reconstr Surg 1982;70:179–183.
174. Levenson SM, Gruber CA, Rettura G, et al. Supplemental vitamin A prevents the acute radiation-induced defect in wound healing. Ann Surg 1984;200:494–512.
175. Howes EL, Briggs H, Shea R, et al. Effect of complete and partial starvation on the rate of fibroplasia in the healing wound. Arch Surg 1933;27:846–858.
176. Haydock DA, Hill GL. Impaired wound healing in surgical patients with varying degrees of malnutrition. JPEN 1986;10:550–554.
177. Thompson WD, Ravdin IS, Frank IL. Effect of hypoproteinemia on wound disruption. Arch Surg 1938;36:500–518.
178. Devereauz DF, Thistlewaite PA, Thibault LF, et al. Effect of tumor bearing and protein depletion on wound breaking strength in the rat. J Surg Res 1979;27:233–238.
179. Williamson MB, Fromm HJ. Effect of cystine and methionine on healing of experimental wounds. Proc Soc Exp Biol Med 1957;80:623–626.
180. Levenson SM, Seifter E. Dynsnutrition, wound healing, and resistance to infection. Clin Plast Surg 1977;4:375–388.
181. Freiman M, Seifter E, Connerton C, et al. Vitamin A deficiency and surgical stress. Surg Forum 1970; 21:81–82.
182. Shapiro SS, Mott DJ. Modulation of glycosaminoglycan synthesis by retinoids. Ann N Y Acad Sci 1981;359:306–321.
183. Cohen BE, Till G, Cullen PR, et al. Reversal of postoperative immunosuppression in man by vitamin A. Surg Gynecol Obstet 1979;149:658–662.
184. Alvarez OM, Gilbreath RL. Effect of dietary thiamine on intermolecular collagen cross linking during wound repair: A mechanical and biochemical assessment. J Trauma 1982;22:20–24.
185. Ehrlich HP, Tarver H, Hunt TK. Inhibitory effects of Vitamin E on collagen synthesis and wound repair. Ann Surg 1972;175:235–240.
186. Fernandez-Madrid F, Prasad AS, Oberleas D. Effect of zinc deficiency on nucleic acids, collagen, and noncollagenous protein of the connective tissue. J Lab Clin Med 82:951–961, 1973.
187. Chvapil M. Zinc and wound healing. In Zederfeldt B, ed. Symposium on zinc. Lund, Sweden: AB Tika, 1974.
188. Lawrence WT, Norton JA, Harvey AK, et al. Wound healing in sarcoma-bearing rats: tumor effects on cutaneous and deep wounds. J Surg Oncol 1987;35:7–12.

189. Chlebowski RT, Heber D. Metabolic abnormalities in cancer patients: carbohydrate metabolism. Surg Clin North Am 1986;66:957–968.
190. Weingweg J, Levenson SM, Rettura G, et al. Supplemental vitamin A prevents the tumor-inducted defect in wound healing. Ann Surg 1990;211:269–276.
191. DuNuoy P, Carrell A. Cicatrization of wounds. J Exp Biol 1921;34:339–348.
192. Grove GL. Age-related differences in healing of superficial skin wounds in humans. Arch Dermatol Res 1982;272:381–385.
193. Sandblom P, Peterson P, Muren A. Determination of the tensile strength of the healing wound as a clinical test. Acta Chirurgica Scandinavia 1953;105:252–257.
194. Cruse PJE, Foord RA. A prospective study of 23,649 surgical wounds. Arch Surg 1973;107:206–210.
195. Goodson WH, Hunt TK. Studies of wound healing in experimental diabetes mellitus. J Surg Res 1977;22:221–227.
196. Prakash A, Pandit PN, Sharma LK. Studies in wound healing in experimental diabetes. Int Surg 1974;59:25–28, .
197. Arquilla ER, Weringer EJ, Nakajo M. Wound healing; a model for the study of diabetic microangiopathy. Diabetes 1976;25(suppl 2):811–819.
198. Mowat AG, Baum J. Chemotaxis of polymorphonuclear leukocytes from patients with diabetes mellitus. N Engl J Med 1971;284:621–627.
199. Bybee JD, Rogers DE. The phagocytic activity of polymorphonuclear leukocytes obtained from patients with diabetes mellitus. J Lab Clin Med 1964;64:1–13.
200. Nolan CM, Beaty HN, Bagdade JD. Further characterization of the impaired bactericidal function of granulocytes in patients with poorly controlled diabetes. Diabetes 1978;27:889–894.
201. Bagdade JD, Root RK, Bugler RJ. Impaired leukocyte function in patients with poorly controlled diabetes. Diabetes 1974;23:9–15.
202. Gottrup F, Andreassen IT. Healing of incisional wounds in stomach and duodenum: The influence of experimental diabetes. J Surg Res 1981;31:61–68.
203. Weringer EJ, Kelso JM, Tamai IY, et al. Effects of insulin on wound healing in diabetic mice. Acta Endocrinol 1982;99:101–108.
204. Yue DK, McLennan S, Marsh M et al. Effects of experimental diabetes, uremia, and malnutrition on wound healing. Diabetes 1987;36:295–299.
205. Howes EL, Plotz CM, Blunt JW, et al. Retardation of wound healing by cortisone. Surgery 1950;28:177–181.
206. Hunt TK, Ehrlich HP, Garcia JA, et al. The effect of vitamin A on reversing the inhibitory effect of cortisone on the healing of open wounds in animals. Ann Surg 1969;170:633–641.
207. Stephens FO, Dunphy JE, Hunt TK. Effect of delayed administration of corticosteroids on wound contraction. Ann Surg 1971;173:214–218.
208. Sandberg N. Time relationship between administration of cortisone and wound healing in rats. Acta Chirurgica Scandinavica 1964;127:446–455.
209. Hunt TK, Ehrlich HP, Garcia JA, et al. Effects of vitamin A on reversing the inhibitory effects of cortisone on healing of open wounds in animals and man. Ann Surg 1969;170:633–641.
210. Shamberger RC, Devereaux DF, Brennan MF. The effect of chemotherapeutic agents on wound healing. International Advances in Surgical Oncology 1981;4:15–58.
211. Lawrence WT, Talbot TL, Norton JA. Preoperative or postoperative doxorubicin hydrochloride (Adriamycin): Which is better for wound healing? Surgery 1986;100:9–12.
212. Peacock EE Jr, Madden JW, Trier WC. Biologic basis for the treatment of keloids and hypertrophic scars. South Med J 1970;63:755–759.
213. Brody GS, Peng STJ, Landel RF. The etiology of hypertrophic scar contracture: Another view. Plast Reconstr Surg 1981;67:673–684.
214. Lawrence WT. In search of the optimal treatment of keloids: Report of a series and a review of the literature. Ann Plast Surg 1991;27:164–178.
215. Edlich RF, Smith OT, Edgerton MT. Resistance of the surgical wound to antimicrobial prophylaxis and its mechanism of development. Am J Surg 1973;126:583–591.
216. Rodeheaver GT, Rye DR, Rust R, et al. Mechanism by which proteolytic enzymes prolong the golden period of antibiotic action. Am J Surg 1978;136:379–382.

217. Rodeheaver G, Bellamy W, Kody M, et al. Bacteriocidal activity and toxicity of iodine-containing solution in wounds. Arch Surg 1982;117:181–186.
218. Siegel RJ, Vistnes LM, Iverson RE. Effective hemostasis with less epinephrine: An experimental and clinical study. Plast Reconstr Surg 1973;51:129–133.
219. Arndt KA, Burton C, Noe JM. Minimizing the pain of local anesthesia. Plast Reconstr Surg 1983;72:676.
220. Christopher RA, Buchanan L, Begalla K, et al. Pain reduction in local anesthesia administration through pH buffering. Ann Emerg Med 1988;17:117–123.
221. Alexander JW, Fischer JE, Boyajian M, et al. The influence of hair-removal methods on wound infections. Arch Surg 1983;118:347–352.
222. Madden H, Edlich RF, Schauerhamer R, et al. Application of principles of fluid dynamics to surgical wound irrigation. Current Topics in Surgical Research 1971;3:85–93.
223. Gross A, Cutright DE, Bhaskar SN. Effectiveness of pulsating water jet lavage in treatment of contaminated crushed wounds. Am J Surg 1972;124:373–377.
224. Hamer ML, Robson MC, Krizek TJ, et al. Quantitative bacterial analysis of comparative wound irrigations. Ann Surg 1975;181:819–822.
225. Schauerhamer RA, Edlich RF, Panek P, et al. Studies in the management of contaminated wounds VII. Susceptibility of surgical wounds to postoperative surface contamination. Am J Surg 1971;122:74–77.
226. Branemark PI, Albrektsson B, Lindstrom J, et al. Local tissue effects of wound disinfectants. Acta Chirurgica Scandinavica 1966;357(suppl.):166–176.
227. Rodeheaver GT, Smith SL, Thacker JG, et al. Mechanical cleansing of contaminated wounds with a surfactant. Am J Surg 1975;129:241–245.
228. Rodeheaver G, Turnbull V, Edgerton MT, et al. Pharmokinetics of a new skin cleanser. Am J Surg 1976;132:67–74.
229. Rodeheaver G, Bellamy W, Kody M, et al. Bacteriocidal activity and toxicity of iodine-containing solutions in wounds. Arch Surg 1982;117:181–186.
230. Custer J, Edlich RF, Prusak M, et al. Studies in the management of the contaminated wound V. An assessment of the effectiveness of pHisoHex and betadine surgical scrub solutions. Am J Surg 1971;121:572–575.
231. Mobacken H, Wengstrom C. Interference with healing of rat skin incisions treated with chlorhexidine. Acta Derm Venereol (Stockh) 1974;54:29.
232. Saatman RA, Carlton WW, Hubben K, et al. A wound healing study of chlorhexidine digluconate in guinea pigs. Fundam Appl Toxicol 1986;6:1–6.
233. Branemark PI, Ekholm R. Tissue injury caused by wound disinfectants. J Bone Joint Surg Am 1967;49:48–62.
234. Kozol RA, Gillies C, Elgebaly SA. Effects of sodium hypochlorite (Dakin's solution) on cells of the wound module. Arch Surg 1988;123:420–423.
235. Lineweaver W, Howard R, Soucy D, et al. Topical antimicrobial toxicity. Arch Surg 1985;120:267–270.
236. Peacock EE Jr. Wound healing and wound care. In: Schwartz SI, ed. Principles of surgery. 5th ed. New York: McGraw-Hill, 1988:307–330.
237. Lowbury EJL, Lilly HA, Bull JP. Methods for disinfection of hands and operation sites. Br Med J 1964;2:531–536.
238. Saggers BA, Stewart, GT. Polyvinyl-pyrrolidone -iodine: An assessment of antibacterial activity. Journal of Hygiene, Cambridge 1964;62:509–518.
239. Haury B, Rodeheaver G, Vensko J et al. Debridement: An essential component of traumatic wound care. Am J Surg 1978;135:238–242.
240. Ordman LJ, Gillman T. Studies in the healing of cutaneous wounds: II The healing of epidermal, appendageal and dermal injuries inflicted by suture needles and by suture material in the skin of pigs. Arch Surg 1966;93:883–910.
241. VanWinkle N, Hastings JC. Considerations in the choice of suture material for various tissues. Surg Gynecol Obstet 1972;135:113–126.
242. George TK, Simpson DC. Skin wound closure with staples in the accident and emergency department. J R Coll Surg Edinb 1985;30:54–56.
243. Golden T. Non-irritating, multipurpose surgical adhesive tape. Am J Surg 1960;100:789–796.
244. Golden T, Levy AH, O'Connor WT. Primary healing of skin wounds and incisions with a threadless suture. Am J Surg 1962;104:603–612.
245. Conolly WB, Hunt TK, Zederfeldt B, et al. Clinical comparison of surgical wounds closed by suture and adhesive tapes. Am J Surg 1969;117:318–322.
246. Edlich RF, Thul J, Prusak M, et al. Studies in the management of the contaminated wound VIII. Assessment of tissue adhesives for repair of contaminated tissue. Am J Surg 1971;122:394–397.
247. Saltz R, Sierra K, Feldman D, et al. Experimental and clinical applications of fibrin glue. Plast Reconstr Surg 1991;88:1005–1015.
248. Jabs AD Jr, Wider TM, DeBellis J, et al. The effect of fibrin glue on skin grafts in infected sites. Plast Reconstr Surg 1992;89:268–271.
249. Mandel MA. Minimal suture blepharoplasty: Closure of incisions with autologous fibrin glue. Aesthetic Plast Surg 1992;16:269–272.
250. Ferguson DJ. Clinical application of experimental relations between technique and wound infection. Surgery 1968;63:377–381.
251. deHoll D, Rodeheaver G, Edgerton MT, et al. Potentiation of infection by suture closure of dead space. Am J Surg 1974;127:716–720.
252. Petry JS, Wortham KA. Contraction and growth of wounds covered by meshed and non-meshed split thickness skin grafts. Br J Plast Surg 1986;39:478–482.
253. Ponten HL. Grafted skin: Observation on innervation and other qualities. Acta Clin Scand Suppl 1960;257:1–78.
254. McGregor IA, Morgan G. Axial and random pattern flaps. Br J Plast Surg 1963;26:202–213.
255. Gimbel NS, Farris W. Skin grafting. Arch Surg 1966;92:554–557.
256. Alvarez OM, Mertz PM, Eaglstein WH. The effect of occlusive dressings on collagen synthesis and re-epithelialization in superficial wounds. J Surg Res 1983;35:142–148.
257. Shuck JM, Pruitt BA, Moncrief JA. Homograft skin for wound coverage. Arch Surg 1969;98:472–479.
258. Robson MC, Krizek TJ, Koss N, Samburg JL. Amniotic membranes as a temporary wound dressing. Surg Gynecol Obstet 1973;136:904–906.
259. Bromberg BE, Song IC, Mohn MP. The use of pig skin as a temporary biologic dressing. Plast Reconstr Surg 1965;36:80–90.
260. Woodruff EA. Biobrane, a biosynthetic skin prosthesis. In Wise, DL, ed. Burn Wound Coverings. New York: CRC Press, Inc, 1984.
261. Salomon JC, Diegelman RF, Cohen IK. Effects of dressings on donor site epithelialization. Surgical Forum 1974;25:516–517.
262. Noe JM, Kalish S. The problem of adherence in dressed wounds. Surg Gynecol Obstet 1978;147:185–188.
263. Noe JM, Kalish S. Wound care. Greenwich, Connecticut: Chesebrough-Pond's, Inc., 1976.
264. Varma AO, Bugatch E, German FM. Débridement of dermal ulcers with collagenase. Surg Gynecol Obstet 1973;136:281–282.
265. Kucan JO, Robson MC, Heggers JP, et al. Comparison of silver sulfadiazine, povidone-iodine and physiologic saline in the treatment of chronic pressure ulcers. J Am Ger Soc 1981;24:232–235.
266. Moncrief JA. Topical therapy for control of bacteria in the burn wound. World J Surg 1978;2:151–165.
267. Geronemus RG, Mertz PM, Eaglstein WH. Wound healing: The effects of topical antimicrobial agents. Arch Dermatol 1979;115:1311–1314.
268. Noe JM, Kalish S. The mechanism of capillarity in surgical dressings. Surg Gynecol Obstet 1976;143:454–456.
269. Winter GD, Scales JT. Effect of air drying and dressings on the surface of a wound. Nature 1963;197:91–92.
270. Adzick NS, Lorenz P. Cells, matrix, growth factors, and the surgeon. Ann Surg 1994;220:10–18.

7 Basic Immunology for Surgeons

Richard J. Rohrer

Introduction

We live in a dangerous world. Microbial invaders from without and defective cells from within present themselves continuously, and stand ready to overrun us. Since the days of the first unicellular organisms in a primal "soup" some 3 billion years ago, defense systems against these constant dangers have been critical to survival. Successful immune defense stratagems have been highly conserved over the course of evolution.

The immune response permeates all activities of surgical importance. In normal individuals, the immune response prevents many surgical conditions outright, especially infections and tumors. The immune response is an important aspect of the first phases of illness and injury. Finally, the immune response is central to the recovery process after surgical intervention, interdigitating with cardiopulmonary and nutritional homeostatic mechanisms.

As immunity (Latin *immunitas*) describes freedom from invasion, it follows that a review of immunology should first lay out the frontiers to be protected, i.e., how "self" vs "nonself" are defined. The active components of the defense mechanism may then be described. Finally, the manner in which these components collectively function is sketched. Special attention is drawn to three major areas of surgical endeavor: shock and trauma, oncology, and transplantation.

The central dogma asserted in this construct is founded upon basic science efforts in many species of animal, especially rodents. While there are many differences between human and other animals, in the interest of clarity, no attempt will be made to highlight them in this manuscript.

As with the more commonly understood military defenses which protect whole societies, few actions of the immune system are "good" in the absolute, teleologically speaking. That is, virtually all defense mechanisms are "double-edged swords." The same agents that save us in one circumstance may harm us in another. Such circumstances of surgical significance will be highlighted as well.

Components of the Immune System

Definition of Self

Before an organism can defend itself against invasion, it must know what turf it is protecting. This is relatively simple for a single-celled organism—the boundary in question is the cell membrane—but is more complex for individual humans. One boundary is made up of epithelial surfaces, skin, gastrointestinal, and respiratory. Another boundary is the endothelial surface that courses throughout the body, the vascular tree. Yet another boundary is apparent at the margins of individual organs or cohesive groups of cells. Finally, there are the boundaries of individual cells—their cell membranes.

Cell surface markers are fundamental to the staking out of turf as "self." Their presence may be purely for the sake of identification, or they may play critical functional roles. Some cell surface markers are species (xeno)-specific. Some markers are unique to a group of individuals within a species (allo-specific). Some markers are completely unique to the individual itself (auto-specific). Some cell-surface markers are organ or function-specific. Examples reach far from the immune system and include breast and gastrointestinal tissue markers. Even for a given individual, the cell surface markers expressed may change over time and, for that matter, during different phases of the cell cycle. This is best exemplified by the changes in many cells from fetal antigens to adult antigens. Because cell surface markers may provoke an immune response in another individual or species (indeed, this is how they most commonly are discovered in the first place), they are often referred to as cell surface antigens.

Figure 7.1. Molecular structures of the Clas I MHC-encoded protein and the class II protein molecule are similar; the molecules also share similar sequences of amino acids. The molecules are characterized by loops made up of about 70 amino acids within each chain; sulfur atoms at each end of the loop are joined by covalent bonds. Class I proteins are expressed on the surface of every nucleated cell in higher vertebrates, in association with the non-MHC-encoded protein beta-2-microglobulin. Class II proteins are expressed only on the surface of selected cells, such as the β cells. The highly schematic diagrams are not drawn to scale. From Marrach P, Kappler J. The T-cell and its receptor. Sci Am 1986;254: 36. Reprinted by permission.

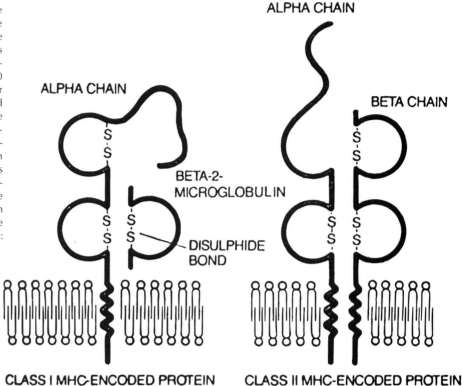

CLASS I MHC-ENCODED PROTEIN   CLASS II MHC-ENCODED PROTEIN

Cell Surface Antigens

Cell surface antigens are generally glycoproteins which protrude through the lipid-rich cell membrane. They are coded-for by DNA in the nucleus of individual cells, constructed from mRNA templates on ribosomes in the cellular cytoplasm, and transported to the cell surface. Under certain circumstances they may detach and float through the interstitial or intravascular spaces. Thus, the expression of cell surface markers is universally a dynamic process, with new surface markers being produced, expressed, and shed continually.

More specific are the familiar ABO markers on the surface of red blood cells. In humans, the A and B antigens, as well as a host of others (Lewis, Kell, etc.), protrude from the RBC membrane and define subgroups within the human species. A common proteinaceous moiety attached to the cell membrane is coupled with a variable carbohydrate moiety. They are present in many other tissues as well, including vascular endothelium. This is an ancient system of self definition; ABO glycoprotein antigens appear to be distant relatives of bacterial surface antigens. The development of anti-blood group antibodies (anti-A in an "O" individual) early in life may be related to bacterial exposure in the neonate, with formation of cross-reactive antibody. Many primates share ABO antigens with humans.

Yet more specific are the major histocompatibility (MHC) antigens. In the human they were first detected on white blood cells and were therefore termed human leucocyte antigens (HLA). They are present on many white blood cells and tissues. They are coded-for on the short arm of chromosome 6. They constantly turn over and, like other cell surface markers, may be bound or soluble.

For descriptive purposes, HLA antigens may be divided into two classes based on structure—so-called class I and class II antigens (Fig. 7.1). Class I antigens are expressed on the surfaces of all nucleated cells; the known class I antigens in the human are labeled A, B, and C. Whereas class I antigens are largely just descriptive of "self," the class II HLA antigens are functional as well as descriptive. Class II antigens are accordingly more restricted in their distribution: under normal conditions they are present only on the surfaces of specialized immune cells. In the human, they are labeled the D or "D-related" (Dr) antigens. In the immune response, the Dr antigens are thought to be the most important HLA participants, followed by HLA-B and HLA-A; HLA-C is relatively unimportant. Even though class II antigen expression is normally restricted, all cells contain the genetic hardware for expression of this antigen. Under special circumstances, such as those involving tissue injury from ischemia, there may be "up regulation" of HLA expression, and class II antigen may be found on the surface of cells from which it is usually absent. This may best be viewed as part of the viable cell's attempt to protect itself from "collateral damage" because of nonspecific inflammation about the nonviable cells.

Each of the HLA antigens have multiple variations.

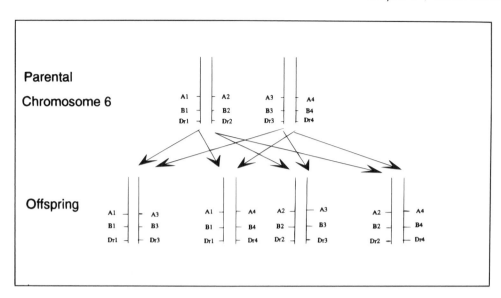

Figure 7.2. Two parents contribute one haplotype each to every offspring, yielding four possible outcomes.

All are proteins which bear structural resemblance to immunoglobulin (described below), but they differ functionally. Notably, class II antigen displays, at its outermost extent, a prominent fold that can be shown three-dimensionally by radiographic crystallography. This fold is known as the "peptide binding groove" and is critical for the functional capacity of this antigen (see *macrophages* below). A host of so-called "minor" histocompatibility surface markers exist as well, which are much less well-defined.

HLA markers are passed from parent to offspring via standard Mendelian genetics. For all chromosomes, including number 6, an individual inherits one maternal strand and one paternal strand. Each strand is referred to as a haplotype. Evidently, each offspring will share one haplotype with each of his parents. Among offspring from the same set of parents, one may calculate that the likelihood that any individual will share both haplotypes with a sibling is 25%, one haplotype 50%, and no haplotypes 25% (Fig 7.2). By their nature, identical twins will share all cell surface markers, including HLA; fraternal twins will follow the inheritance previously described.

Given the fact that every individual inherits a complete set (A,B,C, and Dr) of antigens from each parent, and that there are numerous but finite variants of each, the HLA system confers on man a high degree of individuality, which contrasts with the individuality conferred by the ABO system. Whereas the statistical likelihood that two random humans will share ABO type is about one in ten, the likelihood of sharing HLA type is one in several million.

In addition to HLA cell surface antigens, lymphocytes also possess cell surface molecules which aid in lymphocyte functions, and others which may not be functional in themselves, but serve to distinguish one functional subpopulation from another within the same individual. They are all glycoproteins, and should currently be referred to by the "common determinant" (CD) nomenclature, though references persist to the older "T" and "B" terminology.

Defense Against Nonself

Earth has always been a dangerous place to live. Defense against invasion is therefore an ancient, and highly important, evolutionary attribute. Some defense mechanisms are relatively primitive, whereas others are highly advanced. It appears that, in the evolutionary process, advanced host defenses appeared about the same time that the capacity for organ regeneration was lost, i.e., around the time of evolution from amphibian to reptile.

Toxic Secretions

Perhaps the most ancient method of organismal defense is the secretion of substances which are chemically toxic to other organisms in the neighborhood. Secretion of penicillin by the penicillium mold is a prominent example, and may be thought of, loosely, as part of the mold's immune defenses. The human commercial potential of such substances in the pharmaceutical industry has been and still is enormous.

In humans, secretion of directly toxic chemical substances by most organs and tissues is limited; the antibacterial acid environment of the stomach is a familiar example. Most other epithelial defense systems use mucous secretion and mechanical action to bolster the barrier function.

More recently, the formation of nitric oxide (NO) by cells not normally considered part of the immune system has attracted attention. NO has many effects, including smooth muscle relaxation (vasodilatation) and neurotransmission. However, as a free radical, it is also a potent inhibitor of DNA synthesis. Its formation by vascular endothelial cells and hepatocytes has been offered as an example of nonspecific protection from microbial invasion. Neutrophils and macrophages (see below) also secrete NO as a direct attribute of their immune function.

Most of the human immune response derives from more specialized cellular functions and interactions.

Macrophages

Perhaps the most ancient cellular defense function is phagocytosis; it can be demonstrated easily in very primitive unicellular organisms. This function is performed in humans by the macrophage (or its monocyte counterpart). This cell is of mesenchymal origin, and arises in any individual from an original bone marrow stem cell. It may be freely circulating in the intravascular compartment, migrating more slowly through the lymph and the interstitial space, or virtually stationary within tissues. Kupffer cells in the hepatic sinusoids, for example, are macrophages adapted to an important defensive role in the liver.

As nucleated cells, macrophages express class I MHC molecules on their surface; as highly-specialized immune cells, they express class II MHC molecules. In addition, they also express other recognition and function molecules, including the functional antigen B7-2 (see *T cells*, below).

As the pliable macrophage cell membrane encounters foreign substances in the local environment, it invaginates to surround and engulf the object. Once the invader is delivered in a cytosome to the cell cytoplasm, it is degraded by intracellular peroxidases and other enzymes, and neutralized. Macrophages have recently been shown also to contain the enzyme inducible nitrogen oxide synthase (iNOS). This enzyme is able to mediate the oxidation of L-arginine to yield the gaseous free radical, NO, and a byproduct, L-citrulline. Substrates and cofactors are necessary; also, the macrophage must be stimulated for enzyme activity to be induced (Fig. 7.3). The list of potent inducers is growing, and includes endotoxin (lipopolysaccharide), malarial antigen, interferon gamma (IFN-g), tumor necrosis factor (TNF), and interleukin 1 (IL-1) (see *cytokines*, below), alone or in combination. In the presence of these substrates, cofactors, and inducers, macrophages produce relatively large amounts of NO (in comparison to the NO produced in the vascular endothelium and in neurons). The half-life of this highly-reactive substance varies from seconds to hours, depending on its association, or lack thereof, with a carrier substance. It is likely that NO acts intracellularly upon phagocytized particles in the pericellular interstitium upon invading organisms, and at distant sites, when bound to one or more carrier proteins. Once present at the site of invasion, macrophage-derived NO has two major effects. Prominently, microvascular vasodilatation occurs, thus preserving local tissue perfusion. Subsequently, NO diffuses across the membrane of target cells, inhibiting that cell's ribo-

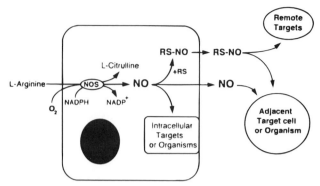

Figure 7.3. The synthesis and fate of NO in cells. Nitric oxide (NO) is produced by the enzyme NO synthase (NOS). The NADPH provides a source of electrons, and molecular dioxygen is incorporated into NO and citrulline, the coproduct of NO formation. Once formed, NO can diffuse to targets within the cell, in the extracellular space, or in adjacent cells or organisms. Nitric oxide, which normally is short-lived, may form stable adducts by interacting with thiol groups on carrier or storage proteins (RS). These stable RS-NO may then have local or remote actions. From Billiar T. Nitric oxide: novel biology with clinical relevance. Ann Surg 1995;221:339. Reprinted by permission.

nucleotide reductase, the rate-limiting enzyme of DNA synthesis.

Beyond simple destruction of foreign particles or organisms, macrophages may specially reprocess certain of the breakdown products of phagocytosis. Fragments of foreign protein may be bundled together with a newly formed class II antigen molecule on its way to the macrophage cell surface. In the bundling process, fragments of degraded protein come to reside in the peptide binding groove of the class II molecule. When the fragment is exteriorized with the new HLA molecule, it faces outward where it may be recognized more easily as a foreign antigen by other elements of the immune system. This process is known as "antigen presentation."

Macrophages also are important in that they secrete IL-1 (see below). IL-1, like the other interleukins, is a polypeptide which, in hormonal fashion, stimulates the immunologic function of responding cells which encounter it.

Natural Killer Cells

Another primitive line from the original bone marrow stem cell is a lymphocyte (non-T, non-B), the natural killer (NK) cell. NK cells are particularly active in the tumor cell response. They demonstrate spontaneous tumoricidal properties when exposed to tumor cells and, unlike T and B lymphocytes, do not require recognition of MHC molecules or antigen processing. How they recognize tumor cells is unclear. They kill tumor cells by incorporating a lipophilic protein into the target cell membrane, which causes increased cell wall permeability, cell swelling, and finally, cell destruction.

NK cells also produce a variety of cytokines, including interferon alpha and gamma, and B-cell growth factor.

Granulocytes

The granulocyte plays an important, though relatively nonspecific, role in immune homeostasis. Named for their histochemical staining properties, the three main lines are polymorphonuclear neutrophils (PMN's), eosinophils, and basophils. All are derived from the same bone marrow stem cell. As nucleated cells, they express class I MHC molecules, however, they do not express class II antigens. In addition, they carry on their surface a number of molecules important for their functioning, including adhesion and interaction with other cells. The best-known of these is the leucocyte function-associated (LFA) antigen (CD 18). These white blood cells carry granules of toxic substances, such as peroxidases; they also contain chemotactic agents that attract cellular elements of the coagulation process, macrophages, and fibroblasts. Finally, granulocytes are also a source of kallikreins, enzymes which act upon free-floating kininogens in the plasma to produce kinins, the best-known of which is bradykinin. Bradykinin and its kin have a pronounced histamine-like effect on tissues, leading to marked vasodilatation and increased vascular permeability. When appropriately stimulated, granulocytes spill or secrete these substances initiating local inflammation in a relatively indiscriminate fashion.

B Lymphocytes

Named for their site of origin in the chicken, the bursa of Fabricius, these cells play an important intermediary role in immune defense. In man, the bursa equivalent is likely the fetal liver or bone marrow. Once produced, they migrate to lymph nodes and spleen, where they appear to remain in residence. As nucleated cells, they express MHC class I molecules on their cell surface. As specialized cells of the immune system, they also express MHC class II molecules. In addition, they display a variety of B cell-specific markers, known as B 1 through B 8, through which various lines of B cells may be identified immunohistologically. Finally, they display immunoglobulin on their surface.

When appropriately stimulated, the B lymphocyte differentiates into plasma cells. These smaller cells, with cytoplasm containing abundant ribosomes on the endoplasmic reticulum, are "factories" with a single mission: to produce a specific antibody.

Immunoglobulin

Antibodies produced by B lymphocytes and plasma cells take the form of immunoglobulins (IG). Immunoglobulins are proteins of unique structure, composed of heavy and light peptide chains (Fig. 7.4). The "root" of the heavy chain complex is constant in its structure among individuals of the same species, and is referred to as the "constant fragment," (Fc) (Fig. 7.5). The portion of an immunoglobulin molecule where light chains are

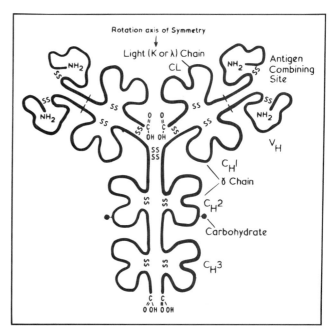

Figure 7.4. Schematic Diagram of a Molecule of Human IgG, showing the two light (κ or λ) chains and two heavy (γ) chains held together by disulfide bonds. The constant regions of the light (CL) and heavy (C_H1, C_H2, and C_H3) chains and the variable region of the heavy chain (VH) are indicated. Loops in the peptide chain formed by intrachain disulfide bonds (C_H1, and so forth) comprise separate functional domains. From Nossal G. Current concepts: immunology. The basic components of the immune system. New Engl J Med 1987;316;1320. Reprinted by permission.

complexed with heavy chains at the site where the antibody will bind to its target is designated the "antibody-binding fragment" (Fab). A myriad of possibilities exist for antigen to specific antibody to be made because the Fab moiety is highly variable in its discrete structure. Over 100 genes code for specific segments of the variable portions of heavy and light chains, leading to millions of potential IG specificities. As complex and pluripotential as they are, it may come as a surprise to note their

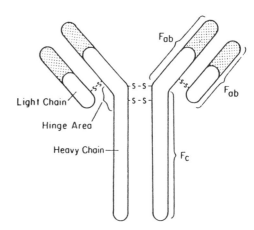

Figure 7.5. Representation of the characteristic Y-shape of a molecule of IgG. The dotted areas indicate the variable regions of the molecule, and the white areas indicate the constant regions.

evolutionary antiquity: even worms produce immuno-globulins.

There are five general immunoglobulin classes: IgM, IgG, IgE, IgA, and IgD. IgM is the first antibody formed after exposure to common microbial antigens, followed by the more durable IgG. IgE figures prominently in immediate hypersensitivity reactions by binding to and activating specialized eosinophils, the mast cells. IgA is secreted in saliva, tears, and breast milk, and thus augmenting resistance to infection in these fluids. IgD is found on the surface of immature B lymphocytes, and its function is uncertain. Immunoglobulins may be soluble or bound to a cell's surface.

The main functions of immunoglobulin are to provide opsonization and to activate complement. Opsonization occurs when the Fab fragment of an immunoglobulin binds to its associated antigen, such as an invading organism. Subsequent macrophage and monocyte phagocytosis of the antibody-coated microorganisms is markedly enhanced. Complement fixation occurs when the antibody-antigen complex triggers the complement cascade, described below.

We are all born with certain natural xenoantibodies (antibody against the MHC and other antigens of different species). In addition, we may acquire further antibodies through exposures later in life. As a result of bacterial exposures as a neonate, humans acquire a multitude of antimicrobial antibodies early in life. Many antigens may closely resemble one another. In these cir-

cumstances, cross reactivity may occur between one antibody and multiple antigens. As noted previously, the carbohydrate moieties of ABO antigens closely resemble capsular carbohydrates of certain bacteria. This likely is the source of cross reacting anti-blood group antibody (i.e., anti-A and anti-B in a blood group O individual, anti-B in a blood group A individual, etc.). When exposed to other human MHC antigens (via pregnancy, blood transfusion, or organ transplantation) antibodies may be formed against the HLA series as well.

Portions of immunoglobulin may, as specific proteins, serve as antigens for the formation of yet other antibodies (usually in a different species). When the constant (Fc) portion of an immunoglobulin serves as the antigen, the immunoglobulin formed against it is referred to as an anti-isotypic antibody. Because of the constancy of the Fc fragment, such an antibody will react with all immunoglobulins of the same class from the same species. When the variable (Fab) portion of an immunoglobulin serves as an antigen, the immunoglobulin formed against it is referred to as an anti-idiotypic antibody. Anti-idiotypic antibodies are highly specific for the Fab fragment against which it was formed.

Complement

An antigen-antibody complex may initiate the complement cascade via the "classic" pathway. Substances such as endotoxin may, in the absence of immunoglobulins, initiate the cascade via the alternate pathway (Fig

Figure 7.6. The complement system. The complement system consists of three families of proteins. Two of these, the classical pathway of activation and the alternative pathway of activation, cause the cleavage of C3 into two fragments, C3b and C3a. These fragments have important biologic activities. In addition, C3b, together with elements of the classical pathway (C4b, C2a) or the alternative pathway (Bb, properidine) forms enzymes (C5 convertases) that cleave C5, the initial member of the terminal family of proteins. Cleavage of C5 leads to the formation of the membrane attack complex that can cause osmotic lysis of cells. From Paul W. The immune system: an introduction. In: Paul W, ed. Fundamental immunology. New York: Raven Press, 1984:3–22. Reprinted by permission.

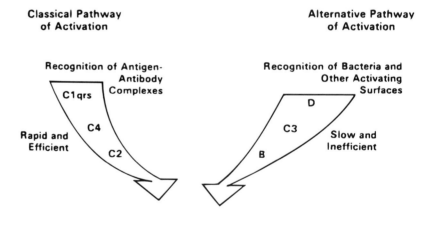

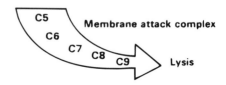

7.6). Both pathways converge with the activation of C3. The sequential activation of proteases, which defines the complement cascade, eventually results in a tight cluster of proteins known as the membrane attack complex (MAC). The MAC is capable of adhering to the target cell membrane and rendering it porous, thereby causing osmotic cell rupture.

Aside from the directly cytotoxic MAC, the proteins of the complement cascade have a variety of other immunologic functions. These include vasodilatation and chemotactic properties, of special importance with regard to neutrophil and eosinophil function in inflammation. The complement cleavage products with the greatest inflammatory activity are C3a and C5b. In addition, the complement cascade provides yet another source for both enzyme and substrate, leading to the production of bradykinin. In the normal host, this potent cascade is kept in check by a regulatory protein, C1 inhibitor.

Dendritic Cells

Derived from a bone marrow stem cell progenitor, dendritic cells are highly-specialized antigen presenting cells with no effector function. They reside primarily in the intercellular and interstitial space but, particularly after having encountered antigen, will migrate through lymphatics to lymph nodes and the spleen. There they migrate to T-cell rich areas to present their antigen.

T Lymphocytes

The T lymphocyte is named for its site of origin, the thymus, and is one of the most sophisticated and important elements of the immune response. T cells derive from a fetal stem cell in the thymus and, before release from the thymus, undergo an extensive process of elaboration and deletion. Maturing T cells are "taught" to recognize "self" MHC antigens and become tolerant of them. Any T cells failing to exhibit tolerance to self are eliminated in a process called clonal deletion. Failure of this system is one factor in autoimmune disease.

As a nucleated cell, it carries MHC class I antigen on its surface. As a specialized immune cell, it also carries class II antigens. In addition, it expresses a variety of cell-specific and functional cell surface markers, several of the series CD 1–14, LFA (CD 18), and CD 28.

Three broad classes of T cells include helper T cells (Th), which amplify the cellular immune response; cytotoxic T cells (Tc), which effect target cell killing; and suppressor T cells (Ts), which buffer the immune response. All T cells express CD3 on the cell surface. Tc and Ts express CD8, whereas Th does not; conversely Th expresses CD4, whereas the other two do not. Through quantitative analysis of lymphocytes bearing these antigens, one index of immunologic competency can be calculated, the CD4/CD8 ratio.

A most important structure on its surface is the T cell receptor (Tcr). It is located on the cell surface geographi-

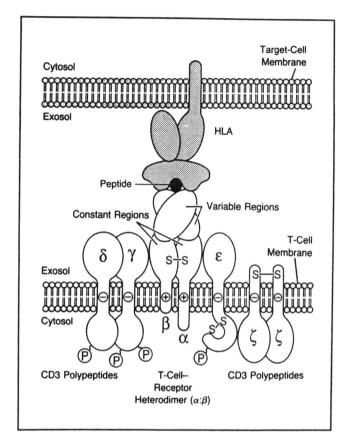

Figure 7.7. Interaction of HLA and the T-cell-receptor complex. The alpha and beta polypeptide chains of the T-cell receptor form a hetero dimer linked by a disulfide bond (S-S) and anchored in the T-cell membrane. The hetero dimer recognizes and binds to peptide associated with an HLA molecule on the surface of a presenting cell. The nonopolymorphic CD3 polypeptides (designated gamma, delta, epsilon, and zeta) are assembled together with the T-cell-antigen receptor and are probably involved in signal transduction. P denotes phosphorylation site. From Krensky A, Weiss A, Crabtree G, et al. Mechanisms of disease: T lymphocyte-antigen interaction in transplant rejection. New Engl J Med 1990; 322:510. Reprinted by permission.

cally close to a CD3 antigen, and a CD28 antigen is not far away. The Tcr has a relatively flat, outward-facing surface. This "antigen-recognition platform" of the Tcr is the critical interface for peptide in the binding groove of macrophage MHC class II molecules; indeed the precise alignment of MHC class II antigen with a protein fragment in the peptide binding groove is the signal event in antigen presentation (Fig. 7.7).

When appropriately stimulated via the Tcr, a signal is transduced to the T cell nucleus. Messenger RNA is elaborated, coding for cytokines and cytokine receptors, which greatly amplify the immune response.

Cytokines

Various cytokines produced by T cells, macrophages, and other specialized cell lines include interleukin (IL) 1 through 13, tumor necrosis factor (TNF), and interferon (IFN) alpha and gamma (Table 7.1). TNF and IL-1 appear to be phylogenetically ancient. These original cyto-

Table 7.1.
Cytokines

Cytokine	Major Sources	Major Functions
IL-1	Macrophages	Promotes phagocytic function and PMN adherence; lymphocyte activation; "endogenous pyrogen"
IL-2	Th cells	Stimulates T cell proliferation and differentiation; stimulates B cell proliferation
IL-3	T cells, myelomonocytes	Hematopoietic growth factor
IL-4	T & B cells, mast cells, macrophages	Induces differentiation of TH cells; induces differentiation of B cells
IL-5	T cells	Stimulates proliferation and differentiation of B cells and eosinophils
IL-6	Monocytes, macrophages, T cells	Stimulates epithelial cell, fibroblast, and B cell proliferation, hepatocyte acute phase protein synth.
IL-7	Stromal cells, thymus	Stimulates early B cell production and thymocytes
IL-8	Monocytes, fibroblasts, endothelial cells	Stimulates granulocyte movement through vascular endothelium, and degranulation
IL-9	Lymphocytes, monocytes	T cell growth factor; mast cell enhancing factor
IL-10	T cells, macrophages	Inhibits monocyte/macrophage function; suppresses inflammatory cytokines; enhances B cell proliferation
IL-11	Lung fibroblasts, marrow stromal cells	Promotes several cell lines; inhibits adipocytes
IL-12	Macrophages, B cells	Stimulates differentiation of Th cells
TNF-alpha	Monocytes, macrophages, NK cells, Kupffer cells	Promotes PMN adherence to endothelium; stimulates fibroblast production of PGE2; stimulates release of multiple other cytokines from lymphocytes
TNF-beta	Monocytes, macrophages	Similar to TNF-alpha; in addition stimulates B cell proliferation
IFN-gamma	T cells	Promotes macrophage and monocyte differentiation
TGF-alpha	Fibroblasts, epithelial cells	Stimulates production of epithelial cells, endothelial cells, and fibroblasts
TGF-beta	Lymphocytes, macrophages, fibroblasts	Inhibits lymphocyte production and PMN adherence, stimulates fibroblast collagen synthesis
Plt-derived GF	Endothelial cells, plts	Stimulates fibroblast and sm. muscle cell production
Plt activ. factor	PMN's, endothelial cells	Promotes platelet degranulation, PMN function

kines may have been elaborations of pheromones, those potent peptides that promote attraction between diverse insects. Cytokines have their intended effect when they reach a target cell with the appropriate cell surface receptor.

Clinically, the most important cytokines are IL-2 and IL-6; the most important receptors produced are IL-2 receptors (which may be soluble or bound). Though they may derive from ancient pheromone peptides, cytokines as a group represent the modern communications hardware of the most advanced element of the immune system, the T cell. Prominent functions include the switching "on" of genes in target cells and chemotaxis of other effector cells.

Immunophysiology of Shock and Sepsis

Maintenance of homeostasis during the stress of injury is one of the most basic of bodily functions, strongly conserved in the evolutionary process. The initial response is dominated by cardiorespiratory and neurologic factors. Shortly after, however, metabolic and immunologic pathways become active.

Even in bland ischemic (hypotensive and/or hy-

poxic) or mechanical injuries, the tissue repair process recruits immunologic help. Gaps in the microvascular endothelium appear, and white blood cells migrate into the interstitial space. As affected parenchymal cells die, they are liquefied in the process of sterile inflammation and are cleared by macrophages using phagocytosis and NO production. Surviving and regenerating cells, perhaps to avoid collateral damage in the inflammatory process, up-regulate their expression of HLA antigens. As survivors wave "flags" of self-identity, macrophages are signaled that these are cells under repair, not be cleared away. In later phases of inflammation, depending on the tissue and severity of injury, fibroblasts are drawn by chemotactic factors and lay down collagen in the process of scarring.

However, injury frequently is not bland. Breaks in epithelial barrier function occur either intentionally (as in surgical interventions) or accidentally. Such breaks inevitably allow ingress of microbes. The front lines of the resistance are manned by macrophages and preformed antibodies. If the host has encountered an organism (or one like it) previously, specific (or cross reacting) IgG antibody will bind to the capsule of the invader. The organism, thus opsonized, will be cleared via the lymphatic to the lymph nodes and spleen. In addition, local macrophages phagocytize and destroy invaders, processing their substructural elements and presenting them as antigens for further immune action. Thus a contaminated injury site may be kept free of infection and converted to a bland injury.

When tissue injury is great, or the microbial inoculation great, local defenses may be overwhelmed, resulting in sepsis. Because of their broad interface with the outside world and potential for dense colonization, this is especially true for the pulmonary system and gastrointestinal tract. Pulmonary alveolar macrophages and Kupffer cells are thus frequently charged with a major defense role in the seriously ill patient.

The release of vasoactive substances in the immune response—especially NO and TNF—is a double-edged sword. While maintenance of tissue perfusion is cytoprotective, an excess of vasodilatation may cause systemic hypotension and secondary deterioration of other organ function. While increased capillary permeability may allow greater access to the interstitium for leucocytes, concomitant edema may impair organ function and healing. Nonetheless, on balance, the effect of these substances would appear to be beneficial; to date, blockade of the immune response in the sepsis syndromes has failed to show improvement in outcomes. Much current research involves the study of novel chemical (NSAIDs) and biologic agents (monoclonal antibodies) to blunt the adverse effects of the inflammatory response while sparing the beneficial effects. Anti-endotoxin, anti-TNF, and IL-1 receptor antagonist are examples. While they are effective in laboratory models and showing modest promise in clinical studies, none have been proven clearly effective in humans. Similarly, blockade of NO synthesis has thus far yielded adverse consequences when experimental animals are subsequently challenged with endotoxin. At this point, no agents have been shown to be capable of selectively blocking the adverse effects of vasoactive inflammatory substances while preserving the beneficial effects.

Maintenance of nutritional parameters, especially in severe injury and sepsis, is critical for the ongoing immune response, and constitutes the only true "immunoenhancement" tool at the clinician's disposal. For the sake of mucosal integrity and the Kupffer cell function, nutrition should preferably be maintained via the enteral route. From the immunologic perspective, antibiotics fill an important adjunctive role, without intrinsically enhancing immune activity.

Immunophysiologic Aspects of Oncology

In the process of DNA replication, mistakes are frequent. In the epithelial cell population, which experiences massive turnover during the course of a lifetime, it is particularly remarkable that errors in proliferation aren't more common. Part of the answer lies at the sur-

face of the abnormal cell. As cells are transformed from normal to malignant, a variety of changes in their cell surface marker population become apparent. If a virus is the causative agent, viral antigens may be expressed. If the DNA of the malignant cell operates at a more "primitive" level, a variety of fetal antigens may appear. Immune recognition of altered cell surface antigens may be extremely important in the tumor surveillance process. Indirect evidence for this may be afforded by the increased skin cancer and lymphoma rates in patients taking immunosuppressive medication. Diagnostically, the generation of monoclonal antibodies against such tumor cell surface markers has allowed advances in detection and classification of tumors.

Natural killer (NK) cells attack tumor cells directly (see previously mentioned NK cells). Though first characterized *in vitro*, little is known of how this system functions *in vivo*.

In addition, T cells are involved in continuous tumor surveillance. When an abnormal (read "nonself") cell surface marker is encountered, the cell may be attacked as if it were an outside invader. In general, this response tends to be more pronounced at a primary tumor site than at a metastatic site. Tumors of viral origin appear to be more immunogenic than tumors that arise spontaneously. Many tumor surface antigens that are detected in laboratory assays may, in fact, elicit a humoral or cellular immune attack *in vitro*. Unfortunately, this is often associated with little or no immune response *in vivo*. One explanation for this may lie in the observation that one of the first cell lines to detect some tumors is the Ts cell. Tc function, in this circumstance, is suppressed before it can even begin. Experimentally, it is possible to selectively destroy Ts cell populations, in which case enhanced host anti-tumor immunity becomes evident.

Macrophages, drawn to the scene by the abnormal tumor antigen, may mount an attack in which NO production is central. In vitro study of macrophage tumoricidal activity demonstrate that tumor killing is lost if NO production is inhibited.

Several lines of oncologic immunomodulation are being pursued. *Immunoenhancement* refers to the administration of agents such as IFN, TNF, and various colony-stimulating or growth factors in the hope of augmenting the native immune response to tumor. *Passive immunotherapy* refers to the administration of exogenous anti-tumor antibody. The antibody may either be directly active against the tumor cell, or be coupled with some more toxic substance. In the latter instance, the antibody uses its specificity to locate and adhere to tumor, whereas the toxic substance (e.g., ricin toxin, diphtheria toxin, or Pseudomonas exotoxin) accomplishes the killing. *Active immunotherapy* involves the elution of tumor antigens from tumor specimens removed surgically, followed by reintroduction of them to the host in hopes of eliciting a more productive immune response against any remaining tumor. Finally, *adoptive cellular immuno-*

therapy combines these technologies. NK cells (or Tc cells) are isolated from tumor specimens or peripheral blood, activated by lymphokines in vitro, and reintroduced into the host. Usually, supplemental IL-2 is administered as well to provide further immunoenhancement. To date, all such interventions are solely investigational.

Many tumor cells, especially lymphomas, express abundant, highly specific immunoglobulin on the cell surface. This has allowed the development of anti-idiotypic antibodies against the specific tumor immunoglobulin and therefore the cell line. Thus far, however, monoclonal antibody immunotherapy has only proven temporarily effective for patients with certain lymphomas. The most promising solid tumors for immunotherapy appear to be melanoma and renal cell carcinoma.

Thus, the mainstay of medical therapy for most cancers remains relatively nonspecific cytotoxic chemotherapy and radiation therapy. The host immune response is relegated to aiding in the healing after surgical therapy, and cleaning up after medical therapy.

Immunophysiology of Organ and Tissue Transplantation

Transplantation for end-stage organ failure has become a frequent event. By the year 2000, it is projected that nearly 50,000 organ transplants will be completed in the United States and Europe combined, and nearly 10,000 more in other parts of the world. Kidney transplants are the most voluminous, accounting for just over half of the total organ transplants completed. Liver and heart transplants, combined, account for one-third, and the remainder is comprised of pancreas, lung, small bowel, and various combination transplants. The limiting factor in organ transplantation is donor availability. Tissue transplants, including heart valves, corneas, skin, and a variety of bone and connective tissue products, do not require heart-beating donors and thus have even greater growth potential.

The source of the donated organ has implications for subsequent recipient immunophysiology. Donors may be live or cadaveric. In the former, donors are considered "living-related" if they are first degree relatives (parent, sibling, offspring) of the recipient, and "living-unrelated" if anything else (generally spouses, relatives by marriage, and friends). For cadaveric donors, death may have been pronounced by neurologic criteria (brain death with persistent cardiac function and organ perfusion) or cardiac criteria (with cold preservation of organs as soon as possible after cessation of cardiac function).

With all donors, variable degrees of MHC matching are accomplished. Transplants between identical twins,

the happiest immunologic circumstance, are rare for obvious reasons. One quarter of sibling transplants are between haploidentical individuals, sharing all six of the most important (paired A, B, and Dr) MHC antigens, as well as an undetermined number of so-called "minor" histocompatibility loci. With computerized matching and a sharing arrangement, approximately 5% of cadaveric kidney transplants in the United States is now between unrelated individuals who just happen to share all six MHC antigens (so-called "six-antigen match," or "zero-antigen mismatch"). In these cases, though, there is probably little sharing of minor histocompatibility loci.

The beneficial effect of matching donors and recipients is clear-cut in kidney transplantation for the combinations described above. In situations where the patient to receive the organ is critically ill (i.e., heart and liver transplantation), logistical factors may take precedence over the beneficial immunologic effects of a favorable match.

Before organ transplantation, attention must be paid to the potential for untreatable hyperacute (humoral) rejection caused by the presence of preformed antibodies. Rejection due to preformed xenoantibody is avoided by the simple expedient of using only human donors. Rejection due to preformed anti-ABO antibody is avoided through matching (with rare exception) donor and recipient blood groups by the rules of classic blood group compatibility. Finally, for all kidney transplants and some heart transplants, rejection due to preformed anti-MHC antibody is avoided by performance of a lymphocyte (donor cells plus recipient serum) crossmatch. Liver grafts appear to be rather tolerant of anti-MHC antibody, and if a lymphocyte crossmatch is done at all, the results are noted only retrospectively.

If an organ is transplanted in the face of preformed antibodies in the recipient, the expected result is immediate hyperacute rejection. The preformed antibody binds to its target antigen on the surfaces of vascular endothelial cells and graft parenchymal cells. Circulating complement is fixed. In the vascular compartment, the normally "anticoagulant" environment of the endothelium is changed to a "procoagulant" environment. Fibrin and platelets are attracted to the endothelium, and thrombosis occurs. The graft, momentarily pink and healthy, becomes violaceous, and infarction occurs within a few minutes. In the parenchyma, complement fixation initiates the complement cascade, culminating in the formation of a "membrane attack complex" (MAC). The parenchymal cell membrane is breached, there is unrestricted flux of anions and cations into and out of the cell, and dies secondary to osmotic injury. No known treatment exists for hyperacute rejection, hence the emphasis upon prevention.

Hyperacute rejection remains the Achilles heel of xenotransplantation. As the recipient immune reaction appears to be primitive and powerful, the most successful

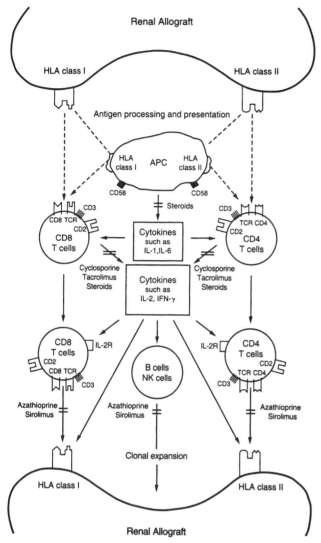

Figure 7.8. The Anti-Allograft Response. This schematic representation of HLA, the primary stimulus for the initiation of the anti-allograft response, shows the participation of cell-surface proteins in antigenic recognition and signal transduction, the contribution of the cytokines and multiple cell types to the immune response, and the potential sites of action (arrows with hatching) of immunosuppressant agents. HLA class I includes the HLA-A, B, and C antigens, and HLA class II includes the HLA-DR, DQ, and DP antigens. APC denotes antigen-presenting cell, TCR T-cell receptor, IL interleukin, IL2R IL-2 receptor, IFN-γ interferon-γ, and NK natural killer. From Suthanthiran M, Strom T. Medical progess: renal transplantation. New Engl J Med 1994;331:365. Reprinted by permission.

research efforts in this area center upon genetic manipulation of donor species-specific antigens to avoid complement fixation altogether, rather than simply dampen it.

Most transplant rejection, however, is cell-mediated. In the unmodified host reaction, antigen recognition is the first step (Fig 7.8). Any recipient Tc cells having prior exposure to donor class I antigen, or recipient Th cells having prior exposure to donor class II antigen, become activated at reexposure. More typically, in the absence of prior exposure to donor antigen, breakdown products

of the injured and dying donor cells are recognized as foreign and engulfed by macrophages. Engrafted organs undergo variable preservation injury, and thus are subject to both the shedding of MHC antigen from disrupted cell membranes, and the up regulation of MHC antigens in cells undergoing repair and mitosis. Thus organs with relatively greater preservation injury—perhaps because of donor hypotension or hypoxia, or prolonged cold or warm ischemia times—are brighter targets for immune response than those with relatively less preservation injury.

As donor proteins are broken down in the macrophage cytoplasm, fragments are incorporated into newly-assembled recipient class II (Dr) antigen bound for the macrophage cell surface. As described earlier, it binds to the peptide binding groove. As a recipient Th draws near, the antigen-recognition platform interfaces with the Dr/peptide complex, and the donor antigen is presented. Simultaneously, the CD 28 cell surface molecule of the recipient Th interacts with the B7-2 surface marker of the macrophage in a process termed costimulation. Costimulation appears to provide a second pathway for Th activation and thus enhances the alloimmune response.

Signal transduction through the Th cell cytoplasm follows. This is a complex series of events involving calcium fluxes, phosphorylation, and enzyme activation (kinases, phosphatases, and isomerases). Because of its low cytoplasmic concentration, activation of the enzyme calcineurin (a serine-threonine phosphatase) is the rate-limiting step in Th cell signal transduction. Once the signal passes to the Th nucleus, however, the net result is the turning on of the IL-2 promoter gene, and the resultant production of IL-2 and IL-2R.

Once Th lymphocytes are activated, the immune response enters a lymphocyte proliferation phase. Interleukin-2 stimulates the proliferation of Tc cells and induces sensitized B cells to differentiate into plasma cells for the production of alloantibody.

In the unmodified transplant immune response, graft destruction follows. Cytotoxic T cells attack donor cells bearing the donor class I antigen, whereas antibody may attack at any cell surface antigen. More granulocytes and macrophages are drawn by chemotactic factors, and the donor cell lytic process progresses. Macrophage production of NO in the rejection process may have paradoxical effects. While the free radicals may clearly damage graft cells, they also appear to suppress local lymphocyte proliferation. It seems likely that macrophage-derived NO will one day be seen as an immunoregulatory substance as well as a toxic agent.

If a humoral element to the otherwise predominantly cell-mediated rejection exists, as in so-called "accelerated" rejection, there may be vascular thrombosis and hemorrhage into the interstitium of the graft.

Since this sequence would occur in all cases except that of the identical twin donor-recipient combination,

Table 7.2.
Immunosuppressive Agents

Agent	Mechanism of Action
Cyclosporine (CSA)	Inhibits IL-2 production by Th cells
Tacrolimus (FK-506)	Inhibits IL-2 production by Th cells
Azathioprine	Inhibits DNA synthesis, lymphocyte proliferation
Mycophenolate mofetil	Inhibits DNA synthesis, lymphocyte proliferation
Glucocorticoids (prednisone, methylprednisolone)	Inhibits DNA and RNA production; margination of lymphocytes; decreased PMN and macrophages chemotaxis and function
Sirolimus (rapamycin)	Inhibits IL-2 action
Brequinar	Inhibits DNA synthesis
15-deoxyspergualin (DSG)	Inhibits lymphocyte maturation and function
Antithymocyte globulin (ATG)	Binds to surface of T cells, inhibiting proliferation and function
Monomurab (OKT3)	Binds to surface of T cells, inhibiting proliferation and function

modulation of the immune response is essential for success. Whereas the historical transplant literature is replete with novel immunosuppressive attempts, from thoracic duct drainage to total lymphoid irradiation, modern immunosuppression rests largely upon the use of a variety of chemical and biological agents.

Chemo immunosuppression is the centerpiece of transplant management. Cyclosporine (CSA), tacrolimus (FK506), azathioprine, prednisone, and methylprednisolone are all commonly used agents. Mycophenolate mofetil is a newer, recently approved drug (Table 7.2). Sirolimus (rapamycin), brequinar, and 15-deoxysperguialin are other promising chemical agents with immunosuppressive properties. Similar to combination chemotherapy for cancer, the use of two or three agents simultaneously for prophylaxis of transplant rejection is now routine. The fundamental principle is to use agents with different mechanisms of action to inhibit the immune response at several different steps. This allows for customization of dosage regimens, depending on the immunosuppressive needs of and the toxicity experienced by the individual patients.

Biologic agents also have a secure immunosuppressive role in the transplant recipient. Antithymocyte globulin (ATG) and monomurab (OKT3) monoclonal antibody are the most commonly used. Both are antibody (globulin) preparations produced by first immunizing non-human animals (usually horses, goats, rabbits, or mice) with human lymphocytes, then culling and purifying the immunoglobulin fraction of the serum. Whereas ATG is a polyclonal preparation containing antibodies with many different specificities, OKT3 is a very

pure—monoclonal—preparation of murine IgG specific for the human CD3 (formerly T3) antigen. Both cause diminution in the circulating T cell population and may be either for "induction" immunosuppression or treatment of established rejection. In the former situation, the biological agent is administered for 3–14 days immediately after the transplant surgery in hopes of averting rejection altogether. In the latter, it is administered only after rejection has occurred and lymphocytes are in the proliferative phase.

Complications of over immunosuppression include infection (especially with cytomegalovirus) and neoplasia (especially skin cancer and lymphoma). A host of potential individual side effects also exists for each agent, including tremor, leucopenia, cataracts, and avascular necrosis of long bones. Cyclosporine and tacrolimus are nephrotoxic, and require close monitoring. However, in most transplant recipients, the quality of life is very good. With the best of surgical and immunosuppressive management techniques, one-year graft survival rates are between 80% and 90%.

REFERENCES

1. Beck G, Habicht GS. Primitive cytokines: harbingers of vertebrate defense. Immunol Today 1991;12:180.
2. Harvell CD. The evolution of inducible defense. Parasitology 1990;100:S53.
3. Murrach P, Kappler J. The T cell and its receptor. Sci Am 1986;254:36.
4. Samuelsson BE, Breimer ME. ABH antigens: some basic concepts. Transplant Proc 1987;19:4401.
5. Billiar TR. Nitric oxide—novel biology with clinical relevance. Ann Surg 1995;221:339.
6. Hibbs, JB Jr, Taintor RR, Vavrin Z. Macrophage cytotoxicity: role for L-arginine deiminase and imino nitrogen oxidation to nitrite. Science 1987;235:473.
7. Hoffman RA, Langrehr JM, Simmons RL. Nitric oxide synthesis: a consequence of alloimmune interaction. Xenobiotica 1994;2:5.
8. Pannen BHJ, Robotham JL. The acute-phase response. New Horizons 1995;3:183.
9. Pinsky MR. A unifying hypothesis of multiple systems organ failure: failure of host defense homeostasis. J Crit Care 1990;5:108.
10. Abraham E, Jesmok G, Tuder R, Albee J, et al. Contribution of tumor necrosis factor to pulmonary cytokine expression and lung injury after hemorrhage and resuscitation. Crit Care Med 1995;23:1319.
11. Bone RC, Balk RA, Fein AM, et al. A second large controlled clinical study of E5, a monoclonal antibody to endotoxin: Results of a prospective, multicenter, randomized, controlled trial. Crit Care Med 1995;23:994.
12. Robertson FM, Offner PJ, Ciceri DP, et al. Detrimental hemodynamic effects of nitric oxide synthase inhibition in septic shock. Arch Surg 1994;129:142.
13. Theuer CP, Pastan I. Immunotoxins and recombinant toxins in the treatment of solid carcinomas. Am J Surg 1993;166:284.
14. Chang AE, Geiger JD, Sondak VK, et al. Adoptive cellular therapy of malignancy. Arch Surg 1993;128:1281.
15. Takiff H, Cook DJ, Himaya NS, et al. Dominant effect of histocompatibility on ten-year kidney transplant survival. Transplantation 1988;45:410.
16. Kahan BD. Cyclosporine. N Engl J Med 1989;321:1725.
17. Suthanthiran M, Strom TB. Renal transplantation. N Engl J Med 1994;331:365.
18. Brayman KL, Stephanian E, Matas AJ, et al. Analysis of infectious complications occurring after solid-organ transplantation. Arch Surg 1992;127:38.

8

CHAPTER

Oncology

Eugene A. Woltering | Walter D. Holder, Jr. | James A. Edney | Brett Sheppard

Tumor Immunology—Humoral Aspects

Introduction

Surgery occupies a pivotal role in the curative and palliative therapy of solid tumors and is an important adjunct in the care of lymphoproliferative malignances. Unfortunately, the best surgical intervention may be thwarted by the lack of clinically relevant information concerning the oncologic process. That is, screening, surgery, and follow-up could be more selective and focused if surgeons knew which patients were at greatest risk for developing cancer and which subset of patients were at greatest risk for recurrence following curative resection. In addition, the availability of tumor-specific adjunctive therapy would provide a means to be both more selective in the conduct of the resection and possibly broaden the indications for the metastectomy (resection of metastasis) or cytoreductive (debulking) surgery. Advancements in molecular biology and genetic techniques have provided a catalyst to address these fundamental problems. The process leading to neoplasia is now seen in terms of specific alterations in oncogenes and subsequent changes in the expression of growth factors or their receptors. Moreover, the process of metastasis formation is believed to be under similar genetic regulation. Future refinements in our knowledge should allow for the rapid diagnosis of the underlying cause of malignancy and provide improved predictive ability in determining the interval and the location of recurrences. In the future, surgical oncology will use molecular biology to an increasing degree. Understanding these tools will enable surgeons to improve therapeutic decision making, will enhance their communication with medical on-

cologists and basic scientists, and will improve patient care (1).

Normal Molecular Machinery

The normal chromosomal constitution of the human somatic cell is a diploid state of 46 chromosomes. By convention, the short arm of the chromosome is designated p and the long arm is termed q. Chromosomes consist primarily of deoxyribonucleic acid (DNA), which associates with positively charged proteins termed histones. The human genome is estimated to be on the order of 100,000 genes (2).

Mitosis is the process of cellular division that apportions new chromosomes equally to daughter cells. Normal mitosis is necessary to maintain the diploid state. The cycle of division involves two coordinated events: DNA replication and then division into daughter cells. The cell cycle is subdivided into four broad periods. G_1 (gap) is the interval from the previous division to the beginning of DNA synthesis. Next is S, or the period of active DNA synthesis. This is followed by G_2, which is the interval between DNA duplication and nuclear division, and M (mitotic), when chromosomes are separated into each daughter cell. The duration of the cell cycle and of each period is variable, depending on the cell type. The typical cycle takes 10 to 30 hr; S, G_2, and M take about 10 hr, and G_1 varies considerably. Nondividing cells such as mature fibroblasts will exit the cell cycle after the M phase. Such cells stop further DNA synthesis and are in the G_0 phase.

Alteration of any portion of the cell cycle by oncogenic mitogens may cause mutations. Errors in mitosis may cause structural chromosomal changes and usually involve the exchange of material between two or more chromosomes (translocation), deletions of DNA, or rearrangement of loci (inversion). Rearrangements, such as the Philadelphia chromosome, a marker for chronic myelocytic leukemia (CML), were some of the first abnormalities discovered (3).

Following division, the flow of information in human cells is transferred from the DNA sequence to ribonucleic acid (RNA), a process called transcription. The RNA messages are then used to create functional proteins in a process known as translation. Nuclear DNA is configured in a double helix and composed of specific sequences of four nucleotides: the two purine bases, adenine (A) and guanine (G), and the two pyrimidine bases, thymine (T) and cytosine (C). In the complementary strands of the helix, A will pair (bond) only with T, and G only with C. Each triplet of bases—known as a codon (e.g., ATT)—on the DNA molecule specifies a particular amino acid. Thus it is the precise order of the nucleotides or codons which determines the specificity of the genetic code (4).

Transcription of information coded in the DNA sequences is initiated by an RNA polymerase that uses the DNA strand as a template to build a complementary messenger RNA (mRNA). RNA, unlike DNA, is a single-stranded moiety with ribose substituted for deoxyribose and uracil (U) substituted for thymine. Thus the DNA codon CTT would correspond to the mRNA triplet GAA. mRNA then migrates into the cytoplasm and binds to ribosomal RNA (rRNA): mRNA now acts as a template for the translation of the original codon. To accomplish this, a specific cytoplasmic transfer RNA (tRNA) binds to the mRNA triplet and then combines with the specific amino acid it coded for. Continual waves of multiple, specific tRNA will then assemble a specific protein (4).

This process is dynamic: because there are a limited number of pathways of response, there must be mechanisms of regulation which determine the appropriate types and amounts of proteins expressed. The genetic machinery must be flexible enough to alter its response to the requirements of wound healing or the catabolism of sepsis. Regulation of gene expression is accomplished through four general categories. The first is regulation of RNA transcription. Certain genes become activated or deactivated, and this alters their availability for transcription. Methylation of the nucleotide (DNA methylation) is one mechanism proposed for this type of control. Another proposed mechanism is unwinding of the chromosome to uncover DNA, making it available for transcription. What normally activates genes and what outside regulators are able to control cell behavior are areas of intense research. The second category of regulation is the control of mRNA processing. This includes alterations in the way mRNA is transported to the ribosome and changes in the cellular environment that alter mRNA stability and thus change its half-life and availability for transcription. The third mechanism is translational regulation. These mechanisms are poorly understood but are suspected to involve the timing of translation and the rate of translation. Finally, posttranscriptional modification of already expressed proteins is an easily accessible mechanism. Changes in the rate of cleavage of inactive to active proteins, biochemical alteration of proteins (phosphorylation and glycosyla-

tion), or a change in the transport of proteins are all regulatory switches that may be altered.

Gene regulation and final expression involve multiple levels of regulation and feedback loops. Each one of the steps is also open to modification by oncogenes or their products. The hallmarks of a malignant cell are hyperproliferation, diminished growth factor requirements, overexpression of growth factors, and loss of anchorage-dependent growth (normal cells require contact with a substratum to grow, whereas malignant cells can grow without attachment to a substrate). These changes are associated with malignancy and are the result of alterations in one or more of the feedback loop genes or regulator controls. Our challenge, then, is to identify aberrant molecular function or behavior and to develop specific interventions.

Technology

Technologic breakthroughs have increased the pace of molecular biology. Knowledge of some of the more common techniques is necessary to augment the understanding and application of the results of relevant studies to surgical care.

Flow Cytometry

Flow cytometry is an optical-based technique that uses a fluorescent dye to stain cells so that specific fluorescent spectra can then identify unique categories of cells. For most cell kinetic studies, acridine orange or propidium iodide dye is used. The binding of these dyes is proportional to cellular DNA content. Once stained, single-cell suspensions are placed in the fluorescence-activated cell sorter (FACS). The cells are then directed into a single file and flow past a detector which measures the light scattered by each cell and the intensity of the cell's fluorescence. Using a FACS, up to 1000 cells per minute may be analyzed. FACS-directed analysis can determine ploidy status and the proliferative indexes of any population. Quiescent (G_1) cells will have a constant diploid amount of DNA (2N), whereas cells with increased DNA content (4N) must be in either S or G_2/M phase. Most tumors will contain both diploid and aneuploid subsets. Aneuploidy is present if there is a second G_1 peak in addition to the normally seen G_1 peak. The ratio of DNA content of tumor to the normal diploic G_1 peak may then be determined; this is known as the DNA index. A normal DNA index is 1.0, thus aneuploidy is any deviation from this.

The S phase fraction (the proliferative index) is based on the ratio of S phase cells to the total number of cells. A normal proliferative index is less than 10%. A higher S phase fraction is associated with accelerated tumor growth. Currently, flow cytometry data have been used in prognostic estimation. That is, tumors with aneuploidy, an elevated S phase, or an abnormal DNA index may need additional therapy. Flow cytometry is also useful for determining receptor status on small amounts of breast tissue and recently has been shown to be reliable in diagnosing lymphoma on fine-needle aspirates (5,6).

Blots

The ability to divide DNA into small, reproducible segments, using DNA restriction enzymes, provides the foundation for blots. Restriction enzymes recognize specific four to eight nucleotide base pair sequences and will cleave DNA only at these specific sequences, which allows the production of multiple copies of gene fragments for study from a particular population. The fragments are then separated by gel electrophoresis. Southern blots transfer the gel electrophoresis product onto a nylon or nitrocellulose filter (the blot), preserving and exposing the nucleotide bases. These bases are then exposed to a specific radioactive nucleic acid sequence known as the probe. The blotted fragments of DNA are complementary to and hybridize with the probe (hybridization is the process of reassociation or annealing of complementary strands to reform a two-stranded structure). The location of the hybridized fragments on the filter is then demonstrated by autoradiography. This technique is sensitive enough to determine the presence of a DNA sequence occurring only once in the human genome and can be obtained from a small tissue sample (4). A variation of this technique, the Northern blot, detects mRNA. Similarly, the Western blot is useful for the detection of specific DNA-binding protein. Blots, therefore, identify an oncogene, quantify its amount, and estimate its activity by locating specific mRNA and encoded proteins. Thus specific gene defects or gene overexpression may be found linked to specific tumors, which may provide an opportunity to design specific therapies. For example, *int-2/hst-1* protooncogenes have been identified in esophageal squamous cell carcinoma. Their copresence correlates significantly with a decreased survival rate. Thus blots done on surgical specimens may dictate the need for aggressive adjunctive therapy (7).

Restriction Fragment Length Polymorphisms

The use of restriction fragment length polymorphisms is a refinement of restriction endonuclease techniques and has become a powerful tool in sorting out specific genetic alterations seen in some inheritable diseases. Polymorphism refers to the variations in the pattern of DNA fragments obtained when the DNA of different patients is cleaved by multiple specific restriction enzymes. Because the enzymes are sequence dependent, a change in sequence at a restriction site will yield DNA fragments of different sizes. These fragments are termed restriction fragment length polymorphisms (RFLPs). If a polymorphic DNA region is near an aberrant gene, then that region may serve as a genetic marker in the kindred of the proband (8). RFLP analysis currently is

facilitating the search for genetic markers for cancer predisposition and prognosis. For example, DNA polymorphisms of the cytochrome P-450$_{IAI}$ gene have been correlated significantly with the development of squamous-cell lung cancer (9). Polymorphisms of the L-*myc* oncogene have also been shown to correlate with the metastatic potential of lung cancer (10). Thus RFLP analysis may identify a subgroup of patients at a higher risk for neoplasia. This would allow for more efficient and earlier surgical intervention.

Transfection and Transformation

Genes involved in carcinogenesis (oncogenes) can be identified by the techniques of transfection and transformation. NIH murine fibroblast 3T3 cells are used commonly. These cells grow in a normal, regulated fashion until an oncogene is introduced or transfected. Cells are said to be transfected when an oncogene is introduced by microinjection of a specific viral vector. Transfected cells then lose their contact inhibition and form small piles of cells, termed focus formation. Once transfected cells lose the ability to regulate growth, they are transformed. Transformed cells can then be injected into murine models, where a solid tumor is evidence of transformation in vivo. Moreover, DNA from transformed cells may be cleaved with restriction enzymes and inserted into viral (phage) DNA. This transformed DNA replicates along with the phage DNA, and when the phage is lysed after infecting a new cell, the viral coat is destroyed and the inserted oncogene remains. The original phage colony harboring the oncogene is then cultured within that cell, providing enough DNA to sequence and identify (4).

Polymerase Chain Reaction

Initially conceived in 1983 by Mullis, polymerase chain reaction (PCR) provides a method for the detection and rapid amplification of minute amounts of unique DNA segments. This technique became automated after the development of a heat-stable DNA polymerase from the thermophilic bacteria *Thermus aquaticus*. This polymerase is known as the *taq* polymerase. PCR amplification is based on three basic steps that repeat in cycles. Step one is denaturation of the DNA to be studied by raising the temperature to near 90° C. The next step is cooling to allow annealing of nucleotide primers to the denatured DNA strands. Primers are chosen specifically so that they will bind to DNA sequences on either side of the DNA that is to be amplified. The third step is primer extension, in which DNA polymerase makes a new copy of the DNA to be amplified. This process is known as extension. Once this step is completed, the temperature is increased again. The newly copied DNA sequences denature and the cycle repeats. Amplification can occur up to several hundred thousand times in a few hours. Thus a specific gene may be amplified from a single original sequence, and subsequently, it can be rapidly studied (11). This technique has replaced the more cumbersome technique of RFLP in some studies (12).

PCR has proven useful in detecting minimum residual disease in marrow and blood samples of lymphoma patients. Specific chromosomal alterations were detected in patients after treatment that identified a group of patients with subclinical disease (13). Similar results were obtained in patients with chronic myelogenous leukemia after bone marrow transplantation (14). PCR has also been able to detect estrogen receptors (ER) in 10-mg samples of breast tumor. Moreover, mutated ER has been identified in ER-negative patients, which may account for the loss of ligand binding (12). Thus PCR should allow earlier intervention in patients believed cured of disease and hopefully improve their survival. Current PCR analysis of ER is approximately 1000-fold more sensitive than current techniques and may change adjuvant therapy decisions for some women with breast cancer. Moreover, it may yield important information on mutated ER forms, allowing manipulation of gene products to achieve a more favorable receptor status.

Molecular Players

Oncogenes

In 1910, Rous reported a "viral" transmissible agent for sarcoma in the Plymouth Rock hen. Subsequent study demonstrated that it was not a viral agent, but a gene acquired by rearrangement or mutation from the normal hen genome after viral infection. The implication of the study was that normal cells may have preexisting genes with latent oncogenic potential. This potential is expressed when the cells undergo specific genetic alteration.

Normal host genes are termed protooncogenes. Only the mutated gene, called the oncogene, has the potential to induce or unsuccessfully suppress oncogenesis. When oncogenes are isolated from viral material, they carry the prefix *v*. When the similar gene is isolated from host DNA, it is designated *c*. Thus the terms *v-src* and *c-src* describe a similar oncogene found in both the viral and hen DNA. Oncogenes derived from a specific tumor or tissue types are designated by a capital letter indicating that tissue type, i.e., L-*myc* is a *myc* oncogene derived from a lung tumor, whereas N-*myc* is derived from a neuroblastoma. Oncogenes are composed of two broad types: dominant and recessive. Dominant oncogenes cause gain of a function and overexpression of the gene or its product. The loss of a recessive oncogene results in the loss of a function. Recessive oncogenes are also called anti-oncogenes or, more commonly, tumor-suppressor genes.

Dominant Oncogenes. Dominant oncogenes are subdivided into four major classes: *(a)* oncogenes from protooncogenes that encode for growth factors; *(b)* oncogenes from proto-oncogenes that encode for membrane or intracellular receptors; *(c)* oncogenes that cause a deviation from the normally encoded pathways for intracellular signaling; and *(d)* oncogenes that act in the nucleus by altering normal transcription factors.

Growth Factors. One oncogene that comes from a gene and encodes growth factors has been identified. This is the *sis* oncogene, which codes for platelet-derived growth factor (PDGF). This oncoprotein is a homodimer identical to the *B*-chain of the normal PDGF. Normal PDGF can be in one of three states: a homodimer of two A chains, a homodimer of two B chains, or a heterodimer of one A and one B chain. All chains cross-react with the same receptor and have similar activity. When the c-*sis* oncogene, located on chromosome 22, was linked to a specific promotor sequence, it was found to be capable of transforming cells. The importance of the *sis* oncogene in human malignancy is not clear. Increased levels of mRNA from tissues expressing the c-*sis* and PDGF have been documented in tissue specimens from osteosarcoma, fibrosarcoma, Ewing's sarcoma, and glioma (15). These observations have lead some investigators to suggest that c-*sis* alters cellular metabolism so that production of PDGF becomes an absolute requirement for continued cell life. These cells may then undergo transformation as a result of the abnormal, continued presence of PDGF.

Membrane and Intracellular Receptors. Oncogenes that encode for membrane receptors with intrinsic protein tyrosine kinase activity include c-*fms*, which encodes for the colony-stimulating factor 1 (CSF) receptor, *erb* B2, which encodes for epidermal growth factor receptor, and *erb* A, which encodes for the intracellular receptor for thyroid hormone.

Studies of the c-*fms* oncogene point to a specific sequence deletion that is responsible for the initiation of oncogene potential (16). The c-*fms* protooncogene has been localized to the q arm of chromosome 5, and some patients with hematologic diseases have this deletion. Activation of the c-*fms* oncogene may cause overexpression of the receptor for CSF. This, coupled with normal secretion of CSF, would induce uncontrolled proliferation of myeloid cell lines. More recently, coexpression of c-*fms* mRNA and CSF has been correlated with ovarian cancer and other malignancies. The role of CSF in nonhematologic malignancies is not known, but CSF can stimulate epithelial malignancies in vitro (17).

The v-*erb* B oncogene was described originally in association with avian erythroblastosis virus (AEV). The oncogene v-*erb* has been demonstrated to encode for a mutated epidermal growth factor (EGF) receptor. This receptor is capable of activation without binding to EGF or other ligands. Thus either overexpression of the normal receptor or a mutation in the normal receptor could augment hyperproliferation of cells with an activated v-*erb* B oncogene. Overexpression of the *erb* B2 oncogene has been documented recently in breast cancer tissue, and the presence of *erb* B2 was found to correlate with a five-fold reduction of survival in breast tumors of otherwise good nuclear grade (9).

The *erb* A oncogene, derived from the intracellular thyroid hormone receptor, appears to function in normal cells as a transcription factor. Although this oncogene does not have a direct transforming effect, it does cooperate with *erb* B in inducing thyroid cell transformation (18). To date, *erb* A has not been implicated in oncogenesis. However, deletion in the p arm of chromosome 3 in patients with small-cell lung cancer is believed to be the loci for c-*erb* A. This deletion is nearly universal in lung cancer and is also found in approximately 85% to 90% of patients with renal-cell carcinomas. Thus the activation of *erb* A may function as a permissive influence in carcinogenesis (19).

Intracellular Transducers. The largest category of oncogenes includes the intracellular transducers; the *ras* family is the predominant member. In general terms, signal transduction functions through one of three major pathways; the phosphatidylinositol system, the protein kinase C system, and the G protein pathway. Activation of one or all of these mechanisms is believed to follow growth factor binding (20).

Phosphatidylinositol Pathway. After growth factor receptor binding, multiple changes in the cellular membrane occur. For example, PDGF activates phosphatidylinositol (PI), which in turn results in a rapid and significant increase in phospholipid turnover. Two distinct kinases are known to function as phosphorylators of PI. Type I phosphatidylinositol kinase yields a 1,3-phosphatidylinositol phosphate (1,3-PIP) and a 1,3,4-phosphatidyl biphosphate (21). Although the precise role of type I kinase is unknown, it is present in some growth factor-stimulated or oncogene-transformed cells. Type I kinase appears to be a requirement for the expression of mitogenesis by some oncogenes (23). Type II phosphatidylinositol kinase results from cleavage of phosphatidylinositol by phospholipase C to form two different intracellular messengers. These are inositol triphosphate (IP_3) and diacylglycerol (DAG). IP_3 releases intracellular calcium, which in turn activates calcium-dependent enzymes and proteins important in mitogenic stimulation. IP_3 also activates protein kinase C (PKC), which provides a way to regulate still another signal transduction pathway. Metabolism of IP_3 is by rapid degradation to act as additional intracellular signals. DAG also activates PKC, and thus activation of PI provides two different loops to regulate the PKC system. DAG is hydrolyzed to arachidonic acid and phosphatidic acid. Arachidonic acid is the precursor to prostaglandin, leukotriene, and thromboxane synthesis. Phosphatidic acid may mimic the action of other growth factors and induce additional type II kinase phosphorylation (23).

Thus overexpression of growth factors or alterations in the growth factor receptor that would cause autoactivation of signal transduction may have profound effects on the cellular machinery. The resulting hyperproliferative drive may simply increase the chance of further errors occurring in any one of the multiple enzymatic steps described above. Moreover, the PI pathway may be influenced not only at the receptor level but at subsequent effector steps as well. The v-*crk* oncogene has recently been shown to encode for oncoproteins homologous to phospholipase C. Thus activation of this oncogene would cause production of IP_3 and DAG without requiring growth factor receptor binding (24).

Protein Kinase C. The family PKC of protein serine-threonine kinases may play a central role in cellular transduction and proliferation. As previously discussed, PKC is now known as the intracellular target for tumor promoters such as phorbol ester, which mimic the actions of DAG. Unlike DAG, which disappears in seconds to minutes, tumor promoters cause a sustained activation of PKC. Activated PKC phosphorylates the receptor of EGF. This causes a decrease in the binding of epidermal growth factor and functionally down regulates the EGF receptor. Sustained activation of PKC will deplete PKC so that paradoxically the cell will lose the ability to down regulate the EGF receptor. This can cause uncontrolled proliferation. PKC also appears to be involved in the activation of the oncogenes c-*fos* and c-*myc* (25). Moreover, the catalytic domain of PKC is also highly homologous to the c-*raf* kinases, which may be expressed after DNA rearrangement. In addition, PKC overexpression has been demonstrated to induce transformation in normal cells (26). Taken together, this work suggests that PKC overexpression, regardless of proximate cause, will contribute to the transformed phenotype.

G proteins and ras Oncogenes. G proteins are defined by their ability to bind guanosine 5'-triphosphate (GTP). G proteins are composed of both G stimulatory (G_s) and the G inhibitory (G_i) proteins. Each type is comprised of three subunits. The classic example of G_s protein signal transduction is the beta-adrenergic system. Epinephrine binds to a stimulatory receptor, which is coupled to G_s. Binding causes a conformational change in G_s. That is, the α subunit releases guanosine 5'-diphosphate (GDP) and binds GTP. This binding induces a second conformational change, which causes the α-GTP complex and then goes on to activate adenylate cyclase. Many α-GTP complexes are formed from each epinephrine found, which enables amplification of the signal. Activation of adenylate cyclase is terminated by the action of GTPase, which hydrolyzes GTP back to GDP. The α-GDP unit then forms with the β- and γ-subunits. Activation of adenylate cyclase proceeds to cyclic adenosine monophosphate (cAMP) synthesis, which in turn activates other protein kinases (27).

G_i proteins share the same β- and γ- subunits but have different α-subunits. When an inhibitory hormone (e.g., prostaglandin E_1) binds to a receptor coupled to

G_i, conformational changes also occur. The G_i α-subunit binds GTP and disassociates into G_i α-GTP and G_i B-T-complexes. The G_i α-GTP complex binds directly to adenylate cyclase to inhibit it. Moreover, the G_i β-γ-complex can also bind to the G_s α-subunit and prevent the G_s protein from becoming activated. G protein activation also plays a pivotal role in adrenal corticotropic hormone (ACTH) stimulation of cAMP-dependent protein kinase activity and may also participate in the coupling of receptors to the PI pathway. Thus all three signal transduction pathways may be inter-regulated (28,29).

The *ras* oncogenes have significant homology with G_s proteins and bind guanine nucleotides. They are also localized on the cytoplasmic membrane similar to G proteins. The transforming potential of *ras* is related to point mutations of several amino acids. However, *ras* does not appear to alter the adenylate cyclase system in mammals. The *ras* oncogene does increase GTPase activity by approximately 50-fold. Although this function is unclear, *ras* alteration of GTP hydrolysis may stabilize mutated *ras* proteins in their active state and provide a continuous proliferative signal through the PKC system (30,31). The *ras* oncogenes are the second most commonly expressed oncogenes in human malignancies (31). Recent work suggests that agents which inhibit cholesterol metabolism (e.g., lovastatin) also inhibit *ras* oncogene membrane translocation and second messenger activation (32). The *ras* oncogenes appear to have a role in both early and late carcinogenesis. Lovastatin prevention of *ras* translocation from cytoplasm to the cell membrane could prevent GTPase alteration. This, theoretically, could reduce or eliminate early steps in the process to neoplasia. Thus lovastatin or similar agents could represent chemoprevention agents for malignancy and could find use in prophylactic or adjuvant therapy after the diagnosis of a carcinoma in-situ of the breast or malignancy confined to the mucosa of a colonic polyp.

Nuclear Oncogenes.   All previously discussed oncogenes have encoded for extracellular growth factors or signal transduction receptor changes. Ultimately, oncogenes must impact on the nuclear control of genetic expression. All nuclear oncogenes are believed to function by acting as, or altering, transcription factors.

The c-*jun* oncogene encodes for proteins that function as a component of the human transcription factor AP-1. AP-1 interacts with regulatory genes whose transcription was induced after phorbol ester exposure. Some phorbol esters mimic DAG action. This work suggests that AP-1 is a nuclear component of PKC signal transduction. Oncogenes may cooperate to alter PKC driven transcription. For example, the c-*fos* oncogene also codes for AP-1. c-*jun* and c-*fos* can form intracellular complexes which are capable of binding DNA. However, the *fos* oncogene alone cannot bind DNA. The *jun* oncogene is able to bind DNA, but this binding is greatly enhanced when *fos-jun* heterodimer is formed (33). The

c-*myc* proto-oncogene is located on human chromosome 8. Overexpression of c-*myc* will maintain cellular division in cells that otherwise would have ceased proliferating (through expression of a stimulatory transcription factor) (34).

Recessive Oncogenes.   In contrast to dominant oncogenes, recessive oncogenes are negative regulators of oncogenesis. That is, loss of their function will lead to oncogenesis. Somatic hybridization studies which fuse normal to malignant cells have shown that most hybrids lose their ability to become tumorigenic once exposed to a normal genome. Thus, hybridization of a normal and a malignant cell results in the suppression of tumorigenesis in the malignant cell previously having this capacity. Because this is a function of fusion with a normal genome, this suggests the presence of genes in the normal cell which can function to suppress tumorigenicity. These genes are said to be negative regulators. However, some malignant-normal cell hybrids are able to maintain some expression of their malignant phenotype, suggesting that tumor suppression may be incomplete in some instances. Thus complete tumor suppression may require homozygous alleles for recessive oncogenes, whereas heterozygous alleles provide incomplete protection from tumorigenicity (an allele is one of two or more different forms of a single gene locus). Distinct alleles of the same gene will have unique nucleotide sequences but are capable of driving the same biochemical process but with a different phenotypic expression, i.e., eye color (35,36).

The study of retinoblastoma (Rb) has provided additional insight into tumor suppression. Rb is a pediatric ocular tumor that occurs in both hereditary and sporadic forms. In the hereditary form, tumors are usually bilateral and multifocal and are seen at an early age. In the sporadic form, the tumors are unifocal and unilateral. Patients with the hereditary Rb disorder inherit a mutant allele from one parent, which occurs in the germ cell line. The other allele is still normal at that time. However, during the last months of gestation, a second mutation occurs in the retinal cell, and with the development of homozygous mutant alleles, the disease is expressed. In the sporadic form, both mutations occur in the same somatic cell (37).

The retinoblastoma suppressor gene (Rb_s) has been present in all normal retinal tissue that has been examined, but it is absent or altered in all Rb cells. Deletions of Rb_s have been localized to specific bands of chromosome 13p. Loss of the Rb_s gene not only results in retinoblastoma but induces susceptibility to additional malignancies. Second primaries occur in up to 30% of retinoblastoma patients. These are usually osteogenic or soft tissue sarcomas and are associated with the loss of heterozygosity of Rb_s. Studies have also demonstrated a structural abnormality of Rb_s in small-cell lung cancer and heart and bladder carcinoma patients. This suggests that the loss of Rb$_s$ function may have a role in other primary malignancies (37–40).

The most important tumor-suppressor gene may arguably be p53. This protein, discovered in 1979, is currently believed to be the most frequently mutated gene in human cancers. The normal function of wild type p53 is to regulate cell growth. It acts as a transcription factor and controls the expression of other genes. This mechanism acts through WAF1/Cip1. This gene is activated by p53 and in turn produces a protein, p21, which arrests cell growth. The growth cycle is arrested in mid-phase by p21 binding to cyclin-dependent kinases. p53 may also act on a separate level to help regulate apoptosis (cell death) in cells with altered DNA. Loss of this function after the mutation of p53 permits the unchecked replication of DNA-injured cells (40,41). Mutation, deletion or inactivation of p53 occurs frequently in human cancers of the lung, stomach, and colon (42, 43). Accumulation of p53 in the nuclei of bladder transitional cell carcinoma has recently been shown to significantly and independently increase the risk of recurrence and death. PCR evaluation of p53 in colorectal cancer has also shown diminished p53—independent of staging. Obviously, the study of p53 and its interactions is a promising area for future intervention. Restoration of wild-type p53 and its "downstream" products could restore regulation to abnormal rapidly dividing cells. Until then, p53 evaluation may be one method by which to select patients at high risk for recurrence who would benefit from aggressive adjuvant therapy (44–46).

Growth Factors

Growth factors are polypeptides that modulate cellular function and regulate cellular growth. These proteins are extremely potent, and in extremely small (picogram) quantities are able to induce a specific response. The actual response that does occur depends more on the type and conformation of the growth factor receptor present and the cellular environment than the specific growth factor itself. That is, a unique growth factor may induce several different responses in the same cell, depending on what receptors are available and what the current biochemical status of the cell is. Growth factor receptors are inactive until bound. When bound to ligand, activation of the intrinsic enzymatic activity of the receptor occurs and signal transduction follows. The following discussion focuses on some growth factors that have relevance to surgically-treated solid tumors (46).

Epidermal Growth Factor. EGF was identified in 1962 by its stimulatory action on epithelial cells. It belongs to transforming growth factor-α (TGF-α). From transformation studies, EGF is believed to regulate cell growth in an autocrine or a paracrine fashion. Autocrine stimulation of growth is believed to be important in malignant cell proliferation. That is, if a malignant cell can acquire the capacity to produce the growth factors necessary for cell growth for which it has functional receptors, then it becomes less dependent on other cells that produce the growth factor needed to proliferate. This will, of course, provide a selective (proliferative) survival advantage for that cell. Cancer cells may also achieve autocrine autonomy by modification of the growth factor receptor so that it initiates signaling without ligand or by altering transduction pathways to initiate signaling downstream from the receptor. For example, this may occur with the truncated EGF receptor coded for by *erb* B in which the tyrosine kinase activity is switched on permanently. Paracrine stimulation, i.e., growth factor action, on cell or stroma nearby the cancer cell is equally important.

In the case of EGF, transformed cells will secrete EGF or EGF-like proteins that act as mitogens. Because these cells already have functional EGF receptors that bind to these peptides and possess the ability to make EGF, these cells possess an autocrine stimulatory feedback loop. Thus, the transformed cells are capable of maintaining their transformed phenotype independent of other regulatory mechanisms (47). As noted, v-*erb* expression results in a defective EGF receptor that can be activated without the action of EGF. Overexpression of EGF does occur in some human malignancies and is associated with a poor prognosis (48). EGF receptor expression in breast cancer is known to be inversely related to the presence of estrogen receptors and is associated with a poor prognosis. The presence of EGF receptor has also identified a subset of node-negative breast cancer patients with a poor prognosis and a poor response to hormone therapy. These patients may represent a subset that is able to benefit most from adjuvant chemotherapy (49, 50).

Transforming Growth Factor

TGF-α. TGF binds to the same receptors as EGF and is also capable of inducing transformation. It is thought to be an embryonal peptide that is overexpressed in malignancy. Like EGF, TGF-α functions in an autocrine fashion and will amplify its own expression (51). TGF-α is thought to have a role in the hypercalcemia of malignancy; it recently was shown to have prognostic significance in lung cancer (52). TGF-α is secreted by hormone-sensitive breast cancer cells as they proliferate, and this secretion is blocked by tamoxifen (53). Thus, alteration in the rate of secretion or complete suppression of TGF-α may be useful in the future as a tumor-specific therapy.

TGF-β. TGF-β is produced by a diverse number of normal and malignant cells; its largest sources in humans are platelets and bone. TGF-β binds to a unique receptor. It exists as a homodimer and heterodimer, giving rise to the terms TGF-β, and TGF-β_2. Because this peptide is ubiquitously expressed, control of its activity is thought to be based on the rate of its activation.

The multifunctional biologic action of TGF-β has not

been completely elucidated. It was originally described as a stimulatory factor for anchorage-dependent cell growth in cooperation with EGF and TGF-α in NIH 3T3 cells. However, in normal tissues, TGF-β appears to have a role in maintaining inhibition of cell growth until activated. Most tumor lines secrete TGF-β but appear resistant to its action. Uncontrolled growth in human lung cancer cells has been linked with an inability to activate TGF-β. Thus, the inhibitory action of TGF-β may also be manipulated by tumor cells to enhance their growth. TGF-β-induced changes in extracellular matrix may also decrease matrix stability and thus decrease adhesion. This would provide a selective advantage for already transformed cells that are capable of anchorage-independent growth over normal cells, which otherwise would require a stable matrix for anchorage-dependent growth (54,55).

Fibroblast Growth Factor.   FGF exists in basic (b) and acidic (a) forms and is secreted by a variety of normal and transformed cells. Both forms bind to the same receptor, which has an intrinsic tyrosine kinase activity. FGF stimulates differentiation of mesothelial neuroectodermal tissues, and this activity may give FGFb its role as a potent stimulator of angiogenesis. FGFb can stimulate endothelial cell migration and invasion (56). Recent work has shown that the increased angiogenesis in breast cancer correlates with an increased potential for the development of metastatic disease (57). The use of inhibitors of angiogenesis, such as heparin-steroid combinations or somatostatin analogue, may allow reduction in tumorigenicity and decrease metastasis (58).

The oncogenes *int*-2, *hst*, and *fgf*-5 have been demonstrated recently to share near 50% identical sequences to FGFa and FGFb. These oncogenes are expressed in Kaposi's sarcoma and gastric cancer. Activation of these oncogenes occurs when transcription is altered and results in expression of FGF-like peptide. Interestingly, the oncogenes, but not the native FGF peptides, have signal sequences that allow them to be inserted into the endoplasmic reticulum. Thus, some oncoproteins can usurp the classic secretory pathways to alter intracellular regulation. FGF, then, may represent a potential target to alter tumor metabolism and arrest metastasis (59).

Molecular Biology of Metastasis

Several avenues of research have demonstrated that the development of metastases is not a random event but rather is linked to genetic regulation (60,61). The first line of evidence for the genetic regulation of metastasis is the association of oncogenes with metastases. Transfection studies have shown that the *ras* oncogene induces metastatic potential in many cell types. The *ras*-transfected cells secrete greater amounts of proteases, which are implicated in the metastatic cascade (62). The *ras*-transfected cells do not respond to the normal inhibitory action of TGF-α, rather TGF-β actually stimulates

DNA synthesis in the *ras*-transfected cells. Thus, the cells have an altered response to growth factor, probably secondary to a receptor mutation. Other oncogenes have been incriminated in the induction of metastatic disease. These include *erb* B2 in breast cancer and L-*myc* in neuroblastoma (63,64).

Second, the presence of multiple degradative proteases is associated with increased tumor aggressiveness. Also, tumors that have little ability to lyse fibrin clot are associated with low metastatic potential. Both TGF-β and FGF play an important regulatory role for plasminogen activators and inhibitors. The growth factors EGF, TGF-β, and FGF each enhance the expression of plasminogen activators in cell culture. Thus, oncogenes that encode for overexpression of these growth factors may also induce increased amounts of proteolytic enzyme (65). However, some degradative proteins may function to limit tumor aggressiveness. Increased proteolysis is associated with the metastatic phenotype. Efforts directed against blocking proteolysis or the production of growth factors may therefore cause reversing the metastatic potential of some tumor cells (55).

Third, recent work has identified distinct metastasis-suppressor genes. The first identified, *nm*23, has an inversely proportional expression of metastases in a murine melanoma model (66, 67, 68). The gene *nm*23 codes for the nucleoside diphosphate kinase (NDP). NDP kinases are known to complex with G proteins in cAMP-linked signal transduction. Expression of *nm*23 could then alter second messenger transduction and minimize the oncogene-induced proliferative signal. NDP kinase is also associated with microtube regulation, and *nm*23 may have a role in stabilizing the mitotic spindle, thus decreasing aberrant mitosis. Recently, the presence of *nm*23 was correlated with a negative nodal status and a good prognosis in patients with breast cancer (69). Future manipulation of *nm*23 and other metastatic-suppression genes may allow for reversal or prevention of neoplastic progression.

Selected Applications of Molecular Biology in Surgical Oncology

Breast Cancer

Research continues to be directed towards evaluating molecular markers which may be helpful in determining the clinical behavior of breast cancers. Hopefully, the development of a "report card" of prognostic factors would help decide which women will benefit the most from adjuvant therapies. Additionally, the elucidation of oncogenes in breast cancer may provide focused therapeutic targets for innovative strategies.

Currently, ploidy and S-phase status are useful markers in primary breast cancer. In a study of over 300 women, aneuploid tumors had twice the recurrence rate of similarly staged diploid tumors (70). Sigersmon has studied 367 women with node negative breast cancer and demonstrated that S-phase provided the greatest prognostic information, followed by PR status and tumor size. A subgroup of patients with a four-fold risk of recurrence was identified as having an S-phase of 12% or more, PR less than 10 fmol/mg, and tumor size larger than 2.0 cm (71). Similar findings have been reported by other groups (72, 73).

Flow cytometry may therefore be able to identify distinct subsets of patients who would benefit from intensive adjuvant chemotherapy and for whom the risk/benefit ratio is acceptable. Finally, a recent investigation of 175 pre-menopausal breast cancer patients demonstrated significantly higher tumor proliferation incidences (S-phase) and more frequent aneuploidy in users of contraceptives than in nonusers (74). Thus, women with a high risk for developing breast cancer may wish to use alternative methods of contraception.

The utility of p53 and other oncogenes is confounded by conflicting or inconclusive investigations. Mutations of p53 have been found more frequently in young women with ER-negative node-positive cancers (75, 76). However, the presence of p53 mutations and the expression of c-*erb*-2 have been associated with a poorer prognosis in node-negative patients (77). The co-expression of p53 mutants with other oncogenes may be an epiphenomenon with regard to p53. Progressive co-expression of oncogenes and not the presence of p53 is significantly associated with decreasing survival (78). The overexpression of c-*erb*-2 in vitro confers resistance to tumor necrosis factor, suggesting that oncogene products may produce tumors more resistant to native immune-surveillance mechanisms. Antibodies directed against c-*erb*-2 have significant anti-proliferative action (79).

The recent isolation of the breast cancer susceptibility gene—BRCA1 on the q arm of chromosome 17 has added a new dimension to women's health care. Mutation of BRCA1, a tumor-suppressor gene, accounts for at least 5% of all cases of breast cancer but may not be important in sporadic cases of breast cancer. A similar gene, BRCA2, also causes a familial susceptibility to breast cancer but does not increase the risk of ovarian cancer as does BRAC1 (80). Currently, the detection of BRCA1 has strong implications for counseling in high-risk women. It has not yet yielded new therapeutics but, like p53, is a provocative candidate for intervention.

Gastric Cancer

Mutation of p53 appears to play an early role in the development of intestinal types of gastric cancers. Recent studies have shown a mutation frequency of 41% in intestinal-type tumors, compared to 4% in diffuse types. Moreover, the mutations of p53 in well-differentiated gastric cancers are more frequent at AT pairs, whereas GC to AT mutations are more common in poorly-differentiated tumors. Some authors believe that p53 is an early initiating event in gastric carcinogenics and that full expression of malignancy requires the mutation of other additional oncogene proteins. This, if correct, is similar to the mechanism proposed for colon cancer and may represent a common mechanism for the development of several epithelial malignancies (81, 82).

Recent investigations of allelic losses lend some credence to this perspective. In some geographic areas, patients with familial adenomatous polypepsis are at a significantly higher risk for developing gastric cancer. In one investigation, deletions occurred in one-third of gastric cancers at the MCC (mutated colon cancer) and APC (adenomatous polyposis colic) only in association with p53 mutations (83). The downstream accumulation of other oncogene products may also determine not only the degree of differentiation (82), but also impact on survival. Similar to the breast cancer story, expression of *erb*-B-2 is significantly associated with shortened survival in well-differentiated resected gastric cancers. Further elucidation of these findings may not only define therapeutic targets, but also provide a clearer understanding of gastrointestinal carcinogenesis (84, 85).

Colon Cancer

Evaluation of mitotic index and ploidy status may provide additional prognostic power and guide decision-making in the care of colorectal cancers. Patients with aneuploid tumors or with elevated S-phase have generally had a poorer prognosis. In one study, a low S-phase was associated with an 82% 5 year survival, whereas high S-phase patients had a 43% survival. Similar results have been obtained for ploidy status. Thus, like breast cancer, the development of a "report card" of prognostic factors may help guide decision making on adjuvant therapies (86-88).

Whereas *ras* oncogene mutations are common occurrences in diverse malignancies, overexpression of *ras* has been demonstrated in up to 60% of colon carcinomas, 40% of colonic dysplastic polyps, and 10% of adenomas (1). The degree of expression of *ras* also has been shown to correlate with the depth of bowel wall invasion (89). The *myc* oncogene is also overexpressed in colon cancer and is associated with deletion on the q arm of chromosome 5. In vitro activation of *ras* and *myc* often confers resistance to chemotherapeutics in standard assays (90, 91). More recently, errors in otherwise normal repetitive sequences of DNA (termed minisatellites) have been shown to be involved in the pathogenesis of genetic damage. Using Southern blots, mutation of the minisatellite HRSA1 has been shown to be significantly associated with colorectal carcinomas. Of interest is that HRSA1 is juxtaposed closely to H-*ras*, suggesting that new mutations in HRSA1 may disrupt the expression of proximity proto-oncogenes (92). This may explain the importance of *ras* in human colorectal carcinogens and underscore the importance of studies attempting to block the expression of *ras* with monoclonal antibodies.

Colorectal cancer has been shown to be the result of a clonal progression of hyperproliferation to fully-expressed neoplasia. This is most likely caused by the accumulation of mutated oncogenes rather than their actual order of appearance, although this certainly must have some significance as well. The multistep process of the development of colorectal cancer has been championed by the Vogelstein laboratory. Allelic clones of specific tumor suppression genes are now known to occur. Losses on the p arm of 17 are seen in more than 75% of colorectal cancers and are associated with the progression of adenomas to carcinomas in some patients. The region lost on 17p is now known to be the wild-type p53 moiety. This, in conjunction with *ras* or *myc* overexpression, may be sufficient to abolish tumor suppression and permit carcinogenesis (93, 94).

Major deletions also occur on 18q in over 70% of late adenomas. This deletion is also a tumor-suppression gene designated DCC or deleted in colon cancer. DCC serves as a cell-adherence molecule, and loss of cellular adhesion is a key step in the development of carcinogenesis. 18q deletion is believed to underlie the development of Lynch Syndrome II. This is an autosomal disorder with early malignancy. Reintroduction of cell surface adhesion molecules in vitro reduces the growth rate and tumorinecity of colon cancer cells (94–97). Finally, the gene for familial adenomatous polyposis coli (APC) has been mapped to 5q. Perturbation of APC not only results in Familial adenomatosis polyposis (FAP) and progression to colon carcinoma but is also present in up to 60% of somatic, sporadic colon cancers and adenomas (98). The loss of 5q appears to lead to hyperproliferation and methylation errors which induce mutation of *ras*, leading to adenomas or early carcinoma. Subsequent loss of DCC and loss of cellular adhesion results in a late stage adenoma. Further loss of p53 abrogates tumor suppression and loss of regulatory control, which results in carcinoma (94). Suppression of tumorigenicity with the reintroduction of normal chromosomes 5 or 18 has occurred in vitro and holds the promise for cure of this malignancy with further refinements in gene therapy (99).

Multiple Endocrine Neoplasia

RFLP analysis initially was used to identify families at risk for MEN-2a. This allowed for early intervention if evaluations for medullary thyroid carcinoma or pheochromocytoma were positive. The development and refinement of PCR has provided accurate and reproducible survival for MEN-2a kindreds. Detection of mutations in the RET proto-oncogene now predicts inheritance of MEN-2a. Non-carriers require no further evaluation, whereas carriers positive for RET undergo

prophylactic total thyroidectomy regardless of plasma calcitonin levels (100–102).

Future Considerations

Currently, molecular biology has provided information leading to definitive therapy in patients with MEN-2a and in the surgical care of neuroblastoma in which n-*myc* amplification guides the aggressiveness of surgical resection (103). As our primitive knowledge base expands, the full promise of molecular intervention will also expand. For example, insertion of a normal Rb1 gene in vivo could suppress cellular division in osteocarcinoma, as has been demonstrated in vitro (104). The vehicle to provide this intervention is the further development of gene therapy.

The strategy of gene therapy in cancer research is directed towards reestablishing normal cellular machinery with the insertion of either tumor-suppression genes or genes directed against oncogene suppression. Other strategies may include driving malignant cells into apoptosis or the development of cytokine elaborating genes to kill the malignant cell. Exciting work is under way with retroviral vectors in humans with malignant brain tumors. Experimental work continues to be done in the field with melanoma, lung, colon, and renal malignancies. Recently, recombinant vaccinia virus cytokine vectors have prevented the development of murine breast cancers when used as vaccinations. Thus, in the future we may not only be able to cure some cancers with molecularly engineered vectors, we may prevent their development in the first place (105–107).

Tumor Immunology—Cellular Aspects

Tumor immunology is the study of the antigenic properties of tumor cells, the host immune response to tumor cells, and the interaction between neoplastic cells and the host immune system. Tumor immunology has a functional role in that it not only seeks to delineate tumor cell-host interactions; it tries to develop methods through scientific research whereby the individual's immune system may be enhanced to prevent the development of tumor cells and to eradicate already-established tumor cells (108).

Despite a history exceeding 100 years, the science of immunology has only recently reached a point at which immunological approaches to cancer diagnosis and treatment are feasible. Early attempts to study the immune response in both patients and animals showed the rejection of transplanted normal and tumor tissues in an unpredictable manner. This work led to the discovery of the major histocompatibility complex (MHC) and the development of multiple inbred mouse strains which have subsequently provided the foundation for many tumor immunology studies. Many of the discoveries in tumor immunology have grown from direct observation of tumor biology. The nature of immunoglobulins and immunoglobulin production was derived primarily from observations on multiple myeloma and other B-lymphocyte neoplasms (109). The study of cell surface antigens on lymphoreticular neoplasms has led to a host of surface markers which have been shown to differentiate lymphocytes on a functional basis (110). A variety of lymphokines, cytokines, and previously unknown cells (e.g., NK and LAX cells) have been identified from basic tumor studies (111).

A major function of the host immune system is the detection of neoplastic cells. In the immunosurveillance theory of tumor development, the establishment of clinically significant malignant neoplasms results from an imbalance or deficit in the immune surveillance mechanism, which permits tumor cells to grow.

The tumor cell-immune system interaction is complex. Multiple factors affect this interaction, including alterations in the genetic control of all components of the immune response; inhibition of the immune response because of extremes of age, stress, hormonal imbalance (e.g., hypopituitarism, Cushing's syndrome, myxedema) and immunosuppressive substances (e.g., steroids, antineoplastic agents, cyclosporin); and variations within the tumor itself. These are complex factors that vary from individual to individual and may even vary within the same individual over time. All these factors must be considered in evaluating the immune response to malignancy.

Organization of the Immune System

An outline of the organization and derivation of the cellular components of the immune system is shown in Figure 8.1. All of these cells originate from undifferentiated bone marrow precursor cells, which differentiate into three major categories: lymphoid, myeloid, and a less defined group (often called third population) consisting of non-T, non-B, or null cells (111).

Lymphoid cells further differentiate into T-lymphocytes after interaction with the thymus gland or into B-lymphocytes after interaction with the bursa of Fabricius (in birds) or the bursa equivalent in mammals (possibly the gut associated Lymphoid tissues—GALT). T and B-lymphocytes are morphologically indistinguishable. One of the first means of distinguishing human T from B-lymphocytes was by the ability of T-lymphocytes to bind to sheep erythrocytes. The development of monoclonal antibody technology by Kohler and Milstein (Fig. 8.2) has been a major advance in terms of identifying cell surface antigens which demonstrate leukocyte lineage and function (109). Monoclonal antibodies have been developed that react to cell surface antigens of both T and B-lymphocytes, myeloid, and third population

cells. An international nomenclature for leukocyte antigens detected by monoclonal antibodies has been developed to classify and organize the many monoclonal antibodies and their respective antigens. The cluster differentiation designation (CD) system for representative leukocyte differentiation antigens is shown in Table 8.1. The T-lymphocyte protein that bound sheep erythrocytes was designated CD2. However, the definitive marker for T-lymphocytes is the T-cell receptor antigen (TCR), and an attached portion designated CD3. T-lymphocytes (CD3+, TCR+ cells by definition) have been further categorized into some populations that show helper/inducer functions (CD4) and those that have cytotoxic and possibly suppressor functions (CD8). CD4+ T-lymphocytes recognize antigens in association with MHC class ll molecules, and CD8+ T-lymphocytes recognize antigens in association with MHC class I molecules. In both cases, the presence of MHC and CD class antigens are required for helper or cytotoxic effects to be seen (111,112).

B-lymphocytes are defined as those which have endogenously produced immunoglobulin(s) (antibodies). Table 8.1 lists some of the antigens other than immunoglobulins carried by B-lymphocytes. Most B-lymphocytes also carry MHC class ll antigens that permit interaction with helper T-lymphocytes. B-lymphocytes under the influence of antigen, antigen presenting cells, and helper T-cells produce specific antibodies in five classes: IgA, IgM, IgG, IgD, and IgE. Most peripheral blood B-lymphocytes have both surface IgM and IgD that express unique specificity on each cell. IgG is the most abundant immunoglobulin in the serum and is a major contributor to immunity against a variety of infectious agents. Receptors for IgG are present on monocytes, macrophages, and neutrophils. IgG can fix complement to produce cell lysis. IgA is combined with a secretory protein and secreted actively in multiple body secretions, where it provides protection against surface (inhaled or ingested) pathogens. IgM is the largest of the immunoglobulins (a pentamer), is the initial antibody produced in the primary immune response, and can fix complement. The specific function of IgD is unknown; it may have a B-lymphocyte surface receptor function. IgE is known as the reaginic antibody and has the ability to initiate allergic responses by interaction with mast cells, producing histamine release (111,112).

The ability of T-lymphocytes to react with specific tumor or other antigens and the ability of B-lymphocytes to produce antigen specific antibody is determined by complex random gene rearrangements of V, D, and H genes in B-lymphocytes and similar genes in T-lymphocytes. The stimulus for the expansion of a clone of either antigen specific T- or B-lymphocytes is the presentation of specific antigen to the lymphocytes together with MHC class ll antigens.

The myeloid precursor cells differentiate into megakaryocytes that ultimately produce platelets and nor-

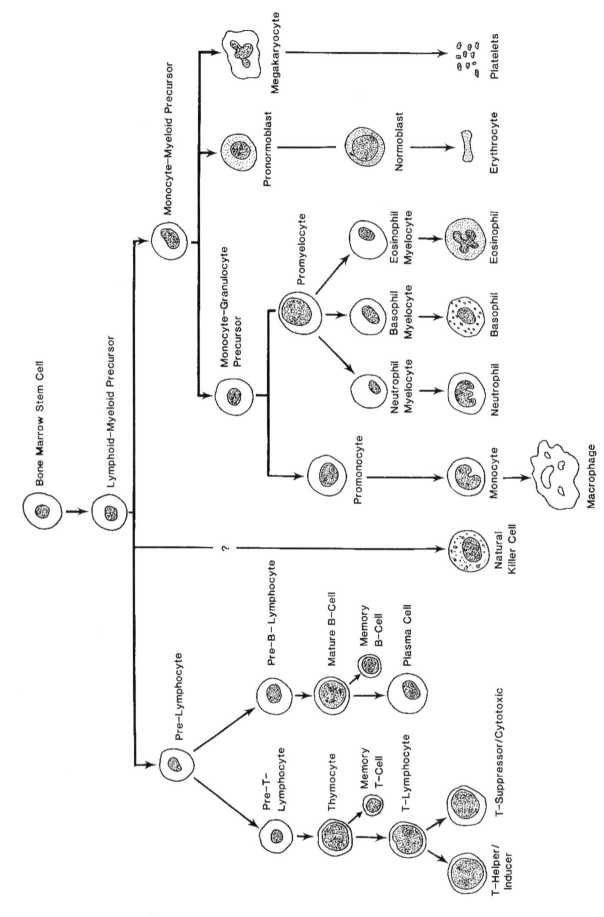

Figure 8.1. Organization and derivation of the immune system cellular components. Modified from Holder W. Current management of lymphomas and Hodgkin's disease. In: Sabiston D, ed. Textbook of surgery update. Philadelphia: WB Saunders, 1989:53–68.

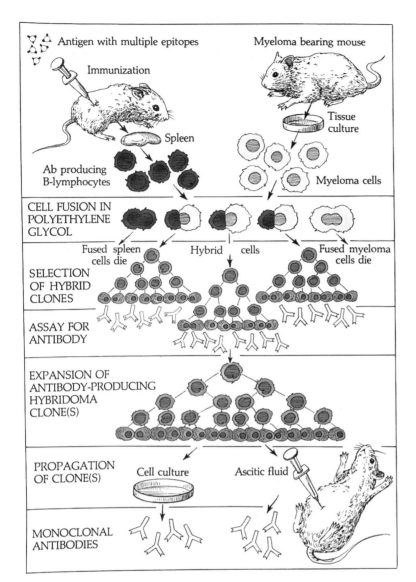

Figure 8.2. Monoclonal antibodies are most frequently produced by immunizing mice with an antigen and then later removing the spleen from the mouse. The splenic B lymphocytes are then fused with a specially selected mouse myeloma cell. The mouse myeloma cell lines most frequently used are ones that will grow indefinitely, do not secrete antibody, and have been selected for an absence of the enzyme HGPRT. Therefore, these cells lack the ability to grow in the presence of hypozanthine, aminopterin, and thymidine (HAT). The mouse lymphocytes have HGPRT and the genetic information to make the specific antibody. Unlike the myeloma cells, they cannot grow in cell culture. The mouse B lymphocytes are fused with the myeloma cells using polyethylene glycol (PEG) and placed into small-cell culture wells containing growth medium and HAT. Only fused cells (hybridomas) composed of a B lymphocyte and a myeloma cell will grow. The resultant cells are tested for specific antibody production. Cells producing appropriate antibody are grown in large batches in culture or injected into mice, where they produce ascites containing large quantities of antibody. From Berner GM. Antibody and immunoglobulins: structure and function. In: Bellanti J, ed. Immunology III. Philadelphia: WB Saunders, 1985;100.

moblasts, which further differentiate into erythrocytes. The myeloid series precursor cells also differentiate into myelocytes that become neutrophils, basophils (mast cells) and eosinophil granulocytes that are primary effector cells of non-specific immune function. The monocyte line of cells functions to break down, process, and present foreign antigens. Included are the macrophages, Kupfer cells, dendritic cells, histiocytes, and related components of the reticuloendothelial system. These cells contain proteases and multiple other enzymes and produce superoxide radicals which effectively kill and digest pathogens and foreign cells.

The third population (non-T, non-B or null cells) are large granular lymphocytes which include natural killer (NK) and lymphokine activated killer (LAK) cells. Many of these cells are CD16+, CD25+, CD3-, and TCR-. However, no specific markers exist for all NK or LAK cells. These cells, through an unknown mechanism, attach to a variety of tumor and virus infected cells and release a pore forming protein (porphyrin) that pro-

duces holes in the cytoplasmic membrane of the target cell causing it to lyse (111,112).

In addition to the cells of the immune system, multiple other circulating factors exist that modulate the immune response through various actions and cell to cell communication. The acute phase proteins include C-reactive protein and related substances, complement, the interferons, and tumor necrosis factors. In addition, there are multiple other mediators of the immune response, including arachidonic acid, the prostaglandins, and the leukotrienes that are beyond the scope of this overview. Lymphokines and other soluble mediators of various immunological functions which have a specific effect on tumor immunity will be discussed below.

Definitions and Terms

The word cancer is a clinical term indicating a malignant new growth. The neoplastic process usually is characterized by the relentless growth of abnormal cells,

Table 8.1.
The CD System of Frequently Referenced Leukocyte Antigens*

Cluster Designation	Representative Antibodies	Identity or Function
T-Lymphocyte		
Antigens		
CD1	Leu 6, OKT6, T6	Cortical thymocytes
CD2	Leu 5, OKT11, T11	All T-lymphocytes, sheep red blood cell receptor
CD3	Leu 4, OKT3, T3	All T-lymphocytes, (T-cell receptor associated)
CD4	Leu 3, OKT4, T4	Helper T-lymphocytes
CD5	Leu 1, OKT1, T101	All T-lymphocytes
CD6	T12	All T-lymphocytes
CD7	Leu 9	? IgM Fc receptor
CD8	Leu 2, OKT8, T8	Suppressor/cytotoxic T-lymphohcytes
B-Lymphocytes and		
Other Antigens		
CD9	BA-2, J2	B-lymphocyte leukemia associated
CD10	CALLA, J5, BA-3	Common acute lymphocytic leukemia antigen, Burkitt's lymphoma, follicular lymphoma
CD11	Leu M5, OKM1	Monocytes, granulocytes, adhesion molecule, complement receptor
CD15	Leu M1	Monocytes, granulocytes, Reed-Sternberg cells
CD16	Leu 11	NK cell and neutrophils
CD19	B4	All B-lymphocytes
CD20	B1	All B-lymphocytes
CD21	B2	Epstein-Barr virus receptor on B-lymphocytes
CD22	Leu 14	Most B-lymphocytes
CD23	MNMG, PL-13	Activated B-lymphocytes
CD24	BA-1	All B-lymphocytes
CD25	Tac	Interleukin-2 receptor
CD45	L-CA, T200	Leukocyte common antigen
CD54	ICAM-1	Adhesion molecule on leukocytes and endothelial cells
CD56	Leu-19	NK and LAK cells
CD71	Transferrin receptor	Activated T and B cells

* The Cluster Designation System was established by the First and Second International Leukocyte Typing Workshops in Paris in 1982 and in Boston, 1984. Additional CD designations continue to be made.

which produces a tumor (mass) that invades and destroys normal tissues and spreads to other areas of the body through multiple routes (e.g., bloodstream, lymphatics, direct spread). The untreated growth of cancer most often results in the death of the host. Cancer begins at a cellular level in a process called malignant transformation. This may be either a single or, more often, a multi-step process. A normal cell is transformed into a malignant one through a variety of mechanisms. The transformation event may occur as a result of exposure to certain viruses, chemicals, radiation and other physical agents, spontaneous random mutations, or gene rearrangements. Considerable evidence exists that transformation occurs much more frequently than does clinical cancer. Transformed cells undergo alterations in their surface composition, which is the basis for immunological recognition. A variety of terms defines the relationship between tumor cells, the host, and various immune components (Table 8.2).

Chemically Induced Tumors

Pott, in the 18th century, observed that there was a high incidence of carcinoma of the scrotum in chimney sweeps, and he related this finding to soot exposure (113). Early in this century, it was found that many polycyclic hydrocarbons and a variety of other manufac-

tured and natural substances could transform cells in tissue culture and also produce cancer in laboratory animals when ingested, injected, or painted on the skin. These agents produced a multiplicity of tumors in terms of their morphology. The experiments of Prehn and Main in 1957 demonstrated that the antigens on methylcholanthrene (MCA) induced sarcomas were tumor specific and could not be detected in other MCA-induced

Table 8.2.
Terms Frequently Used in Tumor Immunology to Define Tumor Cell-host Relationships

Term	Definition
Allogenic	Refers to intraspecies antigenic differences
Anergy	Impaired cell mediated immunity
Autologous	Part of the same individual
Cytokines	Molecules that mediate interactions between cells
Effector Cells	Cells that produce the end effect
Genotype	The genetic characteristics of a cell
Heterologous	Interspecies antigenic differences
Homologous	The same species
Isologous	Identical genetic constitution
Lymphokine	Molecules produced by lymphocytes that mediate interactions between cells
Phenotype	Expressed characteristics of a cell
Syngeneic	Inbred strain with identical genes
Tolerance	Specific immunologic unresponsiveness

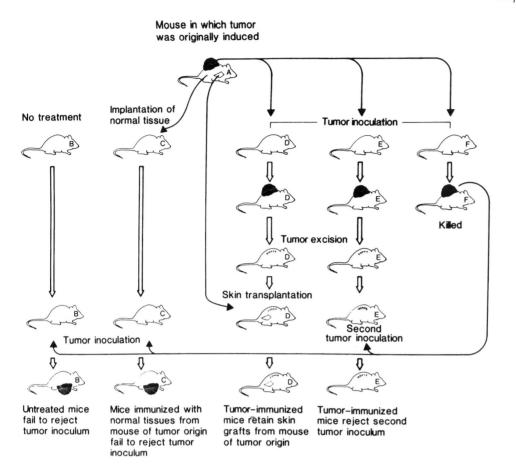

Mouse in which tumor
was originally induced

No treatment

Implantation of
normal tissue

Tumor inoculation

Tumor excision

Killed

Skin transplantation

Second
tumor inoculation

Tumor inoculation

Untreated mice
fail to reject
tumor inoculum

Mice immunized with
normal tissues from
mouse of tumor origin
fail to reject tumor
inoculum

Tumor–immunized
mice retain skin
grafts from mouse
of tumor origin

Tumor–immunized
mice reject second
tumor inoculum

Figure 8.3. Transplantation experiments demonstrating the existence of transplantation antigens on MCA-induced murine sarcomas. Only those mice (E) that had been immunized by previous tumor inoculation and removal rejected the tumor on second tumor inoculation. Tumor immunized mice (D), however, still accepted normal tissue (skin grafts) of the mouse of tumor origin (A) and normal tissues of this mouse (A) did not protect other mice (C) against tumor challenge. Animal F is used simply to store the tumor from mouse A for the period required to immunize other mice (C–E) with normal and malignant tissues. In similar experiments (not shown), the original tumor was removed completely without killing the animal; after an interim period during which the tumor had been stored in a second mouse, the tumor was reimplanted into the original mouse, which now rejected the tumor that once originated from that mouse. This suggested that a mouse can be made immune to its own tumor after it has been removed completely from the animal. From Schreiber H. Tumor immunology. In: Paul W, ed. Fundamental immunology. 2nd ed. New York: Raven Press, 1989:923–956.

tumors or in normal tissues of mice (114) (Fig. 8.3). Also, the tumor cells did not immunize against normal skin grafts from the mouse in which the tumor originated or against other MCA-induced tumors in the same mouse. In addition, no immunization occurred against the tumor by normal mouse tissues. Simply stated, each chemically-induced tumor was immunologically distinct from the normal host cells and from other tumors in the same animal produced by the same chemical carcinogen. Later, it was demonstrated that tumor-specific and tumor-associated antigens could be found on many tumors, including those induced by other chemicals, physical agents, and some spontaneous tumors as well. Small doses of chemical carcinogens do not induce immunity, and tumor viruses are not required for carcinogens to produce tumors. Tumor specific antigens induced by chemical carcinogens tend to be highly immunogenic and can generate antibody and cell mediated immune responses.

Virally Induced Tumors

In contrast to chemically induced tumors, those produced by viruses contain antigens that cross-react with other tumors induced by the same or similar virus, even though they may be histologically different. Oncogenic viruses generally are subdivided into either DNA or RNA types, based upon the nucleic acid they contain

(115). Most cells that become infected with potentially oncogenic DNA viruses are permissive (i.e., they allow virus replication and death of the cell). Some cells do not permit virus replication, but rather incorporate either all or part of the viral DNA into the host genome. These cells and their progeny subsequently carry the viral genetic information indefinitely. Transformation of the cell may result either from a direct triggering of the host genes by the integrated viral DNA or from new proteins induced by the incorporated virus genetic material.

DNA viruses that have been implicated in the production of human tumors include Epstein-Barr virus (Burkitt's lymphoma and nasopharyngeal carcinoma), Hepatitis B virus (hepatocellular carcinoma), Herpes simplex virus type ll (cervical carcinoma), and papilloma virus (cervical carcinoma).

Unlike the DNA viruses, the RNA viruses (often called retroviruses or C-type viruses) tend to elicit a continuous production of virus in cells that they transform. These viruses are infectious and are transmitted from one individual to another. Young and immunosuppressed hosts tend to be particularly susceptible, whereas adults who have a fully functional immune system are more likely to have a reduced incidence of tumor formation and a specific immune reaction to the virus. RNA tumor viruses that have been implicated in the production of human tumors include the human lymphocytotrophic viruses (HTLV) type I (acute T-cell leukemia) and HTLV type ll (hairy cell leukemia). Other studies, which have not been definitive, have implicated RNA viruses in the etiology of several adenocarcinomas, particularly breast.

Oncogenes

A variety of genes, collectively named oncogenes, of either viral or cell origin that can produce transformation of cells in culture have been described. The list of known oncogenes continues to lengthen. Many of these genes code for proteins involved in normal cell regulatory processes, particularly those involving growth, division, and differentiation. The functions of many cellular oncogenes in normal cell growth and development have not been determined. When these genes are activated in an abnormal state (i.e., at an inappropriate time, location, or in an abnormal concentration), transformation will probably occur. Oncogene activation may occur as a result of insertion of a promoter such as a transforming virus, translocation of the oncogene to a site adjacent to an active gene, or after a mutation. Specific oncogene products are being defined (e.g., the *erb* B oncogene is related to the epidermal growth factor receptor and the *sis* oncogene to the platelet derived growth factor) and may be detected by immunological methods. Specific oncogenes are reviewed elsewhere in this chapter.

Tumor Antigens

The characterization of tumor antigens has depended heavily on early research with rodents. A significant advance was the development of genetically identical (isologous) inbred strains and the ability to serially transplant specific tumors within these animals. This provided the first reproducible tumor models for experimental studies. In 1943, Gross found that small doses of tumor cells (in quantities too small to produce tumors) given intradermally into mice would prevent the growth of the same tumor cells, which were capable of producing tumors, given at higher doses (116). These results suggested that tumor cells possessed unique antigens and that immunization against cancer was possible.

Tumor antigens usually are described as either unique or as tumor associated. Unique tumor antigens can be detected only on tumor cells and not on other cells of the host. These antigens appear to be highly specific and limited to a single tumor or may be shared by certain other tumor cells. Tumor associated antigens may be expressed on some normal cells but are expressed at their highest level on tumor cells. Some of these antigens are highly immunogenic, and their presence may induce an immune response, whereas others are poorly immunogenic and produce little or no immune response. The unique characteristics of chemically and virally induced tumor antigens were noted above. The recognition of specific unique tumor antigens is important for targeting the immune response to tumor cells. Unfortunately, few truly tumor specific antigens or antibodies are currently available for diagnostic or clinical studies. Human tumors induced by specific viruses tend to share specific antigens. This finding has contributed to research to develop vaccines specific for the prevention of cancer. This approach has promise, but it remains to be tested in patients at risk of developing cancer. Vaccines against tumor antigens have been used in high risk for recurrence patients and will be described later.

Unlike tumor-specific antigens, tumor-associated antigens greatly predominate in patients with cancer. Table 8.3 lists some of the current clinically important tumor associated antigens. The best characterized tumor-associated antigens are the oncofetal antigens. These are generally not found in the adult or, if present, are at low levels. They occur within the fetus, where their functions are generally unknown. They may be involved with differentiation and lineage specification. The best characterized of the oncofetal antigens are carcinoembryonic antigen (CEA) and alpha fetoprotein (AFP). CEA is found in the developing human colon but is not found in significant levels in the normal adult. It was first described in association with some carcinomas of the colon but has subsequently been found in other tumors such as gastric, pancreatic, and breast cancer, and in inflammatory processes, such as pancreatitis and colitis. An elevated CEA prior to operation is a predictor of a poor prognosis, and a rising serum level of CEA

Table 8.3.
Tumor Antigens that Serve as Diagnostic Markers

Type	Antigen	Tumor
Oncofetal	α-fetoprotein (AFP)	Hepatocellular and testicular carcinomas
	Carcinoembryonic antigen (CEA)	Colorectal, pancreas, gastric, breast, and lung carcinomas
Organ Specific	Prostate-specific antigen (PSA)	Prostate carcinoma
Proliferation Antigen	Tissue polypeptide antigen (TPA)	Breast and gynecologic tumors
Oncogene product	HER2/neu	Breast, ovary, thyroid, lung carcinoma
Monoclonal antibody		
Defined	CA 15-3	Breast carcinoma
	CA 19-9	Colorectal, gastric, pancreas carcinoma
	CA 50	Colorectal, gastric, pancreas carcinoma

after definitive operation is a predictor of recurrence. AFP (an alpha globulin) is found in the developing fetus in the liver and yolk sac cells and is not found in normal adults. Certain patients with hepatocellular carcinoma and germinal tumors, such as non-seminomatous testicular carcinomas, will produce AFP; it can be used as a serologic marker of disease status and a predictor of recurrence. Other tumor-associated antigens include CA 125, neuron specific enolase, prostate specific antigen, CA 19-9, CA 50, and CA 15-3.

There is generally little immune reaction to the tumor associated antigens. Several clinical trials have used antibodies to CEA in therapeutic trials with no consistent benefit. Radiolabeled antibodies to CEA and TAG-72 (and related antibodies) have also been used successfully with intraoperative detectors to remove microscopic deposits of colon carcinoma. The value of this approach in removing residual tumor that would otherwise be undetected appears promising but remains to be determined if this approach adds to disease free and overall survival (117, 118).

Evidence for an Immune Response Against Tumors

Burnett hypothesized that a major role of the immune system was surveillance for the development of neoplastic cells which, when recognized, would be destroyed (119). There are mounting sources of evidence for a significant positive correlation between cancer occurrence and host immune deficiencies. Good (120) and Penn (121) have reviewed the frequency of malignant disease in patients with primary immunodeficiency disorders compared with the general age matched population. The rate of malignancy in a group consisting of x-linked agammaglobulinemia, severe combined immunodeficiency, Wiscott-Aldrich syndrome, combined variable immunodeficiency, and ataxia-telangiectasia had a frequency of malignant disease 10,000 times greater than the general population. In this group, 80% of the tumors involved the lymphatics, and the remaining 20% occurred in the brain, ovary, stomach, and visceral organs.

The incidence of tumors in patients receiving immunosuppressive treatment after organ transplantation is approximately 100 times greater than that observed in the general population of the same age. A particularly susceptible group is patients receiving steroids and azathioprine. More recent studies of patients on steroids and cyclosporin have shown a lower incidence of cancer than those on steroids and azathioprine. These data strongly support the preventative role of the immune system in tumor development.

Further evidence for immune system-tumor interaction comes from data on the spontaneous regression of both primary and metastatic tumors. Choriocarcinoma is characterized by neoplastic proliferation of retained chorionic elements that invade the uterine wall and undergo metastases to distant organs. The tumor that contains antigens of both maternal and paternal origin is rapidly fatal if untreated. This form of malignancy is an example of a human tumor that contains transplantation antigens foreign to the host, but which is not necessarily rejected. A number of reports have shown regressions of metastatic choriocarcinoma after removal of the primary tumor. This regression appears to be on an immunologic basis. Similarly, metastatic neuroblastoma in children is associated with an unusually high incidence of spontaneous regression. Malignant melanoma is perhaps the most common tumor in which spontaneous regression has been noted. Frequently, primary melanomas will have significantly large areas infiltrated with lymphocytes and may even undergo complete regression. Unfortunately, this does not assure the patients will remain disease free, since many of them will later develop metastases.

As an independent variable, tumor infiltration with lymphocytes, when defined by strict criteria, is associated with an improved prognosis compared to tumors which have no evidence of reactivity. This is particularly true in the case of melanoma, breast cancer, and several other tumor types. Several studies have demonstrated the finding of circulating antibody reactive with autologous tumor, positive delayed hypersensitivity skin testing to tumor antigens and tumor cell extracts, and in vitro cell-mediated immunity against autologous tumor cells. These observations of tumor specific immunity have formed the basis for many tumor immunotherapy protocols. Despite the observations that patients with cancer can develop humoral and cell mediated immune responses to their tumors, there is no consensus that these responses play a significant role in the usual cancer patient. Current cancer treatment is based solidly on treatment in three areas: surgery, chemotherapy, and radiation therapy. Immunotherapy has no significant role in the treatment of most cancer patients today, and its use is limited almost solely to research protocols. However, modulation of the immune response against tumors is an important potential treatment modality (122, 123).

Mechanisms by Which the Immune System Kills Tumor Cells

The mechanisms by which antigenically distinct tumor cells are recognized and how they engage in battle with the immune system are complex (Fig. 8.4). The complexity increases as newer studies reveal more details of this intriguing interaction. Tumor cells can be killed in vitro by antibody mediated mechanisms, such as complement mediated antibody cytotoxicity and antibody dependent cell mediated cytotoxicity. These methods of tumor killing are highly effective but are primarily limited to the plasma volume compartment. Some antibody diffuses into the tissues, particularly IgG molecules that are smaller than IgM; this is enhanced by a

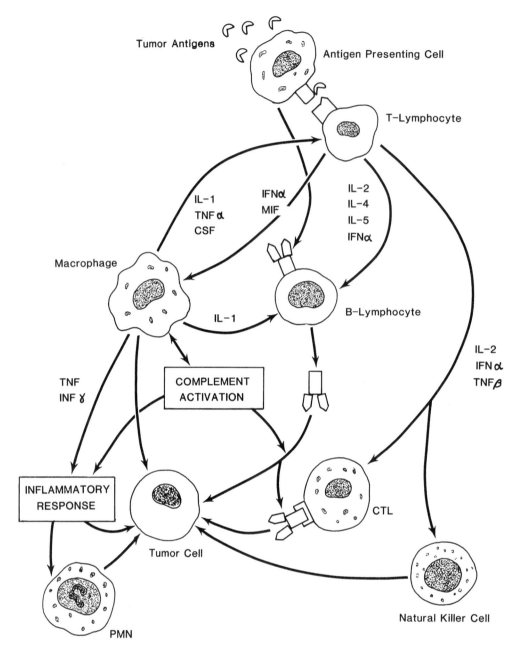

Figure 8.4. Some of the complex interactions between tumor cells and the cells, antibodies and cytokines of the immune system are outlined. *INF*, interferon; *MIF*, migration-inhibition factor; *PMN*, polymorphonuclear leukocyte or neutrophilic granulocyte.

local inflammatory response with an associated capillary leak. Because of these limitations, humoral anti-tumor mechanisms aren't effective much beyond the vascular space. Cell mediated cytotoxicity plays a more important role in vivo.

There are four different types of immune system cells that can kill tumor cells in vitro or in vivo: cytolytic T lymphocytes (CTLs), natural killer (NK) cells, lymphokine activated killer (LAK) cells, and activated macrophages. The ability of CTLs to kill tumor cells has strict limitations. The CTLs must be presensitized to the specific tumor antigen and only when the target antigen is present on cells that also carry MHC Class I antigens. When these criteria are met, the CTL can interact with

the tumor cell and produce lysis. One way of determining this in the research laboratory is to take lymphocytes from peripheral blood or lymph nodes and incubate these with autologous tumor cells which have been labeled with a radioisotope, such as 51-chromium. The lytic action of the lymphocytes (effector cells) against the tumor (target cells) is quantified by measuring the amount of radioisotope released. With the use of appropriate control targets, the CTL activity can be measured accurately. Approximately 30% of patients operated upon to remove tumors display CTL activity against the tumor. Tumor killing can also take place by the induction of apoptosis (programmed cell death) which will be described later.

In humans, there is a group of large, granular lymphocytes which comprise 2% to 5% of peripheral blood lymphocytes. Within this subset are NK and LAK cells. Whether NK and LAK cells are limited strictly to the large granular lymphocyte group is not entirely clear. The biological role of NK cells has not been completely defined. NK cells appear to develop from progenitors under the influence of gamma interferon, and Interleukin-2 (IL-2). In vitro studies of NK cells show a general lack of reactivity against normal cells and a varying but generally positive ability to kill a wide variety of tumor cells, even from diverse species. In contrast with CTLs, NK cells have a broad specificity and do not require the presence of Class I MHC antigens on their target cells.

LAK cells are produced in vitro by incubating peripheral blood leukocytes with IL-2 in an incubator for at least 5 days. The amounts of IL-2 used in the incubation far exceed biological levels. The progenitors of LAK cells appear to be predominantly NK cells. LAK cells show a broader specificity than NK cells against a variety of freshly isolated solid tumors, which often lack NK reactivity. LAK cells also react with many cells in cultures with which NK cells react, generally at higher levels. LAK cells also lack cytotoxicity against normal cells (108,111,121). It is unknown whether LAK cells as defined in vitro exist naturally in vivo.

Macrophages at rest have little cytotoxic ability, but, when activated, undergo biochemical and functional changes that permit them to kill and engulf bacteria, transformed cells, and other foreign material. Macrophages that have been activated can kill tumor cells in a manner that is neither antigen dependent nor MHC restricted. Macrophages can be activated by a number of agents, including lymphokines, antigen-antibody complexes, aggregated IgG, and endotoxin. Macrophages also appear to mediate a number of negative or inhibitory effects on various immune functions.

In addition to producing tumor cell death by cytotoxicity, apoptosis can be induced by a variety of immunologic mechanisms. Apoptosis is a genetic program of cellular self destruction that involves many cells both within the immune system and at other sites to assure that cells die when they should (124). This is a highly important mechanism through embryogenesis and organ development (125). Cell death by apoptosis and cell proliferation maintains the homeostasis of cell numbers in normal tissues. In the thymus, the mechanism of removing auto-reactive thymocytes is the induction of apoptosis triggered by the CD3/T cell receptor complex (126). Both antibody-mediated and lymphocyte-mediated cell killing in many systems involves apoptosis in addition to direct porphyrin mediated killing (127). Cells undergoing apoptosis sustain profound changes, including the development of blebs on the cell membrane, volume contraction, nuclear condensation (pyknosis), and activation of an endonuclease that cleaves the DNA. Regulation of apoptosis continues to

be defined. The *bc1-2* gene on chromosome 18 is characterized as a major repressor of programmed cell death (128). Other genes, including p53, *c-myc*, and *v-abl*, have been shown to induce apoptosis. A variety of growth factors confer a death sparing effect on many normal and neoplastic cells *in vitro*. In addition, FAS antigen, which is found on a variety of cells, particularly T and B cells, has been found to be a mediator of apoptosis. The monoclonal antibody APO-1 recognizes the FAS antigen and, when added to cells possessing FAS, rapidly induces apoptosis (129). Since apoptosis is genetically controlled, defects in the control pathway or inappropriate production of apoptosis suppressing proteins will lead to situations where cells fail to die when they should and may well contribute to the induction of cancer. As apoptosis mechanisms are better understood, many cancer types will be found to have defects in the molecular control of programmed cell death which can potentially be corrected.

Evasion of Immune Destruction by Tumor Cells

Despite the elaborate construction of the immune system with multiple components capable of killing tumor cells, transformed cells may escape destruction and go on to divide and eventually overcome the host. A number of factors have been observed in tumors that facilitate their eluding the immune system.

Sneaking through is a term that characterizes an ability some tumors have to elude the immune system by being poorly antigenic or reside in an area that does not have ready access to immune cells. Thus, the host does not become sensitized to the tumor and allows the tumor to grow and escape detection. Even if the tumor later becomes more immunogenic, it may elude the immune system by virtue of its location and its size.

Induction of tolerance is the acquisition of non-reactivity toward particular antigens. Immunologic tolerance to foreign antigens is an extremely complex phenomenon and remains to be fully delineated. Tolerance may be complete or partial and may involve various components of the immune system. Multiple factors are contributory, and a single mechanism accounting for the generation and maintenance of the tolerance state has not been discovered. Tolerance may be induced by exposure of the antigen in embryonic life. High doses of antigen and particularly persistence of antigen in adult life leads to specific tolerance.

The immune system may be suppressed by *antigen overload*. A variety of tumors produce antigens that are shed from their cell surfaces. The circulating antigen produces a snowstorm effect in that it can bind to receptors on effector cells and prevent their interaction with tumor cells, as well as combining with circulating antibody to form antigen-antibody immune complexes. Some antibodies that bind to tumors are not cytolytic and actually prevent the attachment of the important cytolytic antibodies. These blocking antibodies have been shown in a variety of tumor models to actually enhance the growth of tumors by shielding them from the immune system.

Many tumors, particularly the more virulent types, have sufficient genetic diversity as a result of a high mutation rate that they may escape attack by the immune system. This phenomenon is called *antigenic modulation*. Non-reactive clones of tumor cells grow to replace those destroyed by the immune system, in effect constantly changing the surface antigens depending upon the immune reaction to them.

Some tumors possess the ability to produce host immunosuppression by inhibiting immune function through *specific tumor cell immunosuppression mechanisms*. This includes cytokine secretion, such as transforming growth factor-$\beta2$, which inhibits CTL and NK cell activity, prostaglandin E2 production, which inhibits macrophages, and multiple other mechanisms. In addition, the growing tumor may produce host metabolic effects, anorexia, and immunosuppression on a nutritional basis. Exogenous factors may also contribute to host immunosuppression. Human immunodeficiency virus (HIV) produces the acquired immunodeficiency syndrome (AIDS), causing a defect in the regulation of the host immune response by specifically infecting and killing helper/inducer (CD4 +) T-cells. Other cells are infected by the virus, including macrophages and neural cells. However, the primary immune defect occurs through damage to the helper/inducer subset of T-lymphocytes. Patients with AIDS are able to mount an antibody response to the virus; however, the impaired cellular response leads to overwhelming viral (herpes, cytomegalovirus, etc.), fungal (pneumocystis, etc) and bacterial infections, and to neoplasms including lymphomas and the otherwise rare Kaposi's sarcoma. Exposure to chemical carcinogens increases the rate of malignant transformation of cells to a level which may elude the immune system and cause the development of tumors. Some carcinogens have a direct immunosuppressive effect which facilitates the induction of tumors.

As previously noted, the expression of MHC Class I antigens on the cell surface is essential for the recognition of foreign antigen by CTLs. *Alteration of MHC antigens is* another mechanism of immune system avoidance. Some tumors lack MHC antigens and cannot be killed by CTLs. Other tumors anomalously express MHC antigens, which again prevent their interaction with CTLs. MHC class I and ll induction is enhanced by certain factors used in immunotherapy, including interferons, IL-2, and tumor necrosis factor, and may serve to enhance CTL activity against tumors.

With the study of MHC haplotypes, it is becoming increasingly apparent that certain *genetic factors*, particularly some histocompatibility antigens, are associated with an increased risk of malignancy. Some of the associations include acute lymphoblastic leukemia (HLA-A2),

Hodgkin's disease (HLA-A1), and carcinoma of the breast (Bw35). The precise nature of this association is unknown and may involve both immune and genetic mechanisms.

Immunodiagnosis

Despite the large number of tumor antigens which have been characterized, none have proved to be a universal tumor marker. However, certain antibodies to tumor associated antigens have been produced which are useful in the diagnosis of cancer and the monitoring of patients with cancer. Monoclonal antibody technology (see Fig. 8.2) has provided a continually increasing array of important diagnostic antibodies. For the pathologist, monoclonal antibodies to T cell antigens, intermediate filament, and S-100 proteins have been shown to be tissue type specific and useful to establish the cell lineage of some undifferentiated tumors. Monoclonal antibodies are being increasingly used to detect proteins encoded by oncogenes. An immunochemical method to detect the RAS oncogene protein (P21) may be used to diagnose prostatic cancer and also may provide prognostic information. The Her2/neu oncogene product has been found to be associated with aggressive breast cancer. Some of the more commonly used monoclonal antibodies to tumors associated antigens are listed in Table 8.3.

Immunologic phenotyping of lymphoma cell surface markers is becoming increasingly important, not only for identification of progenitor cells, but also for evaluating the biologic potential of lymphocytes sharing common markers. Also, phenotyping is extremely valuable for evaluating the response to various modes of treatment and in analyzing phenotypic changes that occur in a variety of histologically similar lymphomas. The following are several examples.

Immunologic phenotyping techniques reveal that approximately 75% of non-Hodgkin's lymphoma are derived from T cells, 20% from B cells, and 5% from other cell types. The cells of origin in Hodgkin's Disease appear to have characteristics of B cells (internal immunoglobulin) and myeloid cells (CD15).

Most cutaneous lymphomas (e.g., mycosis fungoides and Sézary syndrome) are shown by immunophenotyping to be helper-inducer T-cells, and most patients with chronic lymphocytic leukemia have a clonal expansion of malignant B-lymphocytes. Other immunodiagnostic tests have valuable prognostic information. Serial measurements of serum IL-2 receptors correlate with the disease activity in hairy cell leukemia, childhood non-Hodgkin's lymphoma, and adult T cell leukemia and lymphoma. The presence of a nuclear proliferation antigen in diffuse large cell lymphomas correlates with a poor prognosis.

Immunotherapy

Immunotherapy is the term used for attempts to alter or enhance the immune system in an effort to bring

Table 8.4.
Classification of Cancer Immunotherapy

Type	Example
Active	
Specific	Tumor cell or tumor antigen vaccines
Nonspecific	Local BCG, Levamisole
Passive	
Specific	Monocolonal antibody or serum treatment, transfer immune cells, RNA, etc.
Nonspecific	Transfer of LAK cells; TNF, IL-2, INF treatment
Indirect	Dietary factors, vitamins, etc. that affect immune system

about an immunologically mediated antitumor effect. The immunotherapy of cancer in patients has three major categories (Table 8.4). Active immunotherapy consists of treatments that are designed to stimulate the patient's own immune system, either specifically against certain tumor antigens or non-specifically with agents that tend to boost the overall immune response. Passive immunotherapy, often called adoptive immunotherapy, refers to the administration of immunologically active components (specific antibodies, etc), essentially in a preformed state, without any requirement for an immune response by the host. Indirect immunotherapy encompasses a broad variety of treatments which have no direct effect on the tumor or immune system, but which may indirectly affect the host response to tumor. This includes dietary manipulations, removal of blocking antibodies, administration of antibodies to angiogenesis factor, vitamin therapy, etc. The agents used in tumor immunotherapy are often referred to as Biotherapeutic Agents or Biological Response Modifiers (BRM).

Active immunotherapy in the form of immunization of patients having established metastatic tumors with killed tumor cells or tumor antigens generally has been ineffective in causing tumor regression. Occasional reports of responses to this form of treatment exist, but they are highly inconsistent. A basic problem with many patients who have metastatic disease is that they are often anergic and unable to elicit an immune response with immunization. In animal systems, immunizations with killed tumor cells or purified tumor antigens prior to tumor challenge have a significant therapeutic effect. This has been much more difficult to demonstrate in patients who have had adjuvant treatment of this kind. Many human tumors are weakly immunogenic, and several methods have been employed to increase their immunogenicity, including the use of neuraminidase to alter the tumor cell surface and potentially unmask hidden tumor antigens. Other approaches have been the modification of the tumor cell by infecting it with immunogenic viruses, such as vaccinia or Newcastle disease virus, or by binding haptens, such as trinitrophenol, to the cells' surfaces. Several authors have reported varying degrees of success in preventing recurrences using these techniques in adjuvant trials in patients with high

risk for recurrence melanoma. The use of BCG as an adjuvant for active specific immunization of patients with melanoma using melanoma cells or antigens has recently yielded some promising results. A vaccine using multiple melanoma antigens (GD2, GM2, O-acetyl GD3, M-TAA lipoprotein, M-fetal glycoprotein, and M-urinary glycoprotein) plus BCG has produced a two-fold increase in survival in stage III melanoma and a three-fold increase in survival in stage IV melanoma patients in a non randomized study (130,131). Improved survival has even been seen in patients with distant metastases (132) and with choroidal melanoma metastases (133). This approach has produced immunological reactivity to several of the melanoma associated antigens (132). The development of an immune response against the ganglioside GM2 in a patient immunization study has been shown to improve survival in a randomized trial in stage III melanoma (134). In addition, antibodies generated against the ganglioside GD3 have been shown to potentiate cytotoxic T cell reactivity and LAK activity against melanoma cells (135,136). From this data, it appears that an immune reaction can be generated against specific melanoma antigens, and this reactivity may be related to improvement in melanoma patient survival.

Nonspecific active immunotherapy has recently been limited primarily to the intralesional administration of BCG for melanoma. This has been effective in producing a local inflammatory response and shrinkage of the injected tumor. Occasionally, satellite lesions have been noted to regress as well. However, visceral metastases do not respond. There has been no prolongation of survival in patients treated in this manner, and the complications include malaise, abscess formation, and systemic BCG infection. Other agents, such as MER (methanol extracted residue of mycobacteria), killed *C. parvum,* and similar bacterial derivatives, have shown little effectiveness when used alone even though they may occasionally induce tumor-reactive antibodies.

Levamisole is an antihelmintic agent that has been used for many years to treat intestinal nematodes in humans and domestic animals. It possesses non-specific immune modulating properties, and as such has been used in a number of adjuvant immunotherapy and chemoimmunotherapy trials. Although there has been some suggestion of improvements in recurrence rates and survivals, these have generally been inconclusive. A report from the Mayo Clinic using adjuvant Levamisole and 5-fluorouracil (5-FU) after surgical resection in patients with Duke's C carcinoma of the colon has shown a statistically significant survival advantage for the treated patients versus those untreated. The response was so significantly impressive that the National Cancer Institute is advising that "no treatment" control groups are no longer justified for Duke's C patients.

Therapy with monoclonal antibodies has yielded promising results. Cytotoxic monoclonal antibodies can be used directly to kill tumor cells, or high affinity antibodies may be used to carry a variety of toxins, drugs, and radioisotopes to produce tumor killing. This methodology has been limited by the use of xenogeneic antibodies (primarily mouse and rat), which quickly induce an antibody immune reaction and also are rapidly consumed by the reticuloendothelial system and concentrated in the spleen and liver. Some success has been achieved in treating patients with B-cell lymphomas, using short courses of specifically designed monoclonal antibodies that react with the lymphoma cell surface idiotype antibodies, which are individually specific for each lymphoma (137). The rapid development of antibodies to the mouse immunoglobulins and the modulation of target antigens continues to be major obstacles in this form of immunotherapy. Since it is not practical to generate monoclonal antibodies for each patient with cancer, efforts are being made to target antigenic determinants which may be shared by several different patients or by several tumor types. Efforts to produce useful human monoclonal antibodies have met with limited success. Antibodies that are currently being studied in clinical trials include TAG-72 and related antibodies, the anticarcinoma antibody 17-1 in metastatic colorectal carcinoma, anti-gangliosides GD3 and GM2 in metastatic melanoma, anti-EGF receptor in hepatocellular carcinoma, and antibodies to CD5, CD19, and CD25 in leukemia and lymphoma, among others.

A number of older forms of adoptive immunotherapy, including the use of immune RNA, thymosin, and transfer factor, have, for the most part, been abandoned because of inconsistent results.

Advances in molecular biology and recombinant DNA technology have permitted the accelerated study of the use of lymphokines and cytokines in the treatment of human cancer. Some of the interactions of various immune system cells and their cytokines are shown in Figure 8.4. The sources and functions of a number of important cytokines is shown in Table 8.5.

Induction of tumor immunity by immunization with genetically altered tumor cells is in its infancy. The development of gene therapy for cancer has recently been reviewed (138). Despite initial promising results, clinical studies to date have not shown significant benefit for the use of genetically transduced tumor cells. Hock et al. demonstrated that tumor cells modified with many of the cytokines, including IL-2, IL-4, IL-7, TNF, or IFNγ, were only slightly superior to irradiated cancer cells as immunogens (139). Also, cells mixed with classical adjuvants were superior to cytokine-modified tumors in their ability to immunize mice against tumors.

Table 8.5.
Some Cytokines that Mediate Immune Responses

Name	Other Names	Source	Function
Interferons			All inhibit viral replication and of some tumors
Alpha	Leukocyte interferon	Leukocyte	
Beta	Fibroblast	Fibroblast	
Growth	Interferon		
Gamma	Immune interferon	Macrophage	
Tumor Necrosis Factors			
Alpha	Cachectin	Macrophage	Lyses some tumor cells, stimulates B-cells
Beta	Lymphotoxin	T-cells	Induces T-cells to produce IL-2
Interleukins			
IL-1	Lymphocyte activating factor	Macrophages, fibroblasts	T and B cell activation
IL-2	T cell growth factor	Activated T cells	Stimulates growth of T, B, NK, and LAK cells
IL-3	Multipotential cell stimulating Factor, mast cell growth factor	Bone marrow pre-B cells	Stimulates growth of pleuripotent hematopoietic and mast cells
IL-4	B cell stimulating factor-1	Activated T and B cells	Stimulates B and some T cell growth
IL-5	B cell growth factor	Activated B cells and eosinophils	Eosinophil differentation and growth
IL-6	B cell stimulating factor-2	Activated B cells	Stimulates growth of B cells and hepatocytes
IL-7	Pre B cell growth	Bone marrow stroma cells, fetal liver	Stimulates growth of B cell precursors and activated T cells
IL-11	No other names	Fibroblasts	Stimulates Ig producing B cells
IL-12	NK and T cell stimulating factor	Activated B cells	Stimulates NK and activated T cell activity and proliferation
IL-13	P-600	T cells	Stimulates growth of activated B cells, induces IgE synthesis
IL-14	High molecular weight B cell growth factor	T cells	Stimulates B cell growth
Colony Stimulating Factors			
GM-CSF	Granulocyte-macrophage stimulating factor	Macrophage	Stimulates growth of granulocytes and macrophages

Interleukin-1 (IL-1) is produced by stimulated macrophages and has many biological activities that are identical to those of tumor necrosis factor-α (Table 8.5). One of the important actions of IL-1 is to induce production of other cytokines, such as TNF, from macrophages and endothelium, IL-6 from fibroblasts, and granulocyte macrophage colony stimulating factor (GM-CSF) from T cells. IL-1 also induces the IL-2 receptor on helper T cells, stimulates the proliferation and differentiation of B cells, and activates NK cells and other macrophages. IL-1 is now being evaluated as an immunotherapeutic agent alone and in combination with other lymphokines in clinical trials.

Interleukin-2 is generated by activated helper/inducer T-cells. It plays an essential role in promoting T cell division and also potentiates B cell growth and the activation of monocytes and natural killer cells. In clinical studies, high doses of IL-2 are used as single agents and to activate NK precursors into lines of LAK cells which are used in experimental cancer therapy. In addition to LAK cell administration, a constant infusion or intermittent administration of IL-2 is required to continue stimulating the LAK cells in patients. IL-2 treatment has significant toxicity, with patients having a syndrome resembling septic shock. It should currently be done only in an institution specializing in this form of treatment. The most significant responses to this form of treatment have been in patients with metastatic renal cell carcinoma and melanoma.

In recent years, clinical studies with IL-2 have shown more limited anti-tumor activity than was anticipated from earlier pre-clinical trials (140). IL-2 is currently only approved by the FDA for good performance status patients with metastatic renal cell carcinoma. The treatment regimen consists of 600,000–720,000 IU/kg (high dose regimen) by 15 minute IV bolus infusion q8h on days 1–5 and 15–19. The overall response rate in 255 patients with renal cell carcinoma was 14%, including complete tumor regression in 4% (141). A large number of trials have attempted to increase the efficacy and decrease the toxicity of IL-2 treatment by patient selection, modification of the dose and schedule, and the addition of other agents. Recent studies suggest that lower dose IL-2 is as effective as higher doses (142). In one report, the combination of lower dose IL-2 (20 $\times$ 106 IU/m2 sub cu) plus interferon alfa (5 $\times$ 106 IU/m2) three times a week produced a 6% complete response and a 19% partial response in 152 patients (143). The addition of LAK cells to high dose IL-2 does not contribute substantially to the response rate (144).

In patients with metastatic melanoma, the high dose q 8 h regimen in 134 patients produced 5 complete responses (4%) and 22 partial responses (16%) (145, 146). However, the responses were durable, lasting considerably longer than would have been expected from responders to chemotherapy. Recently published studies of large series of patients treated with IL-2 with LAK cells have not shown any substantial benefit over IL-2 treatment alone (145,147,148). The addition of TIL (tumor infiltrating lymphocytes with cytotoxic T cell activity) to IL-2 treatment has also been disappointing. The most recent report gives 19 responders out of 79 patients (24%) with metastatic melanoma receiving IL-2/TIL (149). These responses have generally been partial and of short duration. Newer approaches, which are currently being evaluated, include transfecting the TIL with tumor necrosis factor (TNF) gene to increase tumor cell killing by the TIL (150). Currently, the highest response rates reported in the treatment for metastatic melanoma are for regimens combining chemotherapy (usually cisplatin plus DTIC based regimens) with IL-2 alone or IL-2 plus interferon alfa (151, 152). Responses are typically 45%–65%, with 15%–20% complete responses. Although some responses are durable, lasting longer than a year, most responses last between 5 and 7 months. IL-2 is an active agent for cancer treatment, particularly for melanoma and renal cell carcinoma, and its full potential is yet to be determined.

The activities of several other Lymphokines (IL-3, IL-4, IL-5, and IL-6) are also shown in Table 8.5. Many of these, alone or in combination, are potential candidates for use in experimental tumor immunotherapy protocols. Recombinant DNA products of these cytokines are becoming increasingly available and will be considered for use in future studies.

The interferons are a class of unrelated proteins which have antiviral effects. There are three main types: alpha, beta, and gamma, each with multiple subtypes. The antitumor effects of the interferons include increased expression of Class I and Class ll MHC proteins, which facilitate immune system recognition; activation of NK cells and macrophages and stimulation of B lymphocytes; and direct inhibition of viral replication. Interferons alpha and beta seem to exert anti-tumor activity principally by inhibition of cell growth and division. Interferons are produced by several cell types, particularly T cells and macrophages. The interferons are being evaluated in a number of clinical studies for anticancer activity. Gamma interferon is currently approved for use in the treatment of hairy cell leukemia.

Tumor necrosis factor is a third major class of cytokines that have anti-tumor activity. TNF is produced primarily by T-lymphocytes and macrophages secondary to a variety of stimuli, including IL-1, gamma interferon, lipopolysaccharide, viruses, and BCG. In animals receiving intravenous bacterial endotoxin and in patients in septic shock, large quantities of TNFα (cachectin) are produced. In animal models, this protein produces hemorrhagic necrosis of malignant tumors. Human recombinant TNFα has been tested on a variety of tumor cells and has been shown to have a cytolytic effect on approximately one-third, a cytostatic effect on one-third, and no effect on one-third. The factors that make certain tumor cells susceptible to TNF, and the precise mechanism of this effect, is not known. It is currently being tested alone and in combination with other cytokines in a number of clinical trials. TNFα produces a profound cachexia and weight loss through an unknown mechanism.

TNFβ (lymphotoxin) is structurally related to, but distinct from, TNFα. TNFβ can lyse some tumor cells in vitro and is also directly cytotoxic when injected into a tumor. Both of the TNFs stimulate the functional activity of many types of immune effect or cells, including CTLs, NK cells, and macrophages, as well as producing the circulatory collapse and widespread tissue necrosis which can accompany bacterial septic shock. Current studies of cancer immunotherapy combined with genetic engineering at the National Cancer Institute are using TILs into which genes for TNF have been inserted. TILS have a high affinity for tumor cells and should be even more toxic to them by producing TNF.

Colony stimulating factors, particularly granulocyte-macrophage colony stimulating factor (GM-CSF) enhance macrophage tumoricidal activity and stimulate the production of interferon and TNFα by monocytes. The production of GM-CSF is induced by TNFα. The recombinant form of human GM-CSF is used to stimulate hematopoiesis in patients with myelodysplastic syndromes. Currently, the greatest use of the recombinant colony stimulating factors has been to stimulate normal hematopoietic progenitor cells in patients undergoing cancer chemotherapy who have profound bone marrow depression. The colony stimulating factors have been shown to reduce the duration of neutropenia caused by cytotoxic chemotherapy and can accelerate the recovery of the myeloid elements in patients who have undergone high dose chemotherapy followed by autologous bone marrow transplantation. GM-CST use is contraindicated in myelogenous leukemia, which could be exacerbated by this granulocyte stimulator.

Future Directions

Biotechnology continues to advance our knowledge of the immune system and its interaction with cancer. The number of cytokines, growth factors, specific genes, monoclonal antibodies, tumor vaccines, and other active biological agents continues to increase rapidly, almost beyond our abilities to test their activities and evaluate them for clinical utility. Pre-clinical testing is extremely important to define which of many promising biologicals should go into clinical trials for diagnosis, treatment, and imaging. Combinations of biologic treatments together with standard approaches (surgery, chemotherapy, and radiation therapy) appears to have the most benefit for cancer treatment in the future. The ability to genetically engineer human cells by restoring or blocking mutant genes to control cancer and other diseases is in its infancy and will soon be realized.

Epidemiology of Cancer

Cancer epidemiology is the study of the determinants of neoplastic disease and the frequency with which various types of cancers affect differing population groups. The primary thrust of epidemiologic investigation has been to identify specific cancer determinants in the hope that by eliminating them from the population at risk, subsequent tumor development may be prevented.

Cancer epidemiological observations date back to 1700 when Ramazzini determined that breast cancer was more common among nuns than the general population, suggesting that celibacy was a risk factor (153). Paradoxically, in 1842, another Italian, Rigoni-Stern, concluded that endometrial cancer was significantly less common in convents than the general population, concluding in this case that celibacy played a protective role. In 1775, the British surgeon Pott surmised that cancer was an occupational hazard to chimney sweeps. As a result of observations made by subsequent investigators, it was concluded that the combustion products of coal were a factor not only in the development of cancer of the scrotum but of all exposed skin (154). The first report suggesting a connection between tobacco use and the development of cancer was made by Hill in 1761 when he implicated the use of snuff as an etiology for the development of nasopharyngeal cancers. The role of tobacco as a carcinogen was subsequently reaffirmed by von Soemmering, who in 1795 associated pipe smoking with carcinoma of the buccal mucosa (155).

These early epidemiological reports in large part depended on anecdotal observations by physicians who were dealing with groups of individuals with similar cultural or occupational backgrounds. As a result, quantitative data to support these reports were usually lacking. Until the development of the epidemiological study incriminating tobacco as one of the precipitating agents in the development of lung neoplasms, cancer was commonly perceived as simply a manifestation of the degenerative processes associated with aging. These relatively recent epidemiologic studies have been an impetus for not only the initiation of laboratory work to further define the causative agents involved in neoplastic development, but also for the designing of experimental studies in which the suspected cancer-producing agent is either introduced or eliminated from a population group. These experimental studies provide the most compelling evidence for implicating a particular determinant as a carcinogen. These experiments, however, are time-consuming, expensive, and usually only justified after a causal relationship has been established between a disease determinant and a population group by descriptive studies.

Descriptive Studies

The neoplastic process manifests itself in all human groups. Age, sex, race, geography, cultural norms, and sexual habits are but a few of the factors influencing the incidence of cancer. By defining the patterns of disease in population subgroups, descriptive epidemiology has provided insight into the etiology of many cancers. Descriptive epidemiologic studies measure three parameters: incidence, prevalence, and mortality.

Incidence describes the number of new cases of cancer occurring within a population group in a specified period of time.

$$\text{Incidence} = \frac{\text{Number of persons developing a new cancer per unit of time}}{\text{Population at risk}}$$

The unit of time is commonly defined as 1 year, and the rate usually is expressed per 100,000 individuals. The measurement of incidence may be crude (applying to all age groups) or age specific. Because the incidence of cancer within a specific population group varies greatly from young to old, age-specific incidence rates provide much more meaningful information than do crude rates.

Prevalence represents the number of cases, both old and new, existing within a given population at a specific point in time.

$$\text{Prevalence} = \frac{\text{Number of existing cases of carcinoma}}{\text{Population living at that time}}$$

Cancer prevalence depends not only on the incidence but also on the duration of the disease. For example, improvements in adjunctive or palliative management of breast cancer may increase the prevalence of disease while the incidence rate remains constant. Because of the difficulty in determining that nebulous point in time at which the patient may be considered "cured" of cancer, prevalence data are more difficult to ascertain than are incidence data.

The mortality or death rate expresses the frequency with which members of a population die of a cancer. Like incidence data, the mortality rate estimates the probability of an event.

$$\text{Mortality Rate} = \frac{\text{Number of persons dying of cancer in a unit of time}}{\text{Total population living at that time}}$$

Cancer mortality rates are vulnerable to many inaccuracies. Death reporting data usually assign a single cause of death to each reported case. The cause of death of a terminally ill cancer patient may oftentimes incorrectly be assigned to another condition. For many cancers, there may be an obvious disparity between incidence and mortality. For example, nonmelanotic skin cancers may have a case fatality rate less than 1%, whereas for other tumors (e.g., pancreas and lung), the case fatality rate, i.e., the proportion of cancer cases that terminate

in death, may approach unity. In these latter examples, the mortality rate is a valid index of incidence (154).

Deciding which of these three descriptive measures (incidence, prevalence, or mortality rate) is most appropriate for a given situation is contingent on the nature of the specific problem under study. In studying causes of cancer, incidence data usually provide the most useful information. However, as a result of the widespread deployment of the death registration system, mortality data usually are more accessible than incidence rates. Mortality rates may be the data of choice in evaluating the efficacy of various treatment regimens. By combining incidence and mortality data, it is possible to determine the case fatality rate, which is the proportion of cancer cases resulting in death. As mentioned previously, because of the difficulty in defining when a person may be considered cured of a cancer, prevalence data are the most difficult measurement to determine, yet this information is the most useful statistic in planning the long-term need for health care services.

Analytic Studies

Descriptive epidemiologic studies address the distribution of diseases within a population. Analytic studies, however, occupy an intermediate position between descriptive and experimental studies in studying cause-and-effect relationships.

In analytic studies, specific hypotheses are investigated by observation of population groups as opposed to experimental manipulation. Typically, the hypotheses being tested in analytical studies have evolved from observations made from earlier descriptive studies.

Analytic studies are classified as either being of the case control (retrospective) design or cohort (prospective) design. In the case control type study, the population group is identified by disease. The population with a particular disease and a like disease-free group are studied to collect data on exposure to possible causative agents. An example is a study that attempted to associate estrogen use with the development of endometrial cancer. In that study, a group of women with endometrial cancer and a similar group of disease-free controls were interviewed to determine the incidence of the prior use of estrogen in both groups. If the proportion of diseased individuals with exposure to the suspected agent exceeds that of the control group, then it can be surmised that an association may exist. The basic design of a case control study is shown in Table 8.6. If A/(A + C) is

Table 8.6.
Case-Control Study Design

Suspected Etiology Agent	Number of Cases With Disease	Number of Controls Without Disease
With	A	B
Without	C	C

statistically greater than B/(B + D), then a statistically significant association exists between the disease and the suspected agent (4). An estimated relative risk (ERR) of contracting the disease after exposure to the offending agent can be computed as: ERR = AD/BC.

Because of its retrospective nature, a case control study is particularly useful for studying uncommon disease states. For a case control study to arrive at accurate conclusions, the cases under study must be representative of all individuals with the disease process, and the control group must be representative of the nonaffected population. To put this in another way, the prevalence of the hypothesized carcinogen under study must be the same in the control group as it is in the general population. For this reason, hospital-based control studies are particularly vulnerable to the selection bias inherent in the differential probabilities of hospital admission for those individuals with and without the disease who may also have exposure to the risk factor under study. This potential for introduction of bias in selecting either the case group or the control group is one of the potential failings in the retrospective type of study. Case control studies do have the advantage, however, of requiring a smaller study group and a shorter study time than does the cohort design (prospective) study (156).

The cohort design study differs from the case control type in that the population being studied is identified by exposure to a causative agent rather than the disease itself. An example of one such study involved identifying two groups of women who either had or had not been exposed to chest fluoroscopy. These women were followed for a number of years to determine if they eventually developed breast cancer. This study demonstrated a higher incidence of breast cancer in the fluoroscopy group, lending credence to the original hypothesis that fluoroscopy is the cause of breast cancer (157). When studies such as these are based on current exposures and followed for subsequent outcomes, they are termed prospective cohort studies. When they use information based on exposures that have occurred in the past, they are identified as retrospective cohort studies. Cohort studies are especially valuable in determining the risk of developing cancer associated with exposure to agents peculiar to a specific population subgroup (e.g., tobacco users and coal miners).

Cohort studies have the advantage of being able to measure incidence and mortality rates directly, whereas case control studies cannot. Cohort studies are usually less susceptible to the selection biases associated with the case control approach. However, cohort studies, especially those of the prospective design, are time-consuming and expensive undertakings which may involve studying prohibitively large groups of individuals when rare diseases are investigated (155).

Experimental Studies

After analytic studies have suggested a causal relationship between exposure to a suspected carcinogen and subsequent cancer development, experimental studies (referred to as clinical trials in humans) may be conducted to confirm these associations. Experimental studies are designed to either introduce or eliminate exposure to a suspected carcinogen followed by a period of observation to determine the impact, if any, on subsequent cancer development. Obviously, ethical considerations preclude the introduction of a carcinogen within a human population group for the sole purpose of detecting an increase in incidence rates. However, clinical trials are appropriate if they are designed to reduce exposure to a suspected carcinogen (e.g., tobacco and radiation) for the purposes of studying a favorable outcome. After experimental intervention, the follow-up data are analyzed using the cohort design.

The vast number of cancers are not random occurrences. It is the province of epidemiologic study to formulate hypotheses explaining these nonrandom occurrences. The fundamental variables common to most epidemiologic studies are time, place, and person.

The wide fluctuations seen in the incidence of some cancers over time underscores the importance of this factor in the etiology of cancer. For example, in 1930, gastric cancer was the leading cause of cancer death among men in the United States. However, by 1985, although still a disease of significant impact, it had lost its dominant position and fallen to sixth place. During the same period of time, the mortality rate for lung cancer in the U.S. men had increased by a factor of 10, from sixth place to first place (158). This dramatic increase in the incidence of lung cancer is tied closely to the increased use of tobacco over the same period of time. The incidence of pulmonary neoplasms among women has lagged behind their male counterparts; however, because of women's relatively recent increase in the use of tobacco, lung cancer threatens to surpass breast cancer as the leading cause of cancer mortality among U.S. women.

The variable of place is defined by geographic or political boundaries. This factor has served to identify major international differences in both cancer incidence and mortality. The extreme international variation in the incidence of gastric cancer is an excellent example of the importance of this factor. The highest incidence rates for stomach neoplasms are found among Japanese males (90 per 100,000 per year). Latin American countries are intermediate at 45 to 50 per 100,000 per year, whereas rates for gastric cancer in the United States are among the world's lowest (approximately 10 per 100,000 per year) (159).

The study of migration patterns of population groups offers a unique epidemiologic opportunity to observe the roles genetic and environmental factors play in cancer development. In 1972, a study of Japanese natives who had immigrated to Hawaii demonstrated a continued excess risk for stomach cancer in their new homeland, but this risk factor was not passed on to their progeny born in Hawaii (160). However, although gastric cancer risk fell, the Japanese immigrants demonstrated an increased incidence of colorectal neoplasms. Because of the size and specificity of this population group, it was possible to make several observations: (*a*) the investigators noted that more bowel cancer patients than controls had abandoned the practice of eating at least one Japanese-style meal daily, and (*b*) they also concluded that the frequency of beef ingestion correlates with an increased risk for the development of colorectal cancer (160).

In general, the incidence of cancer increases with age. The increased risk with the passage of time may be secondary to exposure to a carcinogenic agent over a prolonged period. Exceptions to the rise in incidence with increasing age are the childhood cancers. Lung cancer demonstrates an initial peak in incidence during early adolescence. This may be secondary to a heightened period of mitotic activity or brief exposure to a carcinogenic agent (161). Breast cancer demonstrates a steady increase in incidence with age, which plateaus in the sixth decade of life and is subsequently followed by a continued increase in frequency. This may be a result of cessation of estrogen production by the ovaries. Another exception to the general increase in frequency of cancers with age is the peak in incidence of Hodgkin's disease in the third decade of life. There may be at least a subgroup of these patients who have an infectious etiology for their cancer (162).

The difference in the incidence of site-specific cancers between the sexes is certainly multifactorial. The preponderance of certain male cancers for a specific anatomic location may be attributed to exposure to carcinogenic factors within the workplace as opposed to differences in the hormonal milieu.

Although environmental factors play a prominent role in cancer genesis, familial clustering suggests that genetic variations do expose the individual to increased susceptibility to specific types of cancer. However, a certain component of the risk which has been attributed to genetics may be the result of common environmental factors (163).

The cause of some tumors is clearly genetic, including susceptibility to skin cancers based on the color of the skin, the relationship between gastric cancer and blood type, and the association between retinoblastoma in patients with xeroderma pigmentosum.

The Surveillance Epidemiology End Results and Mortality data (SEER) Program revealed wide variation in the incidence rates of cancers for different ethnic groups in the United States. Overall, the rates were highest for Hawaiians, whites, and African-Americans, and were lowest for Hispanics and native Americans. Among males, blacks had overall higher rates than whites, 454 versus 371 (expressed as incidence rates per 100,000 population per year) whereas the reverse was true among females—288 for blacks and 301 for whites.

When looking at specific sites, African-Americans demonstrated a higher incidence of pancreas, uterine, prostate, esophageal, and oropharyngeal cancers; their white counterparts had a higher incidence of leukemia, lymphoma, breast cancer, bladder cancer, and malignant melanomas of the skin (164). Although the initial inclination is to implicate genetic factors to explain these differences, it is difficult to separate out the influences of environmental and cultural considerations as explanations for these trends.

The study of cancer epidemiology has shown that nearly all cancers fluctuate widely in incidence, depending on the variables of person, place, and time, and that the variation is intimately associated with genetic and environmental factors. Historically, cancer epidemiologic studies have in large part confined themselves to identifying the gross differences in cancer incidence existing among different subpopulations. The major task lying ahead for the epidemiologist is to expand efforts to identify the precise causes and mechanisms for these variations.

As the world continues to evolve technologically, physicians must accept the fact that new cancer risks will be introduced. It will be the charge of the cancer epidemiologist to quantify the magnitude of these risks so that an informed decision can be made as to whether the potential benefits of these advances justify the risk imposed on the population they are meant to serve.

Staging of Cancer

Tumor staging is a system created for the purpose of identifying where a particular tumor is in its natural evolution. The ideal staging system should serve as a reliable prognosticator of patient outcome, aid in the therapeutic decision-making process, and be universally accepted so that it might be communicated readily to others.

The first cancer staging system was developed for carcinoma of the uterine cervix in 1929 by the League of Nations. In 1932, Dukes, an English pathologist, proposed the staging classification for colorectal carcinoma, which bears his name. Dukes A cases were defined as limited to the rectal wall. Class B described spread to the extrarectal tissue, and class C were those tumors with lymph node metastases. Over the years, the Dukes staging system has undergone numerous refinements. The most widely accepted Dukes revision is the Astler-Coller modification (of 1954).

In the Astler-Coller modification, A cases are confined to the mucosa. B_1 cases are those that penetrate into but not through the muscularis propria. B_2 are those tumors that penetrate the serosa with or without involvement of adjacent organs. C_1 is defined as invasion into but not through the muscularis propria, with involvement of regional lymph nodes. C_2 demonstrates penetration through the serosa and involvement of regional lymph nodes with or without invasion of adjacent organs. Evaluation of the efficacy of the Dukes classification system as a prognosticator of ultimate patient outcome was analyzed in the National Surgical Adjuvant Breast and Bowel Project (NSABP). This study showed that the number of positive nodes was the single most important prognostic indicator for patient outcome. The number of positive nodes is not incorporated in the Dukes staging system. This study presents a compelling argument that any subsequent staging system for colorectal cancer should include the number of lymph nodes involved (165).

In 1943, Denoix from the French Institute Gustave Roussy introduced the TNM classification system. The American Joint Committee on Cancer (AJCC) and the Union Internationale Contre le Cancer (UICC) have embraced this system and expanded it to include a universal staging system specific for all anatomic sites (166).

The TNM system is a classification scheme based entirely on anatomic considerations. It is predicated on the supposition that tumor spread follows an orderly pattern, beginning with the localized tumor (T), which, after progressive growth and local invasion, spreads to regional nodes (N). Left untreated, the neoplasm eventually manifests itself at distant metastatic sites (M). The addition of numbers as subscripts to the three components in the TNM system are used to further define the tumor size or extent of spread. Although descriptive numbers vary between anatomic sites, the following general rules can be made.

Tumor (T)

TX	Primary tumor cannot be assessed
TO	No evidence of primary tumor
Tis	Carcinoma in situ
T1, T2, T3, T4	Numbers indicate increasing size and involvement of adjacent structures
Lymph Nodes	(N)
NX	Regional lymph nodes cannot be assessed
NO	Regional lymph node metastases
N1, N2, N3, N4	Progressive involvement of regional nodes
Metastases	(M)
MX	Presence of distant metastases cannot be assessed
MO	No distant metastases
M1	Distant metastases

Clinical classification of a tumor is based on information obtained before treatment. These data may come as a result of physical examination, imaging studies, or information gleaned at the time of surgical exploration. Pathologic classification, while also dependent on information acquired before therapy, is based primarily on gross and microscopic histologic examination of the removed tumor.

Although the TNM classification system, because of its wide acceptance, is extremely useful, it is not the ideal classification system for all tumor sites. In soft-tissue sarcomas, the histologic degree of cellular differentiation is clearly the single most important prognosticator, whereas for thyroid cancer, patient age is an important predictor of patient outcome.

As the specificity and sensitivity of biologic tumor markers increase and specialized techniques measuring the degree of cellular differentiation and mitotic activity evolve, these factors will certainly have to be incorporated in any staging system (167).

REFERENCES

1. Arbeit JM. Molecules, cancer and the surgeon. Ann Surg 1990; 212:3–13.
2. Brown JM, Harken AH, Sharefkin JB. Recombinant DNA and surgery. Ann Surg 1990;212:178–186.
3. Rowley JD, Aster JC, Sklar J. The clinical applications of new DNA diagnostic technology on the management of cancer patients. JAMA 1993;270:2331–2337.
4. Darnell J, Lodish H, Baltimore D. Molecular cell biology. 2nd ed. New York: Scientific American Books, 1990.
5. Williams NN, Daly JM. Flow cytometry and prognostic implications in patients with solid tumors. Surg Gynecol Obstet 1990; 171:257–266.
6. Sneige N, Dekmezian R, El-Naggan A, et al. Cytomorphologic; immunocytochemical and nucleic acid flow cytometric study of 50 lymph nodes by fine needle aspiration. Cancer 1991;67: 1003–1007.
7. Kitagawa Y, Ueda M, Ando N. Significance of ent-2/hst-1 co-amplification as a prognostic factor in patients with esophageal squamous carcinoma. Cancer Res 51:1504–1508.
8. Lander ES, Botstein D. Mapping complex genetic traits in humans: new methods using a complete RFLP linkage map. Cold Spring Harb Symp Quant Biol 1986;51:49–62.
9. Kawajiri K, Nakachi K, Kazue I, et al. Identification of genetically high risk individuals to lung cancer by DNA polymorphisms of the cytochrome P4501A1 gene. FEBS Lett 1990;263:131–133.
10. Kawashima K, Shikama H, Imoto K, et al. Close correlation between restrictor fragment length polymorphism of L-myc gene and metastasis of human lung cancer to the lymph nodes and other organs. Proc Natl Acad Sci U S A 1988;85:2353–2356.
11. Gibbs RA. DNA amplification by polymerase chain reaction. Anal Chem 1990;62:1202–1214.
12. Fuqua SAW, Falette NF, McGuire WL. Sensitive detection of estrogen receptor RNA by polymerase chain reaction assay. J Natl Can Inst 1990;82:858–861.
13. Lee MS, Chang KS, Cabanillas F, et al. Detection of minimal residual disease cells carrying the t(14;18) by DNA sequence amplification. Science 1987;237:175–178.
14. Gabert J, La Fage M, Maraninchi D, et al. Detection of residual bcr/abl translocation by polymerase chain reaction in chronic myeloid leukemia patients after bone marrow transplantation. Lancet 1989;2:1125–1128.
15. Eva A, Robbins KC, Andersen PR, et al. Cellular genes analogues to retroviral *onc* genes are transcribed in human tumor cells. Nature 1982;295:116–119.
16. Veerbeck JS, Roeroek AJM, Van Den Oviveland AMW, et al. Human c-fms proto-oncogene: comparative analysis with an abnormal allele. Mol Cell Biol 1985;5:422–426.
17. Baiocchi G, Kavanagh JJ, Talpaz M, et al. Expression of the macrophage colony-stimulating factor and its receptor in gynecologic malignancies. Cancer 1991;67:990–996.
18. Weinberger G, Thompson CC, Ong ES, et al. The c-erbA related gene encodes a thyroid hormone receptor. Nature 1986;324: 641–646.

19. Dovovic A, Houle B, kBelouchi A, et al. erb-A related sequence coding for DNA-binding hormone receptor localized to chromosome 3p213 p25 and deleted in small cell carcinoma. Cancer Res 1988;48:683–685.
20. Druker BJ, Mamon HJ, Roberts TM. Oncogenes, growth factors and signal transduction. New Engl J Med 1989;321:1383–1391.
21. Whitman M, Downes CP, Keeler M, et al. Type I phosphatidyinositol kinase makes a novelinositol phospholipid, phosphatidylinositol 3-phophate. Nature 1988; 332:644–646.
22. Kaplan DR, Whitman M, Schaffhausen B, et al. Common elements in growth factor stimulation and oncogenic transformation: 85 (KD) phosphoprotein and phosphatidyl inositol kinase activity. Cell 1987;50:1021–1029.
23. Berridge MJ, Brown (KD), Irvine RF, Heslop JP. Phophoinositides and cell proliferation. J Cell Sci 1985;3:187S–198S.
24. Mayer BJ, Hamagachi M, Harafusa H. A novel viral oncogene with structural similarity to phospholipase C. Nature 1988;332:272–275.
25. Nishizura Y. Studies and prospectives of the protein kinase C family for cellular regulation. Cancer 1989;63:1892–1903.
26. Housey GM, Johnson MD, Hsiao WLW, et al. Overproduction of protein kinase C causes disordered growth control in rat fibroblasts. Cancer Res 1988;52:343–354.
27. Stryer L, Bourne HR. G proteins: a family of signal transducers. Ann Rev Cell Biol 1986;2:391–419.
28. Casey DJ, Gliman, AG. G-protein involvement in receptor-effector coupling. J Biol Chem 1988;236:2577–2580.
29. Berridge JM, Irvine RF. Inositol phophates and cell signaling. Nature 1989;341:197–205.
30. Cooper GM. Onocogenes. Boston: Jones & Bartlett, 1990.
31. Bos, JL. Oncogenes in human cancer: a review. Cancer Res 1989;49:4682–4689.
32. Gibbs JB. Ras c-terminal processing enzymes—new drug targets? Cell 1991;65:1–4.
33. Angel P, Allegroto EA, Okino ST, et al. Oncogene jun encodes for a sequence specific trans-activator similar to AP-1. Nature 1988;322:166–171.
34. Cole MD. The myc oncogene: its role in transformationa and differentiation. Ann Rev Genet 1986;20:361–364.
35. Sager R. Tumor suppression genes: the puzzle and the promise. Science 1989;246:1406–1411.
36. Harris H. The analysis of malignancy by cell fusion: the position in 1988. Cancer Res 1988;48:3302–3306.
37. Lee WH, Bookstin RE, Lee EYHP. Molecular biology of the human retinoblastoma gene, ln: Klein G, ed. Tumor suppressor genes. New York: Marcel Dekker, 1990:169–199.
38. Weichselbaum RR, Beckitt M. Some retinoblastomas, osteosarcomas and soft tissue sarcomas may share a common etiology. Proc Natl Acad Sci U S A 1988;85:2106–2109.
39. Harbour JW, Lai SL, Whang-Peng J, et al. Abnormalities in structure and expression of the human retinoblastoma gene in SCLC. Science 1988;241:353–357.
40. Lee EHYP, To H, Shaw JY, Bookstein R, Scully P, Lee WH. Inactivation of the retinoblastoma susceptability gene in human breast cancers. Science 1988;241:218–221.
41. Finay CA, Hinds PW, Levine AJ. The p53 proto-oncogenes can act as a suppressor of transformation. Cell 1989;57:1083–1093.
42. Culotta E, Koshland DE. p53-molecule of the year. Science 1993;262:1958–1961.
43. Takahashi T, Nau MM, Chiba I, et al. p53: a frequent target for genetic abnormalities in lung cancer. Science 1989;246:491–494.
44. Esrig D, Elmajian D, Croshen S, et al. Accumulation of nuclear p53 and tumor progression in bladder cancer. New England J Med 1994;33:1259–1264.
45. Hamelin R, Laurent-Puig P, Olschwang S, et al. Association of p53 mutations with short survival in colorectal cancer. Gastroenterology 1994;106:42–48.
46. Cross M, Dester TM. Growth factors in development, transformation and tumorigenesis. Cell 1991;64:271–280.
47. Sporn MB, Todaro GJ. Autocrine secretion and malignant transformation of cells. New Engl J Med 1980;303:878–880.
48. Bradley SJ, Garfinkle G, Walker E, et al. Increased expression of the epidermal growth factor on human colon carcinoma cells. Arch Surg 1986;121:1242–1247.
49. Sainsbury C, Frandon JR, Needham GK, et al. Epidermal growth factor receptor status as predictor of early recurrence of and death from breast cancer. Lancet 1987;1:1398–1402.
50. Nicholason S, Richard J, Sainsbury C, et al. Epidermal growth factor receptor (EGFR): results of a 6-year follow up study in operable breast cancer with emphasis on node negative sub group. Br J Cancer 1991;63:146–150.
51. Derynck R. Transforming growth factor alpha. Cell 1988;54:593–595.
52. Tateishj M, Ishida T, Mitsudomi T, et al. Prognostic implication of TGF alpha in adenocarcinoma of the lung. Br J Cancer 1991;63:130–133.
53. Lippman ME, Dickson RB, Geimann EP, et al. Growth regulatory peptide production by human breast carcinoma cells. J Steroid Biochem 1988;30:53–61.
54. Wakefield LM, Smith DM, Masui T, et al. Distribution and modulation of the cellular receptor for transforming growth factor-beta. J Cell Biol 1987;9:95–114.
55. Laiho M, Keski-Oja J. Growth factors in the regulation of pericellular protolysis: a review. Cancer Res 1989;49:2533–2553.
56. Gospodarowicz D, Ferra N, Schweigener L, et al. Structural characterization and biological functions of fibroblast growth factor. Endocr Rev 1987;105:965–975.
57. Weidner N, Semple JP, Welch WR, et al. Tumor angiogenesis and metastasis-correlation in invasive breast cancer. New Engl J Med 1991;324:1–8.
58. Woltering EA, Barrie R, O'Dorisio TM, et al. Somatostatin analogues inhibit angiogenesis in the chick chorioallantoic membrane. J Surg Res 1991;50:245–251.
59. Ruoslahti E, Yama Guchi Y. Proteoglycans as modulators of growth factor activities. Cell 1991;64:867–869.
60. Fidler IJ, Radinsky R. Genetic control of cancer metastasis. J Natl Canc Inst 1990;82:166–168.
61. Muschel R, Liotta LA. Role of oncogenes in metastasis carcinogenesis. 1988;9:705–715.
62. Har JR, Easty D. Identificationn of genes controlling metastatic behavior. Br J Cancer 1991;63:9–12.
63. Palk S, Hasan R, Fisher ER, et al. Pathologic findings from the National Surgical Adjuvant Breast and Bowel Project: prognostic significance of erb B-2 protein overexpression in primary breast cancer. J Clin Oncol 1990;8:103–112.
64. Phillips WS, Stafford PW, Duval-Arnold B, et al. Neruoblastoma and the clinical significance of N-myc oncogene amplification. Surg Gynecol Obstet 1991;172:73–80.
65. Liotta L, Steeg PS, Stetier-Stevenson WG. Cancer metastasis and angiogenesis: an imbalance of positive and negative regulation. Cell 1991;64:327–336.
66. Steeg PS, Bevilacqua G, Kopper L, et al. Evidence for a novel gene associated with lower tumor metastatic potential. J Natl Canc Inst 1988;80:200–204.
67. Stahl JA, Alvero L, Rosengard AM, et al. Identification of a second human nm^{23} gene, nm^{23}-H2. Canc Res 1991;51:445–449.
68. Alvaro L, Flatow U, King CR, et al. Reduced tumor incidence, metastatic potential, and cytokine-responsiveness of nm-23 transfected melanoma cells. Cell 1991;65:25–35.
69. Hennessy C, Henry JA, May FEB, et al. Expression of the anti-metastatic gene nm^{23} in human breast cancer. An association with good prognosis. Natl Canc Inst 1991;83:281–285.
70. Owaimati AA, Robins RA, Hinton C, et al. Tumor aneuploidy prognostic parameters and survival in primary breast cancer. Br J Cancer 1987;55:449–454.
71. Sigurdsson H, Baldetorp B, Borg A, et al. Indicators of prognosis in node negative breast cancer. New Engl J Med 1990;322:1045–1053.
72. Winchester DJ, Duda RB, August CZ, et al. The importance of DNA flow cytometry in node negative breast cancer. Arch Surg 1990;125:886–889.
73. Clark GM, Dressler LG, Owens MA, et al. Prediction of relapse or survival in patients with node negative breast cancer by DNA flow cytometry. New Engl J Med 1989;320:627–633.
74. Olsson H, Ranstam I, Baldetorp B, et al. Proliferation and DNA ploidy in malignant breast tumors in relation to early oral contraceptive use and early abortions. Cancer 1991;67:1285–1290.
75. Caleffi M, Teague MW, Jensen RA, et al. p53 gene mutations and steroid receptor status in breast cancer. Cancer 1994;73:2147–2156.
76. Isola J, Visakorpi T, Holli K, et al. Association of over-expression

of tumor suppression protein p53 with rapid cell proliferation and poor prognosis in node negative breast cancer patients. J Natl Canc Inst 1992;84:1109–1114.

77. Marks JR, Humphney PA, Wu K, et al. Overexpression of p53 and HER:2/neu proteins as prognostic markers in early stage breast cancer. Ann Surg 1994;219:332–341.

78. Bland KI, Konstadovlakis MM, Vezerdis MP, et al. Oncogene protein co-expression. Ann Surg 1995;221:706–720.

79. Vitetta ES, Uhn JW. Monolonal antibodies as agonists. An expanded role for their use in cancer therapy. Cancer Res 1994;54: 5301–5309.

80. Burtness BA. Oncology and Hematology. JAMA 1995;273: 1702–1703.

81. Ranzani GN, Luinetti LS, Padovan, et al. p53 gene mutations and protein nucleus accumulation are early events in intestinal-type gastric cancer but late events in diffuse type. Cancer Epidemiol Biomarkers Prev 1995;4:223–231.

82. Kullman F, McClelland M. Letter to the editor. New Eng. J. Med 1995; 1427–1428.

83. Rhyu MG, Park WS, Jung YJ, et al. Allelic deletions of MCC/APC and p53 are frequent late events in human gastric carcinogens. Gastroenterology 1994 106:1584–1588.

84. Motojima K, Furui J, Kohara N, et al. *erb* B-2 expression in well-differentiated adenocarcinoma of the stomach predicts shorter survival after curative resection. Surgery 1994;115:349–354.

85. Wright PA, Williams GT. Molecular biology and gastric carcinoma. Gut 1993;34:145–147.

86. Scott NA, Rainwater LM, Wieand HS, et al. The relative prognostic value of flow cytometric DNA analysis and conventional clinicopathologic critical care in patients with operable rectal carcinoma. Dis Colon Rectum 1987;30:5513–5520.

87. Bauer KD, Lincoln ST, Vera-Roman JM, et al. Prognostic implications of proliferative activity and DNA aneuploidy in colonic adenocarcinoma. Lab Invest 1987;57:329–335.

88. Kokal WA, Gardine RL, Sheibani K, et al. Tumor DNA content in resectable primary colorectal carcinoma. Ann Surg 1989;209: 188–193.

89. Thor A, Hand PH, Wunderlich D, et al. Monoclonal antibodies define differential *ras* gene expression in malignant and benign colonic diseases. Nature 1984;311:562–564.

90. Maestro R, Viel A, Biocchi M. Correlation between chromosome 5q deletions and different mechanisms of c-*myc* over-expression in human colorectal cancer. Br J Cancer 1991;63:185–186.

91. Nimi S, Nakagawa K, Yokata J, et al. Resistance to anti-cancer drugs in NIH3T3 cells transfected with c-*myc* and/or H-*ras* genes. Br J Canc 1991;63:237–241.

92. Krontiris TG, Devlin B, Karp D, et al. An association between the risk of cancer and mutations in the HRSA1 mini-satellite locus. New Eng J Med 1993;329:517–523.

93. Vogelstein B, Fearon ER, Hamilton SR, et al. Genetic alterations during colorectal tumor development. New Eng J Med 1988;319: 525–532.

94. Fearon ER, Vogelstein B. A genetic model for colorectal tumorogenesis. Cell 1991;61: 759–767.

95. Bresalier RS. Adhesion molecules and gastrointestinal malignancies. Gastroenterology 1994;106:1378–1382.

96. Tanabe KK. Cell adhesion in tumor invasion. Ann Surg Onc 1995; 2:376–377.

97. Lynch HT. The surgeon and colorectal cancer genetics. Case identification, surveillance and management strategies. Arch Surg 1990;125:698–701.

98. Powell SM, Peterson GM, Krush AJ. Molecular diagnosis of familial adenomatous polyposis. New Eng J Med 1993;329:1982–1987.

99. Tanaka K, Oshimura M, Kikuchi R, et al. Suppression of tumorogenecity in human colon cancer cells by introduction of normal chromosome 5 or 18. Nature 1991;349:340–342.

100. Sobol H, Narod SA, Nakamura Y, et al. Screening for multiple endocrine neoplasia type 2a with DNA-polymorphism analysis. New Eng J Med 1989;321:996–1001.

101. Wells SA, Chi DD, Toshima K, et al. Predictive DNA testing and prohylactic total thyroidectomy in patients at risk for multiple endocrine neoplasia type 2a. Ann Surg 1994;220:237–250.

102. Neumann HP, Eng C, Mulligan L, et al. Consequences of direct genetic testing for germline mutations in the clinical management of families with multiple endocrine neoplasia, type II. JAMA 1995;274:1149–1151.

103. Nakagawura A, Ikeda K, Yokoyama T. Surgical aspects of N-*myc* oncogene amplification in neuroblastoma. Surgery 1988;104: 34–40.

104. Huang HJS, Yee JK, Shen JY, et al. Suppression of the neoplastic phenotype by replacement of the RB gene in human cancer cells. Science 1998;242:1563–1566.

105. Gagandeep SP, Poston GJ, Kinsella AR. Gene therapy in surgical oncology. Ann Surg Oncol 1995;2:179–261.

106. Peplinski GR, Tsung K, Whitman E, et al. Construction and expression in tumor cells of a recombinant vaccinia virus encoding human inter-leukin-1 beta. Ann Surg Onc; 1995. 2:151–159.

107. Peplinski GR, Tsung K, Meko J, et al. Prevention of murine breast cancer by vaccination with the tumor cells modified by cytokine-producing recombinant vaccinia viruses. (Submitted for publication.).

108. Schreiber H. Tumor immunology. In: Paul W, ed. Fundamental immunology, 2nd ed. New York: Raven Press,1989.

109. Kohler G, Milstein C. Continuous cultures of fused cells secreting antibody of predefined specificity. Nature 1975;256:495–497.

110. Miller R, Maloney D, Warnke R, et al. Treatment of a B cell lymphoma with monoclonal anti-idiotype antibody. N Engl J Med 1985;306:1349–1363.

111. Brodt P. Tumor immunology—three decades in review. Annual Rev Microbiol 1983;37:447–476.

112. Dawson M, Moore M. Tumor Immunology. In: Roitt L, Brostoff J, Male D, eds. Immunology. 2nd ed. London: Gower Medical Publishing, 1989.

113. Potter M. Percivall Pott's contribution to cancer research. NCI Monograph 1963;10: 1–13.

114. Prehn R, Main J. Immunity to methylcholanthrene induced sarcoma. J Natl Cancer Inst 1957;18:769.

115. Bishop J. Viruses, genes and cancer. ll. Retroviruses and cancer genes. Cancer 1985; 55:2329–2333.

116. Gross L. Intradermal immunization of C3H mice against sarcoma that originated in animal of the same line. Cancer Res 1946;3:326.

117. Sears H, Herlyn D, Steplewski Z, et al. Effects of monoclonal antibody immunotherapy in patients with gastrointestinal adenocarcinoma. J Biol Resp Mod 1984;3:138–150.

118. Arnold MW, Schneebaum S, Berens A, et al. Radioimmuno–guided surgery challenges traditional decision making in patients with primary clorectal cancer. Surgery 1992;112:624–630.

119. Burnet F. The concept of immunological surveillance. Prog Exp Tumor Res 1970;13:1.

120. Good R. Recognition and management of immunodeficient disorders. Vox Sang 1986;51 (Suppl Z):1–13.

121. Penn I. Tumors of the immunocompromised patient. Ann Rev Med 1988;39:63–73.

122. Rosenberg S, Lotze M, Muul L, et al. A progress report on the treatment of 157 patients with advanced cancer using Iymphokine activated killer cells and recombinant interleukin-2 or high dose interleukin-2 alone. N Engl J Med 1987;316:889.

123. Rosenberg S, Packard B, Aebersold P, et al. Use of tumor infiltrating Iymphocytes and interleukin-2 in the immunotherapy of patients with metastatic melanoma. A primary report. N Engl J Med 1988;319:1676.

124. Wyllie AH. Apoptosis: Cell death in tissue regulation. J Pathol 1987;153:313–320.

125. Glucksman A. Cell deaths in normal vertebrate ontogeny. Blot Rev 1951;26:59–62.

126. Murphy KM, Heimberger AB, Loh DY. Induction by antigen of intrathymic apoptosis of CD4+, CD9+ TCRL0 thymocytes *in vivo*. Science 1990;250:1720–1729.

127. Goldstein P, Ojcius DM, Young JDE. Cell death mechanisms and the immune system. Immunol Rev 1991;121:29–65.

128. Vaux DL, Cory S, Adams JM. Bcl-2 gene promotes haemopoietic cell survival and cooperates with c-myc to immortalize pre B cells. Nature 1985:440–443.

129. Trauth BC, Klas C, Peters AMJ, et al. Monoclonal antibody-mediated tumor regression by induction of apoptosis. Science 1989; 245:301–305.

130. Morton DL, Forshag LJ, Hoon DSB, et al. Prolongation of survival in metastatic melanoma after active specific immunotherapy with a new polyvalent melanoma vaccine. Annals of Surgery 1992; 216:463–481.

131. Barth A, Hoon DSB, Forshag LJ, et al. Polyvalent melanoma cell

vaccine induces delayed type hypersensitivity and in vitro cellular immune response. Cancer Res 1994;54:3342–3345.

132. Morton DL, Hoon DSB, Nizze JA, et al. Polyvalent melanoma vaccine improves survival of patients with metastatic melanoma. Ann New York Acac Sci 1993;690:120.

133. Mitchell MS, Liggett PE, Green RL, et al. Sustained regression of a primary choroidal melanoma under the influence of a therapeutic melanoma vaccine. J Clin Oncol 1994;12:396–401.

134. Livingston PO, Wong GY, Adluri S, et al. Improved survival in stage III melanoma patients with GM2 antibodies: a randomized trial of adjuvant vaccination with GM2 ganglioside. J Clin Oncol 1994;12:1036–1044.

135. Hersey P, Schibeci SD, Townsend P, et al. Potentiation of lymphocyte responses by monoclonal antibodies to the ganglioside GD3. Cancer Res 1986;46:6083–6090.

136. Harel W, Shau H, Hadley CG, et al. Increased lysis of melanoma by in vivo elicited human lymphokine activated killer cells after addition of antiganglioside antibodies in vitro. Cancer Res 1990; 50:6311–6315.

137. Miller R, Maloney D, Warnke R, et al. Treatment of a B cell lymphoma with monoclonal anti-idiotype antibody. N Engl J Med 1985;306:1349-1363.

138. Rosenberg SA, Anderson WF, Blaese M, et al. The development of gene therapy for the treatment of cancer. Ann Surg 1993;218: 455–460.

139. Hock H, Dorsch M, Kunzendorf U, et al. Vaccinations with tumor cells genetically engineered to produce different cytokines: effectivity not superior to a classical adjuvant. Cancer Res 1993;53: 714–717.

140. Sznol M, Parkinson DR. Clinical applications of IL-2. Oncology 1994;8:61–75.

141. Atkins MB, Sparano J, Fisher RI, et al. Randomized phase II trial of high dose interleukin-2 either alone or in combination with interferon alfa-2b in advanced reanal cell carcinoma. J Clin Oncol 1993;11:661–670.

142. Yang JC, Topalian SL, Parkinson D, et al. Randomized comparison of high dose and low dose intravenous interleukin-2 for the therapy of metastatic renal cell carcinoma: An interim report. J Clin Oncol 1994;12:1572–1576.

143. Atzpodien J, Hanninen EL, Kirchner H, et al. Multi-institutional home therapy trial of recombinant human interleukin-2 and interferon alfa-2 in progressive metastatic renal cell carcinoma. J Clin Oncol 1995;13:497–501.

144. Rosenberg SA, Lotze MT, Yang JC, et al. Prospective randomized trial of high dose interleukin-2 alone or in conjunction with lymphokine activated killer cells for the treatment of patients with advanced cancer. J Natl Cancer Inst 1993;85:622–632.

145. McCabe MS, Staablein D, Hawkins MJ. The modified group C experience—phase III randomized trials of IL-2 vs IL-2/LAK in advanced renal cell carcinoma and advanced melanoma. Proc Am Soc Clin Oncol 1991;10:213.

146. Parkinson DR, Abrams JS, Wiernik PH, et al. Interleukin-2 therapy in patients with metastatic malignant melanoma: A phase II study. Clin Oncol 1990;8:1650–1656.

147. Dutcher JP, Gaynor ER, Boldt DH, et al. A phase II study of high dose continuous infusion of interleukin-2 with lymphokine activated killer cells in patients with metastatic melanoma. J Clin Oncol 1989;7:477–480.

148. Bar MH, Sznol M, Atkins MB, et al. Metastatic malignant melanoma treated with combination bolus and continuous infusion interleukin-2 and lymphokine activated killer cells. J Clin Oncol 1990;8:1138–1147.

149. Marincola FM, Venzon D, White D, et al. HLA association with response and toxicity in melanoma patients treated with IL-2 based immunotherapy. Cancer Res 52:6561–6566.

150. Marincola FM, Ettinghausen S, Cohen PA, et al. Treatment of established lung metastases with tumor infiltrating lymphocytes derived from a poorly immunogenic tumor engineered to secrete human TNF-α. J Immunol 1994;152:3501–3513.

151. Richards JM, Mehta N, Ramming K, et al. Sequential chemoimmunotherapy in the treatment of metastatic melanoma. J Clin Oncol 1992;10:1333–1343.

152. Buzaid AC, Legha SS. Combination chemotherapy with interleukin-2 and interferon alfa for the treatment of advanced melanoma. Semin Oncol 1994;21:6(suppl 14)23–28.

153. Ramazzini B. De morbis artificum diatriba mutinae. A. Capponi, 1700.

154. Doll R. The epidemiology of cancer. Cancer 1980;45;24–75.

155. DeVita D, Hellman S, Rosenberg S, eds. Cancer: principles and practice of oncology. Philadelphia: JB Lippincott, 1989.

156. Amsel J. Cancer epidemiology, methods and applications. In: Pilch Y, ed. Surgical oncology. New York: McGraw-Hill, 1984: 23–46.

157. Boice J, Monson R. Breast cancer in women after repeated fluoroscopic examination of the chest. J Natl Cancer Inst 1977;59: 823–832.

158. Silverberg E, Luberdra J. Cancer statistics. CA 1989;39:3–20.

159. Muir CS, Nectoux J. International patterns of cancer. In: Schottenfeld D, Fraumeni J, eds. Cancer epidemiology and prevention. Philadelphia: WB Saunders, 1982:119–137.

160. Haenszel W, Kurihara M, Segi M, et al. Stomach cancer among Japanese in Hawaii. J Natl Cancer Inst 1972;49:969–988.

161. Doll R. The age distribution of cancer in man. In: Engel A, Larsen T, eds. Thule international symposia. Stockholm: Nordiska Bokhandelns Forlag, 1968.

162. MacMahon B. Epidemiologic considerations in the staging of Hodgkins disease. Cancer Res 1971;31:1854–1857.

163. Doll R. An epidemiological perspective of the biology of cancer. Cancer Res 1978;38:3573–3583.

164. Young JL, Pollack ES. The incidence of cancer in the United States. In: Schottenfeld D, Fraumeni J, eds. Cancer epidemiology and prevention. Philadelphia: WB Saunders, 1982:132–165.

165. Wolmark N, Fisher B, Wieand HS. The prognostic value of the modifications of the Dukes' C class of colorectal cancer. Ann Surg 1986;203:115–122.

166. Hutter RV, Sobin LH. A universal staging system for cancer of the colon and rectum. Arch Path Lab Med 1986;110:367–368.

167. Beahrs OH, Myers MH. Manual for staging cancer. 2nd ed. Philadelphia: JB Lippincott, 1983.

9 Surgical Infection

Donald E. Fry

Infection is the constellation of clinical manifestations caused by the local inflammatory response that is initiated by microorganisms. Although perceived by clinicians to be a specific response to bacteria, fungi, viruses, or protozoans, the clinical signs and symptoms of the infected state are, in reality, nonspecific inflammatory responses that are elicited with every wound and every injury. It is only because the stimulus of living microorganisms is so great and sustained over time, and the host response so prompt and vigorous, that one associates infection with most inflammatory responses. Indeed, every soft tissue contusion and every laceration elicits the same inflammatory response. However, when bacteria are present, the insult remains active and progressive because bacterial proliferation represents a substantial insult—a sustained injury that drives the inflammatory response until eradication of the microbial stimulus is achieved.

Clinical infection is the biological summation of the numbers of organisms, the intrinsic virulence of the microorganism, the microenvironment of the contaminated tissue, and the responsiveness of the host. An anatomic injury that introduces bacteria into the tissues, whether from a cutaneous laceration or a perforation of the gastrointestinal tract, will be deemed to be clinically infected based on the summation of these variables. Although microorganisms have common features that permit discussion of the prototype bacterium or generic virus, the response from one area of the body to another is different with respect to host response mechanisms. Likewise, environmental issues are different when examining the controlled trauma of a surgical wound to the biologic chaos of a perforated viscus. This chapter summarizes microbial, host, and microenvironmental factors that represent important basic issues in the evolution of clinical infection. With a better understanding of the fundamental variables of infection, a more enlightened approach to therapy can be realized.

Microorganisms

Bacteria

Bacteria are single-cell microorganisms that are considered to be plant cells because of the presence of a rigid cell wall that envelopes the entire organism (Fig. 9.1). Like all cells, whether flora or fauna, the bacterium has a plasma membrane which contains a cytoplasm that has both a variable aqueous and a gel phase. Unlike higher classifications of plant and animal life, the bacterial cell does not contain a nuclear membrane, so the genetic material, while generally segregated in a specific area of the cell, is in immediate proximity to what would be ordinarily considered cytoplasmic components of the cell (1). Bacteria have DNA-type genetic material and generally proceed through the translational and transcriptional processes for phenotypic expression, i.e., protein synthesis. Unlike mammalian cells, bacterial DNA is a single circular structure rather than in strands. Bacterial DNA is attached to an invaginated segment of the plasma membrane, which is referred to as the mesosome. The cell wall-plasma membrane unit of the bacterial cell is an extraordinarily complex structure. Although customarily discussed as separate structural entities, the cell wall and plasma membrane are structurally and functionally integrated and should be discussed as a combined unit. There is a highly variable composition of the cell wall between species of bacteria, and a different physical relationship between the cell wall and the plasma membrane of different strains of bacteria (2,3).

Gram-positive bacteria have a thick cell wall, which is located immediately on the external surface of the plasma membrane (Fig. 9.2). The cell wall is composed of peptidoglycan polymers that are cross-linked by polypeptides to form a rigid protective coat about the

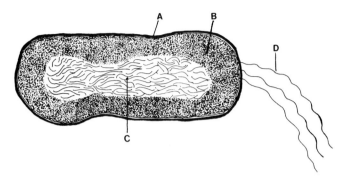

Figure 9.1. A prototype bacterial rod. **A,** cell wall; **B,** cytoplasm, which is rich in ribosomes used in protein synthesis; **C,** nuclear area (bacteria do not have a nuclear membrane); **D,** flagella, which are important in cell locomotion.

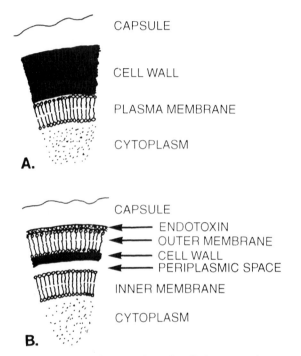

Figure 9.2. Differences between the cell-wall-plasma membrane complex of Gram-positive (**A**) and Gram-negative (**B**) bacteria. The Gram-positive organism has a much thicker cell wall. The Gram-negative bacterium has both an inner and outer membrane around its relatively thin cell wall. Note the periplasmic space between the cell wall and the inner membrane in the Gram-negative bacterium.

microorganism. The cell wall is penetrated readily by solutes, nutrients, and ions. The cell wall serves primarily to protect the cell against unfavorable osmotic changes that would otherwise cause cell swelling and lysis. The lipid bilayer of the plasma membrane contains the necessary enzymes and transport mechanisms that regulate ionic and nutrient access to the cell. The close apposition of the cell wall and the plasma membrane in Gram-positive bacteria essentially provide for no periplasmic space between the two structures.

The Gram-negative bacteria have a far more complex cell wall-plasma membrane structure (see Fig. 9.2). These microorganisms have an outer and inner mem-

brane that has the cell wall interposed in between. The cell wall is of a similar composition to Gram-positive bacteria but is much thinner. The inner membrane is characteristic lipid bilayer, and there is a periplasmic space between the cell wall and the inner membrane (4). Gram-negative bacteria have an outer membrane that makes the microorganism much less easily penetrated by external drugs and other solutes than Gram-positive bacteria (5–7). The outer membrane is a lipid bilayer that has a lipopolysaccharide component known as endotoxin. Endotoxin is an important virulence factor for Gram-negative bacteria. Endotoxin usually contains the lipid A moiety, which is an important component for virulence (8,9). Some strains of bacteria have a lipopolysaccharide of the outer membrane that does not contain the lipid A component (*Bacteroides fragilis*) and results in an attenuated endotoxic effect for these bacterial strains (10).

The outer membrane contains pores that have *porin* proteins which line these microbiologic passages (11). Porin proteins are different in different bacteria and may permit passage or exclude certain macromolecules, depending on the polarity and allosteric properties of both the porin proteins and the potential macromolecules. Because the outer membrane is principally lipid in structure, the porin proteins provide a hydrophilic avenue for access of nutrients, ions, and drugs into the microorganism.

An additional feature of the outer membrane is its immunogenicity, which allows the host to produce antibody specific to outer membrane antigens. Research attention has focused on the common immunogenicity of the lipid A component of endotoxin. This has resulted in the synthesis of antiendotoxin antibodies that presently are being studied for their therapeutic benefits in the treatment of Gram-negative infection (12–14).

Certain strains of bacteria have a capsule that is external to, but contiguous with, the cell wall (15,16). The capsule may be composed of polysaccharide or polyproteins. This capsular coat provides additional protection for the bacterial cell, and the capsule may retard phagocytosis by the host when the bacterial cell is part of an infection. The capsule may protect the bacterial cell from exposure of certain cell-wall-surface antigens, and thus prevent the formation of specific antibody by the infected host. Capsular material may actually serve as a virulence factor in facilitating the infectiousness of the bacterial cell.

The bacterial cell wall may have flagella and pili as external extensions. Flagella may be single and excentrically located at one end of the organism, or they may be multiple (17). The whip-like motion of the flagella provide the bacterial cell with a means of locomotion.

Sex pili are rigid protrusions from the bacterial cell and serve as a means for contact between different microorganisms. These specialized structures serve as conduits for the exchange of genetic material (e.g., plasmids) between bacterial cells and are important in the transfer of resistance among bacterial populations. Only Gram-negative bacteria have sex pili.

Fimbriae and fibrillae are filamentous structures that protrude from the bacterial cell and primarily serve as adhesins to facilitate bacteria to bind to other cells. The adhesion process of bacteria to epithelial cells is an important virulence factor, and fimbriae and fibrillae are important structures that permit bacterial adherence. Fimbriae and fibrillae are found on both Gram-positive and Gram-negative bacteria (18,19). The cytoplasm of the bacterial cell contains the necessary synthetic enzymes and energy-producing systems to maintain viability of the cell. Abundant ribosomes are present to provide the template for protein synthesis. These ribosomes are temperature sensitive and can be bound by specific antibiotics to inhibit protein synthesis. Bacterial cells do not have mitochondria but rather have the apparatus for oxidative phosphorylation on the cytoplasmic surface of the plasma membrane (20).

Fungi

The fungal cell has characteristics that are analogous to the morphology and structure of mammalian cells (21) (Fig. 9.3). The fungal cells may be identified as single cells or may grow in a filamentous fashion, which could be interpreted as a primitive effort at tissue formation because dividing cells actually maintain contact with one another. The continued presence of the cell wall about the fungal cell is the distinctive feature that makes these cells plant life.

Unlike bacteria, the fungal cell has a nucleus that has a nuclear membrane that envelopes the nuclear material of the cell. The genetic material of the fungus is in chromosomal strands rather than the circular configuration of the bacterial cell. Fungi have mitochondria for bioenergy processes. Like mammalian cells, sterols are component parts of fungal plasma membrane.

The cell wall of the fungi is structurally different from bacterial cells. The fungal cell wall does not contain peptidoglycans nor does it contain lipopolysaccharides. The cell wall usually is composed of polysaccharide, which is commonly an N-acetyl-D-glucosamine polymer called chitin. Like bacteria, the cell wall may have a polysaccharide or polyprotein capsule on its external surface. The cell wall serves the role of osmotic control for the fungus in the same way that it serves bacteria.

Fungi are infrequently pathogens in humans. *Candida albicans* is the most frequent clinical isolate and usually is identified in patients that are immunocompromised. Indeed, the fungi have little in the form of exotoxins or structural virulence factors when compared with the many pathogens known to humans.

Viruses

Viruses represent the most primitive form of infectious pathogen. Viruses are distinctly simple in design and are extremely small in size. Viruses were discovered as putative living particles distinct from bacteria because they could not be filtered like bacterial cells (22). Viral particles are 0.02 to 0.30 μm in size, whereas the *Escherichia coli* bacterial cell is a 0.5×2.5 μm rod, the fungal cell is 2 to 3 μm in diameter, and the human erythrocyte is 8 μm in diameter (23).

Viruses are obligate intracellular parasites. They are unable to replicate outside of a host cell. They do not have any intrinsic capability to generate bioenergy and, therefore, must invade and exploit the energy-generating processes of other cells to be able to replicate.

The complete viral microorganism, known as the virion, has only two essential components (Fig. 9.4). The

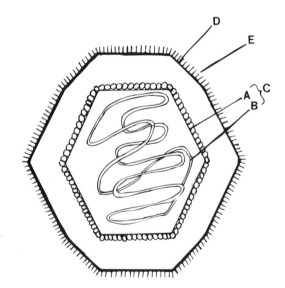

Figure 9.4. A prototype virus. *A,* capsid shell about the nuclear material; *B,* circular strand of genetic material, which is either RNA or DNA but not both; *C,* naked viruses; *D,* outer coat of the virus; *E,* viral spikes, which contain adherence receptors and other enzymes that may mediate virulence.

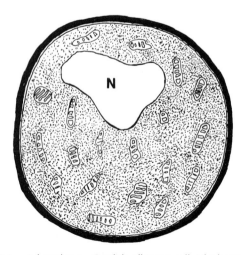

Figure 9.3. A fungal (e.g., *Candida albicans*) cell. Like bacteria, fungi have a cell wall, but unlike bacteria, fungi have a nuclear membrane and mitochondria in the cytoplasm. *N,* nucleus.

virus has a nuclear genetic material that is either DNA or RNA, but not both. DNA viruses usually are double stranded, whereas the RNA viruses may be either single or double stranded. The genome is then encased within a symmetrical protein shell known as the capsid. The composite unit of the capsid with the DNA or RNA genome within is referred to as the nucleocapsid. The capsid serves the purpose of protecting the genome from environmental damage, and it also becomes the means for adherence to host cells that will be infected by the virion. Viruses that have only the nucleocapsid are called naked viruses. The nucleocapsid is either a symmetrical icosahedron or helix (24). All DNA viruses are icosahedral in shape, but RNA viruses may be either icosahedral or helical.

Some viruses may have an additional envelope about the nucleocapsid (25). The protein component of this envelope is derived from the viral genome during the period of intracellular replication. However, the lipid and carbohydrate components are actually from the membranes of the infected cell because viral particles do not have genes for the production of enzymes that are necessary for synthesis of nonprotein structures. The protein components of the envelope structurally appear as spikes. These protein spikes, known in some viral species as peplomers, are analogous to the fimbriae of bacteria and may have specific enzyme activity that contribute to the virulence of the viral microorganism (26).

Infection of the host cell follows a generic pattern, although specific differences can be seen with different viruses (27). Adsorption to the plasma membrane of the cell to be infected occurs first. This is achieved by attachment from the spikes to specific receptor sites on the host cell. Because the envelope of the virus is made of plasma membrane, the fusion of the plasma membrane envelope with that of the host cell effects penetration of the nucleocapsid into the cytoplasm (Fig. 9.5). Naked viruses presumably have binding sites on the capsid surface and are internalized into the infected cell by pinocytosis (Fig. 9.6). Subsequent dissolution of the vacuole releases the nucleocapsid into the cytoplasm. The capsid shell around the viral genome is then digested by enzymes from the host cell's cytoplasm. The viral genome is released, and depending on whether the genome is DNA or RNA, a specific series of events occur.

If the virus is a DNA virus, then the viral genome migrates into the nucleus of the infected cell where RNA polymerase of the host transcribes the viral DNA (28) (see Fig. 9.5). Messenger RNA is similarly produced with translation of viral proteins in the infected cell's cytoplasm. This leads to the synthesis of new viral particles, which are subsequently released with lysis and death of the infected cell. If the infecting virus is an RNA virus, then viral RNA within the host cell cytoplasm can directly become the template for translation of viral particles and the ultimate replication of new viruses (see Fig. 9.6).

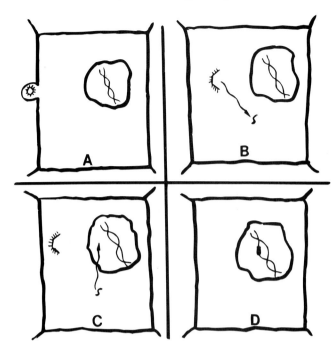

Figure 9.5. The infection process of a cell by a DNA virus that has an outer envelope. **A,** Fusion of the vital envelope with the plasma membrane of the host cell, which results in release of the nucleocapsid within the host cytoplasm. **B,** Disruption of the nucleocapsid within the cytoplasm, which results in the release of nuclear DNA. **C,** Penetration of the viral DNA through the nuclear membrane. **D,** Insertion of the viral DNA into the host cell's chromosome where vital protein can then be transcribed.

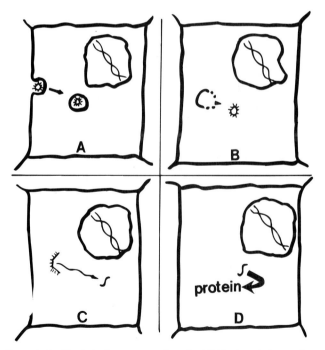

Figure 9.6. The infection process of a naked RNA virus. **A,** Internalization of the naked particle into the infected cell by endocytosis. **B,** Disruption of the vacuole within the host cell cytoplasm with release of the nucleocapsid. **C,** Disruption of the nucleocapsid with release of the viral RNA into the cytoplasm. **D,** The bypass of transcription from the cell nucleus by the viral RNA; translation proceeds from the viral RNA that was released into the cytoplasm from the infecting particle.

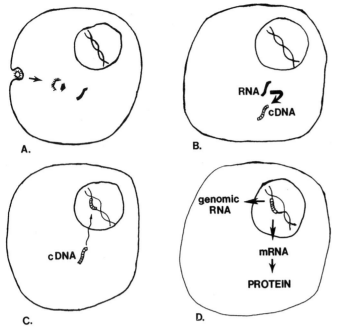

Figure 9.7. Unique feature of the retrovirus group of which HIV is the most notable member. **A,** Cytoplasmic penetration and release of the nuclear RNA from the nucleocapsid. This is similar to the process seen in Figure 9.6. **B,** The RNA becomes the template for the synthesis of a complementary DNA (cDNA) strand within the host cell cytoplasm. **C,** The cDNA then enters the nucleus and becomes integrated into the host DNA. **D,** Like DNA viruses, the transcriptional processes of viral DNA within the host cell's nucleus become the basis for new viral protein synthesis. Genomic RNA is also synthesized from the cDNA, which becomes the nuclear material for new vial particles.

An exception among RNA viruses is the retrovirus group. The retroviruses, the most notable being the human immunodeficiency virus (HIV), have the genetic information to produce reverse transcriptase, which then makes complementary strands of DNA from the viral RNA (29) (Fig. 9.7). The cDNA from the viral RNA then migrates into the infected cell nucleus, and the viral DNA is integrated into the host chromosomes. Viral proteins are then synthesized by the same process that provides transcription and translation for the host cell.

A brief summary of pertinent viral taxonomy for surgeons is provided in Table 9.1 (29). Recently, vital infections have assumed increased interest, not only because of infections that are encountered in the surgical patient, but because of potential occupational risks that may affect the surgeon. The number of pertinent viruses of interest to the surgeon will likely continue to grow.

Virulence Factors

Virulence factors intrinsic to microorganisms are essentially of three types (Table 9.2). Microorganisms may synthesize and secrete biological products that attack

Table 9.1.
The 18 Families of Viruses Known to Cause Infection in Humans

Family	Nuclear Material	Viral Diseases
Poxviridae	DNA	Small pox (Variola)
Herpesviridae	DNA	Herpes simplex
		Varicella/Zoster
		Cytomegalovirus
		EB virus
Adenoviridae	DNA	Mastadenoviruses
Papovaviridae	DNA	Human papilloma virus
Hepadnaviridae	DNA	Hapatitis B
Parvoviridae	DNA	Norwalk virus (Gastroenteritis)
Reoviridae	RNA	Rotavirus and others
		(Fever and Diarrhea)
Togaviridae	RNA	Equine Encephalitis
		Yellow fever
		Dengue fever
		Rubella
Coronaviridae	RNA	Common cold
		Viral pneumonitis
		Gastroenteritis
Paramyxoviridae	RNA	Parainfluenza viruses
		Mumps; Measles
		Respiratory syncytial
Rhabdoviridae	RNA	Vesicular stomatitis
		Rabies

cell populations of the host or attack other homeostatic mechanisms to produce clinical disease. The second group of virulence factors represent structural components of the normal bacterial cell. These structural components, when shed into the environment or when released following the death and lysis of the bacterial cell, have various toxic effects on the host. Finally, the bacterial cell may either secrete enzymes, have cell-structure components, or develop mutational phenotypic changes that make them resistant to antimicrobial chemotherapy. This latter trend among microorganisms is the most important virulence factor presently seen in pathogens.

Exotoxins are produced by many different strains of bacteria, but none are more notable or toxic than the clostridial exotoxins (30). Fulminant cellular necrosis of host cells can be seen with the cytotoxic exotoxins of *Clostridium perfringens* (31). The membrane toxicity of the *Clostridium perfringens* cytotoxin may also provoke hemolysis of red cells. *Clostridium tetani* produces a potent neurotoxin (32), and *Clostridium botulinum* produces a neuromuscular toxin (33). Recently, enteropathogenic toxins from *Clostridium difficile* have represented the most common clostridial infection in the United States. It is associated with gastrointestinal overgrowth of the bacterial strain as a consequence of the influence of systemic antibiotic therapy (34).

Exotoxins are commonly produced by other Gram-positive organisms. Pathogenic Group A streptococci are well known to secrete potent hemolysins when grown on blood agar. Staphylococci are also known to produce hemolysins (35).

Table 9.2.
Summary of the Known Secretory Products of Bacteria that are Identified as Virulence Factors in Human Infection

Virulence Factor	Action	Microorganism
Exotoxins	Cytotoxicity	Clostrium perfringens
	Neurotoxin	Clostridium tetani
	Neuromuscular blockade	Clostridium botulinum
	Enteropathic	
Hemolysins	Lyses red blood cells	Group A Streptococci
		Staphylococcus aureus
Coagulase	Activates coagulation	Straphylococcus aureus
		E. Coli
		Serratia sp.
		Pseudomonas aeruginosa
Leukocidins	Kills phagocytic cells	Streptococcus sp.
		Staphylococcus sp.
Superoxide dismutase	Neutralizes superoxide	Bacteroides fragilis
Catalase	Neutralizes hydrogen peroxide	E. coli
Collagenase	Hydrolyzes collagen	Streptococcus sp.
		Staphyloccus sp.
		Pseudomonas sp.
Hyaluronidase/Heparinase	Hydrolyzes intercellular matrix	Streptococcus sp.
		Staphylococcus sp.
		Clostridium sp.
Filoviridae	RNA	Marburg/Ebola viruses
Orthomyxoviridae	RNA	Influenza A and B viruses
Bunyaviridae	RNA	Unusual fever/encephalitis
Arenaviridae	RNA	Lassa fever
Retroviridae	RNA	Human Immunodeficiency (HIV)
Picornaviridae	RNA	Poliovirus
		Coxsackievirus
		Enterovirus
		Rhinovirus
		Hepatitis A
Caliciviridae	RNA	Gastroenteritis

Staphylococcus aureus produces coagulase as a potent virulence factor. Coagulase provokes coagulation and the precipitation of fibrin within the microenvironment of infection. The resulting fibrin matrix serves to protect the pathogen from phagocytic elements of host defense. Coagulase also provokes intravascular coagulation of the blood supply around the area of infection. This thrombosis commonly leads to the central necrosis within the infectious milieu and results in the characteristic pyogenic character of *Staphylococcus aureus* infections. Although coagulase is identified most notably among staphylococcal species, *E. coli, Serratia* spp., and *Pseudomonas aeruginosa* may also produce coagulase (36).

Gram-positive organisms may actually produce toxins that directly affect phagocytic cells. These leukocidins are seen most commonly as products from *Streptococcus* spp. and *Staphylococcus* spp (37). Bacteria may produce a leukotoxin that is stimulated by the presence of hemoglobin, or the metabolism of hemoglobin by bacteria may produce the toxin. These products appear to be important in the pathophysiology of polymicrobial infections within the intra-abdominal cavity (38).

Selected bacteria may produce various enzymes that affect bacteriocidal mechanisms of phagocytic cells. Superoxide anion is produced and delivered into the phagosome after neutrophil phagocytosis of bacteria. Strains of *B. fragilis* produce superoxide dismutase, which converts superoxide anion to hydrogen peroxide (39). Selected strains of *E. coli* produce catalase, which then reduces the potentially toxic hydrogen peroxide to water (40). The combined effects of superoxide dismutase from *B. fragilis* with the catalase production of *E. coli* represents another potential synergistic relationship that may facilitate the combined virulence of these two strains of pathogens.

Enzymes secreted by certain strains of bacteria may aid the invasion of pathogens into adjacent tissues. Collagenase that is produced by streptococci, staphylococci, and certain *Pseudomonas* spp. are thought to expedite dissection of infection along fascial planes (41). Elastase production would similarly promote microbial invasion. Hyaluronidase and heparinase enzymes are produced by streptococci, staphylococci, and certain clostridial species (40,42). These two enzymes may degrade the intercellular matrix and are of importance in bacterial cellulitis in which organisms are able to progress rapidly through otherwise normal tissues.

Another interesting virulence factor is the secretion of a polysaccharide product by certain strains of *Staphylococcus epidermidis* (43–47). This ''slime'' can actually surround and encase the organism. It appears to facilitate the binding of the *Staphylococcus epidermidis* to foreign surfaces, making it less vulnerable to phagocytic cells. The slime is composed of polysaccharide and has been identified among isolates from infections of peripheral intravascular devices and vascular grafts. This slime coat assumes a certain physical rigidity, which poses some serious problems in attempts to culture the organism.

Structural components of bacteria are clearly virulence factors. The M protein coat of streptococci appears to provide relative protection against phagocytosis (48). It appears to have features that help bind streptococcal pathogens to epithelial cells and may explain the difference in virulence of different strains. Encapsulated bacteria such as *Streptococcus pneumoniae,* meningococcus, and *Haemophilus influenzae* also resist phagocytosis and require opsonization with antibody if hepatic reticuloendothelial clearance of these organisms is to occur (49,50). Of interest, opsonization is not a requirement for splenic clearance of blood-borne encapsulated bacteria, a function that is thought to be critically deficient in the patient who has undergone splenectomy.

The polysaccharide capsule of *B. fragilis* has been studied extensively and assumes considerable significance in the virulence of these organisms (51). If present, the organism has increased virulence as an abdominal infectious pathogen (52). The capsule retards phagocytosis and may actually be leukotoxic. It is clearly associated with the pathogenicity of intra-abdominal infections. If this polysaccharide capsule material is injected into the rat peritoneal cavity, abscesses result without any viable bacteria being present.

Perhaps the most important structural virulence factor of bacteria is endotoxin. This lipopolysaccharide component of the bacterial outer membrane is a common feature of essentially all Gram-negative enteric bacteria (53,54). Different bacterial species may have chemical variations in the molecular detail of their own endotoxin, but the common lipid A component seems to provide similar biological actions and common virulence features. When the endotoxin molecule lacks the lipid A component, its virulence appears to be lost. Hence, *B. fragilis,* which lacks the lipid A moiety within its endotoxin does not produce the same profound hemodynamic effects as that of *E. coli,* which does contain the lipid A portion of the molecule (55).

Endotoxin has many biologic effects. It provokes macrophages to produce endogenous pyrogen, which causes fever (56). Evidence suggests that endotoxin may directly stimulate the thermoregulatory center in much the same fashion as interleukin-1 (IL-1), without needing the intermediary production of endogenous pyrogen by a macrophage cell (57). Endotoxin activates mechanisms in both the intrinsic and the extrinsic coagulation pathways and is experimentally and clinically associated with the development of disseminated intravascular coagulation (58). Endotoxin provokes platelet aggregation and the subsequent release of platelet-derived vasoactive compounds (59).

Endotoxin is a potent activator of the complement cascade via the alternative pathway (60). This biologic effect of endotoxin is thought to be extremely important in the activation of the inflammatory response secondary to soft-tissue contamination, but it is also thought to have a role in the activation of the systemic septic response.

Endotoxin is a potent stimulant to phagocytic cells and the immune system (61). Endotoxin activates phagocytic cells (both neutrophils and macrophages) via activation of complement through specific cleavage products. These bind directly to receptors on the phagocytic cell plasma membrane. Endotoxin activates macrophages directly and stimulates the synthesis of the numerous cytokine chemical signals. These cytokines have the effect of further activating the inflammatory cascade and also have a modulating effect on cellular and humoral immunity. Endotoxin seems to activate neutrophils directly through the CD14 receptor (62) and has been shown to be immunogenic. Sequential administrations of endotoxin produces tolerance in the experimental animal (63). This feature of endotoxin will be further discussed as a potential treatment modality in the septic patient.

Endotoxin has myriad other effects. Although they have extensively studied endotoxin, researchers remain unclear about whether endotoxin affects the cell directly or whether it is simply a potent stimulus to the release of inflammatory mediators, which in turn are the direct effectors. Nevertheless, endotoxin is indeed a potent virulence factor that accounts for many of the features of Gram-negative infection.

Antibiotic Resistance

The introduction of antibiotics into clinical practice is a major advance in the management of patients with bacterial infections. Antibiotics are designed to slow bacterial growth, thereby allowing the host defenses to eradicate the microorganism. Many antibiotics have bactericidal effects in vitro, although whether microorganisms are killed efficiently in vivo remains a point of debate. Nevertheless, antibiotics have significantly improved the outcome of many infections in terms of both survival and recovery time. Unfortunately, the effectiveness of many antibiotics has been seriously compromised by the development of resistance. It has been the generalized use of antibiotics that has led to antibiotic resistance (64).

Resistance is the ability of a formerly sensitive bacteria to a given antibiotic to proliferate in the presence of the drug. Resistance can evolve quickly and may even develop during the course of therapy in a given patient. Conversely, it can be the accumulative consequences of antibiotics in a specific environment. Thus, antibiotic use in the intensive care unit over time may cause the development of resistant pathogens that then become the resident microflora of that environment. Subsequent nosocomial infections reflect these new resistance patterns. The generalized use of antibiotics in our society has resulted in even community-acquired infections that reflect resistance changes. The resistance patterns to penicillin that have occurred with *Staphylococcus aureus* over the past 30 years validates that the entire world of microbial resistance has been changed by antibiotic use.

Resistance may take several forms. It may be the consequences of the organism developing the synthetic capability to produce a neutralizing enzyme, or it may actually reflect structural changes of the microorganism that may eliminate access to the target for the drug. Resistance appears to be a likely problem that will continue to evolve and potentially threatens the use of antibiotic therapy for patients in the 21st century.

To understand the mechanisms of resistance, it is important first to understand sensitivity determinations and how these determinations are made by the clinical laboratory. Standard, reliable, and reproducible methods to provide clinical determinations of sensitivity and resistance of a given organism to a given antibiotic have been the cornerstones of treatment in clinical infectious disease.

The most accurate quantitative method to determine sensitivity is the serial tube dilution method. The microbial isolate is inoculated into a series of tubes containing either agar or broth, each of which have a defined concentration of antibiotics. One is then able quantitatively to define the concentration of antibiotic at which microbial growth is inhibited or, conversely, the concentration at which bacterial activity is present. The minimum inhibitory concentration (MIC) is the drug concentration at which inhibition of bacterial growth occurs, and the minimum bacteriocidal concentration (MBC) defines the drug concentration at which the bacteria are killed. While quantitatively more accurate, the determination of MIC and MBC are expensive for routine use in the clinical laboratory and are reserved largely for use in research.

The disc-diffusion method is the commonly employed method in the clinical laboratory (65). In this method, a 6-mm disc with a threshold concentration of antibiotic is placed onto a freshly inoculated agar plate with the bacterial strain to be tested. The concentration of the antibiotic in the disc defines the break point for the determination of resistance and sensitivity. Because essentially all microorganisms may be inhibited by all available antibiotics if the concentration is high enough, the disc concentration of the drug must be defined in terms of clinically appropriate concentrations. If an antibiotic provides inhibition of bacterial growth at 600 μg/

Table 9.3.
The Effects of an Increased Inoculum of E. coli Bacteria on the Sensitivities of the Microorganisms to Commonly Employed Antibiotics

Antibiotic	Sensitivities of E. coli at Different Inocula[a]	
	10^5	10^7
Ampicillin	2	8
Carbenicillin	<4	32
Cephalothin	8	64
Amikacin	4	32
Gentamicin	1	16
Kanamycin	4	64
Tobramycin	1	16
Chloramphenicol	4	64
Tetracycline	1	32

[a] The sensitivities are expressed in micrograms per milliliter as determined by the tube dilution technique.

mL concentration but the achievable serum concentration is only 32 μg/mL, then in terms of clinical application, the organism is resistant to the antibiotic.

Another important consideration in antibiotic sensitivity is the inoculum effect. If antibiotic activity is governed by the ability of the drug to bind to a critical number of receptor sites on the microorganism, then the bacterial concentration within the environment is important. Thus, an antibiotic that inhibits the growth of an organism when there are 10^5 bacteria/mL may not inhibit the growth when 10^7 to 10^8 bacteria are present. This concentration-dependent activity of an antibiotic is referred to as the inoculum effect. The impact of bacterial concentration on MIC is illustrated in Table 9.3 (66). For commonly used antibiotics, the inoculum effect may have clinical relevance.

Quantitative assessments generally have defined bacterial concentrations at 10^5 organisms per milliliter of fluid or per gram of tissue for most infections. The notable exceptions to this observation are infection with the presence of necrotic tissue and those infections with a pyogenic character. Concentrations in these settings reach 10^7 to 10^8 bacteria/mL. The need for surgical drainage and debridement of these types of infection is further amplified because concentration-dependent resistance for clinically reported sensitive organisms is a certain contributing cause for antibiotic failure in these settings.

Mechanisms of Antibiotic Action

Each group of antibiotic has different mechanisms of action that presumably exploit a metabolic or structural vulnerability of the sensitive organism. The vulnerability of the target site is different in different species, and thus sensitivity to a given drug differs by species, depending on the presence or exposure of the target site.

Antibiotics that attack the outer envelope of the cell are the most common drugs employed in the treatment of clinical infection. These include the penicillins, cephalosporins, monobactams, and carbapenems, which are referred to collectively as β-lactam antibiotics because they have a common structural feature, illustrated in Figure 9.8.

The β-lactam group of antibiotics are bacteriocidal drugs that inhibit the synthesis of the bacterial cell wall. Because the actual enzyme system responsible for cell-wall synthesis lies within the plasma membrane, it is convenient to think of the actions of this group of antibiotics as involving the entire outer envelope of the cell wall and plasma membrane complex.

Knowledge of cell-wall synthesis is important to understanding the actions of β-lactam antibiotics. A critical component of the bacterial cell wall is a complex peptidoglycan. This peptidoglycan is vitally important to control intracellular osmotic regulation. In Gram-positive organisms, the cell wall may be as much as 50 times thicker than in Gram-negative species.

The synthesis of the peptidoglycan portion of the cell wall has three component features (67,68): (a) The monomer unit of the peptidoglycan is synthesized within the bacterial cytoplasm. (b) The monomer is then transported across the plasma membrane, and the polymer is synthesized by the process of transglycosylation. (c) The new polymer is cross-linked to the old cell-wall

structure in the newly formed daughter cells. This occurs after division of the parent bacterium by the process of transpeptidation.

The enzymes responsible for transglycosylation and transpeptidation are identified within the plasma membrane of the bacterial cell. These enzymes covalently bind penicillins and are collectively referred to as penicillin-binding proteins (PBP). Although initially described for penicillins, these binding sites are potential sites for all β-lactam antibiotics. The binding of antibiotics to these membrane enzymes neutralizes the enzyme activity. Thus replicating bacteria in the face of antibiotics that can bind to PBPs do not have the ability within the new daughter cells to complete the cell wall.

Each species of bacteria has a different constellation of PBPs. The affinity and the consequences of binding for each PBP are different between species. Thus the nomenclature and literature on PBPs can be confusing.

The PBPs for *E. coli* are identified in Table 9.4 (69). Binding of an antibiotic to both PBP-1A and PBP-1B affects transglycosylation and transpeptidation; cell lysis is the consequence. Both sites must have threshold-level binding for the antibiotic effects to occur. Binding of only one site does not injure the micro-organism. Mutants with the loss of either binding site become resistant to a previously effective drug. Binding of PBP-2 creates spherical instead of rod shaped bacterial progeny. *E. coli* mutants without the PBP-2 receptor grow as spheres as well. Spherical *E. coli* spontaneously lyse when fully mature for reasons that are not understood. Binding of PBP-3 causes filamentous growth. Filamentous growth also results in cell death. The binding of other *E. coli* PBPs are not identified as having any biological consequences.

Vancomycin is a non-β-lactam antibiotic that also has as its primary biological activity the inhibition of cell-wall synthesis (70). Vancomycin appears to bind to the plasma membrane, but not through the binding of PBPs. Instead, it interferes with the polymerization of normally synthesized monomer units of peptidoglycan. As with β-lactam antibiotics, vancomycin affects actively dividing cells and requires active cell replication to be effective. Unlike β-lactam antibiotics, vancomycin does affect the growth of protoplasts in culture, which reflects

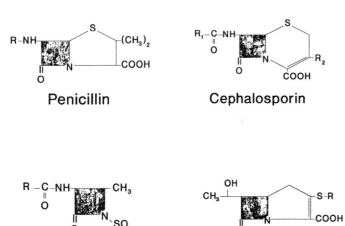

Figure 9.8. The four principal groups of β-lactam antibiotics. The shaded area in each prototype molecule reflects the common lactam ring.

Table 9.4.
Morphologic Changes of E.coli PBP Sites When Bound by β-lactam Antibiotics

PBP	Molecular Weight	PBP-Associated Enzyme Activity	Morphology Seen With Binding
1A	92,000	Transglycosylation Transpeptidation	Cell lysis if 1B is also bound
1B	90,000	Transglycosylation	Cell lysis if 1A is also bound
2	66,000	Transpeptidation	Spherical daughter cells instead of rods
3	60,000	Transglycosylation	Filamentous daughter cells instead of rods
4	49,000	Carboxypeptidation	None known
5	42,000	Carboxypeptidation	None known
6	40,000	Carboxypeptidation	None known

a second mechanism of antibacterial activity, which probably relates to impairment of RNA synthesis.

The antifungal imidazole derivatives affect plasma membrane synthesis and cause lysis of actively dividing cells. The imidazole group of drugs appears to inhibit a demethylation step in the synthesis of lanosterol by binding to one of the cytochrome P-450 enzymes (71). This inhibition results in reduced concentrations of ergosterol, which results in a defective plasma membrane. Synthetic manipulation of the basic imidazole ring has resulted in the compounds of ketoconazole, miconazole, and clotrimazole. These changes have been desirable to reduce potential toxicity by the inhibition of sterol metabolism in humans.

Amphotericin B is another antifungal agent that has the plasma membrane as its primary target, but it does not affect the synthesis of the plasma membrane. Rather, this drug binds to ergosterol, fungisterol, and other sterols in the plasma membrane, which results in alterations of membrane permeability (72). Oxidative damage has also been identified as a potential mechanism of antifungal activity (73). The binding of amphotericin B to sterols poses some problems in that the sterols of mammalian membranes may also be bound, potentially causing some toxicity.

Polymyxin and colistimethate are the last of the outer envelope antimicrobials to be considered here (74). Polymyxin appears to have a detergent effect on the bacterial cell membrane by interacting with the phospholipid component. Plasma membrane injury is thought to cause diffusional loss of intracellular enzymes. This mechanism of action affects resting cells and does not require metabolically active or dividing cells for effect. Binding to plasma membrane poses some toxicity problems because of similar receptor sites on normal tissue plasma membranes.

Certain antibiotics inhibit protein synthesis. Inherent in the effect of such drugs is the ability either to diffuse or to be transported actively into the bacterial cell. The target of these antibiotics is the ribosome (75). The antibiotic binds to the ribosome and inhibits the transcriptional phase of protein synthesis. Chloramphenicol, clindamycin, lincomycin, erythromycin, and tetracycline are drugs that inhibit protein synthesis, but they do not irreversibly bind to the ribosomal target. The reversible nature of binding makes these drugs essentially bacteriostatic in nature. Aminoglycosides irreversibly bind to the ribosome and, therefore, are bacteriocidal.

Several antimicrobial agents have the metabolism of nucleic acids as the primary target. Rifampin (76), the new quinolones (77), and metronidazole (78) inhibit DNA synthesis by binding to the nucleic acid within the nucleus. Antiviral therapy is also targeted at nucleic acid synthesis. Acyclovir, which is the prototype antiviral agent, is a nucleic acid analogue that is incorporated into the new viral genome and has the net effect of preventing new DNA synthesis (79). In addition, the uptake

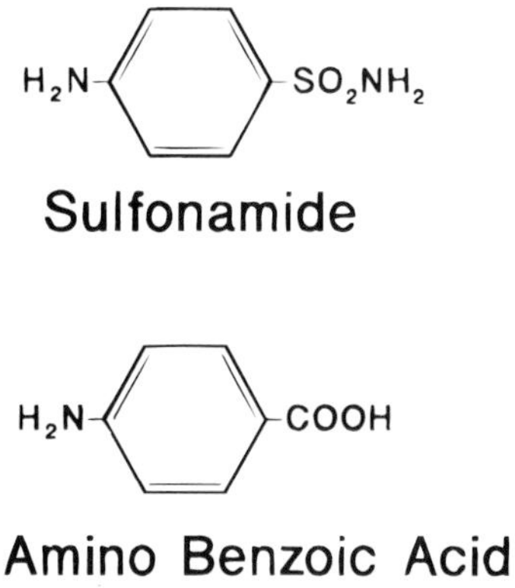

Sulfonamide

Para Amino Benzoic Acid

Figure 9.9. The structural similarities between sulfonamide and *p*-aminobenzoic acid (PABA). Competitive inhibition by sulfonamide of PABA metabolism can be appreciated from these similarities.

of acyclovir also results in its intracellular phosphorylation, which inhibits viral DNA polymerases (80).

Sulfonamides and trimethoprim represent the prototype of the antimetabolite group of antibiotics. Sulfonamides have a metabolic reaction as their target rather than a structural component of the microbial cell. The sulfonamide molecule is a competitive inhibitor of the incorporation of *p*-aminobenzoic acid into tetrahydrofolic acid (81) (Fig. 9.9). This competitive inhibition is a reversible process (bacteriocidal). Trimethoprim is an inhibitor of bacterial dihydrofolate reductase, which is the enzyme step following the one blocked by sulfonamide in folic acid metabolism (82).

Genetics of Resistance

Resistance to antibiotics is the consequence of phenotypic differences between resistant and sensitive strains (83). The phenotypic changes are genetically mediated, although as will be discussed, the genetic material to mediate the phenotypic change can be acquired from the environment or from other bacteria even in the fully mature bacterial cell. The ability to acquire resistance means that resistance of sensitive organisms can occur rapidly, even during a course of therapy.

Intrinsic resistance becomes a characteristic of certain bacteria against certain antibiotics. These bacteria have never had a penicillin-binding protein for a given β-lactam and have always been resistant to these drugs. Certain bacteria may not permit the diffusion or transport of an antibiotic across the cell wall-plasma membrane complex. In this latter group, antibiotics that have ribosomes or nucleic acids as their target sites will not be effective. Intrinsic resistance is constant over time and is commonly used in the clinical laboratory as a means to subspeciate organisms.

Acquired resistance may occur by a variety of different mechanisms. Spontaneous mutation may cause a structural or biochemical change that results in a permanent change in the phenotypic expression of that bacterial cell and its progeny. Mutation may change cell wall-plasma membrane permeability or may change the presentation of plasma membrane receptor sites. Mutations may have metabolic sequelae, such as mutants that increase dihydrofolate reductase production and overcome the growth inhibition from trimethoprim.

Mutation is an infrequent event with a probability of 10^{-7} to 10^{-10} for any bacterial cell during a generation (84). Mutations that affect drug sensitivity are, fortunately, the least common genetic changes that occur spontaneously.

The consequence of a mutation that imparts drug resistance during a course of therapy means that sensitive strains will be eradicated, whereas the resistant strain will proliferate and soon become the predominant isolate. Fortunately, such mutations are infrequent in the management of a given patient; however, the accumulative effect of a mutation over time and the selection pressure created by extensive antibiotic use mean that resistance trends in specialty units with very ill patients is a virtual certainty.

Plasmids represent the most common mechanism for the acquisition of resistance by a bacterial cell (85). Plasmids are extrachromosomal genetic material that can be acquired by a number of different mechanisms and cause phenotypic changes in the bacterial cell. Phenotypic changes that can be acquired from plasmids are identified in Table 9.5. Antibiotic resistance from plasmids may give the bacterial cell the capability to produce neutralizing enzymes that reduce antibiotic effectiveness or may mediate structural changes.

Transduction is one means for a bacterial cell to acquire plasmids (86). Infection of a bacterial cell by a bacteriophage may bring entrapped plasmids with the viral particle. The new genetic material may actually be incorporated into the genome of the bacteria itself. Thus a bacteriophage either may confer resistance by carrying plasmids as new extrachromosomal resistance or may actually introduce a chromosomal change by insertion of its own genome into that of the infected bacteria.

Transformation is the process by which plasmids may be acquired from the environment about the bacterial cell (86). Plasmids are nonchromosomal segments of genetic material that can be internalized within the bacterial cytoplasm and change phenotypic expression of the cell. Death and subsequent lysis of bacteria cause the

release of both chromosomal and extrachromosomal genetic material into the environment. Indeed, plasmids may have been derived originally from the release of chromosomal material that was then assimilated by other microorganisms but was not incorporated into the chromosomal configuration of the recipient microbe.

Direct cell-to-cell transfer of plasmids occurs via the process of conjugation (86). Sex pili of bacteria permit the transfer of genetic material from one bacterium to another and provide the means for plasmid transfer. This is a common mechanism for the transfer of resistance, particularly among the Gram-negative Enterobacteriaceae.

Resistance to β-Lactam Antibiotics

Resistance to β-lactam antibiotics may occur by several mechanisms, but the predominant mechanism is either hydrolysis or enzyme-substrate binding by the enzyme β-lactamase. β-lactamase production in some concentration has been identified in essentially every bacterial species. The enzymes generally work by hydrolysis of the amide bond on the lactam ring, which neutralizes the drug activity. Hundreds of different β-lactamase enzymes have been reported since the initial isolation by Abraham and Chain in 1940 (87).

The near ubiquitous nature of β-lactamase among all bacterial species is secondary to normal chromosomal genetic information. Because β-lactamase actually was identified before the use of antibiotics in clinical practice, its biological role may have been to protect the cell from naturally occurring β-lactam compounds that may have been produced by competing fungal species within the microenvironment. β-lactamase may actually serve a biologic role in the polymerization process of peptidoglycans as part of the normal biosynthesis of the cell wall.

Each β-lactamase enzyme has unique features and activity. Some are active against only penicillins, whereas others are only active against cephalosporins. Of course, some β-lactamases have a more general scope of activity against both groups of drugs. Initially, the activity of β-lactamase enzymes was measured in terms of the rate of hydrolysis of a common substrate, either benzylpenicillin or cephaloridine. More sophisticated systems for classification and characterization of activity are employed, using isoelectric focusing, gene mapping, and other chemical analysis techniques (88,89).

Plasmids have now permitted formerly sensitive strains of bacteria to acquire resistance to β-lactam antibiotics (90). The plasmid mechanism for acquiring resistance via production of this enzyme is a much greater source of resistance than from naturally derived β-lactamase.

The identification of *Pseudomonas* spp. that develop resistance as a function of the ability to produce β-lactamase but produce a form that does not hydrolyze the antibiotic in question raised the issue of alternative

---

Table 9.5.
Phenotypic Changes Mediated by Plasmids in Bacteria

Antibiotic Resistance
Anabolic Pathways
Bacteriophage Resistance
Catabolic Pathways
Detergent Resistance
Gene Transfer
Metal Resistance
Radiation Resistance
Replication Changes

mechanisms of antibiotic neutralization. The nonhydrolytic activity of β-lactamase may be the consequence of the nonreversible binding of the enzyme to the antibiotic with the subsequent formation of an enzyme-substrate complex that neutralizes the drug effect. The antibiotic bound with the enzyme may not be able to bind to the PBPs of the membrane or it may not have its customary effects when bound at the PBP.

Enzyme-antibiotic binding appears to occur from β-lactamases that are derived from the normal chromosome of the bacterial cell. Binding β-lactamase rather than hydrolyzing it appears to be inducible by gene derepression and may be another mechanism for the evolution of resistance during therapy. Because gene expression and control of extrachromosomal plasmids is not thought to be under regulation by repressor genes, β-lactamase induction is believed to be of chromosomal origin. Enzyme-antibiotic binding activity of β-lactamase appears to be less specific than the hydrolysis activity of other β-lactamases. This results in cross-resistance that spans other β-lactam antibiotics as well. This cross-resistance mechanism can actually cause antagonism between two simultaneously used antibiotics, because the induction of β-lactamase by one can provoke resistance to the second (91).

β-lactamases of Gram-positive bacteria are principally those that are identified from *Staphylococcus* spp. Staphylococcal β-lactamase is plasmid derived and has a relatively specific activity against penicillins. It does not have activity against the cephalosporin group of antibiotics. Chemical substitution around the β-lactam ring at the R_1 site in the semisynthetic penicillins of methicillin, oxacillin, and nafcillin has resulted in allosteric inhibition of β-lactamase activity, causing the semisynthetic drugs to have antistaphylococcal activity. When resistance develops to any of the semisynthetic penicillins or to any of the first-generation cephalosporins, resistance develops to all. The so-called methicillin-resistant staphylococci are resistant because of mutations that have changed the PBPs and not because of β-lactamase enzyme activity (92).

The β-lactamases from Gram-negative bacteria are heterogeneous. Resistance may be derived from either plasmids or the bacterial chromosome. Acquired resistance is generally from plasmids, and induced resistance is generally chromosomal in origin. Five classes of β-lactamases found in Gram-negative bacteria have been classified by Richmond and Sykes (93) (Table 9.6).

The β-lactamase from the anaerobic *Bacteroides* spp. represents a sixth class of Gram-negative enzyme that is analogous to the Richmond type I class (see Table 9.6). The β-lactamase from *Bacteroides* spp. is usually chromosomally derived, but plasmid-mediated enzymes have been reported. The β-lactamase of *Bacteroides* spp. has been sensitive to the β-lactamase inhibitors of clavulanic acid and sulbactam. Thus β-lactamase inhibitors have been employed to expand the spectrum of antibiotics

Table 9.6.
Five Types of β-lactamases Classified by Richmand and Sykes

Class	Genetic Location	Principal Substrate	Bacterial Source
I	Chromosome	Cephalosporins	Enterobacter Serratia Pseudomonas
II	Chromosome	Penicillins	Pseudomonas
III	Plasmid	Penicillins and Cephalosporins	E. coli Pseudomonas
IV	Chromosome	Penicillins and Cephalosporins	E. coli Pseudomonas
V	Plasmid	Penicillin	E. coli Pseudomonas

that generally do not have activity against *B. fragilis* (e.g., ampicillin).

Finally, there are non-β-lactamase mechanisms that mediate resistance to β-lactam antibiotics. Particularly in Gram-negative bacteria, mutation-mediated phenotypic changes may impede or prevent the antibiotic from penetrating the outer membrane and gaining access to the target proteins on the plasma membrane. The inability of the antibiotic to penetrate the outer membrane may represent changes in the porin proteins. As noted, changes in the affinity of the antibiotic to the PBPs, synthesis of new PBPs that are not bound by the antibiotic in question, or up regulation of PBP synthesis may cause more binding sites that can be blocked by tolerable concentrations of the drug. Modification of PBPs appears to be the principal mechanism of the evolving resistance of methicillin resistance among *Staphylococcus aureus* and *Staphylococcus epidermidis*.

Resistance to Aminoglycoside Antibiotics

Since 1970, the aminoglycoside group of antibiotics has been the most commonly used antibiotics for the treatment of infections with Gram-negative bacteria. Gentamicin, tobramycin, and amikacin are the aminoglycosides that are most commonly used intravenously. Neomycin is used as an orally administered, nonabsorbed drug for intestinal antisepsis. Streptomycin and kanamycin are parenteral aminoglycosides that are extinct because of toxicity.

The aminocyclitol group of antibiotics have similar mechanisms of action as the aminoglycosides and should be considered here. The prototype drug of this group is spectinomycin. The aminocyclitol antibiotics bind to ribosomes in an irreversible fashion and inhibit protein synthesis. Because there is no competitive inhibition between the aminocyclitols and the aminoglycosides, it would appear that they have different receptor sites on the ribosomes. The aminocyclitols are less toxic and may have a separate transport mechanism that excludes them from the cell populations in which the aminoglycoside display their toxicity.

The aminoglycosides are transported actively into the bacteria's cytoplasm by a transport process that is ATP-dependent. This results in the concentration of the drug within the cell that is significantly greater than that which exists outside the cell. The absence of a transport mechanism excludes the aminoglycosides from the cytoplasm of human cells, except, unfortunately, for the proximal renal tubular and cochlear cells. Although the primary target of aminoglycoside activity is thought to be the irreversible binding to ribosomal sites, the marked bacteriocidal effects of these drugs suggests that other mechanisms of toxicity may be operational.

Resistance to aminoglycosides (and presumably aminocyclitols) can occur by the three following mechanisms: (a) Drug transport into the cell may be impaired by mutations that down-regulate the active transport mechanisms. Fortunately, this mutation is infrequent, because all aminoglycosides apparently use the same transport mechanism, and loss of transport efficiency would cause comprehensive resistance against all aminoglycosides. (b) A mutational loss of affinity for ribosomal binding sites would increase resistance. This mechanism has only been identified with streptomycin but looms as a potential source of resistance for the future. (c) Enzymatic conjugation of the aminoglycoside may occur. Unlike β-lactamase hydrolysis, which occurs external to the cell, aminoglycoside conjugation is an intracellular event mediated by enzymes, which are encoded on plasmids. These enzymes can cause N-acetylation, O-phosphorylation, or O-adenylation of the aminoglycoside and thus neutralizes its intracellular effects (94). All aminoglycosides are vulnerable to this mechanism. Enzymes that are targeted to a specific aminoglycoside do not necessarily cross-react with others; however, because these conjugation enzymes are on plasmids, transfer of resistance to other bacteria is a real concern.

Resistance to Tetracyclines

Tetracyclines are transported actively across the plasma membrane and bind to the 30s ribosome in a reversible and concentration-dependent fashion. This binding blocks the important bonding of tRNA to the mRNA-ribosome complex.

Resistance to tetracyclines appears to be via two plasmid-mediated mechanisms: (a) the active transport of the drug is rendered ineffective; and (b) the bacterial cell may develop the capability to actively eliminate the drug from the cytoplasm, thereby keeping the antibiotic concentrations within the cell suboptimal (95). No known enzyme systems exist to degrade or conjugate tetracyclines. Because mammalian cells do not have the transport mechanism for tetracyclines, the toxicity of this group of antibiotics in humans is minimal.

Resistance to Chloramphenicol

Chloramphenicol, with its highly publicized toxicity (aplastic anemia), has continued to have some use for the treatment of infections involving *Haemophilus influenzae*, meningococcus, and anaerobic pathogens. It is a small molecule and penetrates the central nervous system effectively. Like tetracycline, chloramphenicol is transported into the cell and then binds to the 50s ribosome. The binding is reversible.

Resistance is primarily via the plasmid-mediated production of the enzyme chloramphenicol acetyltransferase (96). The acetylation occurs within the cell cytoplasm. Newer fluorinated chloramphenicol derivatives appear to resist acetylation by this enzyme. Mutant strains of bacteria may have a chromosomally mediated reduction in the transport efficiency of chloramphenicol, which also effectively excludes the fluorinated derivatives as well.

Resistance to Sulfonamide and Trimethoprim

Sulfonamide and trimethoprim are commonly employed together because they have a tandem effect on sequential steps of the biosynthesis of tetrahydrofolate. Sulfonamides inhibit the enzyme dihydropteroate synthetase by competitive inhibition of *p*-aminobenzoic acid, which reacts with aminohydroxy-tetrahydropteridine to form tetrahydropteroic acid. Trimethoprim then blocks the subsequent step by inhibition of the enzyme dihydrofolate reductase.

Resistance to sulfonamides and trimethoprim may occur by four separate mechanisms: (a) the bacterial cell may naturally or by chromosomal mutation exclude the antibiotics from penetrating the cytoplasm; (b) plasmid-mediated alternative enzymes may bypass the sites of inhibition in folate metabolism; and (c) induction of *p*-aminobenzoic acid synthesis may overcome the inhibition achieved by sulfonamide, and probably reflects derepression of chromosomal gene expression (97–99). Enzymatic degradation of one or both of these antibiotics is suspected, but has not been proven.

Resistance to Erythromycin

Erythromycin is transported into the cell and binds to the 50s ribosome. Because there is competitive inhibition with chloramphenicol, these two antibiotics appear to have a common binding site. Binding to the ribosome is reversible.

Resistance is mediated by four mechanisms: (a) there appears to be both a plasmid- and chromosomal-mediated transformation in the ribosomal binding sites; (b) chromosomal mutation may exclude the antibiotic from penetration of the cellular cytomatrix; (c) some evidence suggests that enzymatic removal of the drug from the cell may be a chromosomally mediated mechanism for some resistant mutants (100,101); and (d) an erythromycin esterase that hydrolyzes the drug has been identified (102).

Resistance to Clindamycin and Lincomycin

The lincosamide antibiotics have similar actions to that of erythromycin and chloramphenicol in that they too bind to the 50s ribosome and binding is similarly reversible. Resistance is mediated by both plasmid and chromosomal mutation and follows the same pattern as erythromycin (103).

Resistance to Vancomycin

The evolution of methicillin-resistant *Staphylococcus aureus* and *Staphylococcus epidermidis* has rejuvenated the use of vancomycin. As noted earlier, it inhibits cell-wall synthesis but not through PBPs. Thus, mutational changes that render the semisynthetic penicillins and cephalosporins ineffective do not neutralize the effects of vancomycin.

Unfortunately, resistance to vancomycin appears to be developing. Although not well-studied as yet because of limited numbers of bacterial isolates, three mechanisms appear likely. Drug penetration of a mutationally transformed and more complex cell wall seems to be one likely mechanism. A reduction in the affinity for the vancomycin receptor on the plasma membrane seems even more likely. A reduction in the role of peptidoglycan in the construction of the cell wall is the third proposed mechanism.

Resistance to Metronidazole

Metronidazole penetrates the sensitive bacterial cell, is reduced to a short half-life, toxic intermediate, and then mediates damage to the DNA and other macromolecular structures within the cell. Resistance is rare but is probably the result of delayed bacterial cell penetration or alteration of the reduction process that produces the toxic intermediate (104). Resistance appears to be chromosomally mediated.

Resistance to Other Antibiotics

From the previous discussion, it should be possible to predict the mechanisms that already exist but have not necessarily been defined and are responsible for resistance among those drugs not discussed. Resistance to monobactams is likely to be mediated by β-lactamase. Resistance to the new quinolone antibiotics is likely to be the consequence of the inability of the drug to penetrate the cytoplasm of the bacteria or changes in the nuclear enzyme target (105,106). Acyclovir resistance is likely to be from changes in the viral thymidine kinase or changes in the DNA polymerase (107). By understanding the mechanisms responsible for antibiotic activity, it should be possible to anticipate reasonably the mechanisms of resistance.

Environmentally Mediated Resistance

In vitro determinations of antibiotic resistance are made within the clinical laboratory under ideal conditions. A standardized inoculum of 10^5 bacteria/mL is used. The environment is well-oxygenated, and an optimal neutral pH is employed. There is no protein in the environment to bind the antibiotic and alter drug activity.

The microenvironment of acute bacterial infection is different from that in the clinical laboratory. The bacterial concentrations may be 10^7 to 10^8 organisms/mL (108). An increased concentration of bacteria means that an increased number of target sites are available for the antibiotic and an increased threshold of sites to be bound are necessary for the antibiotic effect. This antibiotic inoculum effect, as discussed previously, likely explains the clinical failures that are encountered when the cultured bacteria are sensitive to the antibiotics employed.

The microenvironment of suppurative infection is anaerobic and acidic (108). Those antibiotics that are transported actively into the bacterial cell (e.g., aminoglycosides) will not be transported into the cell during anaerobiosis by this oxygen-dependent mechanism (109). Similarly, the acid environment affects the proton gradient necessary for aminoglycoside activity. Because the microenvironment is rich in protein exudate from the inflammatory response, necrosis of tissue, and dissolution of phagocytic cells, protein binding is a major issue in neutralizing certain highly protein-bound antibiotics.

The description of high bacterial count, acid pH, anaerobiosis, and high protein concentrations is the environment of pus. Antibiotics in this environment will not be effective. For the surgeon, these considerations underscore that even in the high-tech environment of contemporary medicine, pus still needs to be drained.

Determinants of Infection: The Microenvironment

Because every open soft-tissue injury and every surgical wound has some degree of bacterial contamination, a critical threshold of bacterial numbers is necessary to cause clinical infection. Most surgical and traumatic wounds do not become infected, even though culturable bacteria can be isolated from the wound surface. For a given level of virulence, a specific density of bacteria must be present to create the clinical inflammatory response known as infection.

To produce a clinical infection in subcutaneous fat, the density of bacteria needed would be approximately 10^5 colony-forming units (cfu) per gram of tissue (110). Thus, even a poorly vascularized area, such as subcutaneous tissue, requires large numbers of bacteria to cause clinical disease. The presence of adjuvant factors in the wound may lower the number of necessary bacteria. Silk sutures reduce the threshold of bacterial density by 10^2 to 10^3 to cause infection (111). Bacteria with unusual and potent virulence factors may require relatively few bacteria to cause severe and even life-threatening situations. Such is the case with clostridial gangrene or tetanus following a puncture wound.

Because skeletal muscle is vascularized, it rarely becomes the primary site for infection even in the face of massive contamination. Muscle tissues only become the haven for bacterial infection when the blood supply is compromised. Thus the toxin from *Clostridium perfringens* results in necrosis of muscle, which in turn becomes the growth media for a host of other proliferating bacteria. In necrotizing fasciitis, the advancing line of bacteria moves through the relatively avascular plane of the fascia and only secondarily causes muscle necrosis as the blood vessels, which perforate the fascial layer and perfuse the muscle, are thrombosed.

The threshold of 10^5 bacteria is identified again in other areas. Greater than 10^5 cfu/mL of urine is considered the critical value for conformation of a diagnosis of urinary tract infection (112). Quantitative cultures of 10^5 to 10^6 cfu/mL of tracheal aspirates have been purported to define pulmonary infection, although there remains considerable debate whether tracheal specimens truly reflect the density of bacteria that are present in the lower respiratory tract (113,114).

In other areas, the number of bacteria necessary to cause infection is uncertain. In the peritoneal cavity, the type of bacteria and the presence of adjuvant factors may be more important than the actual bacterial numbers. Because intravascular devices represent a direct conduit into the bloodstream, relatively small numbers of bacteria disseminated via these mechanisms are necessary to cause clinical sequelae.

Adjuvant Factors

Work in the research laboratory clearly illustrates the importance of adjuvant factors. The peritoneal cavity of rodents is virtually impossible to infect without the use of lysed red cells, mucus, or foreign bodies to augment the infectious process. The role of these adjuvant factors is thought to be either stimulation of bacterial proliferation or impairment of host defenses. Adjuvant factors may either be locally active or systemic events.

Among local factors, hemoglobin may be the most potent adjuvant factor. Clot or hematoma within the surgical or traumatic wound reduces the number of bacterial contaminants necessary to cause infection. The mechanism of the adjuvant effect of hemoglobin remains unclear. Polk and Miles suggested that ferric ion derived from hemoglobin degeneration may be a potent growth factor for bacterial proliferation (115). Pruett and

associates concluded after a lengthy series of experiments that bacterial metabolism of hemoglobin produces a leukotoxin that retards phagocytic cells (38). In selected patients with hemolysis, hemoglobin may also be a systemic factor in the exacerbation of septic events.

Foreign bodies reduce the number of bacteria necessary to cause infection. Suture material, vascular grafts, heart valves, and other prosthetic materials increased infection rates in patients. Foreign bodies left in traumatic wounds will become the focus of infection. Perforations of the distal gastrointestinal tract are associated with foreign bodies such as fiber, exfoliated cells, and other debris from the gut to augment the probability of infection. It is unclear what mechanism is responsible for the adjuvantive effects of foreign bodies other than an adverse host defense effect.

Dead tissue remains an important adjuvant. Dead tissue serves both as a substitute for bacterial proliferation and as a haven for bacteria growth, unencumbered by host defense mechanisms. Recently, it has become clear that necrotic tissue is a potent stimulus to the host's inflammatory responses. Thus, clinical infection in wounds is likely to be the consequence of the additive effects of necrotic tissue and bacteria.

Fibrin represents another clinical variable that may be viewed as being either an adjuvant factor for bacterial growth or a positive nonspecific host defense variable. Studies in experimental peritonitis have shown that bacteria imbedded in a fibrin clot will cause abscess and death of experimental animals compared with intraperitoneal bacteria released free into the peritoneal cavity (116). Several publications have demonstrated a beneficial effect of heparin on animal models of peritonitis and have suggested that the salutary effects are secondary to the prevention of the fibrin matrix within the peritoneal cavity (117,118). In addition, because antibiotics generally penetrate the fibrin matrix poorly, the fibrin matrix could protect bacteria from the effects of these drugs. However, the localization effects of fibrin may serve to prevent dissemination of bacteria and in that respect have a positive benefit when bacterial concentrations within the peritoneal cavity are large.

Systemic adjuvant factors may likewise affect local vulnerability to infection and may facilitate the dissemination of bacteria and lead to the septic state. Hypoxemia reduces the availability of oxygen at the interface between the host and the potential pathogens. Molecular oxygen is necessary for the oxidation burst of the neutrophil, which is necessary for the synthesis of reactive oxygen intermediates necessary for intercellular killing of phagocyte and bacteria (Fig. 9.10). Hemorrhagic shock and hypervolemia likewise impair the delivery of oxygen and substrate to the area of injury and contamination. It may also contribute to local infection by impairment of the egress of acid end products of the host-pathogen interaction (119,120). Experimental data have implicated blood transfusion as an immune sup-

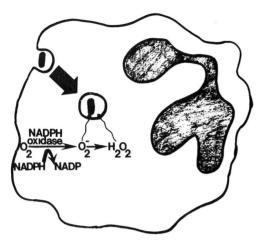

Figure 9.10. The NADPH oxidase pathway generates toxic oxygen intermediates from molecular oxygen with the neutrophil.

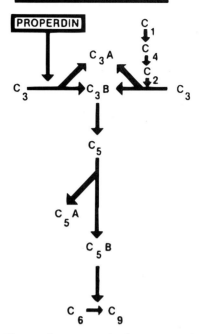

Figure 9.11. The complement cascade. The separate pathways of initiation of complement activation move through either the properdin pathway or the classic pathway.

pressant (121,122). Clinical data have been reported that identify an increased rate of infectious complications with blood transfusion as an independently associated variable (123,124).

Underlying conditions may be systemic variables in the enhancement of bacterial infection. Considerable clinical suspicion has focused on the increased incidence of infections in diabetic patients. Efforts to define specific abnormalities have been inconsistent, and the microvascular disease of diabetes may also contribute to this apparent predisposition to infection (125). Multiple-organ injury has been associated with increased infection morbidity and probably represents the added inflammatory potentiation of tissue necrosis plus bacterial contamination (126).

Malnutrition has been studied exhaustively and appears to affect all components of host responsiveness. A blunted inflammatory response, altered neutrophil functions, and adversely affected delayed hypersensitivity skin testing have all been recognized. What remains less clear is the degree of nutritional repletion necessary to reverse these adversarial parameters. Although delayed hypersensitivity skin tests and in vitro studies of immune function can be reversed by various formulations of nutritional support, clinical data showing improved patient outcome are difficult to identify.

Finally, drugs may represent a systemic variable predisposing to an increased risk of infection. Exogenous steroid use has a generalized dampening effect on all components of host responsiveness to bacteria. Acute and chronic alcoholism has been identified as producing specific abnormalities of host responsiveness. This is important because a high frequency of alcoholism exists among the trauma patient population (127,128).

In summary, adjuvant effects amplify bacterial virulence or repress host responsiveness. The consequence is that fewer bacteria per gram of tissue or per milliliter of body fluid is necessary to trigger clinical infection. Indeed, adjuvant factors may be more important vari-

ables than the actual numbers of contaminating bacteria for identifying clinical infection.

Host Defense

From the perspective of surgical infection, one can categorize host defenses into several distinct components. Nonspecific host defenses are designed to prevent access of microorganisms to the tissues of the host. Nonspecific host defenses can include the glottis mechanism of the airway, which limits contamination of the lung during the process of eating or swallowing, or the integument that serves as a veneer against potential contaminants. Mucins and secretory antibodies become nonspecific mechanisms by preventing bacterial adherence to epithelial cells.

The phagocytic-inflammatory component of host defense represents the initial response to tissue injury and contamination. The role of the phagocytic-inflammatory response is local containment of the contamination and its incipient infection. The complement cascade becomes activated and releases opsonins and chemotactic signals as cleavage products to both attract phagocytic cells and facilitate phagocytic function (Fig. 9.11). Mast cells release inflammatory proteins to flood the injured area with plasma proteins by increasing microvascular permeability. These changes facilitate phagocytic cell access to the area of contamination. Phagocytic cells attempt to eradicate both microorganisms and other adjuvants (e.g., foreign material and dead tissue). Neutrophils are the first phagocytic cells to appear in the area; macrophages appear within 24 hours.

The mobilization of macrophage cells into the evolving inflammation becomes the bridge between the local containment response and the systemic response. The systemic response is associated with fever, which is mediated by the release of IL-1 and other endogenous pyrogens. Other cytokines prime the systemic response by up regulation of acute phase reactants. Fixed macrophages of the hepatic and splenic reticuloendothelial systems become filters to remove microorganisms or microaggregated debris from the systemic circulation. Finally, the macrophage becomes pivotal in presentation of antigen to the lymphocyte, which initiates the immune response. The anti-infective role of the immune response appears limited for bacterial infections.

Thus the host defenses of the patient are pitted against the numbers and virulence potential of the contaminating microorganisms. Adjuvant factors and variables within the microenvironment may impair host defense or facilitate microbial virulence, with the net effect being the amplification of the infectious potential. For a specific contaminating event, infection as an outcome becomes the biological summation of positive host defense mechanisms versus the aggregate negative effects of microbial numbers, virulence, and adjuvant effects.

Specific Infections

The Wound

A wound may be from either a traumatic event or may be a controlled incision. The wound transgresses the skin, which represents the primary nonspecific host defense protection against infection. A laceration or incision results in disruption of blood vessels and devitalization of tissues. Injury and blood vessel disruption cause activation of the complement cascade (129). This in turn activates the coagulation mechanism and the activation of the mast cells. Activation of the mast cell releases an array of inflammatory proteins, including kinins and histamines. The mast cell inflammatory proteins provide for edema formation as capillary permeability changes and protein-rich plasma suffuses the injured area. This imports additional complement and coagulation proteins, which are further activated at the site of injury.

The epicenter of the wound now represents a concentrated area of activated complement cleavage products, activated coagulation proteins, and inflammatory proteins from mast cell release (Fig. 9.12). Diffusion of these activated products into adjacent areas about the perimeter of the injury become chemotactic signals to attract neutrophils into the area.

While chemotactic signals do attract neutrophils into the inflammatory site, these chemical signals mediate changes in the endothelial cell surface and on the surface of the neutrophil (130). Upregulation of P-selectin and E-selectin as adhesion receptors on the endothelial surface of the post-capillary venule results in binding to counter-receptors on the neutrophil, which initiates the rolling or slowing of the neutrophil at the wall of the vessel (131). A constitutively expressed L-selectin receptor on the neutrophil binds to its counterreceptor on the endothelial cell as part of this rolling adhesion event. The "slowed" neutrophil is stopped completely at the endothelial cell surface by the tight binding of the transformed neutrophil integrin (CD11/CD18) receptors on the chemotactically stimulated neutrophil to the constitutively expressed Intercellular Adhesion Molecules (ICAM) of the endothelial cell (132).

The binding of integrins of the neutrophil to the ICAMs of the endothelial cell completes the process traditionally known as margination. The endothelial cell expression of surface Platelet Activating Factor (PAF) apparently serves as a priming signal to the bound neutrophil (133). The process of neutrophil priming puts the phagocytic cell into a state of readiness for rapid response when encountering a second signal (e.g., bacteria, endotoxin). The chemical gradient of chemotactic signals from the epicenter of the inflammatory focus becomes a "beacon" to direct the neutrophil toward the site of provocation.

Following the direction of the chemotactic signals, the neutrophil moves toward the focus of injury by the process of diapedesis (134). The signals stimulating chemotaxis become greater and more concentrated. The process progressively activates more receptor sites on the neutrophil surface to provoke the full state of phagocytic activation. Contact of the neutrophil with opsonized foreign particles activates the process of phagocytosis (135–137). Phagocytosis represents the internalization of the foreign particle to create a phagosome within the cytoplasm of the neutrophil. The phagosome is a sphere of plasma membrane within the cytoplasm of the neutrophil. The phagosome then fuses with lysosomal bodies, which are rich in acid hydrolases and other digestive enzymes, to begin the process of intracellular killing (if the particle is a microorganism) and digestion (138). Reactive oxygen intermediates are secreted actively into the phagosome. These are important participants in the digestion of the internalized particle and the activation of lysosomal enzymes (139).

Circulating monocytes and resident tissue macrophages are similarly drawn into the area of injury by the same chemical signals that resulted in neutrophil migration. The large macrophage cell appears to mobi-

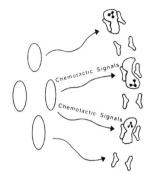

A. Margination

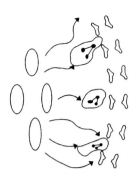

B. Diapedesis and Chemotaxis

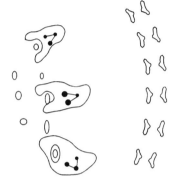

C. Phagocytosis

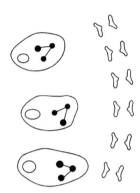

D. Intracellular Killing and Digestion

Figure 9.12. The phases of neutrophil function. **A,** Chemotactic signals form a source of contamination or active infection becomes a siren to initiate neutrophil margination to the endothelial cell at the area of injury. **B,** The chemical gradient of the chemotactic signal results in a directional movement of the neutrophil toward the bacterial source. **C,** The neutrophil then ingests the foreign particle or bacterium via phagocytosis. **D,** Intercellular killing and digestion completes the process.

Table 9.7.
Mediators Responsible For Cell-to-Cell Interactions[a]

Class of Mediator	Definition of Class	Example of Class
Autocrine - Intracellular	A mediator, synthesized within a cell with a target within the same cell	PgE synthesized within muscle cells and then promote proteolysis within same cell
Autocrine - Extracellular	A mediator that is synthesized and released external to that cell, which either has itself or the same cell population as its target.	TNF is released by stimulated macrophages and then stimulates membrane receptors on its own membrane or other macrophages membranes.
Paracrine	A mediator that is synthesized and released to target another cell population in the immediate vicinity.	TNF is released by macrophages and stimulates receptors on adjacent neutrophils.
Endocrine	A mediator that is synthesized and released to target another target site that is remote and requires the chemical signal to travel via the blood stream to reach the effort site.	Interleukin-1 is released by macrophages and travels via the blood stream to stimulate hypothalamic receptors to provoke the febrile response.

[a] Although autocrine, paracrine, endocrine seem to be distinct classifications, a given mediator may fit into more than one category or may actually serve all three functions (e.g., TNF).

lize more slowly; macrophage infiltration does not occur until 24 to 48 hours after the primary inciting event. However, unlike neutrophils, the full activation of the macrophage by complement cleavage products, inflammatory proteins, and foreign particles results in the release of numerous cytokine signals (140), which have important autocrine, paracrine, and endocrine functions (Table 9.7).

The release of IL-1 by the macrophage initiates a systemic response to the injury by endocrine dissemination of this chemical signal (141) (Table 9.8). Locally released IL-1 diffuses into the intravascular compartment and is carried to the hypothalamic area of the brain where specific nuclei are stimulated. Prostaglandin E (PGE) is synthesized and appears to be the effector (final messenger) that diffuses into the central nervous system and provokes the efferent limb of the febrile response (142). Autonomic control results in peripheral vasoconstriction, which serves to reduce heat convection and gives the patient a sense of chilling because of skin coolness. The

Table 9.8.
Effects Stimulated by IL-1

Fever
Neutrophilia
Hypoferremia
Hypozincemia
Hypercupremia
Up regulation: Hepatic acute phase reactants (e.g., C-reactive protein)
Down-Regulation: Hepatic albumin synthesis
Stimulation of Muscle Proteolysis
Increase in Amino Acid Oxidation
Stimulation of Thymocyte Proliferation
Stimulation of Immunoglobulin Synthesis
Modulation of T-Helper/T-Suppressor Cells
Enhancement of Natural Killer Cell Activity
Stimulation of Fibroblasts

centrally mediated shivering response provokes increased heat production. The combined vasoconstriction and shivering responses cause an increased core body temperature.

IL-1 has other effector responses in addition to being an endogenously derived pyrogen (143). IL-1 promotes neutrophilia by mobilization of both the systemic margination reserves of neutrophils and by direct bone marrow stimulation. IL-1 stimulates the up regulation of acute phase reactants by the liver. Increased transferrin production binds iron, reduces circulating serum iron concentrations, and accordingly reduces the availability of this important ion necessary to promote bacterial proliferation. IL-1 up-regulates the hepatic synthesis of C-reactive protein and other acute phase proteins, which are thought to have opsonic functions. IL-1 up-regulates hepatic synthesis of complement components. IL-1 down-regulates the hepatic synthesis of albumin, which, if sustained, will obviously impact serum albumin concentrations. This latter function of IL-1 underscores why serum albumin cannot be used as a measure of nutritional assessment in seriously ill patients—the inflammatory response triggers a down regulation of hepatic albumin synthesis, which is independent of the adequacy of the protein nutritional state.

The stimulated macrophage cell within the wound produces the potent autocrine and paracrine cytokine, tumor necrosis factor (TNF) (144). The release of TNF within the wound injury environment serves the important autocrine function of self-stimulation of the monocytes and macrophages to their full states of activation. This self-stimulated state fully activates the production of a vast array of cytokine and inflammatory protein signals. Although the complete scope of physiologic functions of these cytokine signals remains to be defined, the paracrine function of TNF to stimulate neutrophils to full activation appears to be a critical local function (145). Indeed, one might view the macrophage as being the barometer of the seriousness of a contaminating or wounding event. The full activation of the macrophage means that full mobilization of the inflammatory

response is to follow. The biologic "foot soldier" (known as the neutrophil) is then driven to a frenzy of aggressive phagocytic function when driven by TNF signal. Indiscriminate release of reactive oxygen intermediates and lysosomal enzymes presumably serve the function of environmental digestion and perhaps even the extracellular killing of potential pathogens. This fully activated state of aggressive behavior results in necrosis of tissue, further activation of inflammatory and coagulation proteins, and death of the neutrophil. The end product is known to all surgeons as pus.

This pyogenic response is augmented further by biochemical and physiological events at the perimeter of the wound. The diffusion of the TNF signal and complement cleavage products into the adjacent microcirculation attracts more neutrophils into the inflammatory environment. If the concentration of these chemotactic and activation signals is sufficiently great, then full activation of the neutrophil may actually occur in its marginated state within the intravascular compartment. Full activation with release of reactive oxygen intermediates, and lysosomal hydrolases activates platelets and coagulation proteins. Platelet activation stimulates the production of thromboxane A_2 via the cyclooxygenase-thromboxane synthetase pathway of prostaglandin metabolism (146). This results in (*a*) endothelial damage by the activated neutrophil, (*b*) activation of coagulation, (*c*) activation of platelets, and (*d*) microvasoconstriction. This vasoconstriction leads to microcirculatory thrombosis, which results in central necrosis within the epicenter of the wound. The microcirculatory thrombus about the perimeter also serves a containment function to prevent dissemination of potential pathogens. In the final analysis, the soft-tissue response to wounding and contamination is to contain potential pathogens within the local environment. Local tissue necrosis and suppuration is favored over potential loss of containment, which would threaten the entire host. Indeed, pus is the consequence of a biologically "laudable" function.

Intra-abdominal Infection

Intra-abdominal infection begins as the process of peritonitis, or inflammation of the mesenchymal cell lining of the peritoneal cavity. The process of peritonitis has the distinct phases of contamination, dissemination, inflammation, and resolution or loculation. Peritonitis may occasionally be a primary process, but more commonly, it is secondary to another intra-abdominal disease.

Primary peritonitis is the consequence of peritoneal contamination arising from a remote source and without a fundamental intra-abdominal process. Microorganisms lodge within the peritoneal cavity via either hematogenous or lymphatic spread. Although primary peritonitis secondary to miliary tuberculosis was common in the past, in the modern era, it usually occurs

Table 9.9.
Factors That Favor the Infectious Process and the Host[a]

Factors Favoring Infection	Factors Favoring the Host
Bacterial Inoculum	Dissemination of Contaminant
Endotoxin (e.g., E. coli)	Clearance of Peritoneal Fluid
Capsular polysaccharide	Activation of Complement Cascade
(e.g., B. fragilis)	Deposition of Fibrin
Local Adjuvant Factors	Phagocytosis by macrophages and
Hematoma	neutrophils
Foreign Bodies	Loculation of dense bacterial
Dead Tissue	concentrations
Systemic Adjuvant Factors	
Hypoxemia	
Hypovolemia/Shock	
Steroid Therapy	
Obesity	
Malnutrition	
Diabetes	
Microenvironmental Issues	
Anaerobiosis	
Acidity	
Protein-Rich Environment	

[a] The interactions among these numerous variables underscores the complex nature of intraabdominal infection. Therapeutic measures are designed to reduce bacterial numbers, minimize adjuvant factors, and avoid the microenvironmental issues that favor bacterial proliferation.

in cirrhotics with ascites (147,148). Thus, *Streptococcus pneumoniae* may be the most common pathogen causing primary peritonitis. This occurs as the organism becomes blood borne from a primary pulmonary focus.

Secondary peritonitis is the usual scenario. The process customarily begins with perforation of the gastrointestinal tract and contamination of the peritoneal cavity. Perforation usually occurs secondary to inflammatory or neoplastic processes. Therefore, the peritonitis is a secondary process. The extent, severity, and outcome of the subsequent infection are consequences of the multiple biologic factors (Table 9.9).

An important consideration for predicting the severity of peritonitis is the size of the bacterial inoculum. The inoculum generally will reflect the density of bacteria from that segment of the gastrointestinal tract that perforates. Thus, a perforated peptic ulcer will usually be, at least initially, a sterile, chemical peritonitis. Perforation of a gastric ulcer or a gastric carcinoma will commonly have a significant number of bacteria because of reduced or lost gastric acidity. The organisms will be primarily aerobic Gram-negative rods (149). As perforations occur more distally in the gastrointestinal tract, the bacterial density will progressively increase. The perforated appendix will have 10^6 to 10^7 bacteria per gram of luminal content. The highest bacterial densities will be 10^{10} to 10^{11} bacteria per gram of content in the sigmoid colon. Anaerobic species become greater in number at the distal portion of the intestine, and anaerobic species exceed aerobes by 1000-fold within the sigmoid colon.

Although the actual bacterial count is important in the severity of peritonitis, virulence is also magnified by the presence of adjuvant factors. Food, fiber, and exfoliated cells of the intestinal tract are deposited in the peritoneal cavity with perforation and represent important adjuvant factors that enhance bacterial infection. Blood and hematoma are important adjuvants for infection and are particularly important in those patients that have sustained penetrating abdominal trauma. Dead and ischemic tissue are additional adjuvants.

Contaminants within the peritoneal cavity are disseminated throughout the abdomen by the natural forces of peritoneal fluid movement. Peritoneal fluid accumulates secondary to normal hydrostatic tissue forces. The upright position increases peritoneal fluid formation, whereas recumbent posture allows for fluid clearance. Accumulated peritoneal fluid in the recumbent position has a natural movement toward the diaphragm. With each expiration, a pressure gradient is created that draws peritoneal fluid toward the diaphragm. The fluid is then cleared via the lymphatic fenestrations that are present across the diaphragmatic surface of the peritoneal cavity (150,151). The fluid then passes directly into the lymphatic system. Thus, the human peritoneal cavity is, in reality, a giant lymphocele that communicates directly with the lymphatic system via the thoracic duct. The movement of peritoneal fluid becomes a normal force that disseminates bacteria throughout the peritoneal space (152).

Dissemination of intraperitoneal contaminants can be viewed as having positive nonspecific host defense consequences. Dissemination reduces the density of bacteria. Because the severity of bacterial infections has clearly been associated with the density of bacteria, dissemination is probably of some biologic importance. Dissemination increases the interface between the peritoneal pathogens and phagocytic host defenses. Finally, dissemination with movement of bacteria toward the diaphragm facilitates evacuation of bacteria from the peritoneal cavity.

With seeding of bacteria and other foreign particles into the peritoneal cavity, the inflammatory response is activated. The soft-tissue response within the peritoneum is similar to that seen with the soft-tissue wound described earlier. Resident peritoneal macrophages are activated and release the full array of inflammatory mediators, initiating the process. Complement and mast cell activation cause vascular permeability changes, edema, and recruitment of neutrophils from the systemic circulation into the area of injury. The generalized activation of inflammation results in activation of the coagulation cascade, which results in the formation of fibrin. Fibrin may entrap microorganisms, which has the potentially positive benefit of preventing bacterial invasion of soft tissues but may have the negative effect of insulating the entrapped organisms from phagocytic cells (116).

The bacterial contaminants within the peritoneal cav-

Table 9.10.
Bacteria Cultured from 480 Patients with Acute Peritonitis[a]

Aerobic Isolates	No.	Anaerobic Isolates	No.
Escherichia coli	201	Bacteroides fragilis	131
Streptococci	76	Peptostreptococcus spp.	45
(Nonenterococci)		Clostridium spp.	17
Pseudomonas spp.	56	Fusobacterium spp.	15
Klebsiella spp.	50	Gram negative anaerobes	11
Enterococcus spp.	31	(not otherwise speciated)	
Staphylococcus spp.	31	Eikenella spp.	9
Mixed Enterics (not	22	Propionibacter	4
otherwise		Peptococcus spp.	2
speciated)		Other	8
Enterobacter spp.	18		
Candida spp.	12		
Serratia spp.	12		
Citrobacter spp.	10		
Proteus spp.	8		
Other	12		

[a] A total of 294 cultures were done with only 2.7 microorganisms identified per patient. It was clear from the data of this manuscript that surgeons base antibiotic therapy for the patient with peritonitis upon the presumption of participating bacteria rather than what is reported by the clinical laboratory. Reprinted with permission from: Mosdell DM, Morris DM, Voltura A, et al: Antibiotic treatment of surgical peritonitis. Ann Surg 1991;214:543-549.

Table 9.11.
Location of Intraabdominal Abscesses in 143 Patients

Location of Abscesses[a]	No. of Patients
Subphrenic Space	40
Pelvic Space	35
Subhepatic Space	23
Paracolic Gutter	17
Lesser Sac	16
Subfascial Area	10
Multiple Abscesses	22

[a] Abscesses most commonly occur in those areas of the abdominal cavity that are in a dependent position.
From Tsilibary EC, Wissig SL. Absorption from the peritoneal cavity. Am J Anatomy 1977;144:127–132.

ity are eliminated by two mechanisms. Bacteria are either ingested, killed, and digested by phagocytic cells, or they are removed into the lymphatic system as part of the physiologic clearance of peritoneal fluid. When the density of bacterial contaminants exceed clearance mechanisms, loculation of the contaminants occurs via loculation mechanisms. Fibrin deposition about the perimeter of the dense bacterial collection matures with collagen replacement of the fibrin scaffolding to form the wall of the abscess. The fibrin-collagen barrier protects the host from the consequences of the bacterial dissemination but also shields the septic collection from phagocytic infiltration.

Infection within the peritoneal cavity is usually polymicrobial (Table 9.10). The synergism of aerobic and anaerobic organisms is a major contributor to the pyogenic nature of intra-abdominal infections (153). Gram-negative enteric organisms are particularly virulent, presumably because of the lipopolysaccharide component of the cell wall. B. fragilis does not have a potent lipopolysaccharide cell wall component and appears in most experiments to have minimal pathologic importance. However, a mixture of Gram-negative enteric bacilli with the anaerobic B. fragilis yields synergism, and the resultant infection is considerably greater than would have been anticipated.

The synergism evolves because the aerobic pathogens not only express their own virulence but consume the oxygen of the microenvironment and essentially produce an anaerobic condition for their anaerobic partner. Because bacteria like E. coli are facultative, they can proliferate with or without oxygen. For B. fragilis, the anaerobic conditions permit full expression of its pathologic

potential. Important among its virulence factors is the polysaccharide capsule that retards phagocytosis and promotes a pyogenic response (e.g., dead neutrophils) within the inflammatory environment. This polysaccharide capsule can be shed into the environment and provides protection for B. fragilis's facultative symbiont (51,52). The Gram-negative enteric pathogen is facilitated by the protection afforded by B. fragilis.

The location of abscesses within the peritoneal cavity tends to be the physiologic drainage basins of the abdomen (154,155) (Table 9.11). The two forces that govern the site of the collections of pus are gravity and the movement of peritoneal fluid. Dense collections of bacteria will occur in the subphrenic spaces, the pericolic gutters, and the pelvis because of their dependent locations. Because peritoneal fluid moves toward the diaphragm, obstruction of the egress route of fluid and microorganisms through the diaphragm, secondary to fibrin and other exudative debris, results in subphrenic collections and abscess.

Thus, a complex interaction occurs between the invading microorganisms and nonspecific host defenses. The virulence of the infection process is dictated by the biologic summation of bacterial numbers, intrinsic bacterial virulence, and adjuvant factors within the environment. The summed virulence is pitted against the inflammatory response, which may have intrinsic inborn strengths or weaknesses and may also be compromised by certain systemic influences. Efficient host responsiveness in the face of minimal summed virulence results in resolution of the peritonitis. Overwhelming virulence factors with a compromised host results in fulminant peritonitis and death of the host. Not uncommonly, a biologic stand-off results in abdominal abscess. The inaccessibility of the abscess to host defense mechanisms allows for proliferation. Such abscesses require mechanical intervention to allow resolution of the infection.

Postoperative Pneumonia

Postoperative pneumonia represents a common infection among surgical patients and is the most common infectious complication (if infections of the surgical site

Table 9.12.
Host Defense Mechanisms of the Lung

Host Defense	Mechanism of Action
Glottis/Epiglottis	Prevents aspiration of oropharyngeal fluids and aspiration of ingested food and liquids.
Ciliated Epithelial Cells	Coordinated ciliary motion constantly moves the "carpet" of mucus and other endobronchiolar fluids toward the proximal larger airways for subsequent expectoration by the host.
Mucus	Produced by resident goblet cells within the tracheobronchial tree, mucus provides a vehicle for cilia to expel potential contaminants and also provides a protective layer to prevent bacterial binding to epithelial cells.
Secretory IgA Antibody	Binds to bacterial contaminants and prevents bacteria from then binding to epithelial cells.
Secretory IgG Antibody	Predominantly identified in the distal airways, this antibody serves as an opsonin to facilitate macrophage and neutrophil phagocytosis.
Surfactant/Fibronectin/ C-Reactive Protein	All appear to have non-specific opsonic functions that facilitate the phagocytic clearance of bacteria.
Lactoferrin/Transferrin	Bind iron within the microenvironment of the lung and prevent bacterial growth and proliferation.
Alveolar Macrophage	Represents the primary phagocyte of the alveolar area and becomes the important cell to signal neutrophil invasion of the lung when potential infection is initiated.

are excluded). The gas-exchange surface of the lung is approximately 150 m² (156). Considering that such a large surface area of both tracheobronchial epithelial surface and alveolar surface are at risk for atelectasis, aspiration, and contamination from mechanical ventilatory systems, it is amazing that more postoperative patients do not have pulmonary infection. Postoperative pneumonitis assumes particular importance because of the reportedly high mortality rates, particularly among older patients (157).

Numerous host defense mechanisms exist to prevent infection in the lung (Table 9.12); they have been reviewed in detail elsewhere. The glottis serves as the primary barrier to bacteria or other substances that might provoke an inflammatory response. The endobronchial surface of the tracheobronchial tree is covered by ciliated epithelial cells, which become the target for binding and invasion by potential pathogens. A coating of mucus from goblet and bronchial gland cells becomes a primary barrier to prevent bacterial adherence to the epithelial cells. The coordinated motion of cilia in the lower airway results in the dynamic evacuation of bacteria-laden mucus into the larger proximal airways where it can be expectorated (162,163).

An additional mechanism to prevent bacterial adherence to epithelial cells is the normal secretion of IgA antibodies into the mucus phase that lines the luminal surface of the airway. These nonspecific antibodies bind to specific sites on the bacterial contaminants and appear to prevent bacterial adherence to the epithelial surface of the airway. Nonadherent bacteria are then evacuated via the mucociliary mechanism, or they may be eliminated distally at the alveolar level by macrophage cells. These antibodies are elaborated continuously by submucosal plasma cells and resident lymphocytes within the epithelial lining of the lung. They become a part of the admixture of the mucus coat (164). IgA does not fix complement, nor does it appear to serve a role for microbial opsonization (165).

Several mechanisms do appear to serve primarily an opsonic function. IgG antibody has been identified in greater concentrations in the distally bronchoalveolar areas of the lung. It is probably associated with opsonization (165,166) or even lysis of microorganisms through the activation of complement (167). Surfactant binding to the surface of microbes may facilitate phagocytosis (168). Similarly, fibronectin binding, particularly to *Staphylococcus* spp., may serve an opsonic function (169). Finally, C-reactive protein, and possibly other acute phase reactants that are up regulated via the stress response, may serve an opsonic function (170).

Bacteria have specific needs for certain trace elements and nutrients from their environment. Therefore, nonspecific host defenses that restrict the availability of these trace requirements can be effective in retardation of bacterial growth. Iron is a particularly important element facilitating bacterial growth (115). Most bacteria have their own siderophore mechanisms to bind iron from the microenvironment. Nonspecific host defenses of the lung restrict iron availability by the competitive chelation of iron by lactoferrin within the mucosal secretions of the larger airways and the presence of transferrin within the alveolar secretions (171).

The final intrinsic host defense mechanism of the lung is the alveolar macrophage. These phagocytic cells "patrol" the alveolar space for evidence of potential pathogens at the most distal portion of the airway. Putative pathogens within the alveolar space are phagocytosed promptly (172). Like other macrophages, bacterial growth and proliferation in this space elicits a prompt response of local cytokine release, which ushers the full forces of the inflammatory response. Neutrophils are likewise drawn into the area by the chemotactic signals created upon activation of the macrophage (173). Interleukin 8 (IL-8) appears to be a particularly important neutrophil chemoattractant which is released by the activated alveolar macrophage (174). In addition, IL-8 serves an important endocrine role in promoting systemic neutrophilia. Additional monocytes are mobilized into the evolving inflammatory focus by the production of monocyte chemotactic protein by the alveolar macrophage (175). Eradication of pathogens becomes the ob-

Table 9.13.
Common Isolates from the Lungs of 136 Patients with Postoperative Pneumonia

Pulmonary Pathogens	# Isolates	Comments
Pseudomonas sp.	41	The most common ICU isolate with a resistant antibiotic sensitivity pattern.
Klebsiella sp.	29	Is identified in both nonventilator and ventilator-associated pneumonias.
Staphylococcus sp.	25	Is commonly associated with contamination from the ICU staff. Is a meaningful quality indicator of ICU aseptic management of the entubated patient.
Escherichia coli	24	Commonly seen in both nonventilator and ventilator-associated infections. Generally seen in patients without antecedent antibiotic therapy.
Proteus sp.	18	Usually identified as pathogen in ventilator-associated pneumonia following antibiotics for a non-pulmonary indication.
Enterobacter sp.	16	Can be very resistant pathogens that are usually seen in ventilator-associated patients.
Pneumococcus sp.	13	Usually in nonventilator patients with short hospitalization and no prior antibiotics.
Serratia sp.	10	A ventilator-associated pathogen that tends to be hospital specific.
Group A Streptococci	5	Skin flora contamination of the ventilator equipment.
Hemophilus influenzae	4	Nonventilator-associated pathogen, common in patients with chronic lung disease as an associated variable.

jective in this setting in much the same way that phagocytic cells respond to soft-tissue contamination. Macrophage inflammatory proteins appear to be an important signal to stimulate neutrophil phagocytic activity in the evolving lung infection (176).

Pneumonia in the postoperative period occurs by three separate routes, each of which is discussed here in detail. The common feature of pneumonia, regardless of the clinical setting, is that the host defenses of the lung are compromised, which renders the lung vulnerable to either endogenous colonization or externally introduced bacterial pathogens. The common pathogens of postoperative pneumonias are identified in Table 9.13.

Nonventilator-Associated Pneumonia

The nonventilator-associated pneumonia group is composed of patients with an inadequate minute volume of ventilation. With an inadequate tidal volume per ventilatory cycle and without periodic "sigh" respirations, collapse of multiple segments of alveoli and small airways results in the clinical syndrome of atelectasis. With atelectasis, the normal movement of mucus via ciliary action is compromised, and those bacteria customarily expelled become entrapped in a confined space. Bacterial proliferation begins, and the alveolar macrophage responds by initiating the inflammatory response. Endogenous pyrogens from the alveolar macrophages elicit a systemic febrile response, and similarly the release of IL-1 promotes neutrophilia. Neutrophils migrate to the area of broncho-alveolar collapse and the evolving inflammatory response. Bacterial invasion into adjacent but previously uninvolved areas of lung results in clinical infection as the inflammatory response extends into larger segments of pulmonary tissue.

The postoperative patient has numerous reasons to have a reduced tidal volume. Anesthetic agents and analgesia employed in the immediate postoperative period reduce ventilatory drive and the minute volume of gas exchange. Painful thoracic and abdominal incisions

cause "splinting," i.e., patients avoid deep ventilatory activity. Splinting predisposes to atelectasis, compromised mucociliary function, and invasive infection.

The prevention of nonventilator-associated pneumonia is the correction of the fundamental pathophysiology. The airways and alveoli should be kept expanded by early ambulation, coughing, and deep breathing. Fever within the initial 24 hours of an operation will most commonly be atelectasis. A rapid response by the clinician to atelectasis will reexpand collapsed bronchoalveolar units and abort the evolving infection without the use of systemic antibiotics. Reexpansion of atelectatic segments of lung is associated with lysis of the postoperative fever.

When new infiltrates are identified on the chest roentgenogram, the inflammatory response has become severe enough to make a diagnosis of pneumonia. Treatment of established pneumonia requires continued efforts to restore reinflation of the collapsed airways. In severe or rapidly evolving cases, ventilator support may be necessary because the number of involved pulmonary units may actually compromise systemic oxygenation. Antibiotic therapy should focus on culture-proven bacterial pathogens.

Empirical drug therapy is necessary when culture data are pending or are not available. Although the magnitude and the composition of normal colonization of the healthy human airway remains unclear, the hospitalized surgical patient certainly is colonized. In older patients and in patients with elements of chronic lung disease, normal colonists of the airway include *Streptococcus pneumoniae* and *Haemophilus influenzae*. These become common pathogens for pneumonia in postoperative patients with a limited preoperative hospitalization and no antecedent antibiotic therapy. When preoperative stay has exceeded several days or when patients have received a course of antibiotics, colonization of the respiratory tract will be with more resistant hospital-acquired bacteria. Culture data in this latter group become important in guiding subsequent antibiotic therapy.

It is important to draw the analogy of bronchopneumonia with a pyogenic process anywhere else in the body. The disease is the consequence of bacterial proliferation that arises from within the respiratory tract. The inflammatory response results in purulence that still requires mechanical drainage. In addition to antibiotic therapy, tracheobronchial toilet must be continued to facilitate recovery from postoperative pneumonia. Coughing, expectoration, suctioning, and postural chest physiotherapy remain necessary treatments that are designed to drain the infected lung of the inspissated inflammatory exudate.

Ventilator-Associated Pneumonia

The use of mechanical ventilation in postoperative patients has become commonplace. The ventilator is necessary when patients have had lengthy procedures, massive blood and crystalloid volume administration, blunt chest trauma, or when preexisting lung disease is present. Ventilator support becomes important for the patient but represents a means for increased rates for postoperative pneumonia.

Unfortunately, the ventilator-assisted patient has virtually every host defense mechanism of the lung compromised either by the ventilation process or by the patient's underlying disease. The endotracheal tube eliminates the gross defense of the glottis in allowing oropharyngeal bacteria direct access into the trachea. The balloon-tipped endotracheal appliance may crush the tracheal epithelial lining. Edema of the pulmonary parenchyma may likewise interfere with mucociliary action, and loss of the cough reflex further compromises expectoration of bacteria-laden mucus. Pulmonary bacterial clearance appears to be compromised by pulmonary contusion, steroids, remote infection, shock, and probably by increased lung water. The combination of direct bacterial access through the airway appliance combined with the fundamental disease process of the lung makes pneumonia an unfortunate outcome for many patients.

The prevention of ventilator-associated pneumonia requires efforts to reduce bacterial contamination and vigorous treatment of the underlying process responsible for the ventilator support. Aseptic technique in the placement and management of the endotracheal tube will minimize the early introduction of bacteria into the airway. Minimizing unnecessary volume administration may reduce the risks of tissue edema. Various programs that allow early weaning and extubation may be the most important aspect of prophylaxis. Preventive antibiotics will only change the character of bacterial colonization, thus changing the likely pathogens, but they will not affect the frequency of pneumonia.

The treatment of ventilator-associated pneumonia is difficult. Host defenses are compromised and bacterial pathogens are generally the most resistant organisms characteristic of the surgical intensive care unit. *Pseudomonas* spp., *Serratia* spp., and resistant Enterobacteriaceae are the kinds of bacteria that commonly cause these pneumonias. They require aggressive and often combination drug therapy. Frequent, effective suctioning of the large airways remains important. Tracheostomy may need to be done to facilitate the aggressive suctioning necessary for effective management of secretions.

The penetration of antibiotics into the pulmonary secretions of these patients is problematic. The inflammatory focus has a compromised blood flow secondary to the infection. Penetration of the antibiotics into the area is poor and usually requires high-dose therapy. Antibiotics with synergistic relationships (e.g., penicillins plus aminoglycosides) are commonly employed to optimize the antimicrobial effects within the infection.

Aspiration-Associated Pneumonia

The third category of postoperative pneumonia is aspiration-associated pneumonia. This type of pneumonia may be the consequence of either vomiting and aspiration of gastric contents into the lung, or a more subtle, occult aspiration of oropharyngeal fluids that provide the bacterial inoculum, which may subsequently cause clinical infection.

Gross aspiration pneumonia is initially a chemical pneumonitis. Particulate matter becomes the foreign body adjuvant that fosters bacterial growth and proliferation. Aspiration of unbuffered gastric contents becomes a severe chemical injury of the lung as a sterile inflammatory response is provoked. The chemical pneumonitis from aspiration means that the lung becomes extremely vulnerable to intercurrent bacterial contamination. If the chemical pneumonitis is sufficiently severe, the patient will require ventilatory support, and the scenario of ventilator-associated pneumonia will have been created. Pneumonia in such circumstances is often virulent.

Prevention of aspiration-associated pneumonia requires recognition of the patient at risk. Gross aspiration may be a consequence of altered sensorium and a distended stomach. The altered sensorium is commonly caused by head injury, persistent effects of anesthesia, or postoperative analgesic excess. Elderly post-operative patients may have sensorium changes independent of any of these clinical variables. Gastric distention may be from recently eaten food, as is seen in trauma cases, or it may be from gaseous distention of the stomach. Distention from swallowed air or from active insufflation, such as Ambu bag-associated ventilation, sets the stage for vomiting and gastric acid aspiration. Nasogastric tube decompression of those clinical scenarios seems warranted. Preventive antibiotics given in a futile attempt to prevent bacterial colonization will only cause resistant bacteria, which become the colonists of the acutely injured lung. Treatment of aspiration-associated pneumonia becomes essentially the same as for ventilator-associated infection.

The aspiration of oropharyngeal fluids may occur in postoperative patients, patients that have had nasogastric tubes in place for a sustained period of time, and older patients with a loss in hypopharyngeal sensation. Subtle and occasional aspiration events probably affect all adults but are inconsequential because of the normal paroxysms of coughing that are usually provoked. In seriously ill patients, the cough reflex appears to be less sensitive.

The risk of subtle aspiration of nasooropharyngeal fluids is a problem, and for the seriously ill patient, the colonization of the upper aerodigestive tract may be with resistant hospital-acquired nosocomial pathogens. Prolonged hospitalization and attendant systemic antibiotic therapy increases the risk of resistant colonization.

Prevention of this subtle form of aspiration pneumonia has proven difficult. Oropharyngeal antibiotic pastes have been used and have been reported to be of value. Topical antibiotics invariably lead to enhanced microbial resistance; accordingly, long-term consequences of the routine use of oropharyngeal antibiotics should be suspect for induction of resistance.

Recent concern has focused on alkalinization of the upper digestive tract and its potential consequences for nosocomial pneumonia. Acidification of the stomach is generally viewed as a nonspecific host defense mechanism in that the acid milieu prevents the stomach from becoming a reservoir for bacterial proliferation. Such proliferation of bacteria could potentially cause retrograde colonization of the upper aerodigestive tract and an increase in the incidence of nosocomial pneumonia. Because reduction of gastric acidity has been the goal of prophylaxis for stress-associated gastritis, the use of orally administered antacids and/or systemically administered H_2 histamine antagonists have now been challenged as potentially increasing nosocomial infection rates (177,178). Use of nonalkalinizing agents, such as sucralfate, have now been advocated to reduce resistant bacterial colonization. The scientific basis for this recommendation remains tenuous (Table 9.14), but it deserves further examination.

Postoperative Urinary Tract Infection

Urinary tract infection (UTI) following surgical procedures is usually the consequence of Foley catheterization. The human urinary tract from the pelvis of the kidney to the proximal opening of the urethra at the bladder trigone is sterile. The urethra as the communicating channel to the outside is colonized with small numbers of bacteria at its distal most extent. Encroachment of the sterile confines of the urinary bladder by

Table 9.14.
Prospective Randomized Trial of Sucralfate, Antacids, and H2 Blockade Employed for the Prevention of Stress-associated Mucosal Ulceration, and the Probability of the Patient's Developing Nosocomial Pneumonia

Treatment Group[a]	No. Patients	No. Pneumonia
Sucralfate	61	7 (11.5%)
Antacids	39	9 (23.1%)
H2 Blocker	17	1 (5.9%)
Antacids and H2 Blocker	13	6 (46.2%)

[a] The data indicate that the use of antacids with or without H2 blockage is associated with an increased frequency of nosocomial pneumonia. H2 blockade alone is not associated with an increased rate of nosocomial pneumonia.

the Foley catheter provides the avenue for bacterial colonization.

The host defense of the urinary tract is simple but generally effective (Table 9.15). The constant flow of urine from the kidney to the bladder combined with a functional ureterocystic antireflux mechanism prevents bacterial colonization of the upper tract. However, the presence of stag-horn calculi within the pelvis of the kidney represents a foreign body nidus that will allow bacterial colonization and proliferation, and will effectively overcome the positive host defense effects of urine flow. Similarly, a loss of the antireflux mechanism at the ureterocystic junction means that infection within the bladder may ascend in a retrograde fashion.

The urinary bladder and urethra have numerous host defense mechanisms that prevent infection from occurring. The bladder is lined by transitional epithelium, which resists bacterial binding. The mucus of the urethra has bacteriostatic properties and also secretes IgA to coat would-be pathogens and prevent their binding to epithelial cells (179). Given periodic voiding activity that has the mechanical effects of "flushing" the system, infection is generally an uncommon event (180). For male patients, the 20-cm length of the urethra makes urinary tract infection in the absence of bladder intubation unusual. The shorter female urethra (5 cm) makes retrograde bacterial colonization and urinary tract infection more common.

With placement of a Foley catheter, all host defense mechanisms are breeched. The catheter provides direct access to the lumen of the bladder through a patent tube for contamination from the external world (181,182). The catheter within the urethra erodes and inflames the urethral mucosa and neutralizes the mucin and IgA protective mechanisms (183). The space between the outer wall of the Foley catheter and the urethral mucosa is no longer subject to the cleansing effect of periodic urination. As a result, retrograde migration of bacteria within this biologic dead space sets the stage for proximal proliferation and migration of bacteria around the catheter and into the bladder. In addition, the inflated balloon of the Foley catheter erodes and braids the transitional

Table 9.15.
Host Defense Mechanisms that Prevent Infection within the Urinary Tract

Host Defense Element	Mechanism of Action
Urine Flow	Constant urine flow provides resistance to retrograde migration of bacteria either proximally in the ureters or retrograde within the urethra.
Ureterocystic Anti-reflux Mechanism	The angulation and submuscular course of the ureters when entering the urinary bladder cause a function antireflux mechanism that prevents retrograde urine flow from the bladder.
Transitional Epithelium	The cellular lining of the urinary bladder is resistant to bacterial binding. Injury to the epithelial layer secondary to the Foley catheter is a major factor in increased infection rates secondary to catheter utilization.
Urethral Mucus	Provides a physical barrier to bacterial binding to the mucosal cells of the urethra.
Urethral IgA	Binds to putative bacterial pathogens within the urethra and prevents their binding to epithelial cells both within the urethra itself and potentially within the bladder.
Urethral Length	The male urethra is of sufficient length that retrogrde migration is infrequent in the absence of instrumentation.

epithelium at the trigone and provides the portal of entry for bacteria into the bladder wall.

Finally, bacterial pathogens adhere to the catheter itself and by this means escape being eliminated by the normal process of voiding. Catheters seem to impair the normal function of phagocytic cells that would potentially rid the urinary tract of the unwanted colonization (184,185). As with other indwelling foreign devices, bacteria that colonize the catheter may produce a biofilm that protects the microorganisms from either being mechanically expelled or ingested via the host phagocytic cells (186–188).

The pathogenic bacteria that causes UTI are those that colonize the perineum of the patient. Surface colonization of the skin becomes the colonists of the catheter and the pericatheter space of the urethra. Despite the heavy colonization in the area with anaerobic bacteria, anaerobes are rare pathogens of the urinary tract. This probably reflects the unfavorable oxidation-reduction potential of the bladder lumen for anaerobic growth. Thus *E. coli*, as the predominant aerobic organism of the perineum, is the most common pathogen causing UTI.

Owing to the duration of hospitalization and the use of antibiotics in patients with indwelling Foley catheters, *E. coli* is less predominant in the urinary tract than would ordinarily be expected (Table 9.16). The duration of hospitalization results in competing colonization of the perineum with resistant nosocomial pathogens. Systemic antibiotics will almost invariably provide antimicrobial agent *E. coli* and other common enteric bacteria, which further aids the selection process to favor resistant organisms. Indeed, postoperative patients with greater than 48 hours of prior antibiotic therapy will have a statistically greater probability of having *Pseudomonas* spp. or *Serratia* spp. than *E. coli* in the urinary tract (189).

An understanding of the biology of UTI makes preventive measures easier to comprehend. Aseptic technique in placement of the catheter is obviously important. Anchoring the catheter in place after placement avoids erosion of the balloon on the epithelial lining of the bladder and reduces irritation of the urethra itself. To-and-fro movements of the unanchored catheter will

Table 9.16.
Pathogens Cultured from the Urinary Tracts of 212 Postoperative Urinary Tract Infections in 153 General Surgical Patients

Cultured Pathogen[a]	Pure Culture	Mixed Culture	Total Isolates
E.coli	42	14	56
Klebsiella sp.	22	16	38
Pseudomonas sp.	20	17	37
Proteus sp.	18	12	30
Enterobacter sp.	14	8	22
Enterococcus sp.	6	16	22
Serratia sp.	9	7	16
Citrobacter sp.	4	6	10
Streptococcal sp.	3	6	9
Staphylococcus epidermidis	7	1	8
Providencia sp.	5	0	5
Candida sp.	3	0	3
Total	153	108	256

[a] The pathogens demonstrate a more resistant trend than would normally be seen in community-acquired UTI.

have a sump action and will facilitate the migration of bacteria into the bladder. Obviously, removal of the catheter at the earliest possible time after its purpose has been served is the best way of preventing catheter-induced UTI. Although bladder irrigation with antimicrobial solutions is a common practice in an attempt to prevent UTI, such practices when studied prospectively do not reduce infection rates but certainly do increase the likelihood of resistant pathogens ultimately being cultured (190).

Treatment of established infection is with antibiotic therapy. Because hospital-acquired pathogens are characteristically more resistant to conventional antibiotic choices, culture and sensitivity data are important. Restoration of urine flow is an underdiscussed but important treatment for the patient with a postcatheterization UTI. Urine flow restores normal homeostasis for the bladder and the urethra by the evacuation of microorganisms. Indeed, the truly invasive nature of many so-called UTI in postcatheterization patients is disputable and may only reflect colonization of the urinary bladder (189). Urine flow following catheter removal appears to restore the single most important nonspecific host defense mechanism of the urinary tract.

Table 9.17.
Factors That Promote Infection with Intravascular Device Use

Factor Favoring Infection	Comment
Penetration of Skin	The skin is the most effective of the non-specific host defense mechanisms for the prevention of infection. Subsequent bacterial proliferation around the skin puncture site will readily lead to migration down the catheter tunnel.
Contamination of Catheter and/or Tunnel	Despite careful cleansing of the puncture site, some bacteria are carried down into the soft tissue with placement. Subsequent skin growth and migration down into the tunnel makes infection virtually inevitable and underscores the need for periodic changes of the catheter site.
Foreign Body Effect	The catheter itself results in binding of bacteria. The foreign body also retards phagocytic function and facilitates bacterial proliferation.
Intimal Injury/Clot Formation	The placement of the catheter (not to mention other failed attempts in the immediate area) results in intimal injury of the vessel and clot formation. The clot is ideal for bacterial growth and serves as a ready source of iron.
Hub/Device secondary Contamination	The constant manipulation of the device and with changes of intravenous tubing results in unavoidable contamination of the device at the site of tubing changes. This can lead to secondary migration of bacteria down into the catheter tunnel and resultant infection.

Occasionally, an acute septic event can be encountered in patients following catheter removal. The septic event is most often in postoperative patients, and when it occurs, it is usually associated with acute urinary retention. Stagnant and heavily colonized urine within the urinary bladder after a period of catheterization will cause invasive infection and bacteremia. The inability to void after catheterization, especially among male patients, may result from several sources; among these are underlying spasms from a mild bacterial infection or from obstructive outflow disease (e.g., prostatic hypertrophy). Replacement of the catheter to effect drainage of the infected bladder is an important treatment for these patients in the same way that draining pus is important at any anatomic location.

Intravascular Device Infection

The placement of indwelling devices directly into the vascular tree via percutaneous penetration of the skin has become extraordinarily valuable for the management and monitoring of surgical patients. Peripheral intravenous lines, central venous lines, arterial lines, and Swan-Ganz catheters have become standard and accepted parts of the management of surgical patients. However, the placement of a foreign body conduit into the intravascular compartment poses a major breech to the epidermal protective coating of the human organism and provides a direct avenue for bacterial penetration and dissemination (Table 9.17).

An indwelling intravascular catheter is a wound in the skin that has a foreign body within it. This leads directly into the intravascular compartment. A peripheral intravenous catheter is an excellent example. Soft-tissue trauma is created by the percutaneous puncture, which activates all the elements of inflammation. With the percutaneous puncture, skin bacteria can be injected into the percutaneous tunnel that represents the track from the patient's skin to the venous structure (191–193). Bacteria from the fingers of the individual placing the catheter may actually be the microorganisms that contaminate the tract. These contaminating microorganisms are harbored in the pericatheter space between the external wall of the catheter and the adjacent soft tissue of the tract. The injury created by the trauma of catheter placement, the foreign body itself, and the contaminating bacteria about the catheter establish an inflammatory response in the microenvironment. Eradication of the bacterial contaminant is not achieved by phagocytic activity, as in the case of the phlebotomy puncture, because of the persistent presence of the foreign body.

Another important pathophysiologic event occurs at the site where the catheter actually penetrates the vein. Intimal disruption of the vein and placement of a foreign body in a low-flow structure such as a peripheral vein predispose to the formation of a platelet hemostatic plug and clot formation. If multiple passes of the catheter were attempted before achieving successful catheterization, multiple areas of intimal injury may be present in proximity to the ultimate site of venous cannulation. The indwelling segment of the catheter may also damage the venous endothelium by to-and-fro movements created by normal patient activity. Finally, hypotonic, hypertonic, or otherwise noxious substances within the infusate may damage the venous endothelium and produce thrombosis of the vein. The net consequence of these variables of venous endothelial injury is clot, an ideal situation for bacterial proliferation.

Another important mechanism for catheter contamination involves the care of the puncture site. The skin about the site of percutaneous introduction usually is cleansed, albeit in a superficial and commonly haphazard fashion, at the time of catheter placement. A porous dressing may be placed over the site. Commonly, the gauze dressing is assaulted by fluids. The hub of the catheter usually is handled by a different individual as each new infusion is begun (191,194,195). This results in bacterial contamination and proliferation about the site of the skin puncture and may lead to the migration and proliferation of bacteria down the catheter and into the pericatheter space. Like the Foley catheter infection, the pericatheter space serves as the reservoir for bacterial

Table 9.18.
Pathogens Cultured from the Blood and Semi-quantitative Cultures of the Catheter in 143 Patients with 159 Episodes of Catheter-associated Bacteremia

Cultured Pathogen[a]	No. of Isolates	No. of Suppurative Phlebitis[b]
Staphylococcus aureus	78	23
Staphylococcus epidermidis	33	3
Serratia sp.	18	2
Candida sp.	11	2
Klebsiella sp.	11	4
Enterococcus sp.	8	1
Proteus sp.	6	2
Enterobacter sp.	5	0
Others	6	1
Total	176	38

[a] In 15 cases, multiple organisms were cultured both from the patients' blood and from the catheters themselves.
[b] Suppurative thrombophlebitis were so classified because of the need for the patients to have the vein excised or for local incision and drainage at the catheter site.

proliferation and a source for contamination of the intravascular component of the catheter. If an intravascular clot is present, it too becomes infected. Bacterial proliferation proceeds within this environment that is rich in nutrients (particularly iron), and bacteremia is the consequence.

Thus, it should be no surprise that staphylococcal organisms are the most common bacteremic pathogen associated with intravascular device infections (Table 9.18). *Staphylococcus aureus* and *Staphylococcus epidermidis* represent nearly two-thirds of the pathogens from such devices. In the intensive care unit, the patient that is exposed to the nosocomial pathogens and broad-spectrum antibiotic regimens frequently have a Gram-negative rod contaminating their intravascular device. Central lines seem to have a certain predilection for being contaminated by *Candida albicans* and other *Candida* species.

Prevention and treatment of this problem can then be formulated by understanding the biology of how infection occurs in this setting. Careful cleansing of the skin at the time of placement is of paramount importance. Continued care of the skin site, particularly for central lines and Swan-Ganz lines that will remain in place for a sustained period of time, is essential. Because the real culprit in peripheral catheter bacteremia is the foreign body within the soft-tissue wound, removal and rotation of the catheter site every 48 to 72 hours is of vital importance. Preventive systemic antibiotics will only change the pathogen that will ultimately colonize the puncture site and the catheter. Topical antiseptics and topical antibiotics about the puncture site have not reduced infection rates. Aseptic placement and management, along with rotation of peripheral sites, appears to be the best recourse to prevent intravenous catheter bacteremia.

Treatment of intravenous device-related bacteremia requires a high index of suspicion that the catheter is the culprit. Infected catheters need to be removed and cultured by the semiquantitative technique (196). Appropriate antibiotic therapy needs to be started. The bacteremia associated with Gram-negative organisms tends to be short lived after removal of the catheter, and long-term drug therapy (more than 48 to 72 hours) is probably not justified. Because *Staphylococcus aureus* may cause metastatic infection to heart valves, and because *Candida albicans* may cause metastatic infection to the eye, a full 7 to 10-day course of antimicrobial chemotherapy is necessary for these organisms.

Customarily, the septic response that is triggered by the bacteremia from a device will defervesce promptly after catheter removal. Persistence of the bacteremia may mean that the patient has suppurative thrombophlebitis. The clot within the venous structures at the site of catheter placement can support bacterial growth even after removal of the foreign body. Such situations can develop into intravascular abscesses with continued bacteremia from the site. Excision of the infected vein may be necessary and must be pursued for the patient with persistent bacteremia (197). *Staphylococcus aureus* device infections are notorious for this complication.

Other Infections

Although the infections discussed above clearly represent the majority of infections that are encountered by the surgeon, there are, obviously, others that do occur. Posttraumatic meningitis, suppurative sinusitis, parotitis, and septic arthritis are but a few of the less common but significant infections that can be encountered in the surgical patient.

Posttraumatic meningitis is the consequence of injury that disrupts the bony encasement of the brain and results in contamination of the meninges by organisms. Basilar skull fractures are notorious for allowing microorganisms of the upper aerodigestive tract to contaminate the meninges and the subarachnoid space. Infection is often the result. Binding of bacterial cells to the meningeal cell, bacterial proliferation, and activation of the inflammatory response become the common features that make this infection similar to other infections.

Nosocomial sinusitis is another infection that can be clinically subtle in postoperative patients (198). Chronic nasogastric intubation, which inflames and potentially impairs free drainage from the sinus cavities, combined with antibiotic therapy, which alters the normal colonization, can cause a contamination of static sinus fluids and subsequent acute bacterial infection.

Suppurative parotitis may be seen as a consequence of all the same variables that provoke infection in other tissues. It is likely that suppurative parotitis is the consequence of retrograde migration of bacteria via Wharton's duct into the parenchyma of the parotid salivary gland. It is an uncommon infection, and normal salivary flow possibly removes potential bacterial colonists in the same way that urine flow maintains the relatively

Table 9.19.
Bacterial Pathogens Cultured in 32 Patients with Open Fractures

Open-Fracture Infectious Pathogens[a]	Number[b]
Enterococcus sp.	14
Pseudomonas sp.	11
Klebsiella/Enterobacter	9
Staphylococcus sp.	9
E. coli	2
Serratia sp.	2
Proteus sp.	1

[a] The high frequency of pathogens that would ordinarily be identified as nosocomial bacteria should be emphasized.

[b] The total exceeds 32 because of polymicrobial isolates in selected patients.

sterile environment of the urinary tract. Secretory IgA within salivary secretions prevents binding of pathogenic bacteria to the ductal system of the salivary gland. Under conditions of severe illness, salivary production declines and IgA production may be inadequate. Unfavorable bacterial overgrowth in the mouth allows potential pathogens to infect the parenchyma of the salivary gland.

Septic arthritis can be a complication of an open fracture of any joint. Contamination, binding of bacteria to the surface epithelium, proliferation, and inflammation can cause an active infection. Septic arthritis can even be the consequence of blood-borne contamination and does not always require actual joint injury.

Open fractures can predispose to a major infectious event in trauma patients. An open fracture is a soft-tissue injury that has a broken bone within its midst. The combination of devitalized tissue, hematoma, bone sequestra, and an open avenue for bacterial access creates an ideal environment for bacterial proliferation. Infection may be associated with nonunion of the fracture and, potentially, amputation. Hospital-acquired bacteria appear to be the most common pathogens of these infections and underscore the failure of preventive antibiotics to prevent infections (Table 9.19).

Regardless of the site, a common theme in postoperative infection of any location is injury and contamination. This commonly occurs in the compromise of host defense mechanisms and results in bacterial proliferation and inflammation. Although the clinical presentation of infection assumes the unique feature of the anatomic area affected, the interaction between the host and potential pathogens is generic.

Special Considerations in Surgical Infection

Postsplenectomy Sepsis

Fulminant bacteremia and septic deaths in patients with prior splenectomy were identified as infrequent but serious problems in the 1970s (199–201). The association of these bacteremic deaths with splenectomy changed attitudes about the clinical indications for splenectomy, particularly in patients that had sustained splenic trauma. Conservation of the spleen became a desired objective. Diagnosis of splenic injury without operation and nonoperative therapy became goals of management, particularly for younger patients. Studies were undertaken to elucidate the pathophysiologic consequences of splenectomy.

The splenic reticuloendothelial system has the capability of removing bacterial cells that are poorly or inadequately opsonized from the circulation. Bacteria that gain access to the bloodstream generally are cleared efficiently by the splenic or hepatic reticuloendothelial (RE) cells. Pneumococcus and *Haemophilus influenzae* are encapsulated bacterial strains that likely gain access to the blood via the respiratory tract. These encapsulated bacteria are difficult for the hepatic RE cells to clear if the bacteria have not been opsonized adequately (202). Without specific immunization against the polysaccharide capsule of the specific bacterial strain in blood, opsonization is poor and the spleen rather than the liver is necessary for clearance. Splenectomized patients do not have this clearance capability of poorly opsonized bacteria.

The removal capability for encapsulated bacteria is achieved most effectively by the spleen. An acute IgM response from the white pulp of the spleen after a bacterial challenge results in the release of opsonic antibody to facilitate bacterial clearance by both the liver and the spleen. Loss of the spleen compromises the acute immune production of IgM and is associated with decreased clearance by the RE system (203,204).

An additional host defense mechanism for the spleen is the production of two nonspecific opsonins. Tuftsin appears to facilitate the clearance of bacteria and may also serve as a stimulant to the generalized phagocytic functions of the host (205,206). The spleen is also thought to be a major source for the synthesis of properdin, a protein important in the initiation of the alternative pathway of complement activation. The true significance of the loss of tuftsin remains unclear. The physiologic reserve within the complement cascade is such that splenectomy is probably not that important in increasing the host vulnerability secondary to decreased levels of tuftsin (207,208).

Splenectomy compromises the host. If splenectomy occurs in a preteen or an adolescent, he or she is vulnerable to acute overwhelming sepsis. Despite efforts at conservation, splenectomy remains a necessity for many patients. Methods to prevent this relatively infrequent (< 1%) (200,209) but morbid (death rates of 60% to 70%) (210) complication have been explored. The use of preventive antibiotics has been attempted and remains largely of unproven value. Long-term compliance with the daily administration of preventive antibiotic is unlikely. If compliance is adequate, long-term antibiotic administration is associated with all the problems of modifying the patient's resident microflora and selecting out resistant strains.

The polyvalent pneumococcal vaccine has been employed effectively to reduce the frequency of postsplenectomy sepsis (211,212). This vaccine provides immunization of the host against the 23 most common polysaccharide serotypes of pneumococci. Obviously, it does not provide protection against those serotypes not represented within the vaccine, nor does it provide protection against other bacterial strains (e.g., *Haemophilus influenzae*) that are known to be agents of postsplenectomy sepsis. A new *Haemophilus influenzae* vaccine has been introduced that may increase the scope of protection (213,214). Nevertheless, a risk remains for the splenectomized patient. Patient cognizance of the risk is essential so that immediate antibiotic therapy can be initiated at the first sign of a clinical infection.

Preventive Systemic Antibiotics

The hope that accompanied systemic antibiotic therapy in the 1940s and 1950s was that infection after operative procedures could be prevented. That hope was soon dashed as early efforts to demonstrate the effectiveness of preventive systemic antibiotics proved unsuccessful (215–217).

The classic animal studies of Miles, Miles, and Burke (218) demonstrated that precontamination administration of systemic antibiotics was necessary if prevention of infection was to be achieved. These authors demonstrated that infection could be prevented if antibiotics were given before or at the same time as bacterial contamination. Antibiotics given after contamination were progressively less effective. Antibiotics given more than 4 hours after contamination had no preventive effect.

The failure of preventive systemic antibiotics stemmed from the fact that the antibiotics were not administered before the operative procedure. In the early patient trials that did not show a drug effect, the antibiotics were invariably not given until after the patients were in the recovery room. As a result, active antibiotic was not present within the surgical wound fluid at the time of bacterial contamination. The importance of preoperative administration of the preventive antibiotic requires an understanding of the unique features of the surgical wound.

A surgical incision activates all the biological mechanisms of inflammation that were discussed earlier. Tissue injury activates complement proteins, mast cells, and most important, coagulation of serum proteins to form a fibrin interface across the cut surface of the wound. The process is an active one and occurs continuously, as long as the wound remains open. During the entire period of the procedure, bacterial contamination assaults the wound edges from all potential sources.

Bacteria from the patient's skin, the air of the operating room, the gloves of the surgeon, and endogenous sources are lodged into the wound and become incorporated into the fibrin matrix at the wound interface. With completion of the procedure, the opposite sides of the surgical wound are approximated with sutures to create a fibrin "sandwich," which has varying concentrations of bacteria, depending on the magnitude of intraoperative contamination. Adjuvant factors within the closed wound such as hematoma, dead tissue (e.g., excessive use of the electrocautery), and foreign bodies (e.g., silk sutures) will then amplify the potential virulence of the bacterial contaminants. If summed bacterial numbers plus adjuvant effects exceed the phagocytic functional capacity of the host, then infection results.

If antibiotics are initiated after the wound is closed, they are destined to fail. The fibrin matrix with its entrapped bacteria is relatively impervious to antibiotics. The closed wound is often closed tightly, and this, coupled with wound edema, increases the hydrostatic tissue pressure within the surgical wound. A perimeter of relative ischemia develops in the area of the incision.

The key to successful systemic use of preventive antibiotics is to administer the drug before surgical incision so that adequate antibiotic concentrations may be present within the fibrin matrix as it forms (219). Precise surgical techniques to minimize the quantity of contamination during the procedure, control of adjuvant factors within the wound, and adequate wound concentrations of antibiotic throughout the duration of the procedure will minimize the likelihood of a wound infection.

Finally, the premise that the drug must be present within the wound during the period of fibrin formation and bacterial contamination can be violated by the use of antibiotics that have extraordinarily short biologic half-lives. For example, previous studies with cephalosporin antibiotics have shown that the drugs are present for about two half-lives within the surgical wound following systemic administration (220,221). Antibiotics with short half-lives must be redosed at that interval to maintain drug concentration in the surgical wound. It is desirable to use longer half-life antibiotics to cover the complete duration of the operative procedures so that redosing will not be necessary. When lengthy procedures are contemplated, a schedule for antibiotic redosing should be planned in advance to minimize the risks of unprotected periods of contamination.

Antibiotic Pharmacokinetics

Another important factor that results in poor biologic effect of antibiotic therapy, even when the microorganisms are sensitive to the drug employed, is antibiotic pharmacokinetics. The presumption of all systemic antibiotic treatment is that the drug reaches the site of infection in concentrations adequate to achieve an antimicrobial effect. This goal of therapy assumes that the dosing

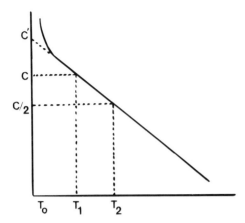

Figure 9.13. A standard antibiotic clearance curve from the serum of an adult patient. Drug concentration is measured to $\log_{10}$ on the ordinate and time is measured on the abscissa. At T_0, the peak antibiotic concentration is achieved, which rapidly enters the linear clearance curve. Extrapolation to the ordinate gives the serum concentration. This allows the computation of the volume of distribution. The time interval for the concentration to decline from point C to C/2 equals $T_2 - T_1$. The time it takes for the serum drug concentration to decline by 50% is the biologic elimination half-life.

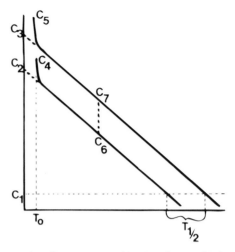

Figure 9.14. The effects on serum kinetics of an antibiotic caused by doubling its dose. Drug concentration is on the ordinate, and time is on the abscissa. Doubling the dose of the antibiotic doubles the peak concentration from C_4 to C_5 and the T_0-equilibrated concentration from C_2 to C_3. The drug concentration at any point in time is increased by one half-life, from C_6 to C_7. If C_1 represents the threshold of antibacterial action of the antibiotic, then doubling the dose increases antibacterial action by only one half-life.

schedule is appropriate. To understand dosing schedules, fundamental knowledge of the dynamics of drug distribution and elimination is essential (222–226).

When an antibiotic is administered intravenously, the drug is distributed rapidly throughout the central pool. The central pool represents the plasma volume and the freely diffusible area of the extracellular fluid volume. The antibiotic then proceeds through a secondary equilibration phase as the drug is distributed into cells and into other less readily reached areas of body fluid. Drug distribution into different tissues varies, depending on extracellular water content, intracellular water content, adipose content, and whether the drug is freely transported across cell membranes and tissue barriers. For example, certain drugs readily pass across the blood-brain barrier and others do not. Access of a drug to the cerebrospinal fluid has obvious consequences to the total volume of water into which a drug is distributed. The volume of distribution reflects the theoretically maximum volume of body water to which a given drug has access and is extrapolated from a kinetic clearance plot (Fig. 9.13). The volume of distribution may be low and approximates only the extracellular water volume when a drug is highly protein bound and is excluded from the intracellular compartment. Paradoxically, the volume of distribution may exceed total body water and reflects the binding of the drug to interstitial or intracellular sites that are not in equilibrium with the central pool.

When the equilibrated concentration is achieved, the antibiotic concentration in the central pool is at a steady rate. As drug elimination occurs either via excretion or metabolism, a reduction of central pool concentration results. The rate of concentration decline follows a semi-logarithmic linear pattern (see Fig. 9.13). Drug elimination is thus described as the biologic elimination half-life. The half-life is the time required for the drug concentration to decline by 50%. The dosing interval for an antibiotic is determined by the number of half-lives that occur before the drug concentration declines below the target concentration required to achieve the desired effect.

Concern about the adequacy of drug dosing can cause surgeons to double the dose in an effort to get better therapeutic benefits. The consequence of doubling the dose is illustrated in Figure 9.14. Because the area under the elimination plot of an intravenously administered antibiotic represents the bioavailability of the drug, doubling the dose means that the area under the curve will be doubled. At most, the peak equilibrated concentration of the antibiotic will be doubled. Because the elimination half-life is relatively constant across multiple drug doses, doubling the peak concentration will only extend the drug dosing interval by one half-life. For long half-life antibiotics, the extended duration of drug presence about the threshold concentration might extend the dosing interval in a clinically relevant way. For short half-life drugs, doubling the dose not only tends to increase peak concentration, but also has minimal benefits for increasing the duration of drug presence in the central pool. The half-life of commonly employed β-lactam antibiotics are listed in Table 9.20.

Another concern about antibiotic use is whether antibiotic concentration at the target site, as opposed to the central pool, is adequate. Figure 9.15 illustrates the theoretical relationships between the central pool and six other tissues. Tissue A might represent the biliary tract,

Table 9.20.
Biological Elimination Half-Lives of Commonly Employed β-lactam Antibiotics

Beta-lactam Antibiotics	Elimination Half-Life[a]
Penicillins	
Penicillin G	30 min
Ampicillin	1 hour
Ticarcillin	70 min
Mezlocillin	55 min
Piperacillin	54–63 min
Cephalosporins	
Cephalothin	35 min
Cefaxolin	1.7–2.0 hours
Cefoxitin	41–59 min
Cefamandole	32 min
Cefuroxime	80 min
Cefonicid	4.5 hours
Cefotetan	3.0–4.6 hours
Cefotaxime	1 hour
Cefoperazone	2 hours
Ceftizoxime	1.7 hours
Ceftriaxone	5.8–8.5 hours
Ceftazidime	1.9 hours
Monobactams	
Aztreonam	1.7 hours
Carbapenems	
Imipenem	2–3 hours

[a] Although much is made about the antimicrobial activity of antibiotics that are selected in patient care, only a limited amount of discussion is focused upon half-life. The half-life of the drug dictates the dosing schedule which may prove to be as important as the antimicrobial activity.

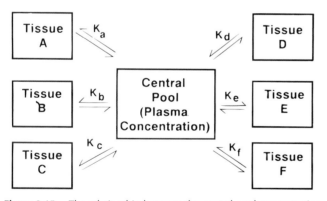

Figure 9.15. The relationship between the central pool concentration and tissue concentrations. The variables that govern tissue penetration by a given antibiotic are complex. Tissue concentrations are not necessarily reflected by plasma measurements.

where the drug in question is excreted into the bile and bile concentrations are actually higher than concurrent central pool concentrations. Tissue B might be the cerebrospinal fluid with essentially no identified concentration. Tissue C might be the subcutaneous tissue, and if the drug were lipophilic, antibiotic concentration might persist at significant concentrations long after the central pool concentration is zero. Tissue D might represent skeletal muscle, which is a well-vascularized tissue without intrinsic fat, and might have drug concentra-

tions that will parallel those in serum. Tissue E might be bone, where the drug is slow to enter but also is slow to exit. Tissue F might represent infected lung tissue, where the inflammatory focus and the central area of the infection is somewhat remote from the nearest functioning microvascular units, with drug concentrations reflecting central pool concentrations but at a suppressed level. Thus, the rationale for increasing drug concentration in the central pool would theoretically increase the gradient of drug delivery into certain areas and might be of therapeutic benefit.

Unfortunately, drug dosing schedules are designed for patients by trials in healthy volunteers. The critically ill surgical patient and the severely injured patient are not represented by healthy volunteers (227–229). First, the volume of distribution of most antibiotics will be dramatically increased in these patients. The so-called third space of injured patients and patients following major operations means that the functional interstitial space is increased dramatically. An increased volume of distribution means that peak concentrations will be less, and the duration of antibiotic concentration above the critical threshold target will be reduced. Second, the elimination half-life may be changed in the critically ill. Intrinsic failure of either kidney or liver function may prolong half-life. Patients with the septic response characteristically have an increased cardiac output and appear to have a corticomedullary redistribution of renal blood flow. The consequences of these changes are a loss of renal concentrating ability and increased secretory elimination of drugs that are eliminated by this mechanism (e.g., aminoglycosides). The consequence may be the reduction of elimination half-life and accelerated renal excretion of the antibiotic. The net effect of physiologic changes mediated by critical illness is that adequate antibiotic concentrations of drugs eliminated by the kidney may be compromised. Suboptimal dosing schedules represent a potential problem for the severely ill patient.

The assumption here has been that sustained antibiotic concentration above the critical inhibitory threshold is important. For some antibiotics this is true, and for others it is probably not valid. Aminoglycosides bind irreversibly to ribosomal proteins. Saturation of binding sites means that a significant postantibiotic effect can be seen. Continued drug effect is identified for a period of hours after the central pool concentration approaches zero. However, for other antibiotics there is minimal or no postantibiotic effect. For example, cephalosporin binding to PBP, particularly in Gram-negative bacteria is reversible. Reduced environmental concentration of the antibiotic results in dissociation of the antibiotic from the PBP. As a result, essentially no postantibiotic effect exists for cephalosporins against gram-negative bacteria.

Vascular Graft Infections

The use of prosthetic implants have become commonplace. The development and use of vascular prosthetic grafts have expanded enormously the surgical management options for patients with severe vascular disease. Prosthetic materials have even achieved a measure of popularity in the management of vascular trauma.

However, the vascular graft poses some special problems with respect to potential for the development of serious prosthesis-associated infections. The graft is a foreign body, and its knitted or woven consistency tends to harbor bacteria once contamination or infection occurs. The grafts are employed necessarily in ischemic tissues that are being revascularized. Revascularization is often attempted when open wounds or distal infection exists. Frequently, antecedent antibiotic therapy may have been necessary, which leaves the patient with resistant bacterial colonization.

The biology of graft infection is similar to wound infection in other settings with the exception that a large foreign body has been used. The surgically dissected wound will have a fibrin matrix which develops like a film across the wound surface. Its quantity is a function of the procedure's duration. Bacteria may be entrapped into this fibrin matrix. When the vascular graft is placed, the activation of the coagulation cascade similarly occurs about the foreign body. A fibrin matrix develops around the entire graft's surface. Contamination during the placement of the graft is entrapped in this fibrin "cast." The foreign body effect reduces the number of bacteria that are necessary to cause clinical infection. Dead tissue about the graft from vigorous dissection or poorly perfused tissue also has a potent adjuvant effect. Retained blood clot augments the process. All the variables are present to favor infection.

It should be obvious that the biologic basis favoring an infectious complication in this setting is compelling. Aseptic technique aimed at reducing bacterial contamination during graft placement is vital. Reduction of other adjuvant factors such as clot, perigraft ischemia, or dead tissue is equally important. The perioperative coverage of the wound with preventive antibiotics has been shown to reduce clinical wound infection and should reduce the probability of graft infection.

Graft infection is fortunately an uncommon event that complicates less than 1% of such procedures. The discharge of pus, thrombosis of the graft, and the development of pseudoaneurysms are common clinical indicators of infection. Graft infections are the consequence of operative contamination, even if the infection is not clinically identified for months or even years later. While seeding of the graft from a secondary source is clearly a possibility, and in patients with distal extremity infections a real concern, operative contamination is by far the most common cause in prosthetic graft infection. *Staphylococcus aureus* has been the traditional patho-

gen of concern for graft infection. These bacteria are present on the patient's skin and in the environmental fallout in the operating room. Gram-negative bacteria can be a particular problem if the patient has had a prolonged preoperative hospitalization or has had a course of antecedent systemic antibiotics.

Staphylococcus epidermidis has become a pathogen of considerable significance in recent years. The resistance of *Staphylococcus epidermidis* to many antistaphylococcal antibiotics has favored its selection on patient skin and in the hospital environment. This organism appears to be the primary pathogen for graft infections that are delayed in clinical presentation. The ability of these organisms to form a glycoprotein matrix about the foreign body surface results in protection of the pathogen from host phagocytosis. It also makes culturing the organism from delayed infections difficult (46,47). Sonication of the infected graft material appears to be an important means of disrupting the glycocalyx and permitting culture of the pathogen from the supernatant (230).

The biological basis for the treatment of graft infection is removal of the foreign body. It is generally unrealistic to think that antibiotics will sterilize infections of prosthetic material. Furthermore, immediate placement of a new prosthetic into the infected environment of the former graft bed seems to be destined for failure in most cases. The options for management require alternate routes to restore perfusion to the tissues that are served by the vascular graft. However, biologic lesions are commonly relearned time and time again. Infections of foreign bodies require removal of the foreign body. Antibiotics have yet to override this fact.

Bacteremia-Septic Response without Infection

In the 1960s, Fine and associates concluded that hemorrhagic shock and potentially other physiologic perturbations were exacerbated, if not primarily mediated, by the release of endotoxins or whole bacteria into the systemic circulation from the gastrointestinal reservoir (231–233). Although initially discredited by Zweifach's (234,235) germ-free rat experiments, the concept of the gastrointestinal reservoir as the source of bacteria or bacterial cell products in a clinical septic condition has now returned to academic scrutiny with a considerable level of interest. Terms such as *persorption* (236,237), *gut origin* sepsis (238), and most popular, *bacterial translocation* (239,240) have emerged to describe this phenomenon. Microbial gastrointestinal translocation appears to be an easily identified experimental observation that remains to be fully defined in terms of its clinical relevance. As a potentially significant clinical event, it is most interesting in that it represents the dissemination of bacteria and bacterial cell products into the systemic circulation, without the provocation of inflammation at the primary site of entry. It is, in essence, bacteremia and the septic response without infection.

There are essentially two requirements for microbial gastrointestinal translocation. First, there must be failure of the intricate gut barrier function that keeps gastrointestinal colonization from being disseminated throughout the body. Second, the hepatic Kupffer cells that ordinarily rid portal blood of all potential toxins and bacteria fail to perform this function. Some endotoxin or whole bacteria may leak into the portal circulation and may occur with normal defecation. Colonic endoscopy, proctoscopy, and intraoperative portal blood cultures have been identified to provoke bacteremia. Occasional portal bacteremia must occur (241–244). Access of portal endotoxins or whole organisms from the gut into the systemic circulation must mean that Kupffer cell function is impaired or that the capacity of these cells to clear organisms and toxins in certain circumstances can be saturated.

The barrier function of the human gastrointestinal tract has both functional and anatomic components. Motility of the intestine is certainly a component part of the intestinal barrier. Propulsion of contents through the intestinal lumen in a distal direction minimizes the period of time that microorganisms are in contact with the mucosa. The in situ proliferation and invasion of bacteria is simply retarded by movement. Loss of this motility function, either by intestinal obstruction or by gastrointestinal ileus, has been associated with bacteremia and the septic response in humans (245).

The anatomic barrier of the intestinal epithelium is obviously an important partition that keeps bacteria and bacterial cell products from entering the lymphatics or bloodstream. Atrophy of the epithelial cells or degradation of the intercellular matrix may be major contributing factors to intestinal microbial translocation.

Concern about cellular atrophy has raised new issues in the design and delivery of nutritional support systems in critically ill patients. Maintenance of the enterocyte and colonocyte now appear to require specific nutrients under circumstances of hypermetabolism and stress. The enterocyte of the small intestine appears to prefer glutamine (246) as an energy substrate, whereas the colonocyte appears to need short-chain fatty acids for oxidation (247). Failure of these two cell populations to receive critical nutrients may lead to epithelial atrophy and may compromise the barrier function of the gut. Because conventional solutions for parenteral nutrition of patients are deficient in both glutamine and short-chain fatty acids, compromise of the gut barrier is thought to be the result of selective nutritional deprivation.

A different school of thought contends that the route of nutritional delivery to the critically ill patient is more important than the composition of the nutrients. Data from experimental thermal injury in rodents have identified jejunal atrophy when nutritional support is provided intravenously (248). Thermally injured rats that received isocaloric, isonitrogenous nutritional support enterally did not sustain the same degree of intestinal atrophy. These experiments suggested that the epithelial cell of the intestine actually derives much of its vital nutrient support from the lumen rather than from the circulation. These data suggest that enteral nutrition, if possible, is essential in the critically ill. Clinical data have been presented that show that reduced rates of nosocomial infection with enteral feeding are comparable to parenteral nutrition. This suggests that translocation of bacteria from the gastrointestinal reservoir may be the source of nosocomial pathogens (249). Whether the gut epithelial cells need specific nutrients during stress or whether the route of protein-calorie delivery is the important issue will require further clinical investigation. Both the composition and the route of delivery of the nutritional support are important considerations.

The intercellular matrix between the apposing cells of the intestinal epithelium is another important consideration in the gastrointestinal barrier. The composition of the intercellular matrix is complex; it is a dynamic structure that is constantly being degraded, resynthesized, and remodeled. Biological stress and protein-calorie malnutrition must certainly increase the porosity of the intercellular matrix and potentially create avenues for the invasion of intraluminal microorganisms. The colonization of the lumen by undesirable microorganisms, either from exogenous contamination or secondary to the influence of broad-spectrum antibiotics, may occur, and they may actually amplify enzymes that digest the intercellular matrix and facilitate the movement of microorganisms out of the lumen.

Another important mechanism that reinforces the biologic barrier of the intestinal tract is retardation of bacterial (or fungal) adherence to the epithelial cells. Considerable evidence suggests that pathologic bacteria must bind to the epithelial cell to express virulence. Pathogenic bacterial cells that are kept from binding to the epithelium are simply propelled downstream by the normal peristaltic function of the gut.

Several mechanisms within the gut inhibit bacterial binding to the epithelium. Goblet cells are found throughout the gastrointestinal tract and produce a complex glycoprotein mucin that is constantly secreted into the lumen. This mucin has bacteriostatic properties that suppress excessive bacterial overgrowth, particularly within the small intestine. This mucin also provides a protective film over the surface of the intestinal epithelium that retards bacterial binding to the lining cells (250).

A second mechanism that retards microorganisms from binding to the epithelium is secretory IgA (251). The gastrointestinal tract has abundant submucosal lymphocytes and mature plasma cells that serve numerous biologic functions. One function is the synthesis of secretory IgA, which is constantly secreted into the lumen of the intestine. This secretory IgA is thought to bind to bacterial cells and block those receptors that mediate their binding to epithelial cells.

A final important barrier that retards binding of microorganisms to intestinal epithelial cells is the normal gastrointestinal flora. The normal colonization of the gut serves to provide antagonism to the growth of bacterial or fungal species that may be potentially injurious to the host. Bacteriocin produced by resident species suppresses the growth of potential pathogens (252,253). Short-chain fatty acids may be toxic to selected unwanted colonists of the intestine (254,255). Lactobacilli can produce hydrogen peroxide, which activates the peroxidase-halide mechanism that suppresses both viral and fungal pathogens (256).

Binding of normal microflora to the epithelial cells of the intestine prevents the binding of potentially pathogenic bacteria. The specificity of this binding by the intestinal colonization of certain animal species is remarkable. For example, the lactobacilli of rats can bind to rat intestinal epithelial cells and block the binding of pathologic organisms. The lactobacilli of birds can serve a similar function. What is truly amazing is that the avian lactobacilli are unable to bind to rat gut cells (257,258). Although the specificity of gut colonization in humans has not been characterized to the extent identified above, the loss of normal colonization because of the use of broad-spectrum antibiotic has led to considerable discussion about the need for selective decontamination of the human gut during critical illness. This technique attempts to eliminate aerobic bacteria and preserve anaerobic species (259). It is unknown if anaerobic microflora are critical to the barrier function of the human gut. A better understanding of the relationship of normal bacterial colonization to the barrier function may have profound consequences for the future design and use of antibiotic therapy.

As suggested above, translocation may be an occasional event, even for a fully intact gastrointestinal barrier. Transient variations in bacterial concentrations within the gut barrier may exceed the threshold of containment even in normal people. Concentration of bacteria within the cecum has been shown to correlate with translocation events in experimental animals (239,240). Increased intraluminal pressure, as with normal defecation, may allow microorganisms or microbial toxins access to the portal circulation.

Liver Kupffer cells prevent these transient portal bacteremias from gaining systemic access to the host and provoking a septic event. The RE function of the liver is efficient and has been shown experimentally to remove 10^4 to 10^5 microorganisms per milliliter of portal blood flow (260). Hepatic reticuloendothelial function probably needs ample opsonic protein to facilitate the removal of blood-borne microorganisms. Thus exhaustion of opsonic proteins may be one mechanism of RE ineffectiveness that could lead to portal bacteremia.

Numerous variables have been experimentally shown to alter hepatic reticuloendothelial efficiency. Corticosteroids, exotoxins, chemotherapeutic agents, and other administered agents have adverse effects on hepatic clearance of microorganisms (260). Shock, hypoxemia, protein-calorie malnutrition, burns, and other perturbations not only are associated events in the provocation of microbial translocation but also impair hepatic Kupffer cell function (261–266).

Patients may have endotoxemia, bacteremia, or fungemia from the gastrointestinal reservoir. The diagnosis of this biologic event remains a diagnosis of exclusion. Despite some good data from human subjects to support bacteremia from the gut as an important event, skepticism remains as to the true clinical relevance of microbial translocation (267). For the clinician who views microbial translocation as a real entity, treatment considerations must focus on the composition of nutritional support, the route of nutritional support, and the appropriate use of broad-spectrum antibiotics in the critically ill patient.

The Septic Response

The primary function of the patient's host defense is to prevent tissue contamination by microorganisms. The primary purpose of the phagocytic-inflammatory response is to eradicate contaminants and, locally, to control infection if contamination of tissue occurs. Unfortunately, the magnitude of the inoculation may overcome the local containment efforts. The severity of the local inflammatory process may be of an extreme order of magnitude, with normally autocrine or paracrine mediators becoming systemic in scope (e.g., TNF). Systemic dissemination of the pathogen or mediators results in the septic response.

Standard definitions for the terms *sepsis*, *septicemia*, *septic syndrome*, and *septic response* have not been given a consensus meaning. The phrase systemic inflammatory response syndrome (SIRS) has recently been used to describe the systemic response to infection and potentially other non-infectious systemic events (268). The elements of SIRS are:

1) Temperature >38°C or <36°C
2) Heart rate >90 beats/min
3) Respiratory rate >20/min or $PaCO_2$ <32 mmHg
4) White blood cell count >12,000/mm^3; or <4000/mm^3; or >10% immature forms

SIRS is considered to be present when two of the above criteria are present. When SIRS is specifically initiated by infection, then the term *sepsis* is employed appropriately. As can be seen in the above criteria for SIRS, these are not particularly severe criteria and are actually fulfilled in the average patient with otitis media or a community-acquired urinary tract infection.

Because the criteria of SIRS are so liberal, the term *septic response* will be used to identify the patient with severe SIRS. The *septic response* refers to those physiologic and biochemical responses that have been identified with systemic manifestations of uncontrolled infection. This represents a nonspecific response of the host to disseminated (*a*) microorganisms or their products from an infected primary source, (*b*) microorganisms or their products without an infected primary source (e.g., bacterial translocation), or (*c*) local inflammatory mediators from an infectious site (e.g., abdominal abscess) or a sterile primary site (e.g., acute pancreatitis) without the participation of microorganisms or their products.

The physiologic and biochemical responses that characterize the septic response are (*a*) the hyperdynamic cardiac parameters, (*b*) a reduced peripheral vascular resistance, (*c*) a narrowed arteriovenous oxygen difference, and (*d*) the evolution of serum lactic levels before hypotension.

The extensive evaluation of injured and septic patients by Siegel and associates (269) has permitted the design of a staging system for the septic response (Fig. 9.16). State A is characteristic of the physiologic stress response. Patients experience a modest elevation of cardiac output and have a modest decline in peripheral vascular resistance. Oxygen consumption is increased and the arteriovenous oxygen difference is normal to slightly increased. Given appropriate volume resuscitation, they do not have increased serum lactate concentrations.

State B represents an exaggerated stress response. Cardiac output may be increased to twice normal levels. The peripheral vascular resistance may be dramatically reduced. The arteriovenous oxygen difference is narrowed, reflecting the presence of abnormal peripheral oxygen use. Total oxygen consumption may be reduced or minimally elevated relative to the increase observed in cardiac output. Lactic acidemia (usually without lactic acidosis) is present.

State C represents the evolution of septic shock. The cardiac output is normal or slightly increased. However, the profound loss of peripheral vascular resistance means that cardiac output cannot meet peripheral demands, and hypotension results. The peripheral abnormality of oxygen use is now compounded by the reduction in perfusion pressure. Marked lactic acidosis results.

State D is the low cardiac output-septic shock state. Left ventricle failure occurs and is associated with increased peripheral vascular resistance. Patients have profound lactic acidosis. There is peripheral abnormality of oxygen consumption, reduced cardiac output, reduced perfusion pressure, and peripheral vasoconstriction. It is commonly a preterminal condition.

The state B patient can be sustained in this exaggerated stress response for a considerable period of time with current support technology. The sustained state B condition sets the stage for the evolution of multiple organ failure, as the peripheral abnormality of oxygen metabolism persists even though cardiac output is elevated and the central perfusion pressure appears to be satisfactory.

Individual patients do not sequentially pass through each of the states of the septic response. The transition from state A to state B requires that the patient has the myocardial reserve to generate the elevated cardiac output to compensate for the loss of peripheral vascular resistance. In those patients that have intrinsic myocardial disease or in the elderly patient, the ability to generate the necessary cardiac output may be lacking. Thus, older patients will commonly decompensate to a state C level with no apparent interval of a state B.

The mechanism of defective peripheral oxygen metabolism in the septic state has been studied extensively. One hypothesis suggests primary cellular defect in oxygen use. This is based on both experimental and clinical observations. Mitochondria seem to be unable to metabolize oxygen and substrate that are presented to the cell. Mitochondria appear to be injured in experimental models of endotoxemia (270,271), although this has been contested by other authors (272). Siegel and associates (269) demonstrated that increases in serum lactate concentration in septic patients occur in an equimolar relationship with increases in pyruvate. They contend that if cellular hypoxia or defective oxygen delivery were the issue, then lactate should increase at a more dramatic rate than pyruvate. They concluded that defective pyruvate dehydrogenase activity results in the inefficient transport of pyruvate into mitochondria. Therefore, the defective oxygen use is actually defective substrate pre-

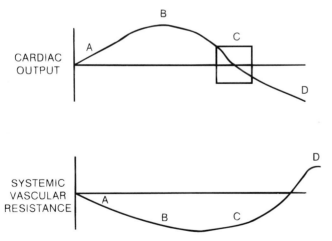

Figure 9.16. The four states of the septic response from the perspective of cardiac output and peripheral vascular resistance. In state A, the cardiac output is elevated modestly and peripheral vascular resistance is modestly diminished. In state B, cardiac output is increased dramatically, whereas vascular resistance is extremely diminished. In state C, cardiac output is in the range of the customarily identified normal values, but because of profound loss of vascular resistance, the patient is identified as in clinical septic shock. State D is congestive heart failure superimposed on the fundamental septic condition. Cardiac output is reduced and peripheral vascular resistance is increased.

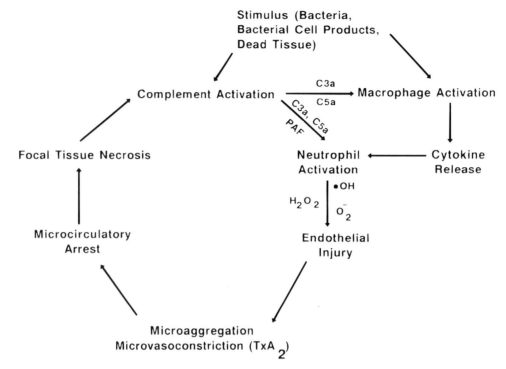

Figure 9.17. Theoretical relationship of multiple variables to explain the microcirculatory hypothesis of multiple organ failure. The biologic stimulus leads to the activated neutrophil state. Adverse interactions between the neutrophil and the endothelial cell cause microvascular injury, which produces a necrotic focus. The focal ischemic injury then becomes the inflammatory focus to recycle the inflammatory process.

sentation to the oxidative phosphorylation mechanism of the cell (273,274).

A second hypothesis focuses on defective nutrient blood flow as the critical issue in the septic response. Experimental studies have demonstrated reduced hepatic and renal blood flow in the face of increased cardiac output. This is associated with a corresponding increase in tissue lactate in affected tissues (275). Interestingly, the systemic lactate:pyruvate ratios rise in unity, as is seen in septic humans. Thus, a selective microcirculatory injury has been hypothesized to explain the septic response.

The microcirculatory hypothesis suggests parallels between the systemic septic response and the biology of the wound (Fig. 9.17). The difference is that the local septic response involves activation of normal local agents and has a beneficial effect, whereas at the systemic level, the effect may not be beneficial. *Systemic* complement activation (268) and *systemic* macrophage activation (277) lead to the systemic activation of the neutrophil. Although the local tissue injury provides a chemotactic signal to focus the direction of the neutrophil, systemic activation results in systemic, non-directed activation. This, in turn, leads to diffuse margination of neutrophils toward endothelial cells. Activation of neutrophils without direction results in the release of reactive oxygen intermediates and lysosomal enzymes, which then creates an inflammatory response. Endothelial injury results in activation of platelets and the coagulation cascade, which leads to thromboxane A_2 release.

A scenario is created wherein a microcirculatory inflammatory lesion is created, which results in a biomechanical plug of neutrophils, platelets, and fibrin. This, combined with the vasoconstrictive effects of thromboxane A_2, results in focal-tissue ischemia (278). The paradox is created wherever hyperdynamic circulation coexists with focal microcirculatory ischemia. The progression of the microcirculatory injury proceeds with time.

The end point of the focal ischemic injury within visceral tissues is focal necrosis. The necrotic focus then becomes the inflammatory stimulus to recycle the entire process. Inflammation begets ischemia, which begets more inflammation. Rapid evolution of the process leads to the state C and state D septic response. Physiologic support leads to the sustained state B condition, which is associated with multiple system organ failure. In essence, those biologic processes that are critical to local containment of infection can become destructive systemic forces.

While the mechanisms which are responsible for the deleterious effects of the septic response remain to be fully elucidated, many newer treatment modalities are being explored. These newer treatment strategies have been designed to neutralize or modulate the mediator and effector systems of the septic response as it is currently understood.

Because endotoxin is recognized as an important activator of sepsis and the septic response, considerable interest has focused on the development of anti-endotoxin antibodies to prevent activation of the process. A human monoclonal antibody (HA-1A) has been studied in septic human subjects, and did not show any overall benefit to the patients studied (279). Patients with gram negative bacteremia did appear to benefit. A second trial has been aborted because of unexplained deaths in the antibody treatment group. A mouse monoclonal antibody (E5) has also been studied in human septic patients. Overall, mortality rates were not improved (280). Anti-endotoxin antibodies do not appear to be a major treatment modality at this time. The failure of this treatment strategy may relate to the multi-factorial nature of the inciting biological stimuli which cause human sepsis, rather than the concept that a single provocative agent (e.g., endotoxin) may initiate the septic response.

Because TNF is viewed by many investigators as one of the principal pro-inflammatory signals of the septic response, therapy to antagonize TNF effects appears to be a rational direction to follow. Monoclonal antibodies against the TNF molecule have been shown to be effective in experimental models of sepsis (281,282). However, human trials with the anti-TNF antibody have failed to demonstrate improved survival (283). A naturally-occurring receptor antagonist to TNF has been identified and shows some experimental promise for treatment (284,285). The experimental data are promising, but clinical trials have not yet been reported.

Another important pro-inflammatory mediator is IL-1. It is thought to amplify TNF effects and to have deleterious pro-inflammatory effects of its own. A receptor antagonist to IL-1 has been identified and has been shown to have positive effects when given to experimental animals with simulated septic events (286–288). Its value in clinical sepsis is currently under investigation.

Many other antagonist therapies have experimental evidence to support potential clinical applications. Complement receptor inhibition has shown some promise in suppressing tissue inflammation from ischemia (289). PAF receptor antagonists have shown benefit in experimental models of sepsis (290,291). Inhibition of prostaglandin metabolism (292,293) and free radical scavengers (294) has also shown favorable experimental promise. Inhibition of nitric oxide production represents yet another strategy (295,296).

Inhibition of neutrophil margination is beneficial in the prevention of inflammatory lesions in ischemia/reperfusion and cold injury. The use of monoclonal antibodies against the CD-18 receptor has been explored in intra-abdominal sepsis (297). However, concern does exist that blockade of margination may cause inability of the host to actually combat a focus of infection (298). Additional studies focusing on the other adhesion molecules are in progress and should be of interest.

Perhaps a more fruitful area of future investigation will be in exploiting the natural counter-inflammatory mechanisms of the host. When a cutaneous abscess is examined, all of the characteristic features of human inflammation can be recognized. When the abscess is drained, natural down-regulatory processes cause curtailment of the inflammation. IL-4, IL-10, and IL-13 are currently recognized as being potential signals that are counter-regulatory to inflammation. Indeed, the use of naturally occurring biological signals to treat the septic condition may prove to be much more effective than all of the synthesized efforts with receptor antagonists and monoclonal antibodies (299).

Summary

The complex interaction among the host, the microbial pathogen, and the microenvironment of infection is becoming better defined. Understanding the mechanisms of antibiotic action and microbial resistance has provided new drugs that are designed to block the resistance mechanism (e.g., clavulanic acid and sulbactam) rather than attack the microorganisms themselves.

Although surgical drainage, debridement, and antibiotic therapy are effective modalities, these treatments have probably reached a point of maximum benefit. Newer treatment modalities should address host modulation, either by facilitation of local containment or by down regulation of the systemic inflammatory response. These newer treatments will require the continued growth of basic information about surgical infection.

REFERENCES

1. Pettijohn DE. Prokaryotic DNA in nucleoid structure. Crit Rev Biochem Mol Biol 1976;4:175–202.
2. Giesbrecht P, Wecke J, Reinicke B. On the morphogenesis of the cell wall of staphylococci. Int Rev Cytol 1976;44:225.
3. Shockman GD, Barrett JF. Structure, function, and assembly of cell walls of gram-positive bacteria. Annu Rev Microbiol 1983; 37:501.
4. Ames GF. Bacterial periplasmic transport systems. Structure, mechanisms, and evolution. Annu Rev Biochem 1986;55:397.
5. Henning U. Determination of cell shape in bacteria. Annu Rev Microbiol 1975;29:45–60.
6. Lugtenberg B, Van Alphen L. Molecular architecture and functioning of the outer membrane of *Escherichia coli* and other Gram-negative bacteria. Biochim Biophys Acta 1983;737:51–115.
7. Nikaido H, Vaara M. Molecular basis of bacterial outer membrane permeability. Microbiol Rev 1985;49:1–32.
8. Luderitz O, Staub AM, Westphal O. Immunochemistry of O and R antigens of salmonella and related Enterobacteriaceae. Bacteriol Rev 1966;30:192–205.
9. Rietschel ET, Gottert H, Luderitz O, Westphal O. Nature and linkages of the fatty acids present in the lipid-A component of salmonella lipopolysaccharides. Eur J Biochem 1972;28:166–173.
10. Kasper DL. Chemical and biological characterization of the lipopolysaccharide of *Bacteroides fragilis* subspecies *fragilis*. J Infect Dis 1976;134:59–66.
11. Benz R. Structure and function of porins from gram negative bacteria. Annu Rev Microbiol 1988;42:359–393.
12. Lachman E, Pitsoe SB, Gaffin SL. Anti-lipopolysaccharide immunotherapy in management of septic shock of obstetric and gynecologic origin. Lancet 1984;1:981–983.
13. Baumgartner JD, McCutchan JA, Van Melle G, et al. Prevention of gram-negative shock and death in surgical patients by antibody to endotoxin core glycolipid. Lancet 1985;2:59–63.
14. Ziegler EJ, Fisher CJ, Sprung CL, et al. Treatment of gram nega-

tive bacteremia and septic shock with HA-1A human monoclonal antibody against endotoxin. N Engl J Med 1991;324:429–436.

15. Costerton JW, Irvin RT, Cheng KJ. The bacterial glycocalyx in nature and disease. Annu Rev Microbiol 1981;35:299–324.

16. Smith H. Microbial surfaces in relation to pathogenicity. Bacteriol Rev 1977;41:475–500.

17. Doetsch RN, Sjoblad RD. Flagellar structure and function in eubacteria. Annu Rev Microbiol 1980;34:69–108.

18. Beachey EH, Ofek I. Epithelial cell binding of group A streptococci by lipoteichoic acid on fimbriae denuded of M protein. J Exp Med 1976;143:759–771.

19. Orskov I, Orskov F, Birch-Andersen A. Comparison of *Escherichia coli* fimbrial antigen F7 with type 1 fimbriae. Infect Immun 1981;34:708–711.

20. Ambrose EJ, Easty DM. Structure and organization of viruses and bacteria. In: Cell biology. Baltimore: University Park Press, 1977:495–528.

21. Shepherd MG, Poulter RTM, Sullivan PA. *Candida albicans:* biology, genetics, and pathogenicity. Annu Rev Microbiol 1985;39:579–614.

22. Dulbecco R, Ginsberg HS. The nature of viruses. In: Davis BD, Dulbecco R, Eisen HN, Ginsberg HS, eds. Microbiology, 4th ed. Philadelphia: JB Lippincott, 1990:769–794.

23. White DO, Fenner FJ. Structure and classification of viruses. In: White DO, Fenner FJ, eds. Medical virology, 3rd ed. New York: Academic Press, 1982:3–34.

24. Tyler KL, Fields BN. Introduction to viruses and viral disease. In: Mandell GL, Douglas RG Jr, Bennett J, eds. Principles and practice of infectious diseases, 3rd ed. New York: Churchill Livingstone, 1990:1124–1134.

25. Wiley DC. Viral membranes. In: Fields BN, ed. Virology. New York: Raven Press, 1985:45–67.

26. Harrison S. Principles of virus structure. In: Fields BN, ed. Virology. New York: Raven Press, 1985:27–44.

27. Simons K, Garoff H, Helenius A. How an animal virus gets into and out of its host cell. Sci Am 1982;246:58–66.

28. Roizman B. Multiplication of viruses: an overview. In Fields BN, ed. Virology. New York: Raven Press, 1985:69–76.

29. Murphy FA. Virus taxonomy. In: Fields BN, ed. Virology. New York: Raven Press, 1985:7–25.

30. Arbuthnott JP. Role of exotoxin in bacterial pathogenicity. J Appl Bacteriol 1978;44:329–345.

31. MacLennan JD. The histotoxic clostridial infections of man. Bacteriol Rev 1962;26:177–276.

32. Bizzini B. Tetanus toxin structure as a basis for elucidating its immunological and neuropharmacological activities. In: Cuatrecasas P, ed. The specificity and action of animal, bacterial and plant toxins. New York: Wiley, 1978:175–218.

33. Simpson LL. Presynaptic actions of botulism toxin and beta-bungarotoxin. In: Cuatrecasas P, ed. The specificity and action of animal, bacterial, and plant toxins. New York: Wiley, 1978:219–239.

34. Taylor NS, Bartlett JG. Partial purification and characterization of a cytotoxin from *Clostridium difficile.* Rev Infect Dis 1979;1:379–385.

35. Wiseman GM. The hemolysins of *Staphylococcus aureus.* Bacteriol Rev 1975;39:317–344.

36. Yoshida K, Takahoshi M, Haga K, et al. Comparison of three blood-clotting substances in *Staphylococcus aureus* strains. J Clin Microbiol 1980;11:293–294.

37. Gilson VM. Leukocytotoxic activity of toxin from the 80–81 strain of *Staphylococcus aureus.* J Bacteriol 1968;95:2409–2412.

38. Pruett TL, Rotstein OD, Fiegel VD, et al. Mechanisms of the adjuvant effect of hemoglobin in experimental infections: VIII. A leukotoxin is produced by *Escherichia coli* metabolism of hemoglobin. Surgery 1984;96:375–383.

39. Tally FP, Goldin BR, Jacobus NV, Gorbach SL. Superoxide dismutase in anaerobic bacteria of clinical significance. Infect Immun 1977;16:20–25.

40. Gesner B, Jenkins C. Production of heparinase by bacteroides. J Bacteriol 1961;81:595–604.

41. Meade J, Mueller C. Necrotizing infections of subcutaneous tissue and fascia. Ann Surg 1968;168:274–281.

42. Meyer K. The biological significance of hyaluronic acid and hyaluronidase. Physiol Rev 1947;335–359.

43. Christensen GD, Simpson WA, Bisno AL, et al. Adherence of

44. Christensen GD, Simpson WA, Bisno AL, et al. Experimental foreign body infections in mice challenged with slime-producing *Staphylococcus epidermidis.* Infect Immun 1983;40:407–410.

45. Christensen GD, Baddour LM, Simpson WA. Phenotypic variation of *Staphylococcus epidermidis* slime production in vitro and in vivo. Infect Immun 1987;55:2870–2877.

46. Bandyk DF, Berni GA, Thiele BL, Towne JB. Aortofemoral graft infection due to *Staphylococcus epidermidis.* Arch Surg 1984;119:102–108.

47. Siverhus DJ, Schmitt DD, Edmiston CE, et al. Adherence of mucin and non-mucin-producing staphylococci to preclotted and albumen-coated velour knitted vascular grafts. Surgery 1990;107:613–619.

48. Fox EN. M proteins of Group A streptococci. Bacteriol Rev 1974;38:57–86.

49. Turk DC. The pathogenicity of *Haemophilus influenzae.* J Med Microbiol 1984;18:1–16.

50. Bornstein DL, Schiffman G, Bernheimer HP, et al. Capsulation of pneumococcus with soluble C-like polysaccharide. I. Biological and genetic properties Cs pnemo coccal strains. J Exp Med 1968;128:1385–1400.

51. Kasper DL, Hayes ME, Reinap BG, et al. Isolation and identification of encapsulated strains of *Bacteroides fragilis.* J Infect Dis 1977;136:75–81.

52. Kasper DL. The polysaccharide capsule of *Bacteroides fragilis* subspecies *fragilis:* immunochemical and morphologic definition. J Infect Dis 1976;133:79–87.

53. Apte RN, Galanos C, Pluznik DH. Lipid A, the active part of bacterial endotoxins including serum colony stimulating activity and proliferation of splenic granulocyte/macrophage progenitor cells. J Cell Physiol 1976;87:71–78.

54. Galanos C, Luderitz O, Rietschel ET, et al. Synthetic and natural *Escherichia coli* free Lipid A express identical endotoxic activities. Eur J Biochem 1985;148:1–5.

55. Fry DE, Kaelin CR, Rink RD. Oxidative metabolism in experimental *Bacteroides fragilis* bacteremia. J Surg Res 1980;28:501–506.

56. Dinarello CA. Interleukin-1 and its biologically related cytokines. Adv Immunol 1989;44:153–205.

57. Skarnes RC, Brown SK, Hull SS, McCracken JA. Role of prostaglandin E in the biphasic fever response to endotoxin. J Exp Med 1981;154:1212–1224.

58. Rivers RPA, Hathaway WE, Weston WL. The endotoxin-induced coagulant activity of human monocytes. Br J Haematol 1975;30:311–316.

59. Horowitz HI, Des Prez, Hook EW. Effects of bacterial endotoxin on rabbit platelets. II. Enhancement of platelet factor 3 activity in vitro and in vivo. J Exp Med 1962;116:619–633.

60. Gewurz H, Shin HS, Mergenhagen SE. Interactions of the complement system with endotoxic lipopolysaccharide: consumption of each of the six terminal complement components. J Exp Med 1968;128:1049–1057.

61. Morland B, Kaplan G. Macrophage activation in vivo and in vitro. Exp Cell Res 1977;108:279–288.

62. Wright SD, Ramos RA, Tobias PS, et al. CD 14 serves as the cellular receptor for complexes of lipopolysaccharide with lipopolysaccharide binding protein. Science 1991;249:1431–1433.

63. Urbaschek B, Ditter B, Becker K-P, Urbaschek R. Protective effects and role of endotoxin in experimental septicemia. Circ Shock 1984;14:209–222.

64. McGowan JE Jr. Antimicrobial resistance in hospital organisms and its relation to antibiotic use. Rev Infect Dis 1983;5:1033–1048.

65. Bauer AW, Kirby WMM, Sherris JC, Turck M. Antibiotic susceptibility testing by a standard single disc method. Am J Clin Pathol 1966;45:490–496.

66. Fry DE, Garrison RN, Trachtenberg L, Polk HC Jr. Bacterial inoculum and the activity of antimicrobial agents. Surg Gynecol Obstet 1985;160:105–108.

67. Waxman DJ, Strominger JL. Penicillin-binding proteins and the mechanism of action of beta-lactam antibiotics. Ann Rev Biochem 1983;52:825–869.

68. Tomasz A. Penicillin-binding proteins and the antibacterial effectiveness of beta-lactam antibiotics. Rev Infect Dis 1986;8(suppl 3):S260–S278.

69. Spratt BG. Penicillin-binding proteins and the future of beta-lac-

tam antibiotics. Journal of General Microbiology 1983;129:1247–1260.

70. Perkins HR, Nieto M. The chemical basis for the action of the vancomycin group of antibiotics. Ann N Y Acad Sci 1974;235:348–363.

71. Vandem Bossche H, Bellens D, Cools W, et al. Cytochrome P-450. Target for itraconazole. Drug Dev Res 1986;8:287–298.

72. Hamilton-Miller JMT. Chemistry and biology of the polyene macrolide antibiotics. Bacteriol Rev 1973;37:166–196.

73. Sokol-Anderson ML, Brajtburg A, Medoff G. Amphotericin B-induced oxidation damage and killing of *Candida albicans*. J Infect Dis 1986;154:76–83.

74. Goodwin NJ. Colistin and sodium colistimethate. Med Clin North Am 1970;54:1267–1276.

75. Pestha S. Inhibition of protein synthesis. In: Weissbach H, Pestha S, eds. Molecular mechanisms of protein synthesis. New York: Academic Press, 1977:467–479.

76. Alford RH. Antimycobacterial agents. In: Mandell GL, Douglas RG Jr, Bennett JE, eds. Principles and practice of infectious disease. New York: Churchill Livingstone, 1990:350–360.

77. Smith JT, Lewin CS. Chemistry and mechanism of action of the quinolone antibacterials. In: Andriole VT, ed. The quinolones. London: Academic Press, 1988:23–81.

78. Goldman P. Metronidazole. N Engl J Med 1980;303:1212–1218.

79. McGuist PV, Furman PA. Acyclovir inhibition of viral DNA chain elongation in herpes simplex virus-infected cells. Am J Med 1982;73(suppl):67–71.

80. Derse D, Cheng Y-C, Furman PA, et al. Inhibition of purified human and herpes simplex-induced DNA polymerases by 9-(2-hydroxyethoxy-methyl) guanine triphosphate. J Biol Chem 1981;256:11447–11451.

81. Miller AK, Buino P, Berglund RM. The effect of sulfathiazole on the in vitro synthesis of certain vitamins by *Escherichia coli*. J Bacteriol 1947;54:9–14.

82. Burchall JJ. Trimethoprim and pyrimethamine. In: Careoran JW, Hahn FE, eds. Antibiotics III. mechanisms of antimicrobial and antitumor agents. Berlin: Springer Verlag, 1975:304.

83. Young FE, Mayer L. Genetic determinants of microbial resistance to antibiotics. Rev Infect Dis 1979;1:55–63.

84. Davies J. Microbial resistance to antimicrobial agents. In: Ristuccia AM, Cunha BA, eds. Antimicrobial therapy. New York: Raven Press, 1984:11–21.

85. Timmis KN, Gonzalez-Carrero MI, Sekizaki T, et al. Biological activities specified by antibiotic resistance plasmids. J Antimicrob Chemother 1986;18:1–2.

86. Sande MA, Kapusnik-Uner JE, Mandell GL. Antimicrobial agents: general considerations. In: Gilman AG, Rall TW, Nies AS, Taylor P, eds. The pharmacological basis of therapeutics, 8th ed. New York: Pergamon Press, 1990:1018–1046.

87. Abraham EP, Chain E. An enzyme from bacteria able to destroy penicillin [Letter]. Nature 1940;146:837.

88. Bauernfeind A. Classification of beta-lactamases. Rev Infect Dis 1986;8(suppl 5):S470–S481.

89. Acar JF, Minozzi C. Role of beta-lactamases in the resistance of gram-negative bacilli to beta-lactam antibiotics. Rev Infect Dis 1986;8(suppl 5):S482–S486.

90. Sanders CC, Sanders WE Jr. Emergence of resistance during therapy with the newer beta-lactam antibiotics: role of inducible beta-lactamases and implications for the future. Rev Infect Dis 1983;5:639–648.

91. Sanders CC, Sanders WE Jr, Goering RV. In vitro antagonism of beta-lactam antibiotics by cefoxitin. Antimicrob Agents Chemother 1982;21:968–975.

92. Malouin F, Bryan LE. Modification of penicillin-binding proteins as mechanisms of beta-lactam resistance. Antimicrob Agents Chemother 1986;30:1–5.

93. Richmond MH, Sykes RB. The beta-lactamases of gram-negative bacteria and their possible physiological role. Adv Microb Physiol 1973;9:31–88.

94. Davies J, Smith DI. Plasmid-determined resistance to antimicrobial agents. Annu Rev Biochem 1978;32:469–518.

95. Benveniste R, Davies J. Mechanisms of antibiotic resistance in bacteria. Annu Rev Biochem 1973;42:471–506.

96. Okamoto S, Suzuki Y. Chloramphenicol-, dihydrostreptomycin-, and kanamycin-inactivating enzymes from multiple drug-resis-

tant *Escherichia coli* carrying episome R. Nature 1965;208:1301–1302.

97. Kabins SA, Panse MV, Cohen S. Role of R-factor and bacterial host in sulfonamide resistance mediated by R-factor in *Escherichia coli*. J Infect Dis 1971;123:158–168.

98. Watanabe T. Infective heredity of multiple drug resistance in bacteria. Bacteriol Rev 1963;27:87–115.

99. Then RL. Mechanisms of resistance to trimethoprim, the sulfonamides and trimethoprim-sulfamethoxazole. Rev Infect Dis 1982;4:261–269.

100. Mao JC-H, Putterman M. Accumulation in gram-positive and gram-negative bacteria as a mechanism of resistance to erythromycin. J Bacteriol 1968;95:1111–1117.

101. Weisblum B, Siddhikol C, Lai CJ, et al. Erythromycin inducible resistance in *Staphylococcus aureus*: requirements for induction. J Bacteriol 1971;106:835–847.

102. Barthelemy P, Autissier D, Gerbaud G, et al. Enzymatic hydrolysis of erythromycin by a strain of *Escherichia coli*. J Antibiot 1984;37:1692–1696.

103. Courvalin P, Ounissi H, Arthur M. Multiplicity of macrolide-lincosamide-streptogramin antibiotic resistance determinants. J Antimicrob Chemother 1985;16(suppl A):91–100.

104. Tally FP, Syndman DR, Shimell MJ, et al. Mechanisms of resistance of *Bacteroides fragilis*. In: Phillips I, Collier J, eds. Metronidazole: proceedings of the Second International Symposium on Anaerobic Infections. London: Royal Society of Medicine and Academic Press, 1979:19.

105. Wolfson JS, Hooper DC. The fluoroquinolones. Structure, mechanisms of action and resistance, and spectrum of activity in vitro. Antimicrob Agents Chemother 1985;28:581–586.

106. Hiraei K, Suzue S, Irikura T, et al. Mutations producing resistance to norfloxacin in *Pseudomonas aeruginosa*. Antimicrob Agents Chemother 1987;31:582–586.

107. Collins P. Viral sensitivity following the introduction of acyclovir. Am J Med 1988;85(suppl 2A):129–134.

108. Fry DE, Garrison RN, Rink RD, et al. An experimental model of intraabdominal abscess in the rat. Advances in Shock Research 1982;7:7–11.

109. Verklin RM, Mandell GL. Alterations of effectiveness of antibiotics by anaerobiosis. J Lab Clin Med 1977;89:65–71.

110. Robson MC, Krizek TJ, Heggers JP. Biology of surgical infection. Curr Probl Surg 1973;3:1–64..

111. Elek SD, Conen PE. The virulence of *Staphylococcus pyogenes* for man: a study of the problem of the wound. British Journal of Experimental Pathology 1957;38:573.

112. Kass EH. Bacteriuria and the diagnosis of infection of the urinary tract. Arch Intern Med 1957;100:709–714.

113. Polk HC Jr. Quantitative tracheal cultures in surgical patients requiring mechanical ventilatory assistance. Surgery 1975;78:485–489.

114. Johanson WG, Pierce AK, Sanford J, et al. Nosocomial respiratory infection with gram-negative bacilli: the significance of colonization of the respiratory tract. Ann Intern Med 1972;77:701–706.

115. Polk HC Jr, Miles AA. Enhancement of bacterial infection by ferric iron. kinetics, mechanisms, and surgical significance. Surgery 1971;70:71–77.

116. Ahrenholz DH, Simmons RL. Fibrin in peritonitis: I. beneficial and adverse effects in experimental *E. coli* peritonitis. Surgery 1980;88:41–47.

117. Hau T, Simmons RL. Heparin in the treatment of experimental peritonitis. Ann Surg 1978;187:294–298.

118. O'Leary JP, Malik FS, Donahue RR, Johnston AD. The effect of minidose heparin on peritonitis in rats. Surg Gynecol Obstet 1979;148:571–575.

119. Miles AA, Niven JSF. The enhancement of infection during shock produced by bacterial toxins and other agents. British Journal of Experimental Pathology 1950;31:73–95.

120. Esrig BC, Fulton RL. Sepsis, resuscitated hemorrhagic shock and "shock lung": an experimental correlation. Ann Surg 1975;182:218–227.

121. Waymack JP, Gallon L, Barcelli U, et al. Effect of blood transfusion on macrophage function in a burned animal model. Curr Probl Surg 1986;43:305–307.

122. Waymack JP, Rapien J, Garnett D, et al. Effect of transfusion on immune function in a traumatized animal model. Arch Surg 1986;121:50–55.

123. Nichols RL, Smith JW, Klein DB, et al. Risk of infection after penetrating abdominal trauma. N Engl J Med 1984;311:1065–1070.

124. Dellinger EP, Oreskovich MR, Wertz MJ, et al. Risk of infection following laparotomy for penetrating abdominal injury. Arch Surg 1984;119:20–27.

125. Robertson HD, Polk HC Jr. The mechanism of infection in patients with diabetes mellitus: a review of leukocyte malfunction. Surgery 1974;75:123–128.

126. Fry DE, Pearlstein L, Fulton RL, Polk HC Jr. Multiple system organ failure: the role of uncontrolled infection. Arch Surg 1980;115:136–140.

127. Klepser RG, Nengster WJ. The effect of alcohol upon the chemotactic response of leukocytes. J Infect Dis 1939;65:196–199.

128. Marr JJ, Spilberg I. A mechanism for decreased resistance to infection by gram-negative organisms during acute alcoholic intoxication. J Lab Clin Med 1975;86:253–258.

129. Wilson DM, Ormrod DJ, Miller TE. Role of complement in chemotaxis. study of a localized infection. Infect Immun 1980;29:8–12.

130. Bevilacqua MP, Nelson RM. Selectins. J Clin Invest 1993;91:379–387.

131. Lawrence MB, Springer TA. Leukocytes roll on a selectin at physiologic flow rates: distinction from and prerequisite for adhesion through integrins. Cell 1991; 65:859–873.

132. Hynes RO. Integrins: versatility, modulation, and signaling in cell adhesion. Cell 1992; 69:11–25.

133. Lorant DE, Patel KD, McIntyre TM, et al. Coexpression of GMP-140 and PAF by endothelium stimulated by histamines or thrombin: a juxtacrine system for adhesion and activation of neutrophils. J Cell Biol 1991; 115:223–224.

134. Wilinson PC. Leukocyte locomotion and chemotaxis: effects of bacteria and viruses. Rev Infect Dis 1980;3:293–318.

135. Stossel TP. Phagocytosis, part 1. N Engl J Med 1974;290:717–723.

136. Stossel TP. Phagocytosis, part 2. N Engl J Med 1974;290:774–780.

137. Stossel TP. Phagocytosis, part 3. N Engl J Med 1974;290:833–839.

138. Elsbach P. Degradation of microorganisms by phagocytic cells. Rev Infect Dis 1980;2:106–128.

139. Babior BM. Oxygen-dependent microbial killing by phagocytes. N Engl J Med 1978;298:659–668.

140. Nathan CF. Secretory products of macrophages. J Clin Invest 1987;79:319–326.

141. Dinarello CA. Interleukin-1 and the pathogenesis of the acute-phase response. N Engl J Med 1984;311:1413–1418.

142. Stitt JT. Prostaglandin E as the neural mediator of the febrile response. Yale J Biol Med 1986;59:137–149.

143. Dinarello CA. Interleukin-1. Rev Infect Dis 1984;6:51–94.

144. Beutler B, Milsark IW, Cerami A. Cachectin/tumor necrosis factor. production, distribution, and metabolic fate. J Immunol 1985;135:3972–3977.

145. Larrick JW, Graham D, Toy K, et al. Recombinant tumor necrosis factor causes activation of human granulocytes. Blood 1987;69:640–644.

146. Hamberg M, Svensson J, Samuelson B. Thromboxanes: a new group of biologically active compounds derived from prostaglandin endoperoxides. Proc Natl Acad Sci U S A 1975;72:2994–2998.

147. Conn HO, Fessel JM. Spontaneous bacterial peritonitis in cirrhosis. variation on a theme. Medicine 1971;50:161–197.

148. Conn HO. Spontaneous bacterial peritonitis, multiple revisitations. Gastroenterology 1976;70:455–457.

149. Nichols RL, Smith JW. Intragastric microbial colonization in common disease state of the stomach and duodenum. Ann Surg 1975;182:557–561.

150. Allen L, Weatherford T. Role of fenestrated basement membrane in lymphatic absorption from the peritoneal cavity. Am J Physiol 1956;197:551–554.

151. Tsilibary EC, Wissig SL. Absorption from the peritoneal cavity: SEM study of the mesothelium covering the peritoneal surface of the muscular portion of the diaphragm. American Journal of Anatomy 1977;149:127–132.

152. Autio V. The spread of intraperitoneal infection: studies with roentgen contrast medium. Acta Chirurgica Scandinavica (Suppl) 1964;123:5–31.

153. Onderdonk AB, Bartlett JC, Louie T, et al. Microbial synergy in experimental intraabdominal abscess. Infect Immun 1976;13:22–26.

154. Alteneier WA, Culbertson WR, Fullen WD, et al. Intraabdominal abscess. Am J Surg 1973;125:70–79.

155. Fry DE, Garrison RN, Heitch RC, et al. Determinants of death in patients with intraabdominal abscess. Surgery 1980;89:517–523.

156. Weibel ER, Taylor CR. Design and structure of the human lung. In: Fishman AP, ed. Pulmonary diseases and disorders, 2nd ed. New York: McGraw-Hill, 1988:11–60.

157. Martin LF, Asher EF, Casey JM, Fry DE. Postoperative pneumonia. determinants of mortality. Arch Surg 1984;119:379–383.

158. Newhouse M, Sanchis J, Bienenstock J. Lung defense mechanisms. N Engl J Med 1976;295:990–997.

159. Newhouse M, Sanchis J, Bienenstock J. Lung defense mechanisms. N Engl J Med 1976;295:1045–1051.

160. Cohen AB, Gold WM. Defense mechanisms of the lung. Annu Rev Physiol 1975;37:325–350.

161. Reynolds HY. Integrated host defense against infections. In: Crystal RG, West JB, eds. The lung: scientific foundations. New York: Raven Press, 1991:1899–1911.

162. Rutland W, Griffin M, Cole PJ. Human ciliary beat frequency in epithelium from intrathoracic and extrathoracic airways. Am Rev Respir Dis 1982;125:100–105.

163. Wong LB, Miller IF, Yeats DB. Stimulation of ciliary beat frequency by autonomic agonists in vivo. J Appl Physiol 1988;65:971–981.

164. Burnett D, Crocker J, Stockley RA. Cells containing IgA subclasses in bronchi of subjects with and without chronic obstructive lung disease. J Clin Pathol 1987;40:1217–1220.

165. Reynolds HY, Kazmierowski JA, Newball HH. Specificity of opsonic antibodies to enhance phagocytosis of Pseudomonas aeruginosa by human alveolar macrophages. J Clin Invest 1975;56:376–385.

166. Reynolds HY, Newball HH. Analysis of proteins and respiratory cells obtained from human lungs by bronchial lavage. J Lab Clin Med 1974;84:559–573.

167. Robertson J, Caldwell JR, Castle JR, Waldman RH. Evidence for the presence of components of the alternate (properdin) pathway of complement activation in respiratory secretions. J Immunol 1976;117:900–903.

168. O'Neill SJ, Lesperance E, Klass DJ. Human lung lavage surfactant enhances staphylococcal phagocytosis by alveolar macrophages. Am Rev Respir Dis 1984;130:1177–1179.

169. Czop JK, McGowan SE, Center DM. Opsonin-independent phagocytosis by human alveolar macrophages. augmentation by human plasma fibronectin. Am Rev Respir Dis 1982;125:607–609.

170. Mold C, Rogers CP, Kaplan RL, Gewurz H. Binding of human C-reactive protein to bacteria. Infect Immun 1982;38:392–395.

171. Reynolds HY, Chretien J. Respiratory tract fluids: analysis of content and contemporary use in understanding lung disease. Dis Mon 1984;30:1–103.

172. Green GM, Kass EH. The role of the alveolar macrophage in the clearance of bacteria from the lung. J Exp Med 1964;119:167–175.

173. Reynolds HY. Lung inflammation. normal host defense or a complication of some diseases. Annu Rev Med 1987;38:295–323.

174. Rodriquez JL. Hospital-acquired gram-negative pneumonia in critically ill, injured patients. Am J Surg 1993; 165(2A Suppl):34S–42S.

175. Katona IM, Ohura K, Allen JB, et al. Modulation of monocyte chemotactic function in inflammatory lesions. Role of inflammatory mediators. J Immunol 1991; 146:708–714.

176. Wolpe SD, Sherry B, Juers D, et al. Identification and characterization of macrophage inflammatory protein 2. Proc Natl Acad Sci U S A 1989; 86:612–616.

177. Driks MR, Craven DE, Celli BR, et al. Nosocomial pneumonia in intubated patients given sucralfate as compared with antacids or histamine type 2 blockers: role of gastric colonization. N Engl J Med 1987;317:1376–1381.

178. Tryba M. The risk of acute stress bleeding and nosocomial pneumonia in ventilated ICU patients: sucralfate vs. antacids. Am J Med 1987;83:117–123.

179. Parsons CL, Greenspan C, Mulholland SG. The primary antibacterial defense mechanism of the bladder. Investig Urol (Berl) 1975;13:72–77.

180. Boen JR, Sylvester DL. The mathematical relationship among urinary frequency, residual urine, and bacterial growth in bladder infection. Invest Urol 1965;2:468–473.

181. Schaeffer AJ, Chmiel J. Urethral meatal colonization in the patho-

genesis of catheter-associated bacteriuria. J Urol 1983;130: 1096–1099.

182. Garibaldi RA, Burke JP, Britt MR, et al. Meatal colonization and catheter-associated bacteriuria. N Engl J Med 1980;303:316–318.

183. Syme R. Epidemic of acute urethral stricture after prostate surgery. Lancet 1982;2:925.

184. Zimmerli W, Lew PD, Walkvogel FA. Pathogenesis of foreign body infection. evidence for a local granulocyte defect. J Clin Invest 1984;73:1191–1200.

185. Zimmerli W, Waldvogel FA, Vaudaux P, et al. Pathogenesis of foreign body infection: description and characterization of an animal model. J Infect Dis 1982;146:487–497.

186. Nickel JC, Grant SK, Costerton JW. Catheter-associated bacteriuria, an experimental study. Urology 1985;26:369–375.

187. Nickel JC, Gristina P, Costerton JW. Electron microscopic study of an infected Foley catheter. Can J Surg 1985;28:50–52.

188. Nickel JC, Ruseska I, Wright JB, et al. Tobramycin resistance of *Pseudomonas aeruginosa* cells growing as a biofilm on urinary catheter material. Antimicrob Agents Chemother 1985;27:619–624.

189. Asher EF, Oliver BG, Fry DE. Urinary tract infections in the surgical patient. Am Surg 1988;54:466–469.

190. Warren JW, Platt R, Thomas RJ, et al. Antibiotic irrigation and catheter-associated urinary tract infection. N Engl J Med 1978; 299:570–574.

191. Maki DG, Ringer M. Evaluation of dressing regimens for prevention of infection with peripheral intravenous catheters: gauze, a transparent polyurethane dressing, and an iodophor-transparent dressing. JAMA 1987;258:2396–2403.

192. Bjornson HS, Colley R, Bower RH, et al. Association between microorganism growth at the catheter insertion site and colonization of the catheter in patients receiving total parenteral nutrition. Surgery 1982;92:720–727.

193. Maki DG, McCormack KN. Defatting catheter insertion sites in total parenteral nutrition is of no value as an infection control measure. Am J Med 1987;83:833–840.

194. Sitges-Serra A, Linares J, Perez JL, et al. A randomized trial on the effect of tubing changes on hub contamination and catheter sepsis during parenteral nutrition. Journal of Parenteral and Enteral Nutrition 1985;9:322–325.

195. Linares J, Sitges-Serra A, Garau J, et al. Pathogenesis of catheter sepsis: a prospective study with quantitative and semiquantitative cultures of catheter hub and segments. J Clin Microbiol 1985; 21:357–360.

196. Maki DG, Weise CE, Sarafin HW. A semi-quantitative method for identifying intravenous-catheter-related infection. N Engl J Med 1977;296:1305–1309.

197. Garrison RN, Richardson JD, Fry DE. Catheter-associated septic thrombophlebitis. South Med J 1982;75:917–919.

198. Caplan ES, Hoyt NJ. Nosocomial sinusitis. JAMA 1982;247: 639–642.

199. King H, Schumacker H. Splenic studies: susceptibility to infection after splenectomy performed in infancy. Ann Surg 1953;136: 239–241.

200. Singer DB. Postsplenectomy sepsis. Perspectives in Paediatric Pathology 1973;1:285–311.

201. Diamond LK. Splenectomy in childhood and the hazard of overwhelming infection. Pediatrics 1969;43:886–889.

202. Krivit W, Giebink GS, Leonard A. Overwhelming post-splenectomy infection. Surg Clin North Am 1979;59:223–233.

203. Frank EL, Neu HC. Postsplenectomy infection. Surg Clin North Am 1981;61:135–155.

204. Krivit W. Overwhelming post-splenectomy infection. Am J Hematol 1977;2:193–201.

205. Eichner ER. Splenic function: normal, too much, and too little. Am J Med 1979;66:311–320.

206. Constantopoulos A, Najjar VA, Wish JB, et al. Defective phagocytosis due to tuftsin deficiency in splenectomized subjects. American Journal of Diseases in Children 1973;125:663–665.

207. Hosea SW. Role of the spleen in pneumococcal infection. Lymphology 1983;16:115–120.

208. Nielson JL, Buskjaen L, Lamm LU, et al. Complement studies in splenectomized patients. Scandinavian Journal of Haematology 1983;30:194–200.

209. Chaikof EL, McCabe CJ. Fatal overwhelming postsplenectomy infection. Am J Surg 1985;194:534–539.

210. Gopal V, Bisno AL. Fulminant pneumococcal infections in "normal" asplenic hosts. Arch Intern Med 1977;137:1526–1530.

211. Smit P, Oberholzer D, Hayden-Smith S, et al. Protective efficacy of pneumococcal polysaccharide vaccines. JAMA 1977;238: 2613–2316.

212. Broome CV. Efficacy of pneumococcal polysaccharide vaccines. Review of Infectious Diseases 1981;3(suppl):582–596.

213. Kafidi KT, Rotschafer JC. Bacterial vaccines for splenectomized patients. Drug Intelligence and Clinical Pharmacology 1988;22: 192–197.

214. Peltola H, Kayhty H, Virtanen M, Makela P. Prevention of *Haemophilus influenzae* type B bacteraemic infections with the capsular polysaccharide vaccine. N Engl J Med 1984;310:1561–1566.

215. Sanchez-Ubeda R, Fernand E, Rousselot LM. Complication rate in general surgical cases: the value of penicillin and streptomycin as postoperative prophylaxis. N Engl J Med 1958;259:1045–1050.

216. Barnes J, Pace WG, Trump DS, Ellison EH. Prophylactic postoperative antibiotics. Arch Surg 1959;79:190–196.

217. Johnstone FRC. An assessment of prophylactic antibiotics in general surgery. Surg Gynecol Obstet 1963;116:1–10.

218. Miles AA, Miles EM, Burke JF. The value and duration of defense reactions of the skin to the primary lodgement of bacteria. British Journal of Experimental Pathology 1957;38:79–96.

219. Polk HC Jr, Lopez-Mayor JF. Postoperative wound infection: a prospective study of determinant factors and prevention. Surgery 1969;97–103.

220. Polk HC Jr, Trachtenberg L, Finn MP. Antibiotic activity in surgical incisions: the basis for prophylaxis in selected operations. JAMA 1980;244:1353–1354.

221. Fry DE, Pitcher DE. Antibiotic pharmacokinetics in surgery. Arch Surg 1990;125:1490–1492.

222. Bodenham A, Shelly MP, Park GR. The altered pharmacokinetics and pharmacodynamics of drugs commonly used in critically ill patients. Clin Pharmacokinet 1988;14:347–373.

223. Benet LZ, Sheiner LB. Pharmacokinetics: the dynamics of drug absorption, distribution, and elimination. In: Gilman AG, Goodman LS, Rall TW, et al, eds. The pharmacological basis of therapeutics, 7th ed. New York: Macmillan, 1985:3–34.

224. Hug CC. Pharmacokinetics of drugs administered intravenously. Anesth Analg 1978;57:704–723.

225. Gibaldi M, Levy G. Pharmacokinetics in clinical practice: 1. Concepts. JAMA 1976;235:1864–1867.

226. Gibaldi M, Levy G. Pharmacokinetics in clinical practice: 2. applications. JAMA 1976;235:1987–1992.

227. Niemiec PW Jr, Allo MD, Miller CF. Effect of altered volume of distribution on aminoglycoside levels in patients in surgical intensive care. Arch Surg 1987;122:207–210.

228. Mitchell PR, Wilson J, Dodek P, et al. Volume of distribution in patients with gram negative sepsis in the ICU [Abstract]. Anesthesiology 1987;67:A126.

229. Klotz U. Pathophysiological and disease-induced changes in drug distribution volume. pharmacokinetic implications. Clin Pharmacokinet 1976;1:204–218.

230. Kaebnick HW, Bandyk DF, Bergamini TM, Towne JB. The microbiology of explanted vascular prostheses. Surgery 1987;102: 756–761.

231. Fine J, Frank ED, Ravin HA, et al. The bacterial factor in traumatic shock. N Engl J Med 1959;260:214–220.

232. Ravin HA, Fine J. Biological implications of intestinal endotoxins. Federation Proceedings 1962;21:65–68.

233. Schweinburg FB, Fine J. Evidence for a lethal endotoxemia as the fundamental feature of irreversibility in three types of traumatic shock. J Exp Med 1960;112:793–800.

234. Zweifach BW. Hemorrhagic shock in germfree rats. Ann N Y Acad Sci 1959;78:315–320.

235. Zweifach BW, Gordon HA, Wagner M, Reyniers JA. Irreversible hemorrhagic shock in germfree rats. J Exp Med 1958;107:437–450.

236. Volkheimer G, Schulz FH. The phenomenon of persorption. Digestion 1968;1:213–218.

237. Volkheimer G, Schulz FH, Beuthin K, Wendlandt H. Persorption of particles. Digestion 1968;1:78–80.

238. Border J, Hassett J, LaDuca J, et al. The gut origin septic states in blunt multiple trauma (ISS = 40) in the ICU. Ann Surg 1987; 206:427–448.

239. Berg RD, Garlington AW. Translocation of certain indigenous bacteria from the gastrointestinal tract to the mesenteric lymph

nodes and other organs in a gnotobiotic mouse model. Infect Immun 1979;23:403–411.

240. Berg RD. Inhibition of Escherichia coli translocation from the gastrointestinal tract by normal cecal flora in gnotobiotic or anti-biotic-decontaminated mice. Infect Immun 1980;29:1073–1081.

241. Eade MN, Brooke BN. Portal bacteremia in cases of ulcerative colitis submitted to colectomy. Lancet 1969;1:1008–1013.

242. Schatten WE, Despray JD, Holden WD. A bacteriologic study of portal vein blood in man. Arch Surg 1955;71:404–409.

243. LeFrock JL, Ellis CA, Turchick JB, et al. Transient bacteremia associated with sigmoidoscopy. N Engl J Med 1975;289:467–469.

244. Dickman MD, Farrell R, Higgs RH, et al. Colonoscopy-associated bacteremia. Surg Gynecol Obstet 1976;142:173–176.

245. Deitch EA. Simple intestinal obstruction causes bacterial translocation in man. Arch Surg 1989;124:699–701.

246. Wilmore DW, Smith RJ, O'Dwyer ST, et al. The gut: a central organ after surgical stress. Surgery 1988;104:917–923.

247. Rolandelli R, Koruda M, Settle R, et al. The effect of enteral feedings supplemented with pectin on the healing of colonic anastomoses in the rat. Surgery 1986;99:703–708.

248. Mochizuki H, Trocki O, Dominioni L, et al. Mechanism of prevention of post burn hypermetabolism and catabolism by early enteral feeding. Ann Surg 1984;200:297–310.

249. Moore FA, Moore EE, Jones TN, et al. TEN versus TPN following major abdominal trauma-reduced septic mortality. J Trauma 1989;29:916–923.

250. McNabb PC, Tomasi TB. Host defense mechanisms at mucosal surfaces. Ann Rev Microbiol 1981;35:477–496.

251. Tomasi TB Jr, Bienenstock J. Secretory immunoglobulins. Adv Immunol 1968;9:1–96.

252. Johanson WG Jr, Blackstock R, Pierce AK, Sanford JP. The role of bacterial antagonism in pneumococcal colonization of the human pharynx. J Lab Clin Med 1970;75:946–952.

253. Sanders E. Bacterial interference: I. its occurrence among the respiratory tract flora and characterization of inhibition of Group A streptococci by viridans streptococci. J Infect Dis 1969;120:698–707.

254. Blacklow NR, Dolin R, Fedson DS, et al. Acute infectious nonbacterial gastroenteritis: etiology and pathogenesis. Ann Intern Med 1972;76:993–1008.

255. Savage DC. Colonization by and survival of pathogenic bacteria on intestinal mucosal surface. In: Britton G, Marshall KC, eds. Adsorption of microorganisms to surfaces. New York: Wiley, 1980:175–206.

256. Klebanoff SJ, Belding ME. Virucidal activity of H_2O_2-generating bacteria. requirements for peroxidase and a halide. J Infect Dis 1974;129:345–348.

257. Fuller R. Ecological studies on the lactobacillus flora associated with the crop epithelium of the fowl. J Appl Bacteriol 1973;36:131–139.

258. Suegara N, Morotomi M, Watanabe T, et al. Behavior of the microflora in the rat stomach: adhesion of lactobacilli to the keratinized epithelial cells of the rat stomach in vitro. Infect Immun 1975;12:173–179.

259. van der Waaij D. Colonization resistance of the digestive tract: clinical consequences and implications. J Antimicrob Chemother 1982;10:263–270.

260. Stone HH, Kolb LD, Currie CA, et al. Candida sepsis: pathogenesis and principles of treatment. Ann Surg 1974;179:697–711.

261. Maejima K, Deitch EA, Berg RD. Bacterial translocation from the gastrointestinal tracts of rats receiving thermal injury. Infect Immun 1984;43:6–10.

262. Baker JW, Deitch EA, Li M, et al. Hemorrhagic shock induces bacterial translocation from the gut. J Trauma 1988;28:896–906.

263. Deitch EA, Winterton J, Li M, et al. The gut as a portal of entry for bacteremia: role of protein malnutrition. Ann Surg 1987;205:681–692.

264. Deitch EA, Berg R, Specian R. Endotoxin promotes the translocation of bacteria from the gut. Arch Surg 1987;122:185–190.

265. Rush BF Jr, Sori AJ, Murphy TF, et al. Endotoxemia and bacteremia during hemorrhagic shock. Ann Surg 1988;207:549–554.

266. Rush BF, Redan JA, Flanagan JJ, et al. Does bacteremia in hemorrhagic shock have clinical significance? Ann Surg 1989;210:342–347.

267. Lanser ME. An experimental phenomenon without clinical sig-

nificance. In: Fry DE, ed. Multiple system organ failure. Chicago: Mosby Year Book, 1992:382–389.

268. American College of Chest Physicians/Society of Critical Care Medicine Consensus Conference. Definition for sepsis and organ failure and guidelines for the use of innovative therapies in sepsis. Crit Care Med 1992;20:864.

269. Siegel JH, Cerra FB, Coleman B, et al. Physiologic and metabolic correlations in human sepsis. Surgery 1979;86:163–193.

270. Schumer W, Das Gupta TK, Moss GS, Nyhus LM. Effect of endotoxemia on liver cell mitochondria in man. Ann Surg 1970;171:875–881.

271. Mela L, Bacalzo LV Jr, Miller LD. Defective oxidative metabolism of rat liver mitochondria in hemorrhagic and endotoxin shock. Am J Physiol 1971. 220:571–580.

272. Fry DE, Siver BB, Rink RD, et al. Hepatic cellular hypoxia in murine peritonitis. Surgery 1979;85:652–661.

273. Vary TC, Siegel JH, Rivkind AI. Clinical and therapeutic significance of metabolic patterns of lactic acidosis. Perspect Crit Care 1988;1:85–132.

274. Vary TC, Siegel JH, Nakatani T, et al. Effect of sepsis on activity of pyruvate dehydrogenase complex in skeletal muscle and liver. Am J Physiol 1986;250:E634–E640.

275. Townsend MC, Hampton WW, Haybron DM, et al. Effective organ blood flow and bioenergy status in murine peritonitis. Surgery 1986;100:205–213.

276. Schirmer WJ, Schirmer JM, Naff GB, Fry DE. Complement activation produces hemodynamic changes characteristic of sepsis. Arch Surg 1988;123:316–321.

277. Schirmer WJ, Schirmer JM, Fry DE. Recombinant human tumor necrosis factor produces hemodynamic changes characteristic of sepsis and endotoxemia. Arch Surg 1989;124:445–448.

278. Asher EF, Rowe RL, Garrison RN, Fry DE. Experimental bacteremia and hepatic nutrient blood flow. Circ Shock 1986;20:43–49.

279. Ziegler EJ, Fisher CJ, Sprung CL, et al: Treatment of gram negative bacteremia and septic shock with HA-1A human monoclonal antibody against endotoxin. N Engl J Med 1991;324:429–436.

280. Greenman RL, Schein RM, Martin MA, et al: A controlled clinical trial of E5 murine monoclonal IgM antibody to endotoxin in the treatment of gram-negative sepsis. The XOMA sepsis study group. JAMA 1991; 266:1097–1102.

281. Beutler B, Milsark JA, Cerami AC: Passive immunization against cachectin/tumor necrosis factor protects mice from the lethal effect of endotoxin. Science 1985; 229:869–871.

282. Tracey KJ, Fong Y, Hess DG, et al. Anticachectin/TNF monoclonal antibodies prevent septic shock during lethal bacteremia. Nature 1987;330:662–664.

283. Abraham E, Wunderink R, Silverman H, et al. Efficacy and safety of monoclonal antibody to human tumor necrosis factor alpha in patients with sepsis syndrome. A randomized, controlled, double-blind, multicenter clinical trial. TNF-alpha MAb Sepsis Study Group. JAMA 1995; 273:934–941.

284. Gatanaga T, Hwang CD, Kohr W, et al. Purification and characterization of an inhibitor (soluble tumor necrosis factor inhibitor) for tumor necrosis factor and lymphotoxin obtained from the serum ultrafiltrates of human cancer patients. Proc Natl Acad Sci USA 1990; 87:8781–8784.

285. Mohler KM, Torrance DS, Smith CA, et al. Soluble tumor necrosis factor(TNF) receptors are effective therapeutic agents in lethal endotoxemia and function both simultaneously as both TNF carriers and TNF antagonists. J Immunol 1993; 151:1548–1561.

286. Ohlsson K, Bjork P, Bergenfeldt M, et al. Interleukin-1 receptor antagonist reduces mortality from endotoxin shock. Nature 1990; 348:550–51.

287. Okusawa S, Gelfand JA, Ikejima T, et al. Interleukin 1 induces a shock-like state in rabbits: synergism with tumor necrosis factor and the effect of cyclooxygenase inhibition. J Clin Invest 1988; 81:1162–1172.

288. Wakabayashi G, Gelfand JA, Burke JF, et al. A specific receptor antagonist for interleukin-1 prevents Escherichia coli-induced shock in rabbits. FASEB J 1991;5:338–343.

289. Weisman HF, Bartow T, Leppo MK, et al: Soluble human complement receptor Type I: in vivo inhibitor of complement suppressing post-ischemic myocardial inflammation and necrosis. Science 1990; 249:146.

290. Chang SW, Fernyak S, Voelkel NF. Beneficial effect of a platelet-activating factor antagonist, WEB 2086, on endotoxin-induced lung injury. Am J Physiol 1990;258:H153–H158.

291. Fletcher JR, DiSimone AG, Earnest MA. Platelet activating factor receptor antagonist improves survival and attenuates eicosanoid release in severe endotoxemia. Ann Surg 1990;211:312–316.

292. Schirmer WJ, Schirmer JM, Townsend MC, Fry DE. Effects of ibuprofen, indomethacin, and imidazole on survival in sepsis. Curr Surg 1987;44:102–105.

293. Schirmer WJ, Townsend MC, Schirmer JM, Fry DE. Imidazole and indomethacin enhance hepatic perfusion in sepsis. Circ Shock 1987;21:253–259.

294. Schirmer WJ, Schirmer JM, Naff GB, Fry DE. Contribution of toxic oxygen intermediates to complement-induced reduction in effective hepatic blood flow. J Trauma 1988;28:1295–1300.

295. Petros A, Bennett D, Vallance P. Effect of nitric oxide synthase inhibitor on hypotension in patients with septic shock. Lancet 1991; 338:1557–1558.

296. Schilling J, Cakmakci M, Battig U, Geroulanos S. A new approach in the treatment of hypotension in human septic shock by NG-monomethyl-L-arginine, an inhibitor of the nitric oxide synthase. Intensive Care Med 1993; 19:227–231.

297. Mileski WJ, Winn RK, Harlan JM, Rice CL. Transient inhibition of neutrophil adherence with the anti-CD 18 monoclonal antibody 60.3 does not increase mortality rates in abdominal sepsis. Surgery 1991; 109:495–501.

298. Sharar SR, Winn RK, Murry CE, et al. A CD 18 monoclonal antibody increases the incidence and severity of subcutaneous abscess formation after high-dose Staphylococcus aureus infection in rabbits. Surgery 1991; 110:213–219.

299. Marchant A, Bruyns C, Vandenabeele P, et al. The protective role of Interleukin 10 in endotoxin shock. Prog Clin Biol Res 1994; 388:417–423.

10 Principles of Pharmacology

Wayne L. Backes / Joseph M. Moerschbaecher

Drug-Receptor Theory

Drugs produce their effects through interplay with existing biochemical and physiologic systems within the body. For example, a drug that influences heart rate or blood pressure acts on the part of the autonomic nervous system that controls that process. Drugs themselves do not have inherent effects. Most drugs exert their effects by binding to specific macromolecules within the body. This interaction initiates a series of biochemical and physiologic changes that culminates in the observed drug response. These macromolecules are known as receptors and are the sites of the initial interaction for the drug. Normally, receptors interact with endogenous compounds in the body. Drugs act by altering the rate at which these normal bodily functions proceed. Drugs do not create novel effects but only modulate the rate of ongoing physiologic processes.

Most drug-receptor interactions fall into three general classifications: (*a*) An agonist is a compound that both binds to and produces an alteration in a receptor, which results in the observed pharmacologic response; (*b*) An antagonist binds to the receptor but, on binding, does not alter the receptor. Antagonists act by inhibiting the effects of agonists; and (*c*) A partial agonist binds to and alters the receptor; however, the resulting response is not as great as that produced by a full agonist.

Most drugs bind to receptors in a reversible manner, which means that the drug can bind freely and dissociate from the receptor molecule. The chemical bonds that are important for reversible drug receptor interactions include ionic bonds, hydrogen bonds, hydrophobic bonds, and van der Waals forces. Ionic bonds are electrostatic attractions between ions of opposite charge. These ionic bonds provide the initial interaction between the drug and receptor. Hydrogen bonds are weaker interactions that further stabilize this initial ionic bond. They are produced by a reciprocal partial ioniza-

tion of both the drug and the receptor molecules. Last, hydrophobic interactions and van der Waals forces provide the final stabilization of the complex. These bonds ultimately control the affinity and also the ability of that particular drug to produce the change in the receptor (1).

Drug receptor interactions are governed by the law of mass action. In an attempt to describe these types of interactions, Clark (2) developed the basis for most of the theories of drug action. The treatment is analogous to the Michaelis-Menten treatment for enzyme kinetic data. The treatment is called the occupancy theory and is based on five assumptions: (*a*) the magnitude of the response is proportional to the number of receptors occupied; (*b*) drug-receptor complex formation is rapid and freely reversible compared with the rate of response; (*c*) one drug combines with one receptor; (*d*) all receptors are identical and equally accessible to the drug; and (*e*) only a small portion of the drug is involved in forming complexes with the receptor molecules (3).

Drug + Receptor $\rightleftharpoons$ Drug-Receptor   Response

According to this model, the drug combines with the receptor, producing a drug-receptor complex. Formation of this complex is the initial interaction that eventually culminates in the pharmacologic response. According to the occupancy theory, the amount of drug-receptor complex is directly proportional to the magnitude of the response; therefore, if the occupancy theory holds and 100% of the receptors are occupied, the maximal response will be attained. In a similar manner, if only 50% of the receptors are occupied, then only 50% of the maximal response will be observed.

Drugs differ in their ability to bind to receptors. This binding is characterized and quantified by use of the dissociation constant (K_d), which is described by equation 2.

$$\frac{[\text{Drug}][\text{Receptor}]}{[\text{Drug} - \text{Receptor}]} = K_d$$

228

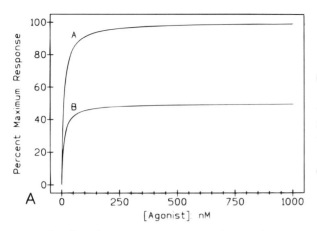

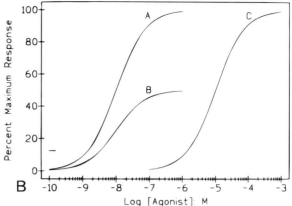

Figure 10.1. The effect of agonist concentration on pharmacologic response. **A,** Linear plot. Curve A represents a full agonist, whereas curve B represents that of a partial agonist. Both drugs in this figure have the same K_d value. **B,** Semilogarithmic plot. Curves A and C represent full agonists that differ in their potencies, whereas curve B represents that of a partial agonist.

The K_d is a measure of the affinity of the drug for the receptor. A tighter drug-receptor complex will have a smaller K_d. Rearrangement of equation 2 yields equation 3, which predicts the pharmacologic effect as a function of drug dose.

$$\text{Response} = \frac{E_{max}\,[\text{Drug}]}{K_d[\text{Drug}]}$$

The relationship between drug dose and response is depicted in Figure 10.1. At the lowest drug doses, a small increase in drug concentration leads to a large increase in the pharmacologic effect observed; however, further increases in drug concentration will lead to a proportionately smaller increase in the drug effect.

Pharmacologists frequently plot such data as the response or the effect observed against the log (dose) as shown in Figure 10.1B. A wide range of concentrations are displayed easily with such a plot, which is particularly useful when drugs that have different affinities for their receptor site are being compared. Two important pieces of information that can be gained from a dose-response curve are the maximal effect (E_{max}) and the ED_{50}. The E_{max} is the maximum possible effect produced by a particular drug as measured on the y axis. As shown in Figure 10.1B, the maximal effect shown for a partial agonist (curve B) is less than that shown for the full agonist (curve A). The ED_{50} is that dose at which 50% of the maximal effect is observed. Determination of the ED_{50} is shown in Figure 10.1B for the full agonist (curve A) and the partial agonist (curve B).

Antagonism

There are two types of antagonism: (*a*) irreversible antagonism, for which the drug covalently binds to the receptor site; and (*b*) reversible antagonism, which is the most common type for therapeutically useful agents. Reversible antagonism can be subdivided further into competitive, or surmountable, antagonism and noncom-

petitive antagonism. As stated previously, antagonists do not act by producing an effect on the receptor themselves, but act by inhibiting the interaction of endogenous agonists with the receptor molecule. Competitive antagonism occurs when both the antagonist and the agonist compete for the same binding site on the receptor molecule. As shown graphically in Figure 10.2, the response to an agonist is affected by the presence of the antagonist by shifting the dose-response curve to the right. In the presence of higher concentrations of antagonist, the dose-response curve for the agonist will be shifted to the right, resulting in an increase in the apparent ED_{50} of the agonist in the presence of the antagonist. The maximal effect produced by an agonist, such as morphine, is not affected by the presence of an antagonist, such as naloxone. The only difference is that a higher dose of morphine is required to produce the maximal response when naloxone is present.

Competitive interactions occur when the binding between an agonist and an antagonist is mutually exclusive. If the agonist is bound to the receptor, then the receptor can be altered, resulting in the pharmacologic response. However, because the antagonist cannot produce an alteration in the receptor, as does an agonist, it acts by blocking agonist binding to the receptor. Therefore, to overcome the effects of the antagonist, higher concentrations of agonist would be required to produce an equivalent response.

With simple noncompetitive antagonism, both agonist and antagonist can bind freely to the receptor; however, each compound binds to its own site (Fig. 10.3B). In the absence of antagonist, the agonist will be able to bind to the receptor site and produce its pharmacologic response. However, antagonist binding to a separate site will inactivate a certain proportion of the receptors, depending on the affinity of the antagonist for the receptor site. The agonist in the presence of antagonist will neither affect the binding of the antagonist to the receptor nor permit a pharmacologic response to be observed in

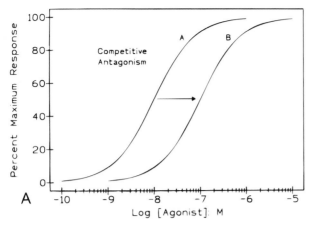

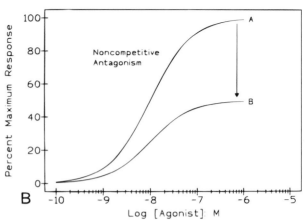

Figure 10.2. Dose-response curves for different types of antagonism. **A,** Competitive antagonism. Agonist dose response in the absence (curve A) and presence of a fixed concentration of competitive antagonist (curve

B). **B,** Noncompetitive antagonism. Agonist dose response in the absence (curve A) and presence (curve B) of a fixed concentration of noncompetitive antagonist.

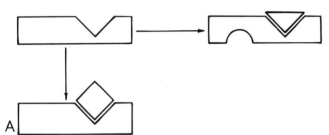

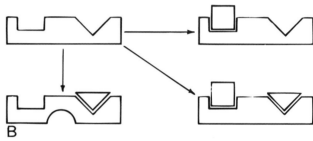

Figure 10.3. Antagonist action. **A,** Competitive antagonism. The receptor molecule can be bound by either agonist (∇) or antagonist (◇), both of which bind to the same site on the receptor molecule. Agonist binding results in a modification of the receptor molecule in such a manner as to elicit the pharmacologic response. The antagonist cannot produce such a change in the receptor but acts by preventing binding of agonist. **B,** Noncompetitive antagonist. In this case, the receptor has two sites,

one that binds agonist and one that binds antagonist. Binding of antagonist (□) does not alter the ability of agonist (∇) to bind; however, when antagonist is present, the agonist cannot produce the modification of the receptor. As a result, the antagonist effectively inactivates a certain proportion of the receptors, and the magnitude of the inhibition depends on the concentration of antagonist present.

those receptors where antagonist is found. As a result, the presence of antagonist will inactivate a certain percentage of the receptors. Further addition of agonist will not overcome the effects of a noncompetitive antagonist. For example, this is why phenoxybenzamine, an irreversibly acting α-antagonist, is used before the surgical excision of a pheochromocytoma. A graphic representation of the effects of a noncompetitive antagonist is shown in Figure 10.2B.

Irreversible antagonism occurs when the antagonist molecule covalently binds to either the active site or a second site. Graphically, either type of irreversible inhibition can look like that shown for simple noncompetitive inhibition (Fig. 10.2B). Differences between irreversible inhibition and noncompetitive inhibition can be identified by more detailed examination.

Behavior of Partial Agonists and Variations in Receptor Response in Different Tissues—Concept of Receptor Reserve

The basic problems with the simplified model described by Clark were: (1) it did not adequately describe

the behavior of partial agonists; and (2) some agonists appeared to produce their effects at less than 100% receptor occupancy. Some effects result because the drug-receptor interaction does not directly lead to the pharmacologic response. Formation of the drug-receptor complex is the initial interaction, triggering a series of events that will eventually culminate in the pharmacologic response. This process is known as signal transduction. The most common mechanisms for signal transduction involve phosphoinositide hydrolysis and calcium mobilization, G proteins, and alterations in the activities of certain regulatory enzymes after phosphorylation by protein kinases. As shown in equation 4, formation of the drug-receptor complex produces an initial response (R_1).

Drug + Receptor $\rightleftharpoons$ Drug-Receptor R_1 Response

As an example, let us assume that the initial response is the mobilization of calcium ion. This then leads to the pharmacologic effect.

Now let us examine the effect of a drug in three different tissues that have differences in receptor density.

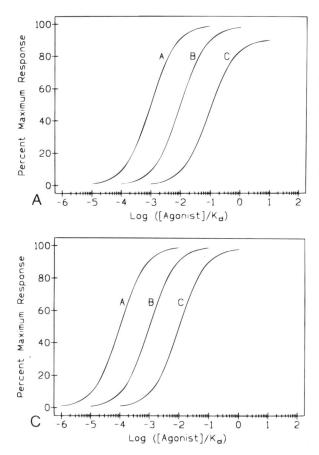

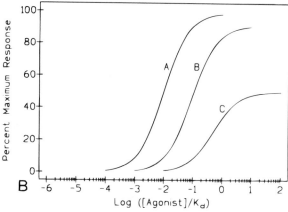

Figure 10.4. Dose-response relationships for agonists with different efficacies under conditions of different receptor densities and reserves. **A,** Curves A, B, and C represent the dose-response curves for agonist X in three tissues with different receptor densities. Drug X obeys the assumptions of occupancy theory in tissue B (where 100% of the receptors are occupied, producing a maximal response) and behaves as a full agonist. In tissue C, which has a lower receptor density, drug X cannot produce as large of a response and behaves as a partial agonist in that tissue. In tissue A, a maximal response is obtained with less than 100% tissue occupancy. **B,** Behavior of drug Y in tissues A, B, and C. Because of the decreased ability of drug Y to modify the receptor (intrinsic efficacy), this drug does not exhibit receptor reserve. It behaves as a full agonist in tissue A and as a partial agonist in tissues B and C. **C,** Agonist Z appears to behave as a full agonist in each tissue because of its larger intrinsic efficacy. The drug exhibits increasing receptor reserve in tissues B and A.

Drug X produces its pharmacologic effect by binding to the receptors in each of the tissues A, B, and C by a process mediated by Ca^{2+} mobilization. Drug X, therefore, produces its effect by binding to the receptors and mobilizing calcium. The released Ca^{2+} then produces the pharmacologic response. Drug X requires a receptor density of 10 receptors per unit area to mobilize sufficient calcium to produce this maximal response. In tissue B (having 10 receptors per unit area), drug X is capable of producing its maximal response by binding to all of the receptors per unit area. However, if drug X is placed in tissue C, where there are only 5 receptors per unit area, sufficient calcium cannot be mobilized to produce the same response seen in tissue B. Drug X behaves as a partial agonist in tissue C, but in tissue B it behaves as a full agonist. However, in tissue A, where the receptor density is 20 receptors per unit area, there are more than enough receptors to mobilize the Ca^{2+} required to produce the maximal response. In fact, in tissue A, the maximal response will be observed when only half the receptors are occupied. Therefore, to produce an equivalent response in tissue A compared with tissue B, lower concentrations of drug X are required. The presence of the receptor reserve found in tissue A will cause a shift in the dose-response curve to the left with respect to the response in tissue B (Fig. 10.4A). This example demonstrates how a drug can behave as a partial agonist in

one tissue (C), a full agonist in another tissue (B), and exhibit receptor reserve in a third tissue (A) (3).

Because agonists differ both in their affinity for receptor site and in their ability to produce the change in the receptor (which results in the pharmacologic response), different drugs can produce different responses in various tissues even though they are binding to the same receptor sites. As an example, drug Y can produce its effects in a manner similar to drug X but may require a receptor density of only 5 receptors per unit area to produce its maximal response. Therefore, drug Y would behave as a full agonist in tissue C (where a receptor density of 5 is observed), and exhibit increasing degrees of receptor reserve in tissues B and A, respectively (Fig. 10.4B). Drug Z, which requires 20 receptors per unit area bound to mobilize sufficient calcium to produce its maximal response, would behave as a full agonist only in tissue A and would behave as a partial agonist in tissues B and C (Fig. 10.4C). These results indicate that the response to a drug depends on both the affinity of the drug for the receptor site and the ability of that drug to stimulate the signal transduction mechanisms. Furthermore, the response of a drug depends on the receptor density present in a particular tissue.

Two terms are generally used to describe drug behavior: potency and efficacy. *Potency* is simply the concentration of drug necessary to produce a response. When less of a drug is required to produce a particular response, it is said to be more potent. A number of factors can affect potency of a drug. The first factor is the affinity of the drug for the receptor. If a drug has a higher affinity (i.e., lower K_d), it is said to be more potent. The potency of a drug can also be affected by the functional relationship between the receptor and response. As described above, the same drug in different tissues has different potencies owing to the presence of receptor reserve in some of the tissues. The final factors that will affect the potency of a drug are pharmacokinetic parameters: absorption, distribution, metabolism, and excretion. Each of these factors will affect the concentration of drug that will get to the receptor site and could, therefore, affect the drug dose required to produce a particular pharmacologic response.

Differences in *efficacy* can be manifest as either differences in the apparent effect of a particular agonist or changes in the apparent potency of a drug. When comparing a full agonist that does not exhibit receptor reserve with a partial agonist, the changes in their efficacy will be reflected by a change in the maximal effect seen with each drug. However, when comparing a drug that exhibits receptor reserve to that same drug in another tissue where receptor reserve is not found, no changes in the maximal effect will be found, although the drug has a different efficacy in the different tissues. These changes will be manifest as a difference in the apparent potency of the drug in these tissues.

Thus far, dose-response curves have been discussed for a single subject. These dose-response curves show the measured magnitude of response from subjects who are administered different doses of a drug. This type of representation is referred to as a *graded dose-response curve*. Because such dose-response curves are for individual subjects, comparisons of the curves among subjects show biologic variation; no two individuals produce exactly the same response at all drug concentrations.

Another method for expressing dose-response data for a population is to assign a quantal response for individuals of a population. An individual is then said to either respond or not to respond. Populations of individuals are then treated with a particular dose of the drug and categorized as either responders or nonresponders. As the concentration of drug is increased, the total number of individuals responding to that drug will also increase. The log of the dose of the drug concentration against the total number of individuals responding will generate a dose-response curve that is called a *quantal dose-response curve*. A quantal dose-response curve can be used to describe the relative effectiveness of a drug in a population of individuals.

No drug produces a single response. For example, aspirin has analgesic effects, antiinflammatory effects, and a variety of adverse effects. Each of these effects would have its own dose-response curves for different dosage ranges. Finally, at high enough doses, the drug would be lethal. Quantal dose-response curves can be used to estimate the relative safety of a particular drug. A term used to estimate the relative safety of a drug is called the therapeutic index. This is equal to the LD_{50} (the dose that produces lethality in 50% of the subjects) divided by the ED_{50}. The larger the therapeutic index, the greater the relative safety of a drug. For example, the barbiturates have a much smaller therapeutic index than do the benzodiazepines.

Absorption, Distribution, Metabolism, and Excretion of Drugs

The pharmacologic response to a drug depends on its concentration at the receptor site; however, the ability of a drug to get to its receptor can be influenced by a number of factors. Once a drug is administered to an organism, it can do a number of things. First, it must be absorbed into the circulation. After absorption, the drug will be distributed. Once in the circulation, it can bind to plasma proteins, accumulate in various tissues reservoirs, or associate at the receptor site where it will produce its pharmacologic effect. The drug can also be eliminated unchanged or can be converted to metabolites, which may be pharmacologically active or inactive. The metabolites can then be excreted (1,4).

Mechanisms of Drug Transport

Drugs differ in their rates of accumulation and elimination from the body owing to differences in their physical properties. To reach their sites of action, drugs must cross one or more biologic membranes, which are composed largely of lipid. These membranes act as primary barriers to drug transport. Therefore, for a drug to get to its site of action, it must either pass around or through these membranes. The body uses a number of different mechanisms for transport of endogenous compounds from one site of the body to another. These processes include passive diffusion, filtration, endocytosis, and carrier-mediated transport. These same mechanisms are used for the transport of drugs to their sites of action and are also involved in their removal from the body (5).

Passive Diffusion

The most common mechanism for drug transport is passive diffusion. This process can be further subdivided into passive diffusion of nonelectrolytes and passive diffusion of weak acids and bases. Passive diffusion occurs when a high concentration of drug exists on one side of a membrane and a low concentration on the other. The drug will then passively transfer through the membrane, a process that will continue until the concentration of drug on both sides of the membrane is equal. Most drugs can transfer across membranes by passive diffusion at least to some extent; however, the rate of transfer by this mechanism differs among drugs. The major factor that appears to control the rate of passive diffusion of nonelectrolytes is the lipid solubility of the drug. A term used to estimate the lipid solubility of a drug is called the partition coefficient (K_p), which is simply the ratio of the concentration of drug in the lipid phase divided by its concentration in the aqueous phase. Therefore, highly lipid-soluble drugs will have larger K_p values. The addition of carbon and hydrogen atoms to a particular drug molecule will have a tendency to increase the partition coefficient for the drug, whereas the addition of polar groups such as hydroxyl, carboxyl, and amino groups will have a tendency to decrease the partition coefficient. Such modifications in the structure of a drug compound alter the rate at which the compounds can transfer by passive diffusion across membranes. This can affect the drug concentration at the receptor and, as a result, the pharmacologic response to a drug.

If all drugs were nonelectrolytes, then the rate of drug transfer would simply depend on the drug's lipid solubility. However, most drugs are electrolytes and have a tendency to ionize in solution. The ability of drugs to ionize has a profound impact on their rate of transfer across biologic membranes. Electrolytes are categorized as either acids or bases. For the sake of this discussion, an acid is a compound that is uncharged when it is in a complex with a hydrogen ion (equation 5).

$$HA \rightleftharpoons H^+ + A^-$$

The types of functional groups that behave as acids are carboxyl, sulfhydryl, and hydroxyl groups. Drugs that behave as bases exhibit ionization characteristics, as illustrated in equation 6.

$$BH^+ \rightleftharpoons H^+ + B$$

In this case, when the drug is in a complex with the hydrogen ion, the complex has a positive charge. The main functional group that undergoes this type of ionization is the amino group that will ionize to $-NH_3^+$.

Different drugs, whether they are acids or bases, will differ in their ability to ionize. For example, some drugs will readily give up their additional hydrogen ion, whereas other drugs will do so less readily. The relative ability of a drug to ionize is defined by its pK. The term pK is defined in the Henderson-Hasselbalch equation as the pH at which a drug would be 50% ionized. For example, a weak acid drug with a pK of 4 is 50% ionized (and 50% un-ionized) in a solution of pH 4. Likewise, a weak acid with a pK of 10 would have equal amounts of ionized and un-ionized species if it were in a solution of pH 10. Remember that the pK indicates the pH at which ionization occurs. Weak acids have pK values

smaller than 7 but also can have pK values greater than 7. Bases can also have pK values anywhere along the pH scale. As the pH of the solution is decreased (the hydrogen ion concentration is increased), the amount of acid in complex will increase as a result of the law of mass action. Because pH and pK are logarithmic functions, each pH unit difference between the pH and pK represents a 10-fold difference in the concentrations of the ionized and un-ionized species. Therefore, if the pH is 3 units lower than the pK value, there is a 1000-fold higher concentration of the un-ionized complexed form of the acid compared with the ionized uncomplexed species. An analogous situation occurs with a base. For example, in a base with a pK of 4 in a solution of pH 2, there will be a 100-fold excess of the ionized complexed species over that of the un-ionized uncomplexed form.

The reason that ionization is important in regard to drug transfer across membranes is that only the un-ionized species can transfer by passive diffusion. For a weak acid (A), the HA species will be the one that transfers by passive diffusion, and for a weak base (B), the uncomplexed species will transfer by passive diffusion. Figure 10.5 illustrates how ionization can alter the transfer of a drug across biologic membranes. In this case, drug A is a weak acid with pK 5 transferring from a solution of pH 1 into a solution of pH 7. The figure shows the equilibrium concentrations of each of these species after transfer has occurred. As previously mentioned, passive diffusion occurs until equal concentrations of the un-ionized species are attained on both sides of the membrane. As a result, the relative amounts of HA on both sides of the membrane will be 1. Because in this example the drug has a pK equal to 5 and is in a solution of pH 1, the relative amount of ionized species will be 0.0001. Once the drug transfers into the pH 7 side of the membrane, it will ionize. The 2 pH unit difference between the pK of the drug and the pH of the solution will produce a 100-fold difference between A^- and HA. As a result, the total amount of drug on the pH 1 side of the membrane will be 1.0001 and the amount of the pH 7 side of membrane will be 101. This illustrates that the ionization of a drug can have a profound influence on the ability of that drug to transfer across a biologic membrane by passive diffusion. This process is called *ion trapping.* An example of the effect of ionization on the transfer of a weak base is shown in Figure 10.5B. The conditions are identical to those shown in Figure 10.5A; the only difference is that the drug is a base rather than an acid. These results show that a weak base under the same conditions as a weak acid will have a greater tendency to accumulate on the side where the pH is lower.

Keep in mind that the ionization characteristics of a drug will affect its rate of transfer across a biologic membrane by controlling the relative amount of un-ionized species that is present. Therefore, a drug that is highly ionized will transfer more slowly because there is a

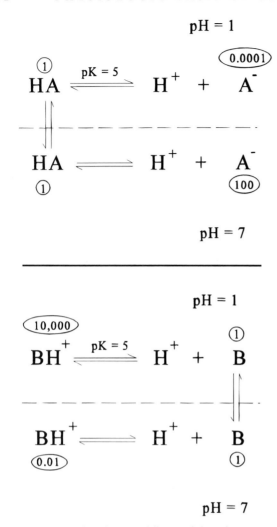

Figure 10.5. Examples of passive diffusion of electrolytes across membranes. **A,** Passive diffusion of a weak acid (pK = 5), when a pH difference exists between the solutions on opposite sides of the membrane. The drug has a tendency to accumulate in the compartment where the drug is most ionized, in this case where the pH = 7 (101:1 for pH 7/pH 1). **B,** Passive diffusion of a weak base (pK = 5) across a membrane with an existing pH differential. The drug accumulates in the compartment where the pH is 1, again where the drug is most ionized.

lower concentration of the readily diffusible un-ionized species. There are, however, cases in which two drugs can have the same pK values and be transferred at different rates; the reason for this occurrence is because of differences in the lipid solubility of these drugs. The more lipid-soluble drug will be transferred more rapidly. In summary, the rate of transfer by passive diffusion depends on the lipid solubility of the drug, whether the drug is an acid or a base, the pK of the drug, and the pH of the surroundings.

Filtration

Filtration is the transfer of drugs either between or into cells through pores. It depends on the existence of a pressure gradient and on the relative size of the compounds with respect to the size of the pore through which filtration is occurring. In general, compounds will pass through or be excluded from the membrane according to their molecular size. If the compounds are similar in size to the pore then there will be resistance to transfer; however, if the compounds are much smaller than the pore, then transfer of the drug depends on the magnitude of the pressure gradient. Sites at which filtration is important include the glomerulus and capillaries (with the exception of capillaries in the central nervous system).

Endocytosis

Endocytosis is the process whereby a drug molecule is engulfed by invagination of a membrane and internalized to produce a vesicle. This process can mediate the transfer of a drug molecule from one side of a membrane to the other. Endocytosis can be divided into pinocytosis and phagocytosis. Many examples of endocytosis have been shown to be receptor-mediated processes for which a ligand binds to the receptor in an area called a coated pit, which is lined by the protein clathrin. The coated pit pinches off eventually to form a vesicle called an endosome. The endosome contains an ATP-dependent proton pump, which will maintain a pH of 5 inside the endosome. Once in the endosome, the receptor and ligand can undergo different fates: (*a*) the ligand can be internalized and the receptor can be returned to the surface; (*b*) both the receptor and ligand can be internalized and targeted for degradation; (*c*) both the receptor and ligand can be transported to the opposite surface of the cell.

Receptor-Mediated Transport

Active transport and facilitated diffusion represent two receptor-mediated transport systems. Active transport is an energy-dependent movement of compounds against the concentration gradient. The primary function of a receptor-mediated process is the transport of endogenous compounds, usually compounds that are charged at physiologic pH. Drugs that are structurally similar to the endogenous compounds can also associate with the transport proteins and can be transported by active transport. Active transport is a unidirectional process in which the drug can accumulate on one side of the membrane. Because a transport protein is required for transfer of the compound, the process is also saturable and requires energy, usually in the form of ATP. As a result, active transport can be inhibited either by structural analogues of the drug or by ATP inhibitors.

Facilitated diffusion is similar to active transport in that it is a receptor-mediated transport process. Facilitated diffusion is also saturable, and drugs can be transported by this process if they can associate properly with the transport protein. Facilitated diffusion differs from active transport in that energy is not required to mediate this process, and facilitated diffusion only occurs down a concentration gradient.

Routes of Drug Administration

A number of routes exist whereby drugs can be administered to an individual. Oral administration is the most common route. It is generally the safest, most convenient, and most economical way to administer drugs. However, oral administration cannot be used in all circumstances. Some drugs are irritating to the gastric mucosa or are destroyed by digestive enzymes or low gastric pH. There are also problems of irregularities with absorption of particular drugs, and many drugs are inactivated by liver or intestinal enzymes. For example, in some individuals, the absorption of phenytoin is negligible, whereas other patients absorb the drug readily. Drugs that are metabolized by hepatic and intestinal enzymes before their distribution throughout the body are said to undergo a first-pass effect. After absorption from the intestine, the blood supply empties directly into the hepatic circulation. Because the liver, and to a lesser extent, intestine are the primary locations of drug-metabolizing enzymes, drugs that undergo extensive metabolism can be largely destroyed before distribution to their sites of action. In compounds that are metabolized extensively, the first-pass effect can be large. For example, an effective oral dose of morphine is approximately six times larger than a standard intramuscular dose.

Parenteral administration usually refers to intravenous, intramuscular, or subcutaneous injection of the drug. The rate of absorption of drugs after intramuscular or subcutaneous injection generally is controlled by a diffusion process in which the rate of absorption will be affected by the surface area of the capillaries at the injection site and the solubility of the drug in the interstitial fluid. The major advantage of both intramuscular and subcutaneous injection is to bypass the first-pass effect of the liver. Subcutaneous administration can be used for drugs that are not irritating to the tissue; it will provide a slow, constant absorption, the rate of which can be altered intentionally. The rate of absorption after subcutaneous administration is fastest if the drug is in aqueous solution. It can be slowed by suspension of the drug in oil and can be further slowed by implanting a solid pellet under the skin. Intramuscular administration provides a more rapid absorption than does the subcutaneous route. The rate of absorption from muscle can also be slowed by suspending the drug in oil.

When drugs are administered intravenously, the absorption process is bypassed. Intravenous administration has several advantages: (*a*) a desired drug concentration in the blood can be attained immediately and accurately; (*b*) the doses can be adjusted according to the patient's response; and (*c*) irritating solutions can be administered, particularly if they are administered slowly. There are, however, disadvantages to intravenous drug administration: (*a*) once a drug has been injected, no absorption process occurs that can be manipulated in the event of overdose; (*b*) drugs cannot be dissolved in oily vehicles; (*c*) drugs cannot be administered that may precipitate constituents of blood; and (*d*) a patent vein must be maintained for continuous injections. In general, intravenous administration must be done slowly with constant monitoring to avoid drug toxicities.

Absorption of Drugs

Absorption is the rate at which a drug leaves its site of administration and enters the general circulation. Anything that affects absorption will affect the drug concentration in the blood and consequently the efficacy and toxicity of a particular drug therapy. A number of factors modify absorption. The first is drug solubility, which is particularly important for orally administered drugs. The more rapidly the drug dissolves, the more rapidly it will be absorbed because it can mix more readily with the aqueous phase at the absorptive site. The second factor that will modify absorption is the concentration of drug at the absorptive site. The rate of transfer by most transport processes depends on the concentration difference between the two sides of the membrane. Therefore, the higher the concentration at the absorptive site, the more rapidly absorption will occur. Blood flow will also affect the rate of absorption by transporting the newly absorbed drug away from the site, thereby maintaining the concentration gradient. Another factor that will affect the absorption of a drug is the area of the absorbing surface. Increases in the absorbing surface lead to an increased rate of absorption. The fifth factor that will affect the absorption of a drug is the route of administration, which has already been discussed (5).

Sites of Absorption Through the Gastrointestinal Tract

When drugs are administered orally, they can be absorbed from a number of sites. The first potential site is the mouth in the case of sublingual administration. The mouth has a small surface area and a pH of about 6. Drugs absorbed from the mouth must be highly lipid soluble and must be potent. Because of the pH of the mouth, certain weak bases can be better absorbed from this site than from the stomach. One of the primary advantages of absorption of drugs from the mouth is that drugs can directly enter the general circulation, avoiding the first-pass effect of the liver. An example of a compound that is absorbed by this mechanism is nitroglycerin, which is often administered sublingually.

The stomach is primarily a digestive organ. It has a rich blood supply and a reasonable amount of surface area. Therefore, the stomach can be a site of absorption for some drugs, particularly weak acids. The pH of the stomach ranges from around 1 to 2, and this low pH can affect the degree of ionization of many drugs and consequently affect the rate of absorption of drugs from this site. In general, weak acids will be absorbed more readily from this site than weak bases. Furthermore, weak bases can accumulate in the stomach even if they are intravenously administered.

The small intestine is the primary site of absorption for most orally administered drugs; it has an extremely large surface area. Although absorption usually is mediated by passive diffusion, it can occur by facilitated diffusion, active transport, endocytosis, or filtration. The pH of the small intestine ranges between 5 and 8; however, in the proximal jejunum, where most of the absorption occurs, the pH is about 5. Both weak acids and weak bases are absorbed better from the intestine than from the stomach, principally because of the extremely large surface area of the small intestine compared with the stomach.

The large intestine has a smaller surface area than the small intestine. Because of the solid nature of the intestinal contents, passive diffusion of drugs is generally restricted from this site; however, the rectum can be used as a site of administration for some drugs. Rectal administration can be used for local conditions such as hemorrhoids, or it can be used for introducing compounds into the systemic circulation. The primary dosage forms are solutions or suppositories. This route is used most often in patients who have nausea or vomiting. Rectal administration also has the advantage of 50% of the blood supply bypassing the liver, therefore circumventing the first-pass effect (5,6).

Drug Absorption Outside the Gastrointestinal Tract

The lung can be used as the site of administration for both local effects, as with albuterol, or for systemic effects, as with general anesthetics. The lung has a large surface area and a high rate of blood flow, which makes it a particularly good site for drug absorption. Drug absorption occurs by simple diffusion, endocytosis, or active transport and avoids the first-pass effect of the liver. Certain disadvantages do exist: (a) administration through the lung is cumbersome; (b) there are difficulties in dosage regulation; and (c) irritation to the pulmonary epithelium can result.

Drugs can be administered through the skin, usually to take advantage of their local effects (e.g., benzocaine for minor burns). In addition, the use of transdermal patches permits the cutaneous absorption of drugs into the systemic circulation for prolonged action (nicotine patches for tobacco dependence). Most drugs enter the skin by passive diffusion, which means that the partition coefficient of the drug and its pK will be important in controlling the rate of its absorption. The outer layer of the skin, the stratum corneum, forms a barrier against rapid penetration of most drugs. This is primarily the result of the low degree of hydration of the cells in this layer, which usually ranges from 5% to 15% but can be increased up to 50% by use of occlusive dressings. The increase in hydration will increase the absorption of drugs from this site. Lipid-insoluble drugs can enter through hair follicles, sweat glands, and sebaceous glands.

Drug Distribution

Drug distribution is the transfer of a drug from the circulation to the interstitial fluid and finally to the tissues of the body. After absorption, drugs will be distributed throughout the vasculature within about 2 to 3 minutes. There are a number of factors that affect their further distribution into the tissues. One factor affecting distribution of drugs is regional blood flow. Different tissues have different rates of perfusion. The heart, liver, and brain are highly perfused tissues; muscle and skin are moderately perfused tissues; and finally, adipose tissue is slowly perfused. The differences in perfusion rates are particularly important for the distribution of lipid-soluble drugs. Because drugs that are extremely lipid soluble are rapidly absorbed by passive diffusion, they will first be distributed into the highly perfused tissues and then are rapidly absorbed from these sites. An example of a drug that follows such a distribution pattern is thiopental, which rapidly produces anesthesia because it arrives at the brain in large concentrations and is then absorbed rapidly. However, as the drug continues to distribute into muscle, skin, and fat, the drug concentration in the plasma decreases. The drug will then transfer back out of the highly perfused tissues (brain) and into the blood. This causes a decrease in the drug concentration in the brain and permits the patient to regain consciousness within a few minutes.

Drug distribution is also affected by the permeability of capillaries. After transport throughout the vasculature, the drug reaches the capillaries and can be transferred either by filtration, passive diffusion, or endocytosis. Driven by filtration, the drug will be transferred across the capillary membranes, primarily by ultrafiltration on the arterial side and by osmotic pressure on the venous side. As a result, the pressure gradient driving the ultrafiltration and the molecular size of the drug will be major determinants controlling the distribution into the interstitial fluid. The size of the capillary fenestrations differ in various tissues and affect the rate of drug transfer. If the drug is lipid soluble, it can be transferred by passive diffusion despite fenestration size. In this case, the degree of ionization and lipid solubility will be important factors controlling the rate of transfer (5).

Once the drug has been transferred across the capillary membranes into the interstitial fluid, it can then be taken up into the tissues. The form of the uptake by tissues depends on the characteristics of the compound.

The distribution of drugs can be restricted by binding to plasma proteins because such binding decreases the free drug concentration in the plasma. The bound portion of the drug cannot reach the receptor site and, therefore, cannot produce its pharmacologic effect. However, the bound drug also cannot be distributed, metabolized, or excreted. The bound drug thus acts as a drug reservoir, which will delay the onset of a drug effect on its initial administration and can prolong drug action once administration of drug is discontinued. These effects depend on (*a*) the affinity of the drug for plasma proteins, (*b*) the drug concentration in the plasma, (*c*) the degree of saturation of the plasma protein-binding sites, and (*d*) the potency of the drug. There are three principal plasma proteins that are involved in drug distribution. Albumin is a plasma protein with a molecular weight of about 68,000; it has one or two high-affinity sites for acidic compounds. Albumin also normally carries fatty acids, so it can also bind lipid soluble drugs, but to a lesser extent. This protein also has many sites for the binding of bases; however, these are low-affinity sites. Lipoproteins comprise the second major group of plasma proteins and have the ability to bind highly lipid-soluble drugs. In general, the binding depends on the lipid content; very low density lipoproteins (VLDL) have a greater ability to bind lipid-soluble drugs than do the low-density (LDL) and high-density lipoproteins (HDL). The third major plasma protein is α_1-acid glycoprotein, which has one high-affinity binding site for basic drugs. This protein is inducible by trauma, injury, or stress, and the protein has a biologic half-life of about 5.5 days. The inducibility of this protein can have a profound effect on the pharmacologic response to a drug. For example, suppose an individual is taking a basic drug that binds to α_1-acid glycoprotein at a level that produces an adequate therapeutic response. If this individual experiences trauma, the level of α_1-acid glycoprotein will be increased, leading to a decreased level of free drug and a diminished therapeutic effect. Maintenance of the proper therapeutic effect under these conditions may require an elevated drug dose. However, suppose a patient is injured (and thus has an elevated α_1-acid glycoproteins level) and several days later is administered a basic drug and an adequate therapeutic response is obtained. When the level of α_1-acid glycoprotein decreases 10 days later, the decrease in the protein level could then increase the free concentration of the drug to the point at which toxic effects may be observed. These examples illustrate how alterations in the level of this plasma protein influence the therapeutic response to a drug (5,6).

Drugs bind with plasma proteins and also accumulate in tissues. There are three basic mechanisms for accumulation in tissues. The first is ion trapping owing to pH differences. For example, cellular pH is about 7, whereas plasma pH is about 7.4. This pH difference can cause the accumulation of certain drugs within the cells, if they are more ionized at 7 than at 7.4. Drugs can also accumulate by binding to intracellular components. For example, iodine can accumulate in the thyroid gland, metals can accumulate in the kidney by binding to metallothionein, and lead can compete with calcium in the bone. The third mechanism for drug accumulation in tissues is partitioning into lipid. Individuals who have been administered a lipid-soluble drug for a long period of time will have a tendency to accumulate such a drug in their adipose tissue. This accumulation is relatively slow because of the low amount of perfusion of this tissue; however, over protracted periods of time, large amounts of a drug can accumulate at that site, particularly if it is extremely lipid soluble. Regardless of mechanism, the major consequence of drug accumulation in tissues will be a delay in the onset of drug action after its administration or a prolongation of the drug effect after termination of its administration.

Physiologic Barriers to Drug Distribution

The capillaries in most organs contain fenestrations that permit the transfer of drugs by filtration. In the brain, however, the capillary endothelial cells and the glial cells are joined by tight junctions, which will prohibit the transfer of drugs by this process. For drugs to enter the brain, they generally must passively diffuse through the cells rather than be filtered among them. Therefore, factors that control passive diffusion of drugs will control whether a drug can be transported into the brain.

Under some conditions, the placenta also provides a barrier to transfer of compounds. In general, the placenta does not prevent transport. If the compounds are lipid soluble, they will be transferred readily from the mother to the fetus. The rate of transport of such compounds thus depends on the drug's pK, its partition coefficient, and whether it binds to plasma proteins. Highly polar or ionized compounds will not cross as readily. Molecular size is also an important determinant for the transfer of water-soluble compounds; those that have molecular weights less than 600 kD freely transfer across the placenta. Compounds that have molecular weights larger than 600 kD cross with increasing difficulty, until the molecular weight exceeds 1000 kd. Such large compounds will not transfer across the placenta.

Excretion of Drugs

Drugs can be excreted from a number of different sites, including kidney, liver, skin, and lungs; however, most excretion occurs from either the kidney or the liver. Renal excretion is the primary route of excretion for most drugs, especially water-soluble drugs. The three major processes are glomerular filtration, passive reabsorption, and tubular secretion.

Glomerular Filtration

Drugs transfer from the glomerulus into the renal tubules by filtration of the blood. This process permits the filtration of substances with the appropriate molecular size, charge, and shape. If the drugs have a molecular weight between 5,000 kD and 75,000 kD, filtration will be increasingly restricted with increasing molecular weight. Compounds with molecular weights greater than 75,000 kD will not be filtered. For drugs with molecular weights in the restricted filtration range (between 5,000 kD and 75,000 kD), both charge and shape will have an influence on glomerular filtration. Charged substances are filtered more slowly than uncharged substances, and globular proteins are filtered more slowly than proteins of random coil. If the drugs are bound to plasma proteins, they generally will not be filtered because of the high molecular weight of the protein-drug complexes.

Passive Reabsorption

About 20% of the blood volume is filtered into the renal tubules as the blood passes through the kidney. Because plasma proteins and other high molecular weight compounds are not filtered through the glomerulus, an osmotic gradient is produced between the blood and the fluid in the renal tubules. As a result, water will have a tendency to transfer from the renal tubules into the blood. Drugs in the renal tubules will then have a tendency to transfer back into the blood by passive reabsorption. Like other passive-diffusion processes, passive reabsorption is controlled by the lipid solubility of the drug, its degree of ionization, and the pH of both the blood and tubular filtrate. If the compound is un-ionized, it will have a greater tendency to be reabsorbed. If the compound is charged, it will tend to be excreted. The pH of the renal tubules can be manipulated therapeutically to increase the excretion of drugs. For example, in the case of overdose with the weak acid phenobarbital, increasing the pH of the urine will cause an increase in the rate of excretion of the drug. This process is called forced alkaline diuresis. The excretion of weak bases sometimes can be increased by acidification of the urine, using ammonium chloride.

Active Tubular Secretion

Strong organic acidic and basic drugs can use the two active secretory systems that are present in the renal tubules for the excretion of certain endogenous compounds. Via these systems, drugs are transferred actively from the blood to the lumen. These systems are not particularly selective, but they do fall into two categories: one for anions and one for cations. The system can exhibit saturation when a high concentration of a drug is present. As with other active-transport processes, the system also requires energy and can be inhibited by competition with other acidic or basic compounds that are eliminated by this mechanism.

Hepatic Excretion

The other major excretory organ is the liver. The hepatic blood capillaries have extremely large fenestrations, which will permit the transfer of most drugs into the interstitial fluid surrounding the hepatocyte. These compounds can be readily taken up into the hepatocyte by either passive diffusion or carrier-mediated transport. Once in the hepatocyte, the drugs can be either excreted into the bile canaliculus or metabolized by the hepatic drug-metabolizing enzymes. Some of these metabolites can then be taken into the bile canaliculus and excreted in bile. Uptake into the bile is mediated by four active-transport systems capable of transporting the following classes of compounds: anions, cations (both of which are similar to those found in renal tubules), bile acids, and neutral organic compounds. After concentrating in the bile, the drugs are then released into the intestine. If the drugs are ionized, they tend to be eliminated in the feces; however, if the drugs are lipid soluble, they can be reabsorbed back into the circulation. This process of uptake from the circulation into the hepatocyte, further uptake and concentration into the bile, release into the intestine, and reabsorption into the circulation is called enterohepatic cycling. This process can prolong the pharmacologic action of some drugs (5–7).

In general, the liver excretes larger compounds than does the kidney. Compounds with molecular weights less than 400 usually are excreted by the kidney; however, as the molecular weight increases, biliary excretion becomes more important.

Although renal and hepatic excretion are the primary routes for excretion of drugs, other sites can be involved. Drugs can be excreted through the lungs. The primary types of compounds that are excreted by this mechanism are gases and volatile liquids. Excretion occurs by simple diffusion across the alveolar membranes and is a major mechanism for excretion of the inhalational general anesthetics. Drugs can also be excreted into sweat and saliva and expressed in breast milk. The primary transport mechanism for their excretion is passive diffusion, for which the partition coefficient, its pK, and the pH in the environment are important. Excretion into the saliva has been shown to be responsible for the drug taste that is observed frequently after intravenous injection of a drug. As stated previously, drugs can also be excreted into breast milk. Generally, drugs will transfer by passive diffusion, and because the pH of milk is about 6.5, weak bases have a tendency to be ion trapped within milk. If the drug binds to plasma proteins, the concentration of the drug in the milk will be decreased. Highly lipid-soluble drugs have a tendency to accumulate in milk fat.

Drug Biotransformation

Most drugs are lipid-soluble substances that are partially ionized at physiologic pH. As a result of their high lipid solubility, large amounts of these drugs have a tendency to be reabsorbed into the general circulation after transport into either the renal tubule or the bile. In fact, some lipid-soluble drugs could not be effectively eliminated within a human's lifetime if the body had to rely solely on renal excretion for elimination. Thus, in addition to normal excretory processes, drug metabolism is a major mechanism by which drug action can be terminated. The process of biotransformation has certain general characteristics. First, it causes a chemical change in the drug, which usually produces more water-soluble metabolites. As a result, the partition coefficient of the drug is altered, causing the metabolites to be excreted more readily. In some cases, the metabolites can be secreted actively by transport systems in the kidney or in the liver. Finally, the pharmacologic activity of a drug usually is terminated by biotransformation reactions.

Biotransformation reactions can be broken into two general categories: (*a*) nonsynthetic, or phase 1, reactions, including oxidation, reduction, and hydrolysis reactions, and (*b*) synthetic, or phase 2, reactions, including conjugation of the drug to endogenous compounds (4). The major enzyme systems involved in biotransformation are found in the liver, but others are found in kidney, lung, and gastrointestinal tract as well as in other tissues. The major enzyme involved in the oxidative reactions of drug metabolism is called cytochrome P450. This enzyme is nonselective and can catalyze the metabolism of compounds having widely diverse chemical structures. Cytochrome P450 cannot act independently, but it is part of an electron-transport chain found in the endoplasmic reticulum, which is required for catalysis. Cytochrome P450 generally catalyzes the hydroxylation of the substrate molecule by inserting one atom from molecular oxygen into the substrate and the other atom issued to form water (Fig. 10.6). Reducing equivalents required for this reaction ultimately originate from NADPH and are transferred through the flavoprotein NADPH⁻ cytochrome P450 reductase. The electrons are then transferred to cytochrome P450. Cytochrome P450 can catalyze a number of reactions in addition to simple hydroxylations, including epoxidation reactions; *N*-, *O*-, and *S*-dealkylation reactions; oxidative deamination; sulfoxide formation; and desulfuration reactions (8).

Cytochrome P450 has a broad substrate selectivity. It can hydroxylate compounds of widely varying structure, including simple hydrocarbons such as benzene and naphthalene up to endogenous compounds such as steroids, fatty acids, and some vitamins. It is responsible for the metabolism of many drugs. The enzyme can also hydroxylate the same substrate at different positions.

There are two basic reasons for the broad substrate selectivity of cytochrome P450. First is that the enzyme has a relatively nonselective active site, which can accommodate a wide variety of different compounds as long as they possess a degree of lipid solubility. The other factor controlling the nonselectivity of the enzyme system is that cytochrome P450 exists in multiple forms, with each isozyme possessing its own substrate selectivity.

A number of other noncytochrome P450 oxidations can also occur. For example, alcohol dehydrogenase is a soluble enzyme that can convert ethanol to acetaldehyde. Aldehyde dehydrogenase is another soluble enzyme that further converts acetaldehyde to acetic acid. Other examples include tyrosine hydroxylase and monoamine oxidase, enzymes that are involved in catecholamine metabolism.

There are three basic types of reduction reaction: azoreduction, nitro reduction, and keto reduction. Enzymes catalyzing these reactions are found either in the microsomes or in the cytosol and in some cases in anaerobic microorganisms found in the ileum and colon.

Practically all organs contain hydrolytic enzymes. They are found in the highest concentrations in the liver, kidney, brain, and plasma. Both esterases and amidases are found in plasma and other tissues and are located primarily in the microsomal fraction of those tissues. Epoxide hydrolase, an enzyme that is involved in the cleavage of the epoxide to a dihydrodiol, is found primarily in the liver and is found in both the microsomal fraction and the cytosol (5).

Conjugation Reactions

Conjugation reactions involve the chemical combination of a drug with an endogenous compound. In general, the drug must have a reactive group or be metabolized to a compound containing a reactive group. Generally, conjugation reactions produce compounds with a reduced pharmacologic activity and a substantially increased rate of excretion. The most common conjugation reaction is the formation of glucuronides, owing to the high availability of glucose, which can form UDP-glucuronic acid. The drug combines with UDP-glucuronic acid through a reaction that is catalyzed by UDP-glucuronyl transferases. This conjugation occurs primarily in the liver but can also occur in the kidney, intestine and lung and, to a lesser extent, in other tissues. UDP-glucuronyl transferases are found in the microsomal fraction. These conjugates can be transferred to the bile and released into the intestine. Once in the intestine, they can be excreted in the feces or, if the glucuronide is susceptible to catalysis by intestinal β-glucuronidase, the compound can be hydrolyzed, which in some in-

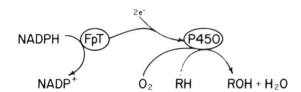

Figure 10.6. The cytochrome P-450 monooxygenase system.

stances will regenerate the parent drug. In this case, the drug can be reabsorbed (enterohepatic cycling). Generally, glucuronides are more water soluble and are usually stronger acids than the parent drug, which accounts for a relatively rapid excretion of the compounds. Glucuronide formation usually abolishes pharmacologic activity.

A primary characteristic of UDP-glucuronyl transferase activity is that it is either low or absent in the fetus and early infant. After birth, these activities increase until they achieve their adult levels. Because of the low levels of these enzymes in newborns, drugs or endogenous compounds that require glucuronidation for elimination can reach toxic levels. A syndrome called kernicterus is found in newborn infants, especially in those that are premature, and is the result of the inability of the liver to conjugate bilirubin to its glucuronide. Bilirubin normally is excreted in the bile as the glucuronide or bound to plasma proteins. However, in infants, the low level of UDP-glucuronyl transferase activity leads to a high level of free bilirubin in the plasma; the bilirubin, in turn, can diffuse across the blood-brain barrier and cause irreversible damage to the central nervous system. Another syndrome, called the gray baby, is a toxic effect resulting from the inability of infants to conjugate chloramphenicol.

Sulfate conjugation is catalyzed by sulfotransferases, which are located in the cytosol of the liver. Sulfate conjugation requires an active sulfate in the form of 3-phosphoadenosine-5'-phosphosulfate (PAPS). Sulfate conjugates are polar and are excreted easily. They require ATP for the formation of activated sulfate. One of the primary characteristics of this system is its saturability, which is caused primarily by the depletion of PAPS. In the event that sulfate conjugation is saturated, many compounds usually eliminated by this process are eliminated by other routes (e.g., glucuronides).

The enzymes involved in N-acetylation reactions are called N-acetyltransferases and can combine an acetate to the drug molecule. The activated endogenous substrate is acetyl-CoA. Genetic studies have demonstrated that both slow and fast acetylators exist. Slow acetylators are homozygous for a recessive gene. These individuals are susceptible to dose-dependent toxicity from drugs that are eliminated via N-acetylation, such as isoniazid.

Methylation reactions are catalyzed by methyltransferases and use S-adenosylmethionine as the activated methyl donor. Methyltransferases are found in the cytosol of many organs, including the liver, lung, and kidneys.

Many drugs can be conjugated with glutathione, a tripeptide that is extremely important for the detoxification of environmental toxicants and chemical carcinogens. The enzymes catalyzing these reactions are called glutathione sulfotransferases. They are found primarily in the cytosol of the liver but can be found at lower levels in lung, kidney, and other tissues. There are multiple forms of glutathione sulfotransferases, which have overlapping substrate specificities (5,6,9).

Factors Affecting Drug Metabolism

Age

Age is a primary factor affecting drug metabolism; greater sensitivity to drugs is observed in the very young and the very old. Although a number of factors change with age, the rate of biotransformation is probably the most important age-related effect. The overall drug metabolizing activity is low in newborns and increases with age. As a result, newborns are more sensitive to the toxic effects of drugs. The elderly are also more sensitive to drugs than are young adults. In elderly patients, the rate of absorption of drugs is decreased because of decreased gastrointestinal motility and decreased blood flow. Distribution is also altered as a result of increases in the amount of body fat, decreases in muscle mass, hyperalbuminia, and decreases in total body water. Metabolism may also decrease owing to decreases in the activity of the drug-metabolizing enzymes as well as decreased blood flow to the liver. Excretion in the elderly can be substantially altered, primarily by a decrease in renal function as an individual ages (5).

Enzyme Induction

A number of the drug-metabolizing enzymes have been demonstrated to be inducible. Induction of glucuronyl transferases and glutathione sulfotransferases has been shown; however, the drug-metabolizing enzymes most susceptible to induction are those of the cytochrome P450 system. As mentioned previously, there are multiple forms of cytochrome P450, and the levels of each isozyme are under genetic control. Exposure to a number of drugs, carcinogens, and other foreign compounds have been shown to increase the levels of particular cytochrome P450 isozymes. Induction of these enzymes not only will accelerate the metabolism of the inducing compound but also will increase the metabolism of other compounds. Some compounds that have been shown to induce cytochrome P450 include phenobarbital, polycyclic aromatic hydrocarbons, and alcohol. In individuals who are exposed to such compounds, the metabolism of certain therapeutically administered drugs could be accelerated, leading to lower plasma levels and a decreased therapeutic response (6).

Other Factors Affecting Drug Metabolism

The drug-metabolizing enzymes are also expressed in a tissue-dependent and species-dependent manner. Tissue-dependent variations in drug metabolism are the result of differential expression of cytochrome P450 isozymes in different tissues. Different P450 isozymes are expressed in different species as well. In most cases, similar enzymes are expressed across species lines; however, these orthologous isozymes may possess different substrate selectivities. Both tissue- and species-dependent differences in expression of these drug-metabolizing enzymes can result either in differences in the rates of metabolism of a particular drug or differences in the metabolic products produced. Such differences may lead to drug toxicity in a particular tissue (because of differences in metabolism in a particular tissue) and to difficulty in extrapolating metabolic data among species.

A number of nutritional factors have also been shown to decrease drug metabolism. Protein deficiency, fat-free diets, and a deficiency in essential fatty acids can all decrease overall drug metabolism. Certain vitamin and nutrient deficiencies have also been shown to decrease drug metabolism, including deficiencies in vitamins A, C, and E; riboflavin; and calcium and magnesium ions. A number of hormones have been implicated in the regulation of drug metabolic activities. Thyroxine and insulin appear to increase drug metabolic activities, and glucocorticoids and testosterone have been shown to alter drug metabolism. Growth hormone appears to increase the activities of some drug-metabolizing enzymes and to decrease the activities of others in experimental animals.

The clinical importance of the drug-metabolizing enzymes is apparent when substantial individual variation in drug metabolism is found among patients. These differences may be caused by genetic variability, differences in exposure to environmental toxicants, or the result of prior drug exposure. Remember that individuals previously exposed to different compounds will not metabolize drugs in a similar manner. As can be seen in cases of metabolic tolerance, prolonged exposure to some drugs alters their metabolism, thereby decreasing the steady-state levels for that drug. These variations in drug metabolism can also lead to drug interactions, for which the presence of one drug or environmental agent can alter the metabolism not only of the parent drug but also of any other drug eliminated by these enzymes. Toxicity from a drug as a result of lower levels of expression of certain drug-metabolizing enzymes or induction of isozymes capable of producing toxic metabolites can also occur (5,6,10).

Clinical Pharmacokinetics

Ultimately, the magnitude of a pharmacologic response is related to the drug concentration at the receptor site. As has been described, the ability of a drug to get to the receptor site is influenced by each of the pharmacokinetic parameters: absorption, distribution, metabolism, and excretion. Clinical pharmacokinetics

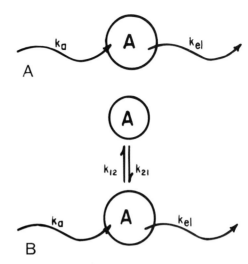

Figure 10.7. Compartmental modeling. **A,** One-compartment model. **B,** Two-compartment model.

permits a quantitative description of the behavior of drugs once they enter the body. It is useful in determining the dosage adjustments that may be required due to altered physiologic states such as aging, renal, or hepatic impairment.

Compartmental Modeling

The fate of a drug in the body can be described by treating the body as a series of compartments into which drugs can transfer. This treatment is called compartmental modeling. In the simplest case, the entire body is treated as a single homogenous compartment (Fig. 10.7A). The drug enters the body at a certain rate, which is governed by the rate constant k_a, known as the absorption rate constant (there is no absorption occurring after intravenous administration). Once the drug enters the body, it is eliminated as regulated by its elimination rate constant k_{el} (5,7).

The behavior of many drugs cannot be explained by a simple one-compartment model. In these cases, the body can be treated as two compartments, a central compartment and a peripheral compartment (Fig. 10.7A). The drug first enters the central compartment controlled by the absorption rate constant k_a. It can then be distributed into the peripheral compartment (based on the rate constant k_{12}) and can be eliminated according to the elimination rate constant k_{el}. Both the elimination of the drug and its distribution from the central to peripheral compartments will continue until the drug achieves a steady state between these compartments. Once the steady state is attained, the drug will continue to be eliminated from the central compartment (controlled by k_{el}). As a result of the decreased drug concentration in the central compartment, the drug will begin to transfer back from the peripheral compartment into the central compartment until elimination of the drug is complete (7).

The physiologic volumes that are represented by the central and peripheral compartments depend on the physical characteristics of the drug. For example, if the drug has a high molecular weight and is water soluble, it will have a tendency to be transferred slowly from the blood into the interstitial fluid. In this case, the blood would represent the central compartment and the remainder of the body would represent the peripheral compartment. In the event that the drug has a low molecular weight and is water soluble, it could readily transfer by filtration into the interstitial fluid but would not be absorbed rapidly into the tissues. For this type of drug, the blood and interstitial fluid would represent the central compartment and the remainder of the body would represent the peripheral compartment. If the drug were very lipid soluble, then passive diffusion into the tissues will occur rapidly. For this type of drug, the blood, the interstitial fluid, and those highly perfused tissues that would first encounter the drug would represent the central compartment. Actually, the body is a multi compartmental model, and each organ or tissue makes up its own compartment. However, many of these organs are typically grouped together, and a one- or two-compartment model can usually adequately describe the behavior of most drugs.

One-Compartment Model

As a drug undergoes the processes of absorption, distribution, metabolism, and excretion, the drug concentration in the blood changes with time. The characteristics of the blood concentration versus time curves are different for different drugs and can be described by the various compartmental models. When a drug that follows a one-compartment model is administered by a single intravenous injection, the drug concentration found at early times is high and continues to decline, as shown in Figure 10.8. The reason for the decrease in

drug concentration is the elimination of the drug by either metabolism or excretion. As is shown in Figure 10.8, when the drug concentration in the blood is high, there is a more rapid rate of elimination, which will tend to level off with time as the drug disappears from the body. The rate of elimination of most drugs depends both on the drug concentration in the body and on the inherent ability of the body to eliminate that drug, as described in equation 7.

$$v = -k_{el}[A]$$

where v represents the rate of disappearance; k_{el}, the elimination rate constant; and [A], the concentration of drug A. Therefore, the elimination rate constant is a characteristic of the particular drug, with higher drug concentrations leading to more rapid elimination. For drugs that follow a first-order disappearance, a plot of the logarithm of the drug concentration in the blood versus time will produce a linear relationship (Fig. 10.8B). The elimination rate constant for a drug can be calculated from Figure 10.8B and is simply the slope of the line. The biologic half-life is the time required to produce a 50% decrease in the drug concentration in the body. This is also a characteristic of the drug and can be determined graphically. The half-life is related to the elimination rate constant as follows: $t_{1/2} = 0.693/k_{el}$.

When drugs are administered by an extravascular route, the drug must first be absorbed into the circulation. During and after absorption of the drug, elimination will occur, usually by a first-order process. Initially, while the absorption process is occurring, the drug concentration in the blood increases, reaches a plateau, and finally decreases. The elimination rate constant can be calculated from this plot in a manner similar to that shown for intravenous administration. The absorption rate constant can also be calculated. The elimination rate constant is a characteristic of the drug and is independent of its route of administration. In other words, a drug given intravenously or by an extravascular route will have the same half-life and the same elimination rate constant (7).

Two-Compartment Model

If a drug follows the two-compartment model and has been administered intravascularly, the curve is no longer linear when plotted on a first-order plot. There are now two phases. Initially, the drug concentration in the blood will be high and will rapidly decrease. At later times, the drug concentration will decrease at a slower rate (Fig. 10.9). After the intravenous administration of drug A (in Fig. 10.7B) into the central compartment, a high concentration of the drug will be present. The drug will then be transferred from the central to the peripheral compartment at a rate determined by the rate constant k_{12} times the concentration of drug A in the central compartment. Early in this process, the drug concentra-

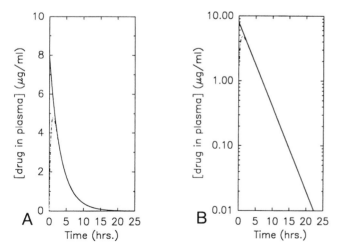

Figure 10.8. Change in drug concentration with time for a drug following one-compartment kinetics. **A,** Linear plot. The solid line represents the change in drug concentration with time after intravenous administration of the drug; the dotted line depicts extravascular drug administration. **B,** Semilogarithmic plot.

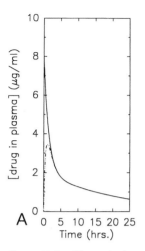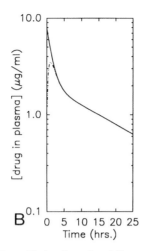

Figure 10.9. Change in drug concentration with time for a drug following two-compartment kinetics. **A,** Linear plot. The solid line represents the change in drug concentration with time after intravenous administration of the drug; the dotted line depicts extravascular drug administration. **B,** Semilogarithmic plot.

tion in the central compartment is high; therefore, the rate of transfer from the central to peripheral compartment will also be high. As this process continues, the drug concentration in the central compartment becomes lower, decreasing the rate of accumulation in the peripheral compartment. In addition, because the drug concentration in the peripheral compartment will continue to increase, the rate of transfer back into the central compartment will increase, depending on the concentration of drug A in the peripheral compartment times its rate constant k_{21}. A steady state will eventually be achieved between the drug in the central and peripheral compartments. While the distribution process is occurring, the drug can be eliminated according to its elimination rate constant k_{el} times the concentration of the drug in the central compartment. Once the steady state is achieved between the central and peripheral compartments, the drug will continue to be eliminated; the rate will depend on the drug concentration in the central compartment. As the drug continues to be eliminated from the central compartment, it can then be transferred from the peripheral into the central compartment. This process continues until the drug is eliminated completely. A graphical representation of what occurs is shown in Figure 10.9. During the early phase, which is called the distribution phase (α), the drug concentration rapidly decreases with time. At later times, the drug concentration decreases at a slower rate, which will continue until the drug is eliminated completely from the body.

The second phase is called the disposition phase (β). It is calculated in the same way that the elimination rate constant is calculated for a one-compartment model and can be determined from the half-life of the drug. The disposition rate constant differs from the elimination rate constant in that the drug is not only being eliminated during this phase but is also being redistributed

from the peripheral to the central compartment. During the α-phase, the primary process responsible for the rapid decrease in drug concentration in the blood is the distribution of the drug from the central to the peripheral compartment. However, during this phase, both the elimination and the redistribution of the drug are occurring. If a drug following a two-compartment model is administered extravascularly, the absorption process is interposed on the pharmacokinetic plot (Fig. 10.9, *dotted line*) (7).

Volume of Distribution

Once a drug is administered, it will be distributed as determined by its physical characteristics. Some drugs may have a tendency to stay in the plasma, others will transfer to the interstitial fluid, and still others will uniformly distribute throughout the body. Furthermore, some drugs have a tendency to accumulate in particular tissue reservoirs. The total volume into which a drug appears to distribute is known as its apparent volume of distribution (V_d). The calculation of volume of distribution is based on the assumption that the drug concentration in the blood is inversely proportional to how extensively the drug is distributed throughout the body. For example, if transfer of a drug to the rest of the body is restricted, it will be retained in the plasma, and a higher drug concentration will be found in the blood. However, if the drug distributes throughout the body, then less will be found in the blood. The apparent volume of distribution for a drug can be calculated after the intravenous injection of a known amount of drug into an individual. The disappearance of drug with time is then plotted on a semilogarithmic plot. One then extrapolates back to time zero to determine what that concentration would have been in the blood before its elimination. The volume of distribution can be calculated as described in equation 8.

$$V_d = \frac{X}{[A]_{t=0}}$$

where X represents the total amount of drug injected and $[A]_t = 0$ is the drug concentration in the body extrapolated to time zero. A drug that tends to stay in the plasma has a volume of distribution of about 5 liters. A drug that transfers into the interstitial fluid and the plasma has a volume of distribution of about 15 liters, and a drug that uniformly distributes throughout the body has a volume of distribution of about 40 liters.

Some drugs have large volumes of distribution. In fact, these volumes can even be larger than the total fluid volume of the body. For example, digoxin has an apparent volume of distribution greater than 700 liters, and the antimalarial drug quinacrine has a volume of distribution of about 50,000 liters. The reason for these extremely large volumes is the binding of the drugs to tissue components. If a drug binds tightly to tissue components, it will tend to accumulate in that tissue, leading to lower drug concentrations in the blood. Because the volume of distribution depends on the amount of drug administered divided by the concentration that is measured in the blood, anything that decreases the concentration in the blood leads to a larger apparent volume of distribution. However, small volumes of distribution are observed if the drug has a tendency to stay in the blood. For example, if a drug binds extensively to plasma proteins, a smaller volume of distribution would be expected (5,7).

Clearance

Clearance is the theoretical volume of blood from which a drug is removed completely in a given period of time. In terms of whole organisms, it may be thought of in relation to the elimination rate constant or in terms of a particular organ, such as the liver or kidney. When referring to the whole organism, the term *total clearance* (Cl_T) is used. One of the simplest ways to calculate the total clearance is shown in equation 9.

$$Cl_T = k_{el} \cdot V_d$$

When clearance is controlled by first-order processes, it is additive. Therefore, the total body clearance is equal to the clearance from the kidney plus the clearance from the liver plus clearance from all other sites.

Multiple Dosing Schedules

In many therapeutic situations, a need exists to maintain a particular steady-state level of a drug. For a drug to be therapeutically effective, a certain minimum concentration must be maintained. Administration of a single dose of the drug may be therapeutically effective for a short time; however, as soon as the drug is administered, elimination begins, leading to a decreased concentration in the blood. Eventually, drug concentrations will drop below the minimum effective concentration. Maintaining therapeutic levels requires continuous administration of the drug.

Continuous Intravenous Infusion

Drugs are sometimes administered by constant intravenous infusion when sustained and carefully regulated drug concentrations must be obtained (Fig. 10.10). In this case, the drug is administered at a constant rate, and the drug is eliminated according to a first-order process. In other words, the rate of elimination of a drug is proportional to the drug concentration in the body. On the initiation of infusion, the drug concentration in the plasma rapidly increases as a result of the slow rate of elimination (see equation 7); however, as the infusion continues, the drug concentration in the plasma increases, leading to an increase in the rate of its elimination. As a result, the concentration will reach a plateau

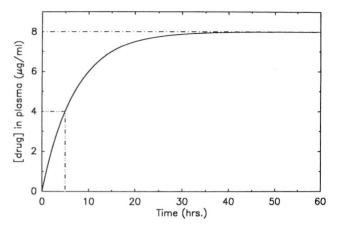

Figure 10.10. Change in plasma drug concentration after intravenous infusion. This drug follows one-compartment kinetics, has a $t_{1/2}$ of 5 hr, and has a steady-state concentration of 8 μg/mL.

(see Fig. 10.10). Eventually, the rate at which the drug is being eliminated is equal to the rate of drug entering the body. At this point, the drug has achieved a steady state. As shown in equation 10, the steady-state concentration (C_{ss}) is equal to the dose rate divided by the total body clearance.

$$C_{ss} = \frac{\text{Dose/Time}}{Cl_T}$$

Therefore, if both the total clearance and the desired steady-state concentration for a drug are known, the infusion rate (dose/time) can be readily calculated.

The time that it takes to achieve steady state is a characteristic that depends on the half-life of the drug. It takes four to five half-lives to achieve a steady-state concentration after multiple drug administration. For example, a drug with a half-life of 5 hours would take about 20 to 25 hours to attain a steady-state concentration. If there is a change in the dose rate, then it will take another four to five half-lives from the point of the change in infusion rate before the steady state is again reached (Fig. 10.11). Therefore, the time required to achieve a steady state depends on the half-life of the drug, whereas the steady-state concentration that is achieved depends on the total body clearance of that drug and the dose rate at which the drug is administered (4,5).

Multiple Dosing

In general, repeated dosing is required to achieve and maintain a desired therapeutic effect. However, intravenous infusions are usually not necessary and in most cases impractical. Therefore, under some circumstances, drugs can be administered by multiple intravenous injection. As is shown in Figure 10.12, a drug being administered according to schedule A will be injected once every four half-lives. In this case, the drug concentration approaches 0 before the next injection. Consequently, there would be little accumulation of drug, and large

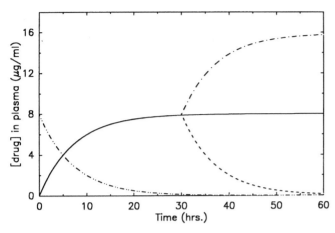

Figure 10.11. The effect of changes in infusion rate on the time required to attain a steady state. The drug depicted has a $t_{1/2}$ of 5 hours and achieves its C_{ss} after 20 to 25 hours (–·–), or four to five half-lives. Another four to five half-lives are required to attain a new steady state after a change in the infusion rate (—). Because the $t_{1/2}$ controls the elimination of a drug after either infusion (– –) or intravenous bolus (–··–), the curves are complementary. At one $t_{1/2}$, either 50% of the C_{ss} is attained (after infusion) or 50% of the drug is eliminated (intravenous bolus).

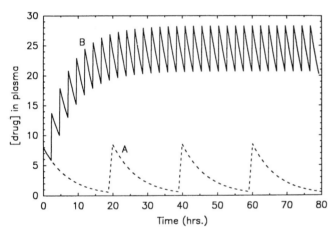

Figure 10.12. The change in plasma drug concentration with time after repeated intravenous injections. The drug was administered once every four half-lives (schedule A) or twice every half-life (schedule B) by intravenous injection. The drug has a $t_{1/2}$ of 5 hours. More frequent administration (shown in schedule B where the dose time is increased) permits accumulation of the drug and decreases the magnitude (on a percentage basis) of the variations.

fluctuations between the maximum and minimum serum drug concentrations are seen. However, if the drug is administered more frequently, as in schedule B, the drug concentration accumulates to a higher steady-state level and the fluctuations (on a percentage basis) are smaller. The magnitude of the fluctuations depends on the frequency of administration with respect to the half-life of the drug. In other words, more frequent administration leads to smaller fluctuations in plasma drug concentrations. As stated previously, the time taken to reach a steady state depends solely on the half-life of the drug. Therefore, if a drug with a long half-life were administered according to the same dosage

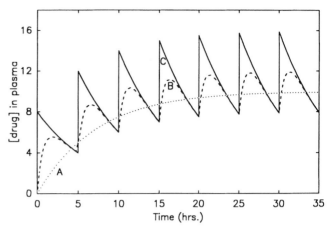

Figure 10.13. Continuous administration of a drug by continuous intravenous infusion (curve A), multiple intravenous injections (curve B), and multiple extravascular administration (curve C).

schedule as a drug with a short half-life, the drug with the long half-life would have a higher degree of accumulation and smaller fluctuations.

In the case in which drugs are administered extravascularly, the drug must first be absorbed into the circulation. Because a finite time is required for absorption to occur, there will be a change in the shape of the curves corresponding to the absorption process (Fig. 10.13). The absorption process actually blunts the sharp changes in drug concentration caused by multiple intravenous injections. The same factors that control selection of a proper dosage schedule for intravenous administration also pertain to extravascular administration of these drugs. Therefore, increasing the frequency of administration will lead to accumulation of the drug and a decrease in the magnitude of the fluctuations. The half-life of the drug still controls the time that it takes for the drug to achieve its steady state (4,5).

In summary, an understanding of pharmacologic principles is important for the rational use of therapeutic agents. Not only is it important to understand the mechanism of action of particular drugs, their therapeutic and adverse effects, but it is also important to understand the factors which may influence the drug concentration at that receptor site. Such information is essential for selection of a therapeutic agent, choice of the proper route of administration and dosage regimen, and for the detection of idiosyncratic reactions which may occur in individual patients.

REFERENCES

1. Neidle EA, Yagiela JA. Pharmacology and therapeutics for dentistry. 3rd ed. St. Louis: CV Mosby, 1989.
2. Clark AJ. The antagonism of acetylcholine by atropine. J Physiol (London) 1926;61:547–556.
3. Ruffolo RR. Important concepts of receptor theory. J Auton Pharmacol 1982;2:277–295.
4. Gilman AG, Rall TW, Nies AS, Taylor P. The pharmacological basis of therapeutics. 8th ed. New York: Pergamon Press, 1990.

5. Craig CR, Stitzel RE. Modern pharmacology. 3rd ed. Boston: Little, Brown, 1990.

6. Pratt WB, Taylor P. Principles of drug action: the basis of pharmacology. 3rd ed. New York: Churchill Livingstone, 1990.

7. Ritschel WA. Handbook of basic pharmacokinetics. Hamilton, IL: Drug Intelligence Publications, 1976.

8. White RE, Coon MJ. Oxygen activation by cytochrome P-450. Ann Rev Biochem 1980;49:315–356.

9. Katzung BG. Basic and clinical pharmacology. 4th ed. Norwalk, CT: Appleton & Lange, 1989.

10. Gonzalez FJ. The molecular biology of cytochrome P450s. Pharmacol Rev 1989;40:243–288.

11 Biostatistics

Alan T. Davis

Assumption

The student believes that the study of statistics constitutes the lowest form of academic masochism and, unless under extreme coercion, would not touch it with a 20-foot pole.

Introduction

Statistics, as defined by Steel and Torrie (1), is "the science, pure and applied, of creating, developing, and applying techniques such that the uncertainty of inductive references may be evaluated." Definitions of this nature send most residents hurtling through plate-glass windows or launching into violent esophageal reflux. In this same vein, one observes that Webster's definition of sadistic is to receive pleasure from inflicting physical or psychological pain on another or others. Hence the term sadistics teacher. (The reader is referred to the glossary at the end of this chapter for other useful terms.)

A far less threatening and more palatable definition is that statistics is "logic or common sense with a strong admixture of arithmetic procedures" (1). This develops an important concept, in that statistics does not involve throwing your good common sense right out the window anytime someone incants in a publication p < 0.05. Contrary to common belief, this is not a signal to run up the white flag, plead shameful ignorance for your former method of conducting surgery, and swear obeisance to the new, statistically verified way. When used correctly, statistics are a powerful tool for the analysis of data. However, they are strictly a mathematical argument for the determination of significance. Depending on how the study was designed, statistical significance does not necessarily imply clinical significance. This will

be a basic tenet throughout the following discussion. In addition, no attempt will be made in this chapter to show the mathematical origins of the tests. You probably do not know how to make an electric drill, but you should know how to use one. Similarly, the emphasis in this text will be on the application of tests, and not on derivation.

Scientific investigations, in general, develop through the following ways (1):

1. A review of facts, theories, and proposals
2. Formulation of a logical hypothesis, subject to testing by experimental methodologies
3. Objective evaluation of the hypothesis on the basis of experimental results

Somewhere between steps 2 and 3, you develop your research design (more on that later). The research design is developed with the intent of using the strongest statistical analysis available. In other words, research design and statistical design are developed concurrently and are plotted and written before one sample is ever taken, be it blood, sweat, or 50-pound chart. If statistics has a bad name, it is from people deciding after the study is over that "oh, my gosh, my golly, this test would be good, but I bet that I can find a really big difference if I massage the data (read: mangle) and use this other test over here." Pretty tempting, eh? Forget it. The path to invalid conclusions is paved by researchers who allow their data and improperly chosen statistics to lead them around by the nose. Besides, if you have your statistics chosen ahead of time, you do not have to worry about what to do when it comes time to analyze the data. This applies, I might add, to proposals in general—once written, they provide a convenient cookbook for your study.

Research Design

There are a wide variety of research designs to choose from, so only the more common types will be identified here. The first four are retrospective designs, whereas the remainder are prospective designs.

Chart Reviews

A chart review implies that the major source for the acquisition of data for a research project is from information recorded in a patient's chart. Thus, the data were acquired in the past, which is why these studies are collectively known as retrospective studies. These studies are also known as "historical studies" or "prospectively impaired studies."

When designing or writing these studies, the time period must be specified, as well as all inclusion and exclusion criteria, i.e., who was allowed into the study, who wasn't, and why. Oftentimes the results of a published study will be of little value to you because the study sample is so different from the patient population that you normally see. The major criticism of retrospective studies is the lack of random allocation of patients to study groups. When reviewing data from a retrospective study, either your own or someone else's data, ask yourself, are the differences shown caused by the treatments, or caused by the patient allocation? For example, perhaps a percutaneous endoscopic gastrostomy (PEG) would appear to be superior to surgical gastrostomy (GAST) or surgical jejunostomy (JEJ), relative to incidence of wound infections. Further analysis, however, may reveal that the PEG was a new procedure during the time period of the study, and therefore only the lower risk patients were given PEGs. This question of allocation is the major point to consider for all retrospective studies. However, some studies can only be accomplished retrospectively. A blanket condemnation of retrospective studies is not intended, but rather a caution as to the limitations of these designs.

Case Report

The case report is the simplest type of study in the literature. It involves the discussion of a finding concerning a single individual. It is primarily a device to draw attention to the readership that the condition in question, although rare, does exist. An improper use of a case report would be to advocate sweeping changes in therapy or treatment of a given condition based on one subject.

Case Series

The case series is similar to the case report but it involves more than one individual. The case series may involve the documentation of a rare disorder in a group of people or may actually be a how-we-do-it study, wherein a given procedure that has been done on a certain number of patients is described and, commonly, advocated. Once again, a study of this type is of informational value only and must not be confused with studies

in which treatments are compared with one another. Although the reader may decide that a new procedure is worth trying after reading a case series, the caution remains that no proof was documented in the study to demonstrate superiority of one method over another.

Case-Control Study

In this retrospective design, patients with two outcomes are compared, relative to some previously acquired risk factor(s). An example would be a review of hospital records to determine the ideal long-term enteral feeding procedure. The question might be whether the type of enteral feeding procedure is a risk factor for aspiration. We could use a case control design by dividing the patients into those who aspirated (the cases) and those who did not (the controls). Then we could look at various feeding procedures as risk factors, such as PEG, JEJ, and GAST.

Retrospective Cohort Study

In the previous example, the subjects were grouped according to outcome. What if we had wanted to group the patients according to the feeding procedure (i.e., PEG, JEJ, and GAST) and determine the frequency of various complications, such as the incidence of aspiration, tube failure, wound complications, and the like? If the study was designed as a retrospective study, this would be a retrospective cohort study. It is worth repeating that in a case control study, the subjects are grouped according to outcome, whereas in the cohort study, the subjects are grouped according to risk factor.

Cross-Sectional Survey

For a cross-sectional survey, a sample of subjects who fit the defined entry criteria (i.e., inclusion and exclusion criteria) are interviewed. An example is a group of 50- to 70-year-old men who are asked whether they have seen a physician or been hospitalized over the last 12 months concerning chest pain. They would also be asked if they exercise 3 or more days a week for at least 30 minutes a day. The objective, obviously, is to link lack of exercise and heart problems. The difficulties, particularly with this study, should also be obvious. Because the study depends totally on subject recall, the accuracy of the recollection is open to question. The influence of confounding variables, such as diet or previous medical history, must also be considered before using this type of design. Depending on the questions being asked, researchers may find that sample size in one group could be absurdly low. Another problem with the cross-sectional survey is that deaths caused by heart disease, even in the age group under study, will not be observed. On the plus side, the study is relatively inexpensive and easy to conduct.

Prospective Cohort Study

In this design, patients are non-randomly assigned to treatments (as in a retrospective cohort study), and prospectively monitored. An example would be the study of the effectiveness of percutaneous contact chole-cysto-lithotripsy (PCCL). Patients could be selected on a volunteer basis to either receive PCCL, or opt for cholecystectomy. Thus, the assignment would be non-random. Complications could be compared between the two groups. Again, whenever there is non-random assignment, the question arises as to whether differences noted in the study are caused by differences between the treatments, or between the patients. Another complicating factor may be that, if one treatment is sufficiently less palatable than the other, the more palatable treatment may be selected much more frequently. It would be like trying to enroll patients into a study on brain tumors. The choice could be between taking a magic, horseshoe-shaped capsule ten times a day, or undergoing brain surgery with a renowned (or maybe even not so renowned) neurosurgeon. There could be a wee tad of bias in treatment selection. An advantage of using this prospective design is the ability to match patients for age and gender. Another advantage over a retrospective design is that all of the data which are of interest can be recorded. Most residents who have been sent off on a glorious chart review have realized quickly that some or all of the variables of interest in present day surgery weren't very interesting at all 10 years ago, as evidenced by their dearth in the charts. Missing data have altered the variables of interest in many a retrospective study, a problem which is avoided easily in the prospective cohort design.

Randomized Controlled Trial

It seems as if there should be a little halo above the words randomized controlled trial (RCT) with, perhaps, a choir in the background, doesn't it? So, what is the big deal about these studies anyway? Most important, as opposed to all of the designs listed above, the subjects are randomly allocated to treatments, i.e., each subject has an equal chance of receiving any treatment. This allows the experimenter to allocate patients, by use of appropriate inclusion and exclusion criteria, such that the groups are as similar as possible, so that any effects noted in the study can be attributed to differences between treatments and not between subjects. This is the preferred situation, in which the experimenter is in control of as much of the study as possible. It is the ideal study design. One of the disadvantages of this design is the expense. Another is that to run the study you must expose subjects to treatments that are possibly either much more harmful than the other treatment or much less beneficial. In some situations, the RCT may be logistically feasible but totally unethical. For these reasons,

cohort and case control studies will continue to have value in the medical literature.

Variables and Randomization

Every experiment needs a hypothesis. For example, let us state that "carnitine is a required nutrient in the diet of the premature infant receiving total parenteral nutrition (TPN)." How would you go about testing this? You could measure weight gain, incidence of cholestasis, plasma and urinary ketones, fatty acid oxidation, respiratory quotient, or urinary dicarboxylic acid output. These are characteristics that can show variability or variation and have been cleverly designated as variables. Variables can be either qualitative or quantitative. It is important to differentiate between these types of variables because they require different types of statistical tests.

Quantitative variables are described as being continuous or discrete. A continuous variable is a value that is only limited by the accuracy of the instrument being used to measure the variable. An example is weight: a person's weight usually is listed as an integer in kilograms or pounds, but the accuracy could be extended to several decimal places if the researcher so desired. A discrete variable is one for which only certain values are possible. An example of this is the number of people in a hospital, which, obviously, cannot be a fraction of a number. Similarly, the spots on a die are discrete numbers. A variation of the continuous and discrete variable is the ratio variable, which is the ratio of two quantitative variables, such as the plasma insulin:glucagon ratio.

Qualitative variables are divided into nominal and ordinal variables. A nominal variable is nothing more than a named category. An example is an individual's favorite ice cream flavor (chocolate, vanilla, or rocky road). In the clinical setting, one often sees this broken down into a yes or no answer, as in survival of the patient or the presence or absence of a complication. When a nominal variable consists of only two categories (such as yes and no), it is also referred to as a dichotomous variable. An ordinal variable usually is seen in ranking scales, such as in injury severity scores. An example is how miserable an individual feels on a particular day, measured on a scale of 1 to 10; 1 might be not miserable at all and 10 could be low-down, dragged-out, dead-duck miserable. Another type of ordinal variable is a visual analogue scale, wherein a patient is asked to mark on a line his or her reaction to pain, scar healing, etc. An example is shown in Figure 11.1.

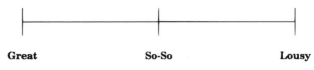

Great   **So-So**   **Lousy**

Figure 11.1. A visual analogue scale.

At first glance, this would appear to be similar to a continuous variable. The only difference is that with continuous variables, the value 10 is 10 times greater than 1. On an ordinal scale, though, this may not be the case. For example, in a pain survey, if 1 means great and 10 means jackhammer headache, 10 obviously means something different than 10 times 1. Thus, the strict mathematical relationship is lacking, which is why a quantitative, continuous variable is different from a qualitative, ordinal variable, and it is also why different statistics are used to analyze these two disparate types of variables.

Back to the original hypothesis. Let us assume that the variable to be measured is plasma ketone body concentration. The original question asks whether there is a carnitine requirement in the premature infant given TPN. The treatment groups, at the very least, will involve one group of babies receiving TPN with carnitine, and one group receiving TPN without carnitine. Now one must determine which babies will receive which treatment. Babies are randomly chosen to receive a randomly chosen treatment.

Why do we bother with all this junk? The primary reason for randomization is to make sure that treatments are distributed over the entire range of the subgroup so that conclusions can be made concerning a larger population. And that is what it is all about. After our study of infants is completed, we will be able to say whether carnitine should be used if any of these little people get premature or need TPN again. What we really want to do, however, is to make a broad statement about any premature infant anywhere in the world who requires TPN. Thus we want our sample—our study group—to be representative of the population, i.e., all premature infants who require TPN.

The process of randomization normally is done using a random number table or a computerized randomization scheme (Table 11.1). One technique, for use in a two-treatment study such as the one proposed here, would be to assign our carnitine treatment to even numbers, and our control group (no carnitine) to odd numbers. Then, very scientifically, we close our eyes, twirl our finger madly, and jab the finger of our choice onto the page holding the random number table. If the number is even, we will start with the carnitine group, and if odd, the control group. Once again, close your eyes, twirl, and jab. Look at the four digit number closest to your finger tip. For example, let's say that, using Table 11.1, my finger landed on the last four digits of the first number of the upper left hand corner (72423). The last four digits are 2423, which means that the randomization will start on row 24 and column 23. Starting from this location (row 24, column 23), and moving in a predetermined path, start recording consecutive two digit numbers between 01 and 50. The first 25 different numbers you record represent the patient numbers that will receive the carnitine treatment. By default, the remaining 25 numbers represent the control subjects. Many other variations on this theme have been used.

The treatment allocation used for this study is called simple random sampling. Let us throw another curve ball into our study, though. Let us assume that the gender of the baby could have an impact on our results. If true, it would be very important to make sure that we have equal numbers of males and females in each group. Now, if we were dealing with a really huge sample size, with a few thousand in each sample, our randomization technique described above would be able to do the job. More often, however, the researcher deals with far smaller sample sizes for a study. With a smaller sample size, it is more likely that we will have differences in the male:female ratio in our two groups. Stratified random sampling is one solution to this problem. In terms of the randomization scheme, instead of randomizing into two groups, we would now randomize into four groups: males receiving carnitine, females receiving carnitine, males not receiving carnitine, females not receiving carnitine. Suggestions on how to analyze an experiment such as this will be described later.

What about other sampling techniques? One popular method, known as sampling with replacement, is to draw numbers from a suitable receptacle, such as an expensive but woefully out-of-fashion tennis shoe. For example, let us say that you have three treatments. You write the three numbers on three pieces of paper and drop them into the shoe. When a patient comes into the unit that matches your inclusion and exclusion criteria, you first obtain informed consent. Then, you reach into the shoe and pull out number three. Your patient will be on treatment three. The number is then put back into the shoe. This ensures that each patient has an equal chance of being entered onto each treatment. The major disadvantage of this technique is that, unless you have a very large sample size, it is unlikely that you will have equal numbers of patients in each group. Thus, this method should be reserved for a large sample size study or for studies in which having equal numbers of subjects per group is not a concern.

How about day of the week? Every other day, you assign patients to either treatment one or treatment two. The problem here is that you may get biased hospital entries on certain days, such as a high number of cases of people on Monday who put off coming in until after the weekend. Thus patient allocation becomes nonrandom. Hospital number? At my institution, the numbers for new patients are all assigned in consecutive order. Consecutive order hardly satisfies the demands for random allocation. Systematic sampling involves picking every kth individual, such as every fifth or sixth patient, and enrolling them in your study. Authoritative sampling is for you power hogs. "I am the omnipotent Dr. Carnitine, and I decree that this baby would be perfect for Rodeocarn, the only carnitine supplement with internal synchronizers. This baby, however, should be placed

Table 11.1.
2500 Random Digits

	00-04	05-09	10-14	15-19	20-24	25-29	30-34	35-39	40-44	45-49
00	72423	83566	11329	25750	12677	91049	52507	00278	73463	60335
01	63166	22293	53406	02630	19100	44506	53877	26050	81764	26368
02	61108	58060	80932	09883	13063	60696	00676	95945	98816	59411
03	43666	91257	06473	32439	05561	76549	82696	59603	82562	81363
04	07792	43006	26578	24397	93911	92004	42253	06448	80347	26124
05	23399	60330	20318	60880	21774	73669	33515	61655	67278	29391
06	67631	65202	21031	03879	61031	88254	49554	78416	48514	99066
07	02543	73555	88540	02155	05018	01220	28172	72855	28434	58925
08	03120	77047	47486	69507	56282	90524	38577	12231	08685	80591
09	00230	78218	79692	83144	78858	72483	09444	23204	35272	45160
10	96754	71426	54287	65424	26662	07719	29242	72539	75303	54562
11	29033	13146	62702	82847	78176	56589	57880	74874	94181	90599
12	55012	18321	18766	31656	22117	31932	46666	08169	24619	36147
13	72194	58859	98711	64737	17375	64688	28403	23949	93769	68982
14	81880	74082	98936	64451	08069	00274	96432	03561	56581	38157
15	74281	30573	60341	39012	96784	73198	35552	91530	25015	71572
16	91961	24027	41554	05439	57111	67064	59754	91349	27927	74402
17	42883	63000	27527	00662	79043	63991	39094	43419	78070	42557
18	39601	02313	87627	06065	65745	31101	68711	75567	69367	84019
19	73359	82594	94437	36134	60067	65873	51669	81390	32264	07821
20	78799	42140	72306	15187	17177	63751	15084	26005	00581	95925
21	72332	88041	99314	25881	13329	72100	35928	80523	38953	86246
22	82371	28231	88556	41286	59242	15858	00773	09763	46328	48205
23	65729	24910	94726	02248	39037	68091	71403	73755	07876	69992
24	53105	29369	94523	85518	34647	11100	08980	05548	96241	84419
25	99935	45604	30101	91641	49666	65322	21112	24906	41697	07832
26	17930	80195	15717	01934	11473	25933	73292	34635	59140	81381
27	89040	53046	87489	31602	23756	81061	75212	23252	44201	14879
28	97678	43333	63509	28179	33755	36657	48266	93272	21095	27726
29	95622	03235	72985	85801	17510	12453	37012	46535	79658	31907
30	71470	02978	61927	17894	91406	56488	41812	90777	42345	39906
31	24572	81408	70885	93947	71517	07744	35280	70503	52658	04697
32	36471	46901	48949	39826	79709	23782	99349	87677	70692	76016
33	00240	77444	09995	94093	91271	40573	00257	41155	93781	29230
34	48489	26192	48519	83375	96198	39637	04961	76620	94731	33415
35	21588	50789	35783	22209	72498	46844	40935	63468	22079	24438
36	87028	02990	45044	01571	91649	20769	36503	11110	87424	74958
37	91676	22673	38591	16721	35016	71308	27670	74107	85872	68503
38	07153	28051	98952	98094	77322	22386	30842	28735	36341	02985
39	69624	38066	33125	24164	59220	06745	78748	44299	08983	55512
40	07477	16514	32063	21476	97638	20046	07097	45045	12435	10477
41	12136	86049	28262	02607	55217	66819	39950	78578	43128	85798
42	17408	73118	61506	55691	17996	72915	30460	86896	86098	55408
43	48827	98302	13907	25099	31077	09226	14101	31238	25579	97852
44	43232	57776	33514	96376	37926	51229	32607	13890	32980	95348
45	66335	16113	52489	75698	63706	54856	09157	19060	84706	55856
46	74650	86636	91280	21186	64657	76728	50815	88405	54003	62553
47	49653	63734	53044	84791	49676	01999	37214	91968	03266	54545
48	27658	41728	04055	91822	47263	75952	88673	12246	37836	42828
49	30070	44406	10734	99867	93491	94030	42803	85920	80060	78450

on control TPN." Authoritative sampling means that The Cheese picks which babies go on which treatment. None of the four treatments listed in this paragraph is adequate for random patient allocation. Randomization via random number tables or computerized randomization schemes ensures true randomization and equal subject numbers per group for any size study. If the sample size is sufficiently large or if having unequal subject numbers per treatment does not bother you, using the sampling with replacement technique is also acceptable.

In practical terms, when reading a prospective, randomized study that uses improper randomization, what are the concerns? The same as those listed for any retrospective study or for the cohort analysis. If a treatment effect is denoted, is it the result of differences in the treatments or between the subjects that comprise the treatments? Thus, improper randomization is not, in and of itself, a reason to trash a study, but it should be a warning flag.

A word about blinding. If you have just devised this randomization scheme, you are no longer blinded. And heaven only knows, only wimp studies are not blinded. Actually, blinding is something that has to be considered on a case-to-case basis. For example, the babies in our study are probably more interested in their critical mass diapers than in placebo effects, and we can safely tell them which treatment group they are in, i.e., the babies will not be blinded. Their sneaky parents are somewhat smarter and should be kept in the dark. However, if the subject is capable of differentiating between treatments, then the subjects need to be blinded. From the investigators' point of view, if our measures of interest (i.e., variables) are all objective (i.e., do not depend on an observer), then the researcher does not need to be blinded. If subjective measures are to be used by the researchers to evaluate the effectiveness of the treatments, then the researchers need to be blinded. If both the subjects and the researchers need to be blinded, you have a double-blind study. In this case, a person outside the study must prepare the randomization scheme. The ultimate study design, applied with one's tongue planted firmly in one's cheek, is the triple-blind study, in which the subjects do not know what they are getting, the residents do not know what they are giving, and the researchers do not know what they are doing (2).

Summarization of Data

So, we have established our design, isolated our variable, and specified the treatment groups—it looks like a good time to hand out some definitions. Let us say that we have decided to sample 50 babies. Another way of putting this is to say that out of all the premature infants on the earth who have been, are, or will be receiving TPN (the population), we are taking a representative sample of 50 (the sample). Somewhere back in your misspent youth, you have no doubt encountered the celebrated and highly renowned bell-shaped curve (Fig. 11.2). The curve, also referred to as the normal distribu-

tion, implies that the variable being studied is symmetrically distributed throughout the population. Populations of quantitative variables that are distributed normally are described by parameters. When we study a sample from this population, we use statistics to describe the sample. A statistic is a guess of the true value of the parameter. Statistics that are used to make reasonable guesses of the true values of parameters are known as parametric statistics. The two primary assumptions for the use of parametric statistics are that the variables in question are quantitative and that the population from which the sample is drawn is distributed normally. The reason for using samples and statistics is that populations, for the most part, are too large to study conveniently.

The center of the bell shaped curve, which divides the distribution into two symmetrical halves, is called the mean, designated μ (parameters are always designated by Greek letters). In the sample, the population mean (μ) is estimated by the sample mean $\bar{x}$. Occasionally, you will see a mean designated as $\bar{y}$, or some other letter with a bar on top, but $\bar{x}$ is the usual representation. The sample mean is calculated by adding up all of the numbers, and dividing by the sample size.

For example, consider the following data set:

$$67.1, 69.0, 65.0, 68.5, 66.9, 69.3; n = 6$$

$$\bar{x} = (67.1 + 69.0 + 65.0 + 68.5 + 66.9 + 69.3)/$$
$$6 = 67.6$$

The assumption was made beforehand that the population from which the sample was derived had a normal distribution (Fig. 11.2). What if the population was distributed nonnormally, as shown in Figure 11.3? In this situation, we note that the population is not described by parameters, and therefore, guesses as to the nature of this population must be made using nonparametric statistics. Ordinal and nominal variables are also analyzed by nonparametric statistics. The two most commonly used descriptors of central tendency in populations not described by parameters are the mode and the median. Consider the following set of data: 1, 2, 3, 4, 7, 7, 7. The mode is the value that occurs most often, which in this case is 7. If we list our values in increasing magni-

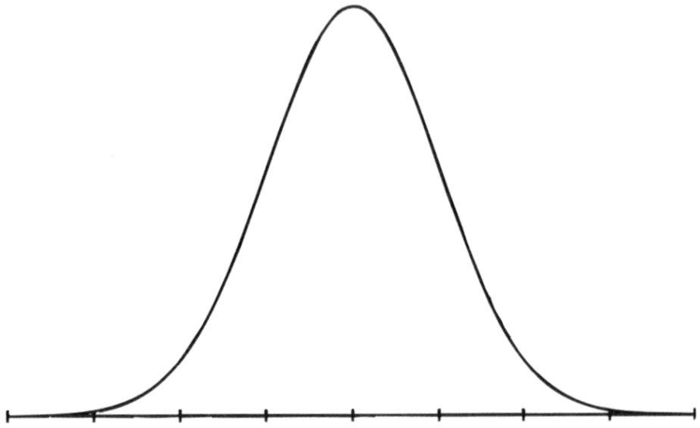

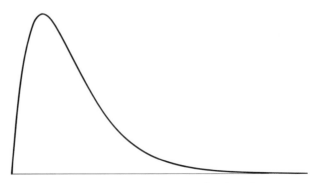

Figure 11.2. The normal distribution.

Figure 11.3. Distribution skewed to the right.

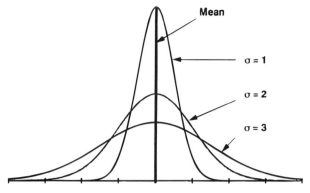

Figure 11.4. Effect of differing variance on the shape of normally distributed populations with the same mean.

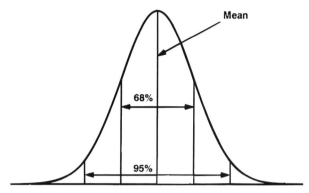

Figure 11.5. Percent of a normally distributed sample encompassed by x̄ ± SD and x̄ ± 2SD.

tude, the median is the value that divides the distribution exactly in half, which in this case is 4. Let us look at another example: 1, 1, 1, 1, 2, 6, 7, 7, 7, 7. In this case, we count four 1's and four 7's. This is a bimodal distribution. The median value lies between 2 and 6, so we add these two values and divide by 2 to arrive at a median of 4. In a normally distributed population, the mean, median, and mode are all equal. The nature and use of nonparametric descriptors and statistics will be discussed later.

For now, let us consider the ramifications of the central limit theorem. Well, actually, it is not as bad as it looks. Basically, it means that you can assume normality of the sampling distribution (and the ability to use parametric statistics on your data), if your sample is sufficiently large. This holds true even if your population distribution is unknown or nonnormally distributed. So, the question becomes, How large is large? Marks (3) notes that with a sample size of 30, almost any distribution—whether it be skewed, rectangular, uniform, or dinosaur shaped—will be amenable to parametric statistics because of the central limit theorem. With this as a premise, let us return to our discussion of descriptors of parameters and statistics.

Reconsider the exemplary data set. The mean for parametric samples defines the midpoint of the data. However, observe the following data:

73.0, 55.2, 66.1, 71.9, 59.2, 80.2; n = 6; x̄ = 67.6

These data have the same mean as the previous data, but here there is a wider spread about the mean (55.2 to 80.2 versus 65.0 to 69.3). Thus, other measures dealing with the variability of the sample are needed. The two most commonly used parametric descriptors of variability are σ^2 and σ, called the variance and standard deviation (SD). The SD is the square root of the variance. The corresponding statistics are s^2 and s.

The standard deviation for the first set of data was 1.6, whereas for the second set of data it was 9.3. Data are usually described as x̄ ± SD. For our two examples, the data are expressed as 67.6 ± 1.6 and 67.6 ± 9.3. Thus we can tell at a glance which sample is more variable. Figure 11.4 depicts the distribution of three nor-

mally distributed populations, all with the same mean, but with different variances. A functional definition is that the range from (x̄ − SD) to (x̄ + SD) encompasses 68% of the sample data, the range (x̄ ± 2SD) encompasses 95%, and the range (x̄ ± 3SD) encompasses 99% (Fig. 11.5).

Another term used to describe sample spread is the standard deviation of the mean, also called standard error, or standard error of the mean (SEM). The parameter is $\sigma_{\bar{x}}$, and the statistic is $s_{\bar{x}}$. The parameter $\sigma_{\bar{x}}$ is the standard deviation of means of all possible groupings of size n from a parent population with standard deviation of σ. The kicker here is that the actual determination of statistically significant differences in parametric statistics involves the use of $s_{\bar{x}}$. We also use $s_{\bar{x}}$ to determine the confidence interval about a mean. For example, for large sample sizes, a 95% confidence interval equals x̄ ± (1.96* $s_{\bar{x}}$). In plain English, this means that we are 95% confident that the population mean lies within this interval.

Data are usually expressed as x̄ ± SD or x̄ ± SEM. The SEM is derived from the SD, as follows: SEM = SD/√n. Thus, the SEM will always be less than the SD. When presenting data, you should always make very clear which measure of variability you are reporting. Note also that a wide data range in a sample can appear very small if the SEM is used. For example, consider x̄ ± SD of 100 ± 120. For a variable such as plasma taurine, this might cause a concern because x̄ ± 1 SD should encompass 68% of the sample, meaning either some poor slob has negative plasma taurine, or your distribution is skewed impressively to the right. However, if your sample size is 100, then your SEM = 120/√100, or 12. Thus, x̄ ± SEM is 100 ± 12. Careful observation of which measure of variability is being used will help you gauge the true range of values observed. As an aside, because of the central limit theorem, even samples as variable as this are amenable to parametric statistics.

What of ordinal data or nonnormally distributed quantitative data? Because we cannot use parameters to describe these data, the variance, SD, and SEM cannot be used. Data must be described as the median or the mode, followed by the range in parentheses. The data set {1, 2, 3, 4, 10, 18, 19}, using the median as our measure of central tendency, would be described as 4 (1–19). This also brings up the question, How do you know if your sample is nonnormally distributed? Any time that you are dealing with all nonnegative or all nonpositive values, and your standard deviation is greater than half of the mean, you should begin feeling uncomfortable about the assumption of normality. In this situation, quantitative data samples should never be analyzed using parametric statistics, unless the sample size is 30 or greater.

One other form of data description used in the literature is to express data as a percentage. For nominal variables, this might be the percentage of wound infection or percentage of intensive care unit (ICU) patients with adult respiratory distress syndrome (ARDS). For quantitative variables, it may involve expressing the value of one treatment as a percentage of another. Although this is a fairly common occurrence, when reading reports, you should remember that 1 of 2 is 50%; of course, so is 2000 of 4000. Sometimes, intentionally or unintentionally, a percentage can obscure the true sample size. When reading a report, make sure that you know the values from which the percentages are calculated. Similarly, when writing, make sure that you provide your readers with the same information.

Significance Testing

Back to our hypothesis: premature infants on TPN require carnitine. Our variable is plasma ketones. First, some perspective. Plasma ketones are a normal by-product of fatty acid oxidation. Abnormal fatty acid use has been hypothesized to be indicated by lowered plasma ketone bodies. Therefore, in the proposed study, two possibilities exist. The first is that the mean plasma concentration of ketone bodies in infants not given carnitine (let us call this $\bar{x}_1$) will be the same as the plasma concentration of ketone bodies in infants receiving carnitine ($\bar{x}_2$). That is, $\bar{x}_1 = \bar{x}_2$. For this study, this is the null hypothesis, which is usually abbreviated H_0. Every study has a null hypothesis, and the null hypothesis always means either that there is no treatment effect or that the effect is of no interest to the researcher. This would be the meaning of the null hypothesis, whether we had 2 or 2000 treatments.

For every experiment, there is always one, and only one, other hypothesis. This is called the alternate hypothesis, and is abbreviated H_A, or H_1. The alternate hypothesis always implies that there is a treatment effect, that something is happening, that the effects of the different treatments are not the same. For the present study, we have three choices for an alternate hypothesis: $\bar{x}_1 \neq \bar{x}_2$; $\bar{x}_1 > \bar{x}_2$; or $\bar{x}_1 < \bar{x}_2$. The choice of the alternate hypothesis will have some impact not only on the wording of the null hypothesis but also on the mechanics of the statistical test. This latter point, related to one-tailed

and two-tailed testing, will be discussed later in this section. For the present, let us choose the alternate hypothesis to be $\bar{x}_1 = \bar{x}_2$. The two hypotheses are usually presented in the following form:

$$H_0: \bar{x}_1 = \bar{x}_2$$

$$H_1: \bar{x}_1 \neq \bar{x}_2$$

Now we are presented with two diametrically opposed hypotheses. We use statistics to test these hypotheses and, in particular, to test the null hypothesis. This process is called significance testing. By accepting the null hypothesis, we have not proved conclusively that it is true, but rather that the evidence acquired in the study is insufficient to reject its validity. Similarly, by rejecting the null hypothesis, we have not proven the alternate, but have accepted the alternate hypothesis by process of elimination. Thus all significance tests are based on H_0, and H_1 is accepted or rejected by default. One added note. The word significant is now one of the official buzzwords of authors everywhere. Its use always implies that significance testing has occurred. If this is not the case, then the word significant should not be used in the report.

Significance testing involves setting limits to protect against two types of error. One is called Type I error. Recall again that we have used a sample to make guesses about the population. A Type I error occurs when we reject the null hypothesis based on our sample, when in the population the null hypothesis is true. The whole point of statistics is to enable us to make observations on a sample, because in most cases, the population is far too extensive for study. What is done to protect against Type I error is to set a probability of acceptable error. This probability, named α, is commonly set at 0.05. This, then, is the origin of the fabled $p < 0.05$. So what does it mean? Simply put, if I say that I reject the null hypothesis at $p < 0.05$, it means that there is less than a 5% chance that I am mistaken. Another way of putting this is to say that the probability that the differences between means is a result of random chance is less than 5%. In addition to its use in significance testing, the α-level is also used before the study begins, in the determination of sample size.

The second type of error is mysteriously called the Type II error. Type II error occurs when the null hypothesis is accepted based on the sample when, in fact, the null hypothesis is false based on the parent population. Once again, a probability of acceptable error is designated. This probability, called β, is usually set at a low level, but higher than α, usually around 0.20. This means that, if we accept the null hypothesis, there is less than a 20% chance that we will be wrong. The β-level is used in sample size determinations. Another term associated with the β-level is power. The power of a study, i.e., the ability to detect differences between groups, is equal to $1 - \beta$.

Sharp minds in the reading audience will note that the chance of a Type II error is commonly set at four times the chance of a Type I error. In other words, we are willing to accept four times the chance of making a mistake in accepting the null hypothesis opposed to rejecting it, i.e., significance testing is slanted toward accepting the null hypothesis. Because of this, only true differences in the data will lead to a rejection of the null hypothesis. If statistics has a bad name, it is through inappropriate application. When the statistical design and experimental design are selected before the study is begun (hint, hint), the statistics at the end of the study provide you with a powerful tool for determining the worth of your data.

Just a little bit longer on the soapbox. I have rather glibly referred to the usual values for α and β, i.e., 0.05 and 0.20, respectively. One can almost discern a radiant aura about these values, as if they had somehow become blessed from above and etched into the fabric of the space-time continuum. Actually, these levels are entirely under the control of the researcher. A word to the wise, however. If you propose to use less stringent α- and β-levels in your study, be prepared to defend those levels, not only in the acquisition of your grant but also when it comes time to present and publish your data.

It was mentioned previously that statistical significance does not always mean clinical significance. However, if you are designing a study, you can set your α-level at such a point that statistical significance does imply clinical significance. For example, in a proposed study of the efficacy of bupivacaine in open wound healing, you determine before the study that for the sample size you will use, if you can determine a significant difference at $p < 0.001$, this will also be clinically significant. Similarly, you can set stringent α- and β-levels to determine a sample size to find a clinically significant result.

To recap: a Type I error involves an error in the testing of the null hypothesis. Type II error means that you have accepted the null hypothesis incorrectly because your sample size was too small. How is sample size determined, anyway? The following, purely for your viewing enjoyment, is a formula to determine sample size in a study of two treatments with nominal variables, such as incidence of wound infection (4).

$$n = (2.8/(P_1 - P_2))^2 * (P_1 (100-P_1) + P_2 (100 - P_2))$$

where n is the sample size; P_1, the rate of infection in patients given placebo; and P_2, the rate of infection in patients given the drug. The factor 2.8 is related to the fact that α- and β-levels were chosen to be 0.05 and 0.20, respectively. Thus the formula will generate a number that delivers the sample size you will need to see a significant difference between groups at $p < 0.05$. Wow, pretty easy, huh, kids? Just plug in P_1 and P_2 and you are off to the races, right? Now is when it would be helpful to have some sinister background music build-

ing up. Think about it. All you need to do to figure out your sample size in a study to determine the percentage of people who get wound infections on either drug or placebo is to plug in the values for the percentage of people who get wound infections on either drug or placebo. Hey, if you know the answer to that one, why run the study?

Oooh, good point. So how do you set up a sample size with this formula? Remember, if you are using this formula, you have not begun the study yet, because you are still designing the study. One way of using this formula is to look over the literature, which you needed to review to write that proposal. Maybe someone has written about a study using a different age group or different gender, or maybe he or she has looked at the same drug in a different surgical procedure or used a different drug in the same procedure. In all of these cases, percentages of wound infection were most likely provided. By plugging in the most relevant information into the formula above, you can arrive at an estimate for your study. Another possibility is to run a pilot study and determine percentages for the larger study based on the pilot. Alternatively, maybe you do not believe the published results from someone else's study, so you want to reproduce the experiment using similar sample subjects and the same sample size. Yet another suggestion would be to use the rate of wound infection currently obtained with the standard of care at your institution. You could then declare a difference in terms of percent improvement, based on what you think would constitute a clinically significant difference.

This is, however, the real world. And just because someone else has published results does not mean that yours will be the same. In addition, the results from the pilot study may not bear any resemblance to the results in your big study. The fact is, however, you have based your estimate of sample size on the best information you had before the start of your study. Only one sample size formula is shown here, but there are others. All of these formulas have the same limitation, i.e., some prior knowledge or educated guess concerning the outcome of the study, whether it be percentage wound infection or variability of plasma ketone bodies, is required.

So let us set up the following scenario. You are at a big national meeting, presenting some data of which you are particularly proud. You have concluded that there is no difference in percent wound infection after biliary surgery between groups treated with antibiotic prophylaxis with either a cephalosporin with a long half-life or a broad-spectrum ureidopenicillin. You are handling the questions in the discussion period quite well, when suddenly, there looms before you a deranged misanthrope with an evil, leering grin. It is obviously a Ph.D. with a hate complex for MD's, but before the guards can throw him or her out, this person slithers to the microphone and sneers, "It appears to me, Doctor, that you have committed a Type II error!" So what has this person said and why has he or she said it to you? Again, a Type II error implies that you have accepted the null hypothesis wrongly. Because the Type II error rate is set by the β-level and because the β-level is only used to determine sample size, you interpret the twisted little misanthrope's remark to mean that your sample size was too small.

What does a poor resident do? You could (a) fix him or her with your evil eye and char the person to foul smelling cinders right on the spot, (b) beg for mercy and swear you will never use a small sample size again, or (c) stand tall in the saddle, defend your study, and win the acclaim of millions. Although choice a has the advantage of ego-inflating gratuitous violence, it might not sit well with your Hippocratic oath. Choice b is loathsome and should be avoided at all costs. Choice c is obvious. Your sample size was chosen for a good reason, and all you have to do is defend your reasons. Let's face it, folks, if you don't have confidence in the validity of your data, you shouldn't be presenting the stuff in the first place. The ultimate answer may lie in the fact that the experimental treatment or drug just is not as effective as you (or some people in the audience) would like for it to be.

What if it is not your study, but someone else's? When the authors of studies accept the null hypothesis, are you really going to take the time to calculate sample size formulas for every article you read to determine whether a Type II error has been committed? For most of you, it will be a pretty frosty day in Brownsville before that happens. That is why for you quick-and-dirty types it is more important to evaluate the α-level and the sample size. In this sense, if the null hypothesis is accepted (at $p > \alpha$), it is up to the reader to determine if the sample size is sufficiently large to warrant the conclusions. That is to say, even though the null hypothesis was accepted, do you believe that the differences noted are clinically significant and would have been statistically significant if a larger sample size had been used?

Some authors have interpreted the preceding statement to indicate that clinically significant events are not always statistically significant. It is preferable to state that if a Type II error has been committed and a clinically significant event may have been obscured, the null hypothesis should be retested. To enact a change in clinical practice based on the presumption that the treatment would have been effective if not for Type II error is asinine. If you believe that there was a Type II error made in a study important to your work, either wait for a better study to be published or conduct the study yourself.

Let us look at the other end of the scale. Suppose someone has presented you with a statistically significant difference at $p < 0.05$. How does that change with sample size? Look at the data in Table 11.2. The variable is diastolic blood pressure, and the values represent the point at which for a given sample size $p < 0.05$. In this example, the variance is held constant for all of the sam-

Table 11.2.
Depiction of the Effect of Sample Size on the Difference Required to Show a Significant Depression in Diastolic Blood Pressure at $p < 0.05$, Using a One-Tailed, Unpaired t Test[a]

Sample Size	Control Blood Pressure (mm Hg)	Treatment Blood Pressure (mm Hg)	Δ (mm Hg)
5	108	96.3	11.7
10	108	100.3	7.7
20	108	102.7	5.3
30	108	103.7	4.3
40	108	104.3	3.7
50	108	104.7	3.3
100	108	105.7	2.3
500	108	107	1
1000	108	107.3	0.7

[a] Standard deviation is held constant at 9.9.

ple sizes. As you can see, the larger the sample size, the smaller the difference required for significance. By the time you get out to 500 individuals in each arm of the study, you can achieve a whopping 1 mm Hg difference and be significant at $p < 0.05$. And you know what the ads say: "Clinically tested by doctors to cause a significant decrease in blood pressure." There is significance and there is significance. Statistics, when applied properly, give you the framework on which to base your clinical decision, using your clinical judgment. Statistics are not an excuse to check your brain at the door.

Let us go back to our original null and alternate hypotheses. Our null hypothesis was that the treatments were equal, whereas the alternate hypothesis stated that they were not equal. Thus, if treatment 1 is either much less or much greater than treatment 2, we will reject the null hypothesis. Mathematically, it can be shown that treatment 1 must be at least 1.96 pooled standard errors greater or less than treatment 2 to see a significant difference. This would be an example of a two-tailed test. The pooled standard error refers to the estimated standard error of the difference between the two sample means. What if the hypotheses had been worded differently? For example, H_0: $\bar{x}_1 \leq \bar{x}_2$ and H_1: $\bar{x}_1 > \bar{x}_2$. To disprove the null hypothesis in this case, treatment 1 would only have to be 1.64 pooled standard errors greater than treatment 2. This constitutes a one-tailed test. Thus, use of a one-tailed test requires a smaller difference to demonstrate statistical significance. There are two catches to this pleasant little scenario. The first is that the decision to use a one-tailed or two-tailed test must have been made as part of the design of the study, i.e., while the proposal was being written. The second catch is that for this particular pair of hypotheses, if treatment 1 is less than treatment 2, the null hypothesis is accepted and no analysis need be done. Before selecting a one-tailed test, you should be sure that you have no interest in results being significant in the reverse direction to your alternate hypothesis. If any doubt exists on this point, a two-tailed test is more appropriate. The most common uses of one-and two-tailed tests are for the *t* test, Fisher's exact test, and Pearson's r (the correlation coefficient), all of which will be discussed later.

Parametric Statistics

Enough, already! Which tests do you use? Let us first concern ourselves with cases for which we want to determine differences between treatments as in our original hypothesis with the two TPN solutions, observing that eminently quantitative variable, plasma ketone body concentration. Let us assume that we are dealing with normally distributed data. Okay, we have a quantitative variable that is normally distributed and we have two treatments—this looks like a job for (dramatic pause) the *t* test! The *t* test (also known as Student's *t* test) is used to determine if differences exist between two (and no more than two!) samples of quantitative data. There are three types of *t* test: *(a)* paired observations, equal variance; *(b)* unpaired observations, equal variance; and *(c)* unpaired observations, unequal variance. For example, paired observations in the present example would be to let each infant, at different time points, have each of the two TPN solutions. This is also called letting each infant be his or her own control. Another use would be with age- and sex-matched individuals, such as in the comparison of bone mineral content in female patients with primary or secondary parathyroidism versus age-matched female control subjects. An example of unpaired observations would be the testing of one cancer therapy in one group of patients and another therapy in another group of unmatched patients. In the third type of *t* test, you assume unpaired observations and unequal variance. Normally, unless there is a wide difference in the variance, one assumes equal variances.

What are the differences between the three tests? The differences lie in the power of the test. In this regard, a paired *t* test has the most power and an unpaired *t* test with unequal variance has the least power. This is based on the fact that, because each subject is his or her own control, there is a reduction in the variability of treatment response. Thus, for a given set of paired data, a *t* test for paired observations will lead you to reject the null hypothesis more often than a *t* test for unpaired observations. In addition to being a more powerful analysis, the paired test also needs less than half the sample size required by an unpaired analysis, when each person is his or her own control. These advantages point out the wisdom of using a paired design and emphasize the importance of creating the research design and statistical design before the study begins. It will not always be possible to use a paired design, but when applicable, its advantages are great. But overall, no matter how great the temptation, no matter what the circumstances, the *t* test can only be used to compare two means of normally distributed, quantitative data, that is to say, two and no more than two!

What if we had wanted to compare more than two TPN solutions? Let us say that we had decided to expand our study, so that we would be testing a control (TPN without carnitine) and two formulas containing two levels of carnitine. Well, we know that a *t* test can be used to compare two, and no more than two, means. With more than two means, for parametric data, we use an analysis of variance (AOV or ANOVA). Simply put, the analysis of variance analyzes the variance between the treatments and within each treatment to determine statistical significance. Variance between the treatments refers to the width of the spread between the treatment means. The greater the spread (i.e., the greater the variance), the more likely it is that a significant difference will be seen, leading to rejection of the null hypothesis. Variance within each treatment refers to the spread within each treatment group. The greater the spread, the more likely that values between treatments will overlap, leading to acceptance of the null hypothesis. Thus a significant analysis of variance will have a high between-group variance and a low within-group variance. The ratio of these two variances, called the F ratio, is the basis for the test. The relevant hypotheses are shown below.

$$H_0: \bar{x}_1 = ... = \bar{x}_n, \text{ where n} \geq 2$$

$$H_1: \text{Inequality; all means are not equal}$$

You should note that the AOV can be used for two or more treatments. A small light clicks on in the dusty recesses of your neuronal vault, and you think, "In that case, why do we even mess with the *t* test then?" Mathematically, the statistical test for the *t* test relies on the *t* statistic, whereas the AOV relies on the F statistic. For two treatments, for a two-tailed *t* test, *t* = F. However, the AOV is not readily applicable to one tailed, two treatment analyses. Also, the *t* test is far easier to calculate, hence the preference for the *t* test for two treatments.

So what is this big deal about not using a *t* test for more than two treatments? Is this more statistical flimflammery, or is there some hard evidence to deter the restive masses? Take a peek at Table 11.3. The table describes the postulated significance level and the actual significance level for multiple mean comparisons. The more treatments you have, the more pair-wise comparisons there are, and the more likely it is that you will make a Type I error, i.e., reject the null hypothesis incorrectly. For example, with 5 means, you would need to run 10 *t* tests to compare all of the means with one another. By rejecting the null hypothesis at the 0.05 level, you would in actuality be taking a 40% risk of making a Type I error among those 10 *t* tests. Why is this? Remember, the default α in most studies is 0.05. This means there is a 1 in 20 chance of making a mistake. But what

Table 11.3.
Evaluation of the Effect of Multiple Testing on the True Chance of Type I Error[a]

Number of Treatments	Number of Tests Required	True p Value[b]
2	1	0.05
3	3	0.14
4	6	0.26
5	10	0.4
10	45	0.9
20	190	1

[a] Modified from Marks RG. Designing a research project. Belmont, CA: Lifetime Learning, 1982.
[b] Assuming a target α level of 0.05.

happens to that 1 in 20 if we make repeated tests on the same set of data? Try this example. A good goal-tender in hockey will stop around 90% of the shots on net. Thus, for any given shot, the odds are fairly high that he or she will stop the puck. However, during a hockey game, after facing 30 shots on goal, the odds are high that at least one goal will be scored. The same is true with multiple t testing (a similar argument holds for multiple testing of two samples for a large number of variables). The more tests you make, the more likely it will be that you make a Type I error. The only problem is that you will not know when or where the error lies. Hence the use of the analysis of variance test, to avoid such uncertainties.

Back to those two hypotheses. Notice that if you reject the null hypothesis, you are accepting the alternate, which only tells you that an inequality exists somewhere. Maybe $\bar{x}_1 = \bar{x}_2 \neq \bar{x}_3$ or $\bar{x}_1 \neq \bar{x}_2 = \bar{x}_3$ or $\bar{x}_2 \neq \bar{x}_3 = \bar{x}_1$ or $\bar{x}_1 \neq \bar{x}_2 \neq \bar{x}_3$. Which is right? Do you, as numerous other researchers have done, use multiple t tests to find the inequality? Well, good, you just do that, and meanwhile why don't you take the rest of this chapter and paper train your new Doberman? Come on, folks, use of a t test after an AOV makes no more sense than using it beforehand. The argument described in the paragraph above still applies. You need to use a fully approved mean comparison procedure.

There are numerous techniques you can use, so this chapter will only cover some of the more popular ones. To begin with, use of these tests is only warranted if an analysis of variance has already been run and the null hypothesis has been rejected. If the null hypothesis was accepted, then just slide on by these procedures, because they are not to be used in that event. With that out of the way, let us look at some techniques.

Okay, you are writing your proposal and have decided on an AOV. Furthermore (let us say you have five treatments), you have decided that if you do reject the null hypothesis, treatments 2 versus 4 and 3 versus 5 are the comparisons you would want to make. No problem. Simply make the decision before the experiment is started to run contrasts. The contrast analysis is done as

a part of the analysis of variance. It is a very powerful tool, but the decision to use contrasts and the determination of which contrasts to run must be made before the experiment has begun. An alternate type of contrast, Bonferroni's t statistic, can also be calculated, provided it is planned before the experiment has begun.

Another technique is the Scheffé's interval. Let us say that you are some hot-shot, big-snot researcher renowned for your eloquent arrogance. You design your study and plan to use analysis of variance. You, however, are so sure that you will accept the null hypothesis that you decide not to use any multiple comparison techniques. But, to your shock, your data show that you must reject the null hypothesis. Like the sludge monkey that you are, you fire your technician for incompetence, then return to your data to try to find a test to use. The Scheffé's is your kind of test. Scheffé's can be used for multiple comparisons between pairs of means, even if you did not decide to use it before the experiment started. In that vein, Scheffé's is also useful for comparing means that were overlooked when you originally set up your contrasts. "But, wait a minute," simpers the obnoxious brown-noser in the front row. "I thought that you said that choosing statistical tests after the study started was illegal!" The Scheffé's test is one of the exceptions, the reason being the low power of the test. By low power, we mean that a comparison that would have shown a significant effect using contrasts may no longer be significant when a Scheffé's test is used.

The first two examples have been extremes. Contrasts assume you know exactly what the interesting comparisons will be, whereas Scheffé's assumes that you were completely taken off guard. For all of us undiscriminating researchers, who do not know which comparisons would be the best for contrasts but who would like to have a powerful method for making all possible comparisons between means, we offer the multiple comparison tests. These abound in the literature, but the ones that pop up frequently include the following:

1. Least significant difference (LSD)
2. Duncan's multiple range
3. Fisher's protected LSD (FPLSD)
4. Student-Newman-Keuls (SNK)
5. Tukey's ω test
6. Waller-Duncan Bayes LSD (BLSD)

All of these tests do the same thing, that is, determine differences between means. The first two procedures carry a relatively high risk of declaring at least one comparison as significant when in fact it is not, and thus are not recommended. The Tukey test is the most conservative of the lot, which is a statistical way of saying it has less power. The BLSD is conservative at low significant F ratios and increases in power as the F ratio becomes greater than 4. The test most frequently used by the author is the SNK.

In the original example—comparing TPN with no

carnitine to two other TPN solutions that have differing carnitine concentrations—the desire of the researcher might be only to compare each of the treatments to a control. Thus comparisons would not be made between the two carnitine treatments but only between each of the carnitine treatments and the control. This is a case for the Dunnett test.

The preceding has been an overview of what is known as a one-way AOV, followed by a multiple comparison procedure. The AOV, however, can be used for any number of treatment comparisons. To make a simple example, suppose that instead of just looking at three TPN solutions containing varying levels of carnitine, we also want to look at differences in plasma ketone body concentrations between males and females. So we have one set of treatments (called Factor A) concerning the TPN solutions and another set of treatments (called Factor B) concerning the gender of the subjects. Any type of AOV involving more than one factor is called a factorial analysis of variance. This particular case is called a two-factor, or two-way, analysis of variance. The AOV generated by these data would determine whether there were effects caused by gender or TPN carnitine concentration. In addition, the test would provide information as to whether an interaction between the two factors occurred during the study. Interaction is best depicted graphically, as shown in Figure 11.6. The upper graph shows the effect on plasma ketone bodies for males and females as a function of carnitine content of the TPN. The slopes for the two curves are very similar. An analysis of variance for this data would show that no interaction existed. The lower graph in Figure 11.6 shows a case in which the lines intersect. This would be a highly significant interaction. In simple terms, it means that the effect

of carnitine addition to the males was the opposite of that seen in the females, i.e., the addition of carnitine had a different effect on the two genders. Although not frequently referred to in reports, the interaction analysis can at times be more revealing than the analysis of the factors themselves.

This concept of factors can be expanded to many levels. For the study defined above, a third set of factors could be age of the child. Thus the analysis of variance is fairly open ended and can accommodate a wide variety of experimental designs. Three other variants of the AOV deserve mention here. When dealing with the *t* test, we spoke of a paired analysis, in which each child would receive each treatment and each subject is his or her own control. The same technique is available in the analysis of variance, and the term for this is blocking. Blocking, as it is used in a clinical study design, means that each subject will receive each treatment. As in the *t* test, when properly used, the use of blocking increases the power of the analysis.

Repeated measures is a buzzword that is found in many clinical studies. For example, imagine a study designed to determine changes in total urinary nitrogen after blunt trauma, using two different drugs designed to decrease muscle protein catabolism. You want to measure urine nitrogen every 24 hours for a 5-day period, and you will obtain the urine from the same patients each day. Thus you will be taking repeated urine measurements from each subject. This is a design for a repeated measures analysis of variance. You will note that only two treatments are proposed here, so that initially it appears that a *t* test would be appropriate. The key term is repeated measures. The AOV will be a much more appropriate, not to mention more powerful, test to use compared with the *t* test.

Let us take yet another popular design, the cross-over study, and apply it to the original study: two groups of infants, receiving TPN with or without carnitine. We know that a paired design will give more power to the study, but we are concerned that time may be a factor. That is, as the babies age, their response to TPN with or without carnitine may differ. One solution may be a cross-over study. In this design, half of the babies would be randomized to receive TPN with carnitine, whereas the other half would receive the control solution. The study would proceed and samples would be collected until, at some predesignated time point, the babies would be switched to the other solution. This is the cross-over. Once again, we are only dealing with two treatments, so it looks like a *t* test. However, the correct and more powerful choice is the AOV.

The *t* test and AOV are called univariate statistics because they determine differences between treatments based on a single outcome variable. When one wants to measure two or more outcome variables that are dependent variables, multivariate statistics are used. With two treatment groups, Hotelling's T^2 is used, and for more

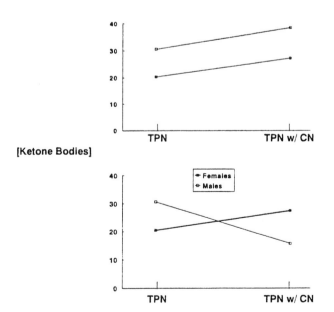

[Ketone Bodies]

Figure 11.6. Top: Depiction of a factorial analysis of variance with a nonsignificant interaction effect. Bottom: Depiction of a factorial analysis of variance with a significant interaction effect.

than two treatments, a multivariate analysis of variance (MAOV or MANOVA) is appropriate. The reader is referred to a more detailed text for additional information concerning these tests. Norman and Streiner (5) recommend the text by Tatsuoka (6), with the proviso that the reader should be familiar with matrix algebra.

The discussion up to this point has centered on the determination of differences between treatment groups. What if you have quantitative, normally distributed data, and you do not want to look at differences, but at relationships? This is a case for linear regression. As you recall from that hellish year in algebra I that your parents forced you to take back when you were too young to know better, $y = mx + b$. The rest, of course, is history. The x is the independent variable, y is the dependent variable, b is the y intercept, and m is the slope.

How is regression analysis used? In the laboratory, it is the basis of the notorious standard curve, by which readings of glucose or free fatty acid concentration can be derived from spectrophotometer readings of optical density of samples. Clinically, it may be used to determine the amount of drug necessary to obtain a desired response. Thus regression can be used to predict the value of a variable based on the value of another variable or other variables. An example taken from the arena of lithotripsy involves the dependence of fragmentation time of gallstones on gallstone weight. As the weight of the gallstone increases, so does the fragmentation time. The equation for the line that describes this relationship is derived by linear regression.

The coefficient of determination is r^2, and r^2 is the proportion of variability that is attributable to the independent variable. The quantity r^2 can vary between 0 and 1. An r^2 approaching 1 indicates that the linear regression equation is a good estimate of the relationship between the points, whereas an $r^2 = 0$ indicates that your data resemble a cluster nebula.

Regression analysis can also be used to demonstrate the degree of association between independent variables. A typical example that has received close scrutiny in the literature in recent years is the relationship between the volume of colonic methane gas and the blood insulin concentration 2 hours after a bolus dose of frijoles (refried beans). Such data could have very important social and political ramifications, so linear regression is used. However, because we are dealing with two independent variables (as opposed to an independent and a dependent variable), we can now test to see how closely the variables are correlated. Pearson's correlation coefficient r is used. The range is $-1 \leq r \leq 1$. Negative numbers infer inverse correlation, i.e., $x \, \alpha \, 1/y$. Values close to 1 or -1 indicate a good fit, and values close to 0 indicate the opposite. The value r can be tested statistically, where the null hypothesis is $r \neq 0$ (no correlation between x and y) and the alternate hypothesis is $r \neq 0$ (correlation between x and y). The test would be two-tailed for these hypotheses. If set up properly when de-

signing the study, the hypotheses can be restated to test for a one-tailed test: $r > 0$ or $r < 0$.

Now, here is an important point. If you accept the null hypothesis (there is no correlation), the regression line should not be drawn. Furthermore, and especially, the regression line should not be displayed in a presentation or a publication, because the line, in and of itself, implies correlation. The usual comeback is, ''But my computer drew a line!'' That's right, it did. Computers, and their software, are wonderfully obedient little marvels. They will do every stupid little thing you tell them to do, and do it very quickly. In this case, a program will gleefully take data that have an r value of 0, and whip out a mighty fine line, complete with coefficients and exponents, suitable for framing. However, just because a computer can do something does not make it right. A computer will also crunch nominal data into a *t* test, but that is not correct either. The weak link in this whole operation is that maniac at the keyboard. If Dr. Loon puts garbage in, most assuredly garbage will come out.

Just to beat it to a miserable, pulsating, pulpy mass, is it legitimate to display the regression line if you also show that the r value is not significant? My personal opinion is no. The visual image has strange, seductive powers, and a picture of a graph showing a line relating two independent variables will always carry more weight than some r value tucked away in the text. If there's no correlation, there should not be a line.

Now, it is a curious circumstance that Pearson's correlation coefficient, when squared, equals r^2, the coefficient of determination. And although r^2 can be used whether you are dealing with two independent variables or an independent and a dependent variable, r can only be used when dealing with two independent variables. Well, that was pretty smooth. Okay, smart guy, how do you know what kind of variable you've got? For the most part, there are two instances when we know that we are dealing with independent and dependent variables. The first occurs when the independent variable is assigned by the researcher. Examples are varying levels of lysine in the diet, varying drug dosages, or even some time interval. The second case is where a known relationship exists between the two variables, such as between blood insulin and glucose concentrations. If the researcher has not assigned one of the variables, and a large body of evidence does not exist to suggest a dependent relationship of one variable on another, then one can safely presume that one is dealing with two independent variables.

That brings us to two very important points. If you are looking at data dealing with two independent variables and the correlation has been shown to be significant, that's great! But, remember that this is still a mathematical argument. With a sufficient sample size, one could show variables to have significant correlation at $p < 0.05$ with an $r = 0.1$ (this is similar to the argument shown in Table 11.2). Squaring this number, to form r^2, gives a value of 0.01. Interpretation of this figure implies that the equation for the line can only account for 1% of the variability associated with the line, i.e., it does a smashingly lousy job of describing the data. This is where your clinical judgment needs to kick in and say that although the correlation has statistical significance, it has little or no clinical significance. In general, if there is any doubt as to the clinical significance of an r value, square it. The value r^2, as mentioned previously, tells you what percent of the variability is accounted for by the line. By this logic, even a seemingly reasonable r value of 0.7 means that the line only accounts for 49% of the variability of the data.

A second major point involving interpretation of correlations deals with the relationship itself. A significant correlation merely implies that the response of two variables, in relation to each other, is predictable. It does not, never has, and never will imply a cause-and-effect relationship. It does not matter if $r^2 = 1.000000$, there is still no cause-and-effect relationship. That is for other experiments and other pieces of data to demonstrate.

So far, we have been talking straight lines. Do not let your mind be constrained by the restrictive linearity that is linear regression. Curvilinear, or nonlinear, regression also exists, and r and r^2 values can be generated just as for linear regression. Thus, although your data are nonlinear, a function (quadratic, cubic, logarithmic, etc.) may yet exist to connect the dots, with the help of our friend, Mr. Computer.

The final type of regression up for discussion is called multiple regression. This technique is indicated if you feel that several independent variables (several different x's) can be used to predict the outcome of another independent variable (y). An example would be the prediction of resting energy expenditure (REE; the y variable) in males, based on age, weight, serum albumin, and a 24-hr total urinary nitrogen excretion (the x variables). Multiple regression not only has an r value for the entire equation but individual r values for each of the component x variables. These give the researcher some indication as to which are the most important in terms of predictive value.

Multiple regression equations can also be formulated using a mixture of qualitative and quantitative variables. However, to use multiple regression, the y variable must be quantitative. One example would be to have gender, or presence or absence of sepsis, in our equation for REE. Because these are nominal variables, dummy variables will have to be ascribed to them. Thus females can arbitrarily be assigned a value of 1, and males a value of 0. Similar assignments could be given for the presence or absence of sepsis, and the multiple regression equation, complete with r values, can be described.

Another procedure, which is best described as a combination of the AOV and regression analysis, is the analysis of covariance (AOCV or ANCOVA). AOCV is used to test for differences between several treatments, in terms of some quantitative, normally distributed variable. The added twist is that the AOCV can correct for some confounding factor, called a covariate. In the presence of a covariate, the use of AOCV provides additional precision and power to the analysis, relative to AOV. For example, look at those babies from our TPN versus TPN plus carnitine study. It was mentioned previously that the age of the infant may have an impact on how he or she responds to supplemental carnitine. One technique that was mentioned to control for this was the cross-over AOV. Another technique that could be used, however, is the AOCV; the covariate is age. Multiple covariates can also be controlled by this procedure.

Nonparametric Statistics

You should know, and I certainly do know, that the preceding has not been an exhaustive list of parametric procedures. However, they are the ones that you will run across most often. What about nonparametric procedures? Let us look at the tests for nominal variables first. Those are the categorical variables (type of organism, presence or absence of wound infection, etc.). For these, there will be no means or standard deviations, only totals in a group. The typical case found in the literature would be a comparison of two treatments. For example, what if, instead of measuring ketone bodies in our premature infant study, we had used incidence of fatty liver as our measure of the usefulness of carnitine? That is, the babies were recorded as having or not having cholestasis. These types of yes-no data (enumeration data, nominal variables) are handled by the use of χ^2 (chi-squared) analysis. Another name for this type of test is a contingency table analysis. The null hypothesis for χ^2 is independence, and the alternate hypothesis is dependence. Do not be misled, the hypotheses really mean the same thing as the hypotheses discussed under parametric statistics. Rejection of the null hypothesis means that there are differences in treatment effect. The most common form of χ^2 analysis is the 2×2 table. This form of χ^2 (2×2 table) is usually expressed as a corrected χ^2, using the Yates correction for continuity.

For example, consider a study of patient-controlled analgesia (PCA) compared with epidural-catheter-injection analgesia (EPI). An observation of the complications revealed that pruritus occurred in 17 of 22 patients receiving PCA and in only 5 of 19 patients receiving EPI. The 2×2 table is shown in Figure 11.7. The analysis would reveal that significant differences did exist between treatment groups.

A 2×2 table is by no means the only form of χ^2 analysis, however. We could just as easily have had a more complex design such as the incidence of nosocomial infections over a 12-month period in five different ICUs in various parts of the country. Another example

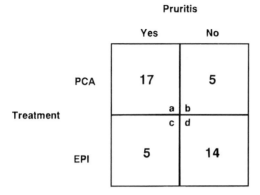

Figure 11.7.   An example of a χ^2 2 × 2 contingency table.

would be to identify which of three different techniques for gallbladder removal are preferred among surgeons from eight different hospitals in a five-state area.

One special note for χ^2. The calculated χ^2 is just an estimate, and as your sample size becomes smaller and smaller, your estimate becomes less accurate, leaving you open to making invalid decisions for rejection or acceptance of the null hypothesis. In a 2 × 2 table, we speak of the four cells in the table. If the expected value(s) for any particular cell in a 2 × 2 table is <5, then the χ^2 method will not be accurate. The formula is as follows:

e_s (expected value) · =

(smallest row total * smallest column total)/sample size

From the analgesia example cited above, e_s = (19 * 19)/41 = 8.8. For this example, the χ^2 is appropriate. For the case of a 2 × 2 table in which e_s is less than 5, Fisher's exact test should be used. Fisher's exact test is accurate for all sample sizes for a 2 × 2 design but usually is reserved for those cases for which a χ^2 test is not advisable. In larger χ^2 designs, such as 3 × 5 or 7 × 3, the general rule of thumb is that if 20% of the cells have an e_s < 5, the χ^2 will not be accurate for the analysis. In cases like these, the researcher only has two choices. The first is to eliminate the offending treatment group, and the second is to use good judgment and combine similar treatments.

So here we go again. In the case of Fisher's exact test, the advice is to use an entirely different test than was proposed originally, whereas in the second case, we are advocating serious postfacto data manipulation. Fisher's exact test is acceptable because it is actually more accurate than the χ^2 test. The reason it has not been used routinely for the large sample sizes in 2 × 2 tables is because the analysis involves a great deal of excited numbers (factorials, for you sophisticated types, like 5!, 10!, and 457!), and when you are doing these puppies by hand, it tends to give you caution. Granted, with the use of a computer, this caveat no longer carries the weight it once did, but Fisher's exact test is still generally reserved for a 2 × 2 table with small sample size.

An additional concern with Fisher's exact test involves the difference between one-tailed and two-tailed tests. Because of the nature of the calculations involved, the χ^2 is always calculated as a two-tailed test. Fisher's exact test, however, can be calculated as a one- or two-tailed test. Therefore, whenever Fisher's exact test is being used in place of the χ^2 owing to small sample size, a two-tailed Fisher's exact test should be used. Conversely, if the original alternate hypothesis called for one treatment to be higher than another treatment in a given direction, nominal variables are involved, and the experimental design is amenable to a 2 × 2 table, Fisher's exact test should be indicated in the proposal as the test to be used.

In the other case, for which the choice is to eliminate data or combine cells, it appears that we are saying that postfacto data manipulation is okay. The reality is that the χ^2 test has limitations. Certainly, no one would predict a large proportion of cells with e_s < 5. This is, however, real life, and things like this happen. We research types just despise going to all the trouble of data gathering and then finding out we have to vaporize some of it. Thus, combining similar treatments under these special circumstances is acceptable. Please, when placed in this situation, use good common sense to make your decision. This has been a repeated theme in this chapter, but it bears restating: numbers, data, and statistical tests are wonderful things, but if you insist on being out to lunch, it's all rather a waste.

Other, more specialized analyses of nominal variables are available. One type of χ^2 analysis is the McNemar test. This is analogous to working with a paired sample. In this situation, a before-and-after determination is made on the same group of subjects. For example, suppose you cornered 100 people and asked them whether they use seat belts. After getting their responses, you herd them into Grand Rounds on a day when a series of horrific automobile accidents, featuring individuals who did not use their seat belts, is going to be presented. After the presentation, you now ask your 100 individuals whether they will use seat belts. The data would then be fitted into a 2 × 2 table and analyzed for significance.

Another specialized χ^2 is the Mantel-Haenzel, which is a nonparametric equivalent of using a covariate, as in the analysis of covariance. As such, it is used in similar circumstances, for example, to control for a confounding variable while discerning the difference between two treatments. Regression analysis for which the y variable is nominal is accomplished using logistic regression. A form of regression analysis in which all of the variables (x and y) are nominal is log-linear regression. An example of the use of logistic regression is to use a variety of x variables to predict survival, which, as mentioned previously, is a nominal variable. Log-linear regression would be used to predict a nominal variable such as survival, if all of the x variables were nominal, such as

Probability of Survival

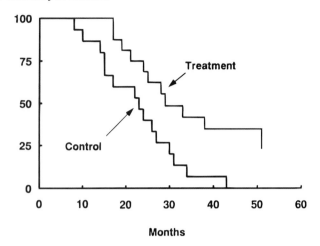

Figure 11.8. Survival curves, generated using the Kaplan-Meier technique.

gender, smoker-non-smoker, incidence of previous heart disease, or presence or absence of sepsis.

Yet another type of analysis for nominal variables that is used frequently in the literature is the life table. Essentially, the life table is a device to determine whether there are differences between treatments in patient survival over time. The analysis takes into account varying factors, such as patients entering the study at different times, patients who leave the study before the end of the study period, and patients who are still survivors by the end of the study. A pair of typical survival curves, using the Kaplan-Meier technique, are shown on Figure 11.8. The null hypothesis is that the two curves are the same, which is the same thing as saying that no treatment effect exists. A variety of statistics are available to analyze these data, depending on how many distributions are to be compared. When the effect of several covariates on survival time is to be assessed, the Cox proportional hazards model is often used. When comparing treatments in a life table, however, keep in mind that the larger the sample size, the smaller the difference that is required to achieve statistical significance. With a sufficiently large sample size, you could have two curves that are virtually identical, and yet the treatments will be statistically significantly different at the $p < 0.05$ level. Thus, having satisfied yourself that there is mathematical significance, you must now use your good clinical judgment to determine if there is also clinical significance.

Ordinal variables are also tested with nonparametric statistics. Nonparametric statistics for ordinal variables are also applicable to nonnormally distributed, quantitative data for small data sets. Ordinal data are commonly referred to as ranked data, i.e., describe your excitement about popular spawning aids for fish, such as fish ladders, on a scale from 0 (least) to 5 (hysterically excited). For most of the more common parametric tests, there is

a corresponding nonparametric test. The major disadvantage of the use of the nonparametric tests is that they are not as powerful as the corresponding parametric test. In other words, with the same set of data, you may detect differences with the latter, but not necessarily with the former. Another disadvantage is that, for some of the more complex AOV designs, no nonparametric equivalents exist. One solution to this dilemma is the use of rankits. Conversion of ranked data, or nonnormally distributed quantitative data that have been converted to ranks, allows the use of parametric statistics on the data. The procedure is described briefly by Gill (7). Yet another solution, similar to the rankits, is the transformation of ranks to fit a normal distribution. An example of this is fitting IQ scores to a normal distribution with a mean of 100.

In general, the nonparametric tests that you will encounter most frequently are the following:

1. The Mann-Whitney U test, also known as the Mann-Whitney, for testing differences between two unpaired treatments
2. The Wilcoxon signed rank test, for testing differences between two paired treatments
3. The Kruskal-Wallis AOV, for testing differences between more than two treatments
4. The Spearman rank correlation, for testing the strength of relationship between two variables

Occasionally, you will read a paper and note that the author has used parametric and nonparametric statistics on the same set of data. When you see this, you should consider that the author knows little or nothing about statistics. Data cannot be both normal and non-normal, ranked and nonranked. Choose one or the other, not both! What of the case for which you determine, before the experiment has begun, to use parametric statistics, and you have nonnormal data? In this situation, it is perfectly legitimate to use the corresponding nonparametric test. A brief rundown of the more popular statistical tests is shown in Table 11.4 . The nonparametric tests for ordinal data are also listed.

Contingency Tables in Diagnostic Testing

As mentioned previously, the χ^2 test is also known as a contingency table analysis. The contingency table has other uses besides the χ^2, however. The specificity and sensitivity of a test are derived from a 2×2 table. The sensitivity is the ability of a test to detect a disease, and the specificity is the ability of a test to determine if no disease is present. The calculations for a 2×2 table for sensitivity and specificity are shown in Figure 11.9. An example is the use of ultrasound in the detection of gallstones. Obviously, the test would only be used if indicated by other signs and symptoms noted on examination. The data are shown in Figure 11.10. Here, the sensitivity and specificity of the test are quite high, at

Table 11.4.
Common Statistical Tests

Study	Quantitative	Nominal	Ordinal[a]
One sample[b]		1. χ^2	1. Kolmogorov-Smirnov
Two unpaired treatments	1. *t* test, equal variances	1. χ^2	1. Mann-Whitney U test
	2. *t* test, unequal variances	2. Fisher's exact test	2. Wilcoxon rank sum test
			3. Kolmogorov-Smirnov
			4. Median test
Two paired treatments	1. Paired *t* test	1. McNemar test	1. Sign test
			2. Wilcoxon signed rank test[c]
Three or more treatments	1. AOV	1. χ^2	1. Kruskal-Wallis AOV
	2. AOV with blocking		2. Friedman's AOV with blocking
	3. Factorial AOV		
Analysis adjusted for covariates	1. AOCV	1. Mantel-Haenzel	
Regression	1. Linear regression	1. Logistic regression	1. Cumulative odds
	2. Nonlinear regression	2. Log-linear regression	2. Continuation ratio
	3. Multiple regression		
Correlation	1. Pearson's *r*	1. Contingency coefficient	1. Spearman rank correlation
			2. Kendell's rank correlation
			3. Kendell's coefficient of concordance

[a] These tests are also appropriate for nonnormally distributed quantitative data of small sample size.
[b] This refers to the comparison of treatment data to some recognized norm or distribution, such as the January to December monthly incidence of cesarean delivery compared with the average of the past 20 years.
[c] This test has more power than the sign test.

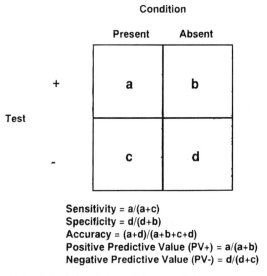

Figure 11.9. Calculations for sensitivity, specificity, accuracy, positive predictive value, and negative predictive value.

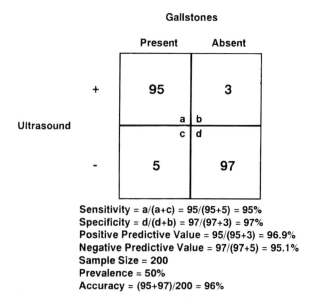

Figure 11.10. Use of ultrasound as a diagnostic test for gallstones when the suspected prevalence of gallstones is high.

95% and 97%, respectively. Another term that occurs in the literature is accuracy, which is the sum of the true positives and the true negatives, divided by the total sample.

Unfortunately, you do not always have the luxury of knowing exactly how many people have the disease of interest. Therefore, an even more useful pair of parameters are the positive predictive value and the negative predictive value. The positive predictive value is the chance of having the disease, if the test results for the disease are positive. Conversely, the negative predictive value is the chance of not having the disease, if the test results are negative. Calculations for these two values

are shown in Figure 11.9. Sample values for the ultrasound example are shown in Figure 11.10.

How are the predictive values and specificity and sensitivity related? In the example in Figure 11.10, the ultrasound has a high probability of detecting the disease and a high positive predictive value. However, this is in a carefully screened group of patients, who would be expected to have a high frequency, or prevalence, of the disease. What about the opposite case? Let us assume that you, in an inexplicable fit of frenzy, begin ordering ultrasounds to test for gallstones on everyone in the greater metropolitan area. Innocent bystanders,

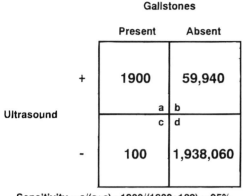

Sensitivity = a/(a+c) =1900/(1900+100) = 95%
Specificity = d/(d+b) = 1,938,060/(1,938,060+59,940) = 97%
Positive Predictive Value = 1900/(1900+59,940) = 3.1%
Negative Predictive Value = 1,938,060/(1,938,060+100) = 99.99%
Sample size = 2,000,000
Prevalence = 0.1%
Accuracy = (1900+1,938,060)/2,000,000 = 97%

Figure 11.11. Use of ultrasound as a diagnostic test for gallstones when the suspected prevalence of gallstones is low.

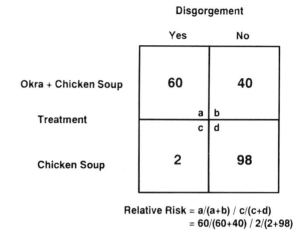

Relative Risk = a/(a+b) / c/(c+d)
= 60/(60+40) / 2/(2+98)
= 30

Figure 11.12. Determination of the relative risk.

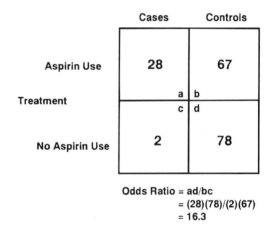

Odds Ratio = ad/bc
= (28)(78)/(2)(67)
= 16.3

Figure 11.13. Determination of the odds ratio.

small children, household pets—no one is safe from your bout of ultrasonophilia. Upon your recovery 12 months later, you notice a preponderance of very sleek sports cars in the radiologists' parking lot, in addition to reams of data. The results might appear as shown in Figure 11.11. Note that the specificity and sensitivity, which are independent of disease prevalence, are the same as in Figure 11.10. However, the positive predictive value is now low (3.1%), whereas the negative predictive value has increased to 99.99%. These changes have occurred because of the change in the prevalence of the disease. Although the prevalence of gallstones in the first example was high as a result of the way that patients were selected, the prevalence was extremely low in the second example. Thus, the positive predictive value has a direct relationship with the prevalence, i.e., as the prevalence increases, the positive predictive value increases. The negative predictive value is indirectly related to the prevalence, i.e., as the prevalence increases, the negative predictive value decreases. Thus, from Figure 11.10, a negative result would indicate no disease was present, and a positive result, owing to its low predictive value, would require additional work to determine if gallstones were present.

Two other concepts that appear in the surgical literature are relative risk and odds ratios. In particular, these values are used often in discussions of cancer and heart disease. Relative risk can be applied in most commonly used designs, with the exception of the case-control study. Relative risk computes the possibility of disease when exposed to a certain agent, relative to the risk of disease when not exposed to the same agent. For a relatively benign example, let us compare a delightful bowl of chicken soup to a bowl of chicken soup that has been tainted with okra, without a doubt the most baneful veg-

etable ever to photosynthesize. These two treatments will be compared, relative to their ability to initiate the disgorgement of gastric material. Subjects will be randomly assigned to both treatments and their responses noted. The results and calculations are shown in Figure 11.12. The risk of disgorgement after ingestion of okra-chicken soup, relative to the chicken soup, is (60/100): (2/100), or 30 times greater. Valuable data for 6-year-olds growing up in the South!

These calculations, however, are not applicable to case-control designs. This is because a much lower incidence of cases exists in the population, relative to the proportion of cases to controls in the study. The odds ratio (also known as relative odds) is used as an estimate of the relative risk. An example of the use of the odds ratio is provided by Hurwitz et al. (8) in their study of the relationship between aspirin usage and Reye's syndrome. The data are provided in Figure 11.13. Note that the calculations for the odds ratio are different from those for the relative risk. The odds ratio indicates that the risk of having Reye's syndrome after salicylate exposure relative to no salicylate exposure was (28/2):(67/78), or 16.3 times greater.

Conclusion

You should realize, of course, that you will not become an expert in statistics after reading this chapter. If you believe that, then you are a living proof of the statement, "A little knowledge is dangerous." Some very complex topics, such as logistic regression or MAOV, were mentioned in a sentence, whereas others, such as discriminant function analysis, have been ignored entirely. The emphasis in this chapter was focused on those experimental designs and techniques that you are most likely to encounter in the literature. What are the major points to remember?

1. Given a sufficiently large sample size, any two treatment groups can be shown to be statistically significantly different. The same holds true for significance in correlation.
2. Statistical significance does not necessarily imply clinical significance.
3. If treatment A versus treatment B has $p < 0.05$, and treatment C versus treatment D has $p < 0.0001$, it does not follow that the difference between C and D is of greater magnitude or importance than between A and B, merely that we are more sure that the difference between C and D is real.
4. When dealing with percentages, remember that 1 of 2 looks the same as 500 of 1000.
5. Correlation between independent variables is indicative of association, not of a cause-and-effect relationship.
6. A *t* test is only used for normally distributed, quantitative variables, with one or two, treatments.
7. A well-designed paper with poorly designed statistics is far superior to a poorly designed paper with well-designed statistics.

Just a few words on that last point. After taking a course in statistics, one usually looks at articles with a different eye. The usual response is to rend papers with slavering jaws and razor-sharp nails, shredding everything to bits, all in the name of improper statistics. Although a great deal of improvement in the proper choice of statistics in journal articles has occurred over the last few years, instances of improper uses of statistics still abound. Nevertheless, if the study design is good, it is a simple matter to disregard invalid p values and to evaluate the means and standard deviations (or nominal or ordinal variables) and still come to your own best guess. Logic and common sense, remember? However, if the experimenter has chosen the wrong control or if the treatment groups have tremendous underlying differences in the patient samples that, in your judgment, are sure to obscure the treatment effects, then it does

not matter how beautiful the statistics are. Repeated measures analysis of variance that uses an ingenious cross-over design with standard errors so low they bring tears to your eyes is not worth a slab of dung if the study design rots. It brings to mind Condon's concept of Type III error—the conclusions are not supported by the data represented (9).

As a closing note, I would like to dissuade the reader from the notion that the purpose of this chapter was to belittle the value of statistics. On the contrary, statistical analysis is an important tool in the ordering and interpretation of data. Its frequent application in the medical literature is a testament to widespread agreement among researchers and reviewers alike as to the importance of statistics. If anything, the purpose of this chapter was to demystify statistics and reinforce the concept that statistics is a tool to assist you in the determination of clinical significance.

GLOSSARY

accuracy—the total number of true positive and true negative values for a test, divided by the total number of tests.

alternate hypothesis—in hypothesis testing, the alternate hypothesis always implies that there is a treatment effect, i.e., that the effects of the different treatments are not the same. It is abbreviated H_A or H_1.

ANOVA—see AOV.

AOV—analysis of variance test, used for testing differences between three or more treatments, if the variable is quantitative and if the samples are normally distributed. The AOV is also abbreviated ANOVA.

case control study—a retrospective comparison of treatments for which the subjects are not randomly assigned.

coefficient of determination—used in regression analysis and abbreviated r^2, the coefficient of determination is the percent of the variability of the data that can be accounted for by the equation for the regression line. The value r^2 can vary between 0 and 1.

cohort analysis—a prospective comparison of treatments for which the subjects are not randomly assigned.

continuous variable—a quantitative variable whose measurement is only limited to the detection limits of the instrument; see discrete variable.

discrete variable—a quantitative variable whose values are limited to discrete numbers. For example, the spots on a die can only be described by whole numbers between 1 and 6 and the number of patients on a floor can only be described by positive whole numbers; see continuous variable.

F—statistic generated by the AOV, for determination of statistical significance.

Hotelling's T^2—a multivariate *t* test used when differences between two treatments in an analysis of more than one dependent, quantitative, normally distributed variable are desired.

MAOV—a multivariate analysis of variance used when differences between more than two treatments in an analysis of more than one dependent, quantitative, normally distributed variable are desired. The MAOV is also abbreviated MANOVA.

mean—a population parameter; the arithmetic average of the quantitative variable in question. The sample mean is commonly abbreviated x̄. This should not be calculated for ordinal, nominal, or nonnormally distributed quantitative variables.

median—in a ranking, from lowest to highest, of all values in a distribution, the median is the middle value, or the average of the two middle values. In a normal distribution, the median is equal to the mean. It is primarily used as a variable descriptor for ordinal or nonnormally distributed quantitative variables.

mode—the value in a distribution that occurs most often; in a normal distribution, the mode equals the mean.

multivariate statistics—required to determine differences between treatments when two or more dependent variables are analyzed; see Hotelling's T^2 and MAOV.

negative predictive value—the chance that an individual will not have the characteristic of interest if the test for that characteristic is negative: $d/(d + c)$.

nominal variable—a qualitative variable that falls into one of several groups, or categories. Yes-no responses are nominal variables, e.g., wound infection and survival.

nonparametric statistic—used for the analysis of ordinal variables and nonnormally distributed quantitative variables, assuming a small sample size.

null hypothesis—in hypothesis testing, the null hypothesis always means that there is either no treatment effect or that the effect is of no interest to the researcher. It is abbreviated H_0.

one-tailed test—used in hypothesis testing for a *t* test or for Fisher's exact test, the alternate hypothesis states that one treatment is greater than another treatment. For Pearson's correlation coefficient, the alternate hypothesis can be either $r < 0$ or $r > 0$.

ordinal variable—a qualitative variable involving scores or ranks, for example, APACHE scores, injury severity scores, and pain scales.

p < 0.05—chance that a true difference between treatments or a relationship between variables does not exist is less than 5%. In this context, 0.05 is equal to α, the Type I error rate.

parametric statistics—used for the analysis of quantitative, normally distributed variables; nonnormally distributed variables may also be analyzed with parametric statistics, providing the sample size is sufficiently large.

Pearson's correlation coefficient—in regression analysis, this is used to determine the strength of association between independent variables. The value for the coefficient r can vary between -1 and 1.

population—all of the subjects in the world who possess the characteristics that are to be studied.

positive predictive value—the chance that an individual will have the characteristic of interest if the test for that characteristic is positive: $a/(a + b)$.

power—the ability to detect differences between treatments or relationships between variables; mathematically, power $= 1 - \beta$.

prevalence—the frequency of occurrence of the characteristic of interest in the sample tested.

qualitative variable—an ordinal (ranks, scales, etc.) or nominal (categorical, yes-no, etc.) variable.

quantitative variable—a continuous (weight, plasma amino acid concentration, etc.), discrete (patients in a hospital, spots on a die), or ratio (insulin:glucagon) variable.

randomized controlled trial—a prospective comparison of treatments for which the subjects are assigned randomly.

randomized sampling—a sampling scheme for which any experimental subject has an equally likely chance of being entered into any of the treatment groups.

rankits—a technique to fit ranked data to a normal distribution for analysis by parametric statistics.

ratio variable—a ratio of two quantitative variables.

regression analysis—used to determine relationships between variables; tests such as the *t* test and the AOV are used to determine differences between treatments.

sample—a subset of the population that will be tested in a study; a good sample is an accurate reflection of the population from which it is drawn.

sensitivity—the ability of a test to detect the characteristic of interest, given that the characteristic of interest is present: $a/(a + c)$.

significance—a statistically significant event occurs when the null hypothesis can be rejected with a probability of error lower than the set significance level.

specificity—the ability of a test to detect the absence of the characteristic of interest, given that the characteristic of interest is not present: $d/(d + b)$.

standard deviation—a population parameter; the square root of the variance. The sample standard deviation is commonly abbreviated SD. The standard deviation is a useful means of expressing variability for a normally distributed, quantitative variable.

standard error of the mean—a population parameter; the standard deviation divided by the square root of the sample size. The sample standard error of the mean is commonly abbreviated SEM. The standard error of the mean is a useful means of expressing variability for a normally distributed, quantitative variable.

statistics—a field of mathematics used to determine if differences between treatments or relationships between variables exist, beyond a reasonable doubt.

stratified random sampling—similar to randomized sampling, but the groups are broken down into subgroups, such as gender or ethnicity. It is commonly used to ensure that the sample reflects the population and that the subject mix of each treatment group is similar.

t test—used for testing differences between two treatments, if the variable is quantitative and if the samples are normally distributed; also called Student's *t* test.

two-tailed test—used in hypothesis testing. For a *t* test or for Fisher's exact test, the alternate hypothesis states that one treatment is not equal to another treatment; for Pearson's correlation coefficient, the alternate hypothesis states that $r = 0$.

Type I error—the chance that the null hypothesis has been rejected incorrectly; the probability of a Type I error is designated as α, which is used for hypothesis testing and sample size estimation.

Type II error—the chance that the null hypothesis has been accepted incorrectly; the probability of a Type II error is designated as β, which is used for sample size estimation and power determination.

Type III error—described by Condon (9); occurs when the conclusions are not supported by the data. Although not a true statistical entity, its existence can be verified by careful literature review.

univariate statistics—required to determine differences between treatments when one variable is analyzed; see *t* test and AOV.

χ^2—used to determine differences between treatments, if the variables are nominal.

REFERENCES

1. Steel RGD, Torrie JH. Principles and procedures of statistics. 2nd ed. New York: McGraw-Hill, 1980.
2. RF. The triple blind test. In: Scherr GH, ed. The best of the Journal of Irreproducible Results. New York: Workman, 1983:96.
3. Marks RG. Designing a research project. Belmont, CA: Lifetime Learning, 1982.
4. Evans M, Pollock AV. Trials on trial. Arch Surg 1984;119:109–113.
5. Norman GR, Streiner DL. PDQ statistics. Philadelphia: BC Decker, 1986.
6. Tatsuoka MM. Significance tests: univariate and multivariate. Champaign, IL: Institute for Personality and Ability Testing, 1971.
7. Gill JL. Design and analysis of experiments in the animal and medical sciences. Vol 1. Ames: Iowa State University Press, 1978.

8. Hurwitz ES, Barrett MJ, Bregman D, et al. Public health service study on Reye's syndrome and medications: report of the pilot phase. N Engl J Med 1985;313:849–857.
9. Condon RE. Type III error. Arch Surg 1986;121:877–878..

SUGGESTED READINGS

Feinstein AR. Clinical biostatistics. St. Louis: Mosby, 1977.
Hulley SB, Cummings SR, eds. Designing clinical research. Baltimore: Williams & Wilkins, 1988.
Ingelfinger JA, Mosteller F, Thibodeau LA, et al. Biostatistics in clinical medicine. New York: Macmillan, 1987.
Marks RG. Analyzing research data. Belmont, CA: Lifetime Learning, 1982.
Michael M, Boyce WT, Wilcox AJ. Biomedical bestiary: an epidemiologic guide to flaws and fallacies in the medical literature. Boston: Little, Brown & Co., 1984.
Sackett DL, Haynes RB, Tugwell P. Clinical epidemiology: a basic science for clinical medicine. Boston: Little, Brown & Co., 1985.
Streiner DL, Norman GR, Blum HM. PDQ epidemiology. Philadelphia: BC Decker, 1986.

CHAPTER

12 Female Reproductive Biology

Keith A. Hansen | Thomas E. Nolan

Female Reproductive Physiology

Introduction

Medical care of the female patient requires a thorough understanding of the normal development and physiology of the reproductive system. The purpose of the human female reproductive tract is to maintain our species by producing oocytes, allowing for fertilization and development of the embryo and fetus. The reproductive system is under a complex series of regulatory mechanisms involving autocrine, paracrine, hormonal, and neuronal systems. Perturbations in any of these systems can result in abnormalities which can mimic or complicate pathophysiologic processes in other organs. This chapter will explore the normal development, growth, and function of the female reproductive system and how it applies to medical care of the female patient.

Embryonic Development

The Ovary

Genetic sex is determined at the time of conception when a spermatozoa fuses with the oocyte in the ampullary segment of the fallopian tube. The spermatozoa has a haploid number of chromosomes with either an X or Y sex chromosome. If the spermatozoa that fertilizes the oocyte has an X chromosome, then the fetus will usually develop along female lines; whereas, if the spermatozoa has a Y chromosome, then the fetus will develop into a male. The human fetus at 4–5 weeks gestation is sexually undifferentiated and has the potential to develop into a normal male or female.

The fetal gonad begins as a thickening along the urogenital ridge overlying the mesonephros consisting of coelomic epithelial cells and underlying mesenchyme. The primordial germ cells begin development in the yolk sac at 4 weeks gestation and migrate by ameboid type movement and differential growth to the urogenital ridge (Fig. 12.1). In the developing ovary, these primordial germ cells undergo a remarkable, exponential increase in numbers through mitosis from a few thousand in early development to over six million at 20 weeks gestational age (Fig. 12.2).

The primordial germ cells continue active development during gestation. Not only are the numbers of cells exponentially increasing by mitosis, but they enter meiosis where they arrest in prophase of the first meiotic division. At this stage, the primordial germ cells become surrounded by a single layer of mesenchymal cells from the urogenital ridge (the future granulosa cells) and form a primordial follicle.

At 16 weeks gestational age, the process of atresia begins to affect germ cells, significantly reducing their total number. By birth, the total number of oocytes has been reduced to about one to two million. The fetal ovary is active throughout gestation and follicles will be stimulated to varying degrees of development during latter stages of gestation, including preantral and antral follicles. However, ovulation does not occur until maturation of the hypothalamic pituitary axis at puberty.

The Uterus

The uterus begins development as two longitudinal infoldings of the coelomic epithelium just lateral to the mesonephros (Fig. 12.3). This forms two tubular structures known as the mullerian ducts, which later fuse to form the uterine body. The distal ends of the mullerian ducts remain unfused to form the fallopian tubes (Fig. 12.4).

The undifferentiated human embryo at 5–6 weeks gestational age has both mesonephric ducts (potential to develop into male internal genitalia) and mullerian ducts. Alfred Jost, in a classic series of experiments,

269

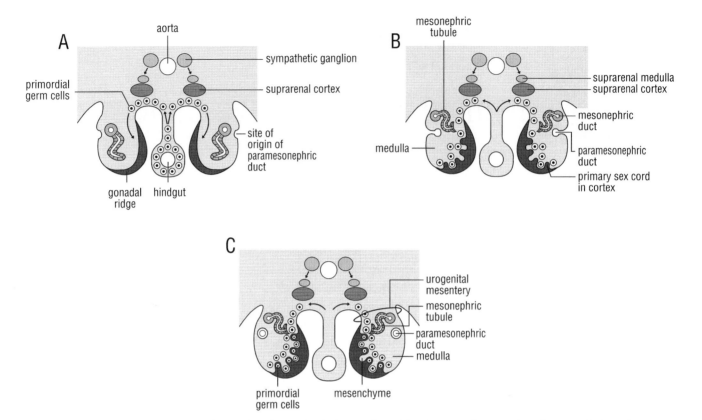

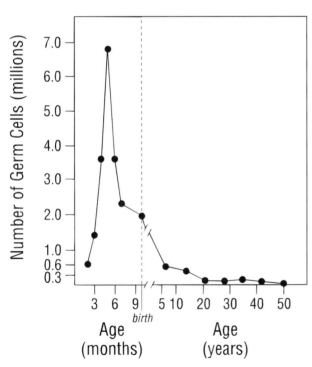

Figure 12.1. **A,** Transverse section through 5 week embryo at level of suprarenal glands. This diagram illustrates migration of primordial germ cells from yolk sac to gonadal ridge. **B,** Transverse section through 6 week embryo. Demonstrating continued migration of primordial germ cells and development of mesonephric duct. **C,** Infolding of paramesonephric (mullerian duct) ducts starting. Reprinted with permission from Moore KL. The developing human: clinically oriented embryology. Philadelphia: WB Saunders Co., 1988.

Figure 12.2. Ontogenetic development of human oocytes. Reprinted with permission from Baker TG, Wai Sum O. Development of the ovary and oogenesis. Clin Obstet Gynecol 1973;3.

demonstrated the dependence of ductal differentiation on gonadal secretions. In the developing male gonad, Sertoli cells produce anti-müllerian hormone, and the Leydig cells secrete androgens. Anti-müllerian hormone is a paracrine hormone that causes ipsilateral regression of the mullerian ducts. Testosterone acts on the developing mesonephric ducts in a paracrine fashion to stimulate their differentiation into epididymis, vas deferens, and seminal vesicles. Anti-müllerian hormone in the male fetus may be involved in descent of the testis into the scrotum. In contrast, the developing female gonad does not produce significant quantities of anti-müllerian hormone, and the mullerian ducts continue development into fallopian tubes, uterine body and the upper part of the vagina. Low levels of androgens produced by the developing ovary are not sufficient to maintain the mesonephric ducts, and they undergo regression. Male development requires the active secretion of steroidal and nonsteroidal molecules from the gonad, whereas female development occurs as the default pathway of sexual differentiation.

Mullerian system development is intimately dependent on normal development of the renal system. Kidney development occurs in stages, and each stage is dependent on normal differentiation of the previous stage. The stages of renal development include the prone-

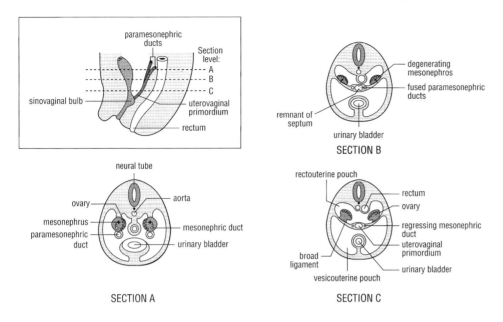

Figure 12.3. Eight-week female fetus. Transverse sections at various levels through mullerian ducts, showing their fusion into a single uterine cavity. Mesonephric ducts undergoing degeneration. Reprinted with permission from Moore KL. The developing human: clinically oriented embryology. Philadelphia: WB Saunders Co., 1988.

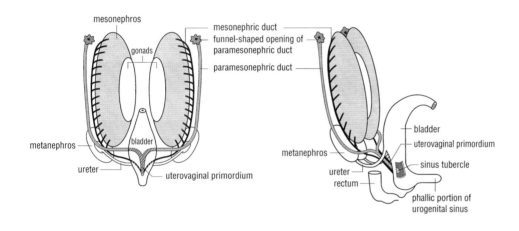

Figure 12.4. Schematic frontal view of 7-week embryo. Illustrating relationship of undifferentiated mullerian and mesonephric ducts to the developing gonad. Reprinted with permission from Moore KL. The developing human: clinically oriented embryology. Philadelphia: WB Saunders Co., 1988.

phros, mesonephros, and metanephros. The close association between renal and genital differentiation explains the association of kidney abnormalities with genital tract abnormalities.

External Genitalia

The external genitalia of male and female embryos is undifferentiated at 5–6 weeks with the potential to develop into either sex's external genitalia, depending on the hormonal milieu. In the male fetus, the testes begin to produce testosterone by 8 to 9 weeks gestational age. Masculinization of the external genitalia can be detected as early as 1 week later, and is completed by 14 weeks gestational age. Masculinization of the external genitalia relies on the conversion of testosterone to dihydrotestosterone by 5-alpha reductase. Dihydrotestosterone results in: (1) enlargement of the genital tubercle which ultimately forms the penis; (2) fusion of the folds of the urogenital sinus which form the penile urethra; and (3) fusion of the labioscrotal folds to form the scrotum.

The female fetus lacks adequate androgen levels, resulting in: (1) the genital tubercle forming the clitoris; (2) the folds of the urogenital sinus forming the labia minora; (3) the urogenital sinus contributing to formation of the lower vagina; and (4) the labioscrotal folds forming the labia majora (Fig. 12.5). If the female fetus is exposed to androgens during development, it can result in variable degrees of masculinization depending on dose, duration, and timing of exposure.

Normal external genitalia development in the male and female fetus depends on appropriate timing and level of exposure to the respective sex steroids. In a male fetus, reduced levels of androgens, either testosterone or dihydrotestosterone, will result in inadequate virilization, resulting in a male pseudohermaphrodite. The degree of genital ambiguity will correlate with the level of androgen to which the fetus is exposed during development. In the female fetus, elevated levels of androgens can result in masculinization of the external genitalia. Similarly, the degree of virilization of the female genitalia correlates with the intensity and length of androgen exposure.

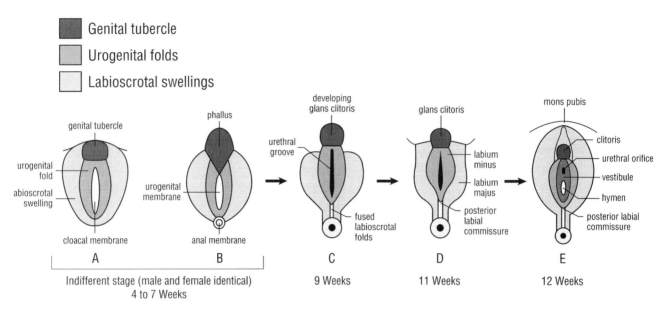

Figure 12.5. External genitalia development from undifferentiated stage to complete development. A&B are at 4–7 weeks gestation. C, D, E are at 9, 11, and 12 weeks respectively. Reprinted with permission from Moore KL. The developing human: clinically oriented embryology. Philadelphia: WB Saunders Co., 1988.

The Neonatal Ovary

The total endowment of germ cells has been reduced from 20 million to 1–2 million by birth. The neonate is separated from the maternal environment at birth, resulting in a fall in circulating steroid levels. This decrease in maternal steroids results in decreased negative feedback on the fetal pituitary gonadotrope with resultant release of gonadotropins, follicle stimulating hormone (FSH), and luteinizing hormone (LH).

In the female fetus, there are increased levels of pituitary and circulating levels of follicle stimulating hormone (FSH) with increased pituitary levels of luteinizing hormone (LH). The male fetus has lower levels of gonadotropins probably related to androgen and inhibin production by the developing testes. Inhibin is a dimeric polypeptide hormone secreted by Sertoli cells, producing a negative feedback effect on FSH secretion by the pituitary gland. After birth, the female neonate has a larger rise in FSH than LH, and this rise will remain for 12 to 24 months. This rise in gonadotropins can stimulate follicular development in the neonatal ovary, resulting in formation of cysts. One of the common causes of abdominal masses in the female neonate is ovarian cysts resulting from gonadotropin stimulation.

Gonadotropin levels remain elevated for 12 to 24 months in the female before reaching a nadir in early childhood which lasts until puberty. These low levels of gonadotropins result from a highly sensitive negative feedback mechanism coexisting with a nonsteroidal central inhibitor of gonadotropin secretion. Despite a quies-

cent hypothalamic pituitary gonadal axis, the ovary continues to show evidence of follicular development and atresia.

Puberty

Puberty is a time of transition from immaturity to a sexually mature adult. This results in numerous physical, hormonal, and psychological changes in an individual. Puberty is usually heralded by onset of a growth spurt, followed by breast budding (median age 9.8 years). The development of the breast usually follows a well defined sequence of events which characterizes the stages of pubertal development (Tanner stages) (Fig. 12.6). The development of axillary and pubic hair, followed by menarche at an average age of 12.8 years are the usual sequence. The development of the ovulatory mechanism with positive feedback is a late event in normal puberty. The usual length of time to complete the pubertal process is 4.5 years for a healthy European girl. Any abnormality in the timing (age at onset or length of time) of puberty may be a sign of a serious underlying disease and needs to be evaluated with a thorough, systematic approach.

The timing of puberty is primarily genetic with significant environmental influences such as nutrition and psychological stresses. Recent studies show a reduction in the mean age of onset of menarche in developing countries, reflecting an improvement in nutrition and general health. A critical weight for the onset of puberty has been hypothesized and probably reflects a shift in body composition to a higher percentage of fat in the

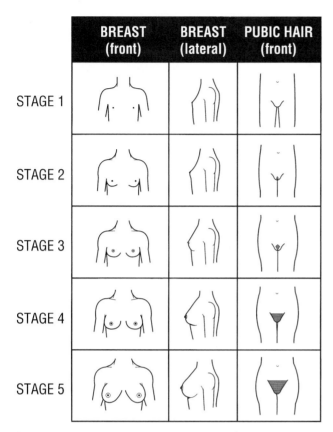

Figure 12.6. Tanner stages of breast and pubic hair in pubertal female. Reprinted with permission from Lee PA. Physiology of puberty. In: Rebar RW, Bremner WJ, eds. Principles and practice of endocrinology and metabolism. Philadelphia: JB Lippincott Co., 1990.

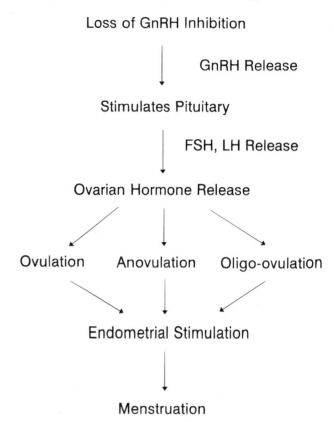

Figure 12.7. The release of the hypothalamus from inhibition both by a decease in sensitivity of negative feedback by steroid hormones and a reduction in the central nonsteroidal inhibitory factor results in GnRH production and secretion. The consequence of this process is maturation of the productive axis.

premenarchal female. The percent body fat has an important role in initiation and maintenance of normal menstrual function during the female's reproductive life. Perturbations (high or low) of the percent fat may disturb ovarian function, resulting in oligo-ovulation or anovulation with an accompanying disturbance in menstruation.

Adrenarche results from increased secretion of adrenal androgens as manifested by the appearance of pubic and axillary hair. These androgens include dehydroepiandrosterone (DHEA), its sulfate, and androstenedione. This increase in androgens first appears at about 6–7 years of age and continues to increase into mid-adolescence (about age 13–15), correlating with an increase in size of the zona reticularis of the adrenal cortex. Adrenarche usually occurs 2 years before the onset of pubertal changes, but is not felt to be a "trigger" for other pubertal changes. The exact initiating event for onset of adrenarche is unknown. This "trigger" mechanism does not appear to involve ACTH or cortisol since these hormones remain stable through the pubertal period of time. Recent evidence supports another pituitary molecule as a possible initiating "trigger," a posttranslational cleavage product of pro-opiomelanocorticotropin (POMC).

Puberty is heralded by activation and maturation of the hypothalamic pituitary gonadal axis which culminates in sexual maturity. During early childhood, pituitary gonadotropins are suppressed to very low levels, thought to be the result of a highly sensitive negative feedback mechanism and an intrinsic central inhibitory influence. Puberty is marked by an orderly decline in the negative feedback mechanism and release from the central inhibitory influence.

The release of the hypothalamic pituitary axis from these suppressive influences releases gonadotrophin releasing hormone (GnRH) from the hypothalamus, which stimulates the release of gonadotropins from the pituitary which interact with the gonad, resulting in production and release of sex steroids (Fig. 12.7). GnRH acts on gonadotrope cells in the anterior pituitary where it induces production of GnRH receptors. By upregulating the GnRH receptors it acts as a "self-primer" and stimulates the synthesis and release of gonadotropins by the gonadotropes. As the gonadotropin levels rise, they increase the production and release of sex steroids by the ovary. This release of sex steroids by the gonad results in the development of secondary sex characteristics in a well-described sequence.

Both sexes have the onset of GnRH pulses initially during sleep. Sleep associated GnRH pulses (measured as LH pulses) are an initial sign of puberty which concurs with onset of LH release in response to exogenous GnRH. The GnRH responsiveness of LH correlates with "awakening" of the hypothalamic gonadotrope axis in the early stages of puberty. As puberty progresses and sex steroids rise, the GnRH pulses extend through the day.

An initial event in puberty is the reduction of negative feedback of estrogen on the hypothalamic pituitary axis resulting in increasing gonadotropin and estrogen levels. This change in hormonal milieu is marked by the onset of secondary sexual characteristics. The development of estrogen-induced positive feedback on the hypothalamic pituitary axis is a late manifestation of puberty and correlates with ovulation. Positive feedback is necessary for normal ovulation to occur and results when the mature pituitary is exposed to elevated levels of estrogen for a prolonged time. A surge of gonadotropins occurs, known as the "LH surge," and is responsible for inducing ovulation.

The onset of menses is usually followed by irregular cycles for a few years consistent with oligo-ovulatory cycles. The menses do not become regular until maturation of the positive feedback mechanism and onset of regular, ovulatory cycles. The onset of positive feedback in the hypothalamic pituitary gonadal axis heralds the onset of regular, ovulatory cycles with the resultant potential for pregnancy.

Precocious Puberty

Precocious puberty is defined as pubertal changes before the age of 8 years and demands a thorough, systemic evaluation. The causes of precocious puberty can be divided into GnRH dependent and independent groups. GnRH dependent precocious puberty is associated with premature maturation of the hypothalamic pituitary axis with the onset of GnRH pulses resulting in gonadotropin and steroid release. GnRH dependent precocious puberty can result in ovulation with the potential for pregnancy. GnRH independent precocious puberty does not result in maturation of the GnRH pulse generator, but is dependent on a peripheral source of gonadal steroids that result in secondary sexual characteristic development (Table 12.1).

Precocious puberty is seen five times more frequently in girls than boys. In 75% of girls, no etiology can be found and is known as idiopathic. The diagnosis of idiopathic precocious puberty is one of exclusion and requires a thorough evaluation. In girls, the younger the patient is on presentation, the more likely she has a pathologic condition.

The most common diagnosis in girls with GnRH dependent precocious puberty is idiopathic. Approximately 7% will have central nervous system lesions that require further evaluation and treatment. Because of activation of the GnRH pulse generator, these patients can

Table 12.1
Etiologies of Precocious Puberty

GnRH Dependent Precocious Puberty
Idiopathic
Sporadic
Familial
CNS disorders

GnRH Independent Precocious Puberty
Gonadal tumors and hyperfunctioning disorders
Ovarian
granulosa cell tumors
granulosa-luteal cell cysts
Ovarian hyperfunctioning syndromes
McCune Albright syndrome
Peutz-Jeghers syndrome
Adrenal tumors and disorders
Adrenal disorders
Congenital adrenal hyperplasia
Adrenal tumors
Adrenal adenomas
Adrenal carcinomas
Exogenous sex steroids
Primary hypothyroidism

ovulate, and reports of early pregnancy document their sexual maturity. The onset of sexual development, however, does not require activation of the GnRH pulse generator with ovulation. Some examples of GnRH independent causes of sexual precocity include ovarian tumors, adrenal tumors, McCune Albright syndrome, and ectopic gonadotropin producing tumors.

McCune Albright syndrome is characterized by Cafe-au-lait spots, polyostotic fibrous dysplasia of bone, and hyperfunction of a number of endocrine systems. One of the most commonly affected endocrine systems in females is ovarian, resulting in precocious development. Other systems that are frequently affected include the thyroid, adrenal, pituitary, and parathyroids. Molecular diagnosis reveals that McCune Albright syndrome is caused by an activating mutation of a G protein.

The workup of precocious puberty should focus on defining the etiology and eliminating the possibility of serious illness. The initial evaluation includes a thorough history and physical examination with detailed historic evaluation of growth and the development of secondary sexual characteristics. Evidence of heterologous sexual development caused by excess androgen secretion in the female should be sought; it may be the first sign of an adrenal tumor or congenital adrenal hyperplasia (CAH). A thorough neurologic, abdominal, and pelvic examination is important to discover signs of tumors involving these organ systems. The patient should also be examined for any signs of systemic illnesses that could result in precocious puberty (McCune Albright syndrome).

Laboratory evaluation of patients should include serum gonadotropins and steroid levels (estradiol, progesterone, 17-hydroxy progesterone, dehydroepiandrosterone sulfate, and testosterone). A GnRH test can be extremely helpful in determining pituitary gonadotropin reserve. Patients with early maturation of the hypothalamic pituitary gonadal axis demonstrate release of gonadotropins on stimulation with GnRH. Important radiologic tests include bone age, imaging of the head with CT or MRI, CT imaging of the adrenals, and pelvic ultrasound. This series of tests can help distinguish GnRH dependent from GnRH independent causes of precocious puberty. Once categorized to the GnRH dependency group, the previously described tests can further characterize the nature and localize the site of excess hormone secretion.

Pubertal Delay

Lack of sexual development may also be a sign of serious illness. The following presentations are signs of potentially serious pathology and demand a rapid, thorough evaluation: (1) lack of onset of menses by age 14 with no signs of secondary sexual characteristics; (2) lack of menses by age 16 regardless of secondary sexual characteristics; or (3) prolonged duration of puberty (>4.5 years). Lack of pubertal development is rare in females and requires an evaluation directed toward abnormalities, including genetic, hypothalamic pituitary, and anatomic (Table 12.2).

The initial evaluation should include: (1) signs of past poor health; (2) evidence of excess exercise or abnormal eating habits; and (3) chronologic height and weight records. The physical examination should include accurate height and weight measurements as well as Tanner staging. Short stature may be the first clue that the subject suffers from: (1) an isolated growth hormone deficiency; (2) global pituitary hormone deficiency; or (3) gonadal dysgenesis. Intracranial disease should be considered, and a detailed neurologic examination is essential.

The laboratory evaluation of patients with delayed puberty includes thyroid function tests, prolactin, gonadotropins, and steroid levels (both gonadal and adrenal). A bone age and skull imaging is important if the patient has low gonadotropins. Patients with high gonadotropins require cytogenetic testing to evaluate for sex chromosome privations.

Gonadotropin levels will help direct the evaluation. Elevated gonadotropin levels are consistent with gonadal deficiency. The most common cause of gonadal deficiency is gonadal dysgenesis caused by a privation of the X chromosome. These patients can vary from a complete absence, mosaic condition, or structural abnormality of the X chromosome. Many patients with gonadal dysgenesis will have a normal 46, XX karyotype. A number of etiologies exist for their gonadal failure, including torsion, inflammation, sickle cell disease, and enzymatic deficiencies. An example of an enzymatic deficiency is 17-hydroxylase deficiency which results in a sexually infantile patient with hypertension and hypokalemia.

Table 12.2.
Etiologies of Delayed Puberty Dependent on Gonadotropin Levels

Elevated Serum Gonadotropins
Chromosomally incompetent ovarian failure
Turner's syndrome
45,X
45,X mosaics (46,XX or 46,XY)
X structural abnormalities
Chromosomally competent ovarian failure
Congenital adrenal hyperplasia
17 alpha-hydroxylase deficiency
Autoimmune oophoritis
Iatrogenic
oophorectomy
radiation therapy
chemotherapy especially alkylating agents
Galactosemia
Idiopathic (vanishing testis syndrome)
Resistant ovary syndrome

Normal or Decreased Gonadotropin Levels
Constitutional delay
Hypopituitarism
Panhypopituitarism
Isolated gonadotropin deficiency (Kallmann's)
Hypothyroidism
Chronic systemic illness
Anorexia nervosa
Sickle cell disease
Thalassemia
Chronic exercise
Hyperprolactinemia
Mullerian anomalies
Mullerian agenesis
Mullerian segmental anomalies
Complete androgen insensitivity

Low gonadotropins can be caused by constitutional delay of puberty or to pathologic conditions. Pathologic conditions include hypothalamic amenorrhea, Kallmann's syndrome, and hyperprolactinemia. In this group of patients, panhypopituitarism and tumors of the pituitary or hypothalamic region should be ruled out. The most common neoplasm is craniopharyngioma, which is a tumor of Rathke's pouch. The treatment for a craniopharyngioma is surgery with possible radiation therapy.

Eugonadal subjects most commonly have mullerian segmental abnormalities like a transverse vaginal septum, complete mullerian agenesis, or androgen insensitivity. Patients with mullerian abnormalities will have 46, XX karyotypes with functional ovaries and a normal distribution of female pubic and axillary hair. Serum testing will show evidence of ovarian function with normal gonadotropins, estrogen and progesterone levels, and female testosterone levels. Subjects with mullerian abnormalities have an increased frequency of renal and skeletal abnormalities. Subjects with complete androgen insensitivity will present with 46,XY karyotypes, functional intra-abdominal testes, and sparse or absent pubic and axillary hair. Serum testing will reveal male levels of testosterone.

Treatment of subjects with delayed puberty is determined by the etiology. Constitutional delay should be treated by reassurance and counseling. If an XY cell line is discovered, gonadectomy is necessary to prevent ovarian neoplasms (most commonly dysgerminomas and gonadoblastomas). Delayed puberty should be treated with hormone replacement therapy to stimulate development of secondary sexual characteristics.

The Ovarian Cycle

The ovary serves important roles in production of gametes and ovarian steroids. The ovary is under complex regulatory mechanisms, with both positive and negative feedback control, resulting in the production of usually one egg per cycle. The human menstrual cycle is divided into three phases: follicular, luteal, and menstrual. The menstrual cycle is a continuum of follicular development, ovulation, and luteinization (Fig. 12.8).

The follicular phase is characterized by a series of events involving feedback mechanisms which allow for the sequential development of a follicle, usually resulting in the release of a single ovum at ovulation.

Primordial follicles are formed initially during embryonic and fetal development from germ cells which arise in the endoderm of the yolk sac. A primordial follicle consists of an oocyte, arrested in the prophase of the first meiotic division, surrounded by a single layer of cells. These will subsequently become functional granulosa cells. The primordial follicle complement is formed by mitotic expansion, reaching maximal numbers in the second trimester of pregnancy. Continual reduction of the number of follicles occurs during the life of the ovary. This process of initiating growth and atresia of follicles continues without interruption until the ovary is completely devoid of follicles (the menopause).

The number of primordial follicles that begin growth in each cycle is unknown, but is related to the total number of follicles remaining in the gonads. The majority of follicles which begin development eventually undergo atresia. The dominant follicle, that follicle which is destined to ovulate, is selected in the first few days of the follicular phase and is dependent on elevations in follicle stimulating hormone in the early follicular phase.

Elevation of FSH follows the late luteal phase reduction in steroids and inhibin. This rise in FSH in the early follicular phase is accompanied by morphologic changes in the follicle, including an increase in the size of the oocyte and a change from flat to cuboidal granulosa cells. Gap junctions also form between the granulosa cells and the oocyte and serve as a mechanism of communication between these cells (allowing for effective paracrine actions). Under the continued stimulatory effect of FSH, the granulosa cells begin to proliferate and transform the primordial follicle into a primary follicle.

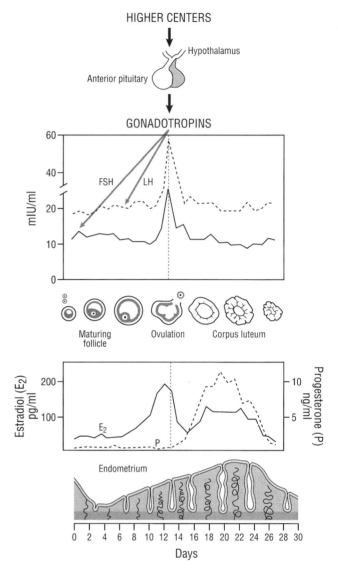

Figure 12.8. Cyclic changes during normal menstrual cycle involving the pituitary, ovary, and uterine endometrium. Reprinted with permission from Danforth DN, Dignam WJ, Hendricks CH, Maeck JVS, eds. Obstetrics and gynecology. Philadelphia: Harper and Row Publishing, Inc., 1982.

Stromal development is also occurring under gonadotropin stimulation resulting in the differentiation of two layers, theca interna and externa, in the primary follicle (Fig. 12.9).

FSH binding to gonadotropin receptors on the developing primary follicle results in proliferation of granulosa cells and steroidogenesis. As the primary follicle continues to enlarge, a membrane develops around the oocyte, the zona pellucida, changing the follicle into a preantral follicle. The preantral follicle depends on continued FSH production, stimulating cell growth and steroidogenesis.

Granulosa cells contain an enzyme with aromatase activity. This activity is stimulated by FSH binding to receptors on granulosa cell membrane. The aromatase enzyme converts androgens into estrogens, thus main-

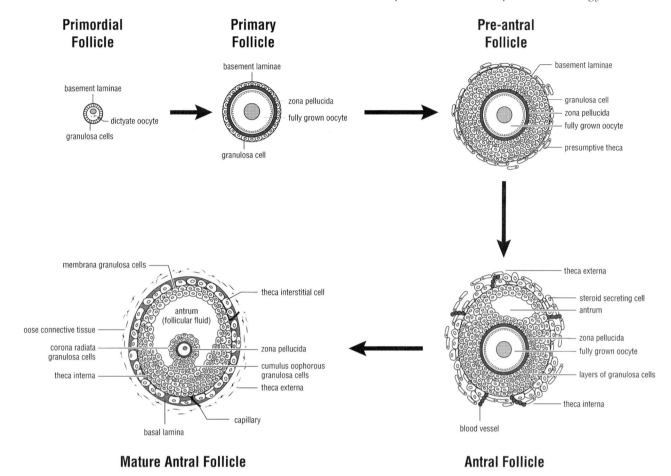

Figure 12.9. Morphologic changes in a developing follicle during a normal follicular phase. Reprinted with permission from Erickson GF, Magoffin DA, Dyer CA, Hofeditz C. The ovarian androgen producing cells: A review of structure/function relationships. Endocrine Reviews 1985;6:371.

taining the estrogenic environment of the follicle. Estrogen and FSH combine to increase the FSH receptor number on granulosa cell membranes, thereby increasing the cellular sensitivity to FSH. This increase in FSH sensitivity allows the cells to continue to respond as FSH levels fall in the latter follicular stage.

The aromatase enzyme is also sensitive to androgen production by theca cells. A low level of androgens stimulate aromatization, whereas higher levels suppress this process. This combination of follicular phase events results in the majority of follicles becoming atretic, with one or a few growing to maturity. Continued growth of the follicle is accompanied by the appearance of fluid around the granulosa cells, eventually forming a cavity within the follicle, transforming the preantral follicle into an antral follicle. The follicular fluid contains FSH, estrogen and other granulosa cell metabolites in relatively high concentrations which bathe the developing oocyte.

Follicular development is a highly integrated process involving effective communication between various compartments of the follicle. A two-cell model has been proposed to explain granulosa cell dependence on thecal cells. In this model, granulosa cells are predominantly FSH dependent, as reflected by FSH receptors on their

surface, whereas thecal cells are predominantly luteinizing hormone (LH) dependent, as reflected by LH receptors on their surface. Thecal cells under the influence of LH convert cholesterol into androgens. The androgens then diffuse to the granulosa layer where they are aromatized into estrogens, thereby maintaining the estrogenic milieu of the follicle.

Conversion from an androgen dependent to estrogen dependent environment marks the selection of the follicle destined to ovulate. This process depends upon the interaction of FSH and estrogen within the follicle and the pituitary gland. Within the developing follicle, FSH and estrogen function to increase FSH receptor number, increasing the gonadotropin sensitivity of the follicle. The increased circulating concentration of estrogen exerts an inhibitory effect upon the pituitary, thereby decreasing circulating concentrations of FSH (classic negative feedback). This combination of events, an increased sensitivity of the dominant follicle and decreased concentration of FSH, selects the follicle destined to ovulate. The ovary supporting the dominant follicle can be distinguished from its counterpart by the fifth day of the follicular phase. In nondominant follicles, the fall in circulating FSH causes atresia (Fig. 12.10).

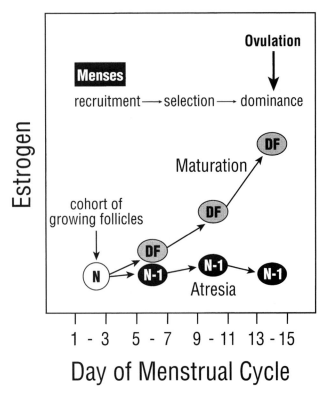

Figure 12.10. Development of a dominant follicle. Illustration of dominant follicle selection during the follicular phase. Reprinted with permission from the American Society for Reproductive Medicine (The American Fertility Society) from Hodgen GD. The dominant ovarian follicle. Fertile Steril 1982; 38:281–300.

The increase in number of granulosa cells in the maturing follicle is accompanied by an increase in vascularity of the theca. The increase in vascularity results in preferential delivery of FSH to the follicle with the greatest blood flow, which can be detected by day 9 of the follicular phase.

Granulosa cells develop LH receptors which allow them to respond to the luteinizing hormone surge at midcycle with completion of development and ovulation. LH receptors first appear in large antral follicles at time of falling FSH levels and increasing intrafollicular estrogen levels. LH receptors form in response to the estrogenic environment and local paracrine events.

Production of gonadotropin releasing hormone by the hypothalamus serves an obligatory role in stimulating release of gonadotropins. Feedback of follicular derived growth factors and hormones "fine tune" the secretion of gonadotropins required to stimulate ovulation. Estrogen, the primary steroidal hormone released from the developing follicle, has both positive and negative feedback effects on the hypothalamic pituitary axis. Estrogen decreases gonadotropin secretion by reducing the secretion and response to GnRH in pituitary cells. The exact mechanism of this negative feedback is unknown. When estrogen reaches adequate concentrations for an extended period of time, a positive feedback mechanism results in robust release of gonado-

tropins from the pituitary gland. This positive effect involves both the hypothalamus and the pituitary gland. In the hypothalamus, estrogen increases the amount of GnRH that is released with each GnRH pulse. In the pituitary gland, estrogen increases the number of GnRH receptors, which results in more gonadotropins being released with each GnRH pulse.

FSH is sensitive to negative feedback, even at low levels of estrogen. LH has a variable response to estrogen; suppression at low levels and stimulation at higher levels. The change from suppression to stimulation occurs when estrogen levels reach an adequate value for a sustained period of time.

The preovulatory follicle responds to different hormones and locally acting growth factors. In the preovulatory follicle, FSH promotes luteinization of the granulosa manifested by enlargement and appearance of lipid inclusions in the cells. Thecal cells simultaneously develop inclusions and become richly vascular. These morphologic changes in the follicle are accompanied by increased production of estrogen and progesterone. Midcycle progesterone production facilitates the LH surge and has a dominant role in production of the FSH surge. The LH surge results after adequate estrogen priming and provides the ovulatory stimulus for the dominant follicle.

Ovulation with the release of a mature oocyte occurs after the LH surge. Ovulation occurs 10 to 12 hours after the LH peak and 34 to 36 hours after the start of the LH surge. Resumption of meiosis and stimulation of a number of proteolytic enzymes, which digest the walls of the follicle, allow the oocyte to release; this occurs after the gonadotropin surge. Ovulation is not an "explosive" event, and studies have shown no increase in intrafollicular pressure before ovulation.

After ovulation, granulosa cells continue to enlarge and develop a vacuolated appearance while becoming the corpus luteum. Thecal cells also contribute to the formation of the corpus luteum. The postovulatory follicle accumulates a yellow pigment known as lutein, hence the name of the corpus luteum. A rapid period of vascularization with ingrowth of capillaries into the granulosa cells occurs immediately after ovulation. The vascularity of the corpus luteum ensures the continued supply of substrates to the metabolically active cells.

The corpus luteum produces ovarian steroids, primarily progesterone and estrogen. The secretion of sex steroids is episodic during the luteal phase and correlates with the pulsatile release of LH. Adequate production of sex steroids depends on adequate follicular growth and gonadotropin receptor formation during the follicular phase. The combination of estrogen and progesterone function to transform the endometrium into an environment which will accept and nurture the developing embryo. A normal menstrual cycle luteal phase is about 14 days (range is 11–17 days). The luteal phase is the most constant part of the menstrual cycle in terms of length. The corpus luteum is programmed to undergo involution in 9 to 11 days after the LH surge, unless rescued by human chorionic gonadotropin (hCG), which is secreted actively by the developing fetoplacental unit. If implantation occurs, hCG maintains the corpus luteum until the ninth to tenth week of gestation.

Pregnancy

Pregnancy is a unique time in ontogeny of the human. A semi-allograft thrives in the center of a potentially hostile maternal immune system. The exact mechanism for this apparent paradox of classical transplant immunology is unknown. Proposed mechanisms include such theories as: (1) the uterus as an immunologically privileged site; (2) production of maternal blocking antibodies; (3) idiotype anti-idiotype antibody networks, and multiple other mechanisms.

Pregnancy is also a unique situation in terms of steroidogenesis when three different interacting systems exist: mother, placenta, and fetus. Each of these units contributes essential nutrients and metabolites to the other while allowing the conglomerate to function as an integrated whole (Fig. 12.11).

Progesterone is synthesized from cholesterol from any source: (1) conversion of acetate to cholesterol; (2) hydrolysis of stored cholesterol esters; or (3) from LDL-cholesterol. Maternal blood LDL-cholesterol is the usual source for progesterone synthesis during pregnancy.

Progesterone, during pregnancy, is produced initially by the corpus luteum which has been rescued by hCG from the syncytiotrophoblast. The developing pregnancy depends entirely on the corpus luteum for progesterone until the seventh week of gestation. From 7 to 10 weeks, both the placenta and corpus luteum are producing progesterone. After 10 weeks, the placenta is the primary source of production. Early miscarriage occurs if the corpus luteum is removed before 7 weeks gesta-

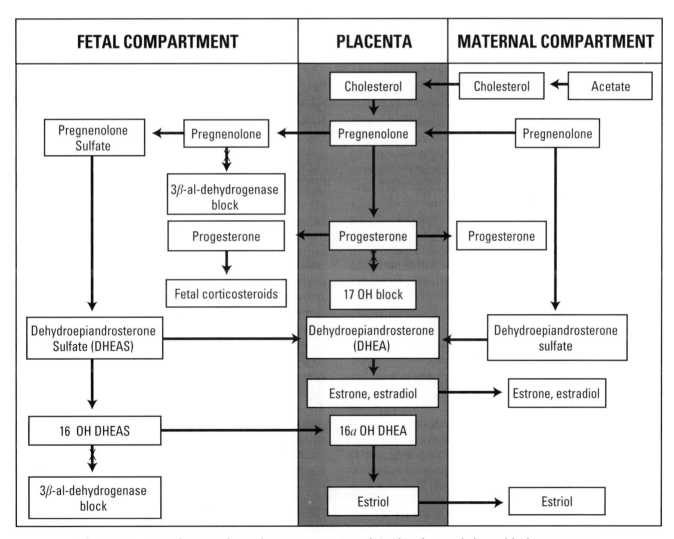

Figure 12.11. Steroidogenic pathways during pregnancy. Interrelationship of maternal-placental-fetal compartments. Reprinted with permission from Reece EA, Hobbins JC, Mahoney MJ, Petrie RH, eds. Medicine of the fetus and mother. Philadelphia: JB Lippincott Co., 1990.

tional age, unless the pregnancy is "rescued" with exogenous progesterone.

Progesterone plays a number of important roles in pregnancy, including preparation and maintenance of the uterine endometrium. The endometrium is thought to suppress maternal immune response to the fetal allograft. Progesterone also supplies the fetus with precursors for the production of glucocorticoids and mineralocorticoids.

Estrogen concentrations are also elevated during pregnancy, but unlike progesterone, estrogen synthesis depends on the production of adequate precursor steroids by the developing fetus. There are three main categories of estrogen produced during pregnancy: estrone, estradiol, and estriol. Estrone and estradiol concentrations in the blood are about one hundredfold greater in pregnancy than in the nonpregnant state, whereas estriol is over one thousandfold greater.

Estrogens depend primarily on the 19-carbon steroid precursors, androgens, for their production. The placenta has a deficiency of $P_{450}17$ enzyme activity, which contains both 17-hydroxylase and 17-20 desmolase activity. Therefore, placental synthesis of estrogen depends on 19-carbon steroid precursors from both maternal or fetal sources. In early pregnancy, androgen precursors come primarily from the mother, whereas later in pregnancy, the majority of 19-carbon precursors come from the fetal adrenal.

The fetal adrenal differentiates at 7 weeks gestation. The thin outer definitive zone can be differentiated from the thick inner fetal zone by 7 weeks. The inner fetal zone is proportionally larger than the adult adrenal gland, rapidly undergoing involution after delivery (Fig. 12.12). Initially, the fetal adrenal develops under the control of hCG, independent of adrenocorticotropic

hormone (ACTH). After midgestation, the secretion of fetal ACTH by the developing hypothalamic pituitary axis assumes greater importance. ACTH is felt to play an obligatory role in steroidogenesis and development of the fetal adrenal but may not be the only control mechanism. Previous studies have suggested a role for prolactin.

Dehydroepiandrosterone sulfate (DHEAS) is the primary 19- carbon precursor secreted by the fetus. The large quantities of estrogen produced during pregnancy inhibit 3 beta-hydroxysteroid dehydrogenase isomerase activity in the fetal adrenal. This inhibition of 3 beta-hydroxysteroid dehydrogenase isomerase results in the fetal adrenal, producing large quantities of delta-5 steroids, DHEA, and DHEAS.

DHEAS secreted by the fetal adrenal may be 16-hydroxylated by the fetal liver to form 16-hydroxy-DHEAS. DHEAS and 16-hydroxy-DHEAS are transported to the placenta, which has an active sulfatase enzyme encoded on the short arm of the X chromosome which will cleave the sulfate moiety from the 19-carbon precursor. DHEAS will then be converted into estrone and estradiol by the placenta, whereas 16-hydroxy-DHEAS will be converted to estriol. Hence, the production of estrogens by the placenta depends intimately on 19-carbon precursors from the fetus transferred to the placenta.

A number of clinical conditions exist in which alterations in fetal adrenal androgen production result in reduced estrogen production. In an anencephalic fetus, the adrenal is small and ill-developed. This does not produce adequate quantities of estrogen precursors, resulting in low estrogen levels. In situations where the fetus is under chronic stress, there will be a lowering of fetal adrenal androgen production resulting in low estrogen production. In the past, estriol was used as a

Figure 12.12. Ontogenetic development of adrenal glands. Note large size of fetal zone during intrauterine life. Reprinted with permission from Reece EA, Hobbins JC, Mahoney MJ, Petrie RH, eds. Medicine of the fetus and mother. Philadelphia: JB Lippincott Co., 1990.

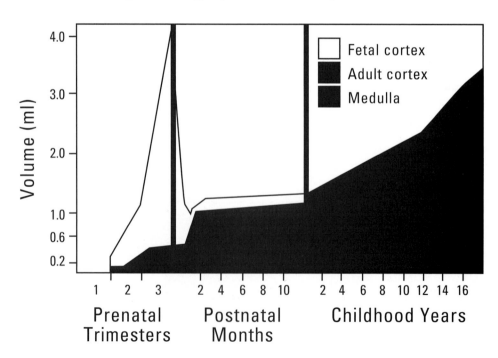

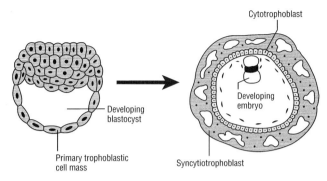

Figure 12.13. A, Human blastocyst. Demonstrating inner cell mass which will develop into the placenta and membranes. **B,** Early embryo illustrating the differentiation of trophoblast into cytotrophoblast and syncytiotrophoblast. Reprinted with permission from Reece EA, Hobbins JC, Mahoney MJ, Petrie RH, eds. Medicine of the fetus and mother. Philadelphia: JB Lippincott Co., 1990.

method of determining fetal well being; however, because of a lack of sensitivity and specificity, this test has been abandoned. Fetal biophysical testing, nonstress test, and ultrasound are the best predictors of fetal well being.

The major protein hormones of pregnancy are produced by the placenta. The cytotrophoblast cell layer of the placenta is composed primarily of single, mononuclear cells which are precursor cells to the syncytiotrophoblast. The syncytiotrophoblast is a syncytium with multinuclei and is most active in hormone production (Fig. 12.13). The placenta releases a number of hormones similar to those produced by the hypothalamus and pituitary, leading to speculation that the placenta has a system of feedback control mechanisms. Hypothalamic hormones expressed in the placenta include corticotropin releasing hormone, gonadotropin releasing hormone, thyrotropin releasing hormone, and others.

Human chorionic gonadotropin (hCG) is a glycoprotein hormone produced by the syncytiotrophoblast of the placenta. The protein hCG is a dimer composed of an alpha and beta chain. The alpha chain of hCG is the same as the alpha chain of a number of pituitary glycoproteins including LH, FSH, and TSH. The beta chains of these molecules are different in structure and presumably are the functional protein moieties. The beta chain of hCG is similar to the beta chain of LH, which accounts for the clinical use of hCG as a substitute for the LH surge in stimulated cycles.

Structural differences in beta subunits of the various glycoprotein hormones has allowed development of highly specific and sensitive immunoassays. The development of a radioimmunoassay for the beta subunit of hCG allows earlier detection of metabolically active placental tissue and pregnancy. Recent developments have included a sensitive radioimmunometric assay directed against the entire hCG molecule, with specific antibodies raised against the alpha and beta subunits. One antibody can be fixed on a solid surface like a microsphere and the other tagged with a detection device, such as a radioactive label for detection.

The concentration of hCG is ≤ 10 mIU/ml at the time of the expected missed menses. This level increases exponentially during early pregnancy until about 10 weeks gestation, when it reaches levels of 100,000 mIU/ml. The exponential increase in hCG levels has led to the clinical axiom that the hCG level should double every 2 to 3 days during the first weeks of a normal gestation. After the hCG level reaches its peak, it decreases and then plateaus for the remainder of pregnancy.

Early in pregnancy, hCG plays a vital role by rescuing the corpus luteum from demise. The corpus luteum will continue to produce progesterone to maintain the uterine endometrium and maintain pregnancy. The developing fetus depends on hCG for stimulation of the fetal testes to produce androgen and stimulation of the fetal adrenal gland.

A number of pathologic conditions exist where hCG concentration can help establish the diagnosis. In early pregnancy, determination of serial hCG levels can predict pregnancy viability. If hCG levels do not increase in a normal progression, then the possibility of an abnormal pregnancy, such as an ectopic gestation or spontaneous abortion, should be considered.

Determinations of hCG are helpful in arriving at a correct diagnosis in a patient suspected of having an ectopic gestation. Ectopic gestation occurs when the pregnancy implants outside the normal intrauterine location, most commonly in the fallopian tube. A negative hCG determination essentially eliminates the possibility of a viable trophoblast and pregnancy. Approximately two-thirds of ectopic pregnancies will have an abnormal rise in serial hCG titers obtained in early pregnancy. The other third will have normal rising titers but may fall or plateau later in gestation.

Pelvic ultrasonography has added an important dimension to diagnosis of an abnormal gestation. A "discriminatory zone" is the hCG level where an intrauterine gestational sac should be detected in a normal gestation. With abdominal ultrasound, the "discriminatory zone" is at 6000-6500 mIU/ml, whereas vaginal sonography has a discriminatory zone of 1000-1500 mIU/ml. The combination of serum hCG level and ultrasonography has proved helpful in the diagnosis of ectopic gestation.

Human placental lactogen (HPL) is also secreted by the syncytiotrophoblast and is composed of a single polypeptide chain with two disulfide bonds. This polypeptide hormone belongs to a group of hormones that also includes growth hormone and prolactin. HPL is produced throughout pregnancy, but tends to increase to high levels in the latter stages of gestation where it correlates with fetoplacental weight. HPL functions by inducing insulin resistance (carbohydrate intolerance) along with increasing IGF-I levels.

Glucose is the primary carbohydrate fuel for the developing fetus and is transported actively by the placenta. The placental hormones, including the sex steroids and HPL, induce a state of insulin resistance in the mother. When glucose levels are elevated (fed state) free fatty acids are stored as triglycerides. When glucose levels fall (fasting state), HPL levels increase, resulting in the mobilization of free fatty acids in the mother. By mobilizing free fatty acids, HPL maintains glucose levels for the developing fetus. Prolonged fasting results in mobilization of maternal adipose tissues and a rise in serum ketone levels. These ketones can be used by the developing fetus but, if persistent, may result in abnormalities in certain developing tissues.

Alpha-fetoprotein is produced primarily by the fetal liver and has no known fetal function. Alpha-fetoprotein is a glycoprotein that resembles albumin and reaches high levels in the fetal circulation. This similarity to albumin has led to hypotheses that it may function as a carrier molecule in the fetal circulation much as albumin does in the adult.

Maternal serum levels of alpha-fetoprotein may be abnormal in a number of abnormal pregnant conditions. Elevated levels of maternal serum alpha-fetoprotein are seen with open neural tube defects, anterior abdominal wall defects, congenital nephrosis, fetal death, multiple pregnancy, fetal maternal hemorrhage, and other less common causes. Data suggest that elevated levels of alpha-fetoprotein of unknown etiology are associated with poor pregnancy outcome. Low maternal serum alpha-fetoprotein levels have been useful in diagnosis of fetal aneuploidy, especially Down's syndrome.

Prolactin is a polypeptide hormone belonging to the growth hormone family which is secreted actively in pregnancy. Prolactin is synthesized and secreted into three compartments during pregnancy: (1) the fetal blood stream; (2) amniotic fluid; and (3) maternal blood stream. Circulating prolactin, whether maternal or fetal, is produced and secreted from the respective pituitary glands and maintains its regulatory pathways, primarily under negative control by dopamine.

Prolactin is also synthesized by decidua and is detected initially soon after decidualization of the endometrium. Prolactin in amniotic fluid is secreted primarily by the decidua which is not under the same control mechanisms as the pituitary. This conclusion results from no change in amniotic fluid prolactin in a patient on dopamine agonist therapy. Amniotic fluid prolactin may play an important role in fluid and electrolyte hemostasis.

A number of polypeptide hormones are produced by the placenta, including human chorionic growth hormone, human chorionic thyrotropin, and human chorionic adrenocorticotropin. These hormones, along with a number of growth factors, play important roles in maternal fetal physiology during pregnancy.

Pregnancy results in a number of hormonal changes in fetal, amniotic fluid, and maternal compartments which help to initiate and maintain pregnancy. These hormonal alterations play an important role in each stage of pregnancy and its successful outcome.

Labor and Delivery

The embryo and fetus are nurtured within the uterine cavity until the developing human reaches maturity and can exist in the extrauterine environment. During the latter stages of gestation, the human uterus begins to episodically contract. These contractions can occur for a period of time but are characterized by a lack of uterine effacement or dilatation. Labor occurs only when the contractions become sufficiently coordinated to cause cervical effacement and dilatation. This change in the cervix allows for the presenting part of the fetus to pass through the pelvis.

The exact mechanism which initiates labor is unknown, however, there are a number of theories which potentially explain it. One intriguing possibility is progesterone withdrawal. In sheep, the withdrawal of progesterone is felt to play a major role in the onset of labor. In humans, systemic progesterone levels do not change before the initiation of labor. The possibility remains of a local decrease in progesterone at the uteroplacental interface resulting in the start of uterine contractions. Another potential etiology for labor is an increase in oxytocin. Oxytocin or Pitocin has been used for a number of years to induce and augment labor, so it is a natural extension to consider it as a cause of labor. In normal labor and delivery, Pitocin levels are only found to significantly increase in the second stage of labor, and hence probably do not play an active initiation role. Investigators have found an increased concentration of oxytocin receptors in the mature uterus. This data supports oxytocin as having a role in labor but not initiating the process.

A unifying concept for the initiation of labor involves communication between the fetal membranes and uterine decidua. The components of this communication network could function together to signal maturity of the fetus and trigger labor. One potential signaling mechanism is prostaglandins, which are formed actively by the decidua and are increased in concentration during normal labor.

Labor is characterized by an increase in the number of oxytocin receptors in the myometrium, increase in myometrial gap junctions, and cervical effacement and dilatation. These changes allow for rhythmic, propulsive uterine contractions which propel the fetus through the bony pelvis.

Labor can be divided into three stages: Stage 1, which involves effacement and dilatation of the cervix; Stage 2, which involves propulsion of the fetus through the bony pelvis; and Stage 3, which starts after delivery of the fetus and ends with delivery of the placenta. Some authors describe a fourth stage which occurs for the first hour after delivery of the placenta.

The first stage can be divided into the latent and active phases. When one analyzes cervical dilatation, it is found to follow a sigmoid curve. The latent phase is that period of time when the cervix is dilatating slowly and ends when it enters the phase of rapid dilatation, which is usually at 4 or 5 cm. The active phase is the linear portion of cervical dilatation and extends from 4 or 5 cm until the cervix is dilated completely at 10 cm. During effacement and dilatation of the cervix, the fetal presenting part will descend slowly into the bony pelvis. Only when the cervix is fully dilated will the second stage of labor begin. This stage of labor is marked by active pushing; the presenting part negotiates the bony pelvis and is delivered. The second stage concludes with the clamping and cutting of the umbilical cord.

The third stage involves the time from delivery of the baby until delivery of the placenta and fetal membranes. This stage usually lasts between 15 and 30 minutes. Some authors describe a fourth stage which is the hour after delivery of the placenta and is marked by a number of physiologic changes, including contraction of the uterus (which reduces blood loss) and a rapid redistribution of maternal circulation.

The average amount of blood lost after a vaginal delivery is about 500 ml and 1000 ml after a cesarean section. A number of etiologies exist for excess blood loss after delivery, the most common including uterine atony, retained placental fragments, and reproductive tract injuries. Less common causes of postpartum hemorrhage include uterine inversion, abnormalities of placentation (placenta accreta), and bleeding diathesis.

Menopause

Menopause is the cessation of menses which occurs at an average age of 52 years in the United States. The climacteric is that period of time marked by waning ovarian function and culminating in ovarian exhaustion. Menopause correlates with the morphologic finding of a few remaining follicles in the ovaries. It is characterized by low gonadal steroids with elevated gonadotropin levels.

The loss of ovarian follicles results in a number of important physiologic changes. First, the lack of responsive follicles results in sterility. Second, it results in the loss of gonadal steroids, both estrogen and progesterone. The loss of estrogen results in increased bone loss in these subjects and, in select individuals, can result in postmenopausal osteoporosis. This loss of estrogen can also result in vasomotor symptoms and the menopausal syndrome of hot flashes, mood swings, irritability, etc. The loss of estrogen also predisposes the individual to

coronary artery disease by altering the plasma lipids and possibly through a direct effect on the coronary arteries. These signs and symptoms of menopause can be reduced with the use of hormone replacement therapy.

Bone Loss

Bone is a metabolically active tissue which is constantly undergoing remodeling, involving the removal of old bone and laying down of new bone. This process is usually under tight control to maintain the integrity of bone and, if anything, interferes with this control mechanism; it will weaken the bone and increase the risk of fracture.

The loss of estrogen at menopause results in loss of overall bone mineral content caused by an accelerated breakdown in bone without an increase in calcium deposition. If allowed to continue unabated, this loss of bone structural integrity results in clinically significant osteoporosis and an increased risk of fractures.

Not all postmenopausal women will develop osteoporosis. A number of risk factors exist which increase a woman's risk. These include being thin, white, a smoker, and having a family history of osteoporosis. However, no risk factor or test exists that can be used to predict which woman will develop osteoporosis. The use of exogenous estrogen can markedly retard this process in postmenopausal women. Calcium supplementation and weight bearing exercise will also improve mineralization and ultimate bone strength.

Unopposed estrogen has been shown to stimulate the endometrium and may result in endometrial carcinoma if used for a prolonged time period. In postmenopausal women who have not had a hysterectomy, it is important to add progesterone to therapy to avoid development of endometrial carcinoma.

Conclusion

The primary purpose of the reproductive tract is to allow for reproduction of our species. Many pathophysiological processes can affect the reproductive system, and the reproductive system may modify the presentation of these same disease processes. Alterations of the reproductive system may also mimic or adversely affect other organ systems, especially intraperitoneal organs. An understanding of the reproductive system is vital to all health care givers caring for women.

This chapter reviews the development, function, and final cessation of the activity of the female reproductive system. This entire process culminates in female reproductive maturity with the ability to carry a pregnancy to its successful completion. After approximately 40 years of ovulatory competence, the ovaries cease functioning. This cessation of function not only results in lack of gamete production but also substantially reduced hormone production. This loss of hormones, specifically estrogen and progesterone, results in menopause and its attendant risks of osteoporosis, heart disease, genitourinary atrophy, and the menopausal syndrome.

GLOSSARY

Cytotrophoblast—single mononuclear cells of the developing placenta which fuse and form syncytiotrophoblast.

Diploid karyotype: 2(n)—condition where a cell contains two complete sets of chromosomes. In humans 46 chromosomes.

Ectopic pregnancy—implantation of a pregnancy outside of the normal intrauterine environment, most commonly in the fallopian tube.

Follicle Stimulating Hormone (FSH)—a dimeric glycoprotein composed of an alpha and beta chain produced by gonadotrophs in the adenohypophysis. Important during folliculogenesis and ovulation.

Human Chorionic gonadotropin (hCG)—a dimeric glycoprotein produced by the syncytiotrophoblast of the placenta which "rescues" the corpus luteum in early pregnancy.

Haploid karyotype (n)—condition where a cell contains one complete set of chromosomes. In the human 23 chromosomes.

Hirsutism—androgen induced excess body and facial hair growth.

Luteinizing Hormone (LH)—dimeric glycoprotein produced by gonadotrophs in adenohypophysis.

Meiosis—cell division occurring in germ cells that reduces chromosome number to the haploid state (2n to n).

Menopause—cessation of menstrual cycles.

Menstrual cycle—cyclic hormonal and anatomic changes which occur in preparation for ovulation and pregnancy. Can be divided into follicular, luteal, and menstrual phases.

Mitosis—cell division in somatic cells that maintains a diploid set of chromosomes (2n to 2n).

Syncytiotrophoblast—multinucleated, syncytium of cells of the placenta which function in the production and secretion of a number of placental hormones.

Virilization—signs of pronounced hyperandrogenemia including temporal balding, deepening of voice, increased muscle mass, and clitoromegaly.

SUGGESTED READINGS

Aloia JF, Vaswani A, Yeh JK, et al. Calcium supplementation with and without hormone replacement therapy to prevent postmenopausal bone loss. Ann Intern Med 1994;120:97.

Baker TG, Sum OW. Development of the ovary and oogenesis. Clin Obstet Gynaecol 1976;3:3.

Bartlemez GW. The phases of the menstrual cycle and their interpretation in terms of the pregnancy cycle. Am J Obstet Gynecol 1957;74:931.

Cohen HL, Eisenberg P, Mandel F, et al. Ovarian cysts are common in premenarcheal girls: a sonographic study of 101 children 2–12 years old. American Journal of Roentgenology 1992;159:89.

Erickson GF, Magoffin D, Dyer CA, et al. The ovarian androgen producing cells: a review of structure/function relationships. Endocr Rev 1985;6:371.

Gambacciani M, Spinetti A, Taponeco F, et al. Bone loss in perimenopausal women: a longitudinal study. Maturitas 1994;18:191.

Jost A, Vigier B, Prepin J, et al. Studies on sex differentiation in mammals. Recent Prog Horm Res 1973;29:1.

Knobil E. The neuroendocrine control of the menstrual cycle. Recent Prog Horm Res 1980;36:53.

Manolio TA, Furberg CD, Shemanski L, et al. Associations of postmenopausal estrogen use with cardiovascular disease and its risk factors in older women. Circulation 1993;88:2163.1.

Midgley AR Jr., Jaffe RB. Regulation of gonadotropins. IV. Correlations of serum concentrations of follicle-stimulating and luteinizing hormones during the menstrual cycle. J Clin Endocrinol Metab 1968;28:1699.

Mikhail G. Hormone secretion by the human ovaries. Gynecol Obstet Invest 1970;1:5.

Mittwoch U, Mahadevaiah S. Comparison of development of human fetal gonads and kidneys. J Reprod Fertil 1980;58:463.1.

Noyes RW, Hertig AW, Rock J. Dating the endometrial biopsy. Fertil Steril 1950;1:3.

Oerter KE, Uriarte MM, Rose SR, et al. Gonadotropin secretory dynamics during puberty in normal girls and boys. J Clin Endocrinol Metab 1990;71:1251.

Rabinovici J, Jaffe RB. Development and regulation of growth and differentiated function in human and subhuman primate fetal gonads. Endocr Rev 1990;11:532.

Reindollar RH, Tho SPT, McDonough PG. Delayed puberty: an updated study of 326 patients. Transactions of the American Gynecologic and Obstetrical Society 1989;8:146.

Schreiber J. Current concepts of human follicular growth and development. Contemporary Obstetrics and Gynecology 1983;26:125.

Simpson ER, MacDonald PC. Endocrine physiology of the placenta. Annu Rev Physiol 1981;43:163.

Tulchinsky D, Hobel CJ. Plasma human chorionic gonadotropin, estrone, estradiol, progesterone and 17 alpha-hydroxyprogesterone in early normal pregnancy. Am J Obstet Gynecol 1973;117:884.

Wilson JD, George FW, Griffin JE. The hormonal control of sexual development. Science 1981;211:1278.

Yen SSC, Vela P, Rankin J, et al. Hormonal relationships during the menstrual cycle. JAMA 1970;211:1513.

13 The Breast

James M. McGreevy | Kirby I. Bland

This chapter reviews the basic science facts that are essential for the clinician to understand breast disorders. To make this presentation readable and usable, it will be neither exhaustive nor comprehensive. The goal of the chapter is to present the basic science of the breast in a fashion that allows the clinician to recall the information easily for use in the practice of surgery.

The Normal Breast

Embryology

The breasts of mammals develop on the ventral aspect of the embryo in longitudinal bands called milk lines (Fig. 13.1). These milk lines extend from the axilla in a curvilinear fashion toward the midline, ending in the inguinal region (Fig. 13.2). Animals bearing multiple pairs of breasts develop these glands in the thoracic and abdominal portion of the milk lines. Humans have only one pair of breasts and develop the organ in the thoracic portion of the milk line. Between 2% and 6% of the human females have an accessory nipple or extramammary collection of breast tissue (1). These extra glands (polymastia) or nipples (polythelia) occur in the milk line. Extra nipples more commonly appear on the chest wall below the breast, whereas extra breast tissue more commonly occurs in the axilla. The milk lines are thickened epithelial bands derived from ectoderm. They begin to appear at the 6th week of gestational age. By 9 weeks, the milk line has atrophied entirely, except in the pectoral region where the breasts develop. As the milk line regresses elsewhere in the embryo, the nipple bud appears. Between 10 and 16 weeks, this nipple bud develops by invagination of the overlying squamous epithelium (Fig. 13.3). As the invading squamous epithelium grows, it sprouts between 10 and 15 longitudinal fingers composed of cells. These epithelial extensions eventually develop into the mammary lobules. As the invading epithelium grows into the mesenchyme, differ-

entiation begins. The mesenchyme forms the smooth muscle of the areola and supporting tissues of the breast as the epithelial cords elongate. Between 20 and 24 weeks gestation, these epithelial cords develop lumens. At 6 months, the lumens of the main epithelial cords extend into the secondary mammary branches. As the embryo approaches term, the mass of the epithelial cords increases fourfold, and lobular-alveolar formation begins at the end of the epithelial cords.

At birth, the breast of the neonate is a branching system of ducts arranged about the nipple with radial symmetry. The 15 to 25 individual mammary units drain into major ducts that converge into a retro areolar ampulla. Each ampulla then opens onto the nipple. At birth, a watery secretion may drain via the nipple, which is called *witch's milk*, or colostrum. The colostrum is primarily water, fat, and cellular debris, which results from secretory activity in the cells of the alveoli (2). This secretion is stimulated by the withdrawal of placental steroids at the time of birth. From infancy until puberty, there is an increase in the supporting stromal structures of the breast and an elongation of the ducts in proportion to the increase in body size; no lobular development occurs before puberty (2).

Gross Anatomy

Topography and Surface Anatomy

The mature female breast varies tremendously in size and shape among individuals, and in the same individual, dramatic differences in configuration occur with pregnancy and advancing age. With pregnancy and lactation, the breast increases in turgor and weight; shape becomes more spherical. After pregnancy, the breast reduces in size and assumes a less round, more flattened, pendulous configuration. With advancing age, the breast substance is replaced with fat such that the elderly female breast is reduced in volume, is less firm, and remains flattened against the chest wall. The principal feature of the surface anatomy of the breast is the nipple and areola. Together they comprise a circular,

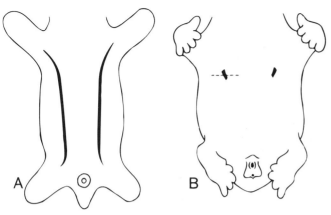

Figure 13.1. The mammary ridges and their regression. **A,** Ventral view of an embryo at the beginning of the fifth week of development (about 28 days), showing the mammary ridges that extend from the forelimb to the hindlimb. **B,** A similar view of the ventral embryo at the end of the 6th week, showing the remains of the ridges located in the pectoral region. From Bland K, Romrell LJ. Congenital and acquired disturbances of breast development and growth. In: Bland KI, Copeland EM, eds. The breast: comprehensive management of benign and malignant diseases. Philadelphia: WB Saunders, 1991:69. Reprinted by permission.

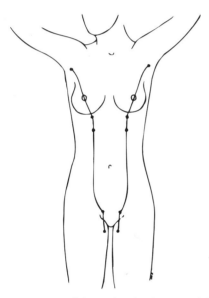

Figure 13.2. Mammary milk line. After development of the milk buds in the pectoral area of ectodermal thickening, the milk streak extends from the axilla to the inguinal areas. At week 9 of intrauterine development, atrophy of the bud has occurred except for the presence of the supernumerary nipples or breast. From Bland K, Romrell LJ. Congenital and acquired disturbances of breast development and growth. In: Bland KI, Copeland EM, eds. The breast: comprehensive management of benign and malignant diseases. Philadelphia: WB Saunders, 1991:70. Reprinted by permission.

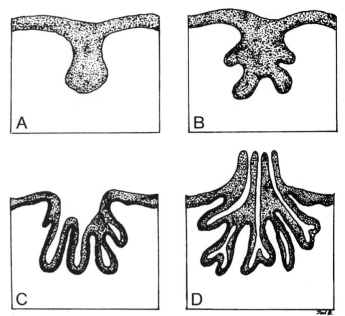

Figure 13.3. Sections through evolutionary development and growth of the mammary bud. **A–C,** Similar sections showing the developing gland at successive stages between the twelfth week and birth. The mammary pit develops, and major lactiferous ducts are present at the end of gestation. **D,** A similar section showing the elevation of the mammary pit by proliferations of the underlying connective tissue forming the nipple soon after birth. From Bland K, Romrell LJ. Congenital and acquired disturbances of breast development and growth. In: Bland KI, Copeland EM, eds. The breast: comprehensive management of benign and malignant diseases. Philadelphia: WB Saunders, 1991:71. Reprinted by permission.

pigmented complex that varies between 2 and 3 cm in size. This area becomes more deeply pigmented and enlarged during pregnancy. The nipple is located in the center of the areola and is raised above the areola for a distance of approximately 1 cm. Less than 10% of normal females have inverted nipples (indention of the nipple complex) (3). The milk ducts open in the base of this

concavity. This normal variant must be acknowledged, because retraction of the nipple can be an early sign of malignancy in those patients who do not have an inverted nipple.

No subcutaneous fat exists directly under the areola. Instead there is a layer of smooth muscle arranged in both a circular and radial fashion. This arrangement produces erection of the nipple and a decrease in the diameter of the areola. Smooth muscle contraction results from both tactile sensory and autonomic sympathetic stimulation. Scattered throughout the areola are elevations of the skin that represent openings of the accessory areolar Montgomery's glands. These glands are an intermediate stage between sweat glands and the mammary glands (2). They do not produce milk but may produce a scant secretion, which often contributes to the moisture of the areola. An increase in size is noted with pregnancy and lactation; these glands diminish after menopause.

Glandular Anatomy

Between 15 and 20 lactiferous ducts are found within the nipple. These ducts coalesce within the nipple such that the actual number of openings may not correlate with the number of breast lobules. The ducts within the nipple dilate to form milk sinuses which extend below

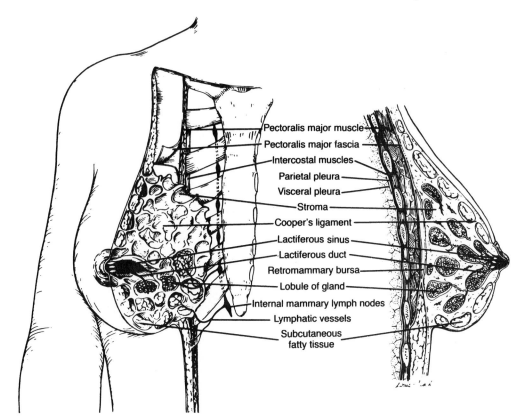

Pectoralis major muscle
Pectoralis major fascia
Intercostal muscles
Parietal pleura
Visceral pleura
Stroma
Cooper's ligament
Lactiferous sinus
Lactiferous duct
Retromammary bursa
Lobule of gland
Internal mammary lymph nodes
Lymphatic vessels
Subcutaneous fatty tissue

Figure 13.4. A tangential view of the breast on the chest wall and a cross-sectional (sagittal) view of the breast and associated chest wall. The breast lies in the superficial fascia just deep to the dermis. It is attached to the skin by suspensory Cooper's ligaments and is separated from the investing fascia of the pectoralis major muscle by the retromammary bursa. Cooper's ligaments form fibrosepta in the stroma that provide support for the breast parenchyma. Between 15 and 20 lactiferous ducts extend from lobules composed of glandular epithelium to openings located on the nipple. A dilation of the duct, the lactiferous sinus, is present near the opening of the duct in the subareolar tissue. Subcutaneous fat and adipose tissue distributed around the lobules of the gland give the breast its smooth contour and, in the nonlactating breast, account for most of its mass. Lymphatic vessels pass through the stroma surrounding the lobules of the gland and convey lymph to collecting ducts. Lymphatic channels ending in the internal mammary (or parasternal) lymph nodes are shown. The pectoralis major muscle lies adjacent to the ribs and intercostal muscles. The parietal pleura, attached to the endothoracic fascia, and the visceral pleura, covering the surface of the lung, are shown. From Romrell L, Bland K. Anatomy of the breast, axilla, chest wall, and related metastatic sites. In: Bland KI, Copeland EM, eds. The breast: comprehensive management of benign and malignant diseases. Philadelphia: WB Saunders, 1991:18(3). Reprinted by permission.

the nipple to become the lactiferous sinuses. Each lactiferous sinus drains between 15 and 20 breast lobules, and each lobule drains between 10 and 100 alveoli (Fig. 13.4). The breast lobules are supported by stromal elements that interdigitate between the lobules to give the breast substance. There is no distinct fascia separating the lobules or encasing the breast parenchyma. Between the breast and the skin is a subcutaneous layer of fatty tissue. The plane between the subcutaneous tissue and the breast substance is well-defined in younger women and may be used as a plane of dissection during mastectomy.

The upper and central portions of the breast are predominantly glandular tissue. The upper-outer quadrant has the largest volume of glandular tissue, which may explain the higher incidence of breast cancer in this area as well as the frequency of pain in this part of the breast caused by proliferative changes (2). The glandular tissue of the upper-outer quadrant extends up toward the axilla in the shape of a tongue. This elongation of breast tissue is called the tail of Spence; it proceeds through the axillary fascia and occasionally into the axilla where it is contiguous with the axillary lymph nodes. If a woman has glandular tissue extending into the axilla, she may experience axillary enlargement during pregnancy or menstruation. Scattered throughout the substance of the breast parenchyma are fibrous thickenings of the stromal connective tissue, which proceed from between the breast lobules and insert in a perpendicular fashion into both the skin and the underlying pectoral fascia. These ligaments, described by Cooper, serve a suspensory function in that they attach the breast to the chest wall and to the skin. When cancer involves these ligaments, they shorten and can result in skin indentation which is recognized clinically as *peau d'orange* (2).

Fascia

Because the breast develops within an envelope of skin and subcutaneous tissue, actual fascia does not invest the breast substance. The organ rests on fascia overlying the pectoralis major muscle. Between the deep layer of the superficial pectoral fascia and the deep pectoral fascia is a potential space referred to as the retromammary bursa (2). This space is evident during mastectomy as this portion of the dissection proceeds quickly and with minimal blood loss.

Another fascial layer of surgical significance is the clavipectoral fascia. This condensation of fascia covers the deep surface of the pectoralis major muscle and envelops the pectoralis minor muscle. It then extends out into the axilla to form a sheath around the axillary vessels. The anterior thoracic vessels and nerves and the cephalic vein pass through the clavipectoral fascia (3). This fascia must be opened sharply to enter the axilla during the course of an axillary lymph node dissection.

Microscopic Anatomy

Before puberty, the epithelium of the ducts within the breast is a two-cell-layered basal cuboidal epithelium, whereas the alveolar lining is a low cylindrical-surface epithelium. With the onset of puberty, sex steroids, especially estrogen, initiate an increase in the number of layers that line both the ducts and the alveoli with the formation of buds and papillae on some of these cells. In the mature nonpregnant breast, there are three cell types in the lining of the ducts: superficial (luminal) A cells, basal B cells, and myoepithelial cells (2).

The A cells of the duct mechanism are involved primarily in milk production. On routine histologic examination, they are dark because of the rich cytoplasmic RNA and reticulum and the many ribosomes within the cytoplasm. These cells can form bridges between themselves and sometimes proliferate into the lumen of the ducts.

The B cells, also called chief cells, are the most abundant cell type lining the duct. These cells have a clear cytoplasm and are not involved in the production of milk proteins. These cells seem to be energy providers for the luminal secretory cells. B cells contain distinctive intracytoplasmic filaments and fibers, which are noncontractile. The filaments of these cells resemble the myofilaments of the myoepithelial cells.

Myoepithelial cells contain actual myofilaments, which insert on the base of the membrane of the cell and perform a contractile function. These cells are located in a basket-like network that surround the alveoli of the small milk ducts. They are stimulated to contract by sex steroids and prolactin. They do not have direct innervation, which allows contraction. With the suckling reflex, oxytocin release from the posterior pituitary results in contraction of the myoepithelial cells such that the milk-filled alveolus is emptied into the smaller milk ducts. As the smaller milk ducts contain a network of myoepithelial cells, milk is evacuated into the larger ductules. No smooth muscle exists around the alveolus or the small milk ducts. These cells decrease in size and number after completion of lactation and are diminished in

number after menopause. As these cells are ectodermal in origin, they resemble their mesodermal counterparts, the smooth muscle cells (2).

Hormone Regulation

Estrogen

Estrogen is the principal hormone responsible for the development of the female breast and for maintenance of the glandular breast elements throughout reproductive life. Estrogen has potent mitogenic effects on mammary epithelium. This steroidal hormone is responsible for the initiation of ductal development as it increases the number of estrogen and progesterone receptors on the mammary epithelial cells (4).

Progesterone

Progesterone, principally of ovarian origin, is responsible for the differentiation of epithelial cells and causes lobular development. This hormone may actually limit proliferation of the tubular system of the glandular breast elements and reduce estrogen binding to membrane receptors (4).

Prolactin

Prolactin is required together with the presence of growth hormone and cortisol for the development of mammary epithelium. This hormone also contributes to the development of the adipose tissue in the breast. Biochemically, it increases the number of estrogen receptors within epithelial cells. Prolactin can act synergistically with estrogen in ductal development and with progesterone in lobulo-alveolar development. This compound is the primary hormone for lactogenesis in late pregnancy and in the postpartum period. It stimulates the differentiation of milk-producing cells and initiates the synthesis of the components of milk in those cells (4).

Other Hormones

The effects of growth hormone, cortisol, and thyroid hormone in the human female breast are not well established. However, each of them initiates a variety of effects on mammary epithelial cells in experimental conditions. The secretion of the primary trophic hormones for the human breast (estrogen and progesterone) is under the control of the neurohormones of the hypothalamus (gonadotropic-releasing hormone, GnRH) and the trophic hormones of the pituitary gland (luteinizing hormone, LH, and follicle-stimulating hormone, FSH; both secreted by the basophilic cells of the anterior pituitary) (Fig. 13.5). Prolactin is secreted by the acidophilic cells of the anterior pituitary gland.

Puberty

With the onset of puberty comes the initiation of the secretion of GnRH, LH, FSH from the anterior pituitary

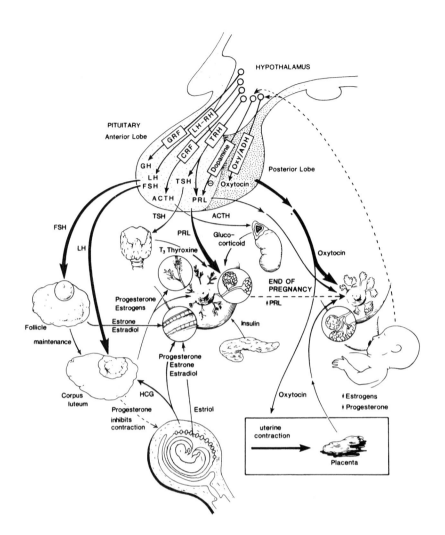

Figure 13.5. Overview of the neuroendocrine control of breast development and function with relationship to gonadotropic hormones of the anterior pituitary and ovary. Basophil secretion of LH and FSH is responsible for ovarian synthesis and release of progesterone and estrogen, respectively. The mammotropic effects of estrogen and progestin initiate myoepithelial and alveolar development. Ductal and stromal enlargement with pregnancy occur as a result of progestin and estrogen secretions in excess from the corpus luteum (first 12 weeks) and thereafter from the placenta. Acidophil cell secretion of prolactin (PRL) is initiated after evacuation of the gravid uterus and is mammotropic to the lobular alveoli. The suckling reflex initiates oxytocin release from the posterior pituitary and is stimulatory to alveolar myoepithelial cells to initiate milk release. Neuroendocrine organs other than the pituitary and ovary secrete hormones (glucocorticoid, GH, insulin, and thyroxine) that are trophic to ductal and glandular maintenance and growth. *GH,* growth hormone; *CRF,* corticotropin-releasing factor; *LH-RH,* luteinizing hormone-releasing factor; *HCG,* human choriogonadotropic hormone; *TRH,* thyrotropin-releasing hormone; *TSH,* thyrotropin.

gland. This event results in estrogen and progesterone release from the ovary. Rising serum levels of estrogen result in breast bud development as the first noticeable event in breast maturation. Estrogen stimulates proliferation of the ductal epithelium, the myoepithelial cells, and the surrounding stroma (4). Progesterone, which is released from the ovary, initiates formation of the secretory components of the mammary epithelium, which is located at the terminal aspect of the ductules. The sex steroids also increase the amount of connective tissue and fat in the breast so that within 2 years of the onset of menses, the breast has assumed a mature spherical configuration.

Menstrual Cycle

The changing serum and tissue concentrations of estrogen and progesterone associated with the menstrual cycle have several effects on the mature female breast, which are outlined in Table 13.1 (2). In the premenstrual phase of the cycle, rising levels of FSH and LH result in elevation of plasma estrogen values. Estrogen values peak in the late follicular phase of the cycle when ovulation occurs. After ovulation, the luteal portion of the cycle begins, estrogen continues to increase above that

seen in the follicular phase of the cycle, and plasma progesterone rises. The elevated plasma estrogen and progesterone tissue concentrations result in an increase in volume of the breast. This increased volume results from water retention, an increase in basement membrane thickness, an increase in alveolar diameter, a stromal infiltration with fluid, lymphoid, and plasma cells, and stimulation of intra alveolar secretion. Consequently, breast volume is greatest in the second half of the menstrual cycle; just before the onset of menses, the size, density, nodularity, and sensitivity of the breast increases. With the onset of menses, tissue volume continuously increases, perhaps related to intra alveolar secretion brought about by sex steroid withdrawal, permitting partial stimulatory action by prolactin. In the postmenstrual period, breast volume decreases with a reduction in alveolar and glandular cell size, a regression of the edema, and a subsidence of the lymphoid inflammatory cell infiltrate. The mammary gland is smallest between the fourth and seventh day of the cycle. This mammary involution results from a fall in plasma levels of estrogen and progesterone after the onset of the menses. This involution is incomplete with each cycle such that mammary growth continues up to the age of 30 to 35 years.

Table 13.1.
Breast Changes During Menstrual Cycle

Phase of Cycle	Effect	Cause	Hormone Control
Pre-Menstrual	Increases in Volume	• Water retention • Basement membrane thickening • Increase in alveolar diameter • Intra-alveolar secretion • Stromal infiltration with fluid, lymphoid and plasma cells	Estrogen Increase
Menses withdrawal	Increase in Volume	• Intra-alveolar secretion	Sex-steroid permitting limited prolactin action
Post-menopausal	Decrease in Volume	• Degeneration of glandular cells • Reduction in alveolar size • Smallest on days 4-7 of cycle	Estrogen withdrawal

Table 13.2.
Breast Changes During Pregnancy

Trimester	Histologic Change
First	• Terminal ductule sprouting • Lobular-alveolar formation begins • Glandular buds invade and replace connective tissue and fat • Alveolar epithelium changes from 2-cell layer to 1-cell
Second	• Ductular proliferation • Increase in lobuloalveolar units • Lymphocytes in connective tissue • Activation of secretory epithelium resulting in colostrum
Third	• Fat droplets in secretory alveolar cells • Filling of alveoli with colostrum • Replacement of connective tissue and fat by lobuloalveolar proliferation

Pregnancy

The changes in the breast induced by pregnancy are summarized in Table 13.2 (2). With the onset of pregnancy, high levels of plasma estrogen and progesterone are secreted by the corpus luteum and are maintained after the twelfth gestational week by the placenta. Plasma estrogen and progesterone values gradually increase throughout all trimesters of the pregnancy; in late gestation, the concentration of prolactin in the serum increases 10-fold. Under the effects of these increasing sex steroids, the areola and nipple become larger, more prominent, and more pigmented. At the microscopic level, sex steroids cause the ducts and lobules to proliferate; these hormones also induce alveolar development.

In the first trimester of pregnancy, lobuloalveolar formation is initiated. The proliferating glandular epithelium replaces resting adipose and connective tissue. The ducts proliferate and branch to begin development of multiple alveoli. In the second trimester of pregnancy, the proliferation of the ductal elements increases. A true lobuloalveolar system develops, and the secretory epithelium becomes active.

In the third trimester of pregnancy, the secretory activity of the epithelium increases. Fat droplets accumulate in the alveolar cells and colostrum fills the alveolar and ductal spaces. Blood flow increases and myoepithe-

lial cells enlarge. In the last weeks of pregnancy, rising prolactin levels induce a limited synthesis of milk fats and proteins.

Menopause

Following withdrawal of the sex steroids with cessation of ovarian function, lobules and ducts in the breast reduce to an atrophic, hypoplastic epithelium. The periductal fibrous tissue becomes more dense, and the lactiferous duct network dilates. Cystic formation occurs as the epithelium in the lobular acini becomes atrophic. There is a loss in total mass of fat tissue within the breast. The end result of these degenerative changes is a decrease in breast volume and a change in shape of the breast from the original lobular structure to a flat, pendulous organ.

Lactation

During pregnancy, sex steroids may cross the placenta and stimulate the fetal breast; 80% to 90% of newborns have nipple discharge (colostral milk) at the time of birth. This secretion comes from the one to two-cell-thick epithelium of the alveoli under the influence of prolactin. With delivery, the sudden withdrawal of the high levels of sex steroids of the placenta from the epithelium of the infantile breast allows prolactin to stimulate the mammary epithelium, producing this witch's milk. This effect reaches a maximum in 4 to 7 days and subsides in 3 to 4 weeks (2) as the circulating hormones are metabolized.

Blood Supply

Approximately 60% of the total breast mass obtains blood supply from the internal mammary artery (3). Ventral branches of this artery (anterior rami mammarii) penetrate the intercostal muscles of the second to the fifth intercostal spaces approximately 1 to 2 cm lateral to the parasternal border. Once these arteries enter the breast, they pass through the breast substance transversely toward the nipple. Extensive collateralizing within the breast occurs via the two other major sources

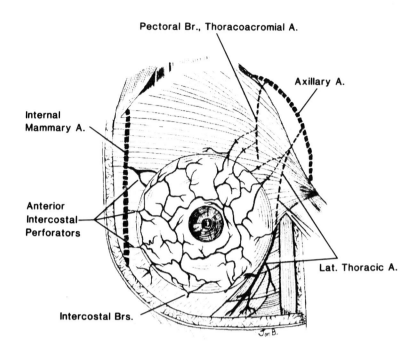

Pectoral Br., Thoracoacromial A.

Axillary A.

Internal Mammary A.

Anterior Intercostal Perforators

Lat. Thoracic A.

Intercostal Brs.

Figure 13.6. Arterial distribution of blood to the breast, axilla, and chest wall. The breast receives its blood supply via three major arterial routes: (*a*) medially from anterior perforating intercostal branches arising from the internal thoracic artery; (*b*) laterally from either pectoral branches of the thoracoacromial trunk or branches of the lateral thoracic artery (the thoracoacromial trunk and the lateral thoracic arteries are branches of the axillary artery); and (*c*) from lateral cutaneous branches of the intercostal arteries that are associated with the overlying breast. The arteries indicated with a dashed line lie deep to the muscles of the thoracic wall and axilla. Many of the arteries must pass through these muscles before reaching the breast. From Romrell L, Bland K. Anatomy of the breast, axilla, chest wall, and related metastatic sites. In: Bland KI, Copeland EM, eds. The breast: comprehensive management of benign and malignant diseases. Philadelphia: WB Saunders, 1991:26. Reprinted by permission.

of blood supply: the lateral thoracic artery and the branches from the intercostal arteries. The lateral thoracic artery originates from the axillary artery proximal to the origin of the subscapularis artery. It passes along the lower border of the pectoralis minor muscle. At approximately the level of the median portion of the muscle belly of the pectoralis minor, the lateral thoracic artery gives off the external mammary artery, which courses ventrally around the muscle belly to supply primarily the upper-outer quadrant of the breast. The lower-outer quadrant of the breast is supplied by branches of the third through fifth posterior intercostal arteries. Other arteries that supply a minor amount of the nutrient blood supply to the breast are the thoracoacromial, subscapular, upper thoracic, and thoracodorsal arteries (Fig. 13.6).

The venous drainage of the breast follows the primary arterial supply. The principal veins are the intercostal veins, which drain to the internal mammary vein; the external mammary vein; and the lateral thoracic vein, which drains into the axillary vein.

There are two other arteries of surgical significance. The first is the thoracodorsal branch of the subscapularis artery. This vessel does not supply blood to the breast but is centrally located within the axillary contents and is contiguous with the central and scapular lymph node groups. Because of its deep location, this vessel can be difficult to control if injured operatively. It lies in close proximity to the long thoracic and thoracodorsal nerves and may be injured during isolation of those structures. A second artery of surgical significance is a large branch of the lateral thoracic artery (see Fig. 13.6), which is the primary blood supply to the pectoralis major muscle. This branch comes directly out of the groove formed by

the pectoralis minor and major muscles approximately 3 to 5 cm below the axillary vein. This large branch enters the pectoralis major in the laterally exposed portion of the muscle belly. If this artery is interrupted, the pectoralis major muscle may undergo severe atrophy.

Lymph Drainage

The axillary lymph nodes that drain the breast are grouped into three levels, defined by their relationship to the pectoralis minor muscle (Fig. 13.7). Level I nodes are those that are lateral to or below the lower border of the pectoralis minor (the external mammary, axillary vein, and scapular lymph node groups). Level II lymph nodes are those that are deep to or behind the pectoralis minor muscle (the central lymph node group and some of the subclavicular nodes). Level III nodes are those that are above the upper border of the pectoralis minor muscle (the subclavicular or apical node group) (Fig. 13.8).

There are four major routes for lymphatic drainage from the breast: the lateral, medial, transpectoral, and retropectoral routes (3). The lateral route is the most important from an operative standpoint. The skin and the majority of the breast drain lymph via the external mammary node group, and lymph flows into the lateral node group thereafter. Subsequent drainage into the proximal aspects of the axilla pass through the subscapular, central, apical, and supraclavicular node groups. Each of these groups are detailed below. The second major route of drainage is the medial route. Lymph from the skin and central and medial parts of the breast follow the major vessels that perforate the intercostal muscles from the internal mammary artery and vein. These lym-

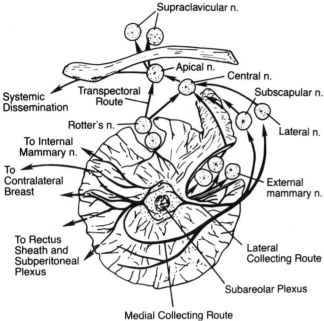

Figure 13.7. Schematic drawing of the breast identifying the position of lymph nodes relative to the breast and illustrating routes of lymphatic drainage. The clavicle is indicated as a reference point. Level I lymph nodes include the external mammary (or anterior) group, the axillary vein (or lateral) group, and the scapular group; level II, the central group; and level III, the subclavicular (or apical) group. The arrows indicate the routes of lymphatic drainage. From Romrell L, Bland K. Anatomy of the breast, axilla, chest wall, and related metastatic sites. In: Bland KI, Copeland EM, eds. The breast: comprehensive management of benign and malignant diseases. Philadelphia: WB Saunders, 1991:28. Reprinted by permission.

phatics drain into the internal mammary lymph node chain. The third major lymphatic drainage route is the transpectoral route. Lymphatics from the retromammary plexus penetrate the pectoralis major muscle to drain into the interpectoral nodes, which are also known as Rotter's nodes. These nodes are located beneath the lateral aspect of the pectoralis major where it forms a groove in contact with the pectoralis minor muscle. Rotter's nodes drain into lymphatics that course along the thoracoacromial artery to the subclavicular group of nodes. A fourth major route of lymphatic drainage from the breast is the retropectoral route. Lymphatics from the superior and internal portions of the breast drain into lymphatics on the lateral and inferior portion of the pectoralis major and minor muscles. These lymphatics eventually terminate in the apex of the axilla and the subclavicular node group. The nodes that drain the lateral aspect of the breast are divided into the following groups.

Axillary Vein Group (Lateral Group). The lateral group is located within level I of the axilla. These veins are the most lateral and numerous group of nodes in the axilla and are located ventral and caudal to the axillary vein. They receive the majority of lymph flow from the arm.

External Mammary Group (Anterior or Pectoral Group). The anterior group is also located in level I of the axilla. These veins are found along the lower border of the pectoralis minor muscle in association with the lateral thoracic vessels. These nodes receive the major portion of the lymph flow from the breast and drain into the central group of axillary lymph nodes.

Figure 13.8. Schematic drawing illustrating the major lymph node groups associated with the lymphatic drainage of the breast. The Roman numerals indicate three levels or groups of lymph nodes that are defined by their location relative to the pectoralis minor. Level I includes lymph nodes located lateral to the pectoralis minor; level II, lymph nodes located deep to the muscle; and level III, lymph nodes located medial to the muscle. The arrows indicate the general direction of lymph flow. The axillary vein and its major tributaries associated with the pectoralis minor are included.

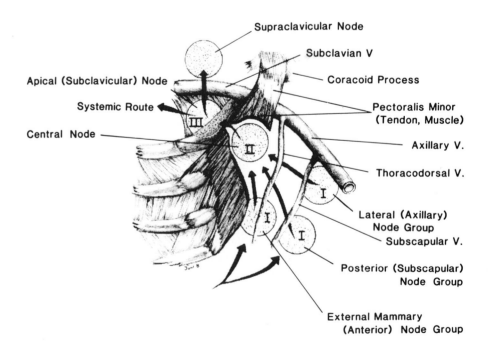

Subscapular (Scapular or Posterior) Group. The subscapular group is also located in level I of the axilla, along the lateral border of the scapula. This group lies on the posterior wall of the axilla in association with the thoracodorsal branches of the subscapular vein. These nodes drain into the central and subclavicular groups.

Central Group. The central group is located in level II of the axilla behind the pectoralis minor muscle wall and is surrounded by fat. These nodes are called the central group because of their location midway between the anterior and posterior axillary line. These nodes are often close to the skin and are, therefore, frequently palpable when they are clinically involved with metastases. They drain into the subclavicular group of nodes.

Subclavicular (Apical) Group. The subclavicular group is located in level III of the axilla at the point where the axillary vein passes under the subclavius muscle to become the subclavian vein. These nodes are the highest and most medial nodes in the axilla and receive lymph from all the other groups of axillary nodes. They drain directly into either the internal jugular vein, the right lymphatic duct, or the thoracic duct.

Interpectoral Group (Rotter's Nodes). Rotter's nodes (named after a German pathologist) are located between the pectoralis major and minor muscles in association with the pectoral branches of the thoracoacromial vessels. Rotter's nodes drain directly into the central and subclavicular groups of nodes.

Innervation

The breast is supplied by both somatic sensory and autonomic innervation. The nipple and areola have abundant somatic sensory and sympathetic autonomic innervation that, when activated, result in contraction of the areola and erection of the nipple (2). Parasympathetic autonomic innervation of the breast exists. Furthermore, the parenchyma of the mammary gland has no innervation (3); lactation is stimulated exclusively by hormonal influences (prolactin). Somatic sensory innervation to the skin overlying the breast has origin from three sources. There are lateral branches of the thoracic intercostal nerves 3 to 7, which supply the skin of the lateral aspect of the breast. Skin of the medial aspect of the breast is innervated from branches of the thoracic intercostal nerves 2 to 6. The superior aspect of the breast is also supplied by branches from the supraclavicular nerve, which arises from the brachial plexus.

Several nerves are of surgical significance during operative procedures on the breast and the axillary contents. The first is the *long thoracic nerve* (respiratory nerve of Bell). This nerve arises from the brachial plexus and passes inferiorly in the medial border of the axilla within a plane dorsal to the axillary vein. The long thoracic nerve is found within the serratus fascia millimeters from the chest wall as it courses to innervate the serratus anterior muscle. Transection of this nerve results in

postoperative disability known as a winged scapula. The second nerve of surgical significance is the *thoracodorsal nerve*. This nerve arises from the posterior cord of brachial plexus and passes inferiorly into the axilla dorsal to the axillary vein. It is usually found in the same plane as that of the long thoracic nerve and approximately 1 to 3 cm lateral to that nerve. The thoracodorsal passes caudally along the lateral border of the axilla for 4 to 7 cm, then turns medially to enter the latissimus dorsi muscle. This nerve is usually exposed in its entire length during an axillary dissection. It can be injured in the lower axilla when the operator feels that the axillary dissection has been completed safely. Additional nerves of surgical significance are the intercostal brachial nerves, which arise from intercostal nerves 2 and 3. These nerves are large and pass directly across (transverse) the axilla through the axillary contents, which are removed in the axillary dissection. They are transected frequently with dissection, resulting in numbness of the upper inner arm. Another nerve of significance during a surgical procedure is the lateral pectoral nerve. This nerve accompanies the lateral thoracic artery into the belly of the pectoralis major muscle. Transection of this nerve will denervate the majority of the pectoralis major muscle and result in significant cosmetic disability with atrophy of this important functional muscle of the chest wall.

Benign Clinical Conditions

Fibrocystic disease is a term that has been used widely in the past but is being replaced appropriately in medical lexicon. The reason for its disuse can be appreciated readily by a consideration of the term's inaccuracy and imprecision. Fibrocystic disease has two definitions, a clinical one and a histologic one. Clinically, the term refers to the presence of palpable lumps in the breast, which fluctuate in size and discomfort with the menstrual cycle. Symptoms become worse with advancing age until menopause, when symptoms cease. Using this clinical definition, at least 50% of females have fibrocystic disease as a normal (physiologic) condition (5). Because the breasts are composed of elements that are remarkably sensitive to sex steroids in terms of their growth and development, changes in size and sensitivity during the cycle are evident. In addition, it is not unusual to have variations in responsiveness to hormonal stimulation that results in variations of tissues density (lumps) between breasts in the same woman and even among quadrants within the same breast. These physiologically induced changes in breast texture and tenderness are so frequent that a precise distinction between clinical disease and physiologic variation is impossible.

Attempts to define fibrocystic disease histologically have been equally problematic. Foote and Stewart (6) attempted to define the pathologic basis of fibrocystic disease by listing five microscopic findings associated with the condition that they referred to as chronic cystic mastitis. Those changes include macrocysts and microcysts, sclerosing adenosis, fibrosis, papillomatosis (epithelial hyperplasia), and apocrine change. Unfortunately, these histological variants are seen frequently in women with or without clinical fibrocystic disease. Love et al. (7) summarized the literature on the subject and noted that 58% of women in eight different autopsy studies had these changes in the normal breast. In addition, women over 70 without an antemortem diagnosis of fibrocystic disease had the histologic changes noted by Foote and Stewart 89% of the time. Furthermore, 69% of the women had histologically confirmed epithelial hyperplasia. Therefore, both definitions are imprecise because the clinical definition fits 50% of the population and the histologic definition applies to 70%. Thus the term *fibrocystic disease* should not be used (7), because of its vague and imprecise connotation. Fibrocystic changes are normal changes expected within the breast that become more evident with aging. The most important task for the surgeon is an understanding of the relationship of fibrocystic change to the risk for developing cancer. The classification shown in Table 13.3 of benign histologic breast conditions has been devised to identify those changes that are associated with the subsequent development of breast cancer (8).

Nonproliferative Lesions

Cysts and Apocrine Metaplasia

Both macrocysts (> 1 cm) and microcysts (< 1 cm) are common in the premenopausal female breast. In an autopsy study of 725 women, 58% had microcysts and 21% had macrocysts (9). The smaller cysts most likely result from lobular involution caused by hormone imbalance. These cysts are lined with cells of apocrine derivation with secretory snouts. The fluid that fills these smaller cysts contains proteins and enzymes that are only found in apocrine epithelium. Also, the lobular component of these microcysts has been demonstrated to contain elastic fiber when stained using immunohistochemical techniques (10). The larger cysts are probably the result of ductal obstruction secondary to sloughed epithelium or from angulation of the duct. Because the processes that produce the cysts are different, one would expect two distinct types of fluid to occupy the cysts. In the macrocyst, the type of fluid is the same as in other cysts that are lined with flattened cells. These cells are nonsecretory with passive barriers through which the cyst fluid equilibrates with the plasma. Macrocystic fluid has a high sodium content and low potassium concentration similar to plasma. They also contain albumin, nonsecretory 75 IgA, and low levels of apocrine cyst proteins. The second type of cyst fluid is that associated with tall columnar cells that have secretory function. This fluid, therefore, has a high potassium concentration, a low sodium concentration, low levels of albumen, and high levels of apocrine cyst proteins. Secretory IgA, epidermal growth factor, and dehydroepiandrosterone sulfate are also found in this fluid.

Cysts tend to be multiple and recurrent. In a study of 352 women followed for 5 years after their initial presentation with a breast cyst, 54% subsequently developed additional cysts, and 12% presented with multiple cysts (11). A total of 10% of cysts that were aspirated in this study refilled to the extent that they became palpable again. The apocrine-lined cysts may be more prone to recur. The presence of breast cysts is not considered to be a risk factor for the development of breast cancer (Table 13.4). However, three epidemiologic reviews suggest a 1.7 to 4.0 times increase in the risk of breast cancer in women with breast cysts (12–14). These reviews did not control for the association of proliferative disorders with breast cysts. Any increase in the risk of breast cancer seen in women with breast cysts is most likely the result of epithelial proliferation, not cystic disease alone.

Table 13.3.
Classification of Benign Histologic Breast Condition

Non Proliferative Lesions

1. Cysts and apocrine metaplasia
2. Duct ectasia
3. Mild epithelial hyperplasia
4. Calcifications
5. Fibroadenoma

Proliferative Lesions

1. Sclerosing adenosis
2. Radical scar and complex sclerosing lesions
3. Moderate and florid epithelial hyperplasia
4. Intraductal papillomas

Atypical Proliferative Lesions

1. Atypical lobular hyperplasia
2. Atypical ductal hyperplasia

Table 13.4.
Relative Risk for Invasive Breast Carcinoma Based on Histologic Examination of Breast Tissue Without Carcinoma

No increased risk (no proliferative disease)
   Apocrine change
   Duct Ectasia
   Mild epithelial hyperplasia of unusual type
Slightly increased risk (1.5–2 times)
   Hyperplasia of usual type, moderate or florid
   Sclerosing adenosis, papilloma
Moderately increased risk (4–5 times) (atypical hyperplasia or borderline lesions)
Atypical ductal hyperplasia and atypical lobular hyperplasia
High risk (8 to 10 times) (carcinoma *in situ*)
   Lobular carcinoma *in situ* and ductal carcinoma *in situ* (noncomedo)

Apocrine metaplasia refers to the transition of the ductal epithelium to the tall columnar cell type with a rounded apical aspect similar to secretory cells in the breast. This metaplastic change is most often found in cysts and has not been confirmed to manifest an increased incidence of breast cancer.

Duct Ectasia

Duct ectasia is a benign condition, resulting in dilatation, periductal inflammation, and fibrosis of the retroareolar ducts just beneath the nipple. A common disorder, it is the presenting complaint of between 1% and 4% of women who present with breast symptoms (15). The incidence of duct ectasia in asymptomatic women has been reported to be as high as 20% to 24% (15). The plasma cell is a predominant feature of the inflammatory process around the ducts, thus the term *plasma cell mastitis* has been applied. Other names for this clinical entity include mammary duct ectasia, periductal mastitis, comedo mastitis, and secretory disease of the breast. This process presents different clinical symptoms manifested at different stages of presentation. The early symptoms are nipple discharge and pain. Late in the course of the disease, the pain becomes more pronounced as the periductal inflammation becomes more profound. Subareolar abscess and mammary duct fistula are other features of this disease in its intermediate stages of development. The late symptoms are those of fibrosis from the periductal inflammation: diminished pain, nipple retraction, mass behind the nipple, skin fixation, and nipple discharge. For obvious reasons, advanced stages of duct ectasia are indistinguishable from ductal adenocarcinoma.

Two theories regarding the development of ductal ectasia are considered. An older theory holds that the genesis of the process is an abnormal dilatation of retroareolar ducts of the nipple. According to this hypothesis, periductal inflammation is caused by extrusion of ductal debris into the periductal stroma across the damaged ductal epithelium. The second theory holds the periductal inflammation as the primary and essential feature of this disorder; ductal ectasia is a result of the destruction of the periductal stroma by the inflammation (15). Duct ectasia is not associated with an increased risk of breast cancer.

Mild Epithelial Hyperplasia

Epithelial hyperplasia refers to an increase in the number of cells in relation to the basement membrane. There are normally two cell layers that line the ducts, thus a thickness exceeding three cells represents hyperplasia. This process presents in a spectrum of mild epithelial hyperplasia to moderate hyperplasia, for which there are five or more cell layers. Finally, florid hyperplasia refers to the process in which ducts are packed with solid sheets of cells. Inflammatory cells may be interspersed with the epithelial cells. In the moderate forms of the disease, the cells can form bridges as they cross the duct. As the hyperplastic cells fill the duct space, they may initiate ductal dilation. Mild to moderate epithelial hyperplasia without cellular atypia is common. These changes may be found in up to 20% of breast biopsies (16). Patients observed to have epithelial hyperplasia without cellular atypia have a slightly increased risk of breast cancer, which is 1.5 to 2.0 times greater than that of the general population.

Calcifications

The widespread application of mammography as a screening modality for breast cancer has resulted in better documentation of the frequency with which microcalcifications occur in the female breast. Approximately 90% to 95% of breast calcifications are associated with benign conditions. Calcium deposits can occur within the ducts or lobules, in the stroma, or within the epithelium. Widely scattered calcium deposits are a common feature with sclerosing adenosis. A total of 5% to 10% of patients in which microcalcifications are identified mammographically will have breast cancer. Although radiographic features may be suggestive of a benign or malignant process, a biopsy is often necessary to establish histology. The characteristics of benign calcifications include long parallel lines that resemble the cast of a blood vessel, the burst or "popcorn" pattern of coarse calcifications within a fibroadenoma, blunt calcifications with radiolucent centers, uniformity of size, and widely dispersed and well-defined deposits without spicules, branches, or comma shapes. Features that are more frequently associated with a malignant process include irregular, poorly defined deposits that have branches, spicules, or comma shapes that are focal in location. These microcalcifications are often identified as five or more densities within 1 cm^2 (17). The absolute number of clustered calcifications is not necessarily of value.

Fibroadenoma

Fibroadenoma is a common clinical entity observed in young women, age 15 to 25. The clinical features of the mass are distinct enough to allow diagnosis by physical examination alone. They are discrete, well-defined, firm, freely movable, and nontender. The mass is composed of elements thought to be derived from the terminal duct lobular unit (18). Fibroadenomas are probably not a true neoplasm but rather an exuberant overgrowth of normal tissue constituents (18). Immunohistochemical and electron microscopic evidence (19) suggest the cell of origin for fibroadenomas may be the fibroblast rather than the myoepithelial cell. In addition, estrogen receptor (ER) and progesterone receptor (PR) are commonly expressed biochemically in fibroadenomas (20). The tumor appears to be sex steroid dependent, a trait it shares with fibrocystic disease. Fibroadenomas can regress, remain the same size, or enlarge. Fibroadenomas will regress with aging, as the incidence of these tumors in mastectomies and at autopsy is low (21).

The cellularity of fibroadenomas have been shown to diminish with aging (22). In a prospective follow-up of 63 patients with 20 fibroadenomas, 31% resolved, 12% became smaller, 25% had no change, and 32% enlarged (18). The risk for breast cancer in patients who have had a fibroadenoma excised is 2–4 times higher than the general population (23). Also, cancer can develop from the epithelial elements of the fibroadenoma stroma; this is an unusual occurrence. Two literature reviews have collected only 96 such cases (24,25). When carcinoma appears in a fibroadenoma, it is usually in older patients (40 to 45 years old) and contained within the fibroadenoma (50%). Half of the cancers are lobular carcinoma-in-situ.

Proliferative Lesions

Sclerosing Adenosis

Sclerosing adenosis, a histologic condition, can present as a painful mass (26) or as an incidental finding in a biopsy done for other reasons. It can be confused microscopically, grossly, and mammographically with cancer. Histologically, this process resembles cancer because there is proliferation of both the stroma and epithelial elements of the terminal duct lobular units in such a manner that cords of epithelial cells are isolated within the stroma. These cords can also be found near nerves and blood vessels. This process is called pseudo infiltration and can resemble invasive adenocarcinoma. In sclerosing adenosis, the normal two-cell layer is maintained in relation to the basement membrane. Therefore, sclerosing adenosis can be distinguished from cancer by electron microscopy as the infiltrating cells of invasive cancer have breached the intact basement membrane of the ductal epithelium (26). The fibrosis (desmoplasia) that occurs with this process distorts the normal lobular architecture in a stellate or whorled pattern that may resemble cancer when examined grossly. This fibrosis may present as a dense opacity on mammography with architectural distortion that is often associated with scattered or clustered microcalcifications. Patients who have sclerosing adenosis on biopsy have a slightly increased risk for development of breast cancer (1.5 to 4.0 times) compared with the normal (index) population (16).

Radial Scar and Complex Sclerosing Lesion

Radial scar and complex sclerosing lesion refer to the same rare pathologic entity. Radial scar is applied to lesions up to 1 cm in size, and complex sclerosing lesion is reserved for lesions larger than 1 cm. The identifying characteristic of these entities is a central scar with proliferating epithelial elements emanating from the center in a stellate fashion. The central sclerosis can be surrounded by various degrees of cystic dilatation, epithelial hyperplasia, apocrine metaplasia, and papillomatosis. This sclerosing process can resemble cancer grossly and mammographically for the same reasons that sclerosing adenosis resembles cancer. There is a slight increase in risk for breast cancer (1.5 to 4.0 times) in patients found to have these lesions on breast biopsy (16).

Moderate and Florid Epithelial Hyperplasia

Moderate and florid epithelial hyperplasia are the most common of the proliferative breast lesions, being identified in 20% of breast biopsies (27). Moderate hyperplasia is defined as cellular proliferation more than three cell layers above the basement membrane. Florid hyperplasia involves many cell layers such that greater than 70% of the duct lumen is filled with cells. The duct is often packed and distended with cells, which can form clefts, papillomas, arches, and bridges within the lumen. The cells have no atypical characteristics. Patients with mild to florid hyperplasia have a slight (1.5 to 4.0 times) increase in risk for breast cancer (16).

Intraductal Papilloma

Intraductal papilloma usually occurs in the lactiferous ducts and sinuses. It commonly presents as bloody nipple discharge and less commonly as a palpable mass. The process results from a neoplastic alteration of epithelial lining of the duct. The tumor (0.5 to 5.0 cm) is attached to the duct wall by a fibrovascular stalk of connective tissue. This stalk branches many times to support a villous pattern of epithelial cells. The entire polyp or papilloma is a discrete tumor that is identified easily by galactogram and occasionally by mammogram. There is an increased risk (1.5 to 4.0 times) of breast cancer in patients with papillomatosis. Multiple papillomas result in higher risk than single papillomas (28).

Atypical Proliferative Lesions

Atypical Lobular Hyperplasia

As with the other proliferative lesions of the breast, the principal reason for identifying and defining atypical hyperplasia is to define the risk of cancer development in a breast with these histologic features. Atypical hyperplasia is identified by similar features that characterize carcinoma-in-situ; however, the histologic changes in atypical hyperplasia are less abnormal than those in carcinoma-in-situ. For this reason, an understanding of the pathologic spectrum of atypical lobular hyperplasia (ALH) begins with the definition of lobular carcinoma-in-situ. Page and Simpson define lobular carcinoma-in-situ as "filling, distortion and distension of more than half of the acini of a lobular unit by a uniform population of characteristic cells" (16). The diagnosis of ALH thus requires that less than half of the acini are completely distended and/or less than half of the acini are filled by the uniform population of characteristic cells (16). This abnormality is associated with a four to five times increased incidence of the development of breast cancer compared with the normal population. A great enhancement in cancer risk is noted for patients who have atypical lobular or ductal hyperplasia and a positive family history. Approximately 20% of these patients develop invasive breast cancer within 15 years of the diagnosis of atypical hyperplasia (28).

Atypical Ductal Hyperplasia

As with the lobular variety, atypical ductal hyperplasia (ADH) is defined as an incomplete expression of the features of ductal carcinoma-in-situ. Page and Dupont (28) define ductal carcinoma-in-situ as two or more ductal spaces that are filled completely with a uniform population of neoplastic appearing cells; there also are intercellular bridges and arches composed of evenly placed, uniform cells (16). ADH has more variants in the histologic patterns of presentation and, therefore, is harder to recognize than ALH. Biopsies that demonstrate ADH often have areas of ductal carcinoma-in-situ, but there are also cells in the involved area that are histologically normal. The hyperplastic cells are oriented properly in regard to the basement membrane and they do not have nuclear abnormalities that are characteristic of the atypical cells (28). Florid epithelial hyperplasia can be confused with atypical ductal hyperplasia. The cancer risk for florid epithelial hyperplasia is much less (1.5 to 2.0 times index) than the risk of atypical ductal hyperplasia (4 to 5 times index).

Inflammatory Lesions

Abscess

Two major types of abscesses are recognized in the breast: periareolar (nonlactational) and puerperal (related to childbirth and breast-feeding). The relative incidence of these two abscesses has changed such that the periareolar variant is now more common than puerperal (29). Benson reports that the number of puerperal breast abscesses seen at the Leeds General Infirmary decreased from approximately 20 per year in 1975 to 5 or less per year in 1987 (29). The most plausible explanation for this change is the prompt recognition of mastitis in lactating women and early treatment with antibiotics. Puerperal mastitis develops in a breast segment when a major duct is obstructed with inspissated milk. The segment becomes engorged with milk, causing mastalgia, swelling, and redness. Bacteria thrive in the stagnant milk, producing a characteristic wedge-shaped abscess, with the base at the edge of the breast and the apex near the nipple. The evolution of the abscess can be aborted if the blocked duct is opened by suckling or if the patient receives antibiotics in early phases of the disease. For

this reason, breast feeding may be allowed to continue in patients with early mastitis as it prevents engorgement and promotes drainage. However, lactation frequently stops spontaneously in patients who develop a puerperal abscess (30). The bacteria commonly involved in puerperal abscess are skin organisms, so the drug of choice is a penicillinase-resistant penicillin. The differential diagnosis for breast abscess in a nonlactating woman includes chronic, recurring periareolar abscess, carcinoma, tuberculosis, inflammatory cysts, and duct ectasia (31). The most common of these disease states is the periareolar abscess. As discussed above, periareolar abscess is commonly associated with primary ductal disease in the lactiferous sinuses. Recurrent periareolar abscess is commonly associated with mammary duct fistula. The recurrence rate for periareolar abscess is 38% (30). The rate is higher once a periareolar abscess has recurred (32). Recurrence is commonly related to the persistence of a fistulous tract from the lactiferous sinuses to the periareolar skin. The tract remains open as a result of granulation tissue and provides a focus for contaminating bacteria to develop an abscess similar to a fistula-in-ano. The management of this problem requires excision of the fistula tract (Fig. 13.9). Table 13.5 contrasts the two major abscesses that commonly occur in the female breast.

Mondor's Disease

Mondor's disease is a nonsuppurative thrombophlebitis of the thoracoepigastric vein. This vein courses along the lateral segment of the breast where it may be exposed to trauma. This process is easy to recognize clinically as a long, linear, tender, cord-like mass located in the lateral anterior aspect of the breast. It is associated with erythema and inflammation. Heparin is not needed; the process is self-limited and resolves within 3 weeks. Heat compresses to the affected site and aspirin therapy are useful to alleviate symptoms.

Hormone Relationship to Benign Breast Disease

Fibrocystic breast disease is usually clinically recognizable before menarche; it ceases with menopause, re-

Table 13.5.
Breast Abscesses

	Puerperal Abscess	Duct Ectasia
Age	< 40 years	> 40 years
Cause	Blocked duct in lactating breast	Ectatic central ducts with inflammation
Location	Peripheral breast	Central breast
Organism	Staphylococcus aureus	Staphylococcus aureus Streptococcus Bacteroides enterococcus
Prognosis	Resolves after drainage	Chronic until ducts excised

Figure 13.9. **A,** Sagittal view of the breast with a periareolar abscess and nipple sinus. **B,** A probe is passed through the sinus tract between the abscess and the nipple. **C,** Extent of excision required to remove the infected sinus tract and correct the nipple inversion when present. **D,** primary closure over a Penrose drain or small Robinson catheter. From Maier WP. Peri areolar abscess in the nonlactating breast. Am J Surg 1982;144: 359–361. Reprinted by permission.

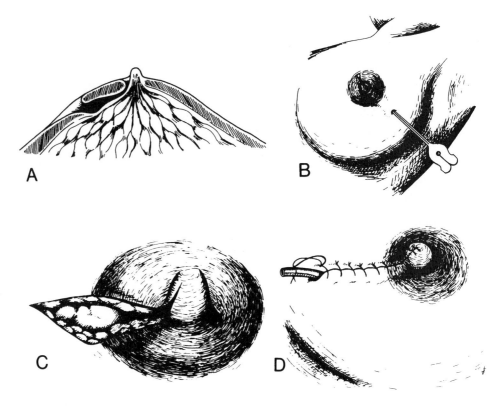

sumes with the institution of postmenopausal hormone replacement (estrogen), and can worsen with use of oral contraceptives. For these reasons, the lumpiness and pain associated with fibrocystic breast changes has been attributed to a hormonal abnormality. The proposed etiology of the entity includes an estrogen excess; progesterone insufficiency; and prolactin, thyroid hormone, or androgen alteration (33). The hyper estrogen theory has never been substantiated with documented increases in plasma or urinary estrogen levels (34). Likewise, a progesterone deficiency has never been established in patients with fibrocystic breast disease (35). Prolactin secretion has been evaluated in patients with benign breast disorders. Although absolute plasma levels are the same as those in normal controls, abnormalities in the chronobiology have also been identified (33). Nocturnal peak values and stimulated levels are higher in patients with fibrocystic changes than in controls (33). It may be that isolated measurements of plasma hormones do not adequately document the influence of sex hormones on the production and maintenance of fibrocystic changes. Tissue homogenates contain higher concentrations of sex steroids than plasma (36). Alterations in the metabolism of sex steroids in the breast microenvironment are possibly responsible for abnormalities seen in patients with proliferative and nonproliferative breast disease.

The Relationship of Silicone to Connective Tissue Disease

The Nurses Health Study cohort was used to evaluate the relationship between silicone breast implants and connective tissue diseases. Among 87,501 women who were eligible for follow up, 516 were confirmed as having definite connective tissue disease and 1,083 as having breast implants. Comparison of these two populations did not find an association between silicone breast implants and connective tissue diseases as defined by a variety of standardized criteria, signs or symptoms of these disease (37).

Gynecomastia

Enlargement of the male breast can occur in the normal course of development and with aging, without an apparent endogenous or exogenous cause. Gynecomastia before puberty is rare, so rare that its occurrence should prompt a search for an endocrinologically active tumor (adrenal or testicular) or enzyme deficiency (11-a-hydroxylase deficiency). The male breast is commonly enlarged in the neonatal period from the influence of placental estrogen. This enlargement regresses within 3 to 6 weeks of age. Puberty is a common time for the male breast to become enlarged and tender. In 60% to 70% of normal males, physiologic gynecomastia occurs within 1 year of the onset of testicular development. Gynecomastia most commonly begins between 12 and 25 years of age, resolves within 12 to 24 months, and is unusual after the age of 20 years (38,39). Breast enlargement and tenderness at the time of adolescence occurs secondary to an increase in serum estrogen relative to serum testosterone (40). Senescent gynecomastia may be a normal developmental occurrence in the elderly male. Niewoehner and Nutter (41) found an incidence of 65%, based on an autopsy study of 214 men. They concluded that palpable bilateral gynecomastia is present in most older men. Its presence correlates with body fat and does not require investigation, unless it is symptomatic, unilateral, or of recent onset. Breast enlargement with advancing age may occur for several reasons: *(a)* a relative decrease in serum total and free testosterone (42); *(b)* increase in serum luteinizing hormone; *(c)* maintenance of a normal serum estrogen; and *(d)* an increase in the conversion of androgen to estrogen by aromatization in peripheral fat stores (43).

Histologically, gynecomastia is composed of elongated major ducts that exhibit branching and proliferation of periductal fibroblastic stroma. In the normal male breast, no branching of the major ducts is evident when epithelial and stromal elements both enlarge proportionately. The ducts in gynecomastia appear to be lined by normal epithelium. Any benign histologic alteration that occurs in the female breast can also be found in the male, with exception of fibrocystic changes, which are extremely rare in the male (44). The increase in epithelial and stromal elements most likely occurs secondary to an increase in the estrogen:progesterone ratio. Prolactin does not seem to have a direct effect on the development of gynecomastia in males. Hyperprolactin states are not associated with gynecomastia. Serum prolactin levels in patients with gynecomastia are normal (45). Prolactin may have an indirect effect on gynecomastia in that it influences the estrogen:androgen ratio (46). Patients with gynecomastia do not have an increased risk for the development of breast cancer. Only Klinefelter's syndrome is associated clearly with an increased risk of breast cancer in the male (47).

The three principal nonphysiologic causes for gynecomastia are estrogen excess, androgen deficiency, and drug effect (40). Estrogen excess in males that results in gynecomastia can occur secondary to several different disorders. Excess estrogen from a gonadal source may occur in true hermaphroditism, germ cell tumors of the testes, and gonadal stromal tumors. The excess estrogen may be produced by nongonadal tumors. Of these, the most common are bronchogenic carcinoma, hepatocellular carcinoma, and adrenal neoplasms. Furthermore, gynecomastia can be associated with hyperthyroidism or hypothyroidism (48) and is most likely the result of an alteration in the metabolism of estrogen (49). Another common clinical cause for gynecomastia is liver disease, mediated by estrogen excess. Cirrhosis, from whatever cause, as well as hemachromatosis and fatty metamorphism may be responsible for this entity. Finally, starvation has also been associated with gynecomastia (50).

The second major nonphysiologic cause for gynecomastia is androgen deficiency. The clinical conditions associated with this mechanism are aging, primary testicular failure (Klinefelter's syndrome), secondary testic-

Table 13.6.
Drugs Associated with Gynecomastia

Drugs with Estrogenic or Estrogen Related Activity
Anabolic steroids (nandrolone, testosterone cypionate)
Clomiphene citrate
Diethylpropion hydrochloride
Diethylstilbestrol
Digitalis
Estrogens
Heroin
Oral contraceptives
Tetrahydrocannabinol (cannabis, marijuana)

Drugs that Inhibit the Action and/or Synthesis of Testosterone
Antineoplastic agents (vincristine, nitrosoureas, methotrexate)
Cimetidine
Cyproterone acetate
D-Penicillamine
Diazepam
Flutamide
Ketaconazole
Medroxyprogesterone acetate
Phenytoin
Spironolactone

Drugs that Enhance Estrogen Synthesis by the Testes
Human chorionic gonadotropin

Drugs with Idiopathic Mechanism for Induction of Gynecomastia	
Amiodarone	Methyldopa
Bumetanide	Nifedipine
Busulfan	Reserpine
Domperidone	Sulindac
Ethionamide	Theophylline
Furosemide	Tricyclic antidepressant
Isoniazid	Verapamil

ular failure (trauma, viral infection, irradiation, and chemotherapy), and renal failure.

The third major cause for nonphysiologic gynecomastia is drug related. A list of medications and hormones that are associated with breast enlargement is given in Table 13.6; these represent an ever-increasing etiologic cause of gynecomastia.

Malignant Clinical Disorders

Abnormal Cell Growth

The most exciting new areas of investigation with respect to breast science are the control (feedback) mechanisms for normal and abnormal cellular growth. These control mechanisms for human breast epithelium remain obscure despite intense work in laboratory animals and in cell culture systems. The regulation of normal growth probably involves hormones and polypeptide growth factors. Growth factors exert autocrine and paracrine effects. These include the stimulation of angiogenesis, stromal proliferation, chemotaxis, and degranulation of monocytes and neutrophils. These growth factors may initiate malignant cell transformation in mammary epithelium when they act in concert with other mitogenic factors, such as inherited genetic factors, chemical carcinogens, ionizing radiation, oncogenic viruses, and other promotional agents. The following discussion will summarize the facts that have been established reasonably or that seem important in the control of human mammary epithelial growth.

Risk Factors for the Development of Breast Cancer

The family history of a patient with suspected breast cancer has taken on new importance. The relative risk of a patient with a first degree relative with breast cancer is 1.5 to 2 times higher than the normal population. This risk is increased, however, if the patient has two affected first degree relatives. In this case, the risk could be 4 to 6 times that of the normal population; the risk is even higher if the relative had bilateral cancer (51). Kinetic factors contributed to an ill defined proportion of breast cancer which may be approximately 5% of all cases. However, the proportion of breast cancer diagnosed before the age of 30 which is related to genetic disorders may be as high as 25% (52). A mutation in one gene, BRCA1, is thought to account for approximately 45% of families with a significantly higher cancer incidence in at least 80% of families with an increased incidence of both early onset breast cancer and ovarian cancer (53). BRCA1 has been mapped and cloned. Hall located the gene to chromosome 17q in 1990 (54). BRCA1 was cloned by a group headed by Mark Skolinck at the University of Utah in 1994 (55). The BRCA1 gene encodes a tumor suppressor gene, which is a protein that acts as a negative regulator of cell growth. Patients with the BRCA1 gene have an extremely high risk of developing breast cancer. That risk exceeds 50% before the age of 50 and 80% by the age of 65 (56). A second gene, BRCA2, has been mapped to chromosome arm 13q (57).

Other risk factors are associated with breast cancer, but to a lesser degree than family history and BRCA1. Recent evidence implicates both alcohol ingestion (58) and fibroadenoma (59) as long-term risk factors.

Estrogen

Since 1980, 24 studies and 3 meta-analyses have failed to consistently demonstrate an increased risk of breast cancer among women who have ever used estrogen therapy (60). One of the largest studies to demonstrate an association between estrogen use and the development of breast cancer is the Nurses Health Study. These investigators also looked at the effect of adding progestins to estrogen therapy in postmenopausal women. They found that risk of breast cancer was increased significantly among women who were currently using estrogen only or estrogen plus progesterone as compared

to postmenopausal women who had never used hormones. This increase was most pronounced in women over the age of 55 and was limited largely to women who had used estrogen therapy for 5 or more years (61).

The profound influence of estrogen in breast development, growth, and maintenance was outlined previously. Because estrogen promotes and stimulates mammary epithelial proliferation and the differentiation of normal epithelium, this hormone contributes to the regulation of neoplastic growth as well. In fact, estrogens function as catalysts for the action of carcinogens in the breast. Women without functioning ovaries do not develop breast cancer. Estrogens act as true tumor promoters (62). Epidemiologic evidence exists for the tumor-promoter role of estrogen. Furthermore, the duration of mammary epithelial exposure to estrogen is proportional to breast cancer risk. Early menarche, late menopause, late age at first full-term pregnancy, and excessive body fat all increase estrogen exposure to enhance the risk for developing breast cancer.

Other evidence in support of a mitogenic role for estrogen is varied. Breast cancer occurs less commonly in men (1% of all breast cancers), oophorectomy before age 30 results in a 70% risk reduction, and dogs who have oophorectomy before the development of the estrus cycle develop breast cancer with less than 1% of the incidence for normal dogs (63). Further indirect evidence for a mitogenic effect for estrogen is that 33% of patients will experience a regression of their breast cancer after oophorectomy or after the initiation of antiestrogen therapy (tamoxifen). Approximately 66% of ER positive tumors will respond to these manipulations (63). Table 13.7 lists the mechanism through which estrogen might exert control on mammary cell growth. Estrogens may initiate the production of locally acting hormones that further influence (regulate) epithelial growth and development. These polypeptide growth factors are capable of initiating the cell cycle in epithelium that would otherwise be at rest (G_0). They may induce the production of other local hormones or growth factors that can induce oncogenes, specifically c-*fos*, c-*myc*, and c-*ras* (62). The specific growth factors that have an effect on mammary epithelium include platelet-derived growth factor (PDGF), epidermal-growth factor (EGF), transforming-growth factor (TGFa), insulin-like growth factor 1 (IGF-1), and somatomedin C. These growth factors will be discussed below.

Estrogen can also influence cell growth by increasing

Table 13.7.
Estrogen and Regulation of Cell Growth

1. Induction of growth factors production
2. Modulation of gene expression
3. Induction of enzymes responsible for DNA synthesis
4. Induction of progesterone receptor
5. Induction of plasminogen activators and collagenolytic enzymes
6. Induction of receptor binding protein for laminin

gene transcription, although the actual genes initiating these molecular events have not been identified. In cell culture, estrogen can induce the production of several enzymes and other proteins involved in nucleic acid synthesis. These include DNA polymerase, the c-*myc* oncogene, thymidine and uridine kinases, thymidylate synthetase, carbamoyl- phosphate synthetase, aspartate carbamoyltransferase, dihydro orotase, glucose 6-phosphate dehydrogenase, and dihydrofolate reductase (62).

Estrogen can also induce the production of the progesterone receptor (PR). The presence of the PR is an indication that the cell's growth is influenced by estrogen. The presence of the PR in breast tumor cells is an indicator of the probability that the tumor will respond to antiestrogen therapy (62). Estrogen also increases the synthesis of plasminogen activators and collagenolytic enzymes. These proteins may function to facilitate cellular invasiveness and, therefore, support cell metastasis. The exact role of these proteins in the regulation of mammary cell growth remains unclear (63). Another estrogen-induced receptor protein in the MCF-7 cell culture line is the receptor-binding protein for laminin. The laminin receptor mediates the attachment of the cells to basement membrane and facilitates the metastatic potential of the cell (62).

Growth Factors

The experimental evidence that locally acting growth factors may play a role in the regulation of normal and abnormal growth in mammary epithelium is new and exciting but thus far unsubstantiated in human studies. Lippman and Dickson (62) suggest that the complexity and variety of mammary growth modulators may provide multiple pathways by which breast cancer growth can be controlled. These include antiligand and antireceptor antibodies, receptor-blocking peptides, and drugs that alter the receptor-ligand interaction. The following growth factors have effects on experimental mammary epithelial cell growth.

Transforming Growth Factor a and Epidermal Growth Factor Families. Human breast cancer cells can produce TGFa. One such line is the MCF-7, which increases synthesis when exposed to estrogen. In addition, antibodies against TGFa or its receptor will retard growth of the MCF-7 cells in culture. Based on this observation, the hypothesis that TGFa is a promoter of breast cancer cell growth is being tested in a phase I clinical trial of anti-epidermal-growth factor (EGF) receptor antibody (62).

Transforming Growth Factor β. This polypeptide promotes differentiation and inhibits growth in most epithelial cells. Normal mammary epithelium stops growing in culture when exposed to TGFβ, and normal mammary duct development is inhibited by local application of TGFβ. This factor is found in human milk (62). Because its actions are antagonistic to those of the other

growth factors, TGFβ may be part of the normal hormonal balance that controls mammary growth. This inhibitory effect may be operative in breast cancer cells that secrete a TGFβ-like factor (60). The role of TGFβ in breast cancer is not yet known. TGFβ may participate in the growth-inhibitory effects of antiestrogen therapy.

Insulin-Like Growth Factor. Insulin-like growth factors 1 and 2, also called somatomedins, are produced by the majority of normal tissues. They are also found in blood and urine (62). In contrast to insulin, which is made only in the pancreas, IGF-1 and IGF-2 polypeptides are synthesized in nearly all organs, including the liver (62). The somatomedins differ from insulin in structure. Insulin has two, disulfide-linked chains, whereas the somatomedins have a single chain (62). IGF-1 is mitogenic for some cultured breast cancer cells. All human breast cancers make an IGF-1-related growth factor (64). And finally, human breast cancer cells in culture increase production of IGF-1 when exposed to estrogen and decrease production when treated with antiestrogens (62).

Platelet-Derived Growth Factor. High concentration of PDGF is found in platelets and in a diverse number of tumors (64). Several human breast cancer cell lines produce a factor with PDGF-related activity. PDGF mediates proliferation of stromal cells (65) and causes the release of prostaglandins I_2 and E_2 (66) to induce fibroblast proliferation, collagen secretion, and production of IGF-1 (67).

Fibroblast Growth Factor. Fibroblast growth factor (FGF) is required for growth of normal mouse mammary cells in culture (68). FGF stimulates neovascularization (69). Human breast cancer cells in culture produce an FGF-related polypeptide (70).

Other Growth Modulation. Many other hormones have growth regulatory activity in normal and malignant mammary cells. A pituitary-derived factor augments the mitogenic effects of estrogen on the MCF-7 human breast cancer cell line (71). Growth hormone-releasing factor from the pituitary may directly inhibit breast cancer cell growth in culture (72), and prolactin stimulates growth in some cell lines (73). Among the many molecules to affect growth of MCF-7 cells in culture, glucocorticoids, iodothyronines, androgens, and retinoids are stimulatory (62); progesterone, somatostatin, interleukins (1 and 6), tumor-necrosis factor, and interferon are inhibitory (62).

Environmental Factors

The environmental forces that are responsible for the large geographic variation in the incidence of breast cancer have not been elucidated. A fivefold difference exists in incidence among Japan (12.1 cases/100,000 women/year), England (54.5 cases/100,000/year), and the United States (57.2 cases/100,000/year) (74). This difference is substantially reduced in first-generation Japanese women raised in the United States (74). The incidence of breast cancer and mortality from the disease are higher in the upper socioeconomic groups (75). This effect of social status seems to be independent of the effects of reproduction factors. The early onset of menses and the early establishment of regular menses are associated with a two to three times increase in breast cancer risk (76). Other reproductive influences that are associated with a decreased risk include early age at the time of first birth, menopause before age 45, and high parity (76). Even though longer exposure to endogenous estrogen seems to be associated with an increased breast cancer risk, epidemiologic studies of patients exposed to exogenous estrogens (hormone replacement or birth control) have not found a significantly increased risk of breast cancer (63). Ionizing radiation increases the risk directly proportional to the dose and inversely proportional to the age at the time of exposure (77). Lactation and breast feeding have a controversial effect on cancer risk. If there is a benefit to breast feeding, it is minimal (78). Alcohol use, smoking and psychological stress have not been associated with an increased risk of breast cancer.

Flow Cytometry

Flow cytometry has been used to identify cancers that have a high likelihood of recurrence. This may be particularly useful in determining which patients with stage I (node negative) breast cancer are likely to develop a recurrence and, therefore, are most likely to benefit from adjuvant chemotherapy. Flow cytometry evaluates the DNA content of a population of cells (approximately 50,000 cells) from a tumor. The ploidy of the tumor is determined by the DNA content of tumor cells in G_0 phase relative to nonmalignant G_0 cells. Diploid tumors are those in which the stem line DNA content is not measurably different from nonmalignant reference cells. Aneuploid tumors are those whose stem line DNA content is altered. The DNA index is the numerical ratio of the mean DNA content of phase G_0 tumor cells to that of normal cells (79). Tumor proliferative activity or index is the percentage of cells in the S and G_2 phases combined (79). Analysis of old breast biopsy specimens by flow cytometry has been correlated with survival and tumor recurrence. Aneuploidy occurs more commonly in ER negative tumors, poorly differentiated tumors, and tumors with nuclear atypia (79). Tumors with a high proliferative index are more likely to be ER negative and poorly differentiated (79). Ewers et al. (80) evaluated 97 stage I and 140 node negative stage II patients. Only 3 of 98 (3%) patients with diploid tumors suffered a relapse at 16 months, whereas 20 of 139 (14%) patients with an aneuploid tumor had recurred. Kallioniemi et al (80) reported a 5-year survival of 95.5% for diploid stage I tumors and 80.2% for aneuploid tumors. In node positive disease, both ploidy and proliferative activity have been linked strongly to clinical outcome (79).

Estrogen Receptor

The ER protein must be present in a tissue, whether it is breast or some other organ, for estrogen to influence development and function. The presence of the ER in tumor cells has clinical implications that will be addressed later, but in general, ER positive tumor cells have retained some of the cell's regulatory mechanism present before the transformation to cancer. Normal breast epithelial cells have specific binding proteins for estrogen, progestins, glucocorticoid, and androgen. The estrogen receptor is most probably located in the nucleus (82) (Fig. 13.10). Three serum proteins bring the estrogen molecule to the target cell: albumin, testosterone-estradiol-binding globulin (TeBG), and corticosteroid-binding globulin (CBG). Estrogen is fat soluble and easily passes into the cell by simple diffusion. Once in the cell, estrogen binds with the receptor protein. The estrogen-ER complex is then incorporated into the nuclear matrix and chromatin (a process known as retention). After nuclear integration occurs, the specific gene affected by the estrogen is activated to produce the specific breast cell protein that characterizes the effect of estrogen on the cell. The exact mechanism by which the estrogen-ER complex interacts with the cell's nucleus is not known.

The clinical usefulness of the ER protein determination in breast tumors is well-established. The presence of the estrogen and progesterone receptors in a breast tumor predicts the effectiveness of hormonal therapy for that tumor. Approximately 53% of ER positive tumors respond to hormone therapy (Table 13.8), compared with only 6% of ER negative tumors (82). The presence of the progesterone receptor enhances the likelihood of hormonal response. The response rate for ER positive and PR positive tumors is 78%; for ER positive and PR negative tumors, 34%; for ER negative and PR negative tumors, 6%; and for ER negative and PR positive tumors, 45% (82). The ER status of male breast cancer also predicts the response to hormonal manipulation, in that 65% of ER positive male breast cancers will respond. A total of 90% of male breast tumors are ER positive; 50% are PR positive (83). Tissues from benign breast processes usually contain less than 10 fmol of ER (ER negative) for each milligram of protein. Wittliff et al. (82) report that 60% to 65% of female breast cancers are ER positive and that 45% to 55% of recurrent and metastatic tumors are ER positive. Approximately 45% to 60% of female breast cancers are PR positive. A study of the tumor registry from Portland Kaiser Permanente noted that between 1975 and 1985, ER negative cancer rose 22%, whereas ER positive tumors increased 131% in the same period (84).

The levels of ER protein in breast cancer vary between

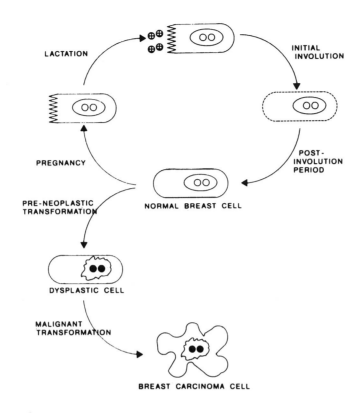

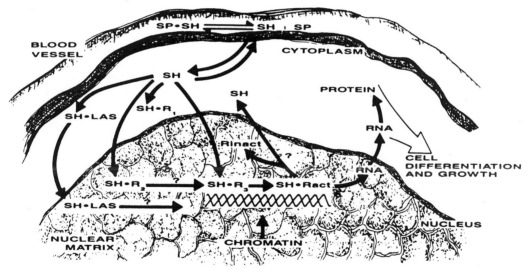

Figure 13.10. Schematic representation of hypothetical intracellular cascade of events following steroid receptor interaction with its receptor in a target cell. Steroid hormones (SH) normally circulate in the blood bound to albumin and certain specific serum proteins (SP) such as TeBG and CBG. As lipid molecules, steroids move across the cell membrane into the cytoplasm in a passive fashion and interact with their intracellular receptor proteins (R) in a reaction exhibiting high affinity and specificity. The exact location of the true receptor protein is unknown, but possibilities include association with the nuclear membrane (R_1), nuclear matrix (R_2), and chromatin (R_3). After association with the steroid, an apparent activation takes place that may involve phosphorylation. The activated steroid hormone-receptor (SHR_{act}) complex associates with acceptor sites in chromatin and stimulates synthesis of nucleic acids and, subsequently, proteins characteristic of the biologic response (differentiation and growth) to the specific steroid hormone. In addition, steroid hormones may be associated with low-affinity sites (LAS) whose subsequent pathway is uncertain. The details of these intranuclear events are presently unclear. However, the presence of the receptor protein in a cell appears to be a prerequisite for response to a steroid hormone stimulus. From Wittliff JL. Steroid receptor analyses, quality control, and clinical significance. In Donegan WL, Spratt JS, eds. Cancer of the breast. 3rd. ed. Philadelphia: WB Saunders. 1988:303–335. Reprinted by permission.

Table 13.8.
Relationship Between Estrogen Receptor Status of Breast Tumor and Patient's Objective Response to Endocrine Therapy

	Estrogen Receptor Status	
Investigator	Responses/ ER$^+$ Tumors	Responses/ ER$^-$ Tumors
Blamey et al.	13/30	5/27
Dao and Nemoto	64/119	4/56
DeSombre and Jensen	39/62	4/108
Maass et al.	64/93	3/76
Manni et al.	68/105	0/12
McCarty et al.	32/58	3/20
Nomura et al.	29/45	0/36
Osborne et al.	70/145	5/53
Paridaens et al.	14/38	0/11
Rubens and Hayward	46/146	5/55
Singhakowinta et al.	20/30	2/25
Skinner et al.	17/30	5/44
Wittliff	46/76	0/44
Total	522/977 (53%)	36/567 (6%)

0 and 6000 fmol/mg protein. No histologic characteristic exists that correlates with the ER level. The ER status of a tumor does not correlate with size, location, nodal status, or clinical stage. Various studies have demonstrated a slight correlation of ER status with several tumor characteristics, including histologic classification, nuclear grade, DNA ploidy, proliferative activity, and lymphocytic infiltration. However, not all authors are in agreement, and additional study is needed (82).

Estrogen receptor status correlates with age. The ER protein quantity is lower and less frequently positive in premenopausal than in postmenopausal women (85). The PR is also found less frequently in younger than older women (86). Tumors tend to lose the estrogen receptor with duration of the tumor and with recurrence (87). Synchronous tumors have a similar ER status 80% of the time (88). Because the ER status varies with the concentration of serum estrogen and progesterone, it follows that hormonal and cytotoxic therapy can alter the ER receptor assay by killing cells containing the receptor or by changing the number of binding sites. Tamoxifen or other hormone treatment should be stopped 3 weeks before a biopsy for the purpose of determining ER status. The ER protein is labile and undergoes degeneration in a warm environment (89,90). Studies on the half-life of ER degeneration have resulted in estimation that varies from 30 minutes to 6 hours. The specimen is best handled by freezing to -70°C within 30 minutes of removal. Although at least 200 mg of tumor should be frozen, 400 to 500 mg is optimal.

Oncogenes

The relationship of oncogenes to breast cancer is undefined. Oncogenes are mutated forms of genes (protooncogenes) that have been transformed from the DNA of host cells. Protooncogenes are most likely involved in the control of normal cell growth and differentiation. When altered in structure and/or function, the protooncogenes become oncogenes, which are thought to contribute to malignant cell transformation (91). Oncogene products that could contribute to carcinogenesis include nuclear proteins that act as transcriptional activators, transmembrane tyrosine kinases that function as growth factor receptors, intracellular serine kinase, tyrosine kinase, and membrane-bound G protein analogues. Overproduction of these proteins may allow the cells to grow more rapidly and develop invasive properties (91). Overproduction occurs through a process called amplification. Amplification is an activation of oncogenes resulting in an excess of DNA template, which leads to an overproduction of oncogene-specific RNA and protein. Amplification and oncogene overexpression have been correlated in certain tumors with aggressive behavior. The first oncogene alteration with clinical significance is the association of the oncogene N-*myc* with more aggressive neuroblastomas (92). Although research may confirm that oncogene amplifications may be a marker for poor prognosis in breast cancer, the evidence at this time does not support this conclusion. Jandrig (93) examined more than 1000 breast cancers for amplification of the oncogene c-*erb* 2. He concluded that the association of this oncogene with a poor prognosis is not convincing. However, Borst and Miller (94) reviewed evidence that oncogene amplification correlates with poor prognosis in breast cancer patients with positive axillary lymph nodes. Some studies have found a significant association between amplification of either c-*myc*, c-*erb* B2, or *int*-2 with a high risk for relapse or poor survival. Despite these reports, the status of oncogenes as outcome predictors continues to be debated (95).

The precise role of the oncogene proteins and the advantage bestowed on a cell as a result of oncogene amplification has not been established in molecular biology. All five oncogenes that have been implicated in breast cancer (*int*-2, c-*erb* B, c-*myc*, c-*Ha-ras*, and *Rb*1) have different cellular functions involving growth and differentiation. In cancers, these oncogenes change their function such that they may contribute to the malignant characteristics of the tumor. The c-*myc* oncogene is commonly rearranged, amplified, or both in human breast cancer (96). Animal data suggest that c-*myc* expression is related causally to the development of breast cancer. Oncogene c-*erb* B, which is analogous to the EGF receptor, is commonly overexpressed in ER negative tumors that portend a poor prognosis and high degree of invasiveness (97). Amplification and protein expression of c-*erb* B has been correlated with the number of positive lymph nodes (64). The *ras* family of oncogenes may contribute to malignant progression (98). Insertion of the v-*ras* H oncogene into MCF-7 cells increased the ability of the cells to invade the basement membrane (99) and increased the production of polypeptide growth factors (100). In spite of this experimental evidence, the precise

Table 13.9.
Steps in the Development of Metastatic Disease

Steps in Metastases	Rate-Limiting Event
1. Primary tumor growth	Angiogenesis
2. Invasion	Secretion of proteolytic enzymes
3. Survival in the circulation embolization	Evasion of host defenses
4. Arrest in organ sites	Specific adhesion to endothelium and basement membranes
5. Extravasation	Secretion of proteolytic enzymes motility factors
6. Growth in the organ environment	Organ-derived factors positive/negative growth regulation

role of oncogenes in any cancer, including the breast, remains conjectural.

Biology of Metastasis

The spread of a cancer from its primary site to distant organs is a complex cascade of incompletely understood biologic events. For a cancer cell to leave the tumor successfully and establish itself as a secondary growth, many stages in the process must be accomplished successfully in sequence. If the cell fails to accomplish any one of a number of the steps in the process of metastases, the cell will not survive. The events of metastases, as described by Price (101), are given in Table 13.9.

Breast tumors appear to be heterogenous populations of cells. Clones of cells from the same tumor have different phenotypes, including karyotype, proteolytic enzymes secreted, hormone receptors, and metastatic potential. Therefore, all cells of a tumor cell line will not have the necessary properties for successful metastasis. This is also important from the standpoint of tumor sampling. A small incisional biopsy may not accurately reflect biochemically or molecularly the entire tumor in terms of receptors, DNA ploidy, etc. And finally, Price points out that heterogeneity is important in terms of tumor kill. Even if a 99.9% kill rate is achieved in a 1 cm^3 tumor, there will be 10^6 residual viable cells to contribute to the viability of the cancer. The understanding of the events that contribute to successful metastasis are just beginning to be defined.

The initial event in metastases is the growth of the primary tumor. The breast cancer cells are able to secrete polypeptides with paracrine and autocrine effects that support growth. One of the most important of these events is angiogenesis. If the tumor is not able to stimulate the growth of new nutrient blood vessels, it will quickly outstrip its blood supply and die. Fibroblast growth factor stimulates angiogenesis (102). As the tumor grows, the next step is invasion of the surrounding stroma and entry into the circulation via blood vessels and lymphatics. This process is facilitated by the secretion of lytic enzymes from the tumor cells. Enzymes produced by human breast cancer cells that could augment local invasion as the tumor grows include such factors as cathepsin D, cathepsin B, plasminogen activator, collagenase, and heparinase (101). The fact that any given tumor secretes these enzymes is not necessarily a

marker for metastatic potential. Some tumors, such as basal cell carcinoma, secrete proteolytic enzymes but have a low incidence of metastasis. This emphasizes the need for a metastatic cancer cell to meet multiple requirements to be successful. In a similar way, mere entry into the bloodstream does not guarantee an established metastasis. In fact, few cells survive hematogenous invasion. Less than 1% of radiolabeled cells placed into the circulation survive for 24 hours, and less than 0.1% become established metastasis (103).

Once the cells are in the blood, several other steps must be accomplished. Cells are destroyed in the circulation by trauma and by activated macrophages. Survival of tumor cells in the blood of the host is enhanced by aggregation of tumor cells into clumps and the specific ability of individual tumor cells to adhere to and penetrate the endothelium (101). The number of tumor emboli entering the blood and the lymphatic systems correlates with the size of the tumor, its duration, and the degree of necrosis and hemorrhage (102).

Once in the lymphatics, the cells pass to regional lymph nodes. In 1894, Halsted (105) described his rationale for the radical mastectomy with his initial report of a remarkably low 6% local recurrence rate at a 2-year follow-up. He thought that hematogenous spread of breast cancer did not occur, but rather the cancer spread by direct extension through the lymphatics (105). He believed that the lymph nodes were actual filters that prevented more distant spread of the disease until they were packed with cancer themselves.

The concept of lymph nodes as barriers to the spread of cancer has been challenged by several pieces of evidence. First, tumor cells can pass directly through lymphatics without nodal arrest when placed into distal lymphatic channels of experimental animals (106). Second, in humans, more proximal lymph node groups may harbor metastatic deposits without evident disease in the more distal groups, indicating that tumor cells can traverse lymph nodes without arrest (107). And finally, National Surgical Adjuvant Breast Project (NSABP) trial B-04 included a subset of patients who did not have an axillary dissection. The other groups in the trial that had an axillary dissection had positive nodes in approximately 30% of the patients. Because the trial was randomized prospectively, it is valid to assume that 30% of the patients in the group that did not have an axillary dissection also had positive nodes. The survival for all patients in this trial is identical in more than 10 years of follow-up (108). Therefore, it does not appear controvertible that positive lymph nodes serve as the source of systemic failure in patients with breast cancer. Based on the NSABP results, the role of the lymph node in breast cancer has been redefined. Instead of barriers to systemic spread of the disease, the nodes most likely serve a role in immunomodulation of the cancer.

Once the neoplastic cells enter the circulation, the next step toward establishment of the successful metastasis is arrest in organ sites. Breast cancer has preference for lung, liver, bone, soft tissue, and brain. These sites are more receptive to breast cancer cell growth because of the presence of a favorable milieu. This idea was called the *soil and seed* theory by Paget (109) in 1889. This theory that cancer cells only grow in organs that are favorable is supported by the recent use of the peritoneovenous shunt in patients with malignant ascites. These patients receive a direct infusion of tumor cell-rich ascitic fluid into the superior vena cava, yet they do not support the growth of these metastatic lesions in every organ (110).

The influences that could contribute to a favorable environment for tumor growth include the ability of the tumor cell to adhere to the capillary endothelium of the organ, the secretion of proteolytic enzymes by either the organ or the tumor cell to enhance the movement of tumor cells into the stroma of the organ, and organ-derived growth-modulating factors. Such local factors most likely control growth and development of the organ as well as tissue repair and, therefore, may enhance growth of the tumor cell (101). It is these differences in the local environment that explain the predilection of ER positive, slow-growing breast metastasis for bone and the tendency for ER negative, fast-growing metastasis to adhere and proliferate in viscera. The polypeptides that have been isolated from some human breast cancers and that could participate in the modulation of metastatic cell growth include TGF, IGF-1 TGFa, and FGF (101).

Chemotherapy

Cytotoxic therapy for node negative disease has evolved from the anatomic, pharmacologic, and molecular biologic considerations for the treatment of breast cancer. The Halstedian view of cancer dissemination by direct extension has been replaced by Fisher's alternative hypothesis that the disease is a systemic one from the beginning (111). This hypothesis attempts to account for systemic failure, which occurs in 25% of node negative patients within 10 years. Clinical evidence suggests that these systemic failures result from established metastases that were present as occult foci at the time of the operation. Systemic disease does not commonly result from showering of tumor cells to the periphery with

tumor manipulation (112). Therefore, perioperative chemotherapy does not address systemic metastasis in the same manner that prophylactic antibiotics address postoperative infection. Even though operative manipulation may initiate systemic spread of cancer cells, early systemic treatment (i.e., before nodal spread) is justified for other reasons. A greater probability of tumor kill exists in smaller tumors, which have, on a percentage basis, a relatively larger volume of mitotically active cells than do large tumors (113).

Another justification for early therapy is the relative infrequency of chemoresistant strains in smaller tumors; consequently, a larger tumor volume would escape kill. Spontaneous mutations occur with neoplastic growth, and larger tumors are more heterogeneous and are more likely to contain one or more drug-resistant subpopulations. Several clinical trials, including the initial NSABP trial, B-01, have demonstrated the clinical uselessness of single-agent chemotherapy (114). NSABP B-01 randomized 826 women after Halsted's radical mastectomy to either adjuvant chemotherapy with thiotepa for 6 months or placebo. No difference in overall survival was observed, but premenopausal women with more than four positive nodes benefited from the chemotherapy (115). Subsequent multidrug trials have confirmed this beneficial effect for premenopausal women with positive lymph nodes at the time of presentation. Adjuvant chemotherapy is less effective for postmenopausal women. This may be related to the greater tumor cell heterogeneity seen in older women, the medical oophorectomy that results from chemotherapy in the premenopausal patient, or the inability of older women to tolerate intense cytotoxic treatment regimens (112).

After demonstration of the efficacy of chemotherapy for premenopausal, node positive patients in several different trials, the possibility of enhancing disease-free survival and overall survival in node negative patients has been evaluated (116). This question was prompted by the high disease recurrence rate in stage I breast cancer and by the demonstrated success of chemotherapy in stage II patients. For instance, in NSABP trial B-06, the tumor recurrence rate was higher in the node negative patients who did *not* receive chemotherapy than in the node positive patients who were treated with melphalan and 5- fluorouracil (117). Three studies of adjuvant chemotherapy have been reported early in their course because of possible positive results. An Intergroup Study and NSABP B-13 and B-14 all have suggested an increase in disease-free survival but no increase in overall survival with various regimens in node negative patients (116,117,118). The treatment-related morbidity and mortality varied with the chemotherapeutic regimen. As these studies approach maturity, the greatest interest will be the subset of node negative patients who are more likely to benefit from adjuvant chemotherapy. Fisher and others (120) have evaluated 950 node negative patients from NSABP B-06 in an attempt to define pretreatment parameters that might predict recurrence. They noted that studies using DNA ploidy, proliferative activity reflected by S phase or thymidine tumor labeling, epidermal growth factor receptor, and *erb* 2 oncogene expression have given inconsistent results. Of the 26 parameters examined, Fisher et al. report that only three correlated with tumor recurrence. These were histologic type, nuclear grade, and race of the patient. Patients with mucinous, tubular, or papillary cancer survived longer than those with typical ductal adenocarcinoma or atypical medullary tumors. Blacks had significantly higher recurrence than whites, but the number of blacks in the study was small. There were 276 paraffin blocks available for flow cytometry. DNA ploidy correlated with nuclear grade but not with survival. In addition, 183 tumors were evaluated for immunohistochemical demonstration of *erb* B2 expression. The authors did note that *erb* B2 expression accurately predicted survival among patients with good nuclear grade.

The duration of adjuvant chemotherapy has been addressed by several studies that have given the same regimen of drugs over different periods of time. Five separate randomized trials seem to support the conclusion that there is little benefit to a course of treatment longer than 6 months (112).

At this time, standard chemotherapy regimens have been defined for certain subsets of breast cancer patients. Carbone (121) summarized the results of 61 trials involving approximately 29,000 women. Results indicate that chemotherapy is effective for premenopausal, node positive (stage II) women with both ER positive and ER negative tumors. Chemotherapy has not been universally effective in postmenopausal patients, with the possible exception of those with ER negative tumors. For postmenopausal patients, the only standard regimen, as outlined by the 1985 Consensus Development Conference on Adjuvant Chemotherapy of Breast Cancer (122), is the use of tamoxifen in stage II, ER positive patients. Node negative, ER negative postmenopausal patients have had an increase in disease-free survival but not overall survival with adjuvant chemotherapy. Tamoxifen may also be added to the regimen of these patients in lieu of, but not in addition to, chemotherapy.

The addition of tamoxifen to chemotherapy does not enhance the effectiveness of the chemotherapy (114). Node positive, ER negative postmenopausal patients have no defined, standard therapy. For stage III disease, combination chemotherapy containing doxorubicin followed by operation and radiation therapy is commonly used (123).

Histologic Types of Breast Cancer

Approximately 85% of breast cancers comprise a group that is identified histologically as invasive ductal adenocarcinoma. More recently, this common histologic type has been called not otherwise specified (NOS) to distinguish it from the less frequent histologic variants with more distinctive histologic characteristics. Those types and their frequency of occurrence are medullary (6%), colloid (2%), Paget's disease (2%), tubular (< 2%), papillary (< 2%), adenoid cystic (< 0.1%), apocrine (< 0.1%), secretory (< 0.1%), and infiltrating lobular carcinoma (5 to 10%). Up to 33% of the invasive ductal adenocarcinomas can be mixed with one or more of the distinct histologic types. A small focus of a histologic subtype within a dominant pattern of NOS does not alter the prognosis. Mixed tumors with a dominant NOS pattern clinically behave as invasive ductal adenocarcinoma. Most of these tumors are moderately to poorly differentiated (Table 13.10).

Paget's disease presents as a crusting erosion of the nipple. It can also be less subtle, presenting with thickening, redness or roughness of the nipple often associated with itching and burning. The histologic diagnosis depends on the presence of the Pagetoid cell in the epithelium. This cell is clear with a large vesicular nucleus and prominent nucleoli (124). The cell can be identified immunohistochemically with carcinoembryonic antigen (CEA) stain. The origins of these cells are controversial; two leading theories are migration of the cells into the epithelium from the tumor and cellular transformation as a result of metaplastic change within the epithelium. This entity is nearly always associated with subareolar invasive or intraductal cancer. In approximately 60% of patients, the associated cancer can be felt on examina-

Table 13.10.
Comparison of Histological Types and Outcome

Histologic Type	Infiltrating Duct Carcinoma	Infiltrating Lobular Carcinoma	Medullary Carcinoma	Mucinous Carcinoma	Papillary Carcinoma
Node Involvement	60%	60%	44%	32%	17%
Crude survival					
5 years	54%	50%	63%	73%	83%
10 years	38%	32%	50%	59%	56%
Actuarial Survival					
5 years	59%	57%	69%	75%	89%
10 years	47%	42%	68%	72%	65%
20 years	38%	34%	62%	62%	65%

tion as a distinct breast mass. Survival with Paget's depends on the stage of the accompanying breast cancer.

Medullary cancer of the breast is bilateral in approximately 20% of patients. This histologic type has one of the fastest growth rates of any breast cancer. Less than 10% of these tumors are ER and PR positive. Approximately 50% are associated with a prominent intraductal component. Despite these characteristics, medullary cancer has a better prognosis than NOS. The gross appearance is softer and bulkier than the usual breast cancer, and it usually presents with a circumscribed, distinct capsule. Cyst formation and hemorrhagic necrosis are common. Microscopically, the tumor contains a dense infiltrate of lymphocytes and plasma cells throughout a uniform, sheet-like growth of large cells with pleomorphic nuclei and frequent mitoses (124).

Tubular cancer is common in younger patients; this tumor is often small (< 1 cm) and has an excellent prognosis because most patients are node negative at presentation (> 90% are stage I) (125). Microscopically, this tumor is characterized by a haphazard array of randomly arranged tubular structures. The important distinguishing histologic feature of this cancer is a single cell layer within the tubular architecture with absence of the basement membrane or myoepithelial cells. This pattern must be present in more than 75% of the tumor to be classified as a tubular cancer.

Colloid cancer is also called mucinous cancer because the cells produce large quantities of mucin pools around the cells. This produces a gelatinous surface on gross inspection. Two-thirds of these tumors are ER positive. This histologic type has a highly favorable prognosis.

Papillary cancer is identified by distinctive, well-defined fibrovascular stalks covered with multilayered epithelium (126). This tumor is associated with a more favorable prognosis than NOS, even when positive nodes are evident (124).

Adenoid cystic cancer is rare in its pure form. The histologic features of this tumor are identical to those of the salivary gland cancer that bears the same name. Axillary metastases are rare, but pulmonary metastasis has been described (127,128).

Apocrine cancer of the breast is exceedingly rare. The histology resembles that of the apocrine glands common to the axillary, anogenital, and groin regions. This can be an aggressive tumor.

Secretory cancer is the most common histologic variant of breast cancer that occurs in children. Metastatic disease is unusual, and local excision is recommended in most cases.

Infiltrating lobular carcinoma is bilateral in at least one-third of patients. It also has a high incidence of multicentricity in the ipsilateral breast. This tumor may produce intracytoplasmic mucin such that some cells have a signet ring-like appearance. Signet ring metastatic deposits can be distinguished from gut tumors with an ER stain. This neoplasm commonly metastasizes to the meninges and serosal surfaces (peritoneum and pleura). The prognosis is similar to the NOS variant.

Grading systems have been described in an effort to classify tumors with reference to the degree of variation from normal histologic patterns. Tumors are graded for nuclear appearance (129) and architectural organization (130). Nuclear grading segregates tumors according to differentiation (124). A well-differentiated tumor has small, uniform round nuclei with few nucleoli and mitoses. Moderately differentiated tumors have an increase in nuclear size, pleomorphism, and chromatin variability. Mitoses are frequent; nucleoli are large and irregular. Poorly differentiated tumors have large nuclei with variable chromatin patterns, prominent nucleoli and frequent, often bizarre, mitotic figures. The architectural grading system is a description of the degree of organization of the tubular-acinar unit (124). Well-differentiated tumors have a prominent tubular pattern. Moderately differentiated tumors have identifiable tubular structures arranged in small groups, nests, or cords. Poorly differentiated tumors have absence of tubular structures, as the cells tend to grow in sheets.

Factors That Predict the Likelihood of Tumor Recurrence

A positive margin is not a good predictor of tumor recurrence (131). The most reliable predictors of tumor recurrence are the size of the primary tumor and the nodal status.

Male Breast Cancer

Breast cancer is an uncommon disease in males. Only 1% of all breast cancers occur in this gender. No clearly defined relationship of gynecomastia to breast cancer exists. Microscopic gynecomastia is so common in older men that it is frequently found in association with cancer. However, no evidence exists to support the concept of a malignant progression from gynecomastia to breast cancer. Hormonal factors may be important, however, in that Klinefelter's syndrome is 20 times more common in male breast cancer patients than the normal population (132). In addition, mumps orchitis in men older than 20 years increases the risk of breast cancer.

Male breast cancer is highly responsive to hormonal therapy. More than 80% of male breast carcinomas are ER positive (133). Approximately 50% of patients respond to hormone manipulation. Orchiectomy, tamoxifen, and aminoglutethimide have been used effectively in therapy, but further study is needed to define optimum hormonal management (134,135). Chemotherapy has been less effective, producing objective responses in approximately 35% of patients with either the Cooper five-drug or doxorubicin-containing combination (136). Despite this hormone responsiveness, the relationship of male breast cancer to estrogen production and sensitivity has not been defined. Studies linking the cancer to hyperestrogenism have not been substantiated (137).

Approximately 85% of male breast cancer is ductal adenocarcinoma; 5% is papillary. Lobular, tubular, and colloid patterns are rare. Paget's disease may occur in males with a presentation and prognosis that are similar to females.

REFERENCES

1. Bland KI, Romrell L. Congenital and acquired disturbances of breast development and growth. In: Bland KI, Copeland EM, eds. The breast: comprehensive management of benign and malignant diseases. Philadelphia: WB Saunders, 1991:69–86.
2. Vorherr H. The breast: morphology, physiology and lactation. New York: Academic Press, 1974.
3. Romrell L, Bland KI. Anatomy of the breast, axilla, chest wall and related metastatic sites. In: Bland KI, Copeland EM, eds. The breast: comprehensive management of benign and malignant diseases. Philadelphia: WB Saunders, 1991:17–35.
4. Keller-Wood M, Bland KI. Breast physiology in normal, lactating and diseased states. In: Bland KI, Copeland EM, eds. The breast: comprehensive management of benign and malignant diseases. Philadelphia: WB Saunders, 1991:36–67.
5. Devitt, JE. Clinical benign disorders of the breast and carcinoma of the breast. Surg Gynecol Obstet 1981;152:437–440.
6. Foote FW, Stewart FW. Comparative studies of cancerous versus noncancerous breasts. I. Basic morphologic characteristics. II. Role of so-called chronic cystic mastitis in mammary carcinogenesis; influences of certain hormones on human breast structure. Ann Surg 1945;121:6–53,197–222.
7. Love SM, Gelman RS, Silen W. Fibrocystic disease of the breast—a nondisease? N Engl J Med 1982;307:1010–1014.
8. Consensus meeting convened by the Cancer Committee of the College of American Pathologists. Is 'fibrocystic disease' of the breast precancerous? Arch Pathol Lab Med 1986;110:171–173.
9. Davies HH, Simons M, Davis JB. Cystic disease of the breast. Relationship to carcinoma. Cancer 1964;17:757–765.
10. Bundred NJ, Walker RA, Miller WA. An immunohistochemical study of the tissue distribution of the breast cyst fluid protein zinc alpha 2 glycoprotein. Histopathology 1987;11:603–610.
11. Hughes LE, Bundred NJ. Breast macrocysts. World J Surg 1989; 13:711–714.
12. Haagensen CD. Diseases of the breast. Philadelphia: WB Saunders, 1986.
13. Jones BM, Bradbeer JW. The presentation and progress of macroscopic breast cysts. Br J Surg 1980;67:669–671.
14. Harrington E, Lesnick G. The association between gross cysts of the breasts and breast cancer. Breast 1987;7:13.
15. Dixon JM. Periductal mastitis/duct ectasia. World J Surg 1989; 13:715–720.
16. Page DL, Simpson JF. Benign, high risk and premalignant lesions of the mamma. In: Bland KI, Copeland EM, eds. The breast: comprehensive management of benign and malignant diseases. Philadelphia: WB Saunders, 1991:113–134.
17. Ennis JT. Diagnostic radiological imaging for breast disease. In: Bland KI, Copeland EM, eds. The breast: comprehensive management of benign and malignant diseases. Philadelphia: WB Saunders, 1991:426–468.
18. Dent DM, Cart PJ. Fibroadenoma. World J Surg 1989;13:706–710.
19. Reddick RL, Shin TK, Saivhney D, et al. Stromal proliferation of the breast: an ultrastructural and immunohistochemical evaluation of cystosarcoma phyllodes, juvenile fibroadenoma. Hum Pathol 1987;18:45–49.
20. Kutten F, Fournier S, Durand JC, et al. Estradiol and progesterone receptors in human breast fibroadenomas. J Clin Endocrinol Metab 1981;52:1225–1229.
21. Foster ME, Garrahan N, Willams S. Fibroadenoma of the breast: a clinical and pathological study. J R Coll Surg Edinb 1988;333: 16.
22. Kern WH, Clark RW. Retrogression of fibroadenomas of the breast. Am J Surg 1973;126:59–62.
23. Dupont WD, Page DL, Parl FF, et al. Long-term risk of breast cancer in women with fibroadenoma. N Engl J Med 1994;331: 10–15.
24. Pick PW, Iossifedes IA. Occurrence of breast carcinoma within a fibroadenoma. A review. Arch Pathol Lab Med 1984;108:590–594.
25. Ozella LV, Gump FE. The management of patients with carcinomas in fibroadenomatous tumors of the breast. Surg Gynecol Obstet 1985;160:99–104.
26. Preece PE. Sclerosing adenosis. World J Surg 1989;13:721–725.
27. Souba WW. Evaluation and treatment of benign breast disorders. In: Bland KI, Copeland EM, eds. The breast: comprehensive management of benign and malignant diseases. Philadelphia: WB Saunders, 1991:715–729.
28. Page DL, Dupont WD. Anatomic markers of human pre-malignancy and risk of breast cancer. Cancer 1990;66:1326–1335.
29. Benson EA. Management of breast abscess. World J Surg 1989; 13:753–756.
30. Benson EA, Goodman MA. An evaluation of the use of stilbestrol and antibiotics in the early management of acute puerperal breast abscess. Br J Surg 1970;57:255–258.
31. Bland KI. Inflammatory, infectious and metabolic disorders of the mamma. In: Bland KI, Copeland EM, eds. The breast: comprehensive management of benign and malignant diseases. Philadelphia: WB Saunders, 1991:87–112.
32. Watt-Boolsen S, Rasmussen NR, Blechent-Toft M. Primary periareolar abscess in the non-lactating breast: risk of recurrence. Am J Surg 1987;153:571–573.
33. Dogliotti L, Orlardi F, Angeli A. The endocrine basis of benign breast disorders. World J Surg 1989;13:674–679.
34. England PC, Skinner LG, Cottrell KR, et al. Sex hormones in breast disease. Br J Surg 1975;62:806–809.
35. Walsh P, Bulbrook RD, Stell PM, et al. Serum progesterone concentration during the luteal phase in women with benign breast disease. Eur J Cancer Clin Oncol 1984;20:1339–1343.
36. Vermeulen A, Deslypere JP, Paridaena R. Steroid dynamics in the normal and carcinomatous mammary gland. J Steroid Biochem Mol Biol 1986;25:799–802.
37. Sanchez-Guerreo J, Colditz GA, Karlson EW, et al. Silicone breast implants and the risk of connective-tissue diseases and symptoms. N Engl J Med 1995;332:1666–1670.
38. Schydlower M. Breast masses in adolescents. Am Fam Physician 1982;25(2):141–145.
39. Carlson HE. Gynecomastia. N Engl J Med 1981;303:795–799.
40. Bland KI, Page DL. Gynecomastia. In: Bland KI, Copeland EM, eds. The breast: comprehensive management of benign and malignant diseases. Philadelphia: WB Saunders, 1991:135–168.
41. Niewoehner CB, Nutter FQ. Gynecomastia in a hospitalized male patient. Am J Med 1984;77(4):633–638.
42. Rubens R, Dhont M, Vermeulen A. Further studies on Leydig cell function in old age. J Clin Endocrinol Metab 1974;39:40–45.
43. Siiteri PK, Macdonald PC. Role extraglandular estrogen in human endocrinology. In: Greep RO, Aswood, eds. Handbook of physiology. Vol. 2. Baltimore: Waverly Press, 1973;7(1).
44. Biagotti G, Kasznica J. Sclerosing adenosis in the breast of a man with pulmonary oat cell carcinoma. Hum Pathol 1986;17:861–863.
45. Turkington RW. Serum prolactin levels in patients with gynecomastia. J Clin Endocrinol Metab 1972;34:62–66.
46. Franks S, Jacobs HS, Martin N, et al. Hyperprolactinemia and impotence. Clin Endocrinol 1978;8:277–287.
47. Schieke O, Visfeldt J, Peterson B. Male breast cancer. 3. Breast carcinoma in association with the Klinefelter's syndrome. Acta Pathol Microbid Seard [A] 1949;81:352–358.
48. Hall PW. Gynecomastia monographs of the Federal Council of the British Medical Association in Australia 1959;2.
49. Chopera IJ, Tulchinsky D. Status of estrogen-androgen balance in hyperthyroid men with Graves disease. J Clin Endocrinol Metab 1974;38:269–277.
50. Jacobs EC. Effects of starvation on sex hormones in the male. J Clin Endocrinol Metab 1948;8:227–232.
51. Harris JR, Lippman ME, Veronesi U, et al. Breast cancer (first of three parts). N Engl J Med 1992;327:319–328.
52. Claus EB, Risch N, Thompson WD. Genetic analysis of breast cancer in cancer and steroid hormone study. Am J Human Gen 1991;48:232–242.
53. Easton DF, Bishop DT, Ford D, et al. Genetic linkage analysis in familial breast and ovarian cancer: Results from 214 families. The Breast Cancer Linkage Consortium. Am J Human Gen 1993;52: 678–701.

54. Hall JM, Lee MK, Newman B, et al. Linkage of early-onset familial breast cancer to chromosome 17q21. Science 1990;250:1684–1689.

55. Miki Y, Swensen J, Shattuck-Eidens D, et al. A strong candidate for the breast and ovarian cancer susceptibility gene BRCA1. Science 1994;266:66–71.

56. King M, Rowell S, Love SM. Inherited breast and ovarian cancer. What are the risks? What are the choices? JAMA 1993;269:1975–1980.

57. Wooster R, Neuhausen SL, Mangion J, et al. Localization of a breast cancer susceptibility gene, BRCA2, to chromosome 13q12-13. Science 1994;265:2088–2090.

58. Graham S. Alcohol and breast cancer. N Engl J Med 1987;1211–1212.

59. Dupont WD, DL Page, Parl FF, et al. Long-term risk of breast cancer in women with fibroadenoma. N Engl J Med 1994; 10–15.

60. Cobleigh MA, Berris RF, Bush T, et al. Estrogen replacement therapy in breast cancer survivors. A time for change. JAMA 1994; 272:540–545.

61. Colditz GA, Hankinson SE, Hunter DJ, et al. The use of estrogens and progestins and the risk of breast cancer in postmenopausal women. N Engl J Med 1995;332:1589–1593.

62. Lippman ME, Dickson RB. Mitogenic regulation of normal and malignant breast epithelium. Yale J Biol Med 1989;62:459–480.

63. Davidson NE, Lippman ME. The role of estrogens in the growth regulation of breast cancer. Crit Rev Oncog 1989;1:89.

64. Dickson RB, Lippman ME. Growth regulation of normal and malignant breast epithelium. In: Bland KI, Copeland EM, eds. The breast: comprehensive management of benign and malignant diseases. Philadelphia: WB Saunders, 1991:363–394.

65. Coffey RJ, Kost LJ, Lyons RM, et al. Hepatic processing of transforming growth factor β in the rat. J Clin Invest 1987;80:705–757.

66. Keating MT, Lewis LT. Autocrine stimulation of intracellular PDGF receptors in v-sis-transformed cells. Science 1988;239:914–916.

67. Clemmons DR, Shaw DS. Variables controlling somatomedin production by cultured human fibroblasts. J Cell Physiol 1983;115:137–143.

68. Hammond SL, Ham RG, Stampfer MR. Serum-free growth of human mammary epithelial cells rapid clonal growth in defined medium and extended serial passage with pituitary extract. Proc Natl Acad Sci U S A 1984;81:5435–5439.

69. Thomas KA, Rios-Comdelloves M, Gremenez-Gallego G, et al. Pure brain-derived acidic fibroblast growth factor is a potent angiogenic vascular endothelial cell mitogen with sequence homology to interlukin I. Proc Natl Acad Sci U S A 1985;82:6409–6423.

70. Halper J, Moses HL. Purification and characterization of a novel transforming growth factor. Cancer Res 1987;47:4552–4559.

71. Dembinski TC, Leung CHK, Shiu RPC. Evidence for a novel pituitary factor that potentiates the mitogenic effect of estrogen in human breast cancer cells. Cancer Res 1985;45:3038–3089.

72. Edne KA, Flanagan CA, Miller RP. Gonadotropin-releasing hormone binding sites in human breast carcinoma. Science 1985;229:989–991.

73. Biswas R, Vonderhaar BK. Role of serum in the prolactin responsiveness of MCF-7 human breast cancer cells in long-term tissue culture. Cancer Res 1987;47:3509–3514.

74. Mant D, Vessey MP. Epidemiology of breast cancer. In: Bland KI, Copeland EM, eds. The breast: comprehensive management of benign and malignant diseases. Philadelphia: WB Saunders, 1991:235–261.

75. Logan WPD. Cancer mortality by occupation and social class 1851–1971. IARC Scientific Publication No 36/OPCS Series SMPS No 44. London: HMSO, 1982.

76. Henderson BE, Pike MC, Casagrande JT. Breast cancer and the oestrogen window hypothesis. Lancet 1981;2:363–364.

77. Howe GR. Epidemiology of radiogenic breast cancer. Prog Cancer Red Ther 1984;26:119–129.

78. McTiernan A, Thomas DB. Evidence for a protective effect of lactation on the risk of breast cancer in young women. Am J Epidemiol 1986;124(3):353–358.

79. Merkel DE, McGuire WL. Ploidy, proliferative activity and prognosis. Cancer 1990;65:1194–1205.

80. Ewers SB, Langstrom E, Baldetorpe B, et al. Flow cytometric DNA analysis in primary breast carcinoma and clinico-pathological correlations. Cytometry 1984;5:408–419.

81. Kallioniemi OP, Blanco G, Alavaikko M, et al. Tumor DNA ploidy as an independent prognostic factor in breast cancer. Br J Cancer 1987;56:637–642.

82. Wittliff JL, Pasic R, Bland KI. Steroid and peptide hormone receptors identified in breast tissue. In: Bland KI, Copeland EM, eds. The breast: comprehensive management of benign and malignant diseases. Philadelphia: WB Saunders, 1991:900–936.

83. Everson RB, Lippman ME, Thompson EB, et al. Clinical correlations of steroid receptors and male breast cancer. Cancer Res 1980;40:991–997.

84. Glass AG, Hoover RM. Rising incidence of breast cancer: relationship to stage and receptor status. J Natl Cancer Inst 1990;82:693–696.

85. Bland KI, Fuchs A, Wittliff JL. Menopausal status as a factor in the distribution of estrogen and progesterone receptors in breast cancer. Surg Forum 1981;32:410–412.

86. Alghanem AA, Hussain S. The effect of age on estrogen and progesterone receptor in primary breast cancer. J Surg Oncol 1985;30:29–32.

87. NIH Consensus Development Conference on steroid receptors in breast cancer. Cancer 1980;46:2759–2963.

88. Allegra JC, Barlock A, Huff KK, et al. Changes in multiple or sequential estrogen receptor determinations in breast cancer. Cancer 1980;45:792–794.

89. Wittliff JL. Steroid binding proteins in normal and neoplastic mammary cells. In: Busch H, ed. Methods in cancer research. Vol. 11. New York: Academic Press, 1975.

90. Ellis LM, Wittliff JL, Bryant MS, et al. Effects of ischemia on breast tumor steroid hormone-receptor levels. Curr Surg 1988;45:312–314.

91. Varmus H, Bishop JM. Introduction. Cancer Surv 1986;5:153–158.

92. Schwab M. Amplification of N-myc in neuroblastoma paradigm for clinical use of an oncogene alteration. Klin Padiatr 1990;202:197–201.

93. Jandrig B. Amplification of oncogenes and disease prognosis. Arch Geschwulstforsch 1990;60:141–148.

94. Borst M, Miller DM. DNA isolation and Southern analysis: a clinician's view. Am J Med Sci 1990;299:356–360.

95. Callahan R. Mutations in human breast cancer: an overview. J Natl Cancer Inst 1989;81:1780–1786.

96. Mariami-Costantini R, Escot C, Theillet C, et al. In situ c-myc expression and genomic status of the c-myc focus in infiltrating ductal carcinoma. Cancer Res 1988;48:199–205.

97. Sainsbury JRC, Farndon JR, Needham GK, et al. Epidermal growth factor receptor status of human breast cancer is related to early recurrence and death. Lancet 1987;1:1938–1402.

98. Ochuchi N, Thor A, Page DL, et al. Expression of the 21,000 molecular weight ras protein in a spectrum of benign and malignant mammary tissues. Cancer Res 1986;46:2511–2519.

99. Albini A, Graf JO, Ketten T, et al. Estrogen and v-ras^H transfection regulate the interaction of MCF-7 breast carcinoma cells to basement membrane. Proc Natl Acad Sci U S A 1986;83:8182–8186.

100. Dickson RB, Kasid A, Huff KK, et al. Activation of growth factor secretion in tumoreginic states of breast cancer induced by 17-beta estradiol or v-ras^H oncogene. Proc Natl Acad Sci U S A 1987;84:837–841.

101. Price JE. The biology of metastatic breast cancer. Cancer 1990;66:1313–1320.

102. Thomas KA, Rios-Comdelloves M, Gremenez-Gallego G, et al. Pure brain-derived acidic fibroblast growth factor is a potent angiogenic vascular endothelial cell mitogen with sequence homology to interlukin I. Proc Natl Acad Sci U S A 1985;82:6409–6423.

103. Fidler IJ. Metastasis: quantitative analysis of distribution and fate of tumor emboli labeled with ^{125}I-5-ioso-2^I deoxyuridine. J Natl Cancer Inst 1970;45:773–782.

104. Fidler IJ, Balch CM. The biology of cancer metastasis and implications for therapy. Curr Probl Surg 1987;24:137–209.

105. Halsted WS. The results of operations for the cure of cancer of the breast performed at the Johns Hopkins Hospital from June 1889 to January 1894. Bull Johns Hopkins Hosp 1894–1895;4:297–350.

106. Fisher B, Fisher ER. Transmigration of lymph nodes by tumor cells. Science 1966;152:1397–1398.

107. Rosen PP, Lesser ML, Kenne DW, et al. Discontinuous or 'skip' metastasis in breast carcinoma. Ann Surg 1986;197:276–283.

108. Fisher B, Redmond C, Fisher ER, et al. Ten-year results of a randomized clinical trial comparing radical mastectomy and total

mastectomy with or without radiation. N Eng J Med 1985;312: 674–681.

109. Paget S. The distribution of secondary growths in cancer of the breast. Lancet 1889;1:571–573.

110. Taren D, Price JE, Kettlewell MGW, et al. Mechanisms of human tumor metastasis studied in patients with peritoneovenous shunts. Cancer Res 1984;44:3584–3592.

111. Fisher BF. Breast cancer management. Alternatives to radical mastectomy. N Engl J Med 1979;301:326–328.

112. Anderson MJ, Kramer BS. Adjuvant systemic therapy for early stage breast cancer. In: Bland KI, Copeland EM, eds. The breast: comprehensive management of benign and malignant diseases. Philadelphia: WB Saunders, 1991:817–842.

113. Griswold DP, Jr. The potential for murine tumor models in surgical adjuvant chemotherapy. Cancer Chemother Rep 1975;5(2): 187–204.

114. Carbone PP. Adjuvant therapy of stage II breast cancer. Cancer 1990;65:2148–2154.

115. Fisher B, Ravdin, Ausman RK, et al. Surgical adjuvant chemotherapy of the breast: results of a decade of cooperative investigation. Ann Surg 1968;168:337–356.

116. Fisher B, Redmond C, Dimitrou N, et al. A randomized clinical trial evaluating sequential methotrexate and 5- fluorouracil for the treatment of node negative breast cancer patients with estrogen receptor negative tumors. N Engl J Med 1989;320:473–478.

117. Fisher B, Redmond C., Poisson R, et al. Eight year results of the NSABP randomized clinical trial comparing total mastectomy and lumpectomy with or without radiation in the treatment of breast cancer. N Engl J M 1989;320:822–828.

118. Fisher B, Costantino J, Redmond C, et al. A randomized clinical trial evaluating tamoxifen in the treatment of patients with node-negative breast cancer who have estrogen-receptor positive tumors. N Engl J Med 1989;320:479–484.

119. Mansour EG, Gray R, Shatila AH, et al. Efficacy of adjuvant chemotherapy in high-risk node-negative breast cancer. N Engl J Med 1989;320:485–490.

120. Fisher ER, Redmond C, Fisher B, et al. Pathologic findings from the National Surgical Adjuvant Breast and Bowel Projects (NSABP). Cancer 1990;65:2121–2128.

121. Carbone PP. Breast cancer adjuvant therapy. Cancer 1990;66: 1378–1386.

122. Abeloff MD, Beveridge RA. Adjuvant chemotherapy of breast cancer—the consensus development conference re-visited. Oncol Williston-Park 1988;2:21–26, 29–33.

123. Swain SM, Lippman, ME. Locally advanced breast cancer. In: Bland KI, Copeland EM, eds. The breast: comprehensive management of benign and malignant diseases. Philadelphia: WB Saunders, 1991:843–862.

124. Pierson KK, Wilkinson EJ. Malignant neoplasia of the breast: infiltrating carcinomas. In: Bland KI, Copeland EM, eds. The breast: comprehensive management of benign and malignant diseases. Philadelphia: WB Saunders, 1991:193–209.

125. Carstens PHB, Greenberg RA, Francis D, et al. Tabular carcinoma of the breast. A long-term follow-up. Histopathology 1985;9: 271–280.

126. Ohuchi N, Abe R, Kasal M. Possible cancerous change in intraductal papillomas of the breast. A 3-D reconstruction study of 25 cases. Cancer 1984;54:605–611.

127. Lim SK, Kovi J, Warner OG. Adenoid cystic carcinoma of the breast with metastasis: a case report and review of the literature. J Natl Med Assoc 1979;71:329–330.

128. Nayer HR. Cylindroma of the breast with pulmonary metastasis. Dis Chest 1957;31:324–327.

129. Black MM, Barclay THC, Hankey BF. Prognosis in breast cancer utilizing histologic characteristics of the primary tumor. Cancer 1975;36:2048–2055.

130. Fisher ER, Gregorio RM, Fisher B, et al. The pathology of invasive breast cancer. A syllabus derived from findings of the NSABP (B-04). Cancer 1975;36:1–85.

131. Solin LJ, Fowble BL, Schultz DJ, et al. The significance of the pathology margins of the tumor excision on the outcome of patients treated with definitive irradiation for early stage breast cancer. Int J Radiat Oncol Biol Phys 1991;21:279–287.

132. Brown P, Terez J. Breast cancer associated with Klinefelter's syndrome. J Surg Oncol 1978;10:413–415.

133. van Geel AN, van Slooten EA, Mavrunae M, et al. A retrospective study of male breast cancer in Holland. Br J Surg 1985;72:724–727.

134. Patel JK, Nemoto T, Dao T. Metastatic breast cancer in males: assessment of endocrine therapy. Cancer 1984;53:1344–1346.

135. Ribeiro G. Male breast cancer: review of 301 cases from Christie Hospital and Holt Raderen Institute, Manchester. Br J Cancer 1985;51:115–119.

136. Lopez M, DiLauro L, Popaldo P, et al. Chemotherapy in metastatic male breast cancer. Oncology 1985;42:205–209.

137. Wilhelm MC, Wanebo HJ. Cancer of the male breast. In: Bland KI, Copeland EM, eds. The breast: comprehensive management of benign and malignant diseases. Philadelphia: WB Saunders, 1991:1030–1033.

CHAPTER

14 The Endocrine System

L. Michael Brunt / John D. Halverson

This chapter is a review of the anatomy and physiology of the endocrine system, using an organ-system approach and including discussion of functional endocrine disorders of importance in surgical practice. Every attempt has been made to integrate the pathophysiologic basis of these functional disorders with their clinical presentation and management.

The Thyroid

Anatomy and Development

The anlage of the thyroid gland first appears embryologically at 3 to 4 weeks of development as a thickening of epithelium in the floor of the pharyngeal gut. The thyroid primordium subsequently migrates caudally, remaining connected with the floor of the pharynx by the thyroglossal duct. This duct normally obliterates and disappears by the end of the second month, marking its origin from the junction of the middle and posterior thirds of the tongue by a small dimple, the foramen cecum. Follicles containing colloid are visible by the end of the third month, at which time concentration of iodide and synthesis of T_4 are apparent. During its descent, the thyroid acquires from the ultimobranchial body parafollicular cells that secrete calcitonin.

Several clinically important developmental abnormalities of the thyroid gland may occur. Complete failure of the thyroid anlage to develop results in absence of the thyroid gland (athyreosis), a rare cause of neonatal hypothyroidism and cretinism. Thyroid tissue also may develop at ectopic sites along the pathway of normal descent of the thyroid gland. Differentiation of thyroid tissue may occur in the setting of a complete arrest in migration (lingual thyroid) or may occur in ectopic suprahyoid or infrahyoid sites and the mediastinum. Lingual thyroid occurs in approximately 1 in 3000 cases of thyroid disease and is the most common site for functioning ectopic thyroid tissue. In about 70% of cases, it

is the patient's only thyroid tissue. Thyroglossal duct cyst is the most common clinically important thyroid developmental abnormality. Thyroglossal cysts arise from persistence of a portion of the thyroglossal duct as a sinus tract or cyst and usually present as midline neck masses that first appear during childhood or adolescence.

The thyroid gland in the adult weighs approximately 20 g, making it the largest of the endocrine organs. It consists of two lateral lobes connected by a narrow isthmus. A pyramidal lobe formed by differentiation of cells of the lower thyroglossal duct into thyroid tissue may sometimes be found at the superior aspect of the isthmus (Fig. 14.1). The isthmus of the gland crosses the trachea just below the cricoid cartilage, and the lateral lobes cover the lower halves of the thyroid cartilages. The right lobe is often slightly larger than the left and tends to enlarge to a greater degree in patients with diffuse goiters. The gland lies deep to the superficial strap muscles of the neck (sternohyoid and sternothyroid muscles) and is related laterally to the sternocleidomastoid muscle and the carotid sheath. It attaches to the cricoid cartilage and tracheal rings by bands of connective tissue termed Berry's ligament.

Histologically, the thyroid is organized into varying sized follicles which are the site of synthesis and secretion of thyroid hormone. The follicles are comprised of a single layer of cuboidal cells which surround a central space that is filled with colloid, containing thyroglobulin. The thyroid cell is polarized such that uptake of iodide occurs at the basal pole and iodination of thyroglobulin takes place at the apical pole. The thyroid also contains the C cells or parafollicular cells which produce calcitonin. In the normal thyroid, the C cells are difficult to see with routine histologic stains but can be identified easily by immunohistochemical staining for calcitonin.

The blood supply to the thyroid (Fig. 14.2) is derived from two main sources: the superior thyroid artery, a branch of the external carotid artery, and the inferior thyroid artery, a branch of the thyrocervical trunk of the subclavian artery. The superior thyroid artery enters the

312

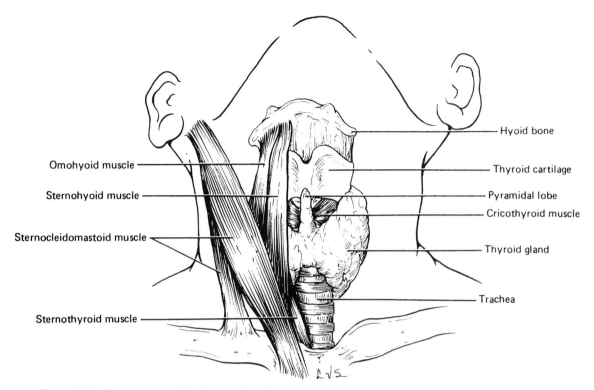

Figure 14.1. Gross anatomy of the human thyroid. From Greenspan FS, Rapoport B. Thyroid gland. In: Greenspan FS, ed. Basic and clinical endocrinology. 3rd ed. Norwalk, CT: Appleton & Lange, 1991:189. Reprinted by permission.

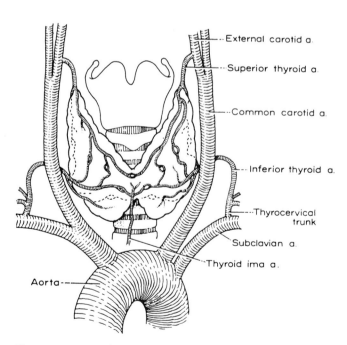

Figure 14.2. Arterial supply to the thyroid gland. The thyroid ima artery is frequently absent. From Tzinas S, Droulias C, Harlaftis N, et al. Vascular patterns of the thyroid gland. Am Surg 1976;42:640. Reprinted by permission.

gland at the superior pole, whereas the inferior artery enters the lateral aspect of each lobe. The thyroidea ima artery is a variably sized vessel that may originate from the innominate artery, the aortic arch, or the lower end of the common carotid artery. It passes upward anterior to the trachea to enter the posterior aspect of the inferior border of the thyroid. Although usually small, it may be a sizable vessel and, if unrecognized, a source of troublesome bleeding during thyroidectomy. This rich vascular network provides the thyroid with a blood flow of 4 to 6 ml/g/min, more than the kidney and 50 times as much as the body as a whole (1). In diffuse thyrotoxic states, thyroid blood flow may reach > 1 liter/min, and this increased flow may be identifiable as a thrill or bruit over the gland.

Blood exits the thyroid via the superior, middle, and inferior thyroid veins. The superior thyroid vein runs parallel with the superior thyroid artery and empties into the internal jugular vein. The middle thyroid vein also drains into the internal jugular vein, but no artery accompanies it. The inferior thyroid veins are the largest and most variable of the thyroid veins. They descend from the inferior poles of the gland to empty into the right and left innominate veins.

The lymph nodes that drain the thyroid (Fig. 14.3) can be categorized according to superior, inferior, and lateral drainage patterns (2). The superior aspect of the isthmus and median aspects of the lateral lobes drain upward into the prelaryngeal (delphian) nodes just

Figure 14.3. Lymphatic drainage of the thyroid gland. From Tzinas S, Droulias C, Harlaftis N, et al. Vascular patterns of the thyroid gland. Am Surg 1976;42:643. Reprinted by permission.

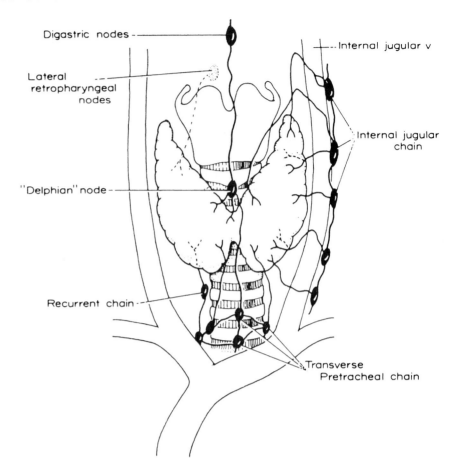

above the isthmus and beyond to the digastric node group. The inferior lymph vessels follow the inferior thyroid veins to drain into the pretracheal and innominate nodes. Lymphatics that drain the lateral lobes course with the vascular supply to drain into the internal jugular, recurrent laryngeal, paratracheal, and paraesophageal lymph node chains. Each of these lymph node groups are common sites of metastatic spread in patients with thyroid carcinoma. Submandibular and mediastinal lymph nodes, however, are rarely involved.

The precise anatomic relationship of the thyroid to the laryngeal nerves must be understood for thyroid surgery to be performed safely. The recurrent laryngeal nerve is a branch of the vagus nerve. On the right side, the recurrent nerve arises from the vagus at the level of the subclavian artery. It then loops from anterior to posterior around the right subclavian artery and passes upward in the tracheoesophageal groove. The left recurrent nerve arises from the vagus at the level of the aortic arch where it loops beneath the ligamentum arteriosum before ascending in a manner similar to the right. The recurrent laryngeal nerve is usually found in the tracheoesophageal groove along the posterior aspect of the thyroid gland (Fig. 14.4). It crosses the inferior thyroid artery at the middle third of the gland and may run behind the artery, between its branches, or in front of it. The nerve often has more than one trunk, each of

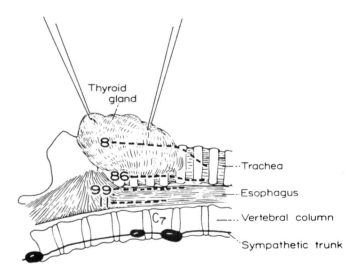

Figure 14.4. Course of the recurrent laryngeal nerve in the normal adult. Lateral view of the course of the recurrent laryngeal nerve at the level of the thyroid gland in 102 cadavers. From Skandalakis JD, Droulias C, Harlaftis N, et al. The recurrent laryngeal nerve. Am Surg 1976;42: 631. Reprinted by permission.

which must be preserved. In approximately 1% of cases, the right nerve is nonrecurrent and enters the larynx directly. A nonrecurrent left nerve is even less common and is usually associated with a right-sided aortic arch. The recurrent nerves penetrate the cricothyroid mem-

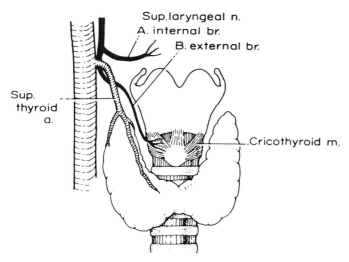

Figure 14.5. Relationship of the internal and external branches of the superior laryngeal nerve, the superior thyroid artery, and the upper pole of the thyroid. From Droulias C, Tzinas S, Harlaftis N, et al. The superior laryngeal nerve. Am Surg 1976;42:636. Reprinted by permission.

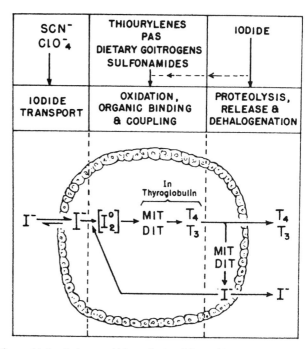

Figure 14.6. Pathway of biosynthesis of thyroid hormone. Shown at the top are inhibitors of the various steps in hormone synthesis. From Ingbar SH. The thyroid. In: Wilson JD, Foster DW, eds. Textbook of endocrinology. 7th ed. Philadelphia: WB Saunders, 1985:686. Reprinted by permission.

brane to form the nerve's terminal branch, the inferior laryngeal nerve. The inferior laryngeal nerve innervates all of the muscles of the larynx except the cricothyroid and supplies sensation to the trachea and subglottic region of the larynx. Unilateral paralysis of the inferior laryngeal nerve from recurrent nerve injury results in paralysis of the vocal cord on that side. The vocal cord becomes bowed outward and can be neither abducted nor adducted. The lack of apposition of the vocal cords produces hoarseness. With time, however, the paralyzed cord may move toward the midline and the voice may improve or even become normal.

The superior laryngeal nerve is a branch of the inferior (nodose) ganglion of the vagus. At the level of the hyoid bone, it splits into internal and external branches (Fig. 14.5). The internal branch provides sensation to the pyriform fossa and laryngeal mucosa above the vocal cords. The external branch innervates the cricothyroid muscle and is of greater surgical importance. It travels with the superior thyroid artery and turns medially to enter the cricothyroid above where the superior thyroid artery branches at the superior pole of the thyroid gland. If the external branch of the superior laryngeal nerve is injured during thyroidectomy, the cricothyroid is paralyzed and the vocal cords cannot be tensed. This results in a loss of timbre and volume in the voice, causing the voice to tire easily and making singing and shouting difficult.

Physiology

The thyroid gland produces two biologically active hormones, L-3,5,3'5'-tetra iodothyronine (thyroxine or T_4) and L-3,5,3'-triiodothyronine (T_3), which are essential for normal growth and development and for regula-

tion of cellular metabolism. Figure 14.6 shows the sequential steps in the biosynthetic pathway for thyroid hormone. Synthesis of thyroid hormone depends on a supply of iodine that comes from dietary sources. In the United States, the average daily intake of iodine is about 500 μg (3). After absorption, iodine is taken up by the thyroid follicular cells by an active transport process. The iodide-trapping mechanism allows the thyroid to store large quantities of iodine (8000 μg and 90% of total body iodine), most of which has been organified. Both thyroid-stimulating hormone (TSH) and organic iodine regulate this process. TSH stimulates iodine uptake, and excess iodide, once it has become organified, inhibits it. The monovalent anions perchlorate and pertechnetate are competitive inhibitors of iodide trapping.

Upon entering the follicular cell, iodine is oxidized and then organified by a process that results in iodination of tyrosine residues on the thyroglobulin molecule to form monoiodotyrosine (MIT) and diiodotyrosine (DIT). This process is catalyzed by the enzyme thyroid peroxidase, which is a membrane-bound glycoprotein of MW 102,000. The formation of the biologically active iodothyronines T_3 and T_4 then proceeds by a coupling reaction involving MIT and DIT. MIT combines with DIT to yield T_3, and two molecules of DIT are coupled to form T_4. TSH positively regulates the organic iodination and coupling process, whereas antithyroid drugs and high concentrations of iodide inhibit it (Wolff-Chaikoff effect). Once organified, iodine is no longer a part of the intracellular pool of iodide and cannot be affected by competitive inhibitors of iodide transport. Two mechanisms regulate secretion of thyroid hormones: (a) a classic feedback loop that involves the pituitary and hypothalamus and (b) an intrinsic thyroid autoregulatory process mediated by glandular content of iodine.

Thyroid-stimulating hormone is a 28,000 molecular weight glycoprotein produced by cells of the anterior pituitary and is the principal agent that modulates thyroid function and thyroid cell growth. TSH exists as a heterodimer that is comprised of α and β subunits. The α subunit is identical to that of two other pituitary glycoprotein hormones (LH and FSH) and human chorionic gonadotropin. The β subunit is unique to TSH and confers its specificity and biologic activity. TSH acts on the thyroid via the TSH receptor and activation of the G protein- adenylate cyclase-cAMP and phospholipase C signaling systems.

TSH has many effects on the thyroid cell. It stimulates all phases of iodide metabolism, including iodine trapping, organification of iodide, iodination of thyroglobulin, and promoting release of T_3 and T_4 from thyroglobulin. It stimulates gene transcription and synthesis of both thyroglobulin and thyroid peroxidase. At higher concentrations, TSH promotes thyroid cell growth and increases thyroid vascularity. In the absence of TSH, thyroid hormone production decreases and atrophy of the gland occurs.

TSH secretion is stimulated by thyrotropin-releasing hormone (TRH) and is inhibited by thyroid hormone. TRH is produced in the supraoptic and paraventricular nuclei of the hypothalamus and is released into the hypophyseal-portal system, through which it is transported to the cells of the anterior pituitary. TRH stimulates both secretion and synthesis of TSH but is not itself affected by the level of thyroid hormones. Inhibition of TSH secretion by thyroid hormones is a function of the rate of secretion of T_4 by the thyroid, serum levels of T_3, and the rate of intrapituitary conversion of T_4 to T_3 (3).

Thyroid hormonogenesis is also regulated in a TSH-independent manner by the availability and glandular content of iodide. Iodide depletion enhances iodide transport and stimulates hormone synthesis. In the presence of excess iodide, however, both iodide transport and hormone synthesis are suppressed (Wolff-Chaikoff effect). In normal individuals, these effects are transient as decreased iodide trapping leads to a decrease in the intraglandular content of iodine and escape from the effect of iodine occurs. Thyroid hormone production is, therefore, regulated closely so that a constant supply of hormone is available to meet the metabolic demands of the individual.

A unique feature of the thyroid gland compared with other endocrine organs is that it contains a large hormone store but has a slow overall hormone utilization rate. This large reserve of thyroid hormone is stored within the thyroglobulin molecule. Most intrathyroidal hormone is in the form of T_4 that may exceed the concentration of T_3 by 10-fold or more. At a T_4 production rate of 80 μg/day, the thyroid has enough reserve to maintain normal hormone levels for 2 to 3 weeks in the event of a block in synthesis. Considering the critical role of thyroid hormone in metabolism and calorigenesis, this provides the organism with an important protective mechanism against hormone depletion.

Thyroglobulin is a 660,000 molecular weight glycoprotein that is virtually the sole constituent of the follicular colloid. As noted previously, the thyroglobulin molecule contains the tyrosine residues, where MIT, DIT, T_3, and T_4 are formed and stored. T_3 and T_4 are subsequently released into the blood by a process that involves endocytosis of thyroglobulin and proteolytic cleavage of T_3 and T_4 by the follicular cell. This process of endocytosis, proteolysis, and release is stimulated by TSH and inhibited by excess iodine and by lithium. Iodine mediates its effect in part by inhibition of TSH-induced stimulation of thyroid adenylate cyclase and by increasing the resistance of thyroglobulin to proteolysis. Despite the efficient storage mechanism of the thyroid, thyroglobulin is detectable in small quantities in the serum of normal individuals. Elevated serum levels of thyroglobulin may be seen in patients with benign or differentiated thyroid tumors. After complete removal of the tumor, thyroglobulin levels return to normal. In patients with differentiated thyroid cancer, thyroglobulin may be useful as a tumor marker to follow patients postoperatively for development of metastatic tumor. Large amounts of thyroglobulin may also be released into the circulation after thyroid surgery and in patients with radiation or subacute thyroiditis.

The pathway for metabolism of thyroid hormone is shown in Figure 14.7 (3). All of circulating T_4 and approximately 20% of T_3 result from direct secretion by the thyroid. The remainder of T_3 comes from peripheral conversion of T_4 to T_3. Approximately 80% of circulating T_4 undergoes extra thyroidal deiodination to T_3 or re-

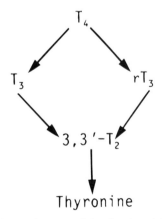

Figure 14.7. Pathway of sequential deiodination of thyroxine to its metabolites. Approximately 90% of the T_4 secreted daily by the thyroid is metabolized through this pathway. Kinetic analysis indicates that approximately 35% of T_4 is converted to T_3 and 40% to rT_3. Reverse T_3 and $3,3'$-T_2 are biologically inactive.

Table 14.1.
Characteristics of Serum Thyroid Hormone Binding Proteins

Protein	MW[a]	Plasma Concentration	Capacity for T_4	Affinity T_4	(M^{-1}) T_3
Thyronine binding globulin	60,000	2 mg/dl	20 μg/dl	2×10^{10}	2×10^9
Thyronine binding prealbumin	50,000	25 mg/dl	250 μg/dl	1.5×10^8	2.5×10^5
Albumin	69,000	4 g/dl	High	1.5×10^6	1×10^7

[a] Molecular weight

From Gavin LA. Thyroid physiology and testing and thyroid function. In: Clark O, ed. Endocrine surgery of the thyroid and parathyroid glands. St. Louis: C.V. Mosby Co., 1985; 7. Reprinted with permission.

verse T_3 (rT_3). Reverse T_3 derives exclusively from T_4 and has little biologic activity. T_3 and rT_3 metabolize to 3,3'-diiodothyronine (3,3'-T_2), which undergoes further deiodination and is excreted in the urine as thyronine. T_3 has approximately three times the biologic activity of T_4. The half-life for T_3 is 3 days and for T_4 is 7 to 10 days. Consequently, patients undergoing thyroidectomy for hyperthyroidism should continue treatment with β-blockade for 2 weeks postoperatively to avoid the untoward effects of residual circulating hormone.

Most circulating thyroid hormone is reversibly bound to three plasma proteins: thyronine-binding globulin (TBG), thyroxine-binding prealbumin (TBPA), and albumin. The extent to which thyroid hormone is bound to these carrier proteins (Table 14.1) is a function of their concentration, binding capacity, and affinity for T_3 and T_4. The high affinity of TBG for T_3 and T_4 makes it the major thyroid hormone binding protein. Virtually no T_3 is bound to TBPA because of the low affinity of interaction between the two. Because protein-bound T_3 and T_4 are biologically inactive, the metabolic state of the patient is determined by the level of free hormone. As most thyroid hormone is protein bound, changes in the plasma concentrations of TBG may affect the total T_4 concentration without altering the serum level of free T_4. In conditions associated with alterations in TBG levels (pregnancy and oral contraceptive use), therefore, free T_4 levels are normal and the patient is clinically euthyroid.

The thyroid hormones exert their metabolic effects at the cellular level after uptake and binding to specific receptors for T_3 in the cell nucleus. There are two T_3 receptor genes (α and β), and the T_3 receptors themselves are members of a family of hormone responsive nuclear transcription factors (4). These T_3 receptors bind to regulatory regions of genes, termed thyroid hormone-response elements, and modify their expression in various tissues in response to stimulation with T_3.

The numerous effects of thyroid hormones on body metabolism are listed in Table 14.2. Thyroid hormone regulates calorigenesis by increasing oxygen consumption and elevating the basal metabolic rate (BMR). It affects protein, carbohydrate, and lipid metabolism and is necessary for normal growth and development. It also increases the sensitivity of the sympathetic nervous system to the effects of catecholamines, which accounts for

Table 14.2.
Actions of Thyroid Hormone

Parameter/ Organ System	Action
Developmental	Essential for normal neural and skeletal development
Calorigenesis	O2 consumption*
	Basal metabolic rate
Intermediary Metabolism	Protein synthesis
	Synthesis/degradation of cholesterol
	Lipolysis
	Glycogenolysis and gluconeogenesis
Cardiovascular	Heart rate and myocardial contractility
Sympathetic nervous system	Sensitivity to catecholamines
	Catecholamine receptors in cardiac muscle
	? Amplification of catecholamine effects at post receptor site
Endocrine	Steroid hormone release
Hematopoietic	Erythropoiesis
	2,3 DPG production
	Maintain hypoxic and hypercapnic drives
Musculoskeletal	Bone turnover
	Urinary hydroxyproline excretion
	Rate of muscle relaxation

* Occurs in all tissues except brain, spleen and testis.

many clinical features seen in patients with hyperthyroidism.

Inhibitors of Thyroid Hormone Synthesis and Secretion

Thionamides

Propylthiouracil (PTU) and methimazole (Tapazole) are members of the thionamide class of antithyroid drugs commonly used in the treatment of hyperthyroidism. These agents act by inhibiting the oxidation and organification of iodine and by blocking coupling of the iodotyrosines MIT and DIT. PTU has the additional effect of inhibiting peripheral conversion of T_4 to T_3. This latter action may be important when a rapid effect is needed in patients with severe thyrotoxicosis. In a small percentage of patients with Graves' disease, long-term remissions may occur after withdrawal of antithyroid medications. PTU is usually administered in a dose of 100 to 300 mg given every 8 hours. Methimazole has the advantage of a single daily dose. Methimazole also crosses the placenta more readily than PTU and should not be used in pregnant patients. The most serious potential side effect associated with thionamide therapy is agranulocytosis that develops in <1% of cases and is usually reversible on cessation of the offending agent.

Iodine

Iodine acts by inhibiting release of thyroid hormone and the organic binding process. This latter action (acute Wolff-Chaikoff effect) is transient, and escape occurs after a few days of therapy. Pharmacologic doses of iodine (> 6 mg/day) are required for the antithyroid effect to occur.

Other Agents

Glucocorticoids suppress the hypothalamic-pituitary-thyroid axis and, in pharmacologic doses, lower serum TSH and T_4 levels. They also lower serum T_3 levels by inhibiting peripheral T_4 to T_3 conversion. Pituitary secretion of TSH is also inhibited by dopamine. Lithium inhibits release of thyroid hormone and may induce goitrous hypothyroidism in susceptible individuals.

Adrenergic antagonists (β blockers) do not inhibit thyroid hormone synthesis, but they are extremely valuable in controlling the peripheral manifestations of increased catecholamine sensitivity in patients with thyrotoxicosis. Propranolol (Inderal) has the added benefit of blocking peripheral conversion of T_4 to T_3.

Tests of Thyroid Function

Serum T_4 and T_3

The initial screening for suspected thyroid disorders should involve measurement of serum total T_4 and the free T_4 index (5). Serum total T_4 assays measure both free and protein-bound hormone. Because changes in total T_4 can result from alterations in either hormone production or hormone binding to serum proteins, an accurate diagnosis of thyroid dysfunction requires measurement of free T_4. Assays directly measuring serum free T_4 are difficult to perform; for most purposes, indirect measurement of free T_4 is adequate. The T_3 resin uptake test is commonly used to measure indirectly the proportion of T_4 that is not protein bound. In this test, radiolabeled T_3 is added to the patient's serum, which is then incubated with an ion exchange resin that competes with the serum-binding proteins for thyroid hormone. As the concentration of free T_4 rises, the availability of unoccupied binding sites on the patient's serum proteins diminishes, and a greater percentage of radiolabeled T_3 is taken up by the resin. Conversely, if the absolute free T_4 concentration is low, more labeled T_3 will be bound by the patient's serum-binding proteins and the resin uptake will be low. The percent tracer bound, therefore, varies inversely with the concentration and affinity of unoccupied binding sites on the serum thyroxine-binding proteins. The product of the percent up-

take and the total serum T_4 concentration gives the free T_4 index, which reflects the absolute concentration of serum free T_4. Measurement of serum total and free T_3 concentrations are not routinely employed in screening but are reserved mainly for the diagnosis of T_3 toxicosis.

Serum TSH and Evaluation of the Hypothalamic-Pituitary-Thyroid Axis

The replacement of a radioimmunoassay for TSH by an ultra sensitive radioimmunometric assay has greatly improved the distinction of euthyroid from hypothyroid and hyperthyroid states (6,7). Measurement of serum TSH has become the primary screening test for the diagnosis of hypothyroidism, and the new assay reliably distinguishes euthyroid subjects from hyperthyroid patients with low or suppressed TSH levels. The sensitive TSH assay is also less affected by nonthyroidal illness and remains unaltered by changes in thyroid hormone binding proteins.

Occasionally, further tests of the functional status of the hypothalamic-pituitary-axis may be indicated. The TRH stimulation test measures the TSH response to an intravenous dose of TRH. Normal subjects should exhibit a rise in serum TSH of 5 to 30 mU/mL that peaks within 15 to 35 min of TRH administration (Fig. 14.8). Patients with hypothyroidism from primary gland failure will exhibit an exaggerated response to TRH, whereas patients with hypothyroidism from pituitary insufficiency will have a subnormal or absent response to TRH.

The T_3 suppression test measures the degree to which the thyroid gland functions autonomously, because T_3 suppresses TSH secretion by the pituitary. Radioactive iodine uptake (RAIU) by the thyroid gland is determined before and after an 8 to 10-day course of T_3 (100 μg/day orally). In normal subjects, the RAIU should be suppressed (< 50% of initial uptake). In patients with an autonomously hyperfunctioning thyroid gland—regardless of the etiology—the RAIU will not be suppressed. In practice, the ultrasensitive TSH assay and the TRH stimulation test have largely supplanted the T_3 suppression test.

Radioactive Iodine Uptake

The radioactive iodine uptake test measures the thyroid content of radioactive iodine after an orally administered dose of ^{123}I (100 μCi). In normal subjects, the percent uptake at 24 hours should be 15% to 30%. ^{123}I is the radioisotope commonly employed because of the shorter half-life and minimal radiation exposure compared with ^{131}I. The RAIU is no longer widely used because of the availability of more precise biochemical tests and the decrease in normal values for RAIU that have occurred because of dietary iodine supplementation. Current use of the RAIU test in the diagnosis of hyperthyroidism is subsequently discussed.

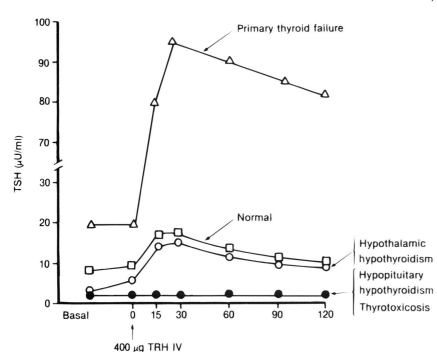

Figure 14.8. TRH stimulation test. The TSH response to 400 mg i.v. of TRH is shown for normal subjects and patients with various thyroid disorders. From DeGroot LJ, Stanbury JB. The thyroid and its diseases. 4th ed. Churchill Livingstone, New York, 1975:230. Reprinted by permission.

Calcitonin

Calcitonin is a 32 amino acid peptide secreted by the parafollicular, or C cells, of the thyroid. Calcitonin radioimmunoassay has been useful for identifying patients with medullary thyroid carcinoma (MTC), a C cell neoplasm of the thyroid. In most patients with MTC, the diagnosis can be established by demonstration of elevated basal plasma calcitonin levels. Patients with MTC, but not normal individuals, also exhibit an increase in plasma calcitonin after intravenous administration of pentagastrin and/or calcium. In cases of familial MTC and the multiple endocrine neoplasia type II (MEN-II) syndrome, provocative testing with calcium-pentagastrin is a sensitive biochemical means for screening patients at risk for the disease and monitoring patients for disease recurrence after thyroidectomy.

Tests for Autoimmune Thyroid Disease

Detection of autoantibodies to thyroid antigens may be useful diagnostically in the evaluation of patients with autoimmune thyroid disorders such as Graves' disease and Hashimoto's thyroiditis. Antimicrosomal antibodies are present in high titer in 95% of patients with Hashimoto's thyroiditis and 80% with Graves' disease. In these conditions, antithyroglobulin antibodies are also detectable but in a lower percentage of cases. Graves' disease is caused by circulating antibodies that bind to and stimulate the TSH receptor on thyroid follicular cells. Originally, a mouse bioassay was used to detect these TSH receptor antibodies. The antibodies detected by this assay were termed long-acting thyroid stimulators (LATS). More recently developed assays for TSH receptor antibody activity have greater sensitivity than the LATS assay and may ultimately prove useful in detecting disease severity and predicting a response to antithyroid medications.

Thyroid Scintigraphy

Imaging of the thyroid with radionuclide agents is sometimes useful in evaluating gland size and identification of hyperfunctioning and hypofunctioning nodules. Hypofunctioning, or cold, nodules are associated with a 15% to 20% incidence of malignancy, whereas functional nodules are usually benign. The two agents most commonly used in thyroid imaging are radioactive iodine and ^{99m}Tc pertechnetate. Both the ^{123}I and ^{131}I radioisotopes are used clinically. ^{123}I has the advantage of a low dose of radiation (30 mrad) and short half-life (12 hr) compared with ^{131}I (500 mrad and a half-life of 8 days). Patients with differentiated thyroid carcinoma in whom screening is done to search for distant metastases, however, should be screened with ^{131}I. Technetium is trapped by the thyroid but not organified and, consequently, has a short half-life (6 hours) and a low associated radiation dose (10 mrad). Unlike radioactive iodine, technetium is not affected by drugs that inhibit organification (propylthiouracil and methimazole). Because of the short half-life and the requirement for earlier imaging, technetium radioactivity may appear in the salivary glands or major vascular structures. Patients with suspected lingual thyroid, ectopic thyroid, or substernal goiter should therefore undergo scanning with ^{123}I.

Hyperthyroidism

Thyrotoxicosis is the clinical state produced by excess circulating thyroid hormone. Table 14.3 demonstrates

Table 14.3.
Symptoms and Signs in 243 Patients with Thyrotoxicosis

Symptom	%	Symptom	%
Nervousness	99	Tachycardia	82
Increased sweating	91	Dyspnea	75
Heat intolerance	89	Weakness	70
Palpitations	89	Increased appetite	65
Fatigue	88	Eye complaints	54
Weight loss	85	Diarrhea	23
Sign	%	Sign	%
Tachycardia*	100	Thyroid bruit	77
Goiter*	100	Eye signs	71
Skin changes	97	Atrial fibrillation	10
Tremor	97		

* Patients with normal pulse rate or absence of a goiter have been observed in some series.
From Williams RH. Thiouracil treatment of thyrotoxicosis; results of prolonged treatment. J Clin Endocrinol 1946;6:3-4. Reprinted with permission.

Table 14.4.
Causes of Thyrotoxicosis

Increased Hormone Production by the Thyroid[a]
Graves' disease
Toxic multinodular goiter
Toxic adenoma
TSH-secreting pituitary tumor
Trophoblastic tumor
Iodine induced (Jod Basedow)

Not Associated with Increased Hormone Production by the Thyroid[b]
Factitious thyrotoxicosis
Subacute thyroiditis
Chronic thyroiditis with transient thyrotoxicosis
Ectopic thyroid tissue (struma ovarii, functioning metastatic thyroid carcinoma)

[a] Associated with increased values of RAIU except for iodine induced hyperthyroidism.
[b] Associated with decreased RAIU values.
Modified from Ingbar S.H. The Thyroid. In: Williams RH ed. Textbook of Endocrinology, 7th ed. Philadelphia: WS Saunders Co., 1985; 743. Reprinted with permission.

the frequency of signs and symptoms in affected organ systems. Elevation of the BMR, increased appetite, heat intolerance, and a slight elevation in body temperature are all manifestations of the accelerated rate of energy metabolism and heat production. The increased rate of protein synthesis and degradation causes increased protein turnover, negative nitrogen balance, weight loss, muscle wasting, and hypoalbuminemia.

Some of the most pronounced features of thyrotoxicosis are seen in the cardiovascular system. Tachycardia is invariably present, and approximately 10% of patients develop atrial fibrillation that may be refractory to medical therapy until control of the thyrotoxicosis is achieved. High output congestive heart failure is sometimes seen, but this occurs primarily in patients with preexisting cardiac disease. Excess thyroid hormone mediates its cardiac effects in part by a direct cardiac stimulatory action and by increasing myocardial sensitivity to the effects of circulating catecholamines by increasing the number of adrenergic receptors in the heart. The latter explains some of the beneficial actions of β-blockade in patients with thyrotoxicosis-related cardiac symptoms.

Table 14.4 lists the various causes of thyrotoxicosis. The most common cause of hyperthyroidism in Western countries is Graves' disease, also known as diffuse toxic goiter (8). An autoimmune basis for the development of Graves' disease is well-established. The pathogenesis involves the production of autoantibodies to the TSH receptor. These thyroid-stimulating antibodies (TSAb) activate adenylate cyclase, which in turn stimulates increased thyroid vascularity, growth, and hormone release. The mechanism of autoantibody formation is unknown but probably results from regulatory abnormalities in both B and T lymphocyte immune responses. Genetic factors also appear to play a role in disease development because an increased incidence exists in relatives of affected individuals. An increase in frequency of HLA-B8 and HLA-DR3 haplotypes has also been observed in Graves' disease patients.

Toxic multinodular goiter (Plummer's disease) is a less common cause of hyperthyroidism; it usually develops slowly over a prolonged period in patients with a long-standing goiter. Toxic multinodular goiter is characterized by multiple heterogeneous autonomously functioning nodules. The role of iodine in the development of this disorder is unclear, but in areas of iodine deficiency and endemic goiter, the administration of iodine may cause hyperthyroidism (Jod-Basedow phenomenon). Toxic adenoma is a much less common cause of hyperthyroidism. The pathogenesis is unknown, but the lesion is a follicular adenoma whose function is not TSH dependent. TSH-secreting tumors of the anterior pituitary are a rare cause of hyperthyroidism. Trophoblastic tumors (hydatidiform mole, choriocarcinoma, and metastatic embryonal carcinoma) induce hyperthyroidism through production of a thyroid stimulator similar to TSH.

Thyrotoxicosis also may occur in the absence of hyperthyroidism from either an increased rate of release of stored hormone (thyroiditis) or from extrathyroidal sources of thyroid hormone. Factitious thyrotoxicosis from the exogenous administration of excess amounts of thyroid hormone usually occurs in patients with psychiatric disorders or medical-paramedical backgrounds. Struma ovarii is an uncommon cause of thyrotoxicosis, which results from excess thyroid hormone production by an ovarian teratoma. Rarely, functioning metastases from thyroid carcinoma may produce enough hormone to cause thyrotoxicosis. Each of these conditions can be differentiated from primary thyroid sources of thyrotoxicosis by the RAIU test.

The concentration of serum free T_4 is increased in the vast majority (95%) of patients with hyperthyroidism. The ultrasensitive TSH assay has greatly facilitated confirmation of the diagnosis because it reliably distinguishes TSH levels in normal individuals (0.3 to 0.5 mU/liter) from the suppressed levels (< 0.1 mU/liter) of hyperthyroid patients. The presence of an elevated serum free T_4 level together with a suppressed serum TSH level establishes the diagnosis. If the serum free T_4 level is normal and the TSH level is low, the patient may have T_3 toxicosis. This may be substantiated by determining that the serum free T_3 level is elevated. In patients with TSH-secreting pituitary tumors, serum T_4 and T_3 levels are elevated and serum TSH is normal or increased. Patients in whom the diagnosis of hyperthyroidism is equivocal may be evaluated further with the TRH stimulation test or the T_3 suppression test. In practice, however, the ultra sensitive TSH assay has obviated the need for more elaborate tests in most patients. Caution must be exercised in evaluating patients who are pregnant or taking oral contraceptives, as the serum total T_4 and T_3 may be elevated because of an increase in the concentration of thyroxine-binding globulin. In the absence of thyroid disease, the serum TSH concentration in such individuals is normal.

Once the diagnosis of hyperthyroidism is established biochemically, the etiology must then be determined. If the patient has a diffusely enlarged goiter and exophthalmos, the diagnosis is Graves' disease and no further tests are necessary. Patients with a nodular thyroid gland should have a radioactive iodine scan. Concentration of iodine in one or more nodules with suppressed uptake in the rest of the gland suggests a toxic adenoma or toxic multinodular goiter. If one of these etiologies is not confirmed, the patient should have a RAIU test. If the uptake is increased, the most likely diagnosis is Graves' disease. If the RAIU is low, the thyrotoxicosis may be the result of thyroiditis or an ectopic or exogenous source of thyroid hormone.

Thyroid Storm

Thyroid storm is a life-threatening complication of severe thyrotoxicosis which requires emergent medical intervention (9). Infection, trauma, and surgery are the usual precipitating events. Fortunately, with improved medical treatment of thyrotoxicosis and better preparation of patients undergoing thyroidectomy, thyroid storm is rarely seen. The clinical manifestations of thyroid storm are those of profound hypermetabolism: fever (which may be extreme), profuse sweating, and marked tachycardia. Congestive heart failure and pulmonary edema may develop. Nausea, vomiting, and abdominal pain are commonly present. The patient appears restless and tremulous and may become delirious and psychotic. If this complication is not recognized and treated, progression to stupor and coma occurs and

death inevitably results. Treatment is directed at correction of the thyrotoxicosis and the precipitating event. Both PTU and inorganic iodide should be administered to block synthesis and to slow the release of thyroid hormone, unless the thyroid storm has occurred after thyroidectomy. Propranolol is given to block adrenergic effects and dexamethasone may aid in inhibiting peripheral conversion of T_4 to T_3. General supportive measures include fever reduction and administration of glucose-containing fluids.

Hypothyroidism

The causes of hypothyroidism include primary thyroid gland failure, pituitary insufficiency, resistance to thyroid hormone, and prior ablative procedures (surgery or radioactive iodine administration). The clinical manifestations of hypothyroidism depend more on severity of the hormone insufficiency and age of onset than on the etiology of the disorder. Thyroid hormone is essential for central nervous system development and for skeletal growth and maturation. In infants, untreated hypothyroidism can cause permanent mental and growth retardation (cretinism). Childhood hypothyroidism is characterized by delayed growth and poor intellectual development. In adults, common symptoms of hypothyroidism include loss of energy, cold intolerance, decreased appetite, weight gain, constipation, muscle aches and stiffness, intellectual lethargy, slowed speech, congestive heart failure, and sexual dysfunction (decreased libido, irregular and heavy menses). Myxedema of the skin, delayed deep tendon reflex responses, bradycardia, and low voltage electrocardiogram (ECG) are frequent accompanying signs. Treatment, consisting of replacement therapy with exogenous thyroid hormone, is highly successful, but it may take several weeks to months for the physical manifestations to disappear.

Measurement of serum T_4 should be the initial screening test in the evaluation of patients with clinically suspected hypothyroidism. The presence of a low serum free T_4 level and elevated TSH establish the diagnosis. Hypothyroidism secondary to pituitary failure is characterized by both decreased serum T_4 and TSH levels and is much less common than primary gland failure. The diagnosis of hypothyroidism in sick patients may be more difficult because of changes in thyroid hormone secretion and alterations in plasma-binding proteins that occur in severe illness. Serum total T_4 and the free T_4 index are frequently depressed in the critically ill, and direct measurement of serum T_4 by equilibrium dialysis may be necessary for accurate assessment of thyroid function. Serum TSH levels should be elevated in hypothyroid sick patients. However, one must be cautious in interpreting TSH results in patients on dopamine or pharmacologic doses of steroids because, in hypothyroid subjects, these agents may suppress TSH levels into the normal range.

The Parathyroids

Anatomy and Development

The parathyroid glands first appear embryologically during the sixth week of gestation. The superior parathyroids arise from the fourth branchial pouch, as does the ultimobranchial body. This latter structure eventually separates from the parathyroid as it joins the thyroid gland to form the C cells. The inferior parathyroids along with the thymus are derived from the third branchial pouches.

Variability in the extent and direction of migration of the parathyroids during development can lead to considerable variation in their anatomic location in the adult (Fig. 14.9) (10,11). The superior parathyroids are usually embedded in fat along the posterior surface of the middle or upper portions of the thyroid lobes posterolateral to the recurrent laryngeal nerve and about 1 cm above the junction of the nerve and the inferior thyroid artery. Occasionally, a superior parathyroid may be found within the substance of the thyroid gland. Other aberrant sites for the superior parathyroids include the tra-

cheoesophageal groove, retroesophageal space, and posterior mediastinum. The inferior parathyroids are located more ventrally than the superior glands, anteromedial to the recurrent laryngeal nerve, and near the lower pole of the thyroid or in the thyrothymic ligament. Because of its embryologic association with the thymus, an inferior parathyroid gland may be found embedded in the thymic tissue in the lower neck. In about 2% of cases, an inferior gland will be located deep within the thymus in the anterior mediastinum. Other aberrant sites for the inferior parathyroids are lateral to the trachea at the level of the lower pole of the thyroid, the carotid sheath, and rarely, the pharyngeal mucosa. Regardless of location, the position of the glands is symmetrical in approximately 80% of cases (11).

Four parathyroid glands are present in most individuals. Studies in which serial embryologic sections have been examined have demonstrated at least four parathyroid glands in every case (12). In an autopsy study of 503 cadavers, Akerstrom et al. (10) found four or more parathyroids in 97% of cases. Supernumerary, or fifth, parathyroid glands, which have been reported in 6% to 13% of cases, may arise from division of one or more of the four main parathyroids during development. Such supernumerary glands are commonly located within the thymus.

The primary blood supply to the parathyroids comes from the inferior thyroid artery, but contributions may

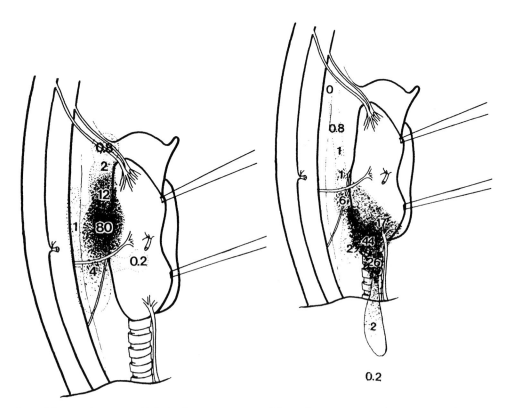

Figure 14.9. Locations of the superior (top) and inferior (bottom) parathyroid glands. The more common locations are indicated by the darker shading. The numbers represent the percentages of glands found at the different locations. From Akerstrom G, Malmaeus S, Bergstrom R. Surgical anatomy of human parathyroid glands. Surgery 1984;95:17. Reprinted by permission.

also be received from the superior thyroid artery or the thyroidea ima artery. The venous drainage is via the superior, inferior, and middle thyroid veins.

Grossly, the parathyroids are oval shaped and each weighs about 40 mg, so that the total combined weight of the four glands rarely exceeds 160 mg. Typically, the lower glands are slightly heavier than the upper glands. The parathyroids are distinguished from adjacent fat and lymph nodes by their red-brown or tan color. Architecturally, the parathyroid glands are composed of cords and sheets of cells arranged within a fatty stroma. The chief cell is the primary cell in the parathyroid that synthesizes and secretes parathyroid hormone (PTH). Oxyphil cells are slightly larger cells than the chief cells and are characterized by a central pyknotic nucleus, eosinophilic cytoplasm, and abundant mitochondria. Oxyphil cells first appear at puberty and increase in number with advancing age, but they rarely make up more than 5% of the total cells in the gland. Water-clear cells are glycogen-laden cells that have a clear cytoplasm. Water-clear cell hyperplasia is a rare cause of hyperparathyroidism.

Physiology

Mineral Metabolism

The principal function of the parathyroid glands and parathyroid hormone is regulation of bone mineralization and maintenance of calcium and phosphate homeostasis. The majority of calcium and phosphate within the body is found in an insoluble form within the skeleton. Calcium, phosphate, and magnesium are also essential for a variety of normal cellular and metabolic processes. The need for precise homeostatic control of these minerals is illustrated by the serious clinical consequences of acute derangements in plasma levels of these ions.

The distribution and body content of calcium, phosphate, and magnesium in the tissues and blood is shown in Table 14.5 (13,14). The average daily intake of calcium is 500 to 1000 mg, most of which is absorbed in the upper small intestine by an active process that is vitamin D dependent. Normal plasma levels of calcium vary slightly among laboratories but generally range from 8.5 to 10.2 mg/dl (2.2 to 2.5 mmol/liter). Plasma calcium is evenly distributed between ionized (46%) and protein-bound (46%) phases, with a smaller percentage (8%) that

is complexed with organic anions. Approximately 80% of protein-bound calcium is complexed with albumin. Protein-bound calcium is not biologically active, and changes in serum protein have little effect on the concentration of the ionized physiologically active fraction. The percentage of total plasma calcium that is protein bound is, however, affected by changes in plasma pH, as hydrogen ion competes with calcium for the same binding site on plasma proteins. This results in an increase in the percentage of ionized calcium in acidosis, whereas in alkalosis, the proportion of ionized calcium ion is decreased.

Extracellular calcium is necessary for the normal activity of a number of physiologic processes, including bone formation, coagulation, and neuromuscular function. Calcium also plays a critical role in a number of intracellular regulatory systems and second messenger pathways, including the cAMP second messenger system.

Calcium is excreted via the urine (100 to 200 mg/day), feces (600 mg/day), and sweat (< 100 mg/day) (13). Normally, the kidney reabsorbs 99% of the filtered calcium load. Consequently, urinary calcium excretion rates of > 500 mg/day are unusual, even in patients with marked hypercalcemia.

Inorganic phosphate deposited in the mineral phase of bone accounts for approximately 85% of total body phosphate. Unlike calcium, phosphate is also distributed widely in nonosseous tissues in both an inorganic form and as a component of cellular macromolecules. These macromolecules include phospholipids and phosphoproteins that are integral components of cellular membranes, nucleic acids, glycogen, and other intermediates of carbohydrate metabolism. Phosphates also serve as substrates for the enzymes of glycolysis, respiration, and the formation of high-energy phosphate bonds (ATP). They are critical for normal muscular contraction and transmission of nerve impulses. Approximately 70% of the daily ingested phosphate is absorbed, primarily in the small intestine. Plasma proteins bind 15% of circulating phosphate, and the remainder either circulates as free ion or is complexed with other cations. Normal serum phosphate levels range from 2.5 to 4.5 mg/dl in the adult and from 5 to 6 mg/dl in children. Serum phosphate levels may vary daily by up to 1.5

Table 14.5.
Body Content and Distribution of Calcium, Phosphate, and Magnesium

		Calcium	Phosphate	Magnesium
Specific tissue distribution	Skeleton	99%	86%	53%
	Exctracellular fluid	0.1%	0.03%	1%
	Cells	1.0%	14%	46%
Total body content*		20–25 g/kg	11–14 g/kg	25 g

* g/kg fat-free tissue (Source reference 16).
Modified from Aurbach GD et al. Parathyroid hormone, calcitonin, and the calciferols. In: Wilson JD, Foster DW eds. Textbook of Endocrinology, 7th ed. Philadelphia: WB Saunders Co., 1985; Reprinted with permission.

mg/dl and are influenced by several factors, including diet, age, and secretion of PTH and other hormones.

Magnesium is the most common divalent intracellular cation and functions in the activation of enzyme systems, cellular metabolism, and neuromuscular electrical activity. Total body magnesium content is 25 g, half of which is in bone and only 1% of which is in the extracellular fluid. Because only 20% of magnesium is protein bound, serum levels (normal range 1.5 to 2.2 mg/dl) are not influenced greatly by changes in serum proteins. The average dietary intake of magnesium is about 300 mg (25 mEq), 50% of which is absorbed. Magnesium is cleared by the kidney in a manner similar to calcium.

Parathyroid Hormone, Calcitonin, and Vitamin D

Parathyroid Hormone. Parathyroid hormone is an 84 amino acid peptide (9400 Daltons) secreted by the parathyroid glands. Serum calcium is the major regulator of PTH secretion, although the precise mechanism of its action on the parathyroid cell is unknown. An inverse relationship exists between the serum calcium level and PTH synthesis-secretion. Increased serum calcium levels inhibit PTH secretion; decreased calcium levels stimulate release. Magnesium also affects PTH secretion in a manner qualitatively similar to calcium, although it is much less potent. Severe hypomagnesemia paradoxically inhibits PTH secretion, probably by interfering with intracellular secretory mechanisms. As a result, hypocalcemia associated with profound hypomagnesemia will not respond to calcium administration until the hypomagnesemia has been corrected. Secretion of PTH is unaffected by serum phosphate levels.

After secretion, the PTH molecule is degraded within minutes into biologically inactive peptides. Full biologic activity resides within the first 34 N-terminus amino acids. Bioactive N-terminus PTH fragments are cleared rapidly from the circulation, whereas biologically inactive C-terminus fragments persist longer in the circulation, especially in the setting of chronic renal insufficiency.

Parathyroid hormone regulates the level of calcium in the extracellular fluid by direct effects on the kidney and bone and, indirectly, via the gastrointestinal tract. In the kidney, PTH increases calcium reabsorption in the proximal convoluted tubule. This effect on calcium clearance is rapid and is associated with increased urinary secretion of sodium, potassium, and bicarbonate. In the skeleton, PTH increases mobilization of calcium from bone to blood in two phases: (a) a rapid phase that results from mobilization of bone in equilibrium with the extracellular fluid and (b) a slow phase that depends on activation of enzymes that promote bone resorption (11). Parathyroid hormone also indirectly increases the rate of calcium absorption from the intestinal tract via its effects on vitamin D. It also regulates phosphate metabolism by increasing renal clearance of phosphate and

increasing release of phosphate from bone. The effects of PTH are mediated via specific receptors in bone and kidney. Binding of PTH to these receptors leads to activation of adenylate cyclase, increased cellular levels of cAMP, and activation of cellular effector systems that induce the appropriate biological effect.

Calcitonin. The principal action of calcitonin is to lower serum calcium by acutely inhibiting osteoclastic bone absorption. Calcitonin also has a phosphaturic effect on the kidneys, which is independent of PTH. Calcitonin secretion is stimulated by low serum calcium levels and is inhibited by increased calcium concentrations. Clinically, calcitonin has been used in pharmacologic doses to lower serum calcium levels acutely in patients with severe hypercalcemia and to treat Paget's disease. However, neither patients with elevated calcitonin levels (medullary thyroid carcinoma) nor patients with calcitonin deficiency (thyroidectomy) have significant alterations in calcium homeostasis. The precise physiologic role of calcitonin in human bone and mineral metabolism is unclear. It may be more important in protecting the skeleton during periods of calcium stress than in maintaining plasma calcium homeostasis.

Vitamin D. The D vitamins (calciferols) are a group of fat-soluble vitamins found in virtually all living plants and animals. Only a few foods (fish liver oils, egg yolk, and liver) contain vitamin D. The principal nutritional source of vitamin D comes from exposure to sunlight. In humans, the precursor for vitamin D_3 (7-dehydrocholesterol) is found in the skin and epidermis. After exposure to ultraviolet radiation, this precursor is converted to vitamin D_3 (cholecalciferol). Vitamin D_3 then undergoes hydroxylation in the liver to form 25-hydroxycholecalciferol (25-OH-D_3) (Fig. 14.10). Approximately 5% to 30% of 25-OH-vitamin D_3 is excreted into the bile and enters the enterohepatic circulation (13). Further hydroxylation in the kidney leads to the formation of 1,25-dihydroxycholecalciferol (1,25(OH)$_2$-D_3),

Site	Vitamin D metabolite
Skin	7-dehydrocholesterol
	↓ ultraviolet radiation
	cholecalciferol (vitamin D_3)
Liver	↓ 25-hydroxylase
	25-(OH)-vitamin D_3
Kidney	↓ 1α-hydroxylase
	1,25-(OH)$_2$-vitamin D_3

Figure 14.10. Metabolic pathway for vitamin D. 1α-hydroxylase activity in the kidney is regulated positively by PTH and is the rate-limiting step in the vitamin D metabolism pathway.

the most potent natural metabolite of vitamin D. Vitamin D acts on the intestine to increase absorption of calcium by stimulating synthesis of a calcium-binding protein that promotes calcium transport across the intestinal cell. Vitamin D also increases, to a lesser extent, intestinal absorption of phosphate and magnesium. It has an antirachitic effect on bone and increases mobilization of calcium and phosphate from bone to blood. Clinically, low circulating $1,25(OH)_2$-D_3 levels are seen in hypoparathyroidism, neonatal hypocalcemia, secondary hyperparathyroidism, rickets, and osteomalacia.

Tests of Parathyroid Function

Biochemical Tests

Measurement of total serum calcium is the most useful screening test for identifying patients with disorders of the parathyroid glands. In most laboratories, the upper limit of normal for serum calcium ranges from 10.2 to 10.4 mg/dl. Patients with moderate to severe hypercalcemia (> 11 mg/dl) should undergo further diagnostic evaluation for hyperparathyroidism. Many patients with mild hypercalcemia (< 11 mg/dl) are found to be normocalcemic on subsequent biochemical evaluations. In patients with mild hypercalcemia, therefore, an elevated serum calcium level should be documented on at least two separate occasions before proceeding with more specific diagnostic tests. Because about 50% of serum calcium is protein bound, changes in serum proteins (albumin) and other anions may significantly affect the total serum calcium level in the blood. Ionized calcium more accurately reflects the physiologic state of calcium homeostasis. Its measurement is a more sensitive test for hyperparathyroidism. However, ionized calcium assays are difficult to perform, and results must be interpreted with a knowledge of the reliability of the assay employed.

Other biochemical abnormalities commonly seen in patients with hyperparathyroidism include hypophosphatemia from the phosphaturic actions of PTH and hyperchloremic metabolic acidosis from increased urinary excretion of bicarbonate. Elevation of the chloride:phosphate ratio to >33 is seen in many patients with hyperparathyroidism but does not distinguish these individuals from patients with hypercalcemia of malignancy. Patients with bone disease from hyperparathyroidism often have an increase in serum alkaline phosphatase. Hypomagnesemia is present in approximately 5% to 10% of patients with primary hyperparathyroidism. If hypocalcemia develops after parathyroidectomy and associated hypomagnesemia exists, the hypocalcemia will be refractory to calcium administration until the serum magnesium level has been normalized.

PTH Assay

Demonstration of an elevated serum PTH level in conjunction with hypercalcemia is diagnostic of hyperparathyroidism in more than 90% of cases. Various types of PTH immunoassays have been used based on the region of the PTH molecule that is recognized (15). The assay of choice is one that measures the intact PTH molecule, which eliminates the problem of detection of inactive fragments of PTH in the circulation associated with region specific PTH assays. The intact PTH assay employs a two-site double antibody technique in which one antibody reacts with the N-terminus of the molecule and the second antibody recognizes the C-terminus region. These two antibodies are bound simultaneously by intact PTH molecules, and the bound antibodies are then detected with either radioactive or chemiluminescent tags. The sensitivity of the intact PTH assay in the detection of patients with primary hyperparathyroidism ranges from 90 to 97%, and the specificity of the assay nears 100%. The intact PTH assay also reliably differentiates patients with hyperparathyroidism from those with hypercalcemia of malignancy. It does not measure the PTH-related protein that has been identified in some malignant tumors (16).

Nephrogenous cAMP

Patients with hyperparathyroidism have increased urinary cAMP levels as a result of PTH-mediated activation of renal adenylate cyclase activity. Increased cAMP production occurs in the renal tubular cells. If measured as a function of creatinine clearance (nephrogenous cAMP), urinary cAMP levels are increased in 90% of patients with primary hyperparathyroidism. However, many patients with malignancies also have increased cAMP excretion. Nephrogenous cAMP determination is currently most useful in evaluating patients with hypoparathyroidism and in identifying states of PTH resistance. Phosphate clearance studies are of no additional value in the diagnostic evaluation of hypercalcemia.

Hyperparathyroidism

Primary Hyperparathyroidism

Primary hyperparathyroidism is the result of excessive secretion of PTH by one or more parathyroid glands. The etiology of hyperparathyroidism in most cases is unknown. A higher than expected incidence of primary hyperparathyroidism has been observed in patients with a previous history of neck irradiation. An altered set point in the level of ionized calcium at which PTH secretion is suppressed has also been demonstrated in patients with hyperparathyroidism, but the role of this physiologic abnormality in initiating the development of hyperparathyroidism is uncertain. Recent molecular studies have begun to identify genetic factors associated with the development of parathyroid gland neoplasms in some groups of patients (17). Parathyroid adenoma-1 (PRAD-1) is a proto-oncogene located on chromosome 11 that is activated in approximately 5%

Pericentromeric Inversion of Chromosome 11 in Parathyroid Adenomas

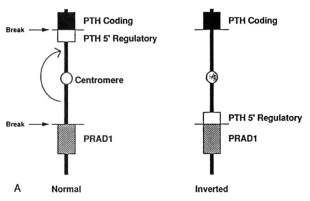

A   Normal   Inverted

PTH / PRAD1 Gene Rearrangement in Parathyroid Adenomas

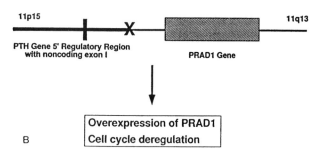

B

Figure 14.11. Schematic illustration of the mechanism of gene rearrangement and overexpression of the proto-oncogene PRAD1 in a subset of parathyroid adenomas. **A,** Pericentromeric inversion of chromosome 11 results in juxtaposition of the PTH gene and the PRAD1 gene. **B,** Molecular structure of the rearranged PTH/PRAD gene complex. The X marks the chromosomal breakpoint between the PTH gene regulatory region from 11p15 and the PRAD1 gene from 11q13. From Habener JF, Arnold A, Potts JT, Jr. Hyperparathyroidism. In Degroot LJ, ed. Endocrinology. Philadelphia: WB Saunders Co., 1995;1044–1057. Reprinted with permission.

of parathyroid adenomas. The product of the PRAD-1 gene is the cyclin protein D1 that affects regulation of the cell cycle. Parathyroid adenomas in which PRAD-1 is activated have undergone tumor-specific DNA rearrangements that juxtapose the regulatory region of the PTH gene (also on chromosome 11) with the coding region of PRAD-1 (Fig. 14.11). This leads to unregulated expression of PRAD-1 in the adenoma cell. The exact mechanism by which increased expression of this gene results in a benign parathyroid neoplasm is unknown. Genetic defects have also been identified in patients with multiple endocrine neoplasia types 1 and 2A, each of which have associated parathyroid hyperplasia and an autosomal dominant inheritance pattern (see section on Multiple Endocrine Neoplasia Syndromes). Mutations in the calcium sensing receptor gene have been identified in patients with familial hypocalciuric hypercalcemia and neonatal severe hyperparathyroidism (18). Abnormal expression of the tumor suppressor gene p53 and inactivation of the retinoblastoma gene have also

Table 14.6.
Differential Diagnosis of Hypercalcemia

Due to Increased Serum PTH
Primary and "tertiary" hyperparathyroidism
Some nonhematologic malignant disease

Not Due to Increased Serum PTH
Drug-induced hypercalcemia (thiazides, furosemide, vitamin D, calcium, vitamin A, lithium)
Granulomatous diseases (sarcoidosis, tuberculosis, berylliosis)
Genetic diseases (familial hypocalciuric hypercalcemia)
Immobilization
"Idiopathic" hypercalcemia
Some nonhematologic malignant diseases
Malignant hematologic diseases
Nonparathyroid endocrine diseases (Addison's disease, hyper- and hypothyroidism)

From Arnaud CD and Kolb FO. The calciotropic hormones and metabolic bone disease. In: Greenspan FS ed. Basic and clinical endocrinology, 3rd ed. Norwalk, CT: Appleton and Lange, 1991;274.

been described in some patients with parathyroid carcinoma.

Patients with primary hyperparathyroidism lack the adaptive mechanisms that normally protect the individual against hypercalcemia. Excessive secretion of PTH with its direct effects on the kidney and indirect actions on the intestine via vitamin D prevents a compensatory increase in urinary and intestinal losses of calcium from occurring. With mild states of hypercalcemia (< 11.5 mg/dl), calcium is reabsorbed efficiently by the kidney, and urinary calcium levels may remain low. With more severe hypercalcemia, however, the renal tubular mechanism is overwhelmed and hypercalciuria results. Decreased renal tubular reabsorption of phosphate leads to increased urinary phosphate excretion and hypophosphatemia. Excess PTH also causes decreased urinary excretion of hydrogen ion and increased excretion of bicarbonate. The hyperchloremic acidosis that results further aggravates the effects of hypercalcemia by increasing the fraction of ionized calcium in the circulation.

Conditions that must be distinguished from hyperparathyroidism in the differential diagnosis of hypercalcemia are shown in Table 14.6. The majority of these disorders can be excluded by a careful history and physical examination, family history, and review of medications (vitamin D, thiazides, alkali, and lithium). The disorders that are most difficult to differentiate from primary hyperparathyroidism are hypercalcemia of malignancy and familial hypercalcemic hypocalciuric hyperparathyroidism.

Hypercalcemia of malignancy is generally characterized by low PTH levels. Patients who present with marked hypercalcemia (calcium > 12.5 mg/dl) or the combination of hypercalcemia and weight loss, anemia, or an elevated erythrocyte sedimentation rate should undergo a careful search for an occult malignancy. The

Table 14.7.
Clinical Manifestations of Hyperparathyroidism

Organ System	Clinical Manifestations
Renal	Polyuria, nocturia, nephrolithiasis, nephrocalcinosis
Musculoskeletal	Proximal muscle weakness, calcific tendinitis, chondrocalcinosis, pseudogout, osteitis fibrosa cystica
Central Nervous System	Impair mentation, loss of recent memory, lethargy, insomnia, emotional lability, depression, somnolence, coma
Gastrointestinal	Anorexia, nausea, vomiting, dyspepsia, constipation
Skin	Pruritus
Ophthalmologic	Band keratopathy
Cardiovascular	Hypertension, heart block

mechanisms of development of hypercalcemia in malignancy are discussed in "Endocrine Manifestations of Nonendocrine Malignancies," below.

Familial hypocalciuric hypercalcemia (FHH), or familial benign hypercalcemia, is a rare condition characterized by asymptomatic or mildly symptomatic hypercalcemia, hypocalciuria, hypermagnesemia, and normal or low PTH levels. This disorder is inherited as an autosomal dominant trait, and the parathyroid glands are usually either normal in size or slightly enlarged. The basis for the development of FHH appears to be mutations in the calcium-sensing receptor gene on chromosome 3 which regulates the parathyroid gland set point and modulates the extracellular calcium concentration (18). Both heterozygous and homozygous forms of these mutations have been identified, and the latter is associated with more severe calcium resistance and hypercalcemia. Patients with FHH are usually asymptomatic and are not rendered eucalcemic by parathyroidectomy.

The clinical features of primary hyperparathyroidism are shown in Table 14.7. With the widespread use of biochemical screening tests, most patients with primary hyperparathyroidism are asymptomatic or have mild, nonspecific symptoms (muscle weakness and fatigue) at the time of diagnosis. The classic findings of osteitis fibrosis cystica with bone cysts and fractures are rarely seen. The principal radiographic sign of osteitis fibrosis cystica is subperiosteal bone resorption, which is best seen in the distal phalanx of the index finger. Other sites for development of subperiosteal erosions include the proximal tibia and femur, distal clavicles, and skull. Nephrolithiasis occurs in approximately 20% to 30% of patients. Extraskeletal calcification from deposition of calcium-phosphate crystals in the soft tissues may occur if the calcium times phosphate solubility product exceeds 70. Calcific tendinitis and chondrocalcinosis with joint pain and nephrocalcinosis with impairment of renal function may result.

Secondary Hyperparathyroidism

Secondary hyperparathyroidism represents an adaptive response to repetitive stimulation of the parathyroid

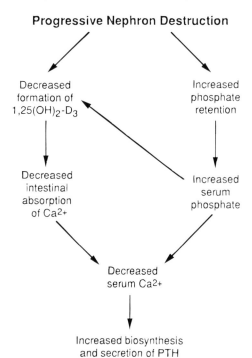

Figure 14.12. Pathogenesis of secondary hyperparathyroidism in chronic renal failure. From Arnaud CD. Hyperthyroidism and renal failure. Kidney Int 1973;4:90. Reprinted from *Kidney International* with permission.

glands by chronically low plasma levels of ionized calcium (19). The parathyroid glands themselves are intrinsically normal in secondary hyperparathyroidism. The most common cause is chronic renal failure. The pathophysiologic basis for the development of secondary hyperparathyroidism is outlined in Figure 14.12. As the glomerular filtration rate decreases to < 40 ml/min, phosphate excretion decreases and the serum phosphate concentration increases. This leads to a transient decrease in serum calcium concentration, which in turn stimulates secretion of PTH by the parathyroid glands. Serum calcium and phosphate levels return to normal as a result of the phosphaturic actions of PTH and mobilization of skeletal calcium. The cycle is progressively repeated with the gradual development of parathyroid hyperplasia and secondary hyperparathyroidism. Decreased intestinal absorption of calcium because of loss of $1,25(OH)_2$-D_3 from the kidney also contributes to the development of hypocalcemia.

The combined effects of increased PTH and reduced vitamin D levels in patients with chronic renal failure produce a complex array of skeletal abnormalities termed renal osteodystrophy. Characteristically, renal osteodystrophy consists of varying degrees of osteitis fibrosa cystica, generalized osteoporosis, osteomalacia, osteosclerosis, and growth retardation (19). The typical lesions of osteitis fibrosa cystica include subperiosteal bone resorption and the formation of bone cysts and cyst-like areas within the bone (brown tumors). Osteosclerosis occurs as a result of an increase in the thickness and number of trabeculae in spongy bone and is responsible for the "rugger jersey" appearance of the spine on plain radiographs. The combined effects of osteitis fibrosa cystica and osteosclerosis may give the skull a mottled, granular (salt and pepper) radiographic appearance. Bone pain with fractures, soft tissue calcification, and pruritus are the predominate clinical manifestations of secondary hyperparathyroidism. Treatment consists of dietary restriction of phosphate (including phosphate-binding antacids), calcium supplementation, and vitamin D therapy. Surgical parathyroidectomy is reserved for patients who develop progressive symptoms or complications on medical therapy.

Hypoparathyroidism

PTH-Deficient Hypoparathyroidism

Hypoparathyroidism may develop either as a result of a deficiency in secretion of PTH or end organ resistance to PTH (pseudohypoparathyroidism) (20). The causes of PTH-deficient hypoparathyroidism are shown in Table 14.8. Injury to the parathyroid glands during surgery accounts for the majority of these cases and is most commonly seen in patients undergoing extensive thyroidectomy for cancer or reoperative parathyroidectomy. The pathophysiologic consequences of PTH deficiency are (a) decreased bone resorption, (b) increased renal clearance of calcium, (c) decreased renal phosphate excretion, and (d) decreased renal production of $1,25(OH)_2$-D_3, which results in decreased intestinal absorption of calcium. Biochemically, these patients are hypocalcemic, are hyperphosphatemic, and have low to absent circulating levels of PTH.

Hypoparathyroidism is characterized clinically by increased neuromuscular excitability, which first manifests itself acutely as paresthesias around the mouth, fingertips, and feet. Progressive hypocalcemia may cause tetany with carpopedal spasms, hyperventilation, and ultimately, convulsions. The alkalosis that results

Table 14.8.
Causes of PTH - Deficient Hypoparathyroidism

Etiology	Basis for PTH Deficiency
Post-Surgical	Loss of all functional parathyroid tissue
Congenital	Congenital absence of parathyroids and thymus (DiGeorge's syndrome)
Idiopathic*	Unknown (? circulating parathyroid autoantibodies)
Functional	Chronic hypomagnesemia

* Idiopathic hypoparathyroidism has been categorized into early and late onset forms. The early onset form of hypoparathyroidism, also termed the "multiple endocrine deficiency-autoimmune-candidiasis syndrome" has a genetic origin and is often associated with circulating parathyroid and adrenal autoantibodies. The late onset form does not have associated autoantibodies, occurs sporadically, and has an unknown pathogenesis. From Arnaud CD and Kolb FO. The calciotropic hormones and metabolic bone disease. In Greenspan FS ed. Basic and clinical endocrinology, 3rd ed. Norwalk, CT: Appleton and Lange, 1991;249-322.

from hyperventilation may worsen the hypocalcemia by increasing the fraction of ionized calcium bound to plasma proteins. Other consequences of long-standing hypoparathyroidism include extrapyramidal neurologic disorders (Parkinsonism), cataracts, prolonged QT interval on ECG, heart block, dental abnormalities, and intestinal malabsorption. The treatment of hypoparathyroidism consists of replacement therapy with oral calcium and vitamin D. Acute hypocalcemia and tetany require emergency treatment with intravenous calcium.

Pseudohypoparathyroidism and Pseudopseudohypoparathyroidism

Pseudohypoparathyroidism is a rare familial disorder characterized by target tissue resistance to PTH, hypocalcemia, and congenital defects in growth and skeletal development. Parathyroid function is normal in these individuals and circulating PTH levels are increased appropriately for the degree of hypocalcemia. The biochemical abnormalities are similar to those seen in patients with surgical hypoparathyroidism, except for the elevated PTH levels. This disorder can also be distinguished from other causes of hypoparathyroidism by the failure of these patients to increase nephrogenous cAMP levels in response to exogenously administered parathyroid hormone. The treatment is the same as for patients with PTH-deficient hypoparathyroidism.

Pseudopseudohypoparathyroidism is characterized by the same skeletal developmental defects as pseudohypoparathyroidism, but it is distinguished by a lack of associated biochemical abnormalities. Serum calcium and phosphate levels are normal and no treatment is necessary.

The Pituitary

Anatomy and Development

The pituitary gland lies within the bony sella turcica (Turkish saddle), which is formed as a recess within the sphenoid bone in the anterior cranial fossa. The pituitary is surrounded by dura. The roof of the sella is formed by a reflection of dura attached to the clinoid processes (the diaphragma sella) (Fig. 14.13). In 10% of patients, the diaphragma sella is very thin, and in 40%, a 5-mm opening is present that may allow pituitary tumors to enlarge into the suprasellar region (21). The floor of the sella is formed by the roof of the sphenoid sinus, which provides surgical access to the pituitary. Laterally, the pituitary is bounded by the cavernous sinus and the carotid artery, and cranial nerves III, IV, and VI cross this sinus just lateral to the sella. The optic chiasm is located 5 to 10 mm above the diaphragma sella and is anterior to the pituitary stalk. The proximity of these

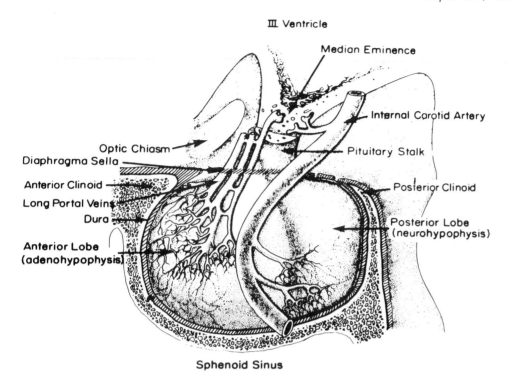

III Ventricle

Median Eminence

Internal Carotid Artery

Optic Chiasm

Pituitary Stalk

Diaphragma Sella

Anterior Clinoid

Posterior Clinoid

Long Portal Veins

Dura

Posterior Lobe
(neurohypophysis)

Anterior Lobe
(adenohypophysis)

Sphenoid Sinus

Figure 14.13. Anatomic relationships and blood supply of the pituitary gland. From Frohman LA. Diseases of the anterior pituitary. In: Felig P, Baxter JD, Broadus AE, Frohman LA, eds. Endocrinology and metabolism. New York: McGraw-Hill, 1981:152. Reprinted by permission of McGraw-Hill, Inc.

structures to the pituitary can cause cranial nerve palsies and visual field defects in patients with pituitary tumors. The pituitary gland normally weighs 500 to 900 mg and measures $15 \times 10 \times 6$ mm (22). The size of the gland may increase twofold in pregnancy.

The pituitary is divided anatomically and functionally into two parts: the adenohypophysis and the neurohypophysis (see Fig. 14.13). The adenohypophysis, derived embryologically from Rathke's pouch, is divided anatomically into the anterior lobe (pars distalis), pars intermedia, and pars tuberalis. In humans, the pars intermedia is indistinct and the anterior lobe, or par distalis, is the main source of pituitary hormone secretion. The neurohypophysis is an anatomic extension of the central nervous system derived from the neural primordia. It consists of the median eminence (infundibulum), the pituitary stalk (infundibular stem), and the posterior lobe (infundibular process).

Pituitary blood flow, which ranges from 0.5 to 0.8 ml/g/min, is the richest blood flow of any organ in the body (23). The adenohypophysis has no direct arterial supply but is supplied by venous blood from long portal veins connecting the median eminence of the hypothalamus and the anterior pituitary. Short portal venous channels from the posterior pituitary also contribute to the blood supply to the anterior lobe. The posterior pituitary receives arterial blood directly from the internal carotid artery via the middle and inferior hypophyseal arteries, which also supply the median eminence of the hypothalamus. Consequently, blood entering the posterior pituitary is outside of the blood-brain barrier. Blood exits the pituitary via the cavernous sinus, which drains into the superior and inferior petrosal sinuses and then

into the jugular bulb and vein. Sampling of inferior petrosal sinus blood for pituitary hormones can be a useful technique for the diagnosis and localization of pituitary tumors, especially in patients with Cushing's syndrome (24).

Physiology

Posterior Pituitary

The posterior pituitary or neurohypophysis secretes two peptides: oxytocin and vasopressin or antidiuretic hormone (ADH) (25). These hormones are each synthesized in axonal cell bodies of the supraoptic and paraventricular nuclei of the hypothalamus. Also synthesized by those hypothalamic neurons are carrier proteins called neurophysins, which bind specifically to the neurohypophyseal hormones. This hormone-neurophysin complex is then transported by the hypothalamic neurons to their termination point on capillaries in the posterior lobe of the pituitary where the active peptide and neurophysin are cleaved and released into the systemic circulation.

The principal action of vasopressin is to promote water absorption in the collecting ducts of the kidney. Increased secretion of vasopressin causes concentration of urine (maximum 1200 mOsm/kg water) and a decline in urine output (to as little as 0.5 ml/min). In the absence of vasopressin, such as occurs in patients with diabetes insipidus, urine osmolality may fall to as low as 30 mOsm/kg water and urine flow may increase to 15 to 20 ml/min. Vasopressin also exerts a constrictive effect on peripheral arterioles elevating blood pressure. Release of vasopressin occurs in response to an increase in plasma osmolality (> 285 mOsm) or decrease in plasma volume of 5% or more.

Oxytocin acts on uterine smooth muscle cells to increase the frequency and strength of contractions and stimulates the myoepithelial cells of the breast to induce milk ejection.

Anterior Pituitary

The anterior pituitary secretes six major hormones: growth hormone (GH), adrenocorticotropic hormone (ACTH), prolactin (PRL), TSH, follicle-stimulating hormone (FSH), and luteinizing hormone (LH). Secretion of these hormones is controlled primarily by hypothalamic hormones synthesized in the arcuate and other hypothalamic nuclei. These hypophyseal hormones are secreted into portal hypophyseal vessels, which connect the median eminence of the hypothalamus with capillary networks that bathe the cells of the adenohypophysis.

Growth Hormone. Growth hormone is a 191 amino acid peptide whose primary function is promotion of linear growth of bone, muscle, and the visceral organs. This growth-promoting action of GH is mediated by the somatomedins, a group of polypeptide insulin-like growth factors synthesized in the liver. Growth hormone acts via the somatomedins to increase amino acid uptake, increase protein synthesis, and decrease protein catabolism by promoting mobilization of fat as a fuel source. Growth hormone also interferes with glucose uptake and carbohydrate use by cells. This causes an increase in glucose levels and stimulation of insulin release. Hypothalamic control of GH secretion is mediated by growth hormone-releasing hormone (GHRH) and somatostatin (growth hormone-inhibitory hormone). A variety of neural, metabolic, and hormonal factors affect the rate of GH secretion. Physiologic stimuli for secretion include stress, exercise, hypoglycemia, and protein depletion. Secretion is episodic with peak secretory episodes occurring during stages 3 and 4 of sleep.

Prolactin. Prolactin is a 198 amino acid peptide whose primary action is stimulation of postpartum lactation. Physiologic stimuli of prolactin secretion include pregnancy, lactation, stress, and exercise. Although physiologic levels of prolactin do not affect gonadal function, hyperprolactinemia from prolactin-secreting pituitary tumors causes hypogonadism in both men and women. Unlike other anterior pituitary hormones, hypothalamic control of prolactin secretion is primarily inhibitory. Dopamine appears to be the principal prolactin inhibitory factor secreted by the hypothalamus. Both TRH and vasoactive intestinal peptide (VIP) stimulate prolactin secretion, although the inhibitory effect from dopamine predominates.

Adrenocorticotropic Hormone. ACTH is synthesized by the corticotroph cells of the pituitary as part of a large precursor molecule—proopiomelanocortin (molecular weight = 28,500). This precursor molecule is processed into several smaller, biologically active amino acid fragments that include ACTH (amino acids 1 to 39), lipotropin (amino acids 1 to 91), and endorphin (amino acids 61 to 91). The principal action of ACTH is to stimulate secretion of glucocorticoids, mineralocorticoids, and androgenic steroids from the adrenal cortex. The most important mediator of ACTH secretion is corticotropin-releasing factor (CRF), produced by the hypothalamus. Corticotropin-releasing factor stimulates ACTH secretion in a pulsatile manner, peaking in the early morning and progressively declining to a nadir in the late afternoon or evening. ACTH secretion is also stimulated physiologically by many types of stress, including pain, trauma, hypoxia, cold exposure, and acute hypoglycemia. Negative feedback control of ACTH release is maintained by cortisol and synthetic glucocorticoids at the level of the hypothalamus and pituitary.

Thyroid-Stimulating Hormone. Thyroid-stimulating hormone is a glycoprotein synthesized by the pituitary thyrotrophs and binds to specific receptors in the thyroid where it stimulates uptake of iodide and synthesis and release of thyroid hormone. TSH secretion is regulated by both stimulatory (TRH) and inhibitory (somatostatin) factors produced by the hypothalamus and by negative feedback inhibition of the hypothalamic-pituitary axis by thyroid hormone.

Gonadotropins. Follicle stimulating hormone and luteinizing hormone are glycoproteins, each of which are composed of an α-subunit and a β-subunit. The α-subunits are identical, and specific biologic activity resides in the β-subunit. The gonadotropins bind specific receptors in the ovaries and testes where they stimulate production of sex steroids and promote gametogenesis. In men, LH stimulates production of testosterone by the interstitial cells (Sertoli cells) of the testis, and FSH stimulates testicular growth. FSH also stimulates the Sertoli cells to produce an androgen-binding protein, which is essential for the development of the high local concentrations of testosterone required for normal spermatogenesis. Both gonadotropins are required for the process of sperm maturation. In women, LH stimulates estrogen and progesterone production by the ovary. The midcycle surge of LH causes ovulation, and continued LH secretion stimulates the corpus luteum to make progesterone. FSH controls maturation of the ovarian follicle, which secretes estrogen under the influence of both FSH and LH.

Secretion of LH and FSH is regulated by the hypothalamic hormone gonadotropin-releasing hormone (GnRH) and by positive and negative feedback mechanisms involving the sex steroid hormones. GnRH is a decapeptide that maintains basal gonadotropin secretion, generates the midcycle surge in gonadotropins necessary for ovulation, and regulates the onset of puberty (22). Secretion of GnRH is pulsatile, with hourly secretory bursts that cause a similar pattern of release of both FSH and LH. Pituitary sensitivity to the effects of GnRH is also increased by estrogen, and rising estrogen levels during the menstrual cycle provide the stimulus for the ovulatory surge in FSH and LH (positive feedback). Secretion of gonadotropins also occurs in response to stress, sexual stimuli, and castration. Stimulation of FSH and LH production is also seen in response to decreased circulating levels of sex hormones in patients with primary gonadal failure (negative feedback).

The Adrenal

Anatomy and Development

The adrenal gland is composed of a cortex and medulla, which have separate embryologic origins. The adrenal cortex arises from the coelomic mesoderm between the fourth and sixth weeks of gestation. The adrenal medulla is derived from cells of the neural crest that also form the sympathetic nervous system and the sympathetic ganglia. Some of these neural crest cells migrate into the adrenal cortex to form the adrenal medulla, but chromaffin tissue may also develop in extra adrenal sites in the para-aortic and paravertebral regions (Fig. 14.14). The most common site for extra adrenal chromaffin tissue is the organ of Zuckerkandl, located adjacent to the aorta near the origin of the inferior mesenteric artery.

The adrenal glands each weigh approximately 4 g and are located in the retroperitoneum along the superior-medial aspect of the kidneys (Fig. 14.15). A fibrous capsule surrounds the glands, which have a yellow appearance because of their high lipid content. The adrenal glands measure 3 to 5 cm in length and width and 4 to 6 mm in thickness. The left gland is slightly larger and thicker than the right. The adrenal glands are highly vascularized and receive arterial blood from branches of the inferior phrenic artery, aorta, and renal arteries. Within the gland, a sinusoidal plexus is formed, which drains into a single, central vein. The right adrenal vein is short and wide and exits the gland medially to enter the posterior aspect of the inferior vena cava. The left adrenal vein exits anteriorly and usually drains into the left renal vein, although it may occasionally enter the inferior vena cava directly. As a result, adrenal venous catheterization is accomplished more easily on the left than on the right.

The adrenal cortex accounts for 90% of total gland weight and is composed of three zones histologically. The outer zona glomerulosa is the exclusive site for aldosterone synthesis, whereas the large central zona fasciculata and inner zona reticularis produce both cortisol and androgens. The cells of the adrenal medulla are polyhedral in shape and are arranged in clumps and cords around blood vessels. Most of the blood supply to the medulla comes from venous blood draining through the

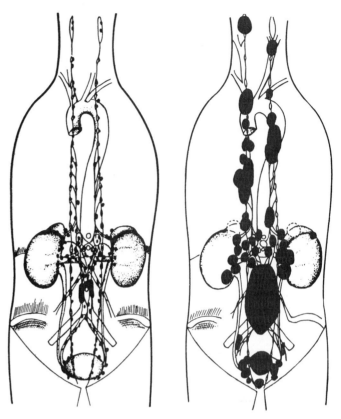

Figure 14.14. Distribution of chromaffin tissue in the newborn compared with distribution of extra adrenal pheochromocytomas. Extra adrenal pheochromocytomas (left) occur in and around the sympathetic ganglia in an anatomical distribution that parallels that of extra adrenal chromaffin tissue in the newborn (right). From Landsberg L, Young JB. Catecholamines and the adrenal medulla. In: Wilson RH, Foster DW, eds. Textbook of endocrinology. 7th ed. Philadelphia: WB Saunders, 1985:935. Reprinted by permission.

cortex. This provides the adrenal chromaffin cells with a high local concentration of cortisol, which induces the enzyme phenyl ethanolamine-*N*-methyltransferase (PNMT) required for conversion of norepinephrine to epinephrine. A direct arterial supply to the adrenal medulla is also present, primarily to cells that predominately secrete norepinephrine. The adrenal medulla is innervated by preganglionic fibers of the sympathetic nervous system.

The Adrenal Cortex

Physiology

The adrenal cortex secretes three major hormones: cortisol, androgens, and aldosterone. The biosynthetic pathway for these hormones and their intermediates is shown in Figure 14.16. Because of the differences in enzymatic activity between the zona glomerulosa and the zona fasciculata and reticularis, the adrenal cortex functions as two separate entities. The zona glomerulosa is the exclusive site of production of aldosterone because it lacks the 17α-hydroxylase enzyme necessary for synthesis of 17α-hydroxyprogesterone and 17α-hydroxy-

Figure 14.15. Schematic representation of the adrenal glands, their location and their blood supply. From Baxter JD. The adrenal cortex. In: Felig P, Baxter JD, Broadus AE, Frohman LA, eds. Endocrinology and metabolism. 2nd ed. New York: McGraw-Hill, 1987: 513. Reprinted by permission of McGraw-Hill, Inc.

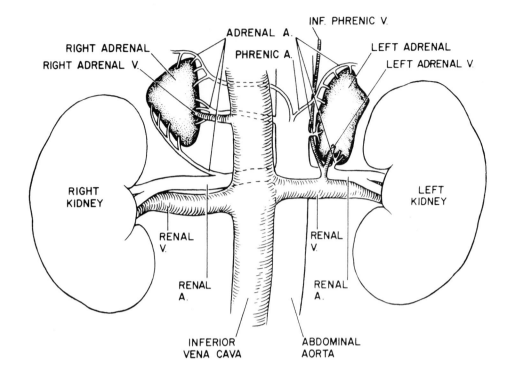

pregnenolone, which are the precursors for synthesis of cortisol and the adrenal androgens. The zona fasciculata and reticularis function as a unit to produce cortisol, androgens, and small amounts of estrogen, but they lack the enzymes necessary for conversion of 18-hydroxycorticosterone to aldosterone. Cholesterol is the precursor from which all adrenal steroids are synthesized. Conversion of cholesterol to pregnenolone is the rate-limiting step in adrenal steroidogenesis and is the major site of action of ACTH.

Glucocorticoids. Secretion of cortisol is regulated by the hypothalamus and pituitary via secretion of CRF and ACTH. Neuroendocrine control of this process is maintained by three mechanisms: (*a*) episodic secretion and the circadian rhythm of ACTH; (*b*) stress responsiveness of the hypothalamic-pituitary-adrenal axis; and (*c*) feedback inhibition of CRH and ACTH secretion by cortisol (26). Cortisol, like ACTH, is secreted in a pulsatile manner, and plasma levels closely parallel those of ACTH (Fig. 14.17). Superimposed on this episodic secretory pattern is a circadian rhythm that results in peak cortisol levels in the early morning and a nadir in the late evening. Physical and emotional stress (trauma, surgery, and hypoglycemia) increase cortisol secretion by stimulating release of CRF and ACTH from the hypothalamus and pituitary, respectively.

Circulating cortisol is more than 90% bound to plasma proteins, 75% which is bound to corticosteroid-binding globulin (CBG) and 15% to albumin. Biologic activity resides in the nonprotein-bound fraction, which has a circulatory half-life of 70 to 120 min. Normal daily production of cortisol is 10 to 30 mg. The liver is the major site of metabolism of cortisol. Two major metabo-

lites are 17-hydroxycorticosteroids and 17-ketosteroids, which are excreted in the urine.

The glucocorticoids exert their effects via their actions on intermediary metabolism and through interactions with a broad range of cells and tissues. Within the cell, these effects are initiated by binding of glucocorticoids to specific cytosolic receptor proteins. The activated glucocorticoid-receptor hormone complex then enters the cell nucleus where it binds to specific hormone-responsive DNA sequences called glucocorticoid-response elements. Glucocorticoid-specific genes are then activated, leading to gene transcription and synthesis of proteins that mediate the glucocorticoid response. The types of proteins synthesized and their ability to stimulate or inhibit other biologic activities varies widely as a result of the differential expression of specific genes in the different cell types (26).

The metabolic effects of the glucocorticoids include stimulation of hepatic gluconeogenesis, inhibition of protein synthesis, increased protein catabolism, and lipolysis of adipose tissue. The increased release of amino acids from muscle protein and release of glycerol and free fatty acids from fat provide the substrates for hepatic gluconeogenesis. In addition, glucocorticoids increase the hepatic response to the gluconeogenic hormones (glucagon and catecholamines) and increase glycogen synthesis. Peripheral uptake of glucose in most tissues (except liver, brain, and red blood cells) is inhibited and may cause hyperglycemia and increased insulin secretion, especially in states of chronic cortisol excess.

Glucocorticoids cause loss of collagen and impair wound healing by inhibition of fibroblast activity. They

STEROID BIOSYNTHETIC PATHWAY

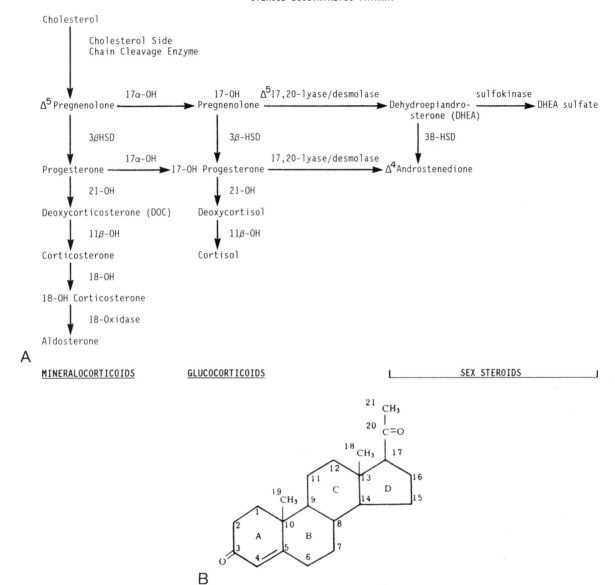

Figure 14.16. **A,** Biosynthetic pathway for adrenal steroid synthesis. *OH,* hydroxylase; *3β-HSD,* 3-hydroxy-Δ^5-steroid dehydrogenase; *17-HSO,* 17-hydroxysteroid oxireductase. From Conte FA, Grumbach MM. Pathogenesis, classification, diagnosis, and treatment of anomalies of sex. In: DeGroot LJ, ed. Endocrinology. 2nd ed. Philadelphia: WB Saunders, 1989:1825. Reprinted by permission. **B,** Basic C21 steroid structure of the adrenocortical steroids. The letters in the formula for progesterone identify the A, B, C, and D rings; the numbers identify the position of each atom within the C21 structure. From Ganong WF. Review of medical physiology. 14th ed. Norwalk, CT: Appleton & Lange, 1989:294.

inhibit bone formation, reduce intestinal absorption of calcium, and induce negative calcium balance, all of which contribute to the development of steroid-induced osteoporosis. Glucocorticoids also have numerous anti-inflammatory actions, which include inhibition of leukocyte mobilization and function, decreased migration of inflammatory cells to sites of injury, and decreased production of inflammatory mediators (e.g., interleukin-1, leukotrienes, and bradykinins). These properties may account for the increased susceptibility to infection of patients who suffer from chronic steroid excess. The glucocorticoids are also essential for cardiovascular stabil-

ity, as evidenced by the cardiovascular collapse that occurs in patients with acute adrenal insufficiency.

Androgens. The adrenal androgens, dehydroepiandrosterone (DHEA) and DHEA sulfate, have minimal direct biologic activity. In the periphery they undergo conversion to the active androgens testosterone and dihydrotestosterone. Increased production of adrenal androgens may occur in patients with Cushing's syndrome, adrenal carcinoma, and congenital adrenal hyperplasia. In normal males, adrenal androgens account for less than 5% of total testosterone production, and so the clinical effects of excess adrenal synthesis

Figure 14.17. Fluctuations in plasma ACTH and gluco-corticoids (11-hydroxy-corticosteroids) throughout the day. Note the greater ACTH and glucocorticoid levels in the morning before awakening. From Krieger DT, Allen W, Rizzo F, Krieger HP. Characterization of the normal temporal pattern of plasma corticosteroid levels. J Clin Endocrinol Metab 1971;32:266. Reprinted by permission of The Endocrine Society.

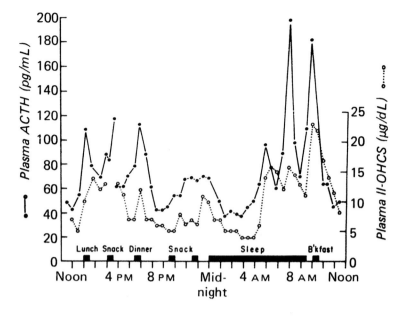

Figure 14.18. Regulation of aldosterone secretion. A fall in blood volume, a fall in blood pressure, or vasoconstriction of the renal arteries produces a decrease in pressure in the afferent arteriole leading to a release of renin from the juxtaglomerular cells and stimulation of the renin-angiotensin-aldosterone axis. ACTH and hyperkalemia also stimulate release of aldosterone. From Bergland RM, Gann DS, De Maria EJ. The pituitary and adrenals. In: Schwartz SI, ed. Principles of surgery. 5th ed. New York: McGraw-Hill, 1989:1566. Reprinted by permission of McGraw-Hill, Inc.

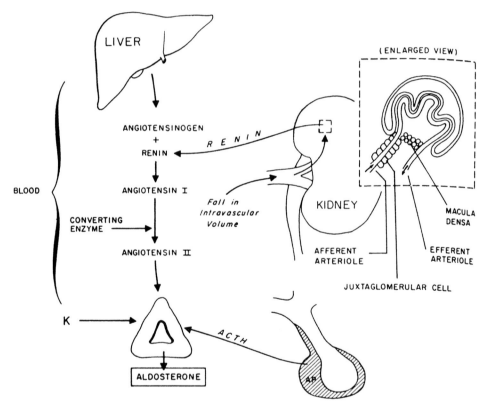

are minimal. In prepubertal boys, however, increased production of androgen may be manifested by the early development of secondary sexual characteristics and penile enlargement. Excess androgen production in women is manifested by the development of acne, hirsutism, virilization, and amenorrhea. Increased production of estrogen causes gynecomastia in men and precocious breast development and menstrual bleeding in women.

Aldosterone. The principal actions of aldosterone are maintenance of extracellular fluid volume and regulation of sodium and potassium balance. The major physiologic regulator of aldosterone secretion is the renin-angiotensin system (Fig. 14.18). The plasma potassium concentration and, to a lesser extent, plasma sodium and ACTH also influence aldosterone secretion. Renin is an enzyme secreted by the juxtaglomerular cells of the kidney in response to decreased pressure in the renal afferent arterioles. Decreases in plasma sodium concentration sensed by osmoreceptors in the cells of the macula densa promote renin release as well. Renin secretion is also stimulated by hyperkalemia and inhibited by potassium depletion. Renin converts angiotensinogen into angiotensin I, a decapeptide that is in turn altered in the lung by converting enzyme to form angiotensin II. Angiotensin II is a potent vasoconstrictor that is important in maintaining blood pressure in response to hemorrhage and hypovolemia. It also directly stimulates cells of the zona glomerulosa to secrete aldosterone. Aldosterone then stimulates renal tubular reabsorption of sodium in exchange for potassium and hydrogen ion secretion. The net effect is fluid reabsorption and expansion of the intravascular volume.

Pathophysiology

Cushing's Syndrome

Signs and Symptoms. Cushing's syndrome refers to the constellation of signs and symptoms that result from chronic glucocorticoid excess. The most common source of Cushing's syndrome is iatrogenic administration of glucocorticoids. ACTH-secreting tumors of the pituitary are the most common cause of spontaneous Cushing's syndrome. Pituitary Cushing's, also termed Cushing's disease, accounts for approximately 70% of all cases of Cushing's syndrome. Ectopic ACTH-secreting tumors comprise 15% of cases and are associated most commonly with small-cell carcinomas of the lung. Primary adrenal tumors (adenomas and carcinoma) account for 15% to 20% of cases.

The clinical symptoms and signs associated with Cushing's syndrome are shown in Table 14.9. Obesity is the most constant feature and is characteristically centrally distributed around the face, trunk, neck, and abdomen. Skin changes occur frequently and include

Table 14.9.
Clinical Features of Cushing's Syndrome

Features	%
Obesity	94
Facial plethora	84
Hirsutism	82
Menstrual disorders	76
Hypertension	72
Muscular weakness	58
Back pain	58
Striae	52
Acne	40
Psychologic symptoms	40
Bruising	36
Congestive heart failure	22
Edema	18
Renal calculi	16
Headache	14
Polyuria-polydipsia	10
Hyperpigmentation	6

From Baxter JD and Tyrrel JB. The adrenal cortex. In: Felig P, Baxter J, Braodus A, et al., eds. Endocrinology and metabolism. New York, NY: McGraw-Hill, 1981; Reprinted with permission.

increased fragility, bruising, and skin striae. Hyperpigmentation is seen most commonly in patients with ectopic ACTH production. Hirsutism from increased secretion of adrenal androgens is frequently present in women, but virilism is uncommon except in patients with adrenal carcinoma. Increased production of adrenal androgens also causes gonadal dysfunction manifested by amenorrhea and infertility. In males, increased production of cortisol may cause decreased libido, reduction in body hair, and testicular atrophy.

There are two essential steps in the laboratory evaluation of patients with Cushing's syndrome: documentation of excess adrenal cortisol production and identification of the source. An outline of the approach to the diagnostic evaluation of Cushing's syndrome is given in Figure 14.19.

Biochemical Screening Tests for the Diagnosis of Cushing's Syndrome

Plasma Cortisol. Because of the episodic nature of ACTH and cortisol secretion, plasma cortisol levels vary greatly with the assay method employed and the time of day that the sample is obtained. Cortisol levels obtained at 4 P.M. are usually about half those obtained at 8 A.M. Patients with Cushing's syndrome lose this diurnal variation in cortisol levels.

Urinary Free Cortisol. The most useful screening test in the evaluation of Cushing's syndrome is measurement of urinary free cortisol. Normally, less than 1% of cortisol is excreted in the urine, but with increased rates of cortisol secretion, corticotropin-binding globulin becomes saturated and free cortisol is excreted. Elevated urinary cortisol levels are present in more than 90% of patients with Cushing's syndrome.

17-Hydroxycorticosteroids and 17-Ketosteroids. Measurement of urinary metabolites of cortisol are less useful in the diagnosis of Cushing's syndrome than plasma and urinary free cortisol levels. 17-ketosteroids are produced from metabolism of both cortisol and androgens. Although they may be elevated in patients with adrenal androgen excess, they are less specific and sensitive than plasma androgen assays.

Low-Dose Dexamethasone Suppression Test. Dexamethasone is a synthetic glucocorticoid with enhanced biologic activity compared with cortisol because of its higher affinity for the glucocorticoid receptor. Dexamethasone suppresses pituitary secretion of ACTH and adrenal production of corticosteroids via feedback inhibition of the hypothalamic-pituitary-adrenal axis. The low dose dexamethasone suppression test is frequently used to establish a biochemical diagnosis of Cushing's syndrome. In the single-dose dexamethasone test, 1 mg of dexamethasone is given orally at 11 p.m. and plasma cortisol measured at 8 a.m. the next morning. Suppression of plasma cortisol to less than 3 μg/dl excludes the diagnosis of Cushing's syndrome. Patients with plasma cortisol levels greater than 10 μg/dl likely have Cush-

Figure 14.19. Diagnostic evaluation of Cushing's syndrome and procedures for determining the cause. From Baxter JD, Tyrrell JB. The adrenal cortex. In: Felig P, Baxter JD, Broadus AE, Frohman LA, eds. Endocrinology and metabolism. 2nd ed. New York: McGraw-Hill, 1987:609. Reprinted by permission of McGraw-Hill, Inc.

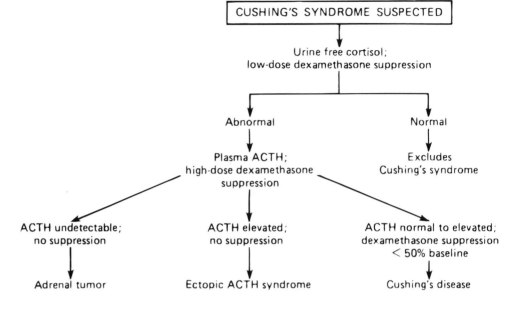

ing's syndrome and require further testing. False negative results with this test are rare, as greater than 98% of patients with Cushing's syndrome have an abnormal response to the overnight dexamethasone test. False positive results occur in approximately 15% of obese patients and 25% of hospitalized chronically ill patients. In the 2-day low-dose dexamethasone test, 24-hour urine collections for 17-hydroxycorticosteroids are obtained before and during the second day of administration of 0.5 mg dexamethasone every 6 hours. This test is cumbersome and time-consuming and requires collection of 24-hour urine specimens. It is associated with both false positive and false negative results and is no longer recommended for the biochemical diagnosis of Cushing's syndrome.

Tests to Determine the Etiology of Cushing's Syndrome

Plasma ACTH. Plasma ACTH levels are used to differentiate ACTH-dependent (pituitary and ectopic ACTH-secreting tumors) from adrenal causes of Cushing's syndrome (Fig. 14.20). In patients with cortisol-secreting primary adrenal neoplasms, ACTH levels are suppressed (< 5 pg/ml). Patients with pituitary Cushing's should have ACTH levels that are normal or moderately elevated (15 to 200 pg/ml). Markedly elevated ACTH levels are often seen in patients with ectopic ACTH-secreting tumors, although some overlap exists with levels seen in Cushing's disease.

High-Dose Dexamethasone Test. The high-dose dexamethasone test is used to distinguish pituitary from nonpituitary causes of ACTH-dependent Cushing's syndrome. The rationale for this test is that supraphysiologic doses of glucocorticoids will suppress the hypothalamic-pituitary axis, ACTH secretion, and cortisol production in patients with ACTH hypersecretion from a pituitary tumor but will not affect cortisol production

in patients with primary adrenal neoplasms or ectopic ACTH-secreting tumors. The single-dose 8 mg dexamethasone test is simpler to perform and more reliable than the 2-day test. A basal level of plasma cortisol is obtained at 8 a.m. on the day before the test. A single 11 p.m. dose of 8 mg dexamethasone is given orally, and plasma cortisol is measured at 8 a.m. the next day. The 2-day high-dose dexamethasone test is performed in a manner identical to the 2-day low-dose test, except dexamethasone is given in a dose of 2 mg every 6 hours and urinary 17-hydroxycorticosteroids are measured. With either test, patients with pituitary Cushing's syndrome should have suppression of plasma or urinary corticosteroids to less than 50% of the basal level, whereas cortisol levels in patients with ectopic ACTH production or primary adrenal tumors are usually unchanged. However, 20 to 30% of patients with mildly increased corticotropin secretion and pituitary Cushing's fail to suppress steroid production to $< 50\%$ of baseline, and some patients with ACTH-secreting tumors do suppress plasma and urine steroids to this level. Therefore, the overall diagnostic accuracy of the high dose dexamethasone suppression test is only 70 to 80% (27).

Inferior Petrosal Sinus Sampling. The most direct method to differentiate pituitary from non-pituitary causes of ACTH-dependent Cushing's syndrome is measurement of inferior petrosal sinus blood for ACTH with and without CRH stimulation (27). This procedure requires a highly-skilled interventional radiologist who can reliably cannulate both inferior petrosal sinuses. Simultaneous measurements of peripheral and bilateral inferior petrosal sinus and plasma ACTH levels are carried out both before and after administration of 100 μg of CRH intravenously. A basal or stimulated inferior petrosal sinus:peripheral ACTH ratio of greater than 2.0 to 3.0 reliably indicates pituitary Cushing's disease, and a gradient less than 1.8 is diagnostic of an ectopic ACTH-

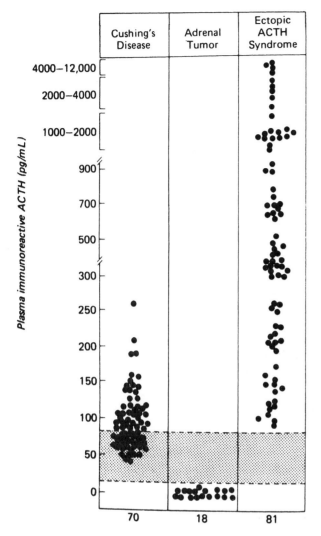

Figure 14.20. Basal plasma ACTH concentrations in patients with spontaneous Cushing's syndrome. From Scott AP, Bloomfield GA, Lowry PJ, Gilkes JJH, Landon J, Rees LH. Pituitary adreno-corticotropin and the melanocyte stimulating hormones. In: Parson JA, ed. Peptide hormones. Baltimore: University Park Press, 1976:266.

secreting tumor (24). This technique may also serve to localize the microadenoma within the pituitary gland if the ACTH gradient lateralizes to only one petrosal sinus. Inferior petrosal sinus sampling is an invasive and costly procedure and should be reserved for patients in whom the diagnosis cannot be made by other means.

Radiologic Tests. Once the biochemical evaluation of the patient with Cushing's syndrome has been completed, radiographic localization of the source of the Cushing's syndrome should be carried out. The most common ectopic ACTH-producing tumors are small cell lung carcinomas or bronchial or thymic carcinoids. The majority of these tumors can be detected by CT scanning or by radionuclide imaging with indium-111 labeled octreotide analogs which detect tumors that express somatostatin receptors. Magnetic resonance imaging of the pituitary will demonstrate an adenoma in 50 to 60% of patients with pituitary Cushing's (28). A computed tom-

ographic scan of the adrenal glands is the preferred localization modality in patients with suspected adrenal Cushing's syndrome. If the results of these studies are negative and the etiology of the ACTH-dependent Cushing's syndrome is still unclear, then bilateral inferior petrosal sinus sampling for ACTH should be carried out because the most likely etiology is an occult pituitary tumor.

Disorders of Excess Adrenal Androgen Production. Adrenal causes of excess androgen production include Cushing's syndrome, adrenal carcinoma, and congenital adrenal hyperplasia. Congenital adrenal hyperplasia refers to a group of autosomal-recessive disorders characterized by defects in the synthesis of cortisol. This impaired production of cortisol stimulates ACTH release, which leads to adrenal hyperplasia and increased production of adrenal androgens and androgen precursors. The most common cause of congenital adrenal hyperplasia is 21α-hydroxylase deficiency. Severe electrolyte and fluid losses may develop in up to 80% of patients with 21α-hydroxylase deficiency because of an associated defect in aldosterone production.

In adults, excess adrenal androgens cause testicular atrophy in males and hirsutism, acne, and irregular or absent menses in women. Virilism in women, from marked excess production of adrenal androgens, is characterized by male pattern baldness, clitoral enlargement, and development of masculine features, including increased muscle bulk and deepening of the voice. The diagnosis of androgen excess is made most accurately by measurement of plasma androgen levels, including DHEA, DHEA sulfate, testosterone, and dihydrotestosterone. Plasma androgens are elevated in approximately 85% of women with hirsutism. Other causes of hirsutism and virilism in women include the polycystic ovary syndrome and androgen-secreting ovarian tumors.

Primary Aldosteronism. Increased production of aldosterone by the adrenal glomerulosa cells results in a syndrome characterized by hypertension and hypokalemia in conjunction with suppression of plasma renin activity (29). Excess aldosterone leads to sodium retention and expansion of the extracellular fluid volume, which feeds back on the renal juxtaglomerular cells and macula densa to shut off renin production. Both potassium and hydrogen ion are excreted in the urine in exchange for sodium, which results in potassium depletion and alkalosis. Movement of hydrogen ion into the cells to replace intracellular potassium also contributes to the alkalosis. Mild glucose intolerance may accompany significant potassium depletion.

The symptoms and signs of primary aldosteronism are nonspecific and include fatigue, weakness, and nocturia. With severe potassium depletion, patients may develop increased thirst, polyuria, and paresthesias. Hypertension is usually present and may be severe, but is rarely malignant.

The diagnosis of primary aldosteronism should be suspected in any patient with spontaneous hypokalemia and hypertension. Patients on a low sodium diet may have a normal serum potassium level, however, because potassium losses decrease as the amount of sodium available for reabsorption in the distal tubule decreases. Patients with a normal potassium level and suspected primary aldosteronism should have a serum potassium determination while on a high sodium diet (1 g sodium for 4 days). Other laboratory features of primary aldosteronism include elevation of serum sodium and bicarbonate levels. The diagnosis is confirmed by demonstrating increased plasma aldosterone levels or increased urinary excretion of aldosterone (normal 5 to 20 μg/24 h), in conjunction with suppressed plasma renin activity. The principal causes of primary aldosteronism are aldosterone-producing adenomas (65%) and idiopathic hyperaldosteronism (35%) from bilateral adrenal cortical hyperplasia. Adrenal carcinoma is an extremely rare cause of hyperaldosteronism. Glucocorticoid-suppressible hyperaldosteronism is another rare cause of primary aldosteronism. This condition is inherited as an autosomal dominant disorder and is characterized by suppression of excessive aldosterone secretion with administration of a glucocorticoid, such as dexamethasone. This syndrome appears to result from a mutational crossover that causes expression of a hybrid gene, encoding aldosterone synthase in the zona fasciculata such that transcription of this gene is regulated primarily by ACTH (30). Elevation of plasma aldosterone in response to increased renin production by the kidney is termed secondary aldosteronism and may be caused by a variety of conditions, including renovascular hypertension, decreased intravascular volume (congestive heart failure, nephrosis, cirrhosis), and Bartter's syndrome.

Adrenal Insufficiency. Adrenal insufficiency occurs most commonly in surgical patients as a result of chronic cortisol administration with suppression of adrenal cortical function. The primary cause of spontaneous adrenal insufficiency is autoimmune adrenal disease. Other causes of adrenal insufficiency include bilateral adrenal hemorrhage, adrenal metastases, and postsurgical after adrenalectomy. Chronic adrenal insufficiency is characterized by hyperpigmentation of the skin, weakness, fatigue, anorexia, weight loss, nausea, vomiting, salt-craving, and hypotension. In patients with inadequate adrenal reserve, the stress of surgery, trauma, infection, or dehydration may precipitate an acute adrenal crisis. Acute adrenal insufficiency is characterized by unexplained vascular collapse with hypotension and shock. Abdominal pain, weakness, depressed mentation, and fever are also commonly present. Patients with unexplained cardiovascular collapse in whom the diagnosis is suspected should be treated empirically with replacement corticosteroids to avoid the lethal consequences of this condition.

Biochemical manifestations of adrenal insufficiency include hyponatremia, hyperkalemia, hypoglycemia, and azotemia, with increased blood urea nitrogen and creatinine concentrations. The diagnosis is confirmed by measurement of urinary or plasma glucocorticoid levels. In patients with partial adrenal insufficiency, determination of adrenocortical reserve with the ACTH stimulation test is necessary to establish the diagnosis. Plasma ACTH levels are often useful in delineating the cause (pituitary versus adrenal) of the adrenal insufficiency. Pituitary-adrenal reserve in patients with adrenal insufficiency can also be assessed with the metyrapone test. Metyrapone inhibits 11β-hydroxylase activity and thereby blocks conversion of 11-deoxycortisol to cortisol. In patients given metyrapone, 11-deoxycortisol production should increase as ACTH secretion increases in response to the decrease in plasma cortisol levels. An increase in 11-deoxycortisol levels (> 7 μg/dl) in response to metyrapone is indicative of normal pituitary and adrenal function.

Adrenal Medulla

The pathway for catecholamine biosynthesis is shown in Figure 14.21. Hepatic synthesis of tyrosine from phenylalanine and dietary sources provide the substrate for catecholamine synthesis. The enzymes necessary for catecholamine synthesis are found in all chromaffin tissues except for PNMT, which is present only in the adrenal medulla, organ of Zuckerkandl, and select central nervous system neurons. High local concentrations of cortisol (as found in the adrenal medulla) are necessary for induction of PNMT activity. Catecholamines are stored in chromaffin granules within the sympathetic nerve terminals and in the cells of the adrenal medulla. Secretion of catecholamines is initiated by release of acetylcholine from preganglionic nerve fibers. Acetylcholine then induces cell depolarization, which results in an influx of calcium into the cell and exocytosis of neurosecretory granules. Secretion of catecholamines occurs in response to a variety of stressful stimuli, including exercise, hemorrhage, surgery, angina or myocardial infarction, hypoglycemia, and anoxia. Upon release, catecholamines rapidly induce their biologic effect and then are metabolized by one of several mechanisms. These include reuptake by sympathetic nerve endings, metabolism by catechol-o-methyltransferase (COMT) and monoamine oxidase, or excretion by the kidney. COMT is the enzyme responsible for metabolism of most circulating catecholamines.

The catecholamines exert their biologic effects by interaction with specific cell-surface receptors. The types of receptors and effects they mediate in the various target tissues are outlined in Table 14.10 (31). The principal physiologic effect of α-receptor stimulation is vasoconstriction. Two types of β receptors exist. The β_1-receptors mediate inotropic and chronotropic stimulation of

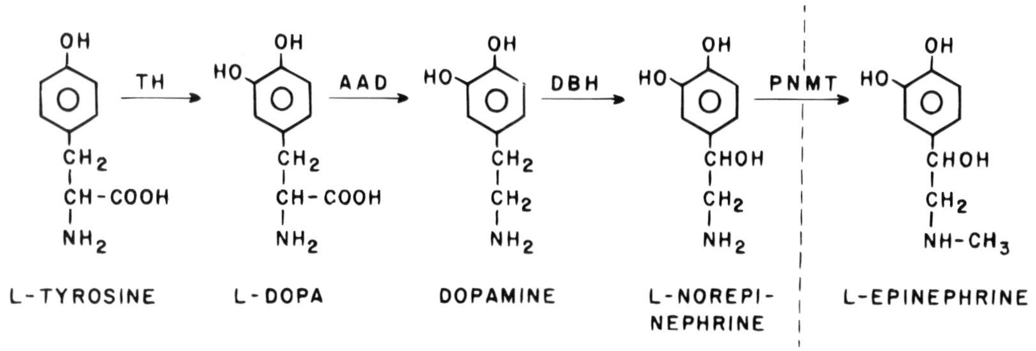

Figure 14.21. Biosynthetic pathway for catecholamines. Tyrosine hydroxylase (TH), aromatic-L-amino acid decarboxylase (AAD), and dopamine-β-hydroxylase (DBH) catalyze formation of norepinephrine from tyrosine. Subsequent formation of epinephrine, catalyzed by PNMT, takes place in the adrenal medulla and in neurons of the central nervous system and peripheral ganglia that use epinephrine as a neurotransmitter. From Bondy PK, Rosenberg LE. Metabolic control and disease. 8th ed. Philadelphia: WB Saunders, 1980:1626. Reprinted by permission.

Table 14.10.
Adrenergic Responses of Selected Tissues

Organ or Tissue	Receptor	Effect
Heart (myocardium)	β_1	Increased force and rate of contraction
Blood vessels	α	Vasoconstriction
	β_2	Vasodilatation
Kidney	β	Increased renin release
Gut	α,β	Decreased motility and increased sphincter tone
Pancreas	α	Decreased release of insulin and glucagon
	β	Increased release of insulin and glucagon
Liver	α,β	Increased glycogenolysis
Adipose tissue	β	Increased lipolysis
Most tissues	β	Increased calorigenesis
Skin (apocrine glands)	α	Increased sweating
Bronchioles	β_2	Dilatation
Uterus	α	Contraction
	β_2	Relaxation

From Goldfien A. Adrenal medulla. In: Greenspan Basis and clinical endocrinology, FS ed. 3rd ed. Norwalk, CT: Appleton and Lange, 1991; 387. Reprinted with permission.

Table 14.11.
Relative Potency of Adrenergic Receptor Agonists

Receptor	Agonist
Alpha	Epinephrine slightly > norepinephrine ≫ isoproterenol
Beta$_1$	Isoproterenol > epinephrine ≅ norepinephrine
Beta$_2$	Isoproterenol > epinephrine ≫ norepinephrine

Modified from Cryer PE. Diseases of the sympathochromaffin system. In: Felig P, Baxter J, Broadus E, et al., eds. 2nd ed. New York: McGraw-Hill, 1987;657. Reprinted with permission.

cardiac muscle, whereas β_2-receptors induce relaxation of smooth muscle in noncardiac tissues, including blood vessels, the bronchi, uterus, and adipose tissue. Catecholamines also affect cellular metabolism by increasing O_2 consumption and heat production. In liver and cardiac muscle, they stimulate glycogenolysis, which serves to increase the availability of carbohydrate for tissue use. In adipose tissue, they induce lipolysis and increase release of free fatty acids and glycerol. Both norepinephrine and epinephrine inhibit insulin secretion. The relative potency of the various catecholamines in stimulating receptor activity is shown in Table 14.11.

Pheochromocytoma

Pheochromocytomas are catecholamine-secreting tumors that arise from chromaffin tissue. The majority of pheochromocytomas (85% to 90%) arise in the adrenal gland, but they may occur in any site where chromaffin tissue is found. Several features of pheochromocytomas are characterized by a 10% frequency of distribution: 10% extra adrenal, 10% bilateral, 10% in children, 10% familial, and 10% malignant. The signs and symptoms of pheochromocytomas are related to the effects of sustained and/or paroxysmal secretion of norepinephrine and epinephrine (31). Paroxysmal attacks from pheochromocytomas often begin as a pounding in the chest from forceful cardiac contractions induced by the β_1-receptor-mediated increase in cardiac output. These symptoms may progress to involve the trunk and head and commonly cause headaches. Hands and feet become cool, moist, and pale from α-receptor-induced peripheral vasoconstriction. Blood pressure may become markedly elevated from the combination of intense vasoconstriction and increased cardiac output. Temperature elevation, flushing, and sweating may result from hypermetabolism and from a reduction in heat loss secondary to peripheral vasoconstriction. Marked anxiety and an impending sense of doom are occasionally present. Most attacks are short-lived (< 15 min duration) but recur frequently. They may be precipitated by physical activity (change in position, exercise, defecation), emotional stress, or may occur spontaneously.

The diagnosis of pheochromocytoma is established by demonstration of elevated levels of urinary catecholamines and metabolites (vanillylmandelic acid and metanephrine). Measurement of plasma catecholamines during an attack may be necessary to establish the diagnosis in the small number of patients with negative urinary studies. Preoperative α-receptor blockade with phenoxybenzamine (Dibenzyline) and expansion of intravascular volume by hydration are essential for intraoperative control of blood pressure during surgical extirpation. Patients with marked tachycardia or arrhythmias may also require β-receptor blockage with propranolol. β-receptor blockade should never be initiated without first achieving α-blockade because a hypertensive crisis can result from unopposed α-stimulation.

Endocrine Pancreas

Cellular Anatomy

The pancreas contains numerous small endocrine glands, called the islets of Langerhans, scattered throughout the exocrine pancreatic tissue. Although the islet cells comprise only 1% of the total pancreatic cell mass, they are richly vascularized, receiving 10% of total pancreatic blood flow (32). Four types of cells—A, B, D, and F—have been identified in normal pancreatic islets. These cells function as major regulators of nutrient metabolism by secretion of glucagon (A cell), insulin (B cell), somatostatin (D cell), and pancreatic polypeptide (F cell). The distribution of these cell types within the various regions of the pancreas is shown in Table 14.12.

Physiology

Insulin

Synthesis of insulin begins with production of the precursor molecule preproinsulin (molecular weight 11,500) in the endoplasmic reticulum of the B cell. Preproinsulin is cleaved to form proinsulin (molecular weight 9,000), which consists of the A and B chains of the insulin molecule and a connecting peptide as shown in Figure 14.22. Proinsulin is transported to the Golgi apparatus and packaged into secretory granules. With maturation of the granule, proinsulin is enzymatically cleaved to form the 51 amino acid insulin molecule and 31 amino acid C-peptide, which are cosecreted by the B cell. Small amounts of proinsulin are also released into the circulation and may be detected by most antisera used in standard immunoassays for insulin. Normally, 12% to 20% of immunoreactive insulin in the bloodstream is accounted for by proinsulin (32).

The insulin molecule (molecular weight 5800) consists of A and B peptide chains linked by two disulfide bridges (see Fig. 14.22). An intra chain disulfide bond also links positions 6 and 11 in the A chain. Circulating insulin has a half-life of 3 to 5 minutes, and about 50% is removed from the circulation by a single pass through the liver.

The normal adult pancreas secretes approximately 40 to 50 units of insulin daily. Basal fasting insulin concentrations in normal subjects average 10 μU/ml but may rise to 100 μU/ml after ingestion of a standard meal. Secretion of insulin by the B cell occurs in response to a variety of physiologic stimuli, including glucose, amino acids, fatty acids, and ketone bodies. The most potent of these stimuli for insulin release is glucose. Within a few minutes of food ingestion, insulin levels rise in response to an increase in glucose levels (Fig. 14.23). Peak insulin levels are reached within 30 to 45 minutes of eating and are accompanied by a rapid decline in blood glucose to near basal levels 90 to 120 minutes postprandially. Several of the gastrointestinal hormones released in response to meal stimulation (gastric-inhibitory polypeptide [GIP], cholecystokinin [CCK], secretin, and gastrin) further augment the rate of insulin secretion by potentiating the effects of glucose on the B cell.

Insulin exerts its biologic activity via both paracrine effects on adjacent islet cells and more distant endocrine effects on liver, muscle, and adipose tissue. Locally, insulin inhibits glucagon secretion by the A cells. Glucagon secretion is further inhibited by somatostatin, which is released from the pancreatic D cells in response to many of the same agents that stimulate insulin secretion.

Table 14.12.
Cell types in the Pancreatic Islets of Langerhans

Cell Types	Approximate % of Islet Volume		Secretory Products
	Dorsally Derived[1] (anterior head, body, tail)	Ventrally Derived[2] (posterior portion of head)	
A cell (α)	20%	<0.5%	Glucagon
B cell (β)	70–80%	15–20%	Insulin, C peptide, proinsulin
D cell (δ)	3–5%	<1%	Somatostatin
F cell (PP cell)	< 2%	80–85%	Pancreatic polypeptide

[1] Arises from embryonic dorsal bud and receives most of blood supply from celiac artery.
[2] Arises from primordial ventral bud and receives blood from superior mesenteric artery.
From Karen JH, Salber PR, Forsham PH, et al. Pancreatic hormone and diabetes mellitus. In: Greenspan FS ed. Basic and clinical endocrinology. 3rd ed. Norwalk, CT: Appleton and Lange, 1991;593. Reprinted with permission.

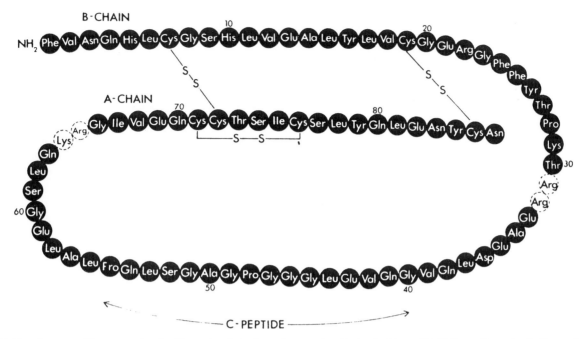

Figure 14.22. Structure of human proinsulin. The molecule is cleaved at amino acids 31 to 32 and 64 to 65 to form insulin and C peptide. From Steiner DF, et al. Structural and immunological studies on human proinsulin. In: Rodriguez RR, Vallance-Owen J, eds. Proceedings of the seventh Congress of the International Diabetes Federation, Amsterdam: Excerpta Medica, 1971:281. Reprinted by permission.

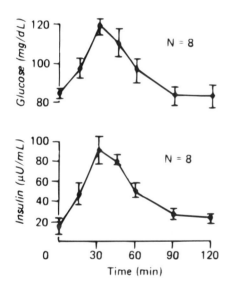

Figure 14.23. Plasma glucose and insulin response to a standard 530 kcal breakfast in normal subjects. From Karam JH, Salber PR, Forsham PH. Pancreatic hormones and diabetes mellitus. In: Greenspan FS, ed. Basic and clinical endocrinology. 3rd ed. Norwalk, CT: Appleton & Lange, 1991:593. Reprinted by permission.

In contrast to the selective stimulation of A and D cells by glucose, ingested amino acids stimulate release of both insulin and glucagon. Consequently, the type of ingested nutrients influences the pattern and rate of islet cell hormone release in response to a meal. The hyperglycemia that results from a predominately carbohydrate meal stimulates insulin secretion, which blunts glucagon release in response to the ingested amino acids. A protein-rich meal, however, results in a rela-

tively greater rate of glucagon secretion because amino acids are potent stimulators of A cells but are less effective in stimulating insulin release in the absence of concurrent hyperglycemia (32). Thus, the carbohydrate:protein ratio of an ingested meal is an important determinant of the secretion rates of these two hormones.

The principal function of insulin is to promote storage of ingested nutrients. Secreted insulin first reaches the liver where it exerts both anabolic and anticatabolic effects. Insulin increases the synthesis and storage of glucagon and promotes both glycogen synthesis and storage and inhibits its breakdown. It stimulates hepatic synthesis of proteins, triglycerides, and formation of very low density lipoproteins. It reduces cellular catabolism by inhibiting gluconeogenesis, ketogenesis, and hepatic glycogenolysis. In muscle, insulin stimulates synthesis of protein and glycogen, whereas in adipose tissue, it promotes storage of triglycerides, increases glucose transport into adipocytes, and inhibits lipolysis. These endocrine effects are detailed further in Table 14.13.

Glucagon

Glucagon is a 29 amino acid peptide (molecular weight 3485) secreted by the A cells. Glucagon has a circulatory half-life of 3 to 6 minutes and is secreted in response to stimulation by amino acids (arginine and alanine), catecholamines, gastrointestinal hormones (CCK, gastrin, and GIP), glucocorticoids, and sympathetic and parasympathetic nerve stimulation. The

Table 14.13.
Endocrine Effects of Insulin

Effects on Liver
Anabolic effects:
Promotes glycogenesis and glycolysis.
Increases synthesis of protein, triglycerides, cholesterol, and VLDL.
Anti-catabolic effects:
Inhibits glycogenolysis, ketogenesis, and gluconeogenesis.

Effects on Muscle
Promotes protein synthesis:
Increases amino acid transport.
Stimulates ribosomal protein synthesis.
Promotes glycogen synthesis:
Increases glucose transport and activity of glycogen synthetase.
Inhibits glycogen phosphorylase activity.

Effects on Fat
Promotes triglyceride storage:
Induces lipoprotein lipase, making fatty acids available for absorption into fat cells.
Increases glucose transport into fat cells, thus increasing availability of α-glycerol phosphate for triglyceride synthesis.
Inhibits intracellular lipolysis.

Modified from Karam JH, Salber PR, Forsham PH, et al. Pancreatic hormones and diabetes mellitus. In: Greenspan FS, ed. Basic and clinical endocrinology. 3rd ed. Appleton and Lange, 1991;598. Reprinted with permission.

major target organ of action of glucagon is the liver, where it stimulates breakdown of stored glycogen and promotes hepatic gluconeogenesis from amino acid precursors and ketogenesis from fatty acid precursors. The major physiologic role of glucagon, therefore, is to provide the organism with a fuel source between meals and during periods of fasting.

Somatostatin

Somatostatin is a 14 amino acid peptide (molecular weight 1640) and derives its name from its growth hormone–inhibitory properties. Somatostatin has been isolated from a number of tissues, including brain, gastrointestinal tract, and pancreas. Secretion occurs in response to the same stimuli that promote insulin release, including glucose, arginine, and other gastrointestinal hormones. The principal function of somatostatin in digestion is to slow movement of nutrients from the intestinal tract into the circulation. It accomplishes this purpose by reducing gastric emptying time, decreasing gastric production of gastrin and gastric acid, decreasing pancreatic exocrine secretion, and reducing splanchnic blood flow. Somatostatin acts in a paracrine manner to inhibit secretion of insulin, glucagon, and pancreatic polypeptide (PP) by islet cells. It inhibits secretion of other nonpancreatic gastrointestinal hormones as well. These properties of somatostatin and the development of a synthetic analogue of human somatostatin (SMS 201–995, or octreotide) have led to its clinical use in the treatment of patients with fistulas of the gastrointestinal

tract and pancreas and patients with unresectable hormone-secreting pancreatic endocrine neoplasms.

Pancreatic Polypeptide

Pancreatic polypeptide is a 36 amino acid peptide (molecular weight 4200) secreted by the F cells, which are located principally in the posterior portion of the head of the pancreas. The physiological action of PP is unknown, but blood levels increase after ingestion of a mixed meal. Elevated circulating levels of PP are frequently present in patients with pancreatic endocrine tumors and may serve as a biochemical marker for the diagnosis of these neoplasms and their response to therapy (33).

Pathophysiology

Tumors of the endocrine pancreas may arise from any of the four major cell types normally present in the islets or from neuroendocrine cells of the pancreas that secrete gastrin, VIP, or neurotensin (Table 14.14) (34). The most common pancreatic endocrine tumors are gastrinomas and insulinomas (35,36). The other tumor types occur much less commonly; only a few cases of somatostatin and neurotensin-secreting tumors have been reported (37). Pancreatic endocrine tumors may occur sporadically or in association with the multiple endocrine neoplasia type I (MEN-I) syndrome. The clinical and diagnostic features associated with the various tumors are shown in Table 14.14. Benign pancreatic endocrine neoplasms are frequently small and may be difficult to localize. Computerized tomography and arteriography are the most useful localization procedures for these neoplasms. If these two studies are negative, selective portal venous catheterization with sampling of the venous drainage beds of the pancreas may provide regional localization.

Multiple Endocrine Neoplasia Syndromes

The multiple endocrine neoplasia syndromes are a group of familial disorders characterized by the development of endocrine neoplasms in multiple sites. The various components of the MEN syndromes and the frequency of their occurrence are shown in Table 14.15 (38,39). The MEN syndromes are each inherited in an autosomal dominant manner with complete penetrance but variable expressivity of the MEN gene. This means that each individual who inherits the MEN gene will exhibit some, but not necessarily all, components of the syndrome. Both sexes are affected with equal frequency, and no racial predilection exists. The genetic defect responsible for MEN-1 has been localized to the long arm

Table 14.14.
Biochemical and Clinical Features of the Major Endocrine Pancreatic Tumors

Tumor	Predominant Peptide	Major Cell Type	Clinical Features	Diagnostic Features
Insulinoma	Insulin	B	Fasting hypoglycemia (glucose < 50 mg/dL) signs of neuroglucopenia & adrenergic discharge	Elevated fasting plasma insulin, failure of insulin suppression in fasting hypoglycemia (insulin/glucose ratio > 0.3)
Gastrinoma	Gastrin	?	Virulent peptic ulcer disease, diarrhea (Zollinger-Ellison syndrome)	Elevated gastric acid output, elevated plasma gastrin, increased gastrin response to intravenous secretin
Glucagonoma	Glucagon	A	Dermatitis (necrolytic migratory erythema), glucose intolerance, diabetes mellitus, weight loss, anemia	Elevated fasting plasma glucagon
Somatostatinoma	Somatostatin	D	Dyspepsia, mild diabetes mellitus, gallbladder disease, steatorrhea, hypochlorhydria	Elevated fasting plasma somatostatin, hyperglycemia without ketonemia
PPoma	PP	F	Not identified (clinically silent)	Elevated fasting plasma PP
VIPoma	VIP	?	Profound secretory diarrhea, hypokalemia, hypochlorhydria, acidosis (WDHA syndrome)	Elevated fasting plasma VIP
Neurotensinoma	Neurotensin	N	Diarrhea, diabetes, weight loss, edema, hypotension (may be indistinguishable from VIPoma)	Elevated fasting plasma neurotensin

WDHA: water diarrhea, hypokalemia, hypochlorhydria.
Modified from Gower WR, Fabri PJ. Sem Surg Oncol 1990;6:98-109. Reprinted with permission.

Table 14.15.
Components of the Multiple Endocrine Neoplasia Syndromes

Syndrome	Component	Frequency
MEN-I	Parathyroid hyperplasia	90%
	Pancreatic islet tumors	80%
	Pituitary tumors	65%
	Other tumors[a]	5–10%
MEN-IIA	Medullary thyroid carcinoma	100%
	Pheochromocytoma	30–40%
	Parathyroid hyperplasia	30–50%
MEN-IIB	Medullary thyroid carcinoma	100%
	Pheochromocytoma	50–90%
	Multiple mucosal neuromas	100%
	Marfanoid body habitus	65%

[a] Includes carcinoids, bronchial adenomas, thyroid adenomas, lipomas, and adrenocortical adenomas.
Source reference 38 and 39.

of chromosome 11 (11q13). A large number of MEN-1 associated tumors have lost one copy of this segment of chromosome 11, which suggests that the responsible gene may be a tumor suppressor gene. Loss of this normal allele thus leaves an individual with only the mutated gene and no functional gene product. The RET proto-oncogene on chromosome 10 has been identified as the gene responsible for both MEN-2A (40,41) and MEN-2B (42). Mutations in the RET proto-oncogene have been identified in patients with Hirschsprung's disease as well. The discovery of these germline mutations in the RET proto-oncogene has allowed the development of presymptomatic DNA testing in kindred members who are at risk for developing MEN-2A and medullary thyroid carcinoma (43,44). Prophylactic thyroidectomy has now been carried out at an early age in

individuals affected with the RET mutation, even if they have normal stimulated plasma calcitonin levels. These recent landmark reports from Wells and colleagues (43) and Lips and associates (44) mark the first time that a genetic test has been used as the sole basis for initiating surgical therapy for a disease.

The mechanism by which the aforementioned genetic defects lead to the development of the MEN syndromes is unknown. The cell types involved in the MEN neoplasms have been postulated to originate in a common embryologic cell precursor in the neural crest or neuroectoderm. Pearse (45) proposed the amine precursor uptake, decarboxylase (APUD) concept to describe the common cytochemical and ultrastructural characteristics of these neural crest derived cells. These APUD cells are characterized by their amine content (dopamine, and 5-hydroxytryptophan) and ability to uptake and decarboxylate precursor amino acids needed in amine synthesis. A total of 40 different endocrine cell types have been included in the APUD nomenclature. However, a defect in neural crest development does not explain the MEN syndromes completely because neither the parathyroids nor pancreatic islet cells are derived from neuroectoderm. Oncogene-related mutational factors may also play a role in the expression of MEN tumors.

The incidence of the various components of the MEN syndromes reflects an average frequency that may vary significantly among different kindreds (see Table 14.15). The clinical and biochemical characteristics of these neoplasms are similar to the features that develop in patients with sporadic endocrine neoplasms of the same organs.

MEN-I

Primary hyperparathyroidism is the most common clinical manifestation of MEN-I. Multiglandular involvement of all four parathyroid glands with hyperplasia is generally present and requires treatment with either subtotal parathyroidectomy or total parathyroidectomy and autotransplantation. The most common pancreatic islet cell neoplasms are gastrin-secreting tumors that cause the Zollinger-Ellison syndrome, followed in frequency by insulinomas. Such patients are rarely cured by surgical resection because of the presence of generalized pancreatic islet cell hyperplasia. If hypercalcemia from hyperparathyroidism is present in patients with the Zollinger-Ellison syndrome and MEN-I, improved control of gastrin-secretion may be achieved by parathyroidectomy. This is probably associated with the observation that hypercalcemia promotes gastrin release from these pancreatic tumors. The most common pituitary tumor seen in this syndrome is a chromophobe adenoma, although prolactin-secreting pituitary tumors are also frequently seen.

MEN-IIA

Medullary thyroid carcinoma is a calcitonin-producing neoplasm of the parafollicular or C cells of the thyroid (see the previous "The Thyroid"). MTC occurs in virtually 100% of patients with MEN-IIA. Hyperplasia of the C cells may precede the development of carcinoma in affected individuals. As discussed previously, calcitonin is a very sensitive biochemical marker for the development of MTC, and provocative stimulation of calcitonin release into the blood by the administration of intravenous calcium and/or pentagastrin is a reliable method for establishing the presence of disease and for monitoring patients after thyroidectomy (46). MTC cells have been shown to synthesize a number of other peptides, including calcitonin gene-related peptide, ACTH, melanocyte-stimulating hormone, VIP, serotonin, substance P, and somatostatin. Carcinoembryonic antigen may also be secreted by MTC cells and can be a useful marker for monitoring patients for disease activity. Pheochromocytomas in patients with MEN-IIA are frequently bilateral and may be preceded by the development of adrenal medullary hyperplasia. Hyperparathyroidism is frequently asymptomatic in these patients and, as with MEN-I, is characterized by generalized parathyroid hyperplasia.

MEN-IIB

Medullary thyroid carcinoma occurs in 100% of patients with MEN-IIB and behaves in a biologically more virulent manner than in patients with MEN-IIA. The incidence of pheochromocytomas is variable, but it has been reported to be 90% in patients who live beyond the age of 20 years (47). The most striking feature of MEN-IIB is the multiple mucosal neuromas that affect the lips, tongue, eyelids, and conjunctiva. Hypertrophied corneal nerve fibers may be seen on slit-lamp examination. Ganglioneuromas in the gastrointestinal tract may cause constipation and cause colonic dilatation and megacolon by an unknown mechanism. A Marfanoid body habitus with long, thin extremities and muscle wasting is often present.

Carcinoid Tumors and the Carcinoid Syndrome

Carcinoid tumors are neuroendocrine tumors that arise in the enterochromaffin or Kulchitsky cells. These cells are a part of the diffuse neuroendocrine system. Kulchitsky cells are found in many tissues, including the crypts of the gastrointestinal tract and the bronchial epithelium. Carcinoid tumors may develop anywhere throughout the gastrointestinal tract and are traditionally classified according to the portion of the embryonic gut from which they are derived (Table 14.16). The most common sites of occurrence, in order of decreasing frequency, are the appendix, ileum, and rectum. Appendiceal and rectal carcinoids are frequently benign whereas most ileal carcinoids are malignant.

Because of their neuroendocrine origin, carcinoid tumors may synthesize and secrete a variety of biologically active substances, including serotonin (5-hydroxytryptamine) (48). The clinical manifestations that result from the release of these humoral mediators into the circulation has been termed the carcinoid syndrome. This syndrome is characterized by flushing, diarrhea, bronchospasm, and endocardial fibrosis of the tricuspid and pulmonic valves. Serotonin is the best documented mediator of the carcinoid syndrome, but other substances (histamine and substance P) are also likely involved. The mediators of the carcinoid syndrome are inactivated after a single pass through the liver. Conse-

Table 14.16.
Biochemical Features and Site of Origin of Carcinoid Tumors

Embryonic Origin	Tumor Site	Secretory Products	Elevated Urinary 5-HIAA Levels
Foregut	Bronchus/Stomach	5-hydroxytryptophan	Yes
Midgut	Small Intestine/Colon	5-hydroxytryptophan and serotonin	Yes
Hindgut	Rectum	None	No

From Roberts LJ, Oates JA. Disorders of vasodilator hormones: the carcinoid syndrome and mastocytosis. In: Wilson JD, Foster DW eds. Textbook of endocrinology. 7th ed. Philadelphia: WB Saunders, Co., 1985; 1363-1378.

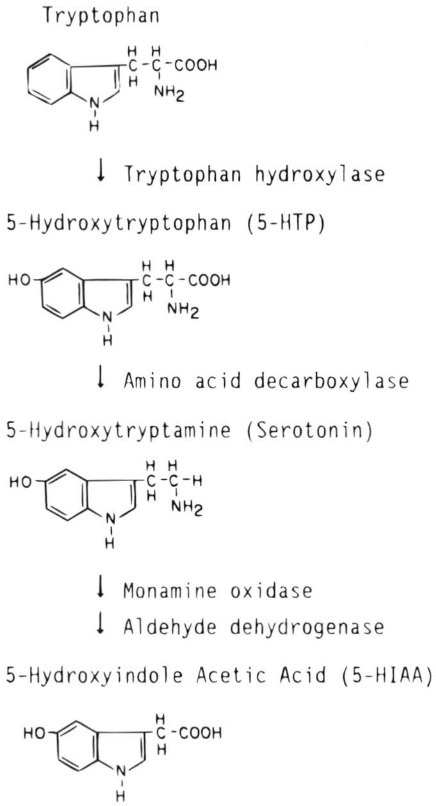

Tryptophan

↓ Tryptophan hydroxylase

5-Hydroxytryptophan (5-HTP)

↓ Amino acid decarboxylase

5-Hydroxytryptamine (Serotonin)

↓ Monamine oxidase
↓ Aldehyde dehydrogenase

5-Hydroxyindole Acetic Acid (5-HIAA)

Figure 14.24. Pathway of serotonin synthesis and metabolism.

quently, the presence of the carcinoid syndrome implies that mediators are being released directly into the systemic circulation. Most cases of carcinoid syndrome, therefore, occur in patients with either hepatic metastases from gastrointestinal tumors or extra abdominal tumors (bronchial carcinoids) that release their mediators systemically. Overall, less than 1% of gastrointestinal carcinoids are associated with the development of the carcinoid syndrome.

The pathway for biosynthesis of serotonin is shown in Figure 14.24. The rate-limiting step in this pathway is conversion of tryptophan to 5-hydroxytryptophan by tyrosine hydroxylase. 5-hydroxytryptophan is converted rapidly by amino acid decarboxylase to 5-hydroxytryptamine (serotonin). Foregut carcinoids generally have low levels of amino acid decarboxylase activity and preferentially secrete 5-hydroxytryptophan (see Table 14.16). After synthesis, 5-hydroxytryptamine is packaged into neurosecretory granules, which then discharge their contents into the circulation. Most circulating 5-hydroxytryptamine undergoes conversion to 5-hydroxyindole acetic acid (5-HIAA) by the actions of monoamine oxidase and aldehyde dehydrogenase and is then excreted in the urine. Measurement of urinary 5-HIAA is the most useful diagnostic test in the evaluation of patients with suspected carcinoid tumors or the carcinoid syndrome. The excretion rate of 5-HIAA in normal subjects is < 10 mg/24 hr.

Endocrine Manifestations of Nonendocrine Malignancies

Ectopic or inappropriate secretion of peptide hormones is one of the most common paraneoplastic manifestations of nonendocrine malignancies. With the exception of the steroid hormones and thyroid hormone, both of which require specialized enzymatic machinery for synthesis, virtually any hormone can be produced in an ectopic manner. In contrast to hormone secretion by normal endocrine cells, ectopic production of hormones by neuroendocrine tumors is usually not suppressible and may predominantly involve secretion of precursor molecules with reduced biologic activity (see "Hypercalcemia of Malignancy" later in this chapter) (49). Neuroendocrine tumors may also secrete peptides that differ in amino acid sequence from the native hormone but retain their physiologic activity. The identification of ectopic hormone production by a neuroendocrine tumor requires fulfillment of the following criteria: (*a*) presence of a tumor and association with a clinical hormone syndrome and elevated circulating hormone levels; (*b*) resolution of hormonal symptoms with treatment of the tumor; (*c*) demonstration of an arteriovenous hormone gradient across the vascular bed of the tumor; (*d*) presence of hormone in the tumor tissue; and (*e*) documentation of synthesis or secretion of hormone by the tumor in vitro or by mRNA analysis (50). The first two criteria are usually sufficient to establish the diagnosis clinically.

Several mechanisms have been postulated to explain the ectopic production of hormones by tumors. First, secretion of active hormone by the tumor correlates with the presence of neurosecretory granules characteristic of cells of the diffuse neuroendocrine system. Originally, these cells were thought to have a common neural crest origin because of their APUD characteristics. However, not all cells with these APUD features are of neural crest origin, and a number of different non-APUD cell tumors also produce hormones in an ectopic manner. The term *neuroendocrine cell* is, therefore, more appropriate for the designation of cell populations with the capability to synthesize and secrete hormonally active products. Second, the altered differentiation or dysdifferentiation hypothesis of Mendelsohn and Baylin (51) proposes that clonal expansion of a primitive cell type that is present in normal tissue at very low frequency may lead to increased expression of hormones in patients with epithelial malignancies. Finally, cell transformation from activation of specific oncogenes within malignant cells may also initiate production of ectopic hormones.

The most common clinical syndromes caused by ectopic production of peptide hormones are shown in

Table 14.17.
Common Ectopic Hormone Syndromes Caused by Non-Endocrine Malignancies

Syndrome	Etiologic Agents	Types of Malignancies
1. Hypercalcemia	1. PTH-related protein	Squamous carcinoma (especially lung)
		Renal cell carcinoma
	2. Local osteolytic factor	Breast carcinoma
	3. Cytokines*	Multiple myeloma, lymphoma
2. SIADH	Vasopressin (ADH)	Small cell lung carcinoma
3. Hypoglycemia	?/IGF-II	Mesenchymal tumors of trunk (soft tissue sarcomas)
		GI tract malignancies
		Carcinoid tumors
		Adrenocortical carcinoma
4. Cushing's syndrome	ACTH	Small cell lung carcinoma
		Bronchial or thymic carcinoid tumors

* Lymphotoxin (tumor necrosis factor-β) in patients with multiple myeloma.
IGF-II: insulin-like growth factor-II.

Table 14.17. In addition, a variety of other hormones may be produced ectopically in patients with neuroendocrine tumors, including human chorionic gonadotropin, growth hormone-releasing hormone, calcitonin, VIP, and erythropoietin.

Hypercalcemia of Malignancy

Malignancy-associated hypercalcemia is the most common endocrine complication of malignancy. It occurs in up to 10% of patients with advanced malignancies and is the most common cause of hypercalcemia in hospitalized patients (49). In 98% of cases, the responsible tumor is identifiable at the time of presentation of the hypercalcemia. Stimulation of bone resorption by local or systemically released tumor products is the principal mechanism by which hypercalcemia of malignancy develops. The biochemical features of hypercalcemia in patients with solid tumors (other than breast carcinomas) is similar to patients with primary hyperparathyroidism: hypercalcemia, hypophosphatemia, and increased nephrogenous cAMP activity. Recently, a parathyroid-related protein with significant N-terminus homology to PTH has been isolated from several of these tumors (16). This PTH-like protein binds to PTH receptors in kidney and bone and has similar physiologic activity to PTH. PTH-related protein does not cross-react with the PTH antisera used in standard PTH immunoassays.

Hypercalcemia in patients with breast carcinoma primarily develops in patients with extensive osseous metastases. The administration of estrogen, androgens, or antiestrogen compounds may precipitate the appearance of hypercalcemia. Production of a local osteolytic factor has been implicated as the etiologic agent. The mechanism of hypercalcemia in patients with multiple myeloma and lymphomas is thought to involve production of hypercalcemia-inducing cytokines.

Syndrome of Inappropriate Antidiuretic Hormone Secretion

Inappropriate secretion of vasopressin, or antidiuretic hormone, is the second most common endocrine

manifestation of malignancy. It occurs in 7% to 8% of patients with small-cell lung carcinoma and results in impaired secretion of free water by the kidneys. This results in symptoms of water intoxication and hyponatremia, including weakness, lethargy, somnolence, and confusion. Profound hyponatremia (< 110 mEq/liter) may cause coma, seizures, and death.

Cushing's Syndrome

Many nonendocrine tumors secrete the precursor molecule for ACTH, proopiomelanocortin. However, most cases of Cushing's syndrome from ectopic ACTH production occur in neuroendocrine cell tumors (small-cell lung carcinoma and carcinoid tumors). This occurs because only neuroendocrine cells are capable of processing and secreting clinically significant amounts of ACTH from proopiomelanocortin. Patients with the ectopic ACTH syndrome do not usually develop the truncal obesity and skin changes typically associated with Cushing's syndrome. Instead, weight loss, muscle weakness, wasting, and hypokalemia are the usual findings.

Hypoglycemia

A number of nonpancreatic islet cell tumors may cause hypoglycemia. Soft tissue sarcomas of the trunk (chest, abdomen, and retroperitoneum) account for 50% of all cases; another 25% are the result of the other tumors listed in Table 14.17. The presence of hypoglycemia together with suppressed plasma insulin levels suggests the diagnosis. The mechanism of hypoglycemia may involve both increased rates of glucose use by the tumor and secretion of humoral factors (insulin-like growth factor 2) with insulin-like effects (52).

REFERENCES

1. Harrison TS. The thyroid gland. In: Sabiston DC, ed. Textbook of surgery. 13th ed. Philadelphia: WB Saunders, 1986:579–619.
2. Tzinas S, Droulias C, Harlaftis N, et al. Vascular patterns of the thyroid gland. Am Surg 1976;42:639–644.
3. Gavin LA. Thyroid physiology and testing of thyroid function. In:

Clark O, ed. Endocrine surgery of the thyroid and parathyroid glands. St. Louis: CV Mosby, 1985:1–34.

4. Brent GA. The molecular basis of thyroid hormone activity. N Engl J Med 1994;331:847–853.

5. Surks MI, Chopra IJ, Mariash CN, et al. American Thyroid Association guidelines for use of laboratory tests in thyroid disorders. JAMA 1990;71:553–558.

6. Nicoloff JT, Spencer CA. The use and misuse of the sensitive thyrotropin assays. J Clin Endocrinol Metab 1990;71:553–558.

7. Toft AD. Use of sensitive immunoradiometric assay for thyrotropin in clinical practice. Mayo Clin Proc 1988;63:1035–1042.

8. Ingbar SH. The thyroid. In: Wilson JD, Foster DW, eds. Textbook of endocrinology. 7th ed. Philadelphia: WB Saunders, 1985:682–815.

9. Greenspan FS, Rapoport B. Thyroid gland. In: Greenspan FS, ed. Basic and clinical endocrinology. 3rd ed. Norwalk, CT: Appleton & Lange, 1991:188–246.

10. Akerstrom G, Malmaeus J, Bergstrom R. Surgical anatomy of the parathyroid glands. Surgery 1984;95:14–21.

11. Wells SA. The parathyroid glands. In: Sabiston DC, ed. Textbook of surgery. 13th ed. Philadelphia: WB Saunders, 1986:620–638.

12. Norris EH. The parathyroid glands and the lateral thyroid in man: their morphogenesis, histogenesis, topographic anatomy, and prenatal growth. Contributions of Embryology 1937;26:247–294.

13. Aurbach GD, Marx SJ, Spiegel AM. Parathyroid hormone, calcitonin, and the calciferols. In: Wilson JD, Foster DW, eds. Textbook of endocrinology, 7th ed. Philadelphia: WB Saunders, 1985:1137–1217.

14. Bringhurst FR. Calcium and phosphate distribution, turnover, and metabolic actions. In: DeGroot LD, ed. Endocrinology. 2nd ed. Philadelphia: WB Saunders, 1989:805–843.

15. Endres DB, Villanueva R, Sharp CF, et al. Measurement of parathyroid hormone. Endocrinol Metab Clin North Am 1989;18:611–629.

16. Broadus AE, Mangin M, Ikeda K, et al. Humoral hypercalcemia of cancer: identification of a novel parathyroid hormone-like peptide. N Engl J Med 1988;319:556–563.

17. Arnold A. Molecular genetics of parathyroid gland neoplasia. J Clin Endocrinol Metab 1993;77:1108–1112.

18. Pollak MR, Brown EM, Wu Chow Y-H, et al. Mutations in the human Ca^{2+}-sensing receptor gene cause familial hypocalciuric hypercalcemia and neonatal severe hyperparathyroidism. Cell 1993;75:1297–1303.

19. Delmez JA, Slatopolsky E. Recent advances in the pathogenesis and therapy of uremic secondary hyperparathyroidism. J Clin Endocrinol Metab 1991;72:735–739.

20. Arnaud CD, Kolb FO. The calciotropic hormones and metabolic bone disease. In: Greenspan FS, ed. Basic and clinical endocrinology. 3rd ed. Norwalk, CT: Appleton & Lange, 1991:247–322.

21. Bergland RM, Gann DS, De Maria EJ. Pituitary and adrenal. In: Schwartz SI, ed. Principles of surgery. 4th ed. New York: McGraw-Hill, 1990:1545–1557.

22. Findling JW, Tyrrell JB. Anterior pituitary gland. In: Greenspan FS, ed. Basic and clinical endocrinology. 3rd ed. Norwalk, CT: Appleton & Lange, 1991:79–132.

23. Lechan RM. Neuroendocrinology of pituitary hormone regulation. Endocrinol Metab Clin North Am 1987;16:475–501.

24. Oldfield EH, Doppman JL, Nieman LK, et al. Petrosal sinus sampling with and without corticotropin-releasing hormone for the differential diagnosis of Cushing's syndrome. N Engl J Med 1991;325:899–905.

25. Ramsay DJ. Posterior pituitary gland. In: Greenspan FS, ed. Basic and clinical endocrinology. 3rd ed. Norwalk, CT: Appleton & Lange, 1991:177–187.

26. Tyrrell JB, Aron DC, Forsham PH. Glucocorticoids and adrenal androgens. In: Greenspan FS, ed. Basic and clinical endocrinology. 3rd ed. Norwalk, CT: Appleton & Lange, 1991:323–362.

27. Findling JW, Doppman JL. Biochemical and radiologic diagnosis of Cushing's syndrome. Endocrinol Metab Clin North Am 1994;23:511–537.

28. Dwyer AJ, Frank JA, Doppman JL, et al. Pituitary adenomas in patients with Cushing's disease: Initial experience with Gd-DTPA-enhanced MR imaging. Radiology 1987;163:421–426.

29. Melby JC. Diagnosis and treatment of primary aldosteronism and isolated hypoaldosteronism. In: DeGroot LJ, ed. Endocrinology. 2nd ed. Philadelphia: WB Saunders, 1989:1705–1713.

30. White PC. Disorders of aldosterone biosynthesis and action. N Engl J Med 1994;331:250–258.

31. Goldfien A. Adrenal medulla. In: Greenspan FS, ed. Basic and clinical endocrinology. 3rd ed. Norwalk, CT: Appleton & Lange, 1991:380–399.

32. Karam JH, Salber PR, Forsham PH. Pancreatic hormones and diabetes mellitus. In: Greenspan FS, ed. Basic and clinical endocrinology. 3rd ed. Norwalk, CT: Appleton & Lange, 1991:592–650.

33. Adrian TE, Uttenthal LO, Williams SJ, et al. Secretion of pancreatic polypeptide in patients with pancreatic endocrine tumors. N Engl J Med 1986;315:287–291.

34. Gower WR, Fabri PJ. Endocrine neoplasms (non-gastrin) of the pancreas. Semin Oncol 1990;6:98–109.

35. Broden G. Insulinoma and glucagonoma. Semin Oncol 1987;14:253–262.

36. Townsend CM, Thompson JC. Gastrinoma. Semin Oncol 1990;6:91–97.

37. Vinik AI, Strodel WE, Eckhauser FE, et al. Somatostatinomas, PPomas, neurotensinomas. Semin Oncol 1987;14:263–281.

38. Cance WG, Wells SA. Multiple endocrine neoplasia type IIa. Curr Probl Surg 1985;22:7–56.

39. Deftos LS, Catherwood BD. Syndromes involving multiple endocrine glands. In: Greenspan FS, ed. Basic and clinical endocrinology. 3rd ed. Norwalk, CT: Appleton & Lange, 1991:725–740.

40. Mulligan LM, Kwok JBJ, Healey CS, et al. Germ-line mutations of the RET proto-oncogene in multiple endocrine neoplasia type 2A. Nature 1993;363:458–460.

41. Donis-Keller H, Dou S, Chi D, et al. Mutations in the RET proto-oncogene are associated with MEN-2A and FMTC. Hum Mol Genet 1993;2:851–856.

42. Lairmore TC, Howe JR, Korte JA, et al. Familial medullary thyroid carcinoma and multiple endocrine neoplasia type 2B map to the same region of chromosome 10 as multiple endocrine neoplasia type 2A. Genomics 1991;9:181–192.

43. Wells SA, Chi DD, Toshima K, et al. Predictive DNA testing and prophylactic thyroidectomy in patients at risk for multiple endocrine neoplasia type 2A. Ann Surg 1994;220:237–250.

44. Lips CJM, Landsvater RM, Hoppener JWM. Clinical screening as compared with DNA analysis in families with multiple endocrine neoplasia type 2A. N Engl J Med 1994;331:828–835.

45. Pearse AGE. Common cytochemical and ultrastructural characteristics of cells producing polypeptide hormones (the APUD series) and their relevance to thyroid and ultimobranchial C cells and calcitonin. Proc R Soc Lond (B) 1968;170:71–80.

46. Wells SA, Baylin SB, Linehan WM, et al. Provocative agents and the diagnosis of medullary carcinoma of the thyroid gland. Ann Surg 1978;188:139–141.

47. Khairi MR, Dexter RN, Byrynski NJ, Johnston CC. Mucosal neuroma, pheochromocytoma and medullary thyroid carcinoma: multiple endocrine neoplasia type 3. Medicine 1975;54:89–112.

48. Engelman K. Malignant carcinoid syndrome. In: DeGroot LJ, ed. Endocrinology. 2nd ed. Philadelphia: WB Saunders, 1989:2649–2657.

49. Strewler GJ. Humoral manifestations of malignancy. In: Greenspan FS, ed. Basic and clinical endocrinology. 3rd ed. Norwalk, CT: Appleton & Lange, 1991:715–724.

50. Baylin SB, Mendelsohn G. Ectopic (inappropriate) hormone production by tumors: mechanisms involved and the biological and clinical implications. Endocr Rev 1980;1:45–77.

51. Mendelsohn G, Baylin SB. Ectopic hormone syndromes: Mechanisms, pathology, and clinical implications. In: Mendelsohn G, ed. Diagnosis and pathology of endocrine diseases. London: JB Lippincott, 1988:641–672.

52. Daughaday WH, Kapadia M. Significance of abnormal serum binding of insulin-like growth factor II in the development of hypoglycemia in patients with non-islet cell tumors. Proc Nat Acad Sci U S A 1989;86:6778–6782.

SUGGESTED READINGS

Brandi ML, Marx JS, Aurbach GD, et al. Familial multiple endocrine neoplasia type I: a new look at pathophysiology. Endocr Rev 1987;8:391–405.

Bravo EL. Evolving concepts in the pathophysiology, diagnosis, and treatment of pheochromocytoma. Endocr Rev 1994;15:356–368.

Brunt LM, Wells SA. Advances in the diagnosis and treatment of medullary thyroid carcinoma. Surg Clin North Am 1987;67: 263–279.

Feldman JM. Carcinoid tumors and the carcinoid syndrome. Curr Prob Surg 1989;26:835–885.

Gavin LA. Thyroid physiology and testing of thyroid function. In: Clark O, ed. Endocrine surgery of the thyroid and parathyroid glands. St. Louis: CV Mosby, 1985:1–34.

Hoet JJ, Remacle C. Organization of the pancreatic islets, with special reference to diabetes, In: DeGroot LJ, ed. Endocrinology. 2nd ed. Philadelphia: WB Saunders, 1989:1247–1262.

Molitch ME. Pathogenesis of pituitary tumors. Endocrinol Metab Clin North Am 1987;16:503–527.

Mozell E, Stenzel P, Woltering EA, et al. Functional endocrine tumors of the pancreas: clinical presentation, diagnosis and treatment. Curr Prob Surg 1990;27:309–386.

Mundy GR. Ectopic production of calciotropic peptides. Endocrinol Metab Clin North Am 1991;20:473–487.

Orth DN. Cushing's syndrome. N Engl J Med 1995;332:791–803.

Ramsay DJ. Renal hormones and endocrine hypertension. In: Greenspan FS, ed. Basic and clinical endocrinology. 3rd ed. Norwalk, CT: Appleton & Lange, 1991:400–406.

Skandalakis JE, Gray SW, Rose JS, Jr. Anatomical complications in general surgery: the neck. New York: McGraw-Hill, 1983:12–36.

Wells SA, Lairmore TC. The multiple endocrine neoplasia syndromes. In: Sabiston DS, ed. Textbook of surgery, 14th ed. Philadelphia: WB Saunders, 1991:590–597.

Yanovski JA, Cutler GB, Jr. Glucocorticoid action and the clinical features of Cushing's syndrome. Endocrinol Metab Clin North Am 1994;23:487–509.

Young WF, Hogan MJ, Klee GG, et al. Primary aldosteronism: diagnosis and treatment. Mayo Clinic Proc 1990;65:96–110.

15 The Cardiovascular System

Lorne H. Blackbourne | Jeffrey T. Cope | Reid W. Tribble | Curtis G. Tribble

Introduction

This chapter is designed to be a review of the basic science of the cardiovascular system written for general surgical residents. It is not intended to be a review for trainees in the disciplines of cardiology or cardiovascular surgical specialties.

Obviously, it is impossible to include every facet of the cardiovascular system in such a review. However, this chapter should allow surgical residents to review the basic scientific principles of the cardiovascular system as it applies to the care of the general surgical patient. A list of selected references follows this chapter, and residents are urged to use these references because they are not only complete but also readable, in-depth sources of information.

Basic Science of the Peripheral Vascular System

Arterial Anatomy

The arteries of the body are divided histologically into three layers. The intima is the layer that contains endothelial cells and, in some places, a single layer of subendothelial smooth muscle cells. Beneath the intima, dividing it from the media, is the internal elastic membrane. The media is the major structural component of the artery containing smooth muscle cells, elastin, proteoglycans, and collagen. The media is separated from the third layer, the adventitia, by the external elastic membrane. When a typical endarterectomy is performed, the cleavage plane is at the level of the external elastic membrane. The blood supply for the inner part of the media comes from direct diffusion from the lumen of the blood vessel wall, and the outer part of the media is supplied by smaller penetrating arteries known as vasovasorum. The third layer, the adventitia, contains elastic tissue, fibroblasts, and collagen, and provides about 60% of the strength of the blood vessel itself.

The Role of Endothelium in the Cardiovascular System

The vascular endothelium is a crucial mediator of vascular physiology. Endothelial cells are involved actively in angiogenesis, coagulation, platelet interaction, inflammation, immune response, synthesis of connective tissue components, metabolic functions and, most importantly, the regulation of vascular tone. The endothelium is, of course, normally non-thrombogenic; therefore, platelets do not adhere to an intact endothelial lining. Platelets do, however, adhere to the basal lamina of vessels denuded of their endothelial coverings. Endothelial cells secrete prostacyclin (PGI2) and nitric oxide (NO), otherwise known as endothelium derived relaxing factor (EDRF). Both of these compounds are active mediators of vasodilatation and potent inhibitors of platelet adhesion and aggregation. Endothelial cells also contribute to anticoagulant properties of the intact vessel via the synthesis of thrombomodulin and protein S, both of which activate protein C, a substance synthesized in the liver that suppresses the actions of factor V and VIII of the coagulation cascade. Heparin sulfate, a component of intact endothelial cell membranes, accelerates the inactivation of thrombin and other coagulation factors by plasma antithrombin III. Furthermore, endothelial cells are involved in thrombolysis through the secretion of urokinase and tissue plasminogen activators.

Recent research has lead to the realization that the vascular endothelium also operates as a critical modulator of vascular tone. Endothelium derived relaxing factors are synthesized and released in response to a host of exogenous vasoactive substances and to physiologically important neurohumoral mediators. These endothelial dependent vasodilators include platelet-derived products such as ADP, ATP, thrombin, and serotonin, as well as local mediators of inflammation, including bradykinin, histamine, and arachidonic acid. Recent research suggests that EDRF is nitric oxide. L-arginine has been identified recently as the likely endogenous precursor of the EDRF.

Regulation of vascular tone is not limited to the endothelium alone. Local mediators, such as adenosine, that control vascular smooth muscle tone independent of the endothelium also play an important role. The inherent differences among vessels and their varying levels of EDRF and responses to endothelial dependant relaxation suggest a highly intricate system in which conduit arteries and resistance arterioles of different organs react to maintain vascular homeostasis and optimal cardiovascular efficiency.

Realize that endothelial dysfunction may occur. This dysfunction can either cause or result from hypertension. Atherosclerosis clearly changes the way endothelial cells respond to various stimuli, sometimes causing paradoxical vasoconstriction under conditions that would ordinarily cause vasodilatation. Endothelial injury may occur during surgical procedures in which clamps are placed outside the lumen of the vessel or catheters are placed inside the vessel. Endothelial dysfunction can also occur in reperfusion of ischemic vascular beds, sometimes with paradoxical responses. In particular, free radicals may inactivate EDRF, allowing counter-balancing vasoconstrictive forces to prevail.

Atherosclerosis

The etiology of atherosclerosis is complex, incompletely understood, and the subject of an enormous amount of research. Basic research centers on the end stage of human atherosclerotic vessels and on the development of atherosclerosis in certain animal models. A great deal of discussion has resulted from large-scale epidemiological studies. However, no single etiology has been identified. The consensus is that atherosclerosis is the end stage response of the vessel wall to injury, which includes such diverse insults as physical injury (balloon catheter denuding of endothelium), ischemia, toxins (tobacco and cholesterol), biologic injury (viruses), mechanical stress (hypertension), and immunological attack (rejection). Four cell types are involved in the response of the vessel wall to injury, including endothelial cells, monocytes, platelets, and smooth muscle cells. Each can release both growth factors and chemoattractants. It seems that one of the earliest events in response to endothelial injury is the attachment of monocytes to the endothelium. Furthermore, platelets may adhere even to minimally injured endothelial cells. These two cell populations may then stimulate intimal proliferative lesions and, subsequently, smooth muscle proliferation.

The histological progression of atherosclerosis begins with intimal thickening. Intimal thickening may reflect an adaptive response of the vessel to increased tension on the vessel wall caused by turbulence. Intimal thickenings have been observed in children and even infants at or near branch points of vessels and may represent local remodeling of the vessel wall related to growth and the associated redistribution of the tensile stresses. Lipid accumulation is not a prominent feature in this type of intimal thickening, and the lumen generally remains regular and normal in caliber. Intimal thickening is not a clear precursor of lipid-containing atherosclerotic plaques, but both processes do occur in similar locations, and intimal thickening is evident in vessels that are especially susceptible to atherosclerosis.

Fatty streaks are the focal patches of fat infiltrating the intima of vessels. They consist of lipid-laden foam cells, which are probably macrophages. These fatty streaks are found with increasing frequency from childhood up into the early adult years. Some seem to resolve at that point, but others may progress to worsening atherosclerotic plaques. There may be a predisposition of the endothelial cells overlying these plaques to disrupt, which then would allow platelet adhesion; this may be the inciting event in the development of a fibrous plaque.

Fibrous plaques are the next stage in the development of typical atherosclerotic lesions. They occur in the immediate subendothelial region and consist of compact and stratified layers of well organized smooth muscle cells. They are covered with a fibrous cap. A necrotic core often lies in the deeper regions of the plaque and contains a variety of forms of lipid. The most advanced lesions, especially those associated with aneurysmal dilatation, consist of dense fibrous tissue and prominent calcium deposits. Calcifications often are found in advanced plaques, and they may be extensive.

The most common sites for these atherosclerotic lesions to develop are at arterial bifurcations or areas of posterior fixation where shearing forces and turbulent flow are the highest. More specifically, locations that are typical for these focal lesions include all of the aortic branches at their origins, the aortic bifurcation, the iliac bifurcation, the common femoral artery bifurcation, the superficial femoral artery at Hunter's canal (where it is fixed) and the common carotid bifurcation.

Basic Hemodynamic Principles

Blood flow in the human circulation can be described in terms of strict hemodynamic principles, which are derived from engineering, mathematics, and physiology disciplines. These principles form the theoretical foundation for the understanding and treatment of vascular disease.

There are three pathologic manifestations of arterial disease: obstruction of the lumen, aneurysmal dilatation, and disruption or dissection of the vessel wall. Arterial obstruction may result from atherosclerosis, thrombi, emboli, fibromuscular dysplasia, trauma, or external compression. The significance of an obstructing lesion depends on where it is situated, the degree of the obstruction, its duration, and the compensatory ability of the body to develop collateral pathways around the lesion. Disruption or dissection of the vessel wall with loss of arterial wall integrity can occur with rupture of an existing aneurysm, hemorrhage into and/or rupture of an atherosclerotic plaque (especially in the aorta), dissection of the arterial wall, or as a result of direct trauma.

The foundation for the understanding of these pathologic events involves some basic principles of hemodynamics. Blood flows through the arterial system in response to differences in total fluid energy. Total fluid energy (E) consists of potential energy and kinetic energy (KE). Potential energy is made up of intravascular pressure (IP) and gravitational potential energy (GPE). Kinetic energy represents the ability of blood to do work on the basis of its motion and is proportional to the density (D) of blood and the square of blood velocity (V).

$$E = IP + GPE + KE$$

$$KE = \frac{1}{2}(DV^2)$$

This concept of the energy of the blood having a pressure component, a kinetic component, and a gravitation component is related to why people hang their legs over the side of the bed when they have ischemic rest pain. They are increasing the energy of the blood in their leg by allowing gravity to help pull the blood down to the most ischemic areas. This concept also explains why patients with marginal blood flow experience pain in their toes after they lie flat in bed.

Bernoulli's principle states that when fluid flows from one point to another, total energy along the stream is constant, provided that flow is steady and no frictional energy losses result. In the circulation, this ideal condition is not present, and a portion of the total fluid energy is lost in moving blood through the arterial circulation as heat. As a vessel gets smaller or a stenosis is present within a vessel, potential energy in the form of pressure converts to kinetic energy in the form of velocity. This phenomenon is seen when one's finger is placed over the end of a garden hose, causing the velocity of the water escaping the end to increase greatly.

Energy losses that occur in flowing blood occur either as viscous losses, resulting from friction between adjacent layers of blood, or as inertial losses, related to changes in velocity or direction of flow. Viscosity describes the resistance to flow that occurs because of the intermolecular attraction between fluid layers. Poiseuille's law describes the viscous energy losses that occur. The law states that the pressure gradient along a tube or vessel is directly proportional to the flow (F), the length of the vessel (L), and the fluid viscosity (v) and is inversely proportional to the fourth power of the radius (r). Simplifying this equation to "pressure equals

flow times resistance" makes it analogous to Ohm's law, which states that pressure is equal to flow times resistance. The predominant factor influencing hemodynamic resistance (R) is the fourth power of the radius.

$$R = \frac{8vL}{\pi r^4}$$

Although the predominant factor in this equation is indeed the radius, the length of the lesion plays an important role as well. As seen in the previous resistance equation, resistance is directly proportional to the length of the lesion. This principle is one reason why a long thin central line has a great deal of resistance compared to a short stubby large bore IV when a patient is given resuscitative fluids or blood rapidly. It also explains why a long area of stenosis in the blood vessel is much more important than a short discrete stenosis.

Occlusive Arterial Disease

The degree of arterial narrowing that is required to produce a reduction in blood pressure or in blood flow is called the critical arterial stenosis. The pressure or energy drop associated with the stenosis is inversely proportional to the fourth power of the radius. Thus, an exponential relationship exists between energy loss or pressure drop and the reduction of lumen size. Furthermore, the pressure drop across a stenosis varies with the velocity given the same radius of the stenosis. In other words, as blood velocity increases, a stenosis that was not impeding flow may become important and cause decreased flow as well as a pressure drop. This has an important clinical implication. A patient may have a 50% stenosis of an artery and have no symptoms at rest at the cardiac output necessary for resting nourishment of the muscle bed distal to the stenosis. If the muscle bed requires increased circulation because of increased metabolic demand (exercise), a huge increase in blood flow occurs because of a decrease in the resistance of the distal runoff bed. The cardiac output and, therefore, the velocity of the blood increase to meet these metabolic demands. A previously marginal stenosis may become critical in the sense that pressure will fall across the stenosis; therefore, flow falls as well. The decrease in flow is linearly related to the increase in pressure gradient. Thus, as a pressure drop across the stenosis increases, flow is similarly decreased across that stenosis. These are the hemodynamic situations that occur in claudication or stable angina.

Generally, significant changes in pressure and flow begin to occur when the arterial lumen has been reduced by 50% of its diameter as reported by arteriography, which correlates with a 75% reduction of cross-sectional area as may be determined intraoperatively, at autopsy studies, or by well-done duplex scanning. Remember that a stenosis that is not significant at resting flow rates may become significant when flow rates are increased.

This fact forms the basis for physiologic testing in the vascular diagnostic laboratory.

There are several other important hemodynamic principles that should be mentioned. As seen from Poiseuille's law, the radius of a stenosis will have a much greater effect on energy losses than its length. Doubling the length of a stenosis will double the energy losses, but reducing the radius by one-half increases the energy loss by a factor of 16. As blood traverses a stenosis, the energy losses that occur with contraction and expansion of the blood as it passes into and out of a stenosis are more significant than the viscous energy losses. These inertial losses of contraction and expansion are independent of the length of the stenosis and are especially prominent at the exit of the stenosis rather than at the entrance. Because energy and, therefore, pressure losses are primarily the result of the entrance and exit effects, separate stenoses of equal diameter are more significant than a single stenosis having the same diameter and a length equal to the sum of the other two. Therefore, multiple subcritical stenoses may have the same effect as a single critical stenosis. Based on this, several points can be made about stenoses in series. When two stenoses are of similar diameter, removal of one will provide only a modest increase in blood flow. If the stenoses have different diameters, removal of the least severe will have little effect, whereas removal of the most severe will improve blood flow dramatically. It makes no difference whether the most severe stenosis is proximal or distal to the least severe because the hemodynamic result is not affected by the sequence of stenoses. These principles apply only to unbranched arterial segments like the internal carotid artery. Thus a patient with tandem lesions, i.e., a severe lesion of the internal carotid artery at the bifurcation and a lesser lesion of the carotid siphon, would be expected to be helped considerably if the proximal cervical carotid lesion were treated with carotid endarterectomy.

When complete arterial obstruction occurs, blood must pass through a network of collateral vessels that bypass the occluded segment. The capacity of the collateral circulation varies according to the level and extent of the occlusive lesion. For example, the collateral flow around an occluded superficial femoral artery through the profunda and into the popliteal can compensate to a large extent for an isolated occlusion of the superficial femoral artery. If, however, an iliac stenosis were added above this, flow would be severely limited through the collateral bed. If the iliac stenosis were removed with direct arterial surgery or transluminal angioplasty, even though the iliac stenosis was not as severe as the superficial femoral artery occlusion, perfusion to the lower leg would be improved because of increased flow through the collateral system. The unvarying principles that concern collateral vessels are that they are always smaller, longer, and more numerous than the replaced artery and that the collateral resistance would always be greater

than that of the original unobstructed artery. Furthermore, the resistance of a collateral system is relatively fixed and cannot change acutely as in the case of a normal artery in which resistance can change to increase or decrease flow.

Aneurysmal Arterial Disease

An arterial aneurysm is defined as an artery that has reached a size two times its normal diameter. Aneurysms occur when the structural components of the arterial wall are weakened. Rupture of an aneurysm occurs when the tangential stress within the arterial wall exceeds its tensile strength. Laplace's law states that tangential arterial wall tension increases as the intravascular pressure and the radius of the vessel increases. The relationship between tangential stress and blood pressure accounts for the importance of avoiding hypertension in patients with aneurysms. Also, the direct relationship between radius and wall tension explains the observed higher incidence of rupture of aneurysms as their size increases.

Venous System

The structure of the venous circulation is considerably different from that of the arterial side of the circulation. Most of these differences are related to the differences in the wall of the vein relative to that of the artery. Furthermore, an important characteristic of many veins is the presence of valves, which are essential for their proper function. The distribution and number of valves correspond to those regions in which the effects of gravity are the greatest. Venous valves have a bicuspid structure with a fine connective tissue skeleton covered by endothelium on both surfaces. Their major function is to ensure antegrade flow of blood and prevent the reflux of blood from proximal to distal veins and from deep to superficial veins.

Because of their structure, veins can undergo large changes in volume with little change in transmural pressure. This enlarged volume with minimal pressure change is called venous capacitance. Veins are actually stiffer per unit of cross-sectional area than arteries when compared at the same distending pressure. This is because of the paucity of elastic tissue and the prominent venous adventitia, which consists mostly of collagen. In the venous system, a wide range of flow rates can be found. In an upright person, venous pressure at the level of the foot exceeds 100 mm Hg. Obviously, at this high pressure, fluid is forced out of the capillaries into the tissue. Some of this fluid may be picked up by lymphatics; however, the single most important element in preventing the accumulation of interstitial fluid is the calf muscle pump. The calf muscle pump produces important changes in venous volume flow rate and flow direction. It lowers the venous pressure in the dependent leg, reduces venous volume in the exercising muscle, and increases venous return. As stated, in a completely stationary upright individual, the venous pressure is high; however, with a single step, the venous pressure within the foot becomes very low and requires several seconds to return to the resting level. When a normal individual walks, the venous pressure remains at a low level throughout the period of exercise. The calf muscle pump empties the local venous system during contraction of the muscle. With relaxation, the veins expand and the venous pressure is lowered because of the functioning valves. If the valves are incompetent, venous pressure becomes increased as blood refluxes past the valves.

Two common manifestations of abnormal venous function are varicose veins and postthrombotic syndrome. Varicose veins occur when incompetent valves in the saphenous system permit reflux of blood from proximal to distal. Progressive incompetence occurs at each valve as the vein dilates. Ultimately, the vein becomes varicose as a result of the constant increase in pressure transmitted through the standing column of fluid.

Postthrombotic syndrome results after an episode of acute deep venous thrombosis (DVT). Factors that are responsible for the development of the postthrombotic syndrome relate mainly to the status of the deep veins below the knee and the perforating veins that connect the superficial and deep venous circulation. When valvular incompetence occurs in both of these areas, high pressures that can be generated by activation of the calf pump mechanism cause increased venous hypertension, not only at rest but also during ambulation. This constant venous hypertension may cause transudation of fibrinogen and coagulation factors into the subcutaneous tissue, which produces a significant barrier to the diffusion of oxygen and nutrients to the skin. This resultant brawny discoloration and occasional skin ulceration is known as venous stasis disease.

The clinician should recognize the two different clinical syndromes associated with the two main types of venous disease: obstructive venous disease and the venous problems associated with valvular incompetence. While it would seem that obstructive venous problems would be a more morbid condition, the reverse is actually true. When no direct communication exists between the large and heavy column of blood from the inferior vena cava all the way down to the foot, the leg will actually accommodate enlarging alternate routes of outflow. Sudden occlusion of an outflow vein is a fairly morbid event, but the gradual occlusion of these types of veins is not nearly as morbid as was once thought. For example, people tolerated ligation of the vena cava fairly well when it was done for chronic pulmonary embolism. Patients tolerate the removal of the superficial femoral vein for use as a conduit elsewhere with minimal subsequent swelling in the leg. In stark contrast to the relatively mild long-term morbidity of this type of venous problem is the situation in which there are pat-

ent veins but no functioning valves between the heart and the ankle. Patients with this anatomical situation generally have morbid venous disease with tensely swollen legs and frequent bouts of venous ulceration on the medial side of their calves and ankles. These patients usually have had prior deep venous thrombosis which has subsequently recanalized with destruction of the valves. These are the patients that will present with noninvasive studies that show no obstructive lesions but obvious venous disease. These are the patients that require much greater attention to the health of the skin in their lower extremities and to compressive therapy in order to minimize edema.

The most severe consequence of venous disease is the unhealthy edema associated with it, particularly focal edema. Focal edema occurs in legs in which incompetent perforators allow the direct pressure of the deep venous system to be transmitted to a superficial site. This can cause ulcerations, particularly on the medial side of the leg known as venous stasis ulcers. These ulcers apparently can form spontaneously, but they may also be the result of trivial trauma that would heal in any other area but cannot heal in the environment of venous hypertension.

The form of therapy for chronic venous insufficiency is the use of elastic support stockings to provide external compression and minimize the amount of edema that occurs during ambulation. Elevation of the legs also helps relieve the symptoms of chronic venous insufficiency by three mechanisms. First, elevation reduces venous pressure by decreasing the effects of gravity. Second, resorption of edema fluid is promoted secondary to decreased hydrostatic pressure. Third, the calf muscle pump will not activate when the limb has been elevated, thus eliminating ambulatory venous hypertension (3).

Basic Cardiac Anatomy

This section on cardiac anatomy assumes that the reader has been acquainted with basic cardiac anatomy. The cardiac conduction system, the coronary arteries, and the cardiac valves will be covered in detail in other sections of this chapter.

Endocardium

Although the endocardium seems like a superfluous structure, it is of great importance to the general surgeon. The endocardium serves as a barrier to infectious agents and has proven important in the structural prevention of endocarditis. The endocardium lines all of the cardiac chambers and the cardiac valves. It is continuous with the lining of all vessels within or connecting to the heart. Human beings can tolerate recurrent bacteremias as often as twice a day and not develop bacterial endocarditis. Animal studies have shown that remarkably high doses of intravascular bacteria are well tolerated. However, if the integrity of the endocardium becomes disturbed, the risk of bacterial endocarditis with bacteremia is increased more than 1000-fold.

Disruption of the endocardium may occur from natural causes, acquired conditions, or from congenital cardiac abnormalities. Deformed cardiac valves will cause repeated abrasion of the valvular endothelium. Extremely narrowed valves or regurgitant valves may also lead to jets aimed at endocardium; such jets have been associated with erosion of the protective lining. Congenital cardiac conditions causing high velocity flow and turbulence, or the jetting of blood, likewise will cause disruption of endocardium.

Iatrogenic interventions that increase the risk of bacterial endocarditis include cardiac catheterization, or the insertion of central venous lines and pulmonary artery catheters. This phenomenon also explains the markedly increased risk of developing bacterial endocarditis in the early period after cardiac surgery. Endocardial injury should be minimized, and when the patient is a risk, prophylaxis for bacterial endocarditis may be necessary.

Epicardium

The epicardium, or visceral pericardium, covers the entire normal heart. When cardiac injuries require closure, the epicardium holds sutures considerably better than does myocardium.

Pericardium

The pericardium is not an inert mass of connective tissue. Scanning electron microscopy shows it to be a highly organized tissue with microvilli and cilia for the production and absorption of fluid and the facilitation of movement across the serosal surfaces. The normal amount of pericardial fluid in an adult is approximately 50 ml.

The pericardium may play an important role as a barrier to inflammation from adjacent structures, particularly the lung. While complete pericardiectomy will not interfere with cardiac function, partial removal of the pericardium in certain locations can leave a situation in which the heart can be subjected to life threatening herniation. Herniation can be a particular problem after intrapericardial pneumonectomy.

A knowledge of certain features of pericardial anatomy plays an important role in interpreting echocardiograms, preventing complications, and improving the efficiency of emergency open chest resuscitation. Understanding this anatomy also offers alternative routes for exposure in operations around the trachea and great vessels.

Because of the pericardial sac attachment to the diaphragm, attempts at open massage of the ventricles during resuscitation generally will be ineffective unless the

pericardium is entered and the hand is placed around the heart within the pericardial sac. Failure to open the pericardium is a common error in emergency resuscitation. In addition, a knowledge of the course of the left phrenic nerve along the posterior lateral margin of the pericardium is important because this must be preserved during emergency pericardiotomy. Knowing that the nerve runs in a vertical fashion generally means that a vertical incision anterior to the area of the nerve will protect this structure.

Occasionally, traumatic injuries to the pulmonary artery or pulmonary veins and to the aorta will require emergency opening of the pericardium to obtain control. Knowing that the left and right pulmonary arteries have short courses within the pericardium is helpful. In addition, it is helpful to know that the pulmonary veins have a short free passage within the pericardial space before exiting. These areas can be exposed for control of these structures.

Pericarditis often presents with a characteristic sharp substernal chest pain, a pericardial friction rub, and electrocardiographic changes with widespread ST segment elevation involving all three standard limb leads and most of the precordial leads. Reciprocal depression usually is found in leads AV_R and V_1. Pericarditis without effusion does not directly affect cardiac function. When an effusion does develop, the occurrence of tamponade depends not only on the volume of pericardial fluid but on its rate of formation. If the effusion has formed slowly, the pericardium may have stretched, and the effect on the heart would be less. When tamponade is present, a paradoxical pulse may develop. This term is actually a misnomer because the pulse amplitude of a normal individual will diminish slightly on inspiration. Thus, a better term would be an "exaggerated" pulse instead of a "paradoxical" pulse. The normal influence of inspiration on cardiac filling is that the negative intrathoracic pressure draws more blood into the right ventricle, whereas the left ventricle transiently receives less blood because blood stays in the lungs, thus the left heart ejects less blood. When cardiac tamponade occurs, this normal slight decrease in pressure with inspiration becomes exaggerated. A decline in systolic blood pressure of 15 mm Hg or more with each inspiration is thought to be definite evidence of a pathologic "paradoxical" pulse. Advanced cardiac tamponade produces Beck's triad, which consists of hypotension, distended neck veins, and muffled heart sounds. Confusion not only exists over the definition of a paradoxical pulse, but there are also questions about the usefulness of the term.

Measuring this physical finding accurately is difficult because it requires a quiet room, a cooperative patient, excellent blood pressure taking skills, and a spontaneously breathing patient. Most frustrating, the finding is inconsistent in trauma. Thus, trying to determine whether a paradoxical pulse is present to help make the diagnosis of tamponade is more useful in the chronic setting, such as after the pericardial effusions, which may be seen in uremia or post pericardiotomy syndrome. Similarly, looking for an enlarged heart shadow on a chest radiograph is an unreliable finding; because the pericardium is stiff and inelastic, it may not be enlarged significantly in acute tamponade. The most reliable clinical findings of tamponade will be hypotension in the setting of increased venous pressure. Echocardiography has been shown to be the simplest diagnostic test beyond these clinical findings to document a pericardial effusion.

Studies of the influence of tamponade on the heart show that the left ventricle itself is markedly resistant to a reduction in its stroke volume by direct compression. Most of the effects produced by tamponade actually are associated with impairment of filling of the left and right atria and the right ventricle. Thus, the overall effect of compression of the other chambers causes impairment of the filling of the left ventricle and subsequent decreased stroke volume and systolic blood pressure. Because the normal stroke volume has been diminished, a compensatory tachycardia then develops. This tachycardia is often insufficient to maintain cardiac output, and a compensatory increase in systemic vascular resistance results. The rise in systemic resistance maintains systemic blood pressure at the expense of cardiac output, cardiac oxygen consumption, cardiac work, and tissue perfusion. When intrapericardial pressure continues to rise, systemic vasoconstriction occurs, and cardiac output diminishes until a shock state exists.

As pericardial fluid volume increases, there is little change in pericardial pressure until a point at which the tension in the pericardium reaches near maximum. At this point, a small increase in pericardial volume produces a rapid increase in pressure. Specifically, the slope of the curve becomes steeper as intrapericardial pressure approaches 14 to 15 mm Hg. This phenomenon also explains why, in the emergency treatment of tamponade, the removal of a small amount of fluid may dramatically increase the blood pressure and cardiac output. Removal of as small a volume as 25 cc can allow enough filling of the heart to significantly increase the output. For instance, if the heart is beating 100 times per minute and pumps 10 cc more per stroke, the cardiac output would be improved by one liter. This small improvement in cardiac output under these sort of dire circumstances can often mean the difference between the patient surviving until definitive treatment can be rendered and the patient dying of cardiac tamponade.

Because the deleterious effect of tamponade predominantly affects right ventricular filling, giving additional intravascular fluids may cause a temporary improvement. Increased preload for the right ventricle increases the volume filling the right ventricle. This increase improves pulmonary venous return. As the left ventricle filling pressure increases, stroke volume increases, as does systolic pressure.

The fact that a state of tamponade produces systemic vasoconstriction to maintain systemic blood pressure also helps explain the increased potential dangers to a patient in tamponade who undergoes general anesthesia. Peripheral vasodilatation is a common side effect of most anesthetic agents and, under these circumstances, causes a rapid loss of blood pressure. This phenomenon explains the wisdom of prepping a patient's chest before the introduction of general anesthesia if a cardiac tamponade has been suspected. This maneuver then permits the rapid decompression of the pericardial space if needed.

The Coronary Circulation

Microcirculation

The coronary perfusion pressure is the pressure that drives blood across the coronary microcirculation. Another approximation of this driving force can be determined by subtracting the central venous pressure from the diastolic blood pressure. This is the gradient across which most of the coronary circulation's blood flow is driven. Thus, as the diastolic blood pressure falls and the central venous pressure (the pressure seen by the coronary sinus) rises, the flow across the coronary microcirculatory bed will lessen. When this driving force is under 25 mmHg, the patient usually will not survive long unless some intervention is rendered to reverse this situation and to improve the coronary perfusion pressure.

The coronary microcirculation is representative of most vascular beds in the body serving muscular tissues. Blood flow through these beds is controlled by a variety of factors. Under conditions of increased oxygen demand or decreased oxygen supply, adenosine is released from most tissues. Adenosine is the nucleoside that results from the breakdown of the high-energy phosphate compounds ATP, ADP, and AMP. It is one of the most potent vasodilators known. Thus, as adenosine is released into the interstitial fluid, the contiguous arterioles are dilated, resulting in increased flow to the area and, therefore, increased oxygen delivery. Other factors may play a role in the vasodilatation associated with ischemia, including the concentration of oxygen, potassium, prostacyclin, and endothelium-derived relaxing factor. There is growing evidence that under conditions of profound and prolonged ischemia, these autoregulatory mechanisms are no longer functional, resulting in irreversible vasoconstriction.

In addition to the metabolic factors noted above, a number of other agents influence coronary blood flow, including physical and neural factors. The majority (about 65%) of coronary blood flow occurs during diastole. Thus, when diastole is shortened by factors such as increased heart rate, nutrient blood flow diminishes. If the end diastolic pressure in the left ventricle is high, flow through the coronary bed will be less, especially in the subendocardial area. Likewise, if the afterload facing the heart is great, the subendocardium will be deprived of blood flow even further during systole. If the diastolic blood pressure is low and the central venous pressure is high, the coronary perfusion pressure can be reduced and coronary blood flow will fall. When sympathetic nerves supplying a nonworking, perfused heart are stimulated, vasoconstriction occurs. However, when sympathetic stimuli exist, the heart works harder and coronary blood flow increases. These changes are influenced primarily by metabolic factors. Cholinergic innervation of the coronary vasculature does not exist. Thus, it is believed that the sympathetic nervous system does not play an important role in regulating coronary artery blood flow (5).

Coronary Arteries and Coronary Arterial Disease

The heart absolutely depends on its coronary blood supply. Normal coronary anatomy normally consists of three primary coronary arteries supplying the left ventricle. The left anterior descending supplies the anterior wall and septum, the circumflex supplies the lateral wall, and the right coronary artery supplies the posterior wall and posterior septum. The coronary system is considered right dominant if the right coronary artery supplies the posterior septum. The right dominant system is present in approximately 85% to 95% of individuals.

The most significant pathologic factor involving coronary arteries is atherosclerosis. Atherosclerosis is a process that is thought to occur in response to chronic vessel injury. The injury response includes endothelial dysfunction, infiltration of the vessel wall with blood-borne elements, vascular smooth muscle cell proliferation, and the accumulation of lipid, resulting in plaque formation. Endothelial necrosis is not necessary for this process; however, alterations in endothelial cell function or increased permeability to macromolecules caused by nondenuding vessel injury are thought to be integral to the atherosclerotic process. Eventual calcification is the end result. Although the processes can be slow, occlusion of vessels can occur acutely, particularly if hemorrhage into a plaque occurs. If an acute occlusion of a coronary vessel occurs, then myocardial cells begin to die after 20 minutes of ischemia. After 60 minutes of occlusion, severe myocardial necrosis can exist, but this degree of necrosis has not been a predictable finding. Much depends on the presence of collaterals around the area of stenosis or occlusion. If the stenosis has occurred gradually, then even an acute occlusion may not cause myocardial damage. However, if only a mild stenosis occurs, followed by an acute occlusion secondary to hemorrhage into a plaque, and collaterals have not developed, then extensive myocardial damage often results. The presence or absence of collaterals explains why the results of thrombolytic therapy can be uncertain. If a patient has much in the way of collaterals, then there will often be no significant myocardial damage after clot lysis. However, if there are minimal collaterals, then major damage can occur despite early thrombolytic therapy.

In the majority of patients who develop coronary stenosis, the process develops slowly. These patients usually report so-called stable angina at initial examination. Although their flow is limited, symptoms develop only during exercise. These patients frequently can be treated medically. Medical therapy usually consists of decreasing myocardial oxygen consumption with beta blockers and increasing coronary flow with coronary dilators such as nitroglycerin. If the pattern is of unstable angina, the patients will have pain at rest. In this situation, the coronary vessels may be more restricted, with less collateral blood supply. In such situations, coronary arteriography best demonstrates the extent of disease and helps to define appropriate therapy.

Invasive therapy for coronary disease is either percutaneous transluminal coronary angioplasty or coronary bypass surgery. Angioplasty has been reserved for the patients with either one- or two-vessel disease and discrete stenoses. Transluminal angioplasty was designed to dilate the coronary stenosis and to provide increased coronary flow. The mechanism by which this occurs remains uncertain. One theory holds that the plaque becomes split by the balloon dilatation and then the process of remodeling occurs, which allows the stenosis to be remodeled by the body's own healing process. Good results are obtained in approximately 66% of patients. The remaining 34% develop restenosis, which can often be retreated. Coronary bypass surgery should be performed in patients with symptoms for whom other therapy has been unsuccessful or is contraindicated (4).

Although the techniques of bypass surgery are not germane here, it is important to understand the difference between vein bypasses and the use of the internal mammary artery (IMA). Vein bypasses provide effective bypass of coronary lesions with a greater than 90% early patency rate. However, vein bypasses may develop a thickened intima and may eventually (after 10 to 15 years) develop atherosclerotic changes in many cases. Although the internal mammary artery has a smaller caliber than a vein, it does provide blood flow analogous to a vein bypass or to a normal coronary artery in the early postoperative period. In the long term, it tends to stay free of atherosclerotic occlusion. The mechanism of this phenomenon has not been completely elucidated.

The IMA does have certain features that may contribute to its long-term patency. The blood supply (vasovasorum) of the IMA is confined to the adventitia and does not penetrate the media. The media is nourished entirely from the lumen. Autopsy studies show that coronary arteries have intimal thickening, which increases in severity with age. The internal mammary arteries appear to be spared from these changes. Human coronary arteries have shown incomplete endothelial cell coverage in contrast to the internal mammary arteries, which are completely covered. Finally, the internal mammary has a thin-walled media with well-differentiated smooth muscle cells compared with the left anterior descending coronary artery, which exhibits multiple defects in the internal elastic laminae and a thickened intimal layer. Taken together, these studies suggest that important histologic differences exist between the IMA and the coronaries and that these differences may play a role in the IMA's resistance to atherosclerosis. When the IMA has been used for coronary artery bypass, long-term patency has been excellent and is in the range of 95% patency at 15 years. Patients with IMA grafts in place also have an increased survival.

Many myocardial infarctions are relatively small and self-limited, and with modern therapy, they have a low mortality. However, a typical example of a larger myocardial infarction is an occlusion of a large left anterior descending artery, which will often cause extensive myocardial damage and may eventually lead to left ventricular aneurysm formation. A left ventricular aneurysm occurs when the damaged wall becomes thinned. The chamber dilates so that when contraction occurs, only a small portion of its volume leaves the ventricle. This causes heart failure and, frequently, arrhythmias. Massive myocardial infarction can also cause cardiogenic shock if more than 40% of the left ventricle has been lost. Myocardial infarctions involving the septum can cause ventricular septal defect. This often is associated with a large left-to-right shunt, right-sided overload, pulmonary edema, and often death. Therapy in this case consists of closing the defect. Finally, infarction can be associated with rupture of a papillary muscle that supports the mitral valve apparatus. This causes severe mitral regurgitation and heart failure. Therapy requires valve replacement (4).

Ischemia and Reperfusion

Ischemic tissue will ultimately progress to cellular death if restoration of blood flow does not occur in a timely manner. However, reperfusion of viable ischemic tissue actually exacerbates cellular injury by inducing a complex cascade of pathophysiologic, biochemical, and morphologic changes. In fact, reperfusion injury is often far more severe than damage incurred during the ischemic period itself. This injury is characterized by cellular edema, intracellular Ca^{2+} overload with subsequent activation of Ca^{2+}-dependent autolytic enzymes, disruption of lipid membranes, and perturbations in mitochondrial structure and function.

Reperfusion injury is a phenomenon with great rele-

vance to the practice of surgery, especially with regard to vascular, cardiac, and transplantation procedures. Each is associated with an obligatory ischemic period followed by restoration of oxygenated blood flow to the ischemic limb, heart, or transplanted organ, respectively. The heart was the first organ discovered to exhibit reperfusion dysfunction. The clinical hallmarks of myocardial reperfusion dysfunction are arrhythmias and impaired ventricular contractile function. This has become known as "myocardial stunning." Any ischemic tissue is susceptible to the deleterious consequences of reperfusion, and some of the manifestations are tissue or organ specific.

Mediators of Reperfusion Injury

Oxygen Free Radicals

The discovery of the detrimental effects of reintroduction of O_2 to previously ischemic tissues led to the suspicion that highly reactive, unstable oxygen metabolites are important mediators of reperfusion injury. These so-called oxygen free radicals, which contain one or more unpaired electrons, are derived from molecular O_2 and include superoxide anion (O_2^-), hydrogen peroxide (H_2O_2), and the extremely potent hydroxyl radical ($\cdot OH$). The rapid generation of these toxic moieties at the onset of reperfusion initiates a series of biochemical processes that causes widespread damage to cellular macromolecules. These processes include peroxidation of lipid membranes, protein degradation, nucleic acid damage, hemoprotein/cytochrome inactivation, and neutralization of nitric oxide. The most damaging effect of oxygen free radicals is lipid peroxidation, which impairs the normal fluidity and permeability of cell membranes, leading to cellular edema, massive Ca^{2+} and Na^+ overload, and cell lysis.

The sources of reactive oxygen metabolites during reperfusion are multiple. Xanthine oxidase, an enzyme that is activated in ischemic endothelial and parenchymal cells and that uses O_2 and hypoxanthine as substrates, is responsible for the majority of superoxide production. Polymorphonuclear cells (PMNs) are also a prolific free radical source, whereas catecholamine oxidation and prostaglandin metabolism are less important mechanisms of reperfusion-associated free radical production. Oxygen free radical scavengers and antioxidants have been shown both experimentally and clinically to ameliorate reperfusion injury by preventing the production of free radicals or by blocking their pathologic effects after they have been synthesized.

Polymorphonuclear Cells (PMNs)

PMNs are also important mediators of reperfusion injury, but they rely on the priming of reperfused tissues by oxygen free radicals for their activation and accumulation. For example, free radicals react with endothelial cells to elicit platelet activating factor (PAF), leukotriene B$_4$(LTB$_4$), and C5A, all of which are chemotactic to neutrophils. In addition, reactive oxygen metabolites induce the expression of the CD11/CD18 complex on the PMN cell surface, the expression of which is a prerequisite to the adherence of PMNs to the microvasculature and their subsequent accumulation in postischemic tissues.

Activated PMNs inflict damage to reperfused endothelial and parenchymal cells in a variety of ways. PMNs release a host of destructive proteolytic enzymes, including elastase, collagenase, gelatinase, lysozyme, and cathepsin G. In addition, as previously mentioned, PMNs are a rich source of oxygen-free radicals by virtue of a superoxide-generating NAD oxidase. Finally, activated PMNs produce substantial quantities of hypochlorous acid, a biologically toxic molecule formed by the activity of myeloperoxidase.

The Endothelium in Ischemia and Reperfusion

Our appreciation of the integral role of the endothelium in reperfusion injury continues to evolve. The complexity of the biologic responses mounted by this cell layer is staggering; until recently, it was thought to be a passive sheet of cells serving only to line the vasculature. A host of mediators formed during reperfusion induces endothelial cells to express intercellular adhesion molecules (ICAM 1 and 2) and endothelial leukocyte adhesion molecule (ELAM). These receptors bind the CD11/CD18 complex on activated neutrophils, thereby facilitating PMN adherence to and migration across the endothelium. In this way, PMNs are able to gain access to the subendothelial parenchymal cells, where they release their destructive enzymes and bioreactive molecules. Endothelial cells also secrete an abundance of soluble factors during reperfusion, including PAF, LTB$_4$, thromboxane A$_2$, and endothelin, the latter of which is the most potent vasoconstrictor known. In combination with decreased endothelial secretion of prostacyclin and the inactivation of the endothelial-derived vasodilator nitric oxide by superoxide, the net deleterious effects of these endothelial factors are vasoconstriction, platelet aggregation, PMN plugging of capillaries, and increased microvascular permeability. The end result is that perfusion of the microcirculation is severely compromised, which manifests as the classic "no-reflow" phenomenon of reperfusion injury.

Cardiac Valves and Valvular Disease

There are four cardiac valves, all of which may be affected by either congenital or acquired cardiac conditions. The valves (aortic, mitral, pulmonic, and tricuspid) have a simple function: cardiac valves permit the unimpeded, unidirectional flow of blood. Only when a valve fails to achieve these two effects does it contribute to any significant alteration in human physiology.

Aortic Stenosis

More than 85% of cases of aortic stenosis are caused by calcification of congenital deformities of the aortic valve, most commonly a bicuspid valve. The other 15% may be caused by senile calcification or to rheumatic valvulitis. Aortic stenosis obstructs outflow from the left ventricle, causing left ventricular hypertrophy and decreasing left ventricular compliance. The obstruction causes significant left ventricular hypertension while maintaining a normal aortic blood pressure. The total effect is a normal driving pressure in the coronary artery while the intramural tension increases markedly. This decreases coronary blood flow and oxygen supply to the left ventricular myocardium, whose oxygen demand is greatly increased because of increased work. Patients with significant aortic stenosis are at risk of sudden death and have a poor prognosis. The typical history of aortic stenosis is a patient with a known cardiac murmur for at least 20 years and the onset of symptoms at the age of 50 or 55. There are only three symptoms of aortic stenosis: chest pain, syncope, and heart failure. The syncope is thought to result from potentially lethal arrhythmias (ventricular tachycardia or self-terminating ventricular fibrillation), leading to a decreased cardiac output and decreased cerebral blood flow. Chest pain results from myocardial ischemia, and congestive heart failure is the end result of the decreased left ventricular compliance. With the onset of any one of the three major symptoms, a patient with aortic stenosis has a 50% probability of dying within 2 years, and 33% of these patients will have sudden death without the progression of symptoms. An increased risk of death also exists when undergoing non-cardiac operations. Aortic stenosis is suspected from hearing a harsh systolic flow murmur over the precordium and is diagnosed easily with 2-D echocardiography. Detailed delineation of the condition can be accomplished at cardiac catheterization. Cardiac catheterization has been accepted as a prerequisite for aortic valve replacement surgery because of the risk of coronary artery disease.

When patients with unrelieved aortic stenosis must undergo noncardiac operations, every attempt must be made to avoid peripheral hypotension, because this leads to further cardiac ischemia. Thus, patients with suspected aortic stenosis should not be treated with vasodilators, especially nitroglycerin. The proper treatment of aortic stenosis in adults is valve replacement.

Mitral Stenosis

About 99% of all cases of mitral stenosis result from rheumatic fever and valvulitis. The consequences of a narrowed mitral valve are atrial hypertension, pulmonary venous obstruction, pulmonary artery hypertension, and an increased pressure load on the right ventricle. In general, the left ventricle remains normal unless previously injured by rheumatic fever or compromised by coronary artery disease.

Patients with mitral stenosis are at risk of developing atrial fibrillation and peripheral emboli. They are sensitive to volume overload, and the infusion of large amounts of colloid may lead rapidly to pulmonary edema. Anything that increases the pulmonary hypertension of these patients may also lead to tricuspid regurgitation and right heart failure.

The natural history of mitral stenosis is protracted. Frequently, the patient will give a 20-or 25-year history of slowly progressive symptoms consisting first of easy fatigability, progressing to dyspnea on exertion, and finally to severe exercise limitation. Until these patients reach a New York Heart Association Class IV status, they are not at high risk of sudden death, but they are predisposed to all the risks of chronic atrial fibrillation and bacterial endocarditis. The proper treatment of late stage mitral stenosis is mitral valve reconstruction or replacement.

Pulmonic Stenosis

Pulmonic valvular stenosis is always the result of congenital heart disease and creates a significant pressure overload for the right ventricle. With time, this usually leads to tricuspid regurgitation or decreased compliance of the right ventricle. Although an uncommon condition, surgical intervention has not been recommended unless the systolic pressure within the right ventricle exceeds 50 mm Hg. Treatment today is balloon valvuloplasty and, in the few unsuccessful cases, open pulmonic valvulotomy.

Tricuspid Stenosis

Tricuspid valvular stenosis has rarely been reported and has generally been ascribed to be the result of rheumatic heart disease.

Aortic Regurgitation

Aortic valvular regurgitation may result from (*a*) bacterial endocarditis, (*b*) traumatic disruption of an aortic leaflet, (*c*) rheumatic valvulitis, (*d*) congenital valvular disease, (*e*) ascending aortic dissection, (*f*) aortoannular ectasia due to Marfan's syndrome or a defect in connective tissue metabolism, or (*g*) idiopathic causes. The exact cause in a given case may not be known. The physiologic consequence is volume overload of the left ventricle, which can remain asymptomatic for many years. As a general rule, leaking valves do not cause symptoms or major physiologic consequences until more than 50% of the systolic forward flow returns to the proximal cardiac chamber during diastole. Thus, aortic regurgitation rarely produces symptoms until the left ventricle constantly ejects more than twice the normal cardiac output. Cardiac compensation occurs through dilatation and hypertrophy. The typical history of aortic regurgitation is that of a cardiac murmur present for 25 to 30 years before the onset of symptoms, often consisting of mild cardiac failure. At that point, the patient generally has a moderately enlarged heart. If the patient is placed on digoxin, the symptoms of heart failure will disappear, and the patient may be carried an additional 3 to 10 years before the symptoms recur. Unfortunately, at that point massive cardiac hypertrophy usually occurs, and the patient has a poor long-term prognosis.

The precise timing of operations for the correction of aortic regurgitation has been debated widely. These patients are not at great risk of sudden death until they develop angina or persistent heart failure.

Mitral Regurgitation

Mitral regurgitation may be caused by (*a*) rheumatic valvulitis (rare), (*b*) dilated mitral annulus, (*c*) stretched or torn chordae tendineae, (*d*) ruptured papillary muscle head or papillary muscle, (*e*) myocardial ischemia, or (*f*) bacterial endocarditis. Mitral regurgitation may cause congestive heart failure.

Acute mitral regurgitation is most likely to result from ruptured chordae or bacterial endocarditis. Myocardial ischemia may cause mitral valve dysfunction and central regurgitation. Thus, the etiology must be determined before proceeding to either cardiac or noncardiac treatment of these patients.

Chronic mitral regurgitation is an insidious condition that produces few symptoms until major cardiac enlargement occurs. These patients are at far greater risk of having permanent underlying myocardial damage and limited cardiac reserve.

There are few palliative steps for the management of acute or chronic mitral regurgitation during noncardiac operations. The most important factors are the avoidance of hypertension and prophylactic measures to prevent bacterial endocarditis.

The treatment of significant mitral regurgitation should be mitral valve replacement or mitral valve repair. Operation should be offered to these patients earlier in the modern era than in the past because now most of these valves can be repaired.

Pulmonic Regurgitation

Pulmonic regurgitation most commonly results from severe pulmonary hypertension and cannot be relieved unless the pulmonary hypertension can be reversed.

Tricuspid Regurgitation

Tricuspid regurgitation usually results from pulmonary hypertension and right ventricular failure, although it may rarely be the result of bacterial endocarditis, especially among illicit drug users. Tricuspid regurgitation can also be associated with long standing mitral regurgitation. Tricuspid regurgitation generally indicates severe right heart failure, and its management is by treatment of right heart failure and pulmonary hypertension if present.

The Perioperative Care of Patients With Cardiac Valvular Disease

Undergoing Noncardiac Surgery

Aortic Stenosis

Aortic stenosis presents a special problem. In aortic stenosis, increases in systemic vascular resistance or the development of systemic hypertension can cause increased myocardial ischemia and failure. However, hypotension decreases the coronary artery filling pressures and may decrease oxygen supply. When patients with aortic stenosis require noncardiac surgery, the placement of a pulmonary artery catheter and direct systemic arterial pressure monitoring are indicated to balance these two extremes.

Bacterial Endocarditis

All patients with native cardiac valvular lesions or prosthetic cardiac valves are at an increased risk for the development of bacterial endocarditis. The introduction of central lines or the performance of any type of operation (clean or dirty) increases this risk. Bacterial endocarditis has been reported widely with minor trauma and endoscopy and other minor operations. These patients must receive appropriate antibiotic prophylaxis before, during, and for appropriate periods after any surgical or traumatic event. Whenever pulmonary artery catheters are positioned, prophylactic antibiotics are indicated until these lines are removed. The American Heart Association has published guidelines for antibiotic prophylaxis against bacterial endocarditis.

Anticoagulants

Anticoagulants are used in all patients with mechanical valves and occasionally for patients with bioprosthetic valves to prevent thrombosis of the valve or systemic embolization. As a general rule, patients with homograft valves need not be placed on long-term anticoagulation. Anticoagulation for patients with mechanical valves is maintained with oral anticoagulants (warfarin sodium) to produce a prothrombin time which is approximately 1.5–2.0 times normal. A more uniform approach to anticoagulation management is to use the International Normalized Ratio (INR) system. Patients with mechanical valves should have their INR main-

tained somewhere in the range between 2.5 and 4.0. The anticoagulation needed is greater if a mitral prosthesis is in place, if atrial fibrillation is chronic, or if the patient has already had a thromboembolic event. Less intensive anticoagulation is appropriate if the patient has an aortic prosthesis (faster flow over the valve) or if a bleeding problem has been present.

Managing the anticoagulation of a patient with a mechanical valve around the time of an elective operation is a challenge. Generally, the best approach would be to have the patient stop taking his or her warfarin for several days, allowing anticoagulation effect to lessen. The patient should then be brought into the hospital and put on continuous IV heparin as the prothrombin time nears normal. Heparin can then be stopped 4 hours before the planned operation because all effects of heparin will in fact be gone in 4 hours. Once the operation has been completed, it is usually safe to resume the heparin anticoagulation 12 to 24 hours after most operations. Oral warfarin should be started soon after the operation has been completed because it will take several days to reanticoagulate the patient. As stated earlier, mitral valve prostheses are at slightly greater risk of causing thromboembolic events than are aortic valves and thus require even more vigilance when anticoagulants are being manipulated.

Untreated Cardiac Valvular Lesions and the Postoperative Care of Patients Undergoing Noncardiac Surgery

All patients with untreated cardiac valvular lesions should be considered at high risk of cardiac complications when other operations are being conducted. The problems of bacterial endocarditis and intraoperative management were noted previously. Assume that all of these patients have compromised myocardial function. The early postoperative period will be managed most easily in a critical care area with the use of a pulmonary artery catheter and direct measurement of systemic arterial pressure. This allows intermittent measurement of cardiac index and of systemic vascular resistance index. Maximum cardiac function will be achieved when cardiac index is maintained above 2.5 liters/min/m^2 and systemic vascular resistance index is maintained below 2200 dynes-sec/cm^5/m^2. If this cannot be accomplished by the use of narcotics and volume replacement, then peripheral vasodilators and inotropic agents should be administered.

Cardiovascular Monitoring

Cardiovascular monitoring is only one aspect of the appropriate care of ill patients, and all data acquired through the use of electronic or electromechanical devices should be correlated with the visual and physical findings before being accepted as valid.

Although cardiovascular monitoring includes palpation, observation, and a clinical assessment of the adequacy of peripheral perfusion, this section will be limited to a discussion of electrical and electromechanical monitoring of cardiovascular variables.

The direct measurement of cardiovascular variables allows the surgeon to separate three basic components of homeostasis: the state of cardiac function, the adequacy of intravascular volume, and the tone of the peripheral and pulmonary vascular systems. By separating these components, the surgeon can usually make rational decisions concerning the need for and the appropriateness of interventions to correct pathologic states. Under many conditions, the inability to separate the various components of the cardiovascular system will lead to faulty diagnosis and inappropriate and less than optimal treatment.

Application

The application of modern technical cardiovascular monitoring is extensive and should not be applied to all patients. The selection of patients who require monitoring significantly relies on the experience and skill of the surgeon. Therefore, only general statements will be made here; the details will be discussed with specific diseases. If observation or tests indicate inadequate or inappropriate cardiac function, tissue or organ perfusion, or abnormalities of intravascular volume, then strong consideration should be given to the application of invasive cardiovascular monitoring.

Inadequate or inappropriate cardiac function may be indicated by irregular cardiac rhythm, tachycardia, or bradycardia. Inadequate perfusion of peripheral tissues or individual organs may be indicated by decreased urinary output, signs of peripheral vasoconstriction, or chemical tests suggesting decreased renal or liver function. Adequacy of the intravascular volume can be assessed indirectly by the filling of the venous system, the general state of peripheral perfusion, and by trends in the hematocrit and hemoglobin.

Intravascular Pressure

For more than a century, various methods have been used for the noninvasive measurement of systemic blood pressure. In ill patients, the measurement of systemic blood pressure by the use of an external pneumatic cuff should always be suspect. Although pressure-measuring systems can be extremely accurate, they are subject to equipment failure and human error in their application. The most accurate measurement of intravascular blood pressure (venous or arterial) is made by the insertion of a fluid-filled tube or a microtransducer directly into a blood vessel. Electromechanical coupling through a transducer converts the mechanical forces of blood pressure to an electrical signal that can be displayed or recorded for monitoring purposes. When fluid-filled monitoring systems are used, small amounts of air within the system or narrowed portions of the catheter system can lead to false readings. A properly positioned and calibrated arterial line is the most accurate form of measuring arterial blood pressure.

The commonly measured intravascular pressures include arterial or systemic blood pressure, central venous pressure or right atrial pressure, pulmonary artery pressure, and pulmonary artery wedge pressure.

Arterial or Systemic Blood Pressure

Arterial blood pressure is a reflection of cardiac pump function, peripheral vascular compliance, peripheral vascular resistance, and intravascular blood volume. By itself, neither a high nor a low arterial blood pressure has any diagnostic meaning. In terms of cardiac function, when systolic arterial blood pressure increases, myocardial oxygen consumption increases and the heart requires an increased end-diastolic resting tension of the myocardium. In turn, this requires an increased left ventricular end-diastolic volume, resulting in an increased left atrial pressure and pulmonary venous pressure. Because the majority of nutrient blood flow in the coronary arteries occurs during diastole, arterial diastolic pressure is an indirect measurement of the driving force that maintains coronary blood flow and myocardial perfusion. High heart rates that reduce the length of diastole or lower arterial diastolic pressures may lead to underperfusion of the myocardium.

Arterial blood pressure is also an indicator of the state of the peripheral vascular system. In elderly patients, when the larger blood vessels are affected by atherosclerosis, rigidity may lead to high peak systolic pressures and low diastolic pressures. However, the behavior of the resistance vessels determines the degree of impedance to flow. If the arterioles are in a high state of tone, impedance may be high and cause an elevation of mean blood pressure.

Central Venous or Right Atrial Pressure

The term *central venous pressure* is used here because of its popularity; however, *right atrial pressure* is a more appropriate term. This measurement determines the right ventricular preload and is a reflection of the adequacy of intravascular volume. In these measurements, it is assumed that the tricuspid valve is normal and, therefore, that the measurement of mean right atrial pressure is a close approximation of the right ventricular end-diastolic pressure.

Pulmonary Artery Pressure

Pulmonary artery pressure is determined by the state of contractility of the right ventricle, the pulmonary arteriolar tone, and the left atrial pressure. As with the left ventricle, increases in pulmonary systolic blood pressure increases oxygen consumption and alters the contractile state of the right ventricle. Pulmonary artery diastolic pressure is an inaccurate reflection of left atrial pressure and left ventricular filling pressure. Pulmonary artery diastolic pressure should only be used as a reflection of left ventricular preload when it has been shown to correlate well with pulmonary artery wedge pressure. This situation does not exist, for example, in pulmonary artery hypertension.

Pulmonary Artery Wedge Pressure

When assessing the adequacy of filling of the cardiac chambers, the true goal is usually to achieve optimal loading of the left ventricle. Exceptional instances exist in which the right side pressures may be more important. These situations include patients with known pulmonary hypertension or right heart failure. The best measure of left-sided filling would be the left ventricular end-diastolic pressure. The left atrial pressure is the best approximation of the left ventricular end diastolic pressure when the left ventricle is relatively normal. However, these pressures are unobtainable without left heart catheters. Therefore, the ability to measure pulmonary artery wedge pressure outside of the cardiac catheterization laboratory was a major advance in cardiovascular monitoring. Properly measured, pulmonary artery wedge pressure is a remarkably accurate measurement of left atrial pressure and, assuming a normal mitral valvular apparatus, it is a close approximation of left ventricular end-diastolic pressure. Left ventricular end-diastolic pressure is a reasonable reflection of the end-diastolic resting tension of the myocardium of the left ventricle. The accurate measurement of pulmonary artery wedge pressure requires the pulmonary artery wave form to disappear with balloon inflation and be replaced by a properly timed wedge wave form, which is the equivalent of a left atrial wave form. An adequate wedge or left atrial wave form should always include a V-wave, which is a positive deflection concomitant with the onset of left ventricular contraction that continues until ventricular relaxation. If a properly timed atrial contraction occurs, an A-wave will be seen during ventricular diastole. Exaggerated V-waves may be caused by a noncompliant left ventricle, atrial contraction after closure of the mitral valve (nodal rhythm), mitral regurgitation, or mitral stenosis.

The pulmonary artery wedge pressure is read most accurately at the "valley" of the ventilatory cycle (end expiration) when the patient is being ventilated. High levels of positive end-expiratory pressure (PEEP) may spuriously raise the pulmonary artery wedge pressure to some degree. This spurious rise occurs especially when levels of PEEP exceed 10 cm of water. A reasonable rule to factor in the effects of PEEP is to subtract half the PEEP level from the measured wedge. In contrast, the pulmonary wedge pressure should be measured at the "peak" of the respiratory cycle (end of inspiration) when the patient is breathing spontaneously.

Substantial risks exist whenever pulmonary artery wedge pressures are monitored. Complications of pulmonary artery catheterization include the possibility of thrombosis of the catheter, valve damage, endocarditis, pulmonary artery rupture, mechanical problems with the catheter such as knots, cardiac arrhythmias, and rupture of the balloon itself. Complete heart block can occur if the patient already has a left bundle branch block because the catheter can cause right bundle branch block. Thus, a catheter capable of pacing should be used in this setting. Several techniques exist for the safe placement of pulmonary artery balloon catheters; however, there is no substitute for caution in the subsequent measurement of wedge pressure. When patients with pulmonary artery balloon catheters are moved intraoperatively or in the postoperative period, the position of the catheter tip repeatedly shifts. If the catheter advances farther into the pulmonary artery than its original placement, subsequent inflation of the balloon can lead to rupture of the pulmonary artery and death. Retraction of the catheter back toward the main pulmonary artery may place it in a position where inflation of the balloon fails to achieve a wedged condition and will require readjustment. A good general rule is that the pulmonary artery catheter should not be advanced past the right heart border on the chest radiograph.

The indication for the use of a pulmonary artery catheter is the need to have precise fluid management of the patient. It is now well known that the ability of even astute clinicians to accurately determine the volume assessment of the patient from the bedside is poor. Thus, if precise fluid management is mandatory, pulmonary artery catheter will probably be required.

When the catheter is being placed, the tracings that one will see first will be the minor irregular deflections reflective of the superior vena cava and the slightly greater deflections seen when the catheter is in the right atrium. The right ventricle tracing will show wide deflections with a very low diastolic pressure and a high systolic pressure. Once the catheter has been advanced into the pulmonary artery, the systolic pressures are the same, whereas the diastolic pressures are higher. The wedge pressure tracing will resemble the right atrial pressure tracing and will be characterized by low systolic pressure with a diastolic similar to the pulmonary artery diastolic. One should never pull the PA catheter back when the balloon is inflated because valvular disruption can occur (Figure 15.1).

Several abnormal waves include the so-called "pseudo wedge" pressure tracing, which is caused by overwedging. This is illustrated in Figure 15.2. An example of a V wave, which results from mitral regurgitation, is illustrated in Figure 15.3.

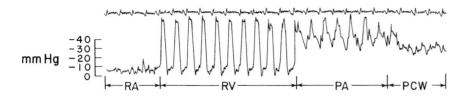

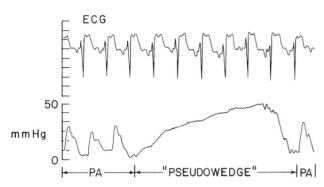

Figure 15.1. Pressure waveforms recorded as pulmonary artery catheter is advanced through right atrium (RA) and right ventricle (RV) into pulmonary artery (PA) and to wedge (PCW) position.

Figure 15.2. Pseudowedge pressure tracing recorded with inflation.

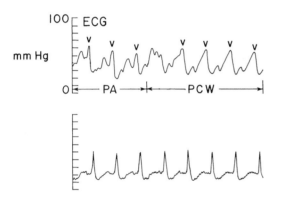

Figure 15.3. V waves in acute mitral regurgitation. V wave can be seen immediately following systolic pulmonary (PA) waveform, but is more prominent on wedge (PCW) waveform. The second wave in PA tracing can be identified as V wave, it peaks at same time following R wave of ECG (0.4 second) as V wave on wedge tracing. Mean wedge pressure is higher than PA diastolic pressure.

Blood Flow

Except in the experimental laboratory, the accurate measurement of blood flow is not possible. Two basic techniques are available for the measurement of cardiac output: the Fick principle and the thermodilution method. Neither technique has an accuracy better than ± 10% even under ideal circumstances, and under most clinical conditions the accuracy is probably little better than ± 15 or 20%. The measurement of cardiac output is presented conventionally as liters per minute. The cardiac index is the cardiac output divided by the body surface area.

$$CO = HR \times SV$$

$$CI = \frac{CO}{BSA}$$

The Fick Principle

The Fick principle can be used to determine blood flow. This principle is based on the use of an indicator to measure the blood flow indirectly. To use this approach, the physician must be able to sample blood going into and out of the system. The blood must also carry an indicator. The indicator could be normal substances like oxygen or other indicators such as dyes, carbon monoxide, or cold crystalloid solutions. It is important to know, or be able to estimate accurately, the total exchange of the indicator (I). The most common direct application of the Fick principle is when the blood flow through the lungs is measured. Thus, when pulmonary blood flow is known, it is assumed to be equal to cardiac output.

The general Fick equation is:

$$\text{blood flow} = \frac{\text{total exchange of indicator}}{\substack{\text{concentration of I entering system} \\ - \text{ concentration of I leaving system}}}$$

When the Fick principle is applied to the lungs, the equation becomes:

$$\text{Cardiac output} = \frac{\text{oxygen consumption}}{\substack{\text{arterial } O_2 \text{ content} - \\ \text{mixed venous } O_2 \text{ content}}}$$

Thus, cardiac output measurement based on the Fick principle ideally requires measurement of the oxygen consumption, arterial oxygen content, and mixed venous oxygen content. It assumes a stable and normal metabolic state. In clinical application, this method may be compromised by several factors. The oxygen consumption is assumed based on tables derived from large numbers of normal individuals and may not reflect the condition of the individual patient. Likewise, the metabolic state is assumed to be normal, which is often not the case. Arterial and venous oxygen content are derived indirectly, either from the partial pressure of oxygen (P_{O_2}) or the colorimetrically determined oxygen content O_2 (saturation), and both methods may introduce sizable errors. When the Fick method is used clinically, the number of assumptions and the potential inaccuracies must be taken into account.

Indicator Dilution Technique

In the indicator dilution technique, a marker of known volume is injected into flowing blood and its concentration measured downstream to determine the volume of blood flowing during a specified time period. The method was first developed using various dyes, the concentration of which could be measured colorimetrically. When dyes were used, it was necessary to withdraw enough blood for measurement in a colorimeter. Because the dyes required several hours to dissipate, they accumulated within the bloodstream, thereby limiting the number of determinations that could be made. Furthermore, as the dyes recirculated, the complexity of the analysis of the indicator concentration increased. Present techniques are based on thermodilution, in which a precisely measured quantity of fluid, the temperature of which is known and is lower than that of the circulating blood (usually room temperature), is injected rapidly into the central venous system, and the variation of the temperature of the blood reaching the pulmonary artery is measured continuously. The greater the magnitude of the temperature drop in the pulmonary artery per unit time, the lower the rate of blood flow, and vice versa. This is the most popular and probably the most accurate technique available clinically, although its accuracy is seldom better than ± 15%. However, technical errors that decrease accuracy include the slow or erratic injection of the indicator, inaccurate measurement of the volume of the indicator, inaccurate measurement of the temperature of the indicator, and improper placement of the pulmonary artery catheter.

Calculated Hemodynamic Variables

Understanding the conversion of cardiovascular measurements to indices and knowing the range of normal indices is important. The importance of indexing certain hemodynamic variables is obvious when the difference in the cardiac output needed for normal function of a 20 kg child as opposed to a 100 kg wrestler is considered. When normal values are reduced to indices, a relatively narrow range of normal values is found. Indexing is conventionally based on body surface area employing standard nomograms. Cardiac output is reported in liters per minute, whereas cardiac index is liters per minute per square meter. When the evaluation of systemic flow is reduced to a cardiac index, the ranges for normal output and changes produced by similar aberrations are fairly close for the small child and large adult.

When measurement of cardiac output became possible, these values could be combined with systemic or pulmonary arterial pressures to determine vascular resistance. The calculation of vascular resistance provides an approximation of the state of vascular tone and has become a critical measurement for the appropriate management of critically ill patients. Vascular resistance is calculated by dividing the pressure difference across a vascular bed by the minute blood flow through that bed. These calculations are, as in the case of peripheral vascular hemodynamics, analogous to Ohm's law. For the pulmonary vascular bed, this resistance (PVR) is the difference between mean pulmonary artery pressure (PA) and mean left atrial pressure (LA) (clinically defined as wedge pressure) divided by cardiac output (CO).

$$PVR = \frac{PA - LA}{CO} \times 80$$

Occasionally, clinicians talk in terms of "Woods units." Woods units are determined by subtracting the wedge pressure from the mean pulmonary artery pressure and dividing by the cardiac output. The most common clinical situation in which this terminology is used is in discussing the degree of patients' pulmonary hypertension before considering heart transplantation. The reason for making this determination is that even a new heart cannot sustain an adequate output in the face of a pulmonary resistance greater than 2.5 or 3 Woods units. Thus, a patient with this type of high, irreversible pulmonary hypertension would require heart-lung transplantation to have a reasonable chance of survival.

Systemic vascular resistance (SVR) is calculated by determining the difference between the mean arterial blood pressure (MAP) and the central venous pressure (CVP) divided by the cardiac output.

$$SVR = \frac{MAP - CVP}{CO} \times 80$$

Although the normal mean pressure ranges vary little from individual to individual, or even between children and adults, cardiac output, as mentioned previously, varies greatly according to the size of the individual. For this reason, resistance index should be used when monitoring patients. Resistance indices (RI) are calculated by substituting the cardiac index (CI) for the cardiac output (2).

$$PVRI = \frac{PA - LA}{CI} \times 80$$

$$SVRI = \frac{MAP - CVP}{CI} \times 80$$

Cardiac Rhythm and Arrhythmias

Normal conduction begins with the sinoatrial (SA) node, which conducts electrical activity through atrial tissue to the atrioventricular (AV) node, down the His bundle, through the Purkinje fibers, finally reaching the ventricles and causing contraction. When arrhythmias occur, they are caused by either problems with impulse conduction or disorders of impulse formation, i.e., automaticity. Impulse conduction problems are the most common cause of arrhythmias. The mechanism is reentry. Reentry occurs when an electrical impulse comes to a branch point in the conduction system and is transmitted unequally down two parallel pathways. When antegrade conduction is blocked in one path, the area beyond the block remains temporally inactivated. Coming down the other path, the unblocked impulse bypasses the blocked region and then, in retrograde fashion, activates the tissue. This can produce a continuous loop of activation. During normal conduction without an antegrade block, the impulses tend to block each other, preventing loop formation. Examples of arrhythmias caused by the reentry mechanism are ventricular tachycardia, Wolff-Parkinson-White syndrome, and atrial flutter.

Supraventricular Arrhythmias

Most supraventricular arrhythmias are responsive to treatment. For example, a patient whose symptom at initial examination is a sinus bradycardia can be treated with a vagolytic anticholinergic agent, such as atropine, to speed up the heart rhythm. Sinus tachycardias can be treated with carotid sinus massage to increase vagal tone and to decrease the speed of the rhythm. However, carotid massage should never be used in persons with atherosclerotic disease because cerebral atheroembolism may occur with carotid manipulation. Beta blockers, such as propranolol, can also be used in these circumstances. Atrial fibrillation is a common rhythm seen after many kinds of surgery. About a third of all the patients who undergo cardiac surgery will have atrial fibrillation some time in their postoperative period. The mechanism of production remains unclear, but atrial fibrillation is often associated with atrial dilatation, hypoxemia, increased catecholamines, and some element of pulmonary disease. Regardless of the cause, the goal of treatment is to slow conduction through the AV node with, for example, digitalis, low dose beta blockade, or calcium channel blockers.

Surgical therapy is possible for certain kinds of supraventricular arrhythmias. Wolff-Parkinson-White syndrome is an arrhythmia that causes tachycardia. The mechanism involves macro reentry, i.e., a specific pathway exists separate from, and bypasses, the normal conduction system. These pathways do not have any conduction delay in them analogous to the atrioventricular node. Thus, impulses from the atria reach the ventricles before the normally conducted impulse, which includes the AV node delay. Evidence for this preexcitation can be found in the electrocardiograms of these patients, in slurring of the initial deflection of the QRS occurs, called a Delta wave. These pathways can be mapped precisely using electrophysiologic techniques. The impulses usually travel in a retrograde fashion during tachycardic episodes. Normal impulses travel through the AV node and then are transmitted rapidly retrograde through these abnormal pathways, resulting in tachycardia. The pathways can be mapped and treated either surgically or with catheter ablation techniques in the electrophysiology laboratory. When the pathway is ablated, the δ-wave should disappear.

Automatic supraventricular tachycardias can also occur; these are arrhythmias that are continuous and related to the firing of a specialized area, usually in the atrium. Often, these constant tachycardias will ultimately cause ventricular dilation and heart failure. They too can be treated surgically by direct ablative techniques or by catheter ablation techniques.

Ventricular Arrhythmias

Ventricular arrhythmias are divided into two basic groups. The first group is ventricular fibrillation, which includes polymorphic ventricular tachycardia. Polymorphic ventricular tachycardia is an irregular-looking rhythm by ECG that is a form of coarse ventricular fibrillation. The mechanisms for the ventricular fibrillation depends on the clinical situation. Ventricular fibrillation is a disorganized arrhythmia of the ventricle and most often occurs on the basis of a metabolic derangement. Less often it is the result of reentry. This derangement can also be caused by ischemia, most notably associated with an acute myocardial infarction. Automaticity in such a case would be related to dying Purkinje fibers or to metabolic changes in the myocardium. Treatment for these kinds of arrhythmias is related to correction of the metabolic abnormality and pharmacologic agents that decrease the sensitization to abnormal impulses. Common drugs used to treat the rate of depolarization are lidocaine and procainamide. Beta blockers may also be useful in treating ventricular ectopy.

Monomorphic ventricular tachycardia is an entirely different arrhythmia. This is a uniform kind of ventricular tachycardia that is often associated with cardiovascular collapse. This arrhythmia often occurs in the first 48 hours after acute myocardial infarction. In this circumstance, it is the result of automaticity. This arrhythmia more commonly occurs later after myocardial infarct and is caused by a reentry mechanism. When the myocardial infarction occurs, some of the tissue is clearly dead and some is absolutely normal. Neither of these kinds of tissue causes arrhythmias. Rather, the injured border zone tissue between the normal and dead tissue provides a substrate for micro reentry. Many unidirectional blocks exist, and as a result, there is an anatomic focus for this arrhythmia. With an anatomic focus, the arrhythmia is less likely to be sensitive to drugs. Frequently, this arrhythmia needs to be treated surgically by endocardial resection of the border zone tissue between the normal and dead endocardium.

The most common clinical arrhythmia is premature ventricular complexes (PVCs). In the face of an acute myocardial infarction or a metabolic derangement, PVCs can lead to ventricular fibrillation. As such, the metabolic derangement needs to be corrected, and PVCs may be suppressed by using lidocaine. However, in the absence of cardiac ischemia, PVCs are a benign arrhythmia. In fact, suppression with drugs often leads to a more malignant form of arrhythmia, ventricular tachy-cardia, or ventricular fibrillation. Although the frequency of the PVCs are often suppressed by treatment, the first PVC seen may lead to the malignant arrhythmia. Therefore, the goal of treating a patient with PVCs is to elucidate and treat the cause.

Electrophysiologic Testing

When a persistent ventricular arrhythmia is present, it should be tested to see if it is inducible or if the arrhythmia occurs in the absence of other precipitating factors. Electrophysiologic testing is performed in the laboratory, using catheters in the ventricle to stimulate the heart. If the arrhythmia can be stimulated using multiple PVCs, then the arrhythmia is certainly of the reentry mechanism, and appropriate therapy can be instituted. In addition, electrophysiologic testing allows for serial drug testing to determine if the arrhythmia can be treated pharmacologically, without taking a chance on empiric drug choices (4). Other treatments for ventricular arrhythmias include endoventricular ablative techniques, which usually involves surgical resection of scar or the use of automatic implantable cardioverter defibrillators.

Cardiac Function

Determinants of Function and Therapeutic Manipulation of Performance

To treat patients with reduced cardiac function appropriately, it is necessary to have an understanding of the physiologic determinants of cardiac function. Such an understanding will allow the appropriate surgical care of acutely ill and chronically debilitated patients undergoing surgical procedures.

There are five basic factors that interact to determine the ability of the heart to function as an effective pump. These factors are also interdependent, and manipulations in one may produce changes in another. They are preload, afterload, electrical state of the heart (rate, rhythm, conduction, etc.), contractility, and compliance.

Preload

The initial filling volume, or pressure, of the left ventricle before contraction determines the sarcomere length and, hence, the muscle performance of individual fibers. The physiologic correlate of the sarcomere length-tension relationship is the Frank-Starling curve. This curve shows that progressive increases in left ventricular filling volume cause progressive increases in ventricular developed pressure until a peak level of function is reached. Additional increases in volume beyond this maximum level do not produce improvements in per-

formance. The anatomic cellular correlate of this physiologic phenomenon describes the stretching of myofibers or muscle cells within the walls of the ventricular chamber such that individual sarcomeres within myocytes increase in length from a resting level of 1.9 μm to a maximum level of 2.2 μm. At 2.2 μm, the overlap of actin and myosin filaments allows the maximum number of cross-bridges between these elements to be formed. This produces the maximum degree of force generation by each cell. Because of the elastic properties of myocardial cells, it is extremely difficult to stretch sarcomeres significantly beyond 2.2 μm under physiologic conditions. In fact, any elongation of sarcomeres beyond 2.2 μm would reduce the overlap of actin and myosin filaments, thereby reducing performance. Thus, the anatomic correlate of the Frank-Starling curve is the ability of the muscle cell to increase force generation as sarcomere length and ventricular filling volumes increase. Increases in volume beyond that which causes optimum sarcomere length will not improve ventricular performance and may be detrimental. Therefore, the preload, filling volume, or pressure in the left ventricle determines the position of the ventricle on the Frank-Starling curve and predicts cardiac performance.

Preload itself depends on the capacitance of the vascular system and the blood volume. Preload can be influenced by volume expansion or contraction and by changes in the capacitance of the venous or arterial circulations. Factors that may reduce venous return to the heart, such as gravitational effects, venodilators, positive pressure ventilation, and positive end-expiratory pressure ventilation, may change preload and, therefore, myocardial performance.

Afterload

Afterload is the arterial resistance against which the heart must overcome to eject blood into the systemic circulation. It is defined as the systemic vascular resistance. The capacitance of the arterial system and the volume of blood contained within the system are the components contributing to peripheral vascular resistance. Thus, change in either arterial capacitance or blood volume will affect afterload. As myocardial functional reserve is reduced by disease, manipulation of afterload may be an important method of improving ventricular performance.

$$SVR = \frac{MAP - RA}{CO \times 80}$$

Where: SVR = systemic vascular resistance, MAP = mean arterial pressure, RA = mean right atrial pressure, and CO = cardiac output.

Since this resistance is the force against which the heart must eject to create forward flow, when the resistance is lowered, the cardiac output should increase.

Two special cases of mechanical afterload manipulation deserve mention: intra-aortic balloon pumps (IABP) and military anti-shock trousers (MAST). The former mechanically decreases afterload while preserving diastolic coronary perfusion pressure by deflating just before systolic cardiac ejection and inflating when the aortic valve has closed. This device is useful for unstable cardiac patients. The latter, MAST suits, elevate central blood pressure primarily by increasing afterload. Unfortunately, the afterload increase is often peripheral to large leaking arterial defects in the setting of central penetrating trauma or ruptured aneurysms. This peripheral increase in afterload is the physiologic equivalent of cross clamping the aorta at the level of its bifurcation. Thus, one must be aware of the effects of this increased afterload on the heart and the aorta or its major branches above this "clamp."

Electrical State of the Heart

Cardiac output is defined by the following equation:

$$CO = HR \times SV$$

$$HR = \text{heart rate}; SV = \text{stroke volume}$$

Thus, increases in heart rate are directly related to increases in cardiac output. However, as heart rate increases beyond 90 beats/min, the total cardiac output may actually begin to decrease. Stroke volume decreases at faster heart rates because the heart cannot fill as completely. Therefore, as heart rate increases beyond 90 beats/min, the total cardiac output may actually decrease as stroke volume begins to decrease at a faster rate than heart rate increases.

Considering the effect of cardiac rhythm on ventricular performance is also important. Sinus rhythm itself, with the coordinated initial depolarization of the atrium followed by depolarization of the ventricle, has an important influence on myocardial performance. In fact, as ventricular compliance decreases, the "atrial kick" provided in normal sinus rhythm has an even more important contribution to cardiac output, approaching a 25% increase. Thus, not only is heart rate a determinant of cardiac performance, but the coordinated depolarization of the cardiac chambers achieved in sinus rhythm also produces a substantial contribution.

Contractility

The inherent ability of the myocardium to generate force independent of loading conditions is characterized by contractility. The inotropic state of the myocardium can be influenced by endogenous and exogenous catecholamines. An assessment of contractility forces can be obtained by measuring the maximum rate of rise of ventricular pressure over time (dp/dt_{max}). This measurement is a basic reflection of contractility as long as preload conditions are held constant.

Ejection fraction (*EF*) is the ratio of the stroke volume (*SV*), defined as the volume ejected by the ventricle in systole, to the end-diastolic volume (*EDV*).

$$EF = SV/EDV$$

Ejection fraction is a useful indicator of ventricular function. Normal ejection fraction is greater than 65%. Although it depends on preload and afterload conditions, ejection fraction can be used to evaluate and compare contractility at baseline.

Compliance

Left ventricular compliance (*C*), or the relationship between the filling pressure (*P*) and chamber volume (*V*), is an indicator of the ease of ventricular distensibility.

$$C = \Delta V/\Delta P$$

Myocardial ischemia, edema, hypertrophy, amyloidosis, restrictive cardiomyopathies, pericardial disease, and pericardial tamponade decrease ventricular compliance. As compliance decreases, the ventricle becomes stiffer and less distensible. This may produce less diastolic filling and decreased cardiac performance.

Measurement of Cardiac Performance

Cardiac index is the most frequently used parameter of myocardial performance in surgical patients. Normal cardiac index ranges between 2.5 and 4.5 liter/min/m². Two clinically applicable methods of determining cardiac output are based on principals of metabolite transport and indicator dilution (8). These concepts are reviewed previously in additional detail.

Pharmacologic Interventions

Sympathomimetic Amines

The primary cardiac effects of the sympathomimetic amines (catecholamines) are mediated by way of β-adrenergic receptors. These agents produce an increase in myocardial contractility, an increase in the frequency of pacemaker discharge in the SA and AV nodes, and an increase in AV node conduction velocity. These agents also produce effects on the vascular system through α- and β-adrenergic receptors. The vasoconstrictor response is mediated by α-adrenergic receptors, and the vasodilator response is mediated by β-adrenergic receptors. The relative potencies of the various sympathomimetic amines on adrenergic receptors are shown in Table 15.1.

The β-receptor activity of dobutamine is much more important than its α-adrenergic effects. At infusion rates of 5 μg/kg/min, dobutamine acts primarily as a positive inotropic agent by increasing myocardial contractility. Dobutamine has more of a chronotropic effect than dopamine. Dobutamine also reduces peripheral vascular resistance by stimulating the beta receptors in the

Table 15.1.
The Relative Potencies and Sites of Influence of the Sympathomimetic Amines

Sympathomimetic Amines Agent	Vascular		Cardiac
	α	β	β
Dobutamine	—	+ +	+ +
Dopamine[a]	+ +	+ +	+ +
Epinephrine	+ +	+ +	+ + + +
Norepinephrine	+ + +	—	+ + +
Isoproterenol	—	+ +	+ + +

[a] Dopamine produces mesenteric and renal vascular dilatation by activating dopaminergic receptors. It also acts on α- and β- receptors directly and can cause the release of endogenous norepinephrine.

peripheral vasculature. After beginning at an initial dose of dobutamine, increases in dosage are titrated to hemodynamic and clinical improvement.

The effects of dopamine are mediated by three different receptors at low, intermediate, and high dose levels of drug treatment. Thus, a dose-dependent action of this drug occurs on the renal vasculature, heart, and peripheral vasculature. At low doses (1 to 5 μg/kg/min), dopamine has a primary effect on stimulating dopaminergic (D_1) receptors in the renal and mesenteric vasculature. This effect is predominantly vasodilation, resulting in augmentation of renal blood flow.

As intermediate levels of dopamine dosage are achieved in the range of 5 to 10 μg/kg/min, the effect is primarily on increasing cardiac contractility and heart rate through the β_1-receptors.

As high levels of dopamine infusion are reached (10 μg/kg/min), a significant degree of peripheral vasoconstriction results as α-adrenergic receptors are activated. This activation causes a significant elevation of systemic vascular resistance. Maintenance of renal vasodilation is lost at these high infusion rates. This drug also has an arrhythmogenic effect, especially at these high doses.

Epinephrine is a potent α- and β-adrenergic agent with a significant inotropic effect on myocardial contractility. It is also associated with significant α-agonist activity and can increase peripheral arterial vascular tone with all of the potentially negative effects seen with decreased peripheral perfusion. Epinephrine is started at a dose of 1 μg/min and can be increased as high as 5-10 μg/min, although these higher doses are rarely used.

Norepinephrine is an extremely potent α-agonist and can be used as a potent pressor agent. Dosage frequently begins in the range of 1 μg/min and can be titrated to increase systemic blood pressure. This agent causes increased activity of all α-receptors with significant elevations in arterial resistance. It may produce marked decreases in coronary, renal, and peripheral perfusion.

Isoproterenol has a pure β-adrenergic effect. Its clinical use is usually restricted to situations such as bradyarrhythmias for which enhancement of heart rate and condition are desirable. It is also a potent pulmonary vasodilator.

Digitalis Glycosides

Digoxin is the most widely used clinical digitalis glycoside. It has a positive inotropic effect on myocardial performance. The effects of digoxin are related to its ability to increase the intracellular calcium available to the contractile apparatus. This effect is achieved by binding with sarcolemmal sodium potassium ATPase and thus blocking the active transport of sodium in exchange for potassium. The increased accumulation of sodium within the cell leads to an increased concentration of calcium through the sodium-calcium ion-exchange mechanism. Digitalis-containing compounds also slow conduction through the AV node and can be of therapeutic value in treating supraventricular tachycardias.

Digoxin has significant interactions with quinidine, verapamil, and amiodarone, which cause its concentration in the blood to be increased. Remember that the pharmacokinetics of digoxin are such that the equilibration is not achieved until 6 to 8 hours after an oral or intravenous dose. Thus, serum levels should be measured after equilibration has occurred.

Digitalis preparations can cause toxicity. The most important effects are ventricular arrhythmias. The most typical digitalis-induced rhythm is junctional tachycardia. This rhythm is a wide complex rhythm originating high in the conduction system (near the "junction" of the atrioventricular node and the His bundle). Ordinarily, a rhythm originating at this level would have a rate of about 40 beats per minute. In digitalis toxicity, this rate is usually 80 to 120 beats per minute. Digitalis toxicity can also be manifested by systemic signs and symptoms, such as gastrointestinal distress and visual changes like seeing greens and yellows. Digitalis toxicity is more likely to be seen when the patient's levels of potassium or magnesium are low.

Vasodilators

Nitroprusside is a pure smooth muscle vasodilator that affects all vascular beds, including the arterial, venous, and coronary circulations. Treatment is usually initiated at a dose of 0.5 μg/kg/min and is titrated upward for an appropriate response in arterial pressure. Nitroprusside is an extremely effective agent when afterload reduction is required. Its effects are transient and can be reversed rapidly by reducing dosage or stopping the drug.

Despite its apparent beneficial effect, some evidence suggests that nitroprusside infusion in patients with significant myocardial ischemia can produce a *steal* phenomenon in which coronary blood flow is directed away from the areas of ischemia. Thus, this agent may not be desirable in such patients.

Nitroprusside is metabolized to cyanide. The cyanide can be metabolized into thiocyanate by the liver and excreted by the kidneys. With normal kidneys, its $t_{1/2}$ is 4 days. However, patients with renal failure may develop thiocyanate toxicity, manifested by tremors, hypoxia, nausea, disorientation, and hypothyroidism. This complication rarely occurs when the drug is used for less than 48 hours. The toxicity can be reversed by infusion of hydroxocobalamin, which converts thiocyanate into cyanocobalamin (vitamin B_{12}).

Nitroglycerin is also a smooth muscle vasodilator, with effects on the coronary and peripheral circulation. Nitroglycerin has a dose-dependent differential action. It acts primarily on veins at low to moderate dosages. At higher dosages, dilatation of the systemic arterial vasculature occurs.

The therapeutic usefulness of nitroglycerin in patients with ischemic coronary artery disease occurs as a result of coronary arterial vasodilation. In addition, a reduction in preload occurs, which produces a decrease in myocardial oxygen consumption. Nitroglycerin is given intravenously with a dose beginning at 50 μg/min and can be titrated upward as required. Oral, sublingual, and dermal forms of this medication are available. Tachyphylaxis to nitroglycerin may develop over time. Options for reestablishing vascular effects include terminating use of the drug for a period of time and treatment with N-acetylcysteine.

Amrinone and milrinone are phosphodiesterase inhibitors. They appear to inhibit myocardial cyclic adenosine monophosphate phosphodiesterase activity, producing an increase in the cellular concentrations of cyclic adenosine monophosphate (cAMP). Amrinone and milrinone thus have positive inotropic effects: they increase ventricular performance and also appear to act on vascular smooth muscle to produce vasodilation. Administration of amrinone has been associated with thrombocytopenia.

The calcium channel blockers can be used for the treatment of angina pectoris, supraventricular tachycardia, and hypertension. By inhibiting the flux of calcium through myocardial channels, they produce a negative inotropic effect. Furthermore, calcium-dependent activity at the pacemaker cells of the sinus and AV nodes is reduced and causes sinus bradycardia and prolonged AV conduction. These agents produce a vasodilatory action on the coronary and peripheral arterial vasculature by directly interfering with calcium-induced smooth muscle contraction. They also appear to have an antivasospastic activity on the coronary vasculature. Many calcium channel blockers are currently available, and they vary in the relative degree of cardiac effect and peripheral vascular effect.

Angiotensin-converting enzyme (ACE) inhibitors interfere with the pulmonary conversion of angiotensin I to angiotensin II. Angiotensin II is an extremely potent vasoconstrictor and also promotes adrenal gland release of aldosterone. This, in turn, produces systemic vasculature volume expansion through increased renal reabsorption of sodium. The ACE inhibitors have an important role in modifying the renin-angiotensin-aldosterone system. ACE inhibitors produce a significant reduction in systemic vasculature resistance by producing vasodilation and diminishing plasma volume. Treatment with these agents may produce hyponatremia and hyperkalemia. Captopril and enalapril are two commonly used ACE inhibitors.

Captopril is effective in the treatment of congestive heart failure and hypertension. The advantage of this agent is that it has less of the quality-of-life side effects produced by other antihypertensive agents that work on the central nervous system. Captopril reduces blood pressure by reducing preload and afterload, and it tends preferentially to maintain flow to the kidneys. Adverse effects associated with this drug include neutropenia, agranulocytosis, rise in serum creatinine, metallic taste, skin rash, proteinuria, angioedema, a persistent cough, and dysgeusia. Captopril is excreted by the kidneys, and increases in creatinine associated with initiation of captopril treatment may suggest a preexistent renal artery stenosis.

Enalapril is an ACE inhibitor with a prolonged duration of action because it requires metabolic conversion in the liver for activation. Enalapril may have a reduced number of side effects relative to captopril because enalapril is a nonsulfhydryl-containing molecule. The sulfhydryl moiety is thought to be a source of many of captopril's side effects. However, enalapril does retain some of the side effects of captopril such as neutropenia, angioedema, and cough. Many other ACE inhibitors are now becoming available.

Mechanical Assist Devices

Although the vast majority of patients requiring supportive measures for decreased ventricular function respond to conservative medical measures, a small percentage of patients do require more aggressive treatment for survival. A number of mechanical devices are now available for use in such patients. The intraaortic balloon pump (IABP) was the first widely used device for support of the failing heart and is still a mainstay of mechanical ventricular support. However, new left ventricular assist devices (LVAD) are becoming available, and technology in this area is progressing rapidly. The ultimate form of ventricular assistance may be some form of total artificial heart.

The IABP supports the circulation by implementing the concept of counterpulsation. This theory suggests that the rapid expansion of vascular volume during diastole and the rapid reduction of vascular volume during systole can augment ventricular function significantly. This mechanism provides increased diastolic blood pressure, which causes improved coronary and peripheral perfusion during diastole. It also produces decreased afterload during systole, which causes improved cardiac performance and reduced myocardial work. The initial attempts at implementing this theory were unsuccessful because of technical difficulties with the rapid infusion and removal of blood. However, the idea of an intravascular balloon that inflates during diastole and deflates during systole was found to be technically easier to implement than blood manipulation. The IABP works by two actions. First, the rapid inflation of a balloon in the descending aorta early in diastole (firing on the T wave) causes improved diastolic pressure and increased coronary and peripheral perfusion. This mechanism depends on a competent aortic valve. Second, just before systole (deflating on the R wave), the IABP rapidly deflates and lowers afterload, thereby producing improved myocardial performance by reducing peripheral resistance.

The IABP remains the mainstay of mechanical support for the failing myocardium. Although the IABP is an effective means of mechanically augmenting ventricular performance, it depends on at least some remaining left ventricular function. In end stage of left ventricular failure, the IABP is of little value.

The LVAD is capable of supporting the entire systemic and/or pulmonary circulation when ventricular performance is severely compromised. A variety of devices have been developed as LVAD pumps. These include roller pumps, centrifugal (vortex) pumps, and pneumatic pulsatile pumps. Each system has its inherent advantages and disadvantages and represents the development of newer technologies.

Congenital Heart Disease and Its Physiological Consequences

Congenital heart disease remains an important public health problem in the United States, with an incidence of 8/1000 live births. In the United States, seven times as many children will be born with congenital heart disease as will develop rheumatic heart disease in their lifetime. Therefore, it is probable that every general surgeon will encounter patients who also have treated or untreated congenital heart disease. The decision-making process for therapy and the methods of treatment may require marked alteration because of cardiac abnormalities.

Arterial Desaturation

Arterial desaturation is most often caused by right-to-left shunting and failure of a portion of blood to pass through the pulmonary circuit. Occasionally, severe heart failure may cause interstitial pulmonary edema and lead to decreased alveolar capillary transport of oxygen. The degree of tissue hypoxia depends on both the hemoglobin level and the degree of intracardiac mixing and pulmonary blood flow. Increasing the fraction of inspired air (FI_{O2}) usually has relatively little effect on tissue oxygenation unless, under special circumstances, it alters the degree of intracardiac mixing.

It might be thought that increasing the hematocrit would increase the oxygen-carrying capacity, and this is true to some extent. The natural response to arterial desaturation is the development of secondary polycythemia, which in and of itself may lead to intermittent diffuse intravascular coagulation and its consequences. A specific diagnosis is extremely important if it becomes necessary to operate on a cyanotic patient with congenital heart disease. When the anatomy is understood, the development of a rational plan for management is possible.

Ventricular Overload

In congenital heart disease, the ventricles or atria may be subjected to unusual stress. Atrial physiology and pathology are poorly understood; however, the consequences of unnatural ventricular stress are better understood and are known to complicate noncardiac surgery. Irreversible damage to the myocardium can occur when the ventricles are required to develop and maintain unusually high systolic pressures for a protracted period of time. Such conditions may include the effect of ventricular septal defect on the right ventricle, mitral stenosis on the right ventricle, coarctation of the aorta, aortic valvular stenosis, or pulmonic valvular stenosis. The natural response of the heart is to develop myocardial hypertrophy; however, when this hypertrophy is maintained for a long period of time, the ventricle becomes noncompliant and ventricular failure develops. Once permanent damage has occurred, correction of the cause may not reverse the loss in compliance.

Also important is the marked increase in oxygen demand by the myocardium whenever it is required to perform under conditions of increased afterload. These patients are more likely to develop sudden myocardial ischemia and arrhythmias than patients without myocardial hypertrophy.

Inadequate Cardiac Output

In the infant, many congenital conditions appear as irreversible shock; however, these generally occur early in life. Often, patients with less severe abnormalities grow into adolescence or adulthood and exhibit only symptoms of decreased exercise tolerance. These symptoms may be associated with a marked limitation in cardiac output. If present, this may increase the risks of noncardiac operations significantly and limit the patient's ability to recover rapidly from trauma or surgery.

Pulmonary Artery Hypertension

Pulmonary artery hypertension, in its simplest terms, indicates high blood pressure within the pulmonary artery and by definition exists when the mean pulmonary artery blood pressure exceeds 30 mm Hg. In many congenital cardiac conditions, pulmonary artery hypertension is a natural consequence. For example, long-standing atrial septal defect or ventricular septal defect can lead to pulmonary hypertension. The individual with a congenital cardiac condition since birth may tolerate pulmonary artery hypertension well, considering that in utero the muscle masses of the right and left ventricle are equal and that the musculature of the pulmonary and systemic vasculature are similar.

The cause of pulmonary artery hypertension must be determined to have a reasonable plan for its management. The cause may be increased pulmonary vascular resistance, increased pulmonary blood flow, or pulmonary venous obstruction.

Increased Pulmonary Vascular Resistance

Determining whether the increased pulmonary vascular resistance is fixed or dynamic is important. Dynamic increases in pulmonary vascular resistance can be controlled by pulmonary vasodilators (such as nitroglycerin, isoproterenol, nitroprusside, etc.) and imply that correction of the congenital cardiac condition may allow pulmonary hypertension to resolve. However, no known pharmacologic agents exist that will control fixed pulmonary hypertension. Fixed pulmonary hypertension is generally the result of long-standing cardiac disease, such as chronic mitral stenosis, large ventricular septal defect over the age of 2 years, cyanotic congenital heart disease with repeated diffuse intravascular coagulation and lysis, and chronic pulmonary embolization.

Increased Pulmonary Blood Flow

When pulmonary hypertension is the result of high pulmonary flow, as occurs with large ventricular septal defect, pulmonary vascular resistance may be normal or only slightly elevated. The use of pulmonary vasodilators may lead to overt, high-output cardiac failure. In fact, the application of small doses of α-agents may be effective in decreasing pulmonary flow and heart failure in some of these patients.

The consequence of untreated long term pulmonary hypertension may be irreversible pulmonary hypertension with consequent right to left shunting if an intracardiac defect exists. This is called Eisenmenger's syndrome.

Classification of Congenital Heart Disease

There are more than 100 anatomical diagnoses for congenital heart disease, and most patients have two or three diagnoses combined. The classification listed below is generally accepted and is relatively simplified. There are only four major categories into which the diseases are classified, and by understanding the basic clas-

sifications, it is relatively easy to understand the condition.

Communications Between the Cardiac Chambers and Great Vessels

Immediately after birth, the pulmonary resistance falls below the systemic resistance. Therefore, any communication between the systemic and pulmonic circuits will cause left-to-right shunting and recirculation of blood. Left and right shunts are not cyanotic lesions. These abnormal communications can occur at the great vessel level (patent ductus arteriosus and truncus arteriosus), at the ventricular level (ventricular septal defect), at the atrial level (atrial septal defect), or as a combination (complete atrioventricular canal). The consequence of this type of shunt is enlargement either of the blood vessels or the cardiac chambers that must carry the increased volume and flow of blood. If the pulmonary resistance is low and the degree of shunt is large, heart failure can result.

Vascular or Valvular Obstructions With or Without a Shunt

A permanently narrowed valve or blood vessel causes increased resistance and requires an increased proximal pressure to maintain the required level of flow. Beginning on the left side of the heart and working backward, it is possible to outline the various causes of obstructing lesions: the obstruction may occur in the aorta (coarctation); at the aortic valve (valvular stenosis); or as a consequence of an abnormal left ventricle (hypoplastic left ventricle; idiopathic hypertrophic subaortic stenosis, IHSS; and mitral valvular atresia). Obstruction may occur within the pulmonary vascular circuit (pulmonary venous stenosis, hypoplastic pulmonary arteries, and pulmonary valvular stenosis). Right ventricular causes include hypoplastic right ventricle and tricuspid atresia. If no intravascular or intracardiac shunts exist, the consequence of valvular or vascular obstruction is the increased stress on the cardiac chamber, which must sustain the increased pressure.

Tetralogy of Fallot

An example of obstruction of cardiac outflow is the obstruction of the right ventricular outflow tract seen in tetralogy of Fallot (TOF). Patients with TOF have muscular bands that partially obstruct blood flow from the right ventricle into the pulmonary artery (in addition to a ventricular septal defect, an overriding aorta, and right ventricular hypertrophy). This right ventricular obstruction is a dynamic obstruction that worsens with increases in myocardial contractility. This phenomena explains the so-called tetralogy spells. Patients with tetralogy of Fallot who have received no medical treatment are always at major risk of the sudden onset of a significant increase in right ventricular outflow tract obstruction, resulting in extreme right-to-left shunting and consequent severe myocardial and cerebral hypoxia. This may be precipitated by endogenous catecholamines, any activity that increases pulmonary resistance (crying and Valsalva maneuver), or the administration of any pharmacologic agents that either increase myocardial contractility (catecholamines, calcium) or decrease peripheral resistance (systemic vasodilators and phlebotomy). The only known effective, nonoperative treatment of cyanotic tetralogy of Fallot is the administration of pharmacologic agents that decrease myocardial contractility (beta blockers or calcium channel blockers). Although patients with tetralogy of Fallot tetralogy are not usually cyanotic at birth; cyanosis often develops later in life.

Transposition of the Cardiac Chambers or Great Vessels

This category of congenital heart disease includes a large number of rare conditions. The one common condition of importance to the general surgeon is dextrotransposition of the great vessels. In this condition, the aorta and its coronary arteries arise from the right ventricle, whereas the pulmonary artery arises from the left ventricle. Survival at birth is impossible unless there is some type of great vessel or intracardiac communication (patent ductus arteriosus, atrial septal defect, or ventricular septal defect). This is a complex condition with unpredictable degrees of intracardiac mixing. As a general rule, all patients with transposition of the great vessels remain cyanotic until they undergo definitive treatment. All infants born with this condition will require some type of interventional therapy and probably cardiac surgery within the first 6 months of life.

Venous Anomalies

Cardiac venous anomalies are remarkably common, but few have physiologic consequences. The most important is anomalous pulmonary venous return in which some or all of the pulmonary veins fail to attach to the left atrium and, instead, return oxygenated blood to the right side of the heart. This generally causes a left to right shunt, but in its mild forms can be asymptomatic. Another venous anomaly is persistence of the embryologic left superior vena cava. The left superior vena cava usually drains into the coronary sinus. Knowledge of this fact can be important when placing central venous lines, pulmonary artery catheters, and coronary sinus cardioplegic catheters.

Natural History and Variability

The natural history of congenital heart disease varies greatly. This relates not only to the dynamic character of certain conditions (tetralogy of Fallot) but also to the natural progression of diseases. Of all of the infants born

with ventricular septal defect, it is thought that more than 50% of the defects will close or become so small as to be inconsequential if the child is managed conservatively. However, of all the children born with transposition of the great vessels, less than 10% will survive to the age of 1 year without surgical intervention. However, coarctation of the aorta may not become evident or be diagnosed until the age of 4 or 5 years. Remarkably, tetralogy of Fallot may remain asymptomatic in 33% of children to the age of 1 year.

Significance for Noncardiac Surgery

Emboli

Any patient with an intracardiac or great vessel shunt has a major risk of either pulmonary or systemic emboli. The meticulous management of all peripheral and central lines is a matter of survival. A small bolus of air lodged in the coronary or cerebral vessel can have lethal consequences. The disruption of a clot from the tips of central catheters can likewise be catastrophic.

Arterial Desaturation

Even small right to left intracardiac shunts will cause major decreases in arterial $P0_2$. This cannot be corrected by increasing FIO_2. If the desaturation is a consequence of dynamic right ventricular outflow obstruction, e.g., tetralogy of Fallot, then the judicious application of beta blockers may be helpful. If the magnitude of an intracardiac shunt is the result of increased pulmonary vascular resistance from alveolar hypoxia or atelectasis, appropriate alterations in ventilation may be indicated. Most important, the surgeon must have an appreciation of the cause of arterial desaturation and the specific anatomy before developing a rational plan of attack.

Bacterial Endocarditis

The preantibiotic history of congenital heart disease indicates that bacterial endocarditis was an important risk for all patients with congenital heart lesions. In general, all patients with uncorrected congenital heart disease should receive prophylactic antibiotics when undergoing noncardiac operations of any type. They should also be considered at risk when they have sustained major trauma or when the placement of temporary central lines becomes necessary. One should refer to the American Heart Association guidelines for appropriate prophylaxis for bacterial endocarditis in the setting of general heart disease.

The Systemic Response to Cardiopulmonary Bypass

Since the inception of the use of cardiopulmonary bypass (CPB) for open heart surgery in 1953, the basic components of the CPB circuit have evolved very little. However, our understanding of the complex physiologic and pathophysiologic consequences of extracorporeal circulation continues to mature. CPB is used most commonly to maintain a bloodless, quiescent field for cardiac surgery. A venous cannula siphons blood via gravity from the right atrium or superior and inferior vena cavae into a venous reservoir. Blood then enters a membrane or bubble oxygenator, which provides oxygen and eliminates CO_2. A heat exchanger serves to control the blood temperature for systemic cooling and subsequent rewarming. Finally, a roller or centrifugal pump returns arterial blood to the systemic circulation by way of an arterial cannula in the ascending aorta or femoral artery. Intense anticoagulation with heparin sodium is required before the institution of CPB to prevent clotting of the patient's blood after exposure to the foreign surfaces of the circuit.

Physiologic Effects

Cardiopulmonary bypass is associated with a number of disruptions in homeostasis which must not necessarily be viewed as pathologic. Whereas some of these physiologic alterations are intentionally established and controlled by the perfusionist, others represent intrinsic physiologic responses of the patient to alterations produced by the CPB.

Perfusion flow rates on CPB generally are maintained at approximately 2 L/min/m², yielding mean perfusion pressures in the range of 50–70 mm Hg. Since such continuous flow rates are believed to adequately perfuse the microcirculation, as evidenced by appropriate mixed venous O_2 levels, most pumps in clinical use today generate nonpulsatile flow.

The hematocrit is normally diluted to approximately 30% during CPB as a result of the use of asanguinous crystalloid and colloid circuit prime. This moderate hemodilution is in fact an asset, as higher hematocrits cause increased viscosity at low temperatures and may thereby compromise perfusion of the microcirculation. Pump prime solutions also produce a marked increase in interstitial fluid volume, which is exacerbated by a CPB-induced increase in microvascular permeability and fluid shifts from the intravascular space. As a result, patients often require large volumes of colloid replacements after cardiac surgery to maintain intravascular volume.

Hypothermia

Most surgeons employ varying degrees of systemic hypothermia during CPB to enhance myocardial and cerebral protection. In general, moderate hypothermia (28–32°C) is considered adequate for coronary artery bypass and valve procedures. However, deep hypothermia to 15°C is required for complex congenital repairs or replacement of the ascending aorta, procedures which mandate the use of low-flow perfusion or circulatory arrest to establish a completely bloodless field. Most patients tolerate even deep hypothermia without any apparent adverse sequelae, as long as rewarming to normothermia is complete before the cessation of CPB. However, rapid fluctuations in systemic vascular resistance are not unusual during the rewarming phase, often necessitating pharmacologic intervention to maintain perfusion pressures within the desired range.

Endocrine Changes

Immediately after the institution of CPB, an abrupt increase occurs in blood levels of renin, angiotensin, aldosterone, antidiuretic hormone, and catecholamines. These levels remain elevated for the duration of CPB. Cortisol decreases initially but reaches supraphysiologic levels by the end of bypass. T_3 and T_4 are decreased significantly throughout the period of CPB and may remain so for several days postoperatively. The mechanisms whereby these endocrine alterations occur are unclear, but nonpulsatile flow has been implicated in some instances.

Pathophysiologic Effects

Most patients tolerate a period of CPB without any apparent untoward effects. However, CPB may incite an unpredictable, adverse systemic response which can culminate in multiple organ dysfunction and thus contribute substantially to cardiac surgical morbidity (Table 15.2). Although many of the mechanisms underlying these complex pathologic responses remain to be elucidated, there is compelling evidence that unphysiologic blood flow patterns, shear stresses, and exposure of blood to nonendothelial surfaces are involved. There seems to be a direct correlation between the duration of CPB and the risk of development of the "postperfusion syndrome." Each of these proposed mechanisms will be discussed separately.

Nonphysiologic Blood Flow Patterns

As discussed previously in this section, most CPB pumps do not provide truly pulsatile blood flow. However, the body's visceral capillary beds may depend on pulsatility for optimal perfusion and autoregulation of nutrient flow. This premise has led to the conclusion that nonpulsatile arterial flow is partly responsible for organ dysfunction after CPB. This argument is especially cogent with regard to "postpump" pancreatitis.

Shear Stresses

Suction lines, the pumping mechanism itself, and turbulence at the end of the arterial cannula may create deleterious shear stresses to which the cellular elements of the blood are particularly sensitive. Red blood cells may be hemolyzed and/or their life spans considerably

Table 15.2.
Organ Dysfunction Associated with Cardiopulmonary Bypass

Systemic	Adverse Effect	Presumed Etiology
CNS	Cerebrovascular accident	Macroembolization (calcium, air, atherosclerotic debris)
		Microembolization (fat, cellular/fibrin aggregates)
		Inadequate cerebral perfusion (watershed)
	Neuropsychiatric changes	Inflammatory mediators
	("postpump delirium")	Inadequate cerebral perfusion
	Depressed consciousness	Inflammatory mediators
		Inadequate cerebral perfusion
	Seizure activity	Any of the above
Pulmonary	Acute lung injury	Reperfusion injury
		Leukosequestration
		Inflammatory mediators
	Pulmonary edema	Increased interstitial fluid
		Increased capillary permeability
Gastrointestinal	Pancreatitis	Nonpulsatile flow, hypoperfusion
	Acalculous cholecystitis	Hypoperfusion
Renal	Acute renal failure	Inflammatory mediators
		Hypoperfusion
Hematologic	Excessive bleeding	Platelet dysfunction
		Hyperfibrinolysis
		Inadequate heparin reversal with protamine sulfate

shortened. In addition, T cell function may remain depressed for several days postoperatively.

Exposure of Blood to Nonendothelial Surfaces

Contact of blood with the artificial surfaces of the CPB circuit may activate a systemic inflammatory cascade, which includes the complement system, coagulation, fibrinolysis, and the kallikrein system. Leukocyte activation and platelet dysfunction also occur. This widespread humoral and cellular activation is the most important pathophysiologic stimulus for the "postperfusion syndrome," the hallmarks of which are increased microvascular permeability, leukocytosis, diffuse interstitial edema, and multiple organ dysfunction.

During CPB, contact of the complement proteins with nonendothelial surfaces activates the alternative pathway, yielding dramatically increased levels of the anaphylatoxins, C3a and C5a. Both of these mediators cause vasoconstriction and increased capillary permeability. In addition, C5a can activate monocytes and neutrophils and induces binding of the latter to the vascular endothelium, resulting in organ dysfunction.

The nonendothelial surfaces of the CPB circuit and exposed collagen from tissue injury cause factor XII activation, which can lead to microthrombi formation, consumption of clotting factors, and subsequent end-organ dysfunction. Furthermore, factor XIIa can activate the kallikrein system, resulting in the eventual elaboration of bradykinin. The effects of bradykinin include increased vascular permeability and vasodilation.

Fibrinolysis is increased during and after cardiopulmonary bypass, although the reasons for this remain unclear. Fibrin degradation products may impair fibrin polymerization and platelet function, and are also capa-

ble of injuring the vascular endothelium. Plugging of fibrin microthrombi in the microcirculation can exacerbate end-organ dysfunction. In addition, fibrinogen adsorbed to the pump circuit activates platelets and can induce platelet thrombi formation.

The total leukocyte count falls immediately after the onset of CPB due to hemodilution, but as bypass progresses, demargination produces a leukocytosis. Complement-activated neutrophils may cause tissue destruction by releasing serine proteases such as elastase, as well as toxic oxygen-derived free radicals. Sequestration of neutrophils in the pulmonary circulation with subsequent activation after cessation of CPB has been implicated in lung reperfusion injury. Additionally, monocytes activated during CPB liberate the inflammatory cytokines: tumor necrosis factor, interleukin-1, and interleukin-6, which may be associated with fever, hypotension, and organ dysfunction after cardiac surgery.

GLOSSARY

Total fluid energy—E = IP + GPE + KE
Total fluid energy *(E)* consists of potential energy and kinetic energy *(KE)*. Potential energy is made up of intravascular pressure *(IP)* and gravitational potential energy *(GPE)*.

Kinetic energy—KE = $\frac{1}{2}(DV^2)$

Kinetic energy *(KE)* represents the ability of blood to do work on the basis of its motion and is proportional to the density *(D)* of blood and the square of blood velocity *(V)*.

Bernoulli's principle—This principle states that when blood flows from one point to another, total energy along the stream is constant, provided that flow is steady and there are no frictional energy losses. Thus, if the stream narrows, the velocity of the stream must increase to keep the total energy of the stream constant at that point. This principle allows Doppler scans to detect arterial stenoses.

Poiseuille's law—$R = \dfrac{8vL}{\pi r^4}$

This law describes the viscous energy losses that occur in a system of moving fluids. The pressure gradient along a tube or vessel is directly proportional to the flow (F) and the length of the vessel (L) as well as the fluid viscosity (v), and is inversely proportional to the fourth power of the radius (r). This relationship is analogous to Ohm's law, which states that pressure is equal to flow times resistance.

Laplace's law—Tension = p × r

Laplace's law defines the tension on the wall of a vessel as being directly proportional to the product (p) and the radius (r) of the vessel.

Coronary perfusion pressure—CPP = DBP − RA

Coronary perfusion pressure (CPP) is defined as the pressure that drives the blood across the microcirculation of the coronary circulation. Since most nutrient blood flow occurs during diastole, the driving pressure is the diastolic blood pressure (DBP). The gradient is determined by subtracting from the diastolic blood pressure the right atrial pressure (RA) which reflects the back pressure on the coronary sinus. The units are mmHg.

Cardiac output—CO = HR × SV

Cardiac output (CO) is defined as the amount of blood pumped per minute. This is determined by the heart rate (HR) and the stroke volume (SV). The units are liters/min.

The cardiac index—$CI = \dfrac{CO}{BSA}$

The cardiac index (CI) is the cardiac output divided by the body surface area (BSA). The units are liters/min/m².

Pulmonary vascular resistance—$PVR = \dfrac{PA - LA}{CO} \times 80$

The pulmonary vascular resistance (PVR) is the difference between the mean pulmonary artery pressure (PA) and the mean left atrial pressure (LA) (pulmonary wedge pressure) divided by cardiac output (CO). The units are dyne · sec · cm⁻⁵.

Systemic vascular resistance—$SVR = \dfrac{MAP - CVP}{CO} \times 80$

Systemic vascular resistance (SVR) is the difference between the mean arterial pressure and the central venous pressure divided by the cardiac output. The units are dyne · sec · cm⁻⁵.

Ejection fraction—Ejection fraction (EF) is the ratio of the stroke volume (SV) to the end diastolic volume (EDV) which reflects the amount of blood ejected by the ventricle during systole. This is calculated easiest using echo cardiography, nuclear medicine studies, or a ventriculogram done at cardiac cath.

$$EF = \dfrac{SV}{EDV}$$

Fick equation—The Fick equation is used to determine total blood flow and is determined by the exchange of an indicator divided by the concentration of this indicator entering the system and the concentration of the indicator leaving the system. When the Fick principles are applied to the lungs, the equation uses oxygen consumption and content.

Cardiac Output—$CO = \dfrac{VO_2}{[CaO_2] - [CVO_2]}$

Oxygen Consumption divided by arterial O_2 content—mixed venous O_2 content (generally the oxygen consumption is approximated from tables of normal values for the type of patient being studied).

REFERENCES

1. Rutherford RB, ed. Vascular surgery. Philadelphia: WB Saunders, 1989.
2. Burton, AC. Physiology and biophysics of the circulation. 2nd ed. Chicago, Year Book Medical, 1972.
3. Bergan JJ, Yao JST, eds. Venous disorders. Philadelphia: WB Saunders, 1991.
4. Hurst JW, Logue RB, Schlant RC, Wenger NK, eds. The heart: arteries and veins. 4th ed. New York: McGraw-Hill, 1978.
5. Berne RM, Levy MN. Cardiovascular physiology. 5th ed. St. Louis: CV Mosby, 1986.
6. Kirklin JW, Barratt-Boyes BG. Cardia surgery: morphology, diagnosis criteria, natural history, techniques, results, and indications. New York: Wiley, 1986.
7. Tribble CG, Nolan SP. Current prosthetic cardia valves: a review. New Dev Med 1988;3(2)47–53.
8. Fozzard HA, Haber E, Jennings RB, et al, eds. The heart and cardiovascular system: scientific foundations. New York: Raven, 1986.

16 The Pulmonary System

Anthony L. Moulton / A. Gerson Greenburg

Introduction

The human body is an aerobic organism. Therefore, the organ responsible for oxygenating the blood that perfuses all of the body—the lung—is pivotal to the function of all the other organ systems. Independent of the efficiency of oxygen delivery (circulatory system) and/or the status of the end organs, dysfunction of the pulmonary system is detrimental to the entire organism. In apparent recognition of its importance, the lung has several unique characteristics: it has a central location; it occupies the greatest volume of any organ in the body; it has a greater surface area and is exposed to the external environment more than any other organ except the skin; it is the lightest organ per volume; its arterial vessels have a unique histology; it receives 100% of the cardiac output (plus bronchial blood flow) at the lowest perfusion pressure of any organ; and most importantly, it receives desaturated arterial blood and returns oxygenated pulmonary venous blood.

We will clarify the physiology of the lung with respect to the function of these unique characteristics. By describing the anatomy, the mechanics of ventilation, the physiology of gas exchange, and adaptation to physiologic alterations and disease, an appreciation of the basic underlying physiology will be attained.

A list of abbreviations, terms, and normal values is compiled in Appendix A. Commonly used formulas for ventilation and respiration are included in Appendix B.

Anatomy

Airways

Tracheobronchial Tree

To understand the function of the lung, the anatomy of the entire respiratory system must be considered. The

upper airway—the nose, mouth, pharynx, and trachea—acts as a passageway for air entering the lungs. These organs heat, cool, humidify, or filter the air. The nasal hairs remove particles greater than 10 μ, with smaller particles removed farther down the respiratory tree. As part of the inspiratory sequence, the tongue must move forward. The glottis and epiglottis protect the airway from aspiration of pharyngeal contents, and the vocal cords also guard the entrance into the trachea. Proper function of the upper airway depends on an unobstructed upper pathway and complex neuromuscular mechanisms, the details of which are beyond the scope of this chapter.

The trachea bifurcates into left and right bronchi, with progressive branching into smaller units to form three lobes on the right and two on the left. There are 18 bronchopulmonary segments, 8 on the left and 10 on the right (Fig. 16.1). There are 23 generations of airways. The first 16 (the conducting zone) serve simply as passageways; these constitute a "dead space" which is ventilated but serves no respiratory functions. Gas exchange occurs in the last seven generations (the respiratory zone). The airways can be divided into three major groups based on location and histology (Fig. 16.2). The trachea, major lobar bronchi, and segmental bronchi comprise the first group. They have cartilaginous walls with little smooth muscle. The columnar epithelium from the nose to the respiratory bronchioles produces mucus that covers the cilia. The cilia beat synchronously at 1000 to 1500 cycles/min and move particles 2 μm to 10 μm in diameter at a rate of 16 mm/min. Kartagener's syndrome is characterized by the absence of mucus production and ciliary mobility; these patients have chronic sinusitis and bronchiectasis. Bronchiectasis is a condition in which the bronchi are dilated and a loss of ciliary action occurs. Secretions pool and become infected. It may be associated with hemoptysis. Goblet cells secrete mucins and other bronchial secretions that contain IgA, which helps maintain the mucosa. IgA is also immunologically active and helps resist infection.

The second group of airways is composed of the

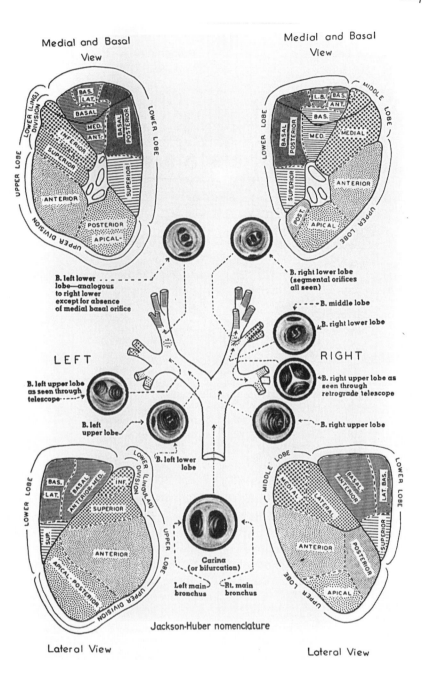

Figure 16.1. Anatomy of the major airways and pulmonary segments. From McVay CB. Surgical anatomy. 6th ed. Philadelphia: WB Saunders, 1984. Reprinted by permission.

membranous bronchioles and terminal bronchioles. These do not contain cartilage, and they have a relatively large amount of smooth muscle, particularly the terminal bronchioles. These are innervated by the autonomic nervous system and contain muscarinic receptors that cause bronchoconstriction with cholinergic stimulation. β_2-adrenergic receptors are also present and produce bronchodilation, but they are not innervated. A normal circadian rhythm exists with morning bronchoconstriction and evening bronchodilation, which may explain why patients with airway diseases more frequently develop respiratory distress in the mornings. Recently, additional innervation mediated by vasoactive intestinal polypeptide (VIP), which produces bronchodilation, has

been identified. The VIP half-life is only 2 min; therefore, it has limited effect. Prostaglandin derivatives also play a role. Prostacyclin, produced by the vascular endothelium, is a vasodilator and bronchodilator and stabilizes membranes. Thromboxane, produced by platelets, is a vasoconstrictor and bronchoconstrictor. Resting plasma levels of these compounds are low, but both are elevated with sepsis and may contribute to adult respiratory distress syndrome (ARDS). Recently identified leukotrienes (e.g., leukotrienes C_4 and D_4) can be potent bronchoconstrictors. Cool temperatures also induce bronchoconstriction.

The third group of airways consists of the last seven generations of respiratory bronchioles, alveolar ducts,

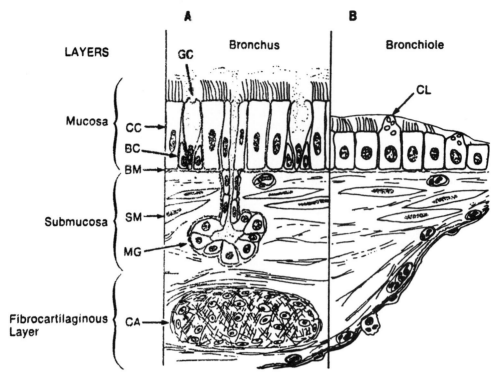

Figure 16.2. Schematic diagram of components of airway wall. **A** is at level of large airways (trachea and bronchi), whereas **B** is at level of small airways (bronchioles). *CC,* ciliated columnar epithelial cell; *GC,* goblet cell; *BM,* basement membrane; *BC,* basal cell; *SM,* smooth mus- cle; *MG,* mucous gland; *CA,* cartilage; *CL,* clara cell. Adapted from Wei- bel ER, Burri PH. Funktionelle Aspekte der Lungemorpholicie. From Weinberger SE. Principles of pulmonary medicine. Philadelphia: WB Saunders, 1992. Reprinted with permission.

Table 16.1.
Airway Numbers and Dimensions

Name	Number	Diameter (mm)	Cross-Sectional Area (cm²)
Trachea	1	25	5
Main bronchi	2	11–19	3.2
Lobar bronchi	5	4.5–13.5	2.7
Segmental bronchi	19	4.5–6.5	3.2
Subsegmental bronchi	38	3–6	6.6
Terminal bronchi	1,000	1.0	7.9
Terminal bronchioles	35,000	0.65	116
Terminal respiratory bronchioles	630,000	0.45	1,000
Alveolar ducts and sacs	4×10^6	0.40	17,000
Alveoli	300×10^6	0.25–0.30	700,000 (surface area)

From Sommers SG, ed. Pathology annual. Vol. 3. New York: Appleton- Century-Crofts, 1968. In Weinberger SE. Principles of pulmonary medi- cine. Philadelphia, WB Saunders, 1992. Reprinted by permission.

and alveoli. In this region, gas exchange occurs. The tra- chea eventually divides into 300 million alveoli, with an increase in cross-sectional area from 5 cm² to 11,800 cm². The total surface area of all alveoli is more than 7 m² (the size of a tennis court) (Table 16.1). With the much greater cross-sectional area in the more distant airways, the velocity of the flow of air is greatly reduced, allowing greater time for diffusion of gases between the alveoli and capillaries (Fig. 16.3).

The Acinus

An acinus is the basic functional respiratory unit. It includes all the structures in the third group of airways, from the respiratory bronchioles onward. All of these are contained in the final 5 mm of the airways (Fig. 16.4). Approximately 130,000 of these acini exist, each of which trifurcate into three orders of respiratory bron- chioles, three orders of alveolar ducts, and 17 alveolar sacs. This yields a total of 2,300 alveoli per acinus.

The terminal air sacs are the alveoli that are in inti- mate contact with a rich capillary network. They vary in size, depending on anatomic location; they are larger in the more negative pleural pressure areas at the apex of the chest cavity. There are two major types of alveolar epithelial cells. Type I cells, the major lining cells, are large, flat, squamous cells with cytoplasmic extensions and are primarily responsible for gas exchange. They are unable to reproduce themselves.

Type II granular pneumocytes do not participate in gas exchange. They are thicker, but they can produce new alveolar epithelial cells (Fig. 16.5A). In addition, type II alveolar epithelial cells secrete surfactant, a sur- face tension-lowering phospholipid film that acts chemi- cally like a detergent. Surfactant lines the alveolus and helps prevent alveolar collapse. By LaPlace's law, the distending pressure (P) to overcome the surface tension (T) is inversely proportional to the radius (r), $P = 2T/r$. Therefore, as the alveolus gets smaller, the surfactant

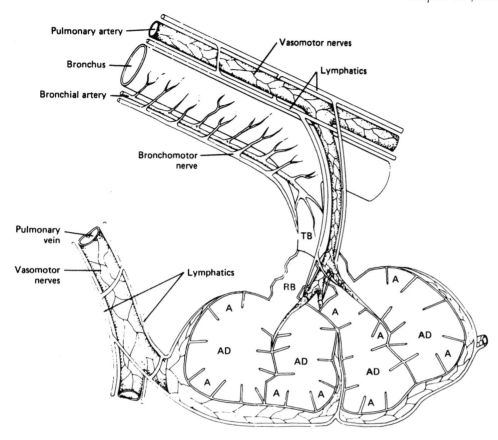

Figure 16.3. Structure of the lung. *A,* alveolus; *AD,* alveolar duct; *RB,* respiratory bronchiole; *TB,* terminal bronchiole. From Staub NC. The pathophysiology of pulmonary edema. Hum Pathol 1970;1:419. In Ganong WF. *Review of medical physiology.* 15th ed. Norwalk, CT: Appleton & Lange, 1991. Reprinted by permission.

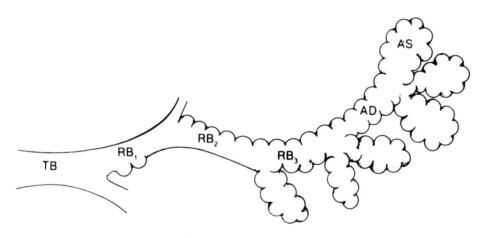

Figure 16.4. Schematic diagram of most distal portion of respiratory tree. Each terminal bronchiole (*TB*) supplies several generations of respiratory bronchioles (RB$_1$ through RB$_3$), which have progressively more respiratory (alveolar) epithelium lining their walls. Alveolar ducts (*AD*) are lined entirely by alveolar epithelium, as are alveolar sacs (*AS*). The region of lung distal to and supplied by terminal bronchiole is termed acinus. From Sommers SC, ed. Pathology annual. Vol. 3. New York: Appleton-Century-Crofts, 1968. In Weinberger SE. Principles of pulmonary medicine. Philadelphia: WB Saunders, 1992. Reprinted by permission.

Figure 16.5. **A,** Electron photomicrograph of a human lung, showing a pulmonary capillary adjacent to an alveolar sac. The capillary contains a neutrophil (*GR*). EP1, type I pulmonary epithelial cell; *EN,* endothelial cell; *N,* nucleus of endothelial cell; *J,* junction between two endothelial cells. From Weibel ER. Lung cell biology. In: Fishman AP, ed. Handbook of physiology. Vol. 1, sec. 3. The respiratory system. Bethesda, MD: American Physiological Society, 1985:47–91. Reproduced in Ganong WF. *Review of medical physiology.* 15th ed. Norwalk, CT: Appleton & Lange, 1991. Reprinted by permission. **B,** Schematic diagram of normal alveolar structure. Type I and type II epithelial cells are shown lining alveolar wall. Type I cells are relatively flat and are characterized by long cytoplasmic processes. Type II cells are cuboidal and have cytoplasmic lamellar bodies (*L*), the source of surfactant. Two capillaries, with capillary endothelial cells (*C*) and erythrocytes (*RBC*) in the capillary lumen are shown. Interstitial space (*IS*) is the relatively acellular region of the alveolar wall. *A,* alveolar space. From Weinberger SE. Principles of pulmonary medicine. Philadelphia: WB Saunders, 1992. Reprinted by permission. **C,** Relative blood pressures in systemic and pulmonary circulation. From Ganong WE. *Review of medical physiology.* 15th ed. Norwalk, CT: Appleton & Lange, 1991. Reprinted by permission. **D,** Both inhaled nitric oxide (NO) and endogenous NO interact with guanylate cyclase (GC) to produce vasodilation. NO is inactivated in blood vessel lumen by hemoglobin (Hb). cGMP = cyclic guanosine monophosphate; GTP = guanosine triphosphate; Mb—yoglobin; NO$_2$–itrogen dioxide; R-SNO = S-nitrosothiol; SH = sulfhydryl. In Lunn RJ. Inhaled nitric oxide therapy. Mayo Clin Proc 1995;70:249.

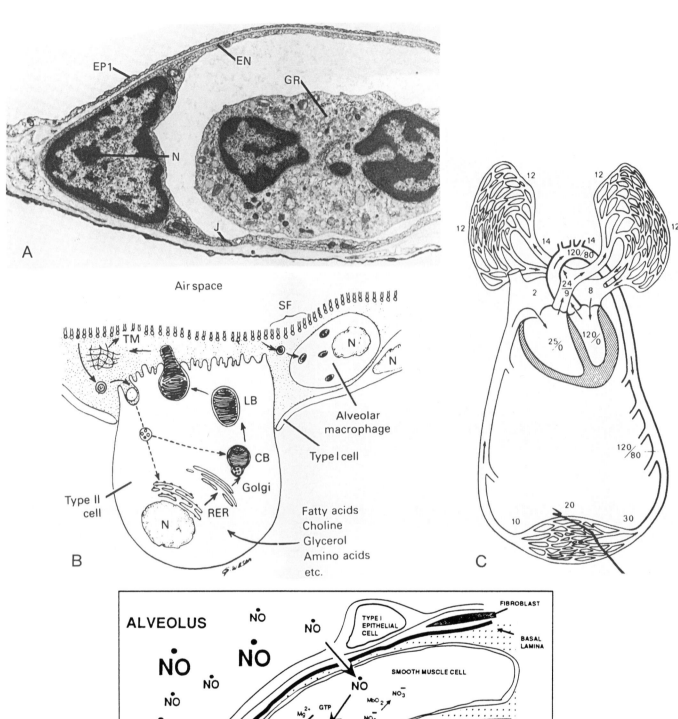

Air space

SF

TM

N

N

Alveolar
macrophage

Type I cell

LB

CB

Golgi

RER

Type II
cell

N

Fatty acids
Choline
Glycerol
Amino acids
etc.

A

EP1

EN

GR

N

J

B

C

12   12

12   12

14   14

120/80

24/9

2   8

25/0   120/0

120/80

10   20   30

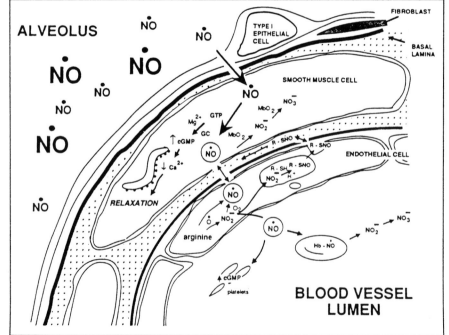

ALVEOLUS

NO

NO

NO

NO

NO

NO

NO

NO

TYPE I
EPITHELIAL
CELL

FIBROBLAST

BASAL
LAMINA

SMOOTH MUSCLE CELL

NO

NO₃⁻

Mg²⁺   GTP

GC

↑ cGMP

MbO₂

NO₂⁻

↓ Ca²⁺

NO

MbO₂

R - SNO   R - SNO

RELAXATION

R - SH   R - SNO

NO₂⁻   H⁺

ENDOTHELIAL CELL

NO

↑ O₂

NO₂

arginine

NO

Hb · NO

NO₂⁻   NO₃⁻

↑ cGMP

platelets

BLOOD VESSEL
LUMEN

becomes more concentrated, and its effect on lowering the surface tension becomes more critical as a means of keeping the alveolus open. Surfactant is produced as intracellular lamellar inclusions that are extruded into the alveolar lumen as tubular myelin, which then spreads as a film over the alveolar surface (see Fig. 16.5B). Surfactant also helps to counterbalance the hydrostatic pressure of blood, thereby preventing pulmonary edema. Without surfactant, unopposed surface tension would result in a 20 mm Hg force pushing fluid from the blood into the alveolus. The lungs themselves have a tendency to collapse, but their elastic recoil inward is counteracted by an outward chest wall elastic recoil. When surfactant is absent or deficient, as in premature infants, or when it is deactivated, as in drowning or in the presence of excess alveolar fluid, alveolar collapse and respiratory distress may ensue. Surfactant levels are increased by thyroid hormone and glucocorticoids. They are decreased in respiratory distress syndrome, with acute pancreatitis, with occlusion of the bronchi or pulmonary artery, with high oxygen levels, and in smokers. Synthetic surfactant is now available and can be administered when clinical evidence of deficiency exists. The incidence of the bronchopulmonary dysplasia (fibrosis) of prematurity has been reduced dramatically because of the introduction of surfactant therapy for selected infants.

The alveoli also contain pulmonary alveolar macrophages that phagocytize particles <2 μm. These come through the interstitium of the capillaries along with plasma cells, lymphocytes, and mast cells. Mast cells contain heparin, histamine, lipids, and polypeptides. These cells may contribute to certain allergic reactions. Polymorphonuclear leukocytes are present in the alveoli only in pathologic states; their presence in broncho-alveolar lavage (BAL) specimens is significant, and the distribution of cell types may be diagnostic.

In addition to surfactant, the lung is metabolically active in other ways, as shown in Table 16.2. Prostaglan-

Table 16.2.
Metabolic Activity of the Lung

Synthesized and used in the lungs
  Surfactant
Synthesized or stored and released into the blood
  Prostaglandins
  Histamine
  Kallikrein
Partially removed from the blood
  Prostaglandins
  Bradykinin
  Adenosine nucleotides
  Serotonin
  Norepinephrine
  Acetylcholine
Activated in the lungs
  Angiotensin I, Angiotensin II

From Ganong WF. *Review of medical physiology.* 15th ed. Norwalk, CT: Appleton & Lange, 1991. Reprinted by permission.

din is produced by the lung and released into the pulmonary veins in response to stimulation produced by stretching of the lung and the pulmonary veins; it also is removed and deactivated in the pulmonary artery. Angiotensin-converting enzyme comes from the pulmonary capillary endothelium. This enzyme converts angiotensin I to angiotensin II and also deactivates bradykinin. This deactivation occurs despite a short circulation time (0.75 sec through the lungs). The lungs also are responsible for removing a number of vasoactive substances, including serotonin and norepinephrine; although epinephrine, dobutamine, oxytocin, vasopressin, and angiotensin II pass through the pulmonary circuit unchanged. There also are fibrinolysins present in the lungs that, when activated, result in lysis of clots in the pulmonary arterial vessels.

The Pulmonary Circulation

The lungs are unique in that they receive the entire cardiac output from the right ventricle into a distensible low-pressure system. The pulmonary arteries progressively branch, roughly following the branches of the airways, into a network of capillaries that bathe the alveoli where gas exchange occurs. The pulmonary veins join progressively, frequently in the loose connective tissue and interlobar spaces. They do not follow the bronchial anatomy as closely as the pulmonary arterial distribution.

The pulmonary circulation is a high-flow, low-pressure (normally mean pressure at approximately 15 mm Hg) system with a transpulmonary gradient between the pulmonary artery and pulmonary vein of only 7 to 8 mm. This is in counterdistinction to the approximately 90 mm Hg difference between the arterial and central venous pressures in the systemic circulation. The lung may contain up to 20% of the total body blood volume, although only 10% of that volume is in the capillaries (see Fig. 16.5C). The velocity of flow through the capillary bed depends on cardiac output; however, a red cell passes through the alveolar-capillary gas exchange area in 0.3 to 0.8 seconds.

In response to exercise, pulmonary circulation increases. Pressures remain low, secondary to dilation of the pulmonary arteries and recruitment of additional vessels. As the lung expands by increased ventilation, additional vascular beds also are opened. With maximal stretch, however, capillary resistance could actually increase. This situation is almost never reached clinically. The thin-walled arteries contain smooth muscle that dilates in response to parasympathetic stimulation with acetylcholine, β-sympathetic receptor stimulation (epinephrine and norepinephrine), bradykinin, prostaglandin E_1 (PGE$_1$), and prostacyclin. They constrict with α-receptor stimulation, histamine, serotonin, thromboxane A_2, and prostaglandin F and E, and hypoxemia. Like other arterial vessels, pulmonary arteries produce an endothelium-derived relaxing factor (EDRF) which results in vasodilation. This has been identified recently as nitric oxide (NO) (Fig. 16.5D). This may have important clinical implications for the treatment of pulmonary hypertension, and inhaled NO may produce selective pulmonary vasodilation.

The ability of pulmonary vascular resistance to facilitate increased pulmonary blood flow at low pressure means that a tremendous pulmonary vascular reserve exists; thus, partial airway or vascular occlusion or the loss of a significant portion of lung can be tolerated reasonably well, especially in the absence of parenchymal disease.

The low pulmonary arterial pressure and transpulmonary gradient means that gravitational changes can be important in distribution of blood flow. In an upright person, hydrostatic pressures in both the pulmonary arteries and veins progressively rise, going from the apex to the base, although alveolar distending airway pressures are higher at the apex (Fig. 16.6). Blood flow increases linearly from the apex to the base, related to the balance between arterial, venous, and alveolar pressures. Flow in the apex is minimal because of low perfusion pressures. It may be virtually nonexistent if alveolar pressures increase above perfusion pressure. In the midportion of the lung, pulmonary venous pressures are lower than alveolar pressures, so pulmonary blood flow is determined by the difference between the arterial and alveolar pressures. At the base of the lung, arterial and venous pressures both exceed alveolar pressure, so blood flow is determined by the gradient between the

pulmonary arterial and pulmonary venous pressures. Thus, elevations in left ventricular and diastolic pressures (LVEDP) that increase left atrial pressure can elevate pulmonary venous pressure, slowing flow and inducing lower lobe "congestion." In its severest form, pulmonary edema can develop.

The bronchial arteries that arise from the aorta or upper intercostal arteries are the other source of blood supply to the lung. They supply all the major airways up to the terminal bronchioles and account for 0.5% to 2.0% of the cardiac output. Most of the bronchial venous return is via bronchial veins into the azygous, hemizygous, and intercostal veins. A small fraction of this venous blood empties directly into the pulmonary veins, causing a "physiologic shunt." This explains the usual 97% O_2 saturation of arterial blood because pulmonary venous blood in the absence of ventilatory or respiratory pathology should be 100% saturated. Mismatches of ventilation and perfusion, or diffusion abnormalities, also result in pulmonary venous blood desaturation. These are called real or pathologic shunts and will be discussed in subsequent sections. The lung primarily receives desaturated systemic venous blood, on which it depends for nutrition. It can tolerate loss of its arterial (bronchial) blood supply without significant dysfunction, as superbly demonstrated in the recent lung and heart-lung transplant experience.

Thorax

Twelve bilateral ribs, the vertebrae, and the sternum, along with the scapulae and clavicles, form the bony

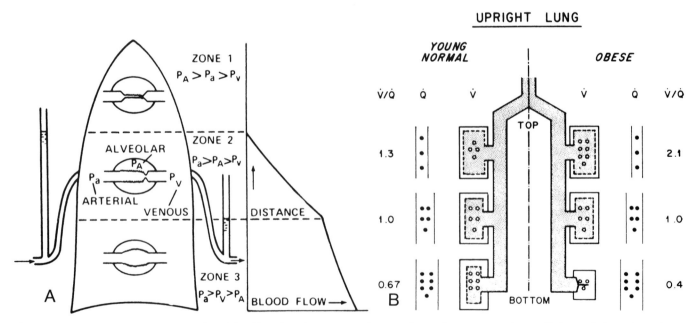

Figure 16.6. **A,** Diagrammatic representation of the effect of gravity on the distribution of blood and ventilation, with greater ventilation at the apex and greater blood flow at the bases. From West JB. Respiratory physiology—the essentials. 4th ed. Baltimore: Williams & Wilkins, 1990. Reprinted by permission. **B,** The effect of obesity that impairs diaphrag-

matic excursion and accentuates the ventilation-perfusion mismatch. From Pontoppidan H, et al. Adv Surg 1970;4:163. In Wolde W, Smith PK. Preoperative assessment of pulmonary function. In Sabiston DC, Spencer FC. Surgery of the chest. 5th ed. Philadelphia, WB Saunders, 1990. Reprinted by permission.

thoracic cage in which the lungs, heart, and great vessels are encased and protected. Pulmonary function depends intimately on these structures. The thorax serves as a rigid protective cage for the lungs. This rigidity maintains an intrathoracic space in which a negative pressure is created by the outward elastic recoil of the curved ribs and cartilages, and changes in the configuration of the thoracic cavity serve as the respiratory pump. The primary respiratory muscles are the diaphragm and the intercostal muscles, although other muscle groups in the neck (the scalene and the sternothyroid and sternohyoid muscles), chest wall (pectoralis and serratus anterior), and the abdomen (rectus abdominis and oblique) may become accessory in higher levels of ventilation and compensatory in diseases for which there is decreased compliance of the lung or muscular weakness. The diaphragm is innervated by the phrenic nerve that arises from roots C3—C5.

The Pleura

The lung and the inner thorax are covered with the visceral and parietal pleura, respectively. These are single layers of mesothelial cells that contain blood vessels, lymphatics, and connective tissue. The pleural space lies between these two layers. The pleura may extend from the apex of the thorax, above the first rib, and may lay reflected deep in the costophrenic and costomediastinal spaces to allow for increased volume with maximal inspiration (Fig. 16.7). The parietal pleura, but not the visceral pleura, has pain fibers. The pleura's main function is lubrication, allowing slippage of these surfaces with normal respiratory motions. The pleura also has absorptive capabilities, mostly from its lymphatics that can resorb up to 500 ml/day. The usual volume of pleural fluid is only 5 to 15 ml, but a turnover of 1 to 2 liters occurs daily. This fluid is usually produced by the visceral pleura and absorbed by the parietal pleura. As in most interstitial spaces, fluid can collect in the pleural space in response to increased hydrostatic pressure (congestive heart failure), decreased oncotic pressure (hypoalbuminemia or anemia), inflammation, infection, or lymphatic obstruction (usually malignant, although posttraumatic, septic, or operative injury to the thoracic duct is also possible).

Normal Ventilation

The bony thorax, primarily because of curvature of the ribs, has a resting *outward* elastic recoil force. The lung, with its cartilaginous and fibrous tissue as well as the surface tension of the alveoli prone to collapse, has a resting *inward* elastic recoil force. The delicate balance between these opposing forces is the basis for normal ventilation mechanics.

Normal ventilation is involuntary and mediated by the respiratory center in the medulla, primarily in a dorsal nucleus and in a ventral group of nuclei (Fig. 16.8). No definite pacemaker cells have yet been identified to explain the rhythmic nature of normal ventilation. Voluntary ventilation is mediated by the cerebral cortex via corticospinal tracts. The efferent neurons from the pons and medulla are in the white matter of the spinal cord between the lateral and ventral corticospinal tracts. All of the nerves concerned with inspiration join in the ventral horns of C3 through C5, in the phrenic motor neurons, or in the external intercostal motor neurons, which can be found in the ventral horns throughout the thoracic spinal cord. Dysfunction of any of these neural pathways, by either local inflammation, trauma, tumor, or systemic disease, can impair the ability to create an effective negative inspiratory effort.

Inspiratory and expiratory muscles typically are alternately inhibited and stimulated (Fig. 16.9). Inspiratory neurons are located primarily in the dorsal nuclei group of the medulla. Expiratory neurons are at either end of the ventral group of nuclei, with additional inspiratory neurons in its midportion. Both are influenced by receptor afferents from the airways and the carotid and aortic bodies. Chemoreceptors located bilaterally in the carotid bodies and in the aortic bodies near the aortic arch are composed of type I and type II glomus (sustentacular). Receptors in the ventrolateral medulla are stimulated to increase ventilation by increased CO_2, or a decrease in pH. The carotid body cells are affected primarily by hypoxemia. In general, the respiratory minute volume is proportional to the metabolic rate. The effective stimuli are mediated by CO_2. Elevated CO_2 levels stimulate an increased rate and depth of inspiration, with a resultant rise in minute volume, whereas low CO_2 levels decrease the respiratory drive. In addition, there are medullary chemoreceptors that respond to cerebral spinal fluid (CSF) pH, which is primarily related to the amount of dissolved CO_2 in serum. This pH change could reflect CO_2 changes of respiratory or metabolic origin.

As long as the pleural space within the bony thorax remains inviolate, the lung remains inflated to varying degrees at all times. The delicate balance between the two opposing recoil forces results in a slightly negative resting intrathoracic pressure of approximately 5 cm H_2O relative to the atmosphere. This prevents collapse of the alveoli.

In response to stimuli from the respiratory centers, the inspiratory phase of normal spontaneous ventilation is initiated by the contraction of the respiratory muscles, primarily the diaphragm, but also the external intercostal muscles. This creates an increase in the negative intrathoracic pressure. With stimulation of the phrenic nerve (C3—C5), the diaphragm contracts and flattens; on deeper inspiration, the ribs can be raised anteriorly and upward, rotating on their articular surfaces with the

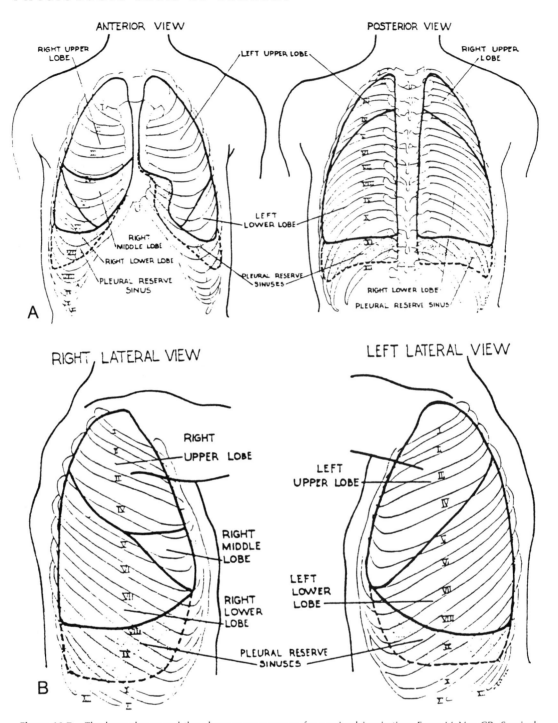

Figure 16.7.   The bony thorax and the pleura reserve spaces for maximal inspiration. From McVay CB. Surgical anatomy. 6th ed. Philadelphia, WB Saunders, 1990. Reprinted by permission.

spinous processes of the vertebra. This action expands the intrathoracic volume, making the negative intrathoracic pressure even more negative relative to the atmosphere. Negative pressures as high as 80 mm Hg can be generated with maximal respiratory effort. When diaphragmatic contraction is combined with relaxation of the glottis, the anterior motion of the tongue, and the opening of the vocal cords, an influx of air into the airways occurs to equalize or offset the negative intrathoracic pressure (Fig. 16.10). Inspiration ceases when the

alveolar pressure equals atmospheric pressure (i.e., a gradient of 0).

Expiration is purely passive. Relaxation of the inspiratory muscles and the elastic recoil of the chest wall will produce a positive alveolar pressure that forces air out the airways. Expiration ceases when the inward recoil pressure of the alveoli equals the resting outward recoil forces of the chest wall. During forced expiration, additional air may be exhaled by contraction of the expiratory muscles, which makes the pleural pressure posi-

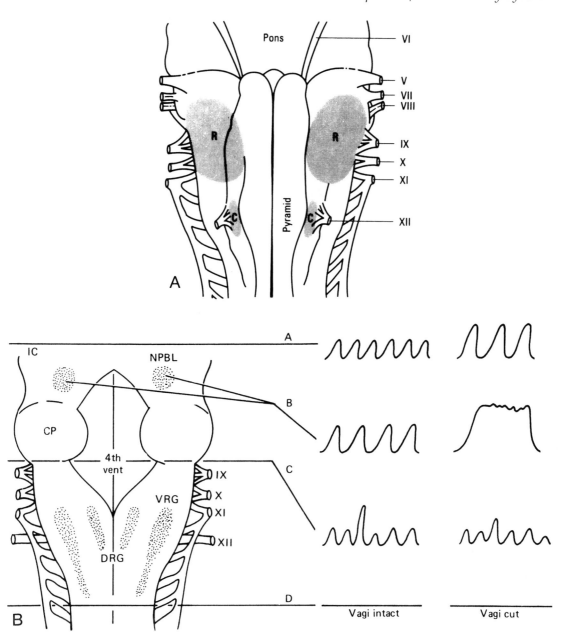

Figure 16.8. **A,** Rostral *(R)* and caudal *(C)* chemosensitive areas on the ventral surface of the medulla. **B,** Respiratory neurons in the brainstem. Dorsal view of brainstem, cerebellum removed. The effects of various lesions and brainstem transections also are shown. The spirometer tracings at the right indicate the depth and rate of breathing. *DRG,* dorsal group of respiratory neurons; *VRG,* ventral group of respiratory neurons; *NPBL,* nucleus pontabrachialis (pneumotaxic center), *4th vent,* fourth ventricle; *IC,* interior colliculus; *CP,* middle cerebellar peduncle. Modified from Mitchell RA, Berget A. State of the art; review of neural regulation of respiration. Am Rev Respir Dis 1975;111:206. In Ganong WF. Review of medical physiology. 15th ed. Norwalk, CT: Appleton & Lange, 1991. Reprinted by permission.

tive. For maximal respiratory volumes, accessory neck, chest, and abdominal muscles can be recruited.

The inherent rhythm of breathing is the result of complex interactions in the dorsal and ventral respiratory groups of the medulla that mediate the depth and the rate of breathing in response to a number of different stimuli (see Fig. 16.9). The pneumotaxic center in the pons is responsible for alternating between inspiration and expiration. There are stretch receptors within the lung that produce feedback signals to shut off inspiration (the Hering-Breuer reflex). These same stretch re-

ceptors indicate the degree of deflation and signal the respiratory center to initiate inspiration. As previously noted, chemoreceptors also exist in the carotid and aortic bodies that respond primarily to changes in oxygen and carbon dioxide tensions. Other chemoreceptors in the ventral lateral medulla are pH sensitive and can, in response primarily to altered CO_2 levels, initiate a ventilatory effort.

Knowledge of the various lung volumes and their changes associated with the cycles of ventilation is essential to understanding basic respiratory physiology.

Figure 16.9. Schematic representation of neural feedback mechanism for control of ventilation. From Fishman AP, ed. Handbook of physiology. Vol. 1, sec. 3, The respiratory system. Bethesda, MD: American Physiological Society, 1969. Reprinted by permission.

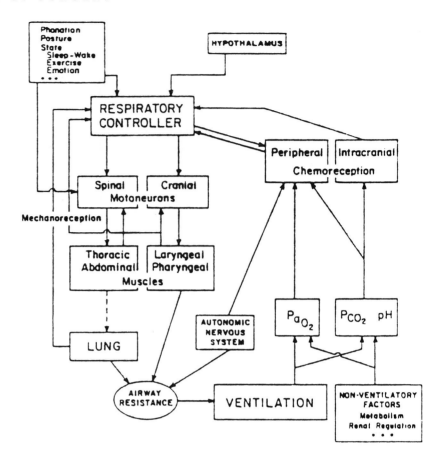

Many of them are useful, clinically measured, parameters. These volumes are shown in Figure 16.11, which demonstrates most of the commonly used volume parameters measured in pulmonary function studies. The total lung capacity (TLC) represents the volume of air that can be contained in the lungs at maximal inspiration with expansion of all the alveolar and airway spaces. Tidal volume (TV) is the volume of air in each breath with normal ventilation. The vital capacity (VC) represents the greatest amount of air that can be forcibly inhaled or exhaled. Residual volume (RV) represents the volume remaining after a maximal expiration. The inspiratory reserve volume (IRV) represents that volume above the usual tidal volume that can be achieved with maximal inspiratory effort. The combination of the normal tidal volume and the inspiratory reserve volume is called the inspiratory capacity (TV + IRV = IC). In a similar way, the additional volume that can be forced out of the lungs with maximal expiratory effort is called the expiratory reserve volume (ERV), and the combination of this with the residual volume is called the functional residual capacity (RV + ERV = FRC). In an average-sized adult, the total lung capacity is approximately 6 liters, a normal tidal volume is approximately 800 to 1000 ml (100 ml/kg), and the inspiratory capacity represents slightly less than half of the total lung capacity.

As noted previously, a large volume of air from the trachea out to the terminal bronchioles (the conducting zone) is not involved actively with gas exchange. This volume is known as physiologic dead space. It is composed of anatomic dead space, the volume of air remaining in the airways at the end of inspiration (usually 150 to 180 ml or 2 ml/kg), and alveolar dead space, which is the amount of air in alveoli that is not perfused. Alveolar dead space is variable and depends on the depth of inspiration, the patency of the airways, the adequacy of perfusion to the ventilated portions of lung, and the diffusion capacity of the lung parenchyma.

A balance between respiratory frequency and tidal volume is necessary to achieve optimal ventilation. Hyperventilation as a response to an excessive amount of CO_2 in the blood increases the respiratory volume, removing (called blowing off) CO_2. This usually causes a normal pH but may produce respiratory alkalosis. If one assumes equilibrium of the alveolar CO_2 with the arterial blood (Pa_{CO2}), measurement of exhaled CO_2 (Pe_{CO2}) can provide an assessment of the relative proportion of dead space and alveolar ventilation, reflected by the following equation:

$$V_D/V_T = \frac{Pa_{CO2} - Pe_{CO2}}{Pa_{CO2}}$$

The ratio of dead space ventilation (V_D) to total ventilation (V_T) is usually less than 0.4. In weaning a patient from a ventilator, a ratio of greater than 0.6 frequently is associated with failure to ventilate spontaneously.

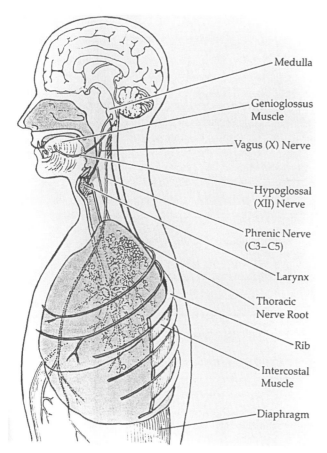

Figure 16.10. Normal ventilatory neural pathways include the medullary respiratory center, stimulating the phrenic nerve (cervical nerves C3–C5) to produce diaphragmatic contraction and the segmental thoracic nerves to stimulate the intercostal muscles. Just before this happens, the hypoglossal nerve (XII) activates the genioglossus muscle, which moves the tongue forward, and the vagus nerve (X) stimulates the vocal cord abduction. Coordination of these is essential to effective ventilation. From Ingram RH, Jr, Fanta CH. Lung function and its assessment. In: Scientific american medicine. Sec. 14, respiratory medicine. New York: Scientific American, 1991:3. Reprinted by permission.

Minute Ventilation

Minute ventilation (V_E) is the total amount of air moved per minute and is the product of the tidal volume and the respiratory rate, $V_E = V_T \times RR$. This is a combination of the volume of air in the dead space and in the functional alveoli. The relative proportion of dead space ventilation and effective alveolar ventilation varies in a number of physiologic and pathologic situations. Although it is difficult to measure directly the amount of effective alveolar ventilation, the high-solubility and high-diffusion capability of CO_2 relative to O_2 means that the arterial P_{CO2} levels are inversely proportional to the effectiveness of alveolar ventilation. A balance between respiratory frequency and tidal volume is necessary to achieve full alveolar expansion. For a given minute ventilation, the higher the respiratory frequency, the less effective the alveolar ventilation. This is because most of the respiratory effort is expended in moving air through the physiologic dead spaces. At the same minute volume, slow and deep inspirations result in more alveolar ventilation. This is the rationale for postoperative spirometry and deep-breathing exercises used to prevent or reverse postoperative atelectasis.

Many of these physiologically important airway volumes are difficult to measure clinically. Vital capacity can be measured by simple spirometry, but this measure does not include the residual volume and hence does not reflect functional reserve capacity or the total lung capacity. Measurement of these volumes requires inhalation of an inert gas, such as helium or xenon, and calculation of a washout curve. The amount of dilution seen in the expired gases reflects the overall pulmonary airway volume. However, in patients with large areas of lung that do not communicate or exchange air with the airways (e.g., bullae), falsely low lung volumes may be derived. In those situations, body plethysmography, in which pressure and volume changes with the patient in an airtight box, are recorded. Such elaborate tests may be necessary to measure lung volumes. These more sophisticated diagnostic tests are reserved for complicated clinical problems.

Routine pulmonary function tests (PFT) measure the more important clinical entities. The best measure of overall ventilatory function is the maximal voluntary ventilation (MVV). This is the largest volume of air that can be moved in and out of the lungs in 1 minute. The MVV reflects not only lung volume capacity but also airway resistance, and it provides a measure of muscle strength and stamina (aerobic conditioning). In the normal adult, it is usually 125 to 170 liters/min. Flow measurements also are clinically important and provide critical data about airway resistance (Fig. 16.12). The forced vital capacity (FVC) measures the volume of air that can be exhaled with maximal expiratory effort after a single full inspiration. The forced expiratory volume (FEV) measures the maximum volume exhaled. When the exhalation is complete, the forced vital capacity (FVC) and the total forced expiratory volume (FEV) are the same. More commonly, however, FEV is measured over defined time periods. The volume exhaled within the first second (FEV_1) and the ratio FEV_1:FVC are important clinical measurements of airway resistance and are commonly used to make therapeutic decisions. Reductions in FEV_1:FVC reflect significant airway obstruction that may be related to spasm, secretions, compression, or an intraluminal mass. Therapy may entail bronchodilators, mucolytic agents, suctioning, bronchoscopy, relief of airway compression (as in vascular rings or extrinsic masses), or removal of an endobronchial mass. Most often, however, a reduced FEV_1 reflects the airway disease of chronic obstructive pulmonary disease (COPD), which may have an active component (bronchospasm) and/or a significant fixed irreversible defect. Therefore, measurements of FEV_1 are obtained usually with and without bronchodilators to help identify therapeutic possibilities.

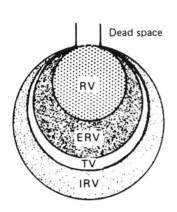

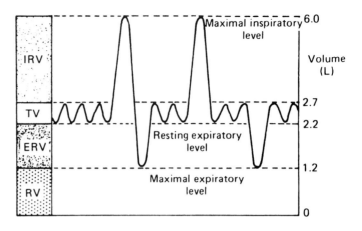

IRV = Inspiratory reserve volume   TV = Tidal volume
ERV = Expiratory reserve volume   RV = Residual volume

Volume (L)				
		Men	Women	
Vital capacity	IRV	3.3	1.9	Inspiratory capacity
	TV	0.5	0.5	
	ERV	1.0	0.7	Functional residual capacity
	RV	1.2	1.1	
Total lung capacity		6.0	4.2	

Figure 16.11. Lung volumes and some measurements related to the mechanics of breathing. The diagram at the upper right represents the excursions of a spirometer plotted against time. Modified from Comroe JH, Jr, et al. The lung: clinical physiology and pulmonary function tests. 2nd ed.: Yearbook, 1962. In Ganong WF. Review of medical physiology. 15th ed. Norwalk, CT: Appleton & Lange, 1991.

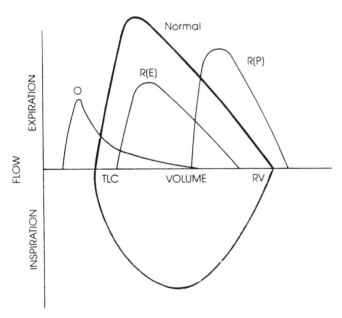

Figure 16.12. Flow-volume curves in different conditions. *O*, Obstructive disease; *R(P)*, parenchymal restrictive disease; *R(E)*, extraparenchymal restrictive disease with limitation in inspiration and expiration. Forced expiration is plotted in all conditions; forced inspiration is shown only for the normal curve. *TLC*, total lung capacity; *RV*, residual volume. From Weinberger SE. In: Principles of pulmonary medicine. Philadelphia: WB Saunders, 1992.

An even more sensitive indicator of airway obstruction is the maximum midexpiratory flow rate (MMFR). This measures the rate of air flow in the midportion of expiration (between 25% and 75% of the forced vital capacity) and also is known as the forced expiratory flow ($FEF_{25\%--75\%}$).

The volume of gas that enters the lung in response to inspiration (natural or artificial) can be measured; the ratio of the volume to the airway pressure, measured in ml/cm H_2O, is defined as compliance. Static compliance is measured at the end of a single inspiration, and dynamic compliance is the continuous relationship of pressure and volume measurements throughout a single breath (Fig. 16.13). The usual adult has a compliance of 100 ml/cm H_2O, normalized per kilogram. Decreased compliance is seen in pathologic states with increased interstitial fluid (e.g., CHF), decreased alveolar volume (e.g., hydrothorax or pneumothorax and elevated abdominal pressure), thickened alveolar walls (as in ARDS), inflammatory mediators and altered vascular permeability, or pulmonary fibrosis (Table 16.3). Loss of compliance may be nonhomogeneous. In a patient on a positive pressure ventilator, therefore, simply increasing ventilatory pressures may only overdistend already inflated alveoli that have normal compliance. Significant overventilation can damage alveoli (barotrauma), increase alveolar capillary permeability, and pulmonary edema.

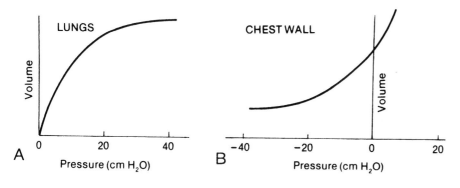

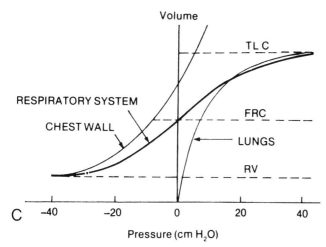

Figure 16.13. Compliance curves, i.e., changes in volume in relationship to pressure in the lungs (**A**), chest wall (**B**), and the overall respiratory system as the balance of recoil pressures within the lung and chest wall change with respiration (**C**). *TLC,* total lung capacity; *FRC,* functional residual capacity; *RV,* residual volume. From Weinberger SE. Principles of pulmonary medicine. Philadelphia: WB Saunders, 1992. Reprinted by permission.

Table 16.3.
Causes of Decreased Ventilatory Compliance

	Decreased Dynamic Compliance	Decreased Static Compliance
Lung	Bronchospasm	Increased tone in small airways
	Pneumothorax	Surfactant impairment
	Stiff lung parenchyma	Atelectasis
	(e.g., edema,	Edema
	fibrosis, ARDS)	Pneumonia
		ARDS
Chest	Edema	Edema
	Muscle spasm	Muscle spasm
	Rib fractures	Rib fractures

Courtesy of Charles Sherman, Miriam Hospital Providence, RI. 1992.

The combination of these ventilatory parameters helps make clinical diagnoses and patient management decisions. With obstructive pulmonary diseases, vital capacity (VC) is reduced and residual volume is increased and may actually result in an increase in total lung capacity. Table 16.4 lists other pulmonary diseases. However, flow measurements, such as FEV_1 and $FEF_{25\%-75\%}$, are more specific indicators of obstructive disease. However, restrictive disease may have normal expiratory air flow, a reduction in vital capacity, total lung capacity, residual volume, and functional reserve capacity. In some patients, the residual volume may actually be increased. The application of these parameters in the evaluation of the respiratory reserve of patients

Table 16.4.
Common Respiratory Diseases by Diagnostic Categories[a]

Obstructive
　Asthma
　Chronic obstructive lung disease (chronic bronchitis and emphysema)
　Bronchiectasis
　Cystic fibrosis
　Bronchiolitis
Restrictive: Parenchymal
　Sarcoidosis
　Idiopathic pulmonary fibrosis
　Pneumoconiosis
　Drug- or radiation-induced interstitial lung disease
Restrictive: Extraparenchymal, Neuromuscular
　Diaphragmatic weakness/paralysis
　Myasthenia gravis[b]
　Guillain-Barre syndrome[b]
　Muscular dystrophies[b]
　Cervical spine injury[b]
Chest wall
　Kyphoscoliosis
　Obesity
　Ankylosing spondylitis[b]

[a] From Weinberger SE, Drazen JM. Disturbances of respiratory function. In: Harvey textbook of medicine. Philadelphia: WB Saunders, 1990:Chap. 201.

[b] Can have inspiratory and expiratory limitation.

Table 16.5.
Criteria of Pulmonary Function for Lung Resection[a]

PFT	Normal	Pneumonectomy	Lobectomy	Wedge/Segment	Inoperable
MVV	>80%	>55%	>40%	>35%	>35%
FEV_1	>2 liters	>2 liters	>1 liter	>0.6 liter	>0.6 liter
$FEV_{25\%-75\%}$	>2 liters	>1.6 liters	>0.6 liter	>0.6 liter	>0.6 liter

[a] From Miller JI, Jr. Physiologic evaluation of pulmonary function in the candidate for lung resection. J Thorac Cardiovasc Surg 1993;2(105):347–351.

Table 16.6.
Pulmonary Function Guidelines That Indicate High Risk of Morbidity and Mortality[a]

Spirometric
1. Maximal breathing capacity <50% predicted
2. Forced expiratory volume in 1 sec <2 liters
Arterial Blood Gases
1. Arterial P_{CO_2} >45mm Hg
2. Hypoxemia is unreliable
Pulmonary Vasculature
1. Pulmonary arterial pressure during temporary unilateral occlusion of left or right main pulmonary artery >30 mm Hg

[a] Modified from Tisi GM. Preoperative evaluation of pulmonary function. Am Rev Respir Dis 1979;119:293. In Wolfe W, Smith PK. Preoperative assessment of pulmonary function. In Sabiston DC, Spencer FC, eds. Surgery of the chest. 5th ed. Philadelphia: WB Saunders, 1990.

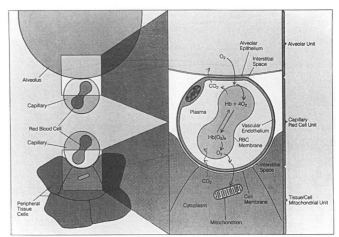

Figure 16.14. Diffusion pathways for O_2 and CO_2 in the lungs, where O_2 uptake and CO_2 release occurs, and in the tissues, where O_2 release and CO_2 uptake occurs. Changes in permeability, tissue fluid, cell wall, and membrane integrity and anatomic relationships can all impact the efficiency of the system. Hung S. Modified from Arturson G, deVerdier CH. Respiratory function of blood. In Arturson G, deVerdier CH. Surgical function of blood. In Burke JF. Surgical physiology. Philadelphia: WB Saunders, 1983:451. In Greenburg AG, Pricolo V. Life threatening acidosis. In Wilmore DW, Brennen MF, Harken AH, et al, eds. Care of the surgical patient. New York: Scientific American Medicine, 1989:1–12.

being considered for major pulmonary resections is evident in the recent work of Craver; this is summarized in Tables 16.5 and 16.6.

Respiration (Blood Gas Exchange)

Once air or the inspired gas mixture reaches the alveoli (ventilation), an exchange of gases must occur with the blood to achieve the purpose of respiration. The pulmonary arteries branch with the airways to form an extensive capillary network so interconnected that, with maximal engorgement, the alveolar walls are almost totally covered with capillaries. Hypoxemia and local acidosis both cause pulmonary arterial constriction, which in turn limits blood flow to poorly ventilated alveoli that optimize overall gas exchange.

Effective oxygenation of the blood implies that elemental oxygen must attach to hemoglobin (Hb) in the red blood cell. The oxygen must pass through a series of layers. These include the alveolar epithelium, alveolar basement membrane, interstitial space, capillary basement membrane, capillary endothelium, plasma, red cell membrane, and the cytoplasm of the red blood cell where it binds with Hb (Fig. 16.14). At room air, some oxygen (about 3%) becomes dissolved in the plasma, but usually, 97% of the effective oxygen transport is bound to Hb.

Hb is a complex protein with four heme moieties, each of which can react with a molecule of oxygen. The affinity for each successive oxygen molecule that is added decreases as the β-chains move closer together. Fully saturated, 1 g Hb binds 1.34 ml O_2. Although the saturation of Hb depends solely on the effectiveness of respiration, the arterial O_2 content (CaO_2) varies with the Hb concentration and is a measure of total oxygen-carrying capacity.

$$Ca_{O2} = Hb\ (g\ \%) \times 1.34 \times O_2\ sat\ (\%) + Pa_{O2} \times 0.0003,$$

$$O_2\ ml/100\ (usually\ 20\ ml\ \%).$$

Blood returning from the lungs is usually about 97% saturated. This reflects a small physiologic shunt, with some of the pulmonary arterial blood going past nonventilated alveoli and the bronchial arterial blood returning into the pulmonary veins. The affinity of Hb for oxygen is represented by the oxygen-Hb dissociation curve (Fig. 16.15). This curve shows the relationship between the arterial P_{O2} content and the degree of oxygen saturation. The curve also demonstrates the physiologic efficiency of Hb. In the normal range of arterial P_{O2} (85 mm Hg), the curve is reasonably flat, and Hb oxygen saturation is reasonably well maintained. A P_{O2} of 60 mm Hg is still associated with 90% Hb saturation. At low P_{O2}, in the range normally found in the venous circulation, large shifts in Hb saturation occur, suggesting

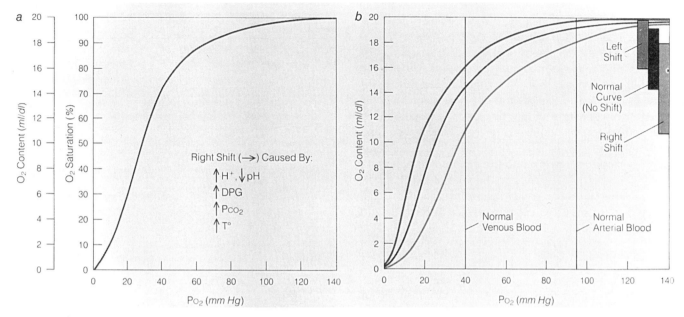

Figure 16.15. The oxygen-Hb dissociation curve, relating P_{o2}, oxygen saturation, and oxygen content. The curve shifts to the right, i.e., Hb has less affinity for oxygen (and therefore releases oxygen more rapidly) under the conditions noted. In the opposite conditions, Hb binds the oxygen more vigorously, i.e., encourages oxygen uptake. Modified from Miller A. Blood acid-base alignment nomogram: scales for pH, PCO_2, base excess for whole blood of different hemoglobin concentrations, plasma bicarbonate, and plasma total-CO_2. Andersen OS. Scand J Clin Lab Invest 1963;15:211. In Greenburg AG, Pricolo V. Life threatening acidosis. In: Wilmore DW, Brennen MF, Harken AH, et al, eds. Care of the surgical patient. New York: Scientific American Medicine, 1989: 1–12.

Hg easily gives up its oxygen in this range. Therefore, an adequate partial tissue pressure of oxygen is maintained.

As noted in the diagram, the oxygen dissociation curve can be shifted by a variety of factors (Fig. 16.15). In response to a lower pH, higher P_{CO2}, elevated temperatures, and increased levels of 2,3-diphosphoglycerate (2,3-DPG), Hb has less affinity for oxygen and, therefore, releases its oxygen to the tissues more easily (i.e., the curve shifts to the right). The response of the oxygen dissociation curve to change in pH is known as the Bohr effect. It is a reflection of the tremendous buffering capacity of Hb, which is about six times more potent than serum proteins. A decreased affinity for oxygen results in increased release of oxygen to the tissues. The resulting deoxyhemoglobin preferentially binds hydrogen ions. The hydrogen ions also form carbamino compounds that create bicarbonate in the plasma. All are exchanged for chloride, resulting in high chloride levels within the red cell cytoplasm (Fig. 16.16). In the alveoli, this process is reversed, with the release of CO_2, which is cleared via the airways.

Anaerobic glycolysis produces 2,3-DPG via the Embden-Myerhoff pathway in response to hypoxia and alkalosis. The new red cell is anaerobic; it does not consume the oxygen it carries. The 2,3-DPG interacts with Hb, resulting in a shift of the oxygen-Hb dissociation curve to right, producing a lower affinity between Hb and oxygen. However, acidosis inhibits red cell glycolysis, which could result in a decrease in 2,3-DPG. The 2,3-

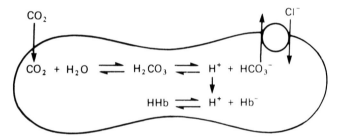

Figure 16.16. The diffusion and transport of CO_2 in the red blood cell. In tissue, CO_2 uptake occurs, and in the lungs, these processes are reversed to release CO_2 into the alveoli to be exhaled. From Ganong WF. Review of medical physiology. 15th ed. Norwalk, CT: Appleton & Lange, 1991.

DPG is increased with exercise (in spite of lactic acid production), at higher altitudes, by anemia, and by chronic hypoxia.

In contrast to the frequent problems with oxygen exchange in a variety of clinical situations, problems with CO_2 gas exchange become clinically important only in advanced pulmonary disease (Fig. 16.16). CO_2 is 20 times as soluble in blood as oxygen, and once dissolved, it rapidly forms carbonic acid. Therefore, it readily diffuses across the alveolar-capillary membranes. The concentration of carbonic anhydrase is high in the red blood cell and helps to decrease CO_2. This exchange occurs within the red cell because carbonic anhydrase is not present in serum. This buffering reaction explains why patients with chronic CO_2 retention usually have a normal pH, with chronically elevated $epHCO_3^-$ (a metabolic alkalosis) compensating for the elevated P_{co2} (a respiratory acidosis). In acute CO_2 retention, however, bicarbonate levels may be normal, and acidosis of varying degrees and consequences may be present. The total arterial blood oxygen (Ca_{co2}) content reflects both dissolved oxygen and the amount of oxygen bound to Hb.

After oxygenation within the lungs, arterial blood is distributed to the body, where dissolved oxygen and oxygen released from Hb diffuse into tissues. The mixed venous blood that returns to the pulmonary artery has a composition that depends on the relationship between blood flow (Q) and oxygen consumption (V_{o2}). This value can be used to calculate a cardiac output (the Fick principle) with the following formula:

$$Q = \frac{V_{O_2}}{Ca_{O_2} - Cv_{O_2}}$$

where Q = blood flow, V_{O_2} = oxygen consumption, Ca_{O_2} = total arterial blood O_2, and Cv_{O_2} = total venous blood O_2.

Therefore, if arterial oxygenation (Ca_{O_2}) remains fairly constant, a fall in the mixed venous saturation (Cv_{O_2}) indicates a fall in cardiac output. Clinically, a mixed venous specimen for oxygen saturation can be used as a "poor man's cardiac output." One must be careful in relying on this calculation because the saturation can depend on Hb level, temperature, pH, systemic oxygenation, and administered O_2, and sampling error can occur. The specimen should be drawn from the pulmonary artery to optimize mixing; therefore, it requires a Swan-Ganz catheter. The presence of pulmonary shunting can substantially alter the results. Catheters that use reflected light beams of various wavelengths to give a continuous on-line oxygen saturation or blood gas reading can reflect trends in oxygenation, which may be more important than absolute numbers.

Variations in Respiration (Physiologic Conditions)

The depth and rate of ventilation respond to a variety of physical and chemical factors, as previously noted. The duration of the expiratory phase is determined by the Hering-Breuer lung stretch reflex. Loss of that autonomic function is known as Ondin's curse. This condition is associated with the bulbar palsy of polio, pseudotumor cerebri, and the Pickwickian syndrome of morbid obesity. A cough may produce alveolar pressures as high as 100 mm Hg. Alveolar pressures may also be increased by bronchospasm, mucus blocking airways, and intrinsic masses or extrinsic tumor masses compressing the airways.

In general, elevated P_{CO2} levels stimulate increases in ventilation by rate and volume changes (Table 16.7). The inability to clear CO_2 adequately (e.g., obstruction to expiration, respiratory depression, and increase in dead space or hypoventilation) may result in hypercapnia and

Table 16.7.
Major Factors Determining Balance Between Ventilatory Supply and Demand[a]

I. Factors limiting ventilatory supply[b]
   A. Respiratory muscle weakness (e.g., fatigue)
   B. Unfavorable length-tension relationship (e.g., due to lung hyperinflation)
   C. Airways obstruction (e.g., asthma)
   D. Restricted obstruction (e.g., pneumonia)
II. Factors raising ventilatory demand[c]
   A. High physiologic dead space:tidal volume ratio ($V_D:V_T$) (e.g., emphysema)
   B. Elevated minute oxygen consumption and hence CO_2 production (e.g., sepsis)
   C. Respiratory quotient (RQ) more than 1.0 (e.g., excessive carbohydrate feeding)
   D. Maintaining arterial P_{CO_2} less than 36 mm Hg (e.g., due to metabolic acidosis)

[a] From Lanken PN. Mechanical ventilatory support. In: Wilson JD, Braunwald E, Isselbacher KJ, et al, eds. Harrison's principles of internal medicine. 12th ed. New York: McGraw-Hill, 1991:1125. Reprinted by permission.
[b] The maximal sustainable ventilation (MSV), which is usually equal to $-\frac{1}{2}$ maximal voluntary ventilation (MVV).
[c] The spontaneous minute ventilation (V_G) needed to maintain a certain arterial P_{CO_2} set by the patient's central neuronal drive. If this V_G is greater than the patient's maximal sustainable ventilation, the patient will develop respiratory muscle fatigue at that V_G.

acidosis. In advanced stages, they are reflected by symptoms of headache, confusion, and eventually CO_2 narcosis and coma. Hypoxemia is also a stimulus to increased ventilation, but it is not as potent a stimulant as is a rise in P_{co2} because deoxyhemoglobin is such a potent buffer. Hypoxemia secondary to hypoventilation increases use of the glycolytic pathway with a concomitant increase in lactic acid production and a decrease in arterial pH. These factors increase respiratory drive. Normalization of the arterial pH decreases the respiratory stimulus from either hypoxia or hypercapnia. In some postoperative patients with metabolic alkalosis, dangerously high CO_2 levels may be tolerated without increased respirations, tidal volume, or minute ventilation. Conversely, mechanical ventilation or hyperventilation with low CO_2 levels (respiratory alkalosis) may mask a significant metabolic acidosis. Adjustments of arterial pH should be undertaken cautiously to avoid altered respiration or minute ventilation.

Imbalances between ventilation and perfusion (ventilation-perfusion mismatches) result in a number of problems and are the major cause of pulmonary dysfunction in the surgical patient. These situations occur when there isn't enough ventilation of an alveolus to completely oxygenate and remove CO_2 from the blood. Alternatively, the alveolus may be ventilated but not perfused, thereby functioning as dead space. Even in the normally ventilated lung, gravitational forces create some ventilation-perfusion mismatch; this occurs because of the increased alveolar pressure in the apices and increased arterial blood pressure in bases of the lungs.

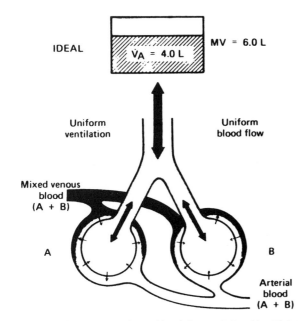

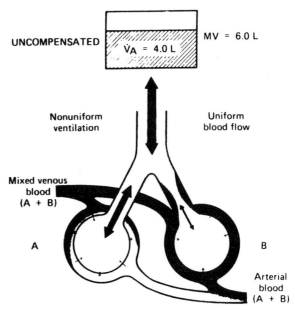

Figure 16.17. Left, Ideal ventilation-blood flow relationship. **Right,** Nonuniform ventilation and uniform blood flow, uncompensated V_A, alveolar ventilation; *MV,* respiratory minute volume. From Comroe JH, Jr, et al. The lung: clinical physiology and pulmonary function tests. 2nd ed. Yearbook, 1962. In Ganong WF. Review of medical physiology. 15th ed. Norwalk, CT: Appleton & Lange, 1991. Reprinted by permission.

In addition, there is the normal physiologic shunt: the bronchial venous blood supply returns to the pulmonary veins without going through the lungs, and the coronary venous blood empties directly into left atrium via Thebesian veins. Both bypass the lungs.

In the normal lung in an upright patient, the volumes of blood flow and ventilation increase from the top to the bottom of the lung. However, the changes in perfusion are greater than the differences in ventilation, so that the ventilation:perfusion ratio is lower at the bottom of the lung and higher at the top of the lung. Diseases that cause increased resistance to oxygen diffusion, e.g., pneumonia and interstitial fibrosis, may lead to more pronounced ventilation-perfusion abnormalities.

The systemic effect of perfusing nonventilated alveoli or bypassing ventilated alveoli is that desaturated blood returns to the pulmonary venous (hence the systemic) circulation, without having been oxygenated (Fig. 16.17). Inasmuch as the rate of oxygen diffusion is significantly less than CO_2, this may result in a clinically significant hypoxemia, although P_{co2} remains normal. This is achieved by compensatory overventilation of some parts of the lung, although ventilation of other portions of the lung remains abnormal. Supplemental oxygen can compensate for some interstitial lung diffusion abnormalities (e.g., atelectasis, pneumonia, and edema), but if a true shunt is present, with desaturated blood completely bypassing the alveoli, as in sepsis, administration of even 100% O_2 will not significantly improve the situation. When compensatory hyperventilation no longer can maintain a normal pH, life-threatening respiratory failure may be present (Table 16.8). The inability to overcome varying degrees of respiratory failure is an indication for mechanical ventilation (Table 16.9).

Table 16.8.
Causes of Respiratory Failure[a]

Location of Disease	Examples
Brain	Sedative overdose
	Cerebrovascular accidents
	Sleep apnea—hypersomnolence syndrome
Spinal cord and muscles	Poliomyelitis
	Myasthenia gravis
	Guillain-Barre syndrome
	Spinal cord trauma, cervical vertebral fracture
	Diffuse myopathy
Chest wall	Rib fracture with flail chest
	Kyphoscoliosis
Upper airways	Vocal cord tumor
	Laryngospasm or edema
	Foreign body
Lower airways and lungs	Bronchitis
	Asthma
	Emphysema
	Severe pneumonias (particularly viral pneumonias such as influenza)
	Adult respiratory distress syndrome
Heart	Pulmonary edema

From *MKSAP v. Syllabus,* 1979. Reprinted by permission.

The other major class of ventilation-perfusion mismatch occurs when significant abnormalities exist in pulmonary perfusion. Table 16.10 lists a wide variety of clinical situations in which this is present. The most common is a pulmonary embolus, in which a clot occludes a branch of the pulmonary artery. The distal lung is deprived of blood flow. Acutely, this means that a portion of the lung is being ventilated but functionally is dead space because no oxygen exchange can take place. This is wasted work of breathing. Although the

Table 16.9.
Conditions Which May Lead to ARDS[a]

1. Diffuse pulmonary infections (e.g., viral, bacterial, fungal, and *Pneumocystis*)
2. Aspiration (e.g., gastric contents with Mendelson's syndrome and water with near drowning)
3. Inhalation of toxins and irritants (e.g., chlorine gas, NO_2, smoke, ozone, and high concentrations of oxygen)
4. Narcotic overdose pulmonary edema (e.g., heroin, methadone, morphine, and dextropropoxyphene)
5. Nonnarcotic drug effects (e.g., nitrofurantoin)
6. Immunologic response to host antigens (e.g., Goodpasture's syndrome and systemic lupus erythematosus)
7. Effects of nonthoracic trauma with hypotension
8. In association with systemic reactions to processes initiated outside the lung (e.g., Gram-negative septicemia, hemorrhagic pancreatitis, amniotic fluid embolism, and fat embolism)
9. Postcardiopulmonary bypass (pump lung, and postperfusion lung)

[a] From Ingram RH Jr. Adult respiratory distress syndrome. In: Wilson JD, Braunwald E, Isselbacher KJ, et al. eds. Harrison's principles of medicine. 12th ed., New York, McGraw Hill, 1991:1125.

Table 16.10.
Pulmonary Perfusion Abnormalities and Their Causes[a]

Type of Impediment	Causes
Intraluminal occlusion	Blood clots (embolic and thrombotic); tumors (in situ and embolic); intrinsic stenotic lesions; emboli of fat, amniotic fluid, or parasites
Extrinsic compression	Hilar or mediastinal tumors, cysts, and fibrotic entrapment
Increased bronchial arterial collateral blood flow	Bronchiectasis and carcinomas
Increased resistance of regional vessels	Hypoxic vasoconstriction and pneumonia
Absence of regional vessels	Bullous lesions and vascular aplasias
Bypass of regional capillaries	Arteriovenous malformations

[a] From Ingram RH Jr. Fanta CH. Lung function and its assessment. In: Scientific American Medicine. Sec. 14, Respiratory medicine. 1991:13. Reprinted by permission.

bronchial artery may provide adequate nutrition in most cases, the distal lung can occasionally infarct, which may be associated with hemorrhage, suppuration, or long-term fibrosis.

If the problem is perfusion of the lung and not ventilation or diffusion, administration of supplemental oxygen does not significantly improve the situation. If, however, oxygenation is adequate, therapy usually consists of heparin and then coumadin anticoagulation. This treatment prevents propagation of further clot and allows for spontaneous thrombolysis. The acute presentation of a pulmonary embolus is often exaggerated by the release of inflammatory agents, e.g., serotonin and histamine, which cause local bronchoconstriction and vasoconstriction. These augment the consequences of the embolus itself and are reversible. If a proximal

Table 16.11.
Factors That Influence Alveolar-Arterial Oxygen Tension Difference[a,b]

1. Right-to-left shunt ($Q_SQ_T \times 100$), i.e., percentage of cardiac output (Q_T) flowing past nonventilated alveoli (Q_S)
2. Arteriovenous oxygen content difference $C(a-v)_{O_2}$.
3. Oxygen consumption (V_{O_2}) $Q_T = V_{O_2}/C(a-v)O_2$
4. Cardiac output (Q_T)
   A. Secondary to change in $C(a-v)_{O_2}$ when oxygen consumption (V_{O_2}) remains constant $Q_T = V_{O_2}/C(a-v)_{O_2}$)
   B. Secondary to redistribution of pulmonary blood flow.
5. Inspired oxygen concentration (uneven distribution plays a greater role when less than 100% oxygen is inspired)
6. Position of the oxygen-hemoglobin dissociation curve (pH, body temperature, red blood cell 2,3-DPG concentration)
7. Position of the arterial point (Pa_{O_2}) on the oxygen-hemoglobin dissociation curve; i.e., above or below full saturation

[a] From Laver MB, Austen WG. Respiratory function: physiologic considerations applicable to surgery. In: Sabiston DC, Jr. ed. Davis-Christopher textbook of surgery. 12th ed. Philadelphia: WB Saunders, 1981.
[b] Not included is the influence of a change in distribution of ventilation or body position as discussed in the text.

enough branch of pulmonary artery is occluded, however, the portion of lung still being perfused may not be adequate to provide sufficient oxygenation to sustain the body's needs. In this situation, more aggressive steps must be taken to reestablish pulmonary perfusion, either by the use of thrombolytic agents (e.g., streptokinase, urokinase, or TPA) or by surgical embolectomy, which is usually reserved for a patient in extreme secondary to cardiogenic shock. This extreme is usually associated with a saddle embolus involving the main pulmonary artery or for chronic pulmonary emboli that have become fibrotic.

Ventilation-perfusion abnormalities may reflect an increased alveolar-arterial (A-a) oxygen gradient. This value is usually about 10 mm Hg, reflecting the physiologic shunt from the bronchial and coronary blood flows. Hypoventilation or low ambient oxygen, seen in high-altitude situations, may result in a normal A-a gradient but low arterial oxygen content levels. A high A-a gradient can reflect ventilation-perfusion mismatches, increased dead space with ineffective ventilation, or an increased arteriovenous shunt, even with a normal alveolar ventilation (Table 16.11).

Response to Exercise

Exercise necessitates coordination between cardiovascular and pulmonary systems. The exact stimulus to increased ventilation is unclear because it occurs even when P_{o2}, P_{co2}, and pH are normal. Psychic and skeletal muscle receptors must play a role. First comes an increase in rate, then depth; both abruptly decrease with cessation of exercise, although they reach basal rates only after the O_2 debt has been repaid. Increased pulmonary blood flow means the oxygen level of the blood reaching the alveoli is lower; the increased gradient leads to increased O_2 uptake. The increases can be impressive, with cardiac outputs going from 5 to 6 liters/min to 20 to 25 liters/min, O_2 consumption from 250 to 4000 ml/min, and CO_2 excretion from 200 to 8000 ml/min.

If O_2 supply is inadequate, anaerobic metabolism takes place with lactic acid production (80% converted to glycogen, 20% metabolized to CO_2 and H_2O). Lactic acid stimulates increased respiration, so the resulting fall in CO_2 (alkalosis) produces respiratory compensation for the metabolic acidosis.

Maximal O_2 uptake is limited by uptake by muscle mitochondria. In exercising muscle, therefore, tissue O_2 levels are low, prompting maximal dissociation of oxyhemoglobin. This release of O_2 from Hg is further enhanced by the increased temperature and 2,3-DPG levels in response to exercise.

Pulmonary Acid-Base Balance

It should be obvious that the adequacy of ventilation is a major contributor to maintenance of the normal acid-base balance by ensuring both adequate oxygenation to metabolically active tissues and the regulation of CO_2 levels. Clinically important states reflect abnormalities in this balance and an awareness of the mechanisms to help direct therapeutic interventions (Table 16.12). Respiratory acidosis is present any time the P_{CO_2} level exceeds normal physiologic levels (usually more than 43 mm Hg). If the diffusion capacity of CO_2 is so high, an elevated P_{CO_2} usually reflects hypoventilation. In certain circumstances, it also can reflect increased dead space or high CO_2 levels in the inspired gas. Respiratory alkalosis is present any time the serum P_{CO_2} level is below normal (less than 37 mm Hg) and usually reflects hyperventilation. These terms apply only to CO_2 levels and do not necessarily indicate the overall patient acid-base

balance because they are usually compensatory metabolic changes that maintain a normal pH (Fig. 16.18). Frequently, metabolic alkalosis exists that serves to counteract the respiratory acidosis, particularly in chronic situations, when the overall pH of the patient is normal. In fact, an arterial pH that is significantly below normal and is associated with an elevated P_{CO_2} is frequently an indicator that the CO_2 retention is acute. This may reflect an acute respiratory problem that mandates emergency intervention. Chronically elevated P_{CO_2} levels, for which there is renal metabolic compensation, are usually well-tolerated and may not (and usually do not) require therapy. Exceptions are patients with advanced obstructive airway disease with a bronchospastic component that requires chronic bronchodilator therapy.

Clinically, chronic hyperventilation is rarely a problem in patients with spontaneous ventilation. It may, however, be a clinically important situation in the patient who is being mechanically ventilated. Abruptly lowering the P_{CO_2} may result in a clinically significant alkalosis with decreased ionization of calcium and an increased susceptibility to cardiac arrhythmias. However, clinical situations may exist in which a respiratory alkalosis is desired, e.g., after head trauma for which efforts are directed toward decreasing cerebral edema by preventing vasodilation. Lowering the CO_2 decreases cerebral blood flow, which may assist in achieving this therapeutic goal.

Pathologic Ventilatory Situations

As noted earlier, the function of the lung depends on a delicate balance between the inward elastic recoil of the lungs and the outward elastic recoil of the chest wall. Normal ventilation is initiated when the negative (outward) pressure in the pleural space is increased, overcoming the inward elastic recoil of the lung, enabling air to enter the airways from the higher atmospheric pressure. Any condition that obliterates or alters the balance between inward and outward forces, either by violation of the integrity of the thorax or the lung or by alteration in the elastic characteristics of either, will adversely affect the ability to ventilate.

Obviously, major obstruction of the upper airways can impede the flow of air into the lungs, even though the lungs and thorax themselves are functioning normally. This may be caused by trauma, tumor, inflammation, foreign body, or secretions. Therapy must be specific for each cause to recreate an unobstructed airway.

Neurologic diseases that affect the chest wall musculature or the diaphragm (e.g., poliomyelitis or phrenic nerve palsy) can adversely affect the patient's ability to expand the intrathoracic space and create sufficient negative intrathoracic pressures to ventilate adequately.

Table 16.12.
Acid-Base Disturbances[a,b]

Condition	P_{CO_2}	pH	HCO_3^-
Normal	36–44 torr	7.36–7.4	23–30 mEq/liter
Respiratory acidosis			
No metabolic compensation			Normal (or)
With metabolic compensation			
Respiratory alkalosis			
No metabolic compensation			Normal (or)
With metabolic compensation			
Metabolic acidosis			
No respiratory compensation	Normal		
With respiratory compensation			
Metabolic alkalosis			
No respiratory compensation	Normal		
With respiratory compensation			

[a] From Wolfe W, Smith PK. Preoperative assessment of pulmonary function. In: Sabiston DC, Spencer FC, eds. Surgery of the chest. 5th ed. Philadelphia: WB Saunders, 1990.

[b] or indicates a greater change from normal than or .

ACID · BASE MAP

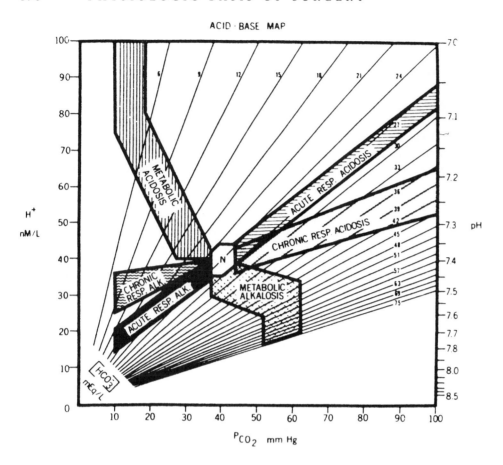

Figure 16.18. Acid-base nomogram, showing the normal compensatory range of pH, Pco$_2$, and HCO$_3^-$ in simple acid-base disorders. Values on the ordinate represent blood H$^+$ concentration (*left*) in nmol/liter (n*M/L*) or pH (*right*). The abscissa is Pco$_2$ in mm Hg. *Diagonal lines* represent isopleths for blood HCO$_3^-$ concentration in mEq/liter (*mEq/L*). Clear area in the center of the graph is the range of normal. From Goldberg M, Green SB, Moss ML, et al. Computer-based instruction and diagnosis of acid-base disorders. A systematic approach. JAMA 1973;223: 269. Reprinted by permission of the American Medical Association, which retains the copyright.

Voluntary or involuntary "splinting," usually secondary to pain, also limits the degree of chest expansion.

Lesions or diseases that result in fibrosis of the chest wall or the lung mean that a greater inspiratory effort is required to expand the lung (decreased compliance). In advanced forms, regardless of the inspiratory effort mounted, these diseases may even limit the maximal capacity of the thoracic cavity to expand.

If a segment of the chest wall becomes unstable, a situation that is almost always the result of trauma, a flail chest, results. In response to the negative intrathoracic pressure created by an inspiratory effort, the affected portion of the chest wall moves paradoxically inward, thereby decreasing the resulting intrathoracic volume and limiting the amount of air brought into the lungs. The underlying lung does not expand and become ventilated. Ultimately, it becomes atelectatic as a result of unopposed inward elastic recoil. This can be exaggerated by splinting, with a further decrease in respiratory effort secondary to pain associated with the rib fractures. If perfusion is maintained to the unventilated portion of the lung, a shunt develops, causing arterial hypoxia and respiratory distress. This distress is proportional to the amount of lung involved and the patient's respiratory reserve. In addition, the atelectatic lung becomes more susceptible to infection. This may compound the overall situation. Pulmonary sepsis with its hemodynamic consequences, particularly if untreated, will increase shunting.

Even in moderately severe cases of flail chest, improving ventilation of the underlying lung can be accomplished by pain control (which may entail intercostal blocks or epidural anesthetics) and aggressive respiratory exercises to reexpand the atelectatic lung and maintain alveolar patency and ventilation. Coughing, deep breathing, incentive spirometers, and even intermittent positive pressure breathing can be used. If these fail, mechanical positive-pressure ventilation may be necessary. This should be considered if an additional element of contusion of the lung or ARDS exists.

Contusion of the lung is the consequence of blunt trauma and is almost always associated with major chest wall injury. It also may be associated with the "blast effect" of penetrating trauma, secondary to a high-velocity missile. Depending on the associated chest wall injury, there may be problems ventilating. The major problem is a diffusion abnormality that interferes with effective gas exchange. In this situation, the alveolus may be ventilated and perfused. The interstitial edema and hemorrhage associated with a pulmonary contusion results in decreased lung compliance and ventilating abnormalities as well. Because of ineffective gas exchange, a functional shunt exists, and the pulmonary venous blood becomes desaturated. Diffusing capacity can be assessed by administration of small amounts of carbon monoxide and measuring the concentration bound to Hb. This must be corrected for the amount of Hb available for binding (the overall diffusing capacity is reduced in the presence of anemia).

Whenever the integrity of the chest wall or the visceral pleura of the lung is disrupted, a communication exists between the pleural space, with its negative pressure, and the atmosphere. Air from the atmosphere will enter the pleural space through the opening in the lung, chest wall, or both. This disrupts the balance between inward recoil of the lung and outward recoil of the chest wall, and the lung collapses, resulting in a pneumothorax. Air continues to enter the pleural space until the lung is completely collapsed. This can result from a spontaneous rupture of the visceral pleura, usually in association with emphysematous bullae. These bullae can be either congenital or acquired. Spontaneous pneumothorax is frequently seen in thin young people who appear otherwise healthy. Some of the patients may have an α-trypsin deficiency. Penetrating trauma is still the leading cause of pneumothorax.

If there is a "ball-valve" mechanism at the site of the air leak, either from the lung or chest wall, air may continue to accumulate in the pleural space with each negative inspiratory effort. It will not be able to exit. Air progressively accumulates in the pleural space, creating positive pressure during expiration. This pushes the diaphragm down and the mediastinal structures toward the contralateral pleural space and becomes a tension pneumothorax. In its extreme, the ipsilateral lung is totally collapsed, the contralateral lung becomes compressed, and venous return to the heart is severely compromised. Decreased return to the heart is directly caused by elevated intrathoracic pressures and physical distortion of the vena cava. In addition, increased thoracic pressure decreases myocardial compliance and decreases cardiac output. This is a life-threatening situation that requires emergency recognition and decompression. A needle into the affected pleural space will allow release of the air under pressure. More definitive therapy for all pneumothoraces entails placement of a catheter or chest tube into the pleural space. This catheter is then connected to a valve or underwater drainage system, which allows for the reestablishment of the negative intrapleural pressure (Fig. 16.19).

Frequently, the source of air entering the pleura (e.g., a needle hole after thoracentesis or lung biopsy) may be only temporary, so the amount of air in the pneumothorax is stable. If the patient is stable and asymptomatic, it may be reasonable to await spontaneous resolution. If a gradient of 60 to 80 mm Hg exists between the air in the pleural space and the levels of the gases in the lung tissue, absorption of the pneumothorax would be expected. Breathing 100% oxygen may speed the resorption.

In the rare situation in which the pneumothorax is large but the source of air entry into the pleural space has been sealed, simple aspiration to eliminate or reduce the pneumothorax may be adequate therapy. This can be per-

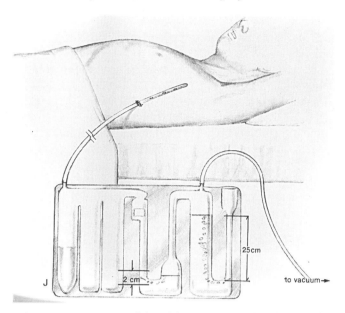

Figure 16.19. Diagram of pleural drainage system. This allows a collection chamber so that accumulating fluid does not alter the hydrostatic pressure necessary to overcome the water seal, although the third chamber regulates the maximal amount of suction that can be delivered to the system as determined by the hydrostatic pressure of the level of fluid in that chamber. From Hood RM. Trauma to the chest. In: Sabiston DC, Jr, Spencer FC, eds. Surgery of the chest. 5th ed. Philadelphia: WB Saunders, 1990:395. Reprinted by permission.

formed with the patient sitting almost upright, with the needle or catheter introduced in the mid-clavicular line via the second intercostal space. This is an extremely unusual situation and requires close observation to be sure the pneumothorax does not reaccumulate.

More frequently, an ongoing source of air leak into the pleural space exists. In this situation, therapy involves placing a catheter or chest tube into the pleural space to evacuate the air. To optimize evacuation of air, the tube ideally should be placed anteriorly and apically. To reestablish the negative intrathoracic pressure necessary to offset the intrinsic inward elastic recoil of the lung, the drainage tube must be connected either to low suction or to some one-way valve system that allows egress of air from the pleural space but prevents its entry into the pleural space. This can be accomplished by the commonly used underwater seal for which the end of the tubing connected to the pleural drain is placed under a level of water. When air in the pleural space exceeds the hydrostatic pressure of the level of water, air bubbles out. On inspiration, fluid is drawn up into the tubing to a level equal to the negative inspiratory pressure generated (the length of tubing between the pleura and the underwater seal prevents aspiration of the underwater seal fluid into the pleural space). If there is also drainage of fluid or blood from the pleural space, a collection chamber needs to be interposed between the pleural drain and the underwater seal compartment. Otherwise, the accumulating fluid would only serve to increase the level of fluid in the underwater seal compartment, thus increasing the hydrostatic pressure that would need to be overcome to allow egress of air from the pleural space.

Most drainage systems, particularly the commercially available ones, also allow application of low suction to the system. This is usually at 15 to 20 cm H_2O pressure, thus slightly higher than the usual resting negative intrathoracic pressure but at a level frequently exceeded by normal inspiratory efforts. This allows fairly normal ventilation of the underlying lung. To ensure that low level of suction and to avoid surges in the amount of suction delivered to the system, the system usually includes a second underwater seal or valve that allows atmospheric air to enter the system (Fig. 16.19).

If the defect in the chest wall is large, usually caused by trauma, an open or sucking chest wound may result in large volumes of air going in and out of the hole in the chest wall in response to respiratory efforts. This neutralizes the pressure and does not allow movement of air through the airways. This can be associated with inadequate ventilation. Mediastinal shift may occur secondary to progressive collapse of the contralateral lung. The life-saving maneuver in this situation should be to cover the sucking chest wall and place a chest tube to allow ventilation of the contralateral lung. Treatment of the pneumothorax on the ipsilateral side will still require insertion of a chest drain, and the chest wall injury will need to be repaired.

In addition to chest wall problems, other major injuries associated with deceleration and blunt thoracic trauma usually involve the heart and major vascular structures. Cardiac contusion or disruption of innominate artery or proximal descending aorta can occur. Rarely, there may be disruption of a major bronchus or the trachea itself. This usually results in a pneumothorax, and when a chest tube is placed, the lung may not reexpand and the air leak may be torrential. In that situation, suction should not be applied to the chest tube, because that will only further impair ventilation. Diagnosis can be confirmed by bronchoscopy. Emergency surgical repair is mandatory.

Even if the chest wall and lung are intact, major collections of fluid (hydrothorax) or blood (hemothorax) may occur in the pleural space. These may prevent expansion of the underlying lung. The lung may then be perfused, but an unventilated lung and a shunt are produced.

Characteristics of pleural effusions are listed in Tables 16.13 and 16.14. Drainage of the fluid is necessary to reverse these effects. If the cause of the fluid can be treated, simple thoracentesis may be adequate, but continued accumulation occurs, insertion of a chest tube will be necessary for adequate drainage. If the fluid continues to be produced and drainage remains high, as is frequently the case with malignant effusions, chemical (e.g., talc, tetracycline, or bleomycin) or mechanical pleurodesis may become necessary. The goal is to create

Table 16.14.
Conditions Associated with Pleural Effusions[a]

Increased	1. Microvascular hydrostatic pressure
	2. Negative intrathoracic pressure
	3. Capillary membrane permeability
	4. Venous pressures
	5. Lymphatic pressures
	6. Inflammation
	7. Peritoneal fluid/pressure
Decreased	1. Microvascular oncotic pressure
	2. Serum protein/albumin
	3. Lung compliance/distensibility
Malignancy	

From Pierson DJ. Disorders of the pleura, mediastinum, and diaphragm. In: Wilson JD, Braunwald E, Isselbacher KJ, et al., eds. Harrison's Principles of internal medicine. 12th ed. New York, McGraw-Hill, 1991:1111.

Table 16.13.
Evaluation of Pleural Fluid[a]

	Transudate	Exudate
Typical appearance	Clear	Clear, cloudy, or bloody
Protein		
Absolute value	<3.0 g/dL	>3.0 g/dL[b]
Pleural fluid:serum ratio	<0.5	>0.5
Lactic dehydrogenase		
Absolute value	<200 IU/liter	>200 IU/liter
Pleural fluid:serum ratio	<0.6	>0.6
Glucose	<60 mg/dL (usually same as in blood)	Variable; often <60 mg/dL
Leukocytes	<1000/mL	>1000/mL
Polymorphonuclear	<50%	Usually >50% in acute inflammation
Erythrocytes	<5000/mL[c]	Variable
Pleural biopsy indicated?	No	Parapneumonic/other acute inflammation: no; chronic/subacute or undiagnosed effusion: yes

[a] From Pierson DJ. Disorders of the pleura, mediastinum, and diaphragm. In: Wilson JD, Braunwald E, Isselbacher KJ, et al., eds. Harrison's Principles of internal medicine. 12th ed. New York, McGraw-Hill, 1991:1111.
[b] Less in hypoproteinemic states.
[c] Assuming atraumatic tap.

an inflammatory reaction between the visceral and parietal pleural that results in fibrous obliteration, so no potential space exists for the fluid to reaccumulate. This action does impose a form of "restrictive" disease on the patient, as it eliminates the normal slippage and parietal and pleural surfaces (see Table 16.9).

In some situations, the pleural fluid accumulation may be chronic, and a fibrous reaction may occur on the surface of the collapsed underlying lung (a pleural "peel") that may preclude the lung's reexpansion even if the pleural effusion was evacuated (Fig. 16.20). Some reactive pleural reaction may resolve with time, but a truly trapped lung under a thick peel will require formal decortication. This situation usually occurs when the pleural effusion is infected (empyema). Simple drainage may prevent sepsis, but cure of the infection will require complete obliteration of the pleural space. Timing is critical; decortication must be performed when the reactive tissue is mature enough to be peeled off the surface of the lung but before too much fibrosis causes obliteration of the plane between the fibrous tissue and the pleural surface of the lung.

Other lesions can interfere with normal ventilation. A lung abscess also adds the problems of actual destruction of lung tissue as well as compression, sepsis, bleeding, and possible rupture into the airway with aspiration into the nonaffected lung. Although abscesses can usually be managed medically and transbronchially with a bronchoscope, external drainage and/or excision of the affected lung may be necessary, particularly if a resistant organism is the cause. If drainage is necessary, contamination of the free pleural space must be avoided or minimized.

Bullous emphysema, usually affecting the upper

lobes, can be associated with α_1-trypsin deficiency but most commonly is associated with smoking and results from disruption of alveolar septa. This results in decreased elastic recoil and increased compliance of the lung. Expansion of the intrathoracic volume (primarily increased anteroposterior diameter) from unopposed outward elastic recoil of the chest wall results in the barrel-chested configuration of the thorax. Recent work suggests that the respiratory difficulty experienced by these patients is caused by the chest wall being maximally expanded at all times, with the diaphragms "flattened" in maximal inspiratory position. Therefore, any inspiratory effort results in minimal air movement. Resection of some of the distended lung, even without gross bullous disease, may allow the chest wall to regain a more normal configuration and restore diaphragmatic mobility. This has led to the recent enthusiasm for "volume reduction" surgery.

Patients with bullous emphysema are at an increased risk for pneumothorax. In other instances, air continues to accumulate in bullae because expiratory airway resistance increases significantly. Greater compression of the normal lung parenchyma occurs, so increased dead space and perfused atelectatic lung is associated with the potential for shunting. The resulting hypoxemia is, therefore, multifactorial. Bullectomy decreases dead space, allows expansion of functional lung parenchyma, and decreases the risk of spontaneous rupture and pneumothorax. Often, when a question of resectability exists in the presence of significant parenchymal disease, a ventilation-perfusion scan may help evaluate operative risk.

If the proposed resection involves a portion of lung that receives little blood supply, it may have little effect on overall postoperative function. However, emphysematous lungs may have perfusion of poorly ventilated segments. Resection will decrease dead space, decrease the work of breathing, and decrease the percentage of shunt.

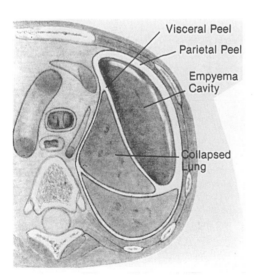

Figure 16.20. Cross-sectional diagram of the thorax, showing an empyema cavity with its fibrous peel, which must be removed to allow complete reexpansion of the lung. If there is just pleural thickening without a definite peel, drainage alone may be sufficient therapy. From Hood RM. Trauma to the chest. In: Sabiston DC, Jr, Spence FC, eds. Surgery of the chest. 5th ed. Philadelphia: WB Saunders, 1990:395.

ARDS (Adult Respiratory Distress Syndrome)

ARDS is a term initially devised in 1967 to describe the syndrome of acute respiratory distress in patients with diffuse interstitial edema, alveolar infiltrates, and decreased lung compliance (<50 ml/cm H_2O) with severe arterial hypoxemia ($Pa_{O_2}/F_IO_2 \leq 150$ without PEEP or ≤ 200 with PEEP). Though histologically similar to the interstitial edema associated with cardiac failure, essential criteria for this definition is normal left atrial or pulmonary capillary wedge pressures. This often follows aspiration, shock, massive volume infusions, or sepsis. It has also been called shock lung, non-cardiogenic pulmonary edema, post traumatic pulmonary insufficiency, or alveolar capillary leak syndrome. Despite recent advances, ARDS still carries a mortality of 40%, with even higher risk in some groups (e.g. 75% in patients > 60 years with sepsis).

The pathophysiology of ARDS and its therapeutic implications have been the subject of intense debate and a vast amount of literature. It has become more apparent that ARDS is often the first manifestation of a systemic inflammatory response that may lead to multiorgan failure. The increased pulmonary capillary permeability may result from endothelial damage by toxins—either inhaled, aspirated, or endotoxins from sepsis. Any or all of the following have also been implicated as contributing to ARDS: complement activation; excessive activation of alveolar macrophages; release of inflammatory mediators such as leukotrienes, thromboxanes, and prostaglandin; and activation of leukocytes with release of free oxygen radicals, proteases, and other cytolytic compounds.

Histology of the pulmonary capillaries may show aggregates of platelets, polymorphonuclear leukocytes and macrophages in the endothelium. Damage to the endothelium promotes accumulation of fluid in the interstitial space and, in advanced cases, the alveoli. This interferes with surfactant and results in alveolar collapse. Because this is non-homogeneous, a patchy pattern of ventilation-perfusion imbalances develops in association with shunting and decreased pulmonary compliance. This worsens problems of oxygenation.

Vast amounts of literature exist regarding attempts at treatment of ARDS, but mechanical ventilation with PEEP is the mainstay of therapy. Addition of surfactant, nitrous oxide, oxygen free radical scavengers, and a wide variety of different ventilator modes have been advocated. The underlying cause of the ARDS, e.g., sepsis, must also be treated. Despite all these advances, the mortality remains high. Even when ARDS does resolve, it does not resolve quickly (usually > 7 to 10 days). Permanent pulmonary fibrosis is probably the result of high oxygen toxicity and barotrauma from the methods of ventilation. Recent modifications in ventilator management of the patient with ARDS have been directed at reducing this iatrogenic component.

Mechanical Ventilation

Except for elective surgery, in which general anesthesia with paralysis is desired, every attempt should be made to allow the patient to ventilate spontaneously. For patients with varying degrees of respiratory distress, aggressive medical and respiratory therapy should be adequate. In advanced respiratory failure, mechanical assistance may be necessary. Unlike spontaneous venti-

lation, in which air enters the lung to compensate for increased negative intrathoracic pressure, mechanical ventilation delivers air under positive pressure against the compliance of the lung (Fig. 16.21).

Endotracheal intubation with mechanical ventilation remains a mainstay of therapy. It is beyond the scope of this chapter to go into all the indications for mechanical ventilation in detail. The purpose of mechanical ventilation is to provide as near normal minute ventilatory volume (MVV) by adjusting ventilator tidal volumes, rates, and inspiratory volumes. Excessive airway pressures must be avoided to prevent "barotrauma" which results in pulmonary edema caused by alveolar cellular damage and increased alveolar capillary permeability (Fig. 16: 22). Ratios of inspiratory and expiratory phases and expiratory airway pressures can also be regulated. The principal modalities of mechanical ventilation are discussed below. Diagrammatic representation of volume and pressure modes of ventilation are shown (Figure 16.23).

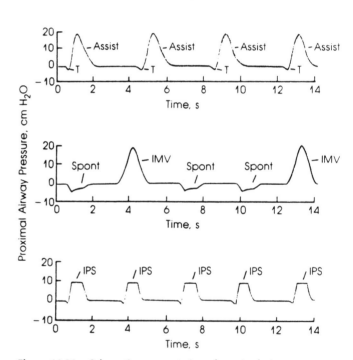

Figure 16.21. Schematic representation of proximal airway pressure waveforms during assisted ventilation and two modes of weaning. **Top,** During mechanical ventilation in the assist mode, the patient triggers each breath by a short inspiratory effort (T) preceding the ventilator breath (Assist) at a rate of 15/min. **Middle,** During synchronized intermittent mandatory ventilation, the patient breathes spontaneously (Spont) at a rate of 20/min also from the ventilator's demand valve and also receives unassisted ventilator-delivered tidal volumes (IMV) at a preset rate of approximately 7/min. The SIMV breaths are synchronized to avoid stacking a ventilator breath on top of a spontaneous breath. **Bottom,** During inspiratory pressure support ventilation, the patient breathes spontaneously at a rate of 20/min from the ventilator's demand valve, as with SIMV, but the inspiratory effort is aided by the ventilator maintaining the proximal airway pressure relatively constant at 10 cm H_2O during the entire inspiration (IPS). From Lanken PN. Mechanical ventilatory support. In: Wilson JD, Braunwald E, Isselbacher KJ, et al. Harrison's principles of internal medicine. 12th ed. New York: McGraw-Hill, 1991.

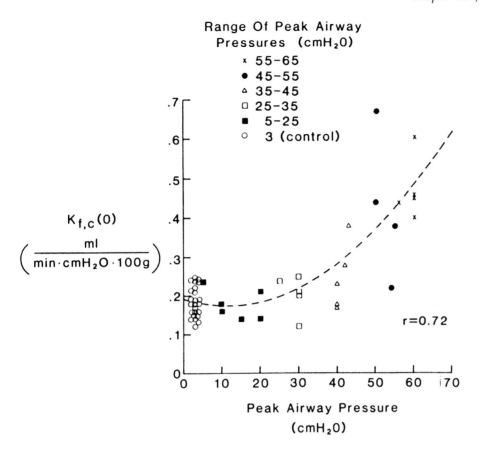

Range Of Peak Airway Pressures (cmH₂O)

- × 55–65
- ● 45–55
- △ 35–45
- □ 25–35
- ■ 5–25
- ○ 3 (control)

$K_{f,c}(0)$

$\left(\dfrac{ml}{min \cdot cmH_2O \cdot 100g}\right)$

r=0.72

Peak Airway Pressure (cmH₂O)

Figure 16.22. Effect of high peak airway pressures on the capillary filtration coefficient K_{fc} of isolated, blood-perfused lobes of dog lungs. The lobes were ventilated at 6 breaths per minute for 20 minutes, with peak airway pressures ranging from 5 to 60 cmH₂O. K_{fc} measured immediately after the challenge remained roughly unchanged up to 40 cmH₂O peak airway pressure and then increased for larger pressures. Range of peak airway pressures in cmH₂O (x)55-65: (●) 45-55; (△) 35-45; (□) 25-35 (■) 5-25; (○) 3 9control). R = 0.72. In Parker JC, et al, Increased microvascular permeability in dog lungs due to high peak airway pressures. J Appl Physiol, 57:1809-1816, 1994.

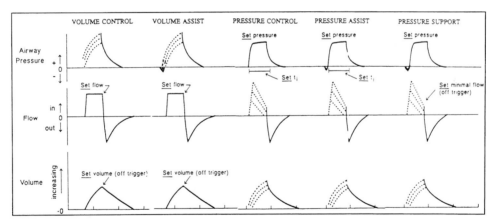

Figure 16.23. Comparison of volume and pressure modes. The *top line* represents airway pressure (+ and—indicate above and below atmospheric pressure), the *middle line* represents gas flow (*in* and *out* indicate flow toward and away from the patient), and the *lower line* represents tidal volume. In volume control mode, or controlled mechanical ventilation (CMV), the tidal volume and inspiratory flow rate are preset. The breath cycles to expiration when the preset tidal volume is reached (off trigger). Airway pressure is variable, depending on lung and chest wall compliance. In volume-assist mode, or assist-control ventilation (ACV), the situation is similar to CMV, except that the patient triggers the breath by generating negative pressure at the start of inspiration. In pressure-control mode, or pressure-control ventilation (PCV), the maximal airway pressure and inspiratory time (tᵢ) are preset. Gas flow rate can be varied, and tidal volume depends on lung and chest wall compliance. In pressure-assist mode, or pressure assist-control ventilation (PACV), the situation is identical except that the patient triggers the breath by generating negative pressure at the start of inspiration. In pressure support mode, or pressure support ventilation (PSV), the situation is similar to PACV, except that the patient is able to increase the delivered tidal volume by continued spontaneous inspiration after the maximal airway pressure has been achieved. The ventilator cycles into expiration (off trigger) when the patient's gas flow declines to about 25% of the peak flow rate. From Sladen et al. Tracheal intubation and mechanical ventilation. In: Sabiston D, Spencer F, eds. Surgery of the chest, 6th ed. Philadelphia, WB Saunders, 1995.

Table 16.15.
Comparison of Advantages and Disadvantages of Four Commonly Used Weaning Techniques[a]

Major Technique	Major Advantages	Disadvantages
T-piece trial	No additional work of breathing needed to open ventilator's demand valve	No exhaled volume monitoring or other alarms No automatic sighs
Continuous positive airways pressure (CPAP) mode, i.e., a CPAP trial	Still connected to ventilator's circuits with full monitor's alarms May lack sighs on some ventilators	Additional work of breathing required to open ventilator's demand valve
Intermittent mandatory ventilation (IMV)	Allows for transition from 100% mechanical to 100% spontaneous ventilation as gradually as desired	Additional work of breathing to open demand valve during spontaneous breaths
	May be tolerated better hemodynamically by patients in left heart failure	Rate of weaning may be slower due to slow step-wise decreases in IMV rate
	May require less bedside personnel compared with T-piece or CPAP trials	May result in less bedside observations than T-piece or CPAP trials
Inspiratory pressure support (IPS)	Low levels of IPS (5–10 cm H_2O) decrease work or spontaneous breathing through artificial airway	Tidal volumes with high levels of IPS will vary if respiratory mechanics change (analogous to a pressure-cycled ventilator)
	High levels of IPS (≥20 cm H_2O) may be more comfortable than assist mode	

[a] From Lanken PN. Mechanical ventilatory support. In: Wilson JD, Braunwald E, Isselbacher KJ, et al., eds. Harrison's principles of internal medicine. 12th ed. New York, McGraw-Hill, 1991:1125.

Table 16.16.
Various Parameters Useful for Weaning from Mechanical Ventilators[a]

Parameter	Value Predicting Failure	Value Predicting Success
I. Respiratory muscle function		
A. Maximal inspiratory pressure	< -20 mm Hg	> -30 mm Hg
II. Ventilatory demand		
A. Spontaneous respiratory rate	>35/min	<30/min
B. Minute ventilation (V_E)	>10 liter/min	< liter/min
C. $V_D:V_T$[b]	≥0.6	<0.4
III. Ventilatory ability		
A. Vital capacity	<10 mL/kg	≥15 m/kg
B. Maximal voluntary ventilation	$<2 \times$ resting V_E	$≥2 \times$ resting V_E
IV. Oxygenation		
A. Intrapulmonary right-to-left shunt	>20%	<20%

[a] From Lanken PN. Mechanical ventilatory support. In: Wilson JD, Braunwald E, Isselbacher KJ, et al., eds. Harrison's principles of internal medicine. 12th ed. New York, McGraw-Hill, 1991:1125.
[b] Physiologic dead space:tidal ratio.

Volume Control

Preset tidal volume is delivered under positive pressure at a fixed rate. This is ideal for paralyzed patients. There is no allowance for any spontaneous inspiratory efforts of the patient.

Assist-Control

In response to a patient's inspiratory effort, a preset tidal volume is delivered. This may be used in weaning after a period of mechanical ventilation. However, an agitated patient who triggers the ventilator inappropriately may hyperventilate with this type of ventilation.

Intermittent Mandatory Ventilation (IMV)

The ventilator will deliver a fixed tidal volume gas at a preset rate that can be varied. However, the patient may also initiate spontaneous ventilation. Oxygen at the desired concentration is available at negligible resistance. This is frequently used as a mode for weaning from the ventilator (Table 16.15).

Mandatory Minute Volume (MMV)

The exhaled volume is measured and the ventilator is triggered only when a preset volume is not achieved by spontaneous ventilation. This also is used as a modality for ventilatory weaning.

Intermittent Positive Pressure Ventilation (IPPV)

Gas flow is initiated by negative inspiratory pressures, and gases are delivered until a preset pressure level is reached. The tidal volume delivered, therefore, depends on airway resistance. This modality is now reserved primarily for delivery of nebulized medications.

Positive End Expiratory Pressure (PEEP)

A valve maintains positive pressure in the airways at all times, including at the end of the expiration. A cuffed endotracheal tube with a tight seal is essential to maintain this pressure. It is designed to maintain alveolar patency when there is a tendency to collapse secondary to increased tissue oncotic pressures or the collection of fluid in the interstitial space. A negative side effect is that PEEP decreases venous return to the heart and may produce hypotension in hypovolemic patients.

High-Frequency Positive Pressure (Jet) Ventilation (HFPPV)

A high-frequency injection of gas forces air back and forth (oscillating) directly in the respiratory tree under relatively low pressures. This minimizes barotrauma to the lung and the hemodynamic consequences of high ventilatory pressures and PEEP. It is generally reserved for patients who fail conventional ventilator support or for special situations, e.g., bronchopleural fistulae with large air leaks. It may be useful intraoperatively to ventilate distal lung parenchyma during resection/reconstruction of the trachea or major bronchi.

Pressure Support (PS)

The patient's inspiratory effort is augmented by the ventilator to a preset positive airway pressure. This decreases ventilatory work and is usually used to help slowly wean difficult patients from the ventilator. Weaning parameters for an average-size adult are listed in Table 16.16. For the patient who is chronically ventilator dependent, tracheostomy may be indicated. Occasionally, by decreasing upper airway dead space, with the resultant decreased work of breathing, the tracheostomy may speed ventilatory weaning.

Appendix A.
Typical Normal Respiratory Parameters

		25 Years 6 Months Male	55 Years 5 Months Female
VC	Vital capacity	5.4 liters	2.4 liters
FRC	Functional residual capacity	4.0 liters	2.2 liters
RV	Residual volume	1.9 liters	1.4 liters
TLC	Total lung capacity	7.3 liters	3.8 liters
FEV_1	Forced expired volume in 1.0 sec	4.4 liters	2.0 liters
FEV_1/VC	FEV_1/vital capacity ratio	80%	75%
$FEF_{25\%-75\%}$	Forced expiratory flow between 25% and 75% of VC	4.6 liters	2.3 liters
Dl_{CO_2}	Diffusing capacity for CO_2	36.0 ml/min/mm Hg	18.0 ml/min/mm Hg
Pa_{O_2}	Arterial partial pressure of O_2	90 ± 10 mm Hg (torr)	
Pa_{CO_2}	Arterial partial pressure of CO_2	40 ± 3 mm Hg	
Ca_{O_2}	Arterial content of O_2	20 ml/100 ml (vol %)	
Cv_{O_2}	Mixed venous content of O_2	15 ml/100 ml	
$C(a-v)_{O_2}$	Arterial-venous O_2 content difference	5 ml/100 ml	
Ca_{CO_2}	Arterial content of CO_2	47 ml/100 ml	
Cv_{CO_2}	Mixed venous content of CO_2	51 ml/100 ml	
Pv_{O_2}	Mixed venous partial pressure of O_2	40 mm Hg	
Pv_{CO_2}	Mixed venous partial pressure of CO_2	46 mm Hg	
pH_a	Arterial pH	7.40 ± 0.03	
HCO_3^-	Arterial blood bicarbonate concentration	24 ± 2 mEq/liter	
BE	Base excess	0 ± 2 mEq/liter	
Pp1	Pleural pressure	-5 cm H_2O at FRC -30 cm H_2O at TLC	
C_T	Compliance of thorax	0.1 liter/cm H_2O	
C_{CW}	Compliance of chest wall	.02 liter/cm H_2O	
C_L	Compliance of lung specific compliance	0.2 liter/cm H_2O 0.06 liter/cm H_2O/liter of FRC	
R_{aw}	Airway resistance	<2.5 cm H_2O/liter/sec	
F_1O_2	Inspired oxygen fraction (room air)	0.21	
P_B	Barometric pressure (sea level)	760 mm Hg	
PA_{O_2}	Alveolar partial pressure of O_2	100 mm Hg	
PA_{CO_2}	Alveolar partial pressure of CO_2	40 mm Hg	
f	Respiratory frequency	10–15/min	

(continued)

Appendix A.
(continued)

		25 Years 6 Months Male	55 Years 5 Months Female
V_A	Alveolar ventilation	4–5 liters/min	
V_E	Total ventilation	6–8 liters/min	
V_T	Tidal volume	500 ml (0.5 liter)	
$V_{D_{anat}}$	Dead space volume (anatomic)	150–200 ml	
$V_D{:}V_T$	Physiologic dead space volume to tidal volume ratio	<0.4	
V_{O_2}	Oxygen uptake	250–300 ml/min	
V_{CO_2}	Carbon dioxide production	200–250 ml/min	
R	Respiratory exchange ratio (V_{CO_2}: V_{O_2})	0.8	
Q_T	Cardiac output (total)	5 liters/min	
Q_S/Q_T	Shunt flow (%)	<5%	
Hb	Hemoglobin concentration	15 g/100 ml	
$P_{50\%}$	Partial pressure of O_2 at 50% saturation of Hb	27 mm Hg	

Appendix B.
Formulas of Ventilation and Respiration

Minute ventilation

$V_E = V_T \times RR$ V_T = tidal volume

  RR = respiratory rate

$V_E = V_D + V_A$ V_D = physiologic dead space

  V_A = alveolar ventilation

Wasted (dead space) ventilation—Bohr equation

$$VD/VT = \frac{P_{A_{CO_2}} - P_{E_{CO_2}}}{P_{A_{CO_2}}}$$

$P_{A_{CO_2}}$ = alveolar CO_2

$P_{E_{CO_2}}$ = expired CO_2

Normal VD/VT = 0.2 − 0.4

Physiologic dead space (VD) = anatomic dead space (conducting airways, usually 150–180 ml or 2 ml/kg) + alveolar dead space (ventilated but not perfused alveoli)

Alveolar Ventilation (assumes equilibrium between alveolar and arterial P_{CO_2})

Arterial blood O_2 content

$Ca_{O_2} = Hb \times 1.34 \times \% - sat + dissolved\ O_2$

O_2 transport = $Ca_{O_2} \times$ C.O. $\times$ 10 (conversion factor)

Shunt (usually measured on 100% O_2)

$$QS/QT = \frac{Cc_{O_2} - Ca_{O_2}}{Cc_{O_2} - Cv_{O_2}}$$

QS = shunt flow

QT = total flow

Cc_{O_2} = capillary O2 content

Ca_{O_2} = arterial O2 content

Cv_{O_2} = mixed venous O2 content

Normal = 3–5%

(Cc_{O_2} assumed to be in equilibrium with alveolar (administered) O_2, i.e., 100)

Henderson-Hasselbalch—defines relationship pH, HCO_3^-; P_{CO_2} pH = 6.1 + log_{10} ((HCO_3^-)/0.03·P_{CO_2})

Appendix C.
Factors in Respiratory Problems

Ventilation
  Airways
    Patency
    Asthma
    COPD
    Bronchiectasis
  Muscle
    Chest wall
    Diaphragm
  Alveoli
    Inflammation
    Infection
    CHF
  Effusions
  Pneumothorax
Perfusion
  Anatomic PA
  RV function
  LV function
  Pulmonary embolus
Primary disease PA
  Wegener's
  Sarcoid
  Pulmonary hypertension

SUGGESTED READINGS

Adrogue HJ, Rashad MN, Grimm AB, et al. Assessing acid-base status in circulatory failure: differences between arterial and central venous blood. New Engl J Med 1989;320:1312.

Agnostini E, D'Angelo E. Statics of the chest wall. In: Roussos C, Macklam PT, eds. The thorax. New York: Marcel Dekker, 1986: 256–296.

American College of Surgeons. I. Lung function and its assessment and VII. Disorders of the thoracic cage. In: Care of the surgical patient. Vol. I. New York: Scientific American Medicine, 1988.

Barnes PJ. Airway neuropeptides: roles in fine tuning and in disease? News Physiol Soc 1989;4:116.

Bartlett RH. Use of the mechanical ventilator. In: Care of the surgical patient. Vol 1. New York: Scientific American Publishers, 1988.

Bierman MI. Respiratory physiology. In: Simmons RL, Steed DL, eds. Basic science review for surgeons. Philadelphia: WB Saunders, 1991: 163–167. Anesthesiology 1994;80:983–991.

Borg U, Stoklosa JC, Siegel JH, et al. Prospective evaluation of combined high frequency ventilation in post trauma patients with ARDS refractory to optimized conventional ventilatory, management. Crit Care Med 1989;17:1129.

Boyd AD, Ribakove GH, Sparaco RJ. Tracheal intubation and mechanical ventilation: The surgeon's viewpoint. In: Sabiston DC, Spencer FC, eds. Surgery of the chest. 6th ed. Philadelphia: WB Saunders, 1995.

Boysen PG, Kirby RR. Practical applications of blood gas measurements. In: Civetta JM, Taylor RW, Kirby RR, eds. Critical care. Philadelphia: JB Lippincott, 1988:311–316.

Celli BR. Respiratory muscle function. Clin Chest Med 1986;7:567.

Cherniak NS, Longobardo GS. Abnormalities in respiratory rhythm. In: Handbook of physiology. The respiratory system. Bethesda, MD: American Physiological Society, 1986;2(3):729–749.

Cooper JD, Trulock EP, Triantafillou AN, et al. Bilateral pneumectomy (volume reduction) for chronic obstructive pulmonary disease. J Thorac Cardiovasc Surg 1995;209:106–19.

Demling RH, Goodwin CW. Pulmonary dysfunction. In: Wilmore DW, ed. Care of the surgical patient. Vol. 1. New York: Scientific American Publishers, 1988.

Dreyfuss D, Saumon G. Lung overinflation: Physiologic and anatomic alterations leading to pulmonary edema. In: Zapol W, Lemaire F, eds. Adult respiratory distress syndrome. New York: Marcel Dekker Inc., 1991.

Esteban A, Frutos F, Tobin M, et al. A comparison of four methods of weaning patients from mechanical ventilation. New Engl J Med 1995;332:345–350.

Fong Y, Moldawer L, Shires G. The biologic characteristics of cytokines and their implication in surgical injury. Surg Gynecol Obstet 1990; 120:363.

Ganong WF. Review of medical physiology. 15th ed. Norwalk, CT: Appleton & Lange, 1991.

Gass GD, Olsen GN. Preoperative pulmonary function testing to predict morbidity and mortality. Chest 1986;89:127.

Glauser FL. Worsening oxygenation in the mechanically ventilated patient. Am Rev Respir Dis 1988;138:458.

Gold WM, Bousey HA. Pulmonary function testing. In: Murray JF, Nadel FA, eds. Textbook of respiratory medicine. Philadelphia: WB Saunders, 1988:611–682.

Goldenheim P, Kazemi H. Cardiopulmonary monitoring of critically ill patients. N Engl J Med 1984;311:717.

Greenfield L, Proctor M. Caval filters: Indications and limitations. In: Pulmonary Perspectives (ACCP) 1995;12:5–6.

Hagg JC. Neutrophil kinetics and lung injury. Physiol Rev 1987;67: 1249.

Hechtman HB, Lekuk S, Alexander F, et al. Humoral mediators in adult respiratory distress syndrome. In: Siegel JH, ed. Trauma: emergency surgery and critical care. New York: Churchill Livingstone, 1987:565–580.

Hickling K, Henderson S, Jackson R. Low mortality associated with low volume pressure limited ventilation with permissive hypercapnia in severe adult respiratory distress syndrome. Intensive Care Med 1990;16:372–377.

Higginbottam T, Otulana BA, Wallwork J. The physiology of heart-lung transplantation in humans. News Physiol Soc 1990;5:71.

Jenkinson S. Lung transplantation for primary pulmonary hypertension: Is it effective? In: Pulmonary Perspectives (ACCP) 1995;12:7–8.

Johnson D, Thomson D, Hurst T, et al. Neutrophil-mediated acute lung injury after extracorporeal perfusion. J Thorac Cardiovasc Surg 1994;107:1193–1202.

Kinasewitz GT, Fishman AP. Pleural dynamics and effusions. In: Fishman AP, ed. Pulmonary diseases and disorders. New York: McGraw-Hill, 1988:2171–2181.

Kollef MH, Schuster DP. The acute respiratory distress syndrome. Review Article (179 ref.) New Engl J Med 1995;332:27–37.

Lai-Fook ST. Mechanics of the pleural space: fundamental concepts. Lung 1987;165:249.

Lessard M, Guérot E, Lorino H, et al. Effects of pressure-controlled with different I:E ratios versus volume controlled ventilation on respiratory mechanics, gas exchange, and hemodynamics in patients with adult respiratory distress syndrome.

Levitsky MG. Pulmonary physiology. 3rd ed. New York: McGraw-Hill, 1991.

Lewis R, Austen F, Soberman R. Leukotrienes and other products of the 5 lipoxygenase pathway. N Engl J Med 1990;323:645.

Lunn R. Inhaled nitric oxide therapy. Mayo Clin Proc 1995;70:247–255.

Marini J. Ventilation of the acute respiratory distress syndrome: Looking for Mr. Goodmode. Anesthesiology 1994;80:972–975.

Mercat A, Craïni L, Teboul J, et al. Cardiorespiratory effects of pres-

sure-controlled ventilation with and without inverse ratio in the adult respiratory distress syndrome. Chest 1993;4:871–875.

Milberg J, Davis D, Steinberg K, et al. Improved survival of patients with acute respiratory distress syndrome (ARDS):1983–1993. JAMA 1995; 273:306–309.

Miller JI. Physiologic evaluation of pulmonary function in the lung resection candidate. J Thorac Cardiovasc Surg, in press.

Murray JF. The normal lung: the basis for diagnosis and treatment of pulmonary disease. 2nd ed. Philadelphia: WB Saunders, 1986.

Namm JF. Applied respiratory physiology. 3rd ed. London: Butterworths, 1987.

Papadakos P. Modes of mechanical ventilation: Pressure versus volume. Controversies in Critical Care 1995;1:1–6.

Petty TL. The use, abuse, and mystique of positive end-expiratory pressure. Am Rev Respir Dis 1988;138:475.

Pingleton SK. Complications of acute respiratory failure. Am Rev Respir Dis 1988;137:1463.

Raffin TA. ARDS: mechanisms and management. Hosp Pract (Off Ed) 1987;22:65.

Rangel-Frausto M, Pittet D, Costigan M, et al. The natural history of the systemic inflammatory response syndrome (SIRS): A prospective study. JAMA 1995;273:117–123.

Ray CS, Sue DY, Bray G, et al. Effects of obesity and respiratory function. Am Rev Respir Dis 1983;128:501.

Rubin B. Airway mucus: it's not just snot. In: Pulmonary Perspectives (ACCP) 1995;12:1–4.

Sahasa K. The pleura. Am Rev Respir Dis 1988;138:184.

Shuck JM, Snow NJ. Injury of the chest wall. In: Mattox KL, Moore EE, Feliciano DV, eds. Trauma. East Norwalk, CT: Appleton & Lange, 1981:321–335.

Siegel JH, Stoklosa JC, Borg U. Cardio respiratory management of the adult respiratory distress syndrome. In: Siegel JH, ed. Trauma: emergency surgery and critical care. New York: Churchill Livingstone, 1987:581–673.

Siegel JH, Giovannini I, Coleman B. Ventilation: perfusion, maldistribution secondary to the hyperdynamic cardiovascular state as the major source of increased pulmonary shunting in human sepsis. J Trauma 1979;19:432.

Sjostrand U. Pneumatic systems facilitating treatment of respiratory insufficiency with alternative use of IPPV/PEEP, HFPPV/ PEEP, and CPPB or CPAP. Acta Anaesthesiol Scand Suppl 1977;64:123.

Sladen RN, Stolp B, MacIntyre NR. Tracheal intubation and assisted ventilation: The anesthesiologist's viewpoint. In: Sabiston DC, Spencer FC, eds. Surgery of the chest. 6th ed. Philadelphia: WB Saunders, 1995.

Slutsky A, et al. Mechanical ventilation. Amer College Chest Physic Consensus Conference. Chest 1993;104:1833–1859. (158 ref.)

Snyder JV, Froese A. Respiratory lung. In: Snyder JV, ed. Oxygen transport in the critically ill. Chicago: Yearbook Medical Publishers, 1987:351.

Taylor AE, Rehder K, Hyatt RE, et al. Clinical respiratory physiology. Philadelphia: WB Saunders, 1989.

Tisi GM. Preoperative evaluation of pulmonary function. Am Rev Respir Dis 1979;119:293.

Tisi GM. The physician and the clinical pulmonary function laboratory. In: Pulmonary physiology in clinical medicine. Baltimore: Williams & Wilkins, 1980:53–73.

Tobin MJ. Respiratory monitoring. JAMA 1990;264:244.

Trinkle JK, Richardson JD, Franz JL, et al. Management of flail chest without mechanical ventilation. Ann Thorac Surg 1975;19:355.

Weinberger S, Weiss JW. Weaning from ventilatory support. New Engl J Med 1995;332:388–389.

Weinberger SE. Principles of pulmonary medicine. 2nd ed. Philadelphia: WB Saunders, 1992.

West JB. Respiratory physiology—the essentials. 4th ed. Baltimore: Williams & Wilkins, 1990.

Wilson JD, Braunwald E, Isselbacher KJ, et al. Principles of internal medicine. 12th ed. New York: McGraw-Hill, 1992.

Wolfe WG, Smith PK. Preoperative assessment of pulmonary function: quantitative evaluation of ventilation and blood gas exchange. In: Sabiston DC, Spencer FC, eds. Surgery of the chest. 5th ed. Philadelphia: WB Saunders, 1990:1–20.

17 The Digestive System

G. Robert Mason / Peter J. Kahrilas / Mary F. Otterson / Ivan M. Lang / Gordon L. Telford,
Susan W. Telford / Sushil K. Sarna / Verne E. Cowles / Timothy R. Koch / Haile T. Debas,
George Gittes / Bernard M. Jaffe / Stanley J. Dudrick / Rifat Latifi / Gilbert A. Castro

Endocrine and Paracrine Control and Function

Historical Perspective and Classification

Understanding of the regulation of intestinal function has progressed dramatically since the late 19th century when Pavlov's tenet of "nervism," that all gastrointestinal function was controlled by nerves, was widely held. In 1902, Bayliss and Starling (1) discovered the first hormone, secretin. This led to a rapid escalation in research in the new field of endocrinology, and the role of hormonal control in the regulation of gastrointestinal function became increasingly appreciated. Other major events in the historical development of gastrointestinal endocrinology are outlined in Table 17.1.

Gastrointestinal peptides may be grouped both by the mode of their delivery to target cells and/or by their chemical structure. Although these peptides were originally referred to as hormones (endocrine agents that are delivered to their target cells via the bloodstream), it has become increasingly apparent that most peptides use other modes of delivery. Many are paracrine agents and are secreted into the interstitial fluid through which they diffuse to reach their target cell locally. Others are neurocrine agents and are secreted by neurons in the enteric nervous system. The latter are particularly numerous and include neurotransmitters, or substances secreted at nerve terminals that reach their receptor by crossing a short junctional gap. Others are secreted into the interstitial fluid through which they diffuse to their target cell. The same peptide may use all modes of delivery. For example, somatostatin may act as an endocrine, paracrine, and neurocrine agent. VIP relaxes gastrointestinal smooth muscle as a neurotransmitter, but it may regulate local blood flow as a paracrine agent. Table 17.2 classifies gastrointestinal peptides according to modes

of delivery, and in Table 17.3, a classification according to structural similarities is given.

Brain-Gut Axis

Many gut peptides are found in the brain. Conversely, several peptides initially isolated from the CNS have been found in the neurons and endocrine cells of the gastrointestinal tract. This dual presence of peptides has given rise to the concept of the brain-gut axis (2). Although somatostatin was discovered in the hypothalamus originally, more somatostatin exists in the gastrointestinal tract than in the brain. Similarly, although CCK was extracted from intestinal mucosa originally, a higher concentration of CCK exists in the brain than in the gut. The functional significance of the brain-gut axis remains to be elucidated. However, CCK may be an important satiety factor, acting centrally. Other peptides have been found to regulate body temperature and blood glucose by acting centrally. The list of peptides included in the brain-gut axis is long and getting longer. Some of the important peptides in this respect are CCK, somatostatin, VIP, substance P, and calcitonin gene-related peptide (CGRP).

Regulation of Release of Gastrointestinal Peptides

The most important stimulant of release of gastrointestinal peptides is food. The composition and pH of food or chyme has significant effects on which peptides are released. Activation of either extrinsic or intrinsic nerves is also important in release (3). Inhibition of release is accomplished by withdrawal of stimuli, the fasting state, negative feedback inhibitory loops, activation of inhibitory neurons, and the action of inhibitory peptides such as somatostatin. The regulation of release of the more important peptides is discussed below.

Gastrin

Release of gastrin is stimulated by vagal stimulation, food in the antrum, and gastric distension. Vagal-stimu-

Table 17.1.
Major Historical Events in Gastrointestinal Endocrinology

Year	Researcher	Discovery
1890	Pavlov	Tenet of "nervism"
1902	Bayliss and Starling	Discovery of secretin (first hormone)
1906	Edkins	Discovery of gastrin
1922	Banting and Best	Discovery of insulin
1928	Roscoe Graham	Insulin-secreting tumor
1928	Ivy and Oldberg	Discovery of CCK
1935	Whipple	"Whipple's triad"
1942	Grossman and Robertson	Gastrin as a hormone
1943	Harper and Raper	Discovery of pancreozymin (PZ)
1955	Zollinger and Ellison	Zollinger-Ellison syndrome
1964	Gregory	Isolation of gastrin
1967	Berson and Yalow	Radioimmunoassay for insulin
1968	Jorpes and Mutt	CCK is the same as pancreozymin
1968	Pearce	Amine precursor uptake and decarboxylation (APUD) theory
1972	Guillemin and Schally	Discovery of somatostatin

Table 17.2.
Classification of Gastrointestinal Peptides

Mode of Delivery	Peptide	Source/Location
Endocrine	Gastrin	G-cells, antrum, duodenum
	CCK	CCK-cells, duodenum, jejunum
	Secretin	S-cell, duodenum, jejunum
	Somatostatin	D-cell, entire GI tract, pancreas
	Insulin	B-cell, islet
	Glucagon	A-cell, islet
	Enteroglucagon	L-Cell, ileum, colon
	Neurotensin	N-cell, ileum, colon
	PYY	L-cell, ileum, colon
	PP[a]	PP-cell, islet
	Motilin	M-cell, duodenum
	GIP	GIP-cell, duodenum
Paracrine	Somatostatin	D-cell, entire GI tract, pancreas
	VIP	neurons, ENS
Neurocrine	VIP	neurons, ENS
	Somatostatin	entire ENS
	GRP	gastric ENS
	CCK	gastric, pancreatic ENS
	CGRP	entire ENS, C-fibers
	NPY[b]	pancreatic ENS, vagus
	SP[c]	C-fibers, entire ENS

[a] Pancreatic polypeptide.
[b] Neuropeptide Y.
[c] Substance P.

Table 17.3.
Families of Gastrointestinal Peptides

Gastrin	Gastrin
	CCK
Secretin	Secretin
	Glucagon
	Enteroglucagon
	VIP
Pancreatic Polypeptide	Pancreatic polypeptide
	PYY
	NPY
CGRP	CGRP
	Islet associated peptide (IAP)/Amylin
	Calcitonin

lated release of gastrin depends on the release of gastrin-releasing peptide (GRP) from nerve terminals and on cholinergic inhibition of somatostatin release. The most important components of food for inducing release of gastrin are polypeptides and amino acids. Neither carbohydrates nor fats stimulate the release of gastrin. Gastric distension releases gastrin by both short and long reflexes involving cholinergic neurons. Acute gastric alkalinization does not release gastrin directly, but potentiates release by chemical or neural stimuli. However, prolonged alkalinization of the antrum (> 8 hours) causes release of gastrin.

Inhibition of gastrin release is accomplished primarily through antral acidification. When antral pH reaches 2.0, gastrin secretion ceases. Antral acidification causes inhibition of gastrin release by stimulating paracrine release of somatostatin from D cells of the gastric antrum. Indeed, somatostatin is an important modulator of gastrin release. A reciprocal relationship exists between the release of gastrin and somatostatin. The release of gastrin is associated with inhibition of somatostatin and vice versa.

Cholecystokinin

The most important site of release of CCK is the duodenum. CCK release is stimulated when polypeptides and amino acids, fat, and hydrochloric acid are present in the lumen of the duodenum.

Inhibition of CCK release is accomplished through negative feedback loops involving trypsin and chymotrypsin in the duodenal lumen and "monitor peptide" in the pancreatic juice. Trypsin acts by digesting CCK-releasing peptide from the duodenal mucosa. The mechanism by which the monitor peptide acts is still unknown.

Secretin

The most important releasor of secretin is duodenal acidification. Secretin release is initiated when the pH in the lumen of the duodenum falls below 4.5. A second releaser of secretin is fat, but this occurs only at high luminal fat concentrations.

Somatostatin

Endocrine release of somatostatin occurs during a meal. The major stimulant is probably the intraluminal fat. Acidification of the gastric and duodenal mucosa also releases somatostatin in isolated-perfused organ preparations. In the intact animal, this release is probably paracrine. Other stimulants of somatostatin release include CGRP and catecholamines. Inhibition of somatostatin release is accomplished by release of acetylcholine from cholinergic neurons.

Pancreatic Polypeptide

Release of pancreatic polypeptide has cephalic, gastric, and intestinal phases. Cephalic release of pancreatic polypeptide is caused by vagal stimulation and is the predominant phase during a meal. The gastric phase is the result of the activation of reflexes, and the intestinal phase is caused by the action of food on the intestinal mucosa. Release of pancreatic polypeptide in response to a meal is reduced significantly after truncal vagotomy and/or antrectomy. Other mechanisms of inhibition of pancreatic polypeptide release are unknown and in some cases may serve as a test for completeness of vagotomy.

Neurotensin, Peptide YY, and Enteroglucagon

Neurotensin, peptide YY (PYY), and enteroglucagon are released from the distal small intestine and the colon by fat. Mechanisms of their inhibition are unknown. Massive small bowel resection leads to hyperenteroglucagonemia.

Motilin

Motilin is released by vagal stimulation, mixed meals, and particularly by fat and intraduodenal alkalinization. Motilin release is inhibited by pancreatic polypeptide and somatostatin.

Glucose-Dependent Insulinotropic Peptide

Glucose-dependent insulinotropic peptide (GDIP) is released from the duodenum and jejunum by triglycerides, micellar fat, and carbohydrates (4). Mechanisms of its inhibition are unknown, but its release is impaired in chronic pancreatitis.

Axonal Transport and Trafficking

Neurocrine regulation of gut function is mediated through intrinsic and extrinsic neurons of the enteric nervous system. These neurons affect other cells by the release of neurotransmitters or neuropeptides from the nerve terminal into the synaptic space (5). These neuropeptides are not synthesized near the synapse. Rather, they are synthesized in the cytoplasm of the cell body surrounding the nucleus, termed the perikaryon, which is separated from the synapse by the length of the axon. In contrast to the synapse and axon, which do not contain ribosomes and therefore do not make proteins, the perikaryon contains ribosome-rich endoplasmic reticulum, which serves to synthesize the neuropeptides. Once synthesized, neuropeptides are shuttled to the cis end of the Golgi apparatus where they are packaged in vesicles. Glycosylation of vesicles occurs in such a way as to define where in the cell they will be delivered. The vesicles destined to be released at the synapse become attached to microtubules that run the length of the axon. This attachment allows the fast transport of vesicles to the nerve terminus as needed. This fast transport travels at 400 mm/day. Large structural proteins not contained within vesicles are transported much more slowly, at 1 to 5 mm/day.

Peptide Hormone Receptors

Peptide hormones and neuropeptides exert their action by binding to membrane-bound receptors (6). Unlike steroid hormones, which pass through the cell membrane because of their lipophilic nature and bind to nuclear receptors, peptide hormones generally do not pass through the cell membrane. Once bound to a membrane receptor, a cascade of intracellular events is initiated, resulting in the cell-specific changes attributable to the peptide hormone. The beginning of the cascade is usually the result of a conformational change in the membrane-bound receptor caused by the specific binding of its ligand. Again, this mechanism differs significantly from steroid hormone pathways in that steroid receptors may directly regulate gene expression by binding to regulatory elements of the DNA. Peptide hormone receptors are membrane bound and, therefore, cannot migrate to the nucleus to directly alter gene expression. They must activate intermediate steps that modify regulation of gene expression.

The structure and function of peptide hormone receptors is an area of active research. Currently, several distinct families of peptide hormone receptors exist, and each member of a family has a different extracellular domain responsible for binding specific ligands. However, all members of a family have the same or similar transmembrane and intracellular domains mediating similar intracellular signaling processes. Three principal families of peptide hormone receptors are known: (*a*) the catalytic receptors (often tyrosine kinases); (*b*) channel-linked receptors; and *(c)* G protein-linked receptors.

Tyrosine Kinase Receptors

Tyrosine kinase receptors have the following characteristic features: (*a*) a unique ligand-binding extracellular domain; (*b*) a conserved transmembrane domain that passes straight through the cell membrane without any redundant folds; and *(c)* a conserved intracellular domain that contains the active tyrosine kinase portion. Receptors for insulin, platelet-derived growth factor, and epidermal growth factor (EGF) are all examples of peptide hormone receptors of this type. Once bound, a conformational change in the receptor occurs that causes the enzymatic portion of the intracellular domain to become active. Dimerization of the EGF receptor may be an example of the conformational change occurring to activate the tyrosine kinase enzyme. The activated enzyme phosphorylates tyrosine residues on specific target proteins, including other enzymes, factors important in regulation of gene transcription, and the tyrosine kinase itself. Without the tyrosine kinase activity of these cells, there are very few tyrosine residues within the cell that are phosphorylated. Thus, binding by these tyrosine kinases receptors can have a large incremental effect on activity of target proteins. Other than autophosphorylation, the specific substrates for the tyrosine kinases are not known. Autophosphorylation leads to positive feedback and up regulation of the receptor. In contrast, endocytosis of the receptor-ligand complex leads to down regulation of the receptor.

Channel-Linked Receptors

These receptors are found most commonly in cells of a neuronal lineage and usually bind specific neurotransmitters. Such receptors undergo a conformational change upon binding the neurotransmitter and thereby allow passage of ions across the cell membrane, usually resulting in changes in voltage potential. This well-characterized mechanism allows for the rapid conduction seen across synaptic junctions.

G Protein

Another family of peptide hormone receptors are the G protein-interacting receptors. These receptors typically are a single-chain polypeptide, consisting of a ligand-specific extracellular domain, a conserved transmembrane domain with redundant folds that cross the cell membrane seven times, and an intracellular domain that interacts with G protein. All β-adrenergic receptors, muscarinic receptors, and several neuropeptide receptors are members of this family. The intracellular domain is located adjacent to the G protein, a G_t-binding-regulatory protein. This G protein is located, in turn, adjacent to a membrane-bound enzyme or ion channel and modulates the activity of the enzyme or channel in response to binding to the extracellular domain of the receptor. In general, receptor binding sets in motion a cascade of intracellular events, initiated by the action of G protein, which ultimately results in altered levels of intracellular messengers, such as cAMP, cGMP, and Ca^{2+}.

The G protein itself is currently under active study. It appears that G protein is a hetero trimer, the α-subunit of which binds to the peptide receptor and activates adenylate cyclase. The β- and τ-subunits combine to form the cell membrane-binding domain. The most commonly associated enzyme with the G protein is adenylate cyclase, which generates cAMP from ATP. The activation of adenylate cyclase by G protein depends on the binding of GTP by G protein. This activation is terminated when the G protein hydrolyzes GTP and releases GMP and inorganic phosphate ion. Cholera toxin specifically inhibits this hydrolysis and therefore leads to the constitutive activation of adenylate cyclase. Similarly, the *ras* oncogene product is a G protein-like molecule, mutations of which can lead to an inability to hydrolyze GTP. The constitutive adenylate cyclase activity leads to cell proliferation and possibly malignancy, rather than the hypersecretion seen in cholera.

Secondary Messengers

cAMP Pathways

Once cAMP is generated from adenylate cyclase, it acts as an intracellular messenger that activates protein kinase A. Protein kinase A, in turn, phosphorylates serine and threonine residues of specific proteins, thereby regulating their activity. The specific proteins phosphorylated by protein kinase A are determined by the tissue. For example, skeletal muscle protein kinase A phosphorylates and activates phosphorylase kinase, which phosphorylates and activates glycogen phosphorylase.

Ca^{2+}

Intracellular levels can increase 10-fold over a few seconds as a result of the strong gradient that exists between the intracellular compartment ($Ca^{2+} < 10^{-7}$ M) and either the extracellular compartment ($Ca^{2+} > 10^{-5}$ M) or the intracellular calcium sequestering compartments (CSC). Like cAMP, calcium is an important intracellular messenger. Normally, the low intracellular calcium levels are maintained by the activity of a Ca^{2+}-ATPase pump on the cell membrane and on the CSCs inside the cell. An important aspect of the intracellular calcium effector pathway is that intracellular magnesium is present at 10^{-3} M and in many ways can behave similarly to calcium. Therefore, specific calcium regulated pathways must be at least 1000-fold selective for Ca^{2+} or Mg^{2+}.

Intracellular calcium is thought to mediate most of its actions by binding to calmodulin, a 150 amino acid polypeptide that frequently makes up more than 1% of total protein in eukaryotic cells. Calmodulin binds four calcium ions with high affinity and, once activated by calcium binding, further binds to and activates other proteins and enzymes in the cell. Termed Ca^{2+}-calmodulin-dependent protein kinases, these target proteins are responsible for the tissue-specific effects of elevated intracellular Ca^{2+} levels.

Inositol Phosphate Pathways

At least 25 different receptors exist that bind peptide hormones and mediate their intracellular effects through phosphatidylinositol (PI). When binding occurs, these receptors change conformation so that their intracellular domain activates a G protein-like protein. This G protein-like protein is adjacent to a membrane-bound phospholipase C, and it activates the enzyme when the receptor binds its ligand. Phospholipase C initiates a cascade of events similar to the cAMP pathway. Phospholipase C cleaves phosphatidylinositol bisphosphate from the inner leaflet of the cell membrane to release inositol-l,4,5-triphosphate and diacylglycerol, both of which may act as intracellular messengers. Inositol-l,4,5-triphosphate directly stimulates the release of Ca^{2+} from intracellular stores (CSCs) by binding to a regulatory protein on the outer membrane of the CSC. This stimulation of Ca^{2+} elevation is modified in three ways: (a) the calcium is systematically pumped out of the cell; (b) inositol-l,4,5-triphosphate is dephosphorylated to terminate the stimulus; and (c) inositol-l,4,5-triphosphate may be phosphorylated to inositol tetraphosphate, which results in a less intense, though greatly prolonged, stimulation of elevated intracellular Ca^{2+}. Experimentally, the effect of inositol-l,4,5-triphosphate can be mimicked using calcium ionophores.

In contrast to inositol-l,4,5-triphosphate, diacylglycerol directly activates protein kinase C. This activation requires the concomitant binding of diacylglycerol and phosphatidylserine, which greatly enhances the affinity of protein kinase C for calcium. When protein kinase C binds calcium, it becomes activated and phosphorylates serine and threonine residues on proteins such as the Na^+/K^+-ATPase pump. The effect of diacylglycerol is terminated by its phosphorylation. The stimulatory effects of diacylglycerol may be mimicked experimentally by phorbol esters that bind to and activate protein kinase C.

Thus, the mechanisms through which extracellular signaling molecules can bind to and initiate an intracellular response are multiple and complex. Superimposed on this complexity is the added complexity of varied levels of ligands, depending on physiologic and pathologic conditions as well as altered sensitivity and efficiency of the target cells.

Examples of Regulated Functions

The major functions of the more important gastrointestinal peptides are given in Table 17.4. Examples of regulated function in motility, secretion, and cell growth are discussed later.

Motility

Sphincters of the Gastrointestinal Tract. Relaxation of the sphincters of the gastrointestinal tract is mediated by the release of VIP from nerve terminals close to the circular muscle fibers. Release of VIP at these sites may also be caused by other peptides. For example, the relaxation of the sphincter of Oddi by such peptides as CCK may have a common effector pathway through the release of VIP (7).

Peristalsis. Peristalsis is brought about by concomitant contraction orally and relaxation aborally to a bolus of food. The proximal contraction appears to be mediated by acetylcholine and substance P. The aboral re-

Table 17.4.
Major Physiologic Functions of Gastrointestinal Peptides

Gastrin	Stimulation of gastric acid secretion
	Stimulation of cell growth
CCK	Stimulation of pancreatic exocrine secretion
	Gallbladder contraction
	Inhibition of gastric emptying
	Growth of acinar cells
Secretin	Stimulation of pancreatic water and bicarbonate secretion
	Stimulation of biliary water and bicarbonate secretion
	Inhibition of gastric acid secretion
	Stimulation of gastric pepsin secretion
Somatostatin	Inhibition of gastric acid, pancreatic exocrine, biliary, and enteric secretions
	Inhibition of secretion of all GI endocrine peptides
	Inhibition of action of all GI peptides
	Inhibition of gastrointestinal motility and gallbladder contraction
	Inhibition of cell growth
	Increased reabsorption of water and electrolytes in the small bowel
Neurotensin	Stimulation of pancreatic secretion
	Vasodilatation
	Inhibition of gastric acid secretion
GIP	Glucose-dependent release of insulin
	Inhibition of gastric acid secretion
Motilin	Inhibition of MMC
	Increased gastric emptying
	Increased pepsin secretion
PP	Inhibition of acid secretion
	Inhibition of pancreatic exocrine secretion
Enteroglucagon	Increased glycogenolysis
	Increased lipolysis
	Increased gluconeogenesis
PYY	Inhibition of gastric acid secretion
	Inhibition of pancreatic exocrine secretion
	Inhibition of MMC

laxation is mediated by VIP. The descending relaxation in the gastrointestinal tract that is so important in coordinated peristalsis is mediated by VIP and is inhibited by somatostatin. This coordinated peristalsis (MMC) normally occurs between meals (8).

Secretion

Parietal cell secretion is activated by cell-surface receptors for gastrin, histamine, and acetylcholine (8). The thought, smell, and taste of food activate vagal centers, resulting in efferent vagal stimulation, causing release of acetylcholine and GRP. Acetylcholine binds to the cholinergic receptor at the parietal cell and leads to calcium-dependent stimulation of acid secretion. Release of acetylcholine within the gastric wall also results in the suppression of somatostatin release, causing the disinhibition of both the parietal cell and the G cell in the antrum. The release of GRP at the G cell causes the secretion of gastrin. A potentiated interaction then occurs between gastrin and acetylcholine at the level of the pari-

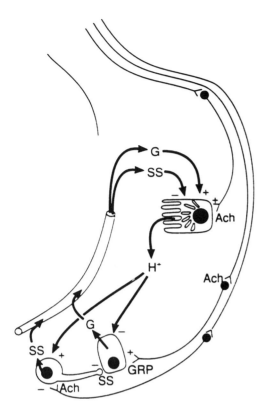

Figure 17.1. Control of acid secretion. Acid production by oxyntic cells in the stomach is controlled by the interplay of neurocrine, endocrine, and paracrine factors acting directly and indirectly on the parietal cell and the G cell. *Ach,* acetylcholine; *SS,* somatostatin; *G,* gastrin. From Debas HT, Mulvihill. Neuroendocrine design of the gut. Am J Surg 1991; 161:243–249.

Table 17.5.
Causes of Hypergastrinemia

I. Increased Production
   A. Gastrinoma (Zollinger-Ellison syndrome)
   B. Loss of negative feedback inhibition
     1) Achlorhydria
     2) Retained antrum syndrome
   C. G-Cell hyperplasia
     1) Postvagotomy state
     2) Inherited syndrome (Pseudo-Zollinger-Ellison Syndrome)
II. Decreased Metabolism or Excretion
   A. Massive small bowel resection
   B. Renal failure

etal cell. The cell regulation of gastric acid secretion is represented schematically in Figure 17.1.

The gastric phase of acid secretion is mediated largely through the release of antral gastrin. Release of histamine also occurs in the parietal mucosa during the gastric phase. Some of the histamine release is the result of the action of gastrin on mast cell-like cells, but other mechanisms of histamine release may also operate. At any rate, the occupation of their respective receptors by histamine and gastrin leads to a potentiated interaction to stimulate acid secretion. Gastrin acts through the inositol-1,4,5-triphosphate and calcium mechanisms, whereas histamine relies on the stimulation of cAMP as the secondary messenger.

Cell Growth

Gastrin, epidermal growth factor, and insulin are important growth factors that also act as gastrointestinal hormones (9). Gastrin is trophic to the oxyntic mucosa. Hypergastrinemia caused by a gastrinoma or G cell hyperplasia leads to hypertrophy of the gastric rugae in the proximal stomach. Conversely, antrectomy results in long-term atrophy of the oxyntic mucosa. The gastrin effect seems to be directed at the gastric stem cells. Chief cells, which produce pepsinogen, do not originate from

stem cells but rather are generated by division of mature chief cells. These cells do not proliferate in response to gastrin.

The proliferative response to gastrin is also seen in the mucosa of the small intestine and colon, and it appears that the mucosal atrophy and loss of disaccharidases seen during fasting can be prevented by exogenous pentagastrin treatment.

EGF, produced by salivary glands and duodenal Brunner's glands, is a potent stimulant of oxyntic and intestinal mucosa proliferation in mature animals and has a beneficial effect on healing of experimental ulcers. It also seems to play a role in growth and maturation of these gastrointestinal mucosae and of the pancreas in the newborn. EGF can act from the luminal surface, consistent with its presence in luminal secretions and with the abundance of EGF receptors on mucosal enterocytes. Trophic actions have also been attributed to CCK in the pancreas, enteroglucagon in intestinal adaptation to resection, and insulin in the general growth and maturation of the gastrointestinal tract.

Pathologic Conditions of Altered Peptide Secretion

Hypergastrinemia

Hypergastrinemia occurs as a result of excessive gastrin production by an endocrine tumor, loss of negative feedback mechanism to antral acidification, G cell hyperplasia, and defective metabolism or excretion of gastrin (10). Table 17.5 summarizes the causes of hypergastrinemia. A distinction between hypergastrinemia caused by gastrinoma and by G cell hyperplasia is made readily by using the secretin and meal-stimulated tests. Secretin causes a paradoxical release of gastrin from gastrinoma but has little effect on gastrin release from the normal antrum or the antrum with G cell hyperplasia. In contrast, a meal results in a comparatively small release of gastrin in patients with gastrinoma (because of excessive acidification of the meal decreasing the normal meal-induced gastrin stimulation) but an exaggerated gastrin response in subjects with G cell hyperplasia.

Chronic Pancreatitis

The decreased entry of pancreatic enzymes into the duodenum of patients with chronic pancreatitis causes increased release of duodenal CCK into the blood. It has been theorized that this increase in CCK causes the pain experienced by patients with chronic pancreatitis. This hypothesis is the basis for enzyme-replacement therapy to control pain in such patients. Such patients may also have pain from their steatorrhea, which may be controlled by enzyme-replacement therapy.

States of Decreased Stimulation of Gallbladder Contraction

Three conditions result in a prolonged decrease in gallbladder contraction, long-term total parenteral nutrition, prolonged somatostatin-agonist therapy, and somatostatinoma. In the first condition, stimulation of CCK release does not occur when oral feeding is suspended. In the second and third conditions, somatostatin causes inhibition of both the release and action of CCK. In all of the conditions, an increased incidence of gallstones is seen. Periodic treatment with CCK or the oral administration of lipids has been recommended to decrease the incidence of cholelithiasis in such patients.

Somatostatin-secreting tumors are rare. They develop in the pancreas and are characterized by a triad of symptoms, including diarrhea with steatorrhea, mild diabetes, and gallstone formation. These symptoms are the result of the inhibitory action of somatostatin on pancreatic exocrine secretion, insulin secretion, CCK secretion, and gallbladder contraction, respectively.

Carcinoid Syndrome

The carcinoid syndrome is characterized by: (a) diarrhea; (b) crampy abdominal pain and borborygmi; (c) flushing; (d) bronchoconstriction; and (e) the development of valvular insufficiency with a high incidence of tricuspid or pulmonic involvement. Serotonin is now thought to be the mediator of the gastrointestinal symptoms, but the cause of the subendocardial fibrosis that leads to valvular incompetence is unknown. The valves in the left heart are protected to a relative degree because the lung degrades serotonin. The vasoactive symptoms are thought to result from the release of kinins and peptides such as tachykinins (substance P and substance K), VIP, and neurotensin. Again, somatostatin agonist therapy is effective in controlling the symptoms of this disease.

Dumping Syndrome

Excessive dumping of chyme into the intestine when the pylorus is removed, destroyed, or bypassed results in characteristic gastrointestinal and systemic symptoms. The early dumping syndrome consists of abdominal pain followed by diarrhea, fatigue, palpitations, sweating, and sometimes flushing. These symptoms are caused both by a reduction in circulating volume owing to osmotic fluid shifts into the gut lumen and by the release of vasoactive amines and peptides (11,12). So-

matostatin agonist therapy has been effective in this condition too.

The late dumping syndrome occurs 2 or more hours after the ingestion of food and is manifested by symptoms of hypoglycemia. Excessive insulin secretion occurs during the meal and this outlasts the initial hyperglycemic response. Somatostatin agonist therapy inhibits the initial hyperglycemia, reduces the release of insulin, and prevents the symptoms of hypoglycemia.

Swallowing and Esophageal Physiology

Swallowing

Swallowing consists of two phases: an oral phase and a pharyngeal phase (13). The oral phase consists of propelling material backward by squeezing the tongue against the palate in an anterior to posterior sequence. The pharyngeal phase begins when the bolus reaches the posterior surface of the tongue, at which time the pharyngeal swallow response is triggered. The pharyngeal swallow response is composed of several closely coordinated actions: (a) elevation and retraction of the soft palate with closure of the nasopharynx (levator veli palatini, tensor veli palatine, and palatopharyngeus muscles); (b) anterior superior displacement of the larynx (mylohyoideus, geniohyoideus, digastricus, stylohyoideus, stylopharyngeus, salpingopharyngeus, and thyrohyoideus muscles); (c) laryngeal closure at the level of the epiglottis, false vocal folds, and true vocal folds (thyroarytenoideus, aryepiglotticus, and oblique arytenoideus muscles); (d) relaxation and opening of the upper esophageal sphincter (cricopharyngeus muscle); and (e) initiation of the pharyngeal contraction that propels the bolus into the open inlet of the esophagus (pharyngeal constrictors, tongue). The functional rearrangement of the pharynx during swallow is shown in Figure 17.2. Swallowing is orchestrated by the swallowing center, which is in the nucleus of the solitary tract and the underlying reticular substance, 2 to 4 mm rostral to the obex (14).

Upper Esophageal Sphincter

The upper esophageal sphincter (UES) functions as an integral part of both the esophagus and the pharynx (15). Viewed in cross-section, the closed sphincter has a slit configuration, with the lamina of the cricoid cartilage comprising the anterior wall and the cricopharyngeus attached in a "C" configuration making up the lateral and posterior walls. Resting pressure within the UES exhibits marked radial asymmetry, with greater pressures recorded anteriorly and posteriorly than laterally. UES pressure is composed of both an active component,

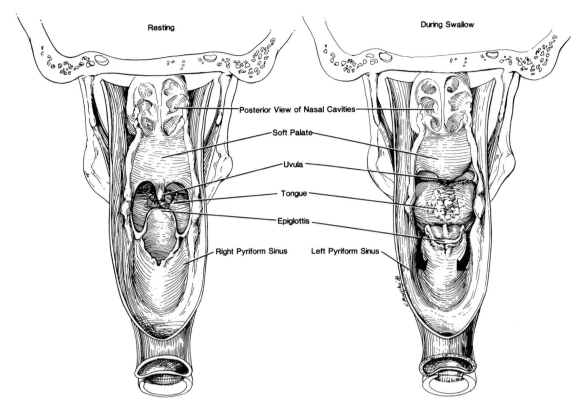

Resting

During Swallow

Posterior View of Nasal Cavities

Soft Palate

Uvula

Tongue

Epiglottis

Right Pyriform Sinus   Left Pyriform Sinus

Figure 17.2. Posterior view of the pharynx with the pharyngeal constrictors cut at the midline and laid open to reveal the anterior pharyngeal wall. The pyriform sinuses can be seen as the spaces between the lateral aspects of the larynx and the pharyngeal constrictors. On the right side is the anatomic configuration during a swallow with the larynx elevated and closed; on the left side, the larynx is in its resting, open position. The *arrows* show the bilateral path taken by swallowed material. From Kahrilas PJ. The anatomy and physiology of dysphagia. In: Gelfand DW, Richter JE, eds. Dysphagia, diagnosis, and treatment. New York: Igaku-Shoin, 1989.

related to cricopharyngeal contraction, and a passive component, attributable to tissue elasticity (about 10 mm Hg). The active component of UES pressure is augmented during inspiration, phonation, emotional stress, and balloon distension of the esophagus. Although controversial, the evidence suggests that acidification of the esophageal mucosa has no effect on UES pressure. UES pressure during sleep and anesthesia in humans is typically about 10 mm Hg. Thus, in the absence of modifying stimuli, passive elasticity maintains closure of the LES.

During swallowing, the UES both relaxes and opens. Video fluoroscopic studies done concurrently with intraluminal manometry have shown that UES relaxation occurs during swallow-associated laryngeal elevation and precedes the opening of the sphincter by about 0.1 sec. Sphincter opening results from traction on the anterior sphincter wall caused by contraction of the suprahyoid and infrahyoid musculature, which also results in a characteristic pattern of hyoid displacement. Sphincter closure coincides with the arrival of the propagated pharyngeal contraction. Upper esophageal sphincter relaxation also occurs as part of the belch reflex. The stimulus triggering UES relaxation during belching is the distension of a long segment of the esophageal body by gas reflux. Thus, the esophageal response to sudden distension of a long portion of the esophageal body is the opposite of balloon distension of a discrete segment.

Esophageal Body

The esophageal body is a 20 to 22-cm long muscular tube composed of striated muscle proximally and smooth muscle distally. Myenteric plexus neurons reside between the longitudinal and circular muscle layers. These enteric neurons are the relay neurons between the vagus and the smooth muscle; their function in the striated muscle esophagus is obscure. Two predominant types of effector neurons exist within the esophageal myenteric plexus. Excitatory neurons mediate contraction of both longitudinal and circular muscle layers via cholinergic receptors. Inhibitory neurons affect predominantly the circular muscle layer via a nonadrenergic, noncholinergic peptide neurotransmitter. The extrinsic innervation of the esophagus is via the vagus nerve. Fibers innervating the striated muscle originate in the nucleus ambiguous and synapse directly on striated muscle neuromuscular junctions. Innervation of the esophageal smooth muscle is provided by the dorsal motor nucleus of the vagus. Sensory nerves in the esophagus are stimulated strongly by esophageal distension, an effect mediated by peptidergic neurons.

Primary peristalsis in the esophagus is initiated by swallowing, whereas secondary peristalsis is elicited at any level of the esophagus in response to luminal distension. A second swallow, initiated while an earlier peristaltic contraction is still progressing in the striated muscle esophagus, causes rapid and complete inhibition of the contraction induced by the first swallow. With a series of swallows at short intervals, the esophagus remains inhibited and quiescent until after the last swallow in the series, when a normal peristaltic contraction occurs. Primary peristalsis is a stripping wave that empties the esophagus from its proximal to distal end (16) (Fig. 17.3). The longitudinal muscle of the esophagus also contracts at the onset of peristalsis; the net effect is a transient shortening of the structure by 2.0 to 2.5 cm.

The physiologic control mechanisms governing the striated and smooth esophageal musculature are distinct. The striated muscle of the esophagus receives exclusively excitatory vagal innervation, and peristaltic contraction results from the sequential activation of motor units in a craniocaudal sequence. The organization of peristalsis in the striated muscle esophagus is subject to control from within the swallowing center of the medulla in much the same way as is the oropharyngeal musculature. Vagal control of the smooth muscle esophagus is more complex. Vagal fibers synapse on myenteric plexus neurons rather than directly at neuromuscular junctions. Vagal fibers going to the smooth muscle fire in succession during primary peristalsis to facilitate activation of the intramural neurons, which are able to organize peristalsis. No vagal activity occurs during secondary peristalsis, confirming that the organization of peristalsis in the smooth muscle is an intramural process. Single fiber recordings have described two populations of vagal fibers going to smooth muscle, those whose activity coincided with deglutitive inhibition and others whose discharge correlated temporally with the onset on contraction at each esophageal segment.

Lower Esophageal Sphincter

Physiologically, the lower esophageal sphincter (LES) is a 3 to 4-cm-long segment of tonically contracted smooth muscle at the distal end of the esophagus. Resting tone of the LES varies among individuals from 10 to 30 mm Hg relative to intragastric pressure. Lower esophageal sphincter pressure is lowest in the postprandial state and highest at night. Intra-abdominal pressure, gastric distension, peptide hormones, various foods, and many drugs affect the LES pressure. Inspiratory augmentation of LES pressure corresponds both temporally and quantitatively with electromyographic activity of the diaphragmatic crux (17). Intrinsic LES tone is found to be equivalent to end expiratory tone,

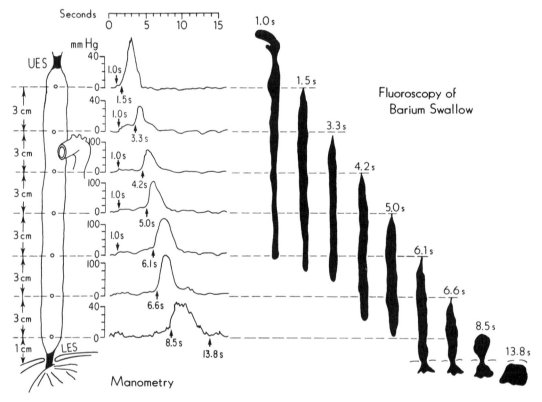

Figure 17.3.   Concurrent manometric and video recording of a barium swallow. The fluoroscopic tracings on the right show the distribution of the barium column at the times indicated above the individual tracings and by *arrows* on the manometric record. A single peristaltic sequence completely cleared the barium bolus from the esophagus. Pharyngeal injection of barium into the esophagus occurs at the 1.0-sec mark. During peristalsis, luminal closure and hence the tail of the bolus passed each recording site concurrent with the onset of the pressure wave. Thus, at 1.5 sec, the contraction had just reached the proximal recording site and barium had been stripped from the esophagus proximal to that point. From Kahrilas PJ, et al. The effect of peristaltic dysfunction on esophageal volume clearance. Gastroenterology. 1988;94:73–80.

suggesting that in normal circumstances, the diaphragm augments LES pressure only during inspiration. The mechanism of LES tonic contraction is not fully understood, but seems to be a physiologic property of the muscle itself rather than of nerves innervating the sphincter. Basal LES tone is inhibited by swallowing, in parallel with the deglutitive inhibition that traverses the smooth muscle esophagus. The process inducing relaxation of the LES is identical to that mediating the inhibitory front along the esophagus. The smooth muscle of the sphincter should be viewed as identical to the adjacent circular muscle, except that it maintains a tonic contraction at rest caused by a myogenic mechanism.

Vagal influence on LES pressure is similar to that in the esophageal body. Vagal stimulation activates both excitatory and inhibitory myenteric neurons. Vagal innervation of the LES includes spontaneously active fibers of two types, those that exhibit a sudden increase with swallowing, abruptly cease firing when the peristaltic contraction arrives, and then resume a spontaneous rate, and others that cease activity with swallowing and resume normal activity when the bolus reaches the stomach. Thus, the LES pressure at any instant reflects the balance between excitatory and inhibitory neural input. Altering the pattern of vagal discharge can result in a swallow-mediated LES relaxation. Another complex phenomenon relating to LES pressure was discovered during investigation into the mechanism of gastroesophageal reflux. Despite adequate LES pressure, normal volunteers periodically exhibit gastroesophageal acid reflux as a result of transient episodes of LES relaxation (18). Transient LES relaxations are also a component of the belch reflex. The frequency at which episodes of LES relaxation occur is increased significantly by gaseous distension of the stomach.

Summary

Swallowing involves an oropharyngeal and esophageal phase. The oropharyngeal phase is enacted by the medullary swallowing center and the striated musculature of the oropharynx and is followed by esophageal peristalsis. The esophagus is a muscular tube with a striated muscle sphincter at the top and a smooth muscle sphincter at the bottom. The upper sphincter relaxes and opens briefly during the pharyngeal swallow. The lower sphincter relaxes during esophageal peristalsis and opens as the bolus is propelled into the stomach.

Gastric Secretion

Morphologic-Functional Relationships

Although acid may be the most important secretory product of the stomach, gastric mucosal cells also pro-

Table 17.6.
The Major Secretory Products of the Stomach

Acid	Parietal Cells	Oxyntic Area
Intrinsic Factor	Parietal Cells	Oxyntic Area
Pepsinogens		
Group I	Chief Cells, Mucous Neck Cells	Oxyntic Area
Group II	Chief Cells, Mucous Neck Cells	Oxyntic Area
	Mucous Cells	Cardia and Antrum
Bicarbonate	Mucous Neck Cells	Oxyntic Area
	Mucous Cells	Cardia and Antrum
Mucus	Mucous Neck Cells	Oxyntic Area
	Mucous Cells	Cardia and Antrum
Gastrin	G Cells	Antrum
Serotonin	Enterochromaffin Cells	Oxyntic Area and Antrum
Somatostatin	D Cells	Oxyntic Area and Antrum

duce and secrete into the lumen several other important molecules. As detailed in Table 17.6, these include mucus, bicarbonate, pepsinogens, intrinsic factor, and small concentrations of such humoral mediators as gastrin, somatostatin, prostaglandins, and serotonin. To synthesize this array of biologically important products, the gastric mucosal glands contain specialized cells, each of which has a specific biosynthetic role.

The stomach has traditionally been subdivided into four anatomic sections: the cardia, fundus, corpus, and antrum. Although subtle microscopic differences exist between the fundus and corpus, these two zones have considerable functional overlap. As a result, they are generally considered together as the oxyntic portion of the stomach, and their glands are referred to as oxyntic or parietal glands. As demonstrated in Figure 17.4, the parietal cells are scattered within the epithelium of the oxyntic glands, the chief cells occupy a basilar portion, and the mucous neck cells are predominately located closer to the faveolus. The epithelium of oxyntic glands consists of approximately 35% parietal cells, 25% chief cells, 20% nonspecific mucosal cells, 10% mucous neck cells, and 10% enteroendocrine cells.

Parietal cells have unique morphologic characteristics that facilitate their specialized role. They are heavily laden with mitochondria, which occupy one-third of the cytoplasm. This attests to the enormous energy requirements for gastric acid secretion. The secretory process is carried out on microvilli of the secretory canaliculi. These organelles are quite abundant and face the gastric lumen. The surface area of the microvilli increases dramatically during stimulation of acid secretion by recruitment of and fusion with adjacent tubovesicles (19).

The chief cells are also well-suited to their secretory role. The prominent endoplasmic reticulum provides a matrix for the synthesis of pepsinogens. The pro-enzymes are stored within zymogen granules near the lu-

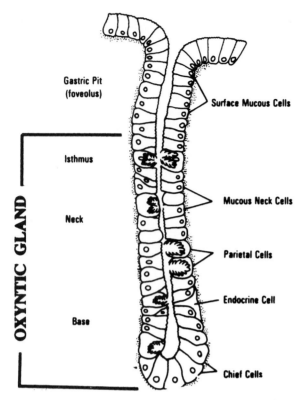

Figure 17.4. Schematic illustration of a typical gastric gland. From Pandol SJ, Isenberg JL. Salivary, gastric, duodenal, and pancreatic secretions. In: West JB, ed. Physiological basis of medical practice. 12th ed. Baltimore: Williams & Wilkins, 1990:652.

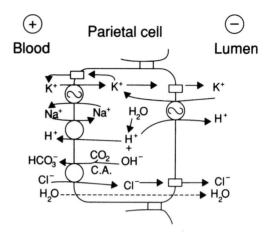

Figure 17.5. A summary of parietal cell transport processes during gastric acid secretion. From LR Johnson. Gastric secretion. In: Johnson LR, ed. Gastrointestinal Physiology. 4th ed. St. Louis: Mosby Year Book, 1991:70.

minal surface of the cells. Release of pepsinogen is thus readily accomplished by exocytosis.

In contrast to the oxyntic area, the antrum contains no parietal cells. Hence, no acid production or release occurs by this portion of the stomach. However, the antrum is the site of G cells. These cells are responsible for gastrin synthesis. G cells are roughly triangular in shape. The narrow portion of the cells contain microvilli that project into the lumen and presumably transmit information regarding lumenal pH and the electrolyte and nutrient conditions to the basally located gastrin-containing granules.

Secretion of Gastric Acid

Physiology

A number of statistics serve to put the secretion of gastric acid in perspective. The oxyntic portion of the stomach contains 1 billion parietal cells. Gastric acid output averages 1 to 2 liters/day. The pH of gastric juice is less than 1.0. Acid is produced in concentrations of 150 to 160 mEq/liter. The gradient in transmembrane hydrogen ion concentrations between the parietal cell cytosol and the gastric lumen is 2.5 million.

Very specialized enzymatic mechanisms have been established to accomplish the ion transport requirements of gastric acid secretion (20). Critical to this pro-

cess are carbonic anhydrase (which catalyzes the reaction of $OH^- + CO_2 = HCO_3^-$) and H^+/K^+-ATPase, Na^+/K^+-ATPase, and HCO_3^-/Cl^- exchanges.

The H^+/K^+-ATPase, a dimer consisting of α- and β-subunits, is responsible for exchanging hydrogen ion for potassium at the secretory canaliculus. The availability of intracellular K^+ at the canaliculus is assured by the Na^+/K^+-ATPase, which pumps sodium out of the parietal cell in exchange for potassium. To maintain intracellular neutrality, chloride is drawn into the parietal cells in exchange for bicarbonate. The extracellular HCO_3^- enters the bloodstream and raises the pH of the gastric venous effluent. Hydrochloric acid and, to a lesser degree, potassium chloride, concentrate at the secretory canaliculus and move through conductive channels into the gastric lumen. This process is illustrated in Figure 17.5.

The overall electrolyte changes during gastric acid secretion are detailed in Table 17.7. The major effects are an increase in chloride secretion and a fall in sodium chloride release by the combined effects of H^+/K^+-ATPase. Water flows passively with the electrolytes in accordance with the osmotic gradients. Because the enzymatic mechanisms are inefficient (e.g., they exchange $2\,K^+$ into the cell in exchange for $3\,Na^+$ out of the cell), a great deal of energy is required. This is derived from ATP synthesized by the mitochondria within parietal cells.

Neurohumoral Control

The studies of Soll and his colleagues (21,22) have resulted in the development of a functional model of the parietal cell with three independent receptors, one each for histamine, gastrin, and acetylcholine (Fig. 17.6). When parietal cell H_2 receptors are occupied by the ligand, adenylate cyclase is activated, converting ATP to cAMP. By a series of subsequent reactions, protein ki-

Table 17.7.
Electrolyte Changes in Gastric Juice During Gastric Secretion

Electrolyte	Change	Mechanism
H^+	Increase from 10 to 130 mEq/L	H^+/K^+ ATPase activity
Na^+	Decrease from 150 to 10 mEq/L	Na^+/K^+ ATPase pumps Na^+ out of parietal cells
Cl^-	Increase from 120 to 160 mEq/L	Cl^-/HCO_3^- exchange, concentrating Cl^- within the parietal cell
k^+	Increase from 10 to 20 mEq/L	Overall effect of Na^+/K^+ ATPase and H^+/K^+ ATPase results in a slight increase in parietal cell K^+

Table 17.8.
Phasic Regulation of Acid Secretion

Physiologic Mechanism	Phases		
	Cephalic	Gastric	Intestinal
Stimulus	Smell and sight of food	Gastric distention, nutrients	Nutrients
Pathway	Vagal neurons, CNS neuropeptides	Topical effect, vagovagal reflexes	Topical effect
Mediators	Neural, acetylcholine, gastrin	Gastrin, acetylcholine	Gastrin, enterooxyntin
Inhibition	Vagotomy, CNS neuropeptides	Gastric acidification, somatostatin	Fatty acids, duodenal acidification
Mediator	Sympathetic activity or inhibitional vagal effects	Inhibitional gastrin release	Competition with gastrin (CCK), enterogastrone (neurotensin, GIP, PYY, and serotonin)

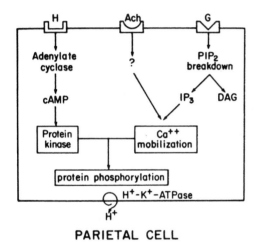

PARIETAL CELL

Figure 17.6. A conceptual model of the parietal cell with independent receptors for gastrin, histamine, and acetylcholine. From Debas HT, Mulholland MW. Drug therapy in peptic ulcer disease. Curr Prob Surg 1989: 26(1):14.

nase C is activated, resulting in protein phosphorylation and stimulation of H^+/K^+-ATPase activity.

The mediators of gastric acid secretion by acetylcholine and gastrin are different from those of histamine, and the final pathways are less well understood. When either or both of these receptors are occupied, phosphoproteins are activated. This results in the breakdown of phosphatidylinositol biphosphate into diacylglycerol and inositol-1,4,5-triphosphate (IP_3). The latter compound mobilizes calcium, increasing the intracellular concentration of this ion. Under these circumstances, calcium ion serves as the second messenger, stimulating a protein kinase (not protein C kinase) and resulting in protein phosphorylation and the subsequent stimulation of the H^+/K^+-ATPase (23).

On a less molecular level, a number of physiologic

mechanisms have been described that stimulate and inhibit gastric acid secretion. These are best described in terms of the phases of secretion. Gastric acid secretion is generally considered to occur in three phases, from the initial cephalic phase through the gastric phase to the final intestinal phase (Table 17.8).

The cephalic phase is mediated predominantly by neural impulses. It is initiated by the sight and smell of food and accounts for as much as 30% of the maximal rate of acid secretion. Although vagotomy abolishes this phase of acid secretion, it is unrealistic to consider this effect as totally mediated via the parietal cell acetylcholine receptor. In fact, vagal stimulation is known to release gastrin, and the gastrin response to sham feeding is 50% of that noted after a protein meal (24). Some evidence also suggests that histamine may play a role in the mediation of all stimulated acid secretion, so its participation in the cephalic phase cannot be disregarded totally.

Neuropeptides have also been implicated in the cephalic phase of acid secretion. The injection of gastrin, thyrotropin-releasing hormone (TRH), and cholecystokinin into the cerebral ventricles has been shown to stimulate gastric H^+ secretion (25). However, intraventricular administration of bombesin, neurotensin, and corticotropin inhibits gastric acid secretion either by abolishing the prostimulatory parasympathetic effects or by inducing sympathetic activity.

The gastric phase of acid secretion is mediated largely by gastrin. In fact, a fairly good correlation exists between the amount of gastrin released by peptones and the amount of acid secreted. Despite this clear role of gastrin, evidence also suggests that local neuronal and vagovagal reflexes also participate in this phase. The three major gastric mechanisms for stimulation of gastric secretion are distension of the stomach, topical application of small peptides and amino acids (particularly phenylamine and tryptophan), and hypercalcemia (26). In contrast, inhibition of gastrin release suppresses the gastric phase of acid secretion. This can be accomplished by duodenal acidification or the administration of somatostatin.

The intestinal phase of gastric acid secretion is so designated because the acid secretory effect occurs long after the nutrients have emptied from the stomach. The stimuli for this phase are similar to those involved in the gastric phase. Gastric acid secretion is associated with the administration of amino acids into the duodenum and proximal jejunum. Although duodenal gastrin appears to be predominantly responsible, it has long been postulated that the proximal intestine secretes enterooxyntin, an intestinal hormone that directly stimulates gastric acid secretion. Unfortunately, no specific enterooxyntin has yet been well characterized.

There are two discrete mechanisms for intestinal phase inhibition of acid secretion. The first involves cholecystokinin, which shares substantial structural homology with gastrin. Because CCK is a weak stimulator of acid secretion, when this duodenal hormone occupies gastrin receptors, it competitively inhibits gastric secretion by displacing the more active ligand, gastrin, from the receptors. The second inhibitory mechanism involves one or more enterogastrones. The most likely humoral candidate for this role is neurotensin, but gastric inhibitory peptide (GIP), PYY, and serotonin have also been implicated (27).

Medications That Inhibit Gastric Acid Secretion

Pharmacologic competitors have been developed for two of the three parietal cell receptors. These agents play an important clinical role in the control of gastric acid hypersecretion.

Clinically, the most important of these are the H_2 receptor blockers. A number of H_2 receptor blocking agents have been developed. Although they effectively inhibit gastric acid secretion, they also inhibit histamine-mediated effects on such diverse organs as the atrium of the heart and the fundus of the uterus (28). These drugs also bind nonspecifically to androgen receptors (29) as well as those on the microsomal oxidase system of the liver, lymphocytes, and central nervous system. The quest for the ideal H_2 receptor blocker will end when an agent is found that binds only to the H_2 receptors on parietal cells.

Until recently, anticholinergics had produced such serious side effects (blurred vision, dry mouth, increased pulse rate, and urinary retention) that they were not clinically useful. The doses tolerated caused only 30% inhibition of gastric acid secretion, 50% of that achieved by H_2 receptor blockers. However, a relatively new agent, pirenzepine, appears to bind selectively only

to M_1 receptors. These are the receptors that are associated with gastric postganglionic cholinergic fibers (30). Because the drug does not interact with the muscarinic receptors on the heart (31), bladder, or eye, this agent is better tolerated than any previous anticholinergic medication. Unfortunately, no effective gastrin receptor blockers have yet been developed.

Regardless of the stimulus or mediator, gastric acid is generated by the proton pump. Thus, an inhibitor of the proton pump would be an effective modality in the control of gastric acid secretion. The first such drug, omeprazole (32), becomes active within the secretory canaliculus only when acid secretion is stimulated. At a pH of 2 or less, omeprazole is protonated, concentrated at the secretory canaliculus, and converted to a sulfonamide. This latter derivative inhibits H^+/K^+-ATPase by covalently binding to sulfhydryl groups of the α-chain of the enzyme. Restoration of acid secretion requires parietal cell biosynthesis of new enzyme, so the half-life of this effect is 12 to 18 hours. Because of its mode of action, omeprazole is specific, but it does create one potential problem. The drug is so effective in abolishing acid secretion that it results in hypergastrinemia, and at least in rats, this hormonal imbalance causes massive proliferation of enterochromaffin cells. Ultimately, these result in the development of carcinoid tumors (33). Fortunately, there have been no reports of omeprazole-induced carcinoids in humans.

Secretion of Other Products

Pepsinogens

Pepsinogens are the proenzyme forms of gastric peptidases. Below pH 2, they become active pepsins by autocatalysis, which occurs when they lose a specific portion of their amino terminus. There are three principal molecular forms: pepsinogen I (synthesized in the oxyntic area), pepsinogen II (which is also synthesized in the antrum and duodenum), and the slow-moving protease (34). Inexplicably, pepsinogens I and II can be identified in the systemic circulation by radioimmunoassay. The synthesis and storage of pepsinogens are similar to that for pancreatic enzymes. Their release is almost entirely by exocytosis. Secreted predominantly by chief cells, the rate of their secretion parallels that of gastric acid.

Intrinsic Factor

Intrinsic factor is a 45,000-dalton glycoprotein whose sole responsibility is the luminal binding of vitamin B_{12} to facilitate its absorption in the ileum. Parietal cell secretion of intrinsic factor occurs via membrane translocation (35). This secretory process parallels that of gastric acid in that it is stimulated by the histamine, gastrin, and acetylcholine receptors. However, in contrast to acid, once all the stored glycoprotein has been released into the lumen, its secretion stops until more of the glycoprotein can be synthesized.

Mucus

Gastric mucus is incredibly viscous and protects the gastric mucosa from peptic or acid digestion by forming a 0.2-mm-thick protective barrier between the lumen and the epithelial surface. These large glycoproteins also provide a lubricated surface that aids in the passage of nutrients and small particles out of the stomach. Gastric mucus is synthesized by mucous cells as glycoprotein mucins.

The principal carbohydrate moieties are oligosaccharides, containing galactose, fructose, and *N*-acetyl-glucose. When mucins are hydrated, the material becomes mucus, which is secreted by exocytosis, rapid apical expulsion, and mucosal cell exfoliation.

Bicarbonate

The other secretion that protects the gastric mucosa is bicarbonate ion (36). Bicarbonate secretion by mucous cells is stimulated by sham feeding and cholinergic agonists. Thus it seems to be produced by the same stimuli that are responsible for acid. Released bicarbonate binds to the epithelial side of the mucus layer and keeps the pH at the surface of the stomach at or close to 7, despite the ongoing acid secretion into the lumen. The exact physiologic mechanisms of gastric bicarbonate secretion are unknown but seem to involve diffusion according to pH gradients, an anion HCO_3^- carrier at the basolateral surface, a glucagon-responsive Cl^-/HCO_3^- exchange, and a prostaglandin (cAMP-sensitive active bicarbonate transporter).

Gastric Motility

All of the major functions of the stomach—storage, digestion, and propulsion of ingested food—require involvement of the contractile activity of gastric smooth muscle. There are many control mechanisms, including myogenic, neural, and chemical components, that coordinate the diverse range of gastric function (37–40).

Myogenic Control

When examined in vitro, smooth muscle cells from different regions of the stomach have unique patterns of electrical activity. In cells from the distal stomach, the resting membrane potential is more negative and unstable than in cells from the fundus. Antral cells spontaneously depolarize. The voltage magnitude of the depolarization is greatest in the most distal stomach, whereas the cycle frequency of depolarization is highest in the mid-stomach (37).

As in the heart, gastric smooth muscle cells with the highest frequency of depolarization entrain and drive the slower cells that surround them. The cells with the highest frequency are two-thirds of the way up, along the greater curvature, and depolarize at 3 cycles/min. This has been called the *pacesetter potential*, or electrical control activity (ECA) (39) (Fig. 17.7).

When release of acetylcholine produces a sufficient change in membrane voltage to open calcium channels, a contraction occurs (37). The electrical correlate of a contraction is electrical response activity (ERA), also called a spike (39). There is a one-to-one relationship between ERA and contraction. Although each oscillation of the pacesetter potential may not result in a contraction, contractions cannot occur more often than the ECA frequency of about three spikes/min (39) (see Fig. 17.7).

Neural Control

There is extrinsic innervation of the stomach. It includes mechanosensitive vagal afferents that respond to passive distension and to antral contraction. Neurol control also includes slow-responding chemosensitive vagal afferents. In addition, mechanosensitive and chemosensitive splanchnic afferents exist. These fibers travel through the mesenteric nerves to prevertebral ganglia before reaching the spinal cord (37).

Vagal efferents are both excitatory and inhibitory. The excitatory efferents are parasympathetic cholinergic fibers that increase both fundic tone and antral contraction, and constrict the pylorus. The inhibitory efferents are noradrenergic, noncholinergic fibers and produce fundic relaxation, inhibit antral contraction, and relax the pylorus. These neurons probably release vasoactive

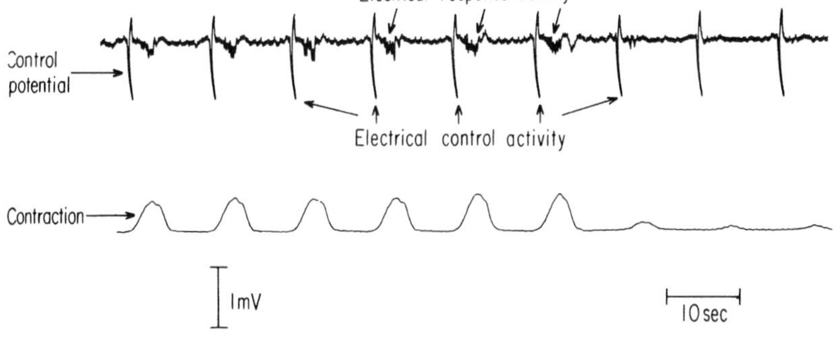

Figure 17.7. Simultaneous myoelectric-contractile recording from the antrum of a dog, illustrating both electrical control activity and electrical response activity. In addition, the 1:1 relationship between ERA and contractions is shown clearly.

intestinal peptide (VIP) as one neurotransmitter. Sympathetic efferents that course through the celiac ganglia may inhibit gastric contractile activity through modulation of intrinsic neurons or through the release of norepinephrine (37).

The intrinsic innervation of the stomach includes both the submucosal and myenteric plexuses. The ability of the stomach to adjust to and continue to function after complete extrinsic denervation is a testimony to the sophistication of the enteric nervous system.

Chemical Control

It is difficult to draw conclusions regarding the role of various hormones in modulating gastric function in the postprandial period. Early studies were performed after ingestion of nonnutrient meals with very high doses of drugs or hormones. These experiments probably have little to do with normal postprandial motility. However, new specific cholecystokinin (CCK) antagonists have been used to demonstrate that CCK does indeed slow gastric emptying after a meal (37).

Fasting Contractile Activity

Because the control mechanisms and contractile patterns of the stomach are so different from those of the small intestine, it is impossible to extrapolate from one to the other. However, in the fasting state, the stomach exhibits cyclic patterns of contractile activity that bear some similarity to the phases of the small intestinal migrating myoelectric (motor) complex (MMC). Because all phases of this cyclic activity start simultaneously in the fundus, corpus, and antrum of the stomach, the contractile activity is called cyclic motor activity (CMA) rather than MMC (39).

Cyclic motor activity is divided into four phases (Figs. 17.8 and 17.9). Phase I is the quiescent state. Gastric phase II activity consists of intermittent contractions that have a smaller amplitude than those of phase III. Gastric phase III is characterized by maximal contractile activity in the stomach and lasts for 10 to 25 minutes. In contrast to what occurs in the small intestine, gastric smooth muscle generally does not contract at its maximal possible frequency. Instead, gastric contractions during phase III occur as groups of two or three contractions, which occur every 1 to 3 minutes. The overall frequency is less than the maximum electrical frequency of 3 cycles/min. Phase IV follows phase III and also consists of intermittent contractions.

Postprandial Motility

The three major functions of the stomach are storage, digestion, and propulsion of ingested food toward the absorptive surface of the small bowel. When food is ingested, the tonic contraction of the proximal stomach is reduced. This allows consumption of food without a dramatic increase in intragastric pressure. The tone of the lower esophageal sphincter tends to increase, although this change depends on the volume and content of the ingested meal.

After the ingestion of solid or semisolid food, the stomach contributes substantially to the breakdown of nutrients which has already begun in the mouth by the process of mastication. This is accomplished through the contraction of the distal stomach (antrum) and the closure of the pylorus. The gastric luminal contents are mixed with gastric exocrine secretions and ground in a process called trituration. Ingested liquids are emptied rapidly from the stomach and are replaced by secreted digestive juices.

As a meal empties from the stomach, the process of spreading the nutrients across the absorptive surface of

Figure 17.8. Cyclic motor activity within the stomach and the MMC in the duodenum are illustrated through the use of extraluminal strain gauge transducers. A small *arrow* designates the end of phase III at each recording site. The location of each strain gauge transducer is indicated at the left of the tracing. **A,** Normal fasting contractile activity; cycling can be seen. **B,** Demonstrates the disruption CMA and the MMC after ingestion of a solid meal. CMA does not resume for approximately 6 hours.

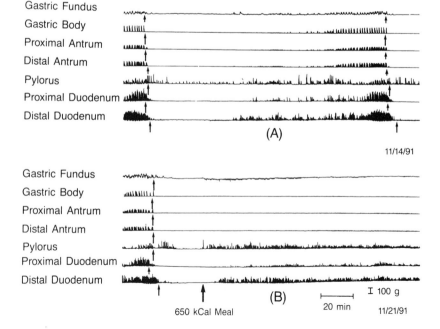

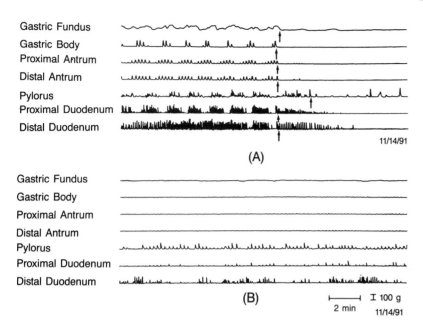

Gastric Fundus
Gastric Body
Proximal Antrum
Distal Antrum
Pylorus
Proximal Duodenum
Distal Duodenum

11/14/91

(A)

Gastric Fundus
Gastric Body
Proximal Antrum
Distal Antrum
Pylorus
Proximal Duodenum
Distal Duodenum

(B)

I 100 g
2 min   11/14/91

Figure 17.9. A less condensed tracing of both fasted and postprandial contractile activity. **A,** Normal phasic contractile activity. **B,** Gastric and duodenal contractile activity 20 minutes after the ingestion of a 650-kcal solid meal (see Figure 17.8 for details).

the small intestine begins. In humans, gastric emptying depends on at least five factors: the content of the meal; gastric tone; antryopyloroduodenal coordination; the transport function of the small intestine; and gravity.

The content of the ingested meal influences the rate of gastric emptying. Fats empty more slowly than do carbohydrates. Liquids empty more rapidly than do solids. Gastric tone seems to be most important in the initial accommodation to the volume of the meal and in the rapid emptying of the liquid portion of a meal. In contrast, antropyloric coordination is responsible for the grinding function of the stomach. Because of this grinding, essentially all nutrients that exit the stomach are either in liquid or semiliquid form. The pyloroduodenal area may play an important role in gastric emptying. Some evidence exists that transport of nutrients along the length of the entire small bowel is important for adequate gastric emptying to occur (40). When the small intestine is exposed to fat, gastric emptying is slowed. Finally, gravity may contribute to the rate of gastric emptying. Gastric emptying of a nonnutrient isotonic liquid is accelerated in the right decubitus position in humans.

In summary, the initiation and modulation of both fasting cyclic motor activity and postprandial gastric contractions appear to be under the control of the enteric nervous system (neuroendocrine control), the central nervous system (neural control), and circulating hormones (chemical control). The maximum frequency and characteristics of gastric contractions are the result of the intrinsic myogenic properties of gastric smooth muscle (myogenic control).

Vomiting

The digestive tract serves two roles in vomiting: a sensory reflex function to determine when emesis should be initiated, and a motor function to assist the emetic process. The sensory reflex function should not be confused with nausea. Although nausea often occurs in close association with vomiting and is a sensation associated with the digestive tract, its relationship with the digestive tract is not well-understood.

Sensory Functions

The digestive tract contains many sensory elements of the vomiting reflex (41). Mechanoreceptors, activated by either pinching the seromuscular layer, rubbing the mucosa, or by the presence of wall distension (or lumen occlusion), have been found in the stomach, jejunum, and ileum. Chemoreceptors, probably located in the mucosa, have a similar distribution and can be activated by various irritants, including hydrochloric acid, cupric sulfate, vinegar, and hypertonic saline. Regardless of the type of receptor, the proximal duodenum and stomach are the most sensitive regions. Delayed gastric emptying and gastric atony have been associated with emesis, but no experimental evidence exists that these altered motor states directly cause vomiting (41).

Both vagus and splanchnic nerves carry afferent fibers from these emetic receptors, but their receptive fields differ and the vagal input may be more important (41). Vagotomy, but not splanchnicectomy, blocks vomiting that is activated by mechanical and chemical stimulation of the stomach. Spinal cord transection at C7-T1, but not vagotomy, blocks ileal obstruction-induced vomiting. In contrast, centripetal electrical stimulation of either the gastric branch of the vagus nerve or the abdominal vagal trunks readily activates vomiting. These receptors also mediate vomiting initiated by peritonitis, x-ray exposure, and cancer chemotherapeutic agents. Vagotomy and splanchnicectomy block these effects, but the nature or specific location of these receptors is not known. X-ray or chemotherapeutic agent-induced emesis may be mediated by serotonin 3 (5-HT$_3$) receptors in the digestive tract (42). The location of these receptors is uncertain because 5-HT$_3$ antagonists do not block cupric sulfate-induced vomiting and 5-HT$_3$ receptors have also been located at central vagal afferent terminals. Receptors in the digestive tract are probably not involved in motion-induced vomiting because abdominal vagotomy and splanchnicectomy do not consistently affect this response (41).

Motor Functions

Vomiting is often defined as the oral evacuation of gastric contents, but this description is inaccurate and incomplete. The physiologic motor events that contribute to a vomit are productive only if there are gastric contents to expel. In addition, regurgitation and belching also result in gastrooral reflux and are controlled by different physiologic mechanisms. Three sets of digestive tract events provide the major motor functions that contribute to vomiting (41–43).

The Gastrointestinal Motor Correlates.   The gastrointestinal motor correlates of vomiting include two distinct and sequential events: a large amplitude contraction that begins at the mid small intestine and propagates retrograde through the gastric antrum (the retrograde giant contraction (RGC)), and a series of moderate amplitude phasic contractions that occur primarily in the lower small intestine (the post-RGC phasic contractions (Fig. 17.10). The RGC begins about 1 minute before vomiting and it propagates at about 8 to 10 cm/sec. The RGC retropels contents of the upper small intestine to the stomach in a single mass movement in preparation for vomiting, but the RGC does not participate in gastrooral reflux during vomiting. The post-RGC phasic contractions last for about 5 to 10 minutes and move the contents of the lower small intestine into the colon in a stripping fashion.

Initiation of the gastrointestinal motor correlates of vomiting is mediated by the vagus nerves (43). The fibers innervating the jejunum pass through the celiac branch of the vagus nerve, reaching the small intestine via the mesenteric nerves. Extrinsic denervation, transection, myotomy, or even mechanical injury of the intestinal wall can block the occurrence of the RGC locally and for a short distance distally (25 to 40 cm) without blocking the orad propagation of the RGC across the dysfunctional segment. These findings indicate that the orad propagation of the RGC is controlled largely by the central nervous system. The vagal fibers that control initiation of these gastrointestinal responses synapse in the enteric nervous system, but the RGC and the post-RGC phasic contractions are mediated by different neuromuscular transmitters. The RGC is mediated by acetylcholine, but the transmitter mediating the post-RGC phasic contractions is unknown (42). Neither response

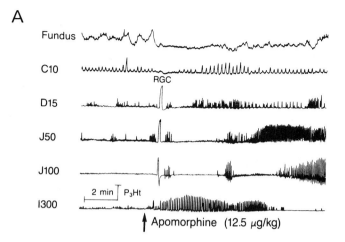

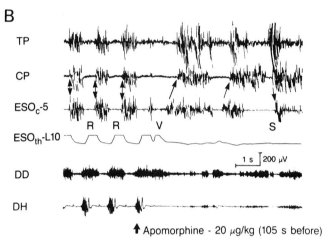

Figure 17.10.   The digestive tract motor responses associated with vomiting. **A,** The gastrointestinal responses recorded using force transducers. **B,** The pharyngoesophageal responses recorded using electromyography. *C,* gastric corpus; *D,* duodenum; *J,* jejunum; *I,* ileum; *P^{3}Ht,* height of phase III of the migrating motor complex; *TP,* thyropharyngeus; *CP,* cricopharyngeus; *ESO^c,* cervical esophagus; *ESOth,* thoracic esophagus; *DD,* diaphragmatic dome; *DH,* diaphragmatic hiatus; *R,* retching; *V,* vomiting; *S,* swallowing. Numbers of recording devices indicate distance from the pylorus (**A**) or cricopharyngeus (**B**).

is mediated by peripheral dopaminergic, adrenergic, serotonergic, or opioid receptors. Under normal physiologic conditions, the gastrointestinal motor correlates of vomiting always occur before retching begins, but they can occur without progressing to retching and vomiting. This suggests that the motor responses controlled by the vomiting center are organized in series (41).

The function of the gastrointestinal motor correlates of vomiting have not been examined experimentally, but some conclusions can be drawn from known physiologic evidence (41,42). One function is to move noxious or poisonous substances from the small intestine to the stomach for expulsion during vomiting or to the colon for expulsion during defecation. An additional function may be to dilute or buffer the acid-peptic gastric juice with intestinal, Brunner's gland, or pancreaticobiliary secretions before expulsion through the esophagus. The relatively unprotected mucosa of the esophagus is prone to injury by the reflux of gastric secretions.

The Esophagogastric Motor Correlates. The lower esophageal sphincter and proximal stomach relax at about the same time the RGC is initiated in the small intestine (see Fig. 17.10). Relaxation of the LES lasts about 2 minutes, but gastric fundic relaxation lasts about 10 minutes. There is no contractile activity of the thoracic esophagus associated with vomiting. Relaxation of both the proximal stomach and LES is mediated by the release of VIP from the vagus nerves (41).

The Pharyngoesophageal Motor Correlates. The pharynx and cervical esophagus exhibit four distinct sets of responses associated with vomiting: (*a*) increased swallowing; (*b*) increased tone before retching; (*c*) rhythmical relaxation and contraction during retching; and (*d*) active reflux during vomitus expulsion (see Fig. 17.10). About 1 minute before vomiting, swallow frequency increases and remains at this level for about 8 minutes. The function of this increased swallowing frequency is unknown, but like the RGC, increased swallowing of saliva may help dilute or buffer gastric secretions before gastroesophageal reflux. Between 10 and 20 seconds before retching, the cervical esophagus contracts in the longitudinal axis. The result of this longitudinal contraction of the cervical esophagus is to pull the relaxed proximal stomach into the thoracic cavity.

After the preparatory functions of the RGC, swallowing and longitudinal contraction of the cervical esophagus have set the stage. Retching begins at the diaphragmatic dome and hiatal fibers and anterior abdominal muscles contract simultaneously (42). During retching, the pharynx and cervical esophagus relax and contract 180° out of phase with contractions of the respiratory muscles. The results of retching are to move the gastric contents into the esophagus. The number of retches activated per vomit varies considerably, depending on the stimulus, stimulus intensity, stomach contents, and probably other undefined factors. The function of retching is unknown, but it may be a method to maximize momentum of the vomitus. During retching, when the LES and proximal stomach are relaxed, effective gastroesophageal reflux may not occur because of the contraction of the hiatal fibers. However, during vomitus expulsion, when contraction of the rectus abdominis and diaphragmatic dome are maximum, the hiatal fibers relax. This relaxation allows the full force of abdominal pressure and gastric elasticity to propel its contents through the proximal stomach and LES to the relaxed esophagus and pharynx. When the vomitus reaches the cervical esophagus, it is prevented from returning to the stomach by a contraction of the cervical esophagus, which propagates retrograde at 10 to 12 cm/sec to the pharyngeal muscles. This esophagopharyngeal retrograde contraction may be responsible for projectile vomiting. Just before this retrograde contraction, the geniohyoid muscle contracts strongly and actively opens the relaxed upper esophageal sphincter. These pharyngoesophageal motor events are probably mediated by cholinergic receptors and controlled by brainstem nuclei as part of the central emetic pattern generator (43). These responses are probably mediated by the pharyngoesophageal nerves, which branch from the vagus just above the nodose ganglia.

Nausea

Mechanical or chemical stimulation of the duodenal, but not gastric or jejunoileal mucosa, can cause nausea. Various changes in digestive tract activity have been associated with nausea, including retrograde movement of intestinal contents, sustained duodenal contractions, the migrating motor complex, delayed gastric emptying, gastric atony, and gastric antral dysrhythmia. However, no experimental evidence suggests that any of these changes in digestive tract activity cause the feeling of nausea (41,42).

Digestion and Absorption

Digestion and absorption of carbohydrates, proteins, and fats occur primarily in the small intestine, although mechanical and chemical processes initiated in the mouth and stomach greatly facilitate their assimilation (44–46).

Digestion or chemical breakdown of food is mediated by hydrolytic enzymes secreted by glandular cells in the oral cavity, chief cells in the stomach, and exocrine cells in the pancreas as well as by hydrolytic enzymes in the brush border of the enterocytes. Digestion is facilitated by bile acids, which aid in the emulsification of lipids and in the solubilization of lipolytic products. The digestive process, which occurs optimally in an acid environment in the stomach, is halted in the intestine by the alkalinizing effect of the bicarbonate secreted by the exocrine pancreas and duodenal epithelium.

Digestion of all three major nutrients involves hydrolysis by specific enzymes. Carbohydrates are hydrolyzed to monosaccharides, proteins to amino acids and small peptides, and triglycerides to free fatty acids and glycerol. Active transport across the small bowel mucosa occurs against concentration gradients for most essential nutrient substrates, including simple sugars (glucose, fructose), electrolytes (sodium, chloride, calcium, magnesium, and iron), amino acids, pyrimidines, long-chain fatty acids, cholesterol, bile salts, folic acid, vitamin B_{12}, and the other water-soluble vitamins (45). The actual site of absorption of a specific nutrient depends somewhat on bowel motility and the intraluminal solute load.

The capacity of the small intestine to absorb nutrients, water, and electrolytes is proportional to the available mucosal surface area. The combination of valvulae con-

Table 17.9.
Gastrointestinal Absorption

Anatomic Site	Nutrient Substrates
Stomach	Water, alcohol
Duodenum	Water, simple sugars, amino acids, free fatty acids, alcohol, vitamins, iron
Proximal jejunum	Electrolytes, carbohydrates, protein, water soluble vitamins
Mid-jejunum	Protein, fat soluble vitamins, fat
Distal jejunum	Bile salts, cholesterol, vitamins, fat
Colon	Water, electrolytes

niventes, intestinal villi, and epithelial brush border greatly increases the total absorptive capacity of the gross anatomic length of the intestine. In addition, there are specialized sites along the gastrointestinal tract at which specific nutrient substrates are absorbed optimally or exclusively (Table 17.9).

Carbohydrate Digestion and Absorption

Dietary carbohydrates consist predominantly of starch, sucrose, and lactose. Other carbohydrates, such as glucose, sorbitol, trehalose, cellulose, hemicellulose, and pectins, comprise about 10% to 12% of dietary carbohydrates (47). Cellulose and hemicellulose are not digestible in humans because of the absence of appropriate enzymes in the gastrointestinal tract. The digestion of starch begins in the mouth with the action of α-amylase secreted by the salivary glands. Amylase hydrolyzes starch into the disaccharide maltose and maltotetrose by disrupting the inner α-1,4-glycosidic bonds. However, some of the starch chains are cross-linked by 1,6-linkages and are thus resistant to the action of amylase and cannot be hydrolyzed. The resultant products formed are α-limit dextrins. Because food is retained in the mouth for only a short time before swallowing, only 3% to 5% of the ingested starch is hydrolyzed in the oral cavity. However, digestion continues in the body and fundus of the stomach until the pH of the gastric contents falls below 4.0, when the action of salivary amylase is inhibited (48). Salivary amylase is not essential for starch digestion except in newborns, in whom pancreatic amylase secretion is insufficient (49).

Before amylase is inactivated by gastric acid secretion, 30% to 40% of the starch reaching the stomach is converted into maltose, isomaltose, and α-limit dextrins. Pancreatic amylase is secreted in the active form and completes the hydrolysis of the remaining starch in the jejunum. The products formed through luminal digestion by amylase, together with the ingested dietary disaccharides (lactose, sucrose, and trehalose), are digested by brush border enzymes, which include maltase, dextrinase, lactase, sucrase, and trehalase. The actions of these enzymes yield glucose, fructose, and galactose (Table 17.10).

Glucose and galactose are transported across the lu-

Table 17.10.
Intestinal Surface Digestion of Dietary Carbohydrates[a]

Carbohydrate Presented

Lactose
Sucrose
Maltose, Maltotriose
Dextrins

Enzyme

Lactase
Sucrase[b]
Sucrase[b] or glycoamylase
Glucoamylase or α-dextrinase
α-dextrinase[c]
Sucrase[b] or glucoamylase

Mechanism of Action

Hydrolysis of β-1, 4-linkage of disaccharide (but not of cellulose)
Hydrolysis of α-1, 4-linkage
Sequential removal of glucosyl residue from nonreducing end
Initial removal of α-1, 4-linked glucose residues from nonreducing end
Cleavage of α-1, 6-linked glucose stub
Hydrolysis of released maltooligosaccharides

Products

Glucose, galactose
Glucose, fructose
Glucose
Oligosaccharide with terminal α-1, 6-linked glucose residues; glucose
Maltooligosaccharides
Glucose

[a] From Gray GM. Carbohydrate absorption and malabsorption. In: Johnson, LR. ed. Physiology of the gastrointestinal tract. New York: Raven Press, 1981;1065.
[b] Having an α-1, 4 glucosidase activity, sucrase is active against maltose and maltotriose (isomaltose).
[c] α-dextrinase is also called isomaltase and cleaves α-1,6 glucoside bonds. It is essential for the removal of the α-1, 6 linked glucose stub from partially hydrolyzed α-dextrins.

minal membrane into the enterocyte by an active transport system in the brush border (49) which uses a common carrier protein that couples the movement of two sugars to one sodium ion (50). Transport of carbohydrates out of the enterocyte into the interstitial space is achieved by sodium-independent carriers that are present in the basolateral membrane. Fructose absorption differs from glucose and galactose absorption because it occurs mainly by facilitated diffusion.

The absorption of hexoses occurs primarily in the duodenum and jejunum and is usually completed as chyme reaches the distal jejunum. Molecules of starch and glucose, although different in size and caloric values, have an identical osmotic effect. Thus, digestion of starch to oligosaccharides and the further breakdown of oligosaccharides to glucose increases the osmolarity in the gut lumen. However, the rapid absorption of monosaccharides after action by brush border enzymes reduces the osmotic pressure and minimizes the potential for drawing fluid into the lumen from the blood. The activity of the brush border enzymes is considerably less in the ileum than in the jejunum.

The capacity of the human small intestine to absorb

free glucose and galactose is enormous, and there appears to be little physiologic control of absorption of these sugars. Normally, the process of carbohydrate absorption is extremely efficient. However, if malabsorption occurs, osmotic diarrhea may result because the carbohydrates remaining in the intestine increase the luminal osmotic pressure. Fermentation of residual carbohydrates by bacteria in the distal ileum and colon further enhances this osmotic effect, adding to net fluid secretion and compounding the diarrhea.

Diarrhea as a result of poor assimilation of carbohydrates is most commonly caused by deficiencies of carbohydrate-splitting enzymes in the intestinal brush border. Lactase deficiency is the most common disaccharidase deficiency and may be associated with long-term intestinal disease or viral enteritis. Intolerance to sucrose and isomaltose is rarely seen because this condition would require the unlikely simultaneous absence of several enzymes that exhibit maltase activity.

Primary absorptive defects that contribute to osmotic diarrhea have also been documented. In cases of glucose and galactose intolerance, patients fed fructose thrive and show no symptoms because fructose is transported by a different mechanism.

Defects in carbohydrate assimilation may be caused by congenital deficiencies in digestive enzymes and transport systems. Poor assimilation may also be related to various disorders of the gastrointestinal tract that cause inflammation, including celiac disease and infections caused by viruses, bacteria, protozoans, and helminths.

Because amylase is ordinarily secreted in tremendous excess, clinically significant deficiencies of this enzyme are very rare, even with pancreatic exocrine deficiency.

Protein Digestion and Absorption

During digestion, proteins undergo degradation into peptides and amino acids. Protein digestion begins with the gastric phase and is influenced by both hormonal and neural factors. Pepsinogen, which is secreted by gastric chief cells in response to ingested meals and low gastric pH, is converted by hydrochloric acid to pepsin, the major gastric protease. Although pepsin is important for breaking down dietary proteins, it is not essential for normal protein digestion and absorption unless pancreatic function is impaired (51). Patients who have undergone total gastrectomy and those with pernicious anemia absorb protein efficiently and maintain positive nitrogen balance if adequate amounts of protein are ingested.

Pepsin is an endopeptidase that has specificity for disrupting peptide bonds involving aromatic l-amino acids (47). Most of the naturally occurring amino acids are l-amino acids, and they are absorbed by different transport systems. When the gastric contents mix with alkaline pancreatic juice in the duodenum, pepsin activ-

ity is terminated, and digestion by pancreatic proteases is initiated. Protein hydrolysis in the intestine results primarily from the action of activated pancreatic enzymes, trypsin, chymotrypsin, and carboxypeptidases. The hydrolysis of proteins to free amino acids and their absorption into the circulation is a stepwise process (52). Gastric hydrolysis of protein yields peptides that stimulate intestinal endocrine cells to release cholecystokinin and secretin, which, in turn, stimulate the pancreas to secrete enzymes and bicarbonate into the intestinal lumen.

The pancreatic endopeptidases (trypsin, chymotrypsin, and elastase) cleave proteins at specific interior peptide bonds, whereas the exopeptidases, mainly carboxypeptidase A and B, sequentially cleave terminal peptide bonds. These pancreatic proteases are secreted in inactive forms and are converted to active enzymes by the combined action of enterokinase, a brush border enzyme, and trypsin. Free amino acids and oligopeptides are the end products of the additive action of endopeptides and exopeptidases. Subsequently, proteases in the brush border contribute to the enzymatic catalytic digestion of the oligopeptides. The brush border oligo peptidases generally cleave the N-terminus amino acids from their substrates and yield smaller peptides.

The final products of protein digestion, amino acids, and dipeptides and tripeptides are absorbed by distinct transport systems (Table 17.11). Whereas protein is absorbed mainly in the form of small peptides and amino acids, the final measurable amino nitrogen in postprandial portal-vein blood is primarily in the form of amino acids (53). Nevertheless, a few small peptides do appear in portal blood after ingestion of protein (54).

Table 17.11.
Intestinal Transport Mechanisms for Amino Acids[a]

Type
Neutral
Dibasic
Dicarboxylic
Amino acids and glycine

Specificity
Aromatic (e.g., tyrosine, tryptophan, phenylalanine) and alipathtic (e.g., alanine, valine, leucine, methionine, serine, glycine)
Diamino acids (e.g., lysine, arginine)
Glutamic acid; aspartic acid
Proline, hydroxproline, glycine

Characteristics
Active transport: very rapid, Na+ dependent
Active: 10% of neutral uptake rate; partially Na+ dependent
Carrier mediated: ? active, partially Na+ derived: rapid
? Active: Na+ dependent; slow; may not be physiologically important because proline and glycine are often absorbed in dipeptide or tripeptide

[a] From Gray GM. Mechanism of digestion and absorption of food. In: Sleisenger MH, Fordtran JS, eds. Gastrointestinal disease: Pathophysiology, diagnosis, management. 3rd ed. Philadelphia: WB Saunders, 1983: 856.

Several transport systems exist for amino acids, but some amino acids (e.g., glycine, proline, and hydroxyproline) may be transported by more than one mechanism. The transport of amino acids across the apical membrane of enterocytes is carrier mediated, sodium dependent, and, characteristically, energy dependent.

Mucosal uptakes of peptides and amino acids are independent processes (52). While oligopeptides apparently can be absorbed by the intestine without first being broken down into individual amino acids, dipeptides and tripeptides are transported actively against a concentration gradient by a separate carrier system. The dipeptide transport propensity is influenced by its structure, including the specific amino acid residues, their position in the carboxyl amino positions, the length of the side chains, and the stereoisomerism. The majority of oligopeptide that are absorbed undergo additional intracellular hydrolysis (55).

The absorption of small peptides may represent a major mechanism for absorption of dietary protein and has important physiologic and clinical implications. For example, consideration of oligopeptide absorption is essential in designing formulas for optimal enteral nutrition.

Absorption of oligopeptides across the brush border occurs more rapidly than the transport of free amino acids. Whereas amino acids are absorbed more rapidly in the proximal intestine, the peptides appear to be absorbed well in both the proximal and distal gut.

Numerous pathologic disorders of the gastrointestinal tract affect protein digestion and absorption and may have subsequent metabolic and nutritional consequences. A marked reduction in the formation of peptides from dietary protein occurs in patients with pancreatic insufficiency. The digestion and absorption of protein is also reduced in celiac disease because of the underlying inflammation that deranges epithelial structure and function. Selective disorders of protein digestion exist, including congenital enterokinase deficiency and trypsinogen-trypsin deficiency. Among selective disorders of amino acid transport, cystinuria (defect in the uptake of basic amino acids) and Hartnup disease (defect in the uptake of neutral amino acids) are well-known.

Resection of long segments of small bowel, or jejunoileal bypass in patients undergoing treatment for obesity, causes protein-calorie malnutrition. This is related to a reduction in amino acid absorption in the functioning jejunum (56). However, dipeptide absorption is not affected significantly by jejunoileal bypass, suggesting a greater resistance of the peptide carrier systems to the effects of malnutrition or to a different spatial distribution in the intestine.

Some diseases are characterized by excretion of proteins from the blood into the gut. They are known as protein-losing enteropathies (57), and include lymphan-giectasia, Whipple's disease, congestive heart failure, and inflammatory bowel disease.

Lipid Digestion and Absorption

The digestion and absorption of lipids, represented by triglycerides or fat, is a complex process that, like protein and carbohydrate digestion and absorption, depends on coordination of the gastric, pancreatic, biliary, and intestinal functions. Unlike carbohydrates and proteins, lipids enter epithelial cells by a sequence of chemical and physical events that render water-insoluble nutrients absorbable in an aqueous phase. Triglyceride assimilation depends on four principal events: (a) secretion and delivery of bile and various lipases to the intestinal lumen; (b) emulsification; (c) enzymatic hydrolysis of ester linkages; and (d) solubilization of lipolytic products within bile salt micelles (47).

Dietary fat, whether of animal or vegetable origin, consists mainly of triglycerides, three long-chain fatty acids attached to a molecule of glycerol (58). Approximately 90% of the fatty acid components in triglycerides consist of palmitic, stearic, oleic, and linoleic fatty acids, each of which contain 16 or 18 carbon atoms. The remaining 10% of fatty acids consist of medium-chain triglycerides composed of 6 to 12 carbon atoms.

The minor lipid components of the diet include phospholipids, sterols, fat-soluble vitamins (A, D, E, and K), and several mostly nonpolar compounds in minute quantities.

Four well-recognized enzymes and one cofactor are involved in the degradation of dietary lipid: lingual lipase, pancreatic lipase with its cofactor colipase, pancreatic carboxylic ester hydrolase, and pancreatic phospholipase A_2 (59).

Lingual lipase hydrolyzes dietary triglycerides in the stomach and is responsible for the presence of 15% to 20% of the free fatty acids in fat recovered from the stomach. This enzyme is stable and functions at acidic pH between 2.2 and 6.0. Lingual lipase acts primarily at the ester linkages in the 1 and 3 positions of triglycerides, producing mainly protonated fatty acid and diglycerides still in the emulsified form. These products are important in promoting the next step in the digestive cycle, i.e., duodenal digestion involving pancreatic lipase-colipase.

The intraluminal phase of digestion of fat continues with the action of pancreatic lipase, which is capable of hydrolyzing triglycerides to 2-monoglycerides and fatty acids. It cannot hydrolyze the ester bond in the 2 position of triglycerides (60). Pancreatic lipase is secreted in an active form, displays optimum activity at pH 8, and remains active at a pH as low as 3. The monoglycerides go unhydrolyzed, which is important for the physical chemistry of fat assimilation. For pancreatic lipase to compete favorably for the glyceride interface, the bile salts must first clear any interfering substances from the interface of the glyceride substrate. Although bile salts inhibit the enzymatic activity of this lipolytic enzyme by physically separating it from its substrate and actually inactivating lipase under physiologic circumstances, this inactivation is prevented by colipase. Colipase, a 102–107 amino acid polypeptide with a molecular weight of 11,000, is secreted by the pancreas as pro-colipase, which is activated when hydrolyzed by trypsin to a 96 amino acid-containing peptide. Colipase binds to lipase and changes its molecular configuration, enabling the lipase to compete with the bile salts for the substrate interface. Lipase and colipase are not abundant within the duodenum during the fasting state. However, the presence of fat stimulates their secretion in large quantities. Once colipase attaches to the oil-water interface, lipase binds to a specific site on the colipase molecule and consequently carries out its catalytic function, breaking down triglycerides. Deficiency of colipase may lead to malabsorption of fat (61).

Phospholipase A$_2$ is secreted in the pancreatic juices as a proenzyme which is activated by trypsin. This enzyme serves as a catalyst for the hydrolysis of the phospholipids, mainly phosphatidylcholine or lecithin, to their lysoform and a free fatty acid (59). Its action extends to both the dietary phospholipids and biliary phospholipids, which are quantitatively more important (62,63). Phospholipase A$_2$ has an absolute requirement for bile salts and calcium in hydrolyzing dietary phospholipids at the 2 position and producing lysophospholipid and free fatty acid.

The second lipid-splitting enzyme in pancreatic juice, similar to lipase, is classified as a carboxylic ester hydrolase. This pancreatic esterase hydrolyzes different types of neutral lipid substrates, including esters of cholesterol, the fat-soluble vitamins A, D, and E, and all three ester linkages of triglycerides. Because of its action on cholesterol esters, it is known as cholesterol esterase. Cholesterol esterase is active against substrates incorporated into bile salt micelles, and its activity depends on the presence of specific bile salts such as taurocholate and taurochenodeoxycholate.

The end products of enzymatic digestion of fat are fatty acids, 2-monoglycerol, and phospholipids disseminated in bile salt solution. Formulation of a mixed micellar solution is a spontaneous and dynamic process involving combinations of bile salts, fatty acids, and monoglycerides. The formation of micelles depends on the types of bile salts present and their concentrations. When a critical micellar concentration is achieved (2 to 5 mM), the molecules aggregate with the lipophilic sites oriented toward the center and with the hydrophilic sites directed outward. The fatty acids and monoglycerides are solubilized in the lipophilic interior of micelles (64). However, diglycerides and triglycerides are too large to be packed into these micelles and thus must undergo further hydrolysis by lipase. Fat-soluble vitamins are solubilized by inclusion in mixed micelles.

Hydrolysis of lipids is rapid in the duodenum. Ninety to 95% of the absorption of fat is completed within the proximal 100 cm of the jejunum. For the products of fat digestion to be absorbed, they must diffuse through two functional barriers, the apical membrane of the intestinal cell and the thin water layer overlying the cell (the unstirred water layer). The diffusion rate depends on the thickness of the unstirred water layer, the concentration gradient across it, and the permeability coefficient of the micelle (65,66). Thus, flux across the unstirred water layer is a function of the concentration gradient over the layer times its permeability (44). Similarly, flux across the membrane is determined by the gradient across the membrane plus the permeability factor. Transport through the unstirred water layer depends on the solubilization of fatty acids in bile salt micelles and is probably the rate-limiting step in the uptake of long-chain fatty acids and other nonpolar compounds such as cholesterol.

It is uncertain where the mixed micelle dissociates, but it likely occurs after the micelle has diffused through the unstirred water layer and contacts the brush border membrane. At the brush border, the bile salts remain within the intestinal lumen, whereas fatty acids, cholesterol, and monoglycerides diffuse into the cytoplasm of the enterocyte. Once within the cytoplasm, fatty acids are transferred to the endoplasmic reticulum. Reesterification to form triglycerides occurs at this point by two different pathways, the monoglyceride acylation and phosphatidic acid pathways. The reformed triglycerides accumulate within the Golgi apparatus and are transported out of the cell across the basolateral membrane as chylomicrons, which enter the central lacteal of the villus. From the lacteals, the chylomicrons pass via larger lymphatic channels, draining the intestine into the thoracic duct and, finally, into the left subclavian vein.

Bile salts generally remain in the intestinal lumen and are absorbed in the distal 100 to 150 cm of ileum by an active process that involves saturation kinetics, is susceptible to metabolic inhibitors, and is sodium dependent (67). Bile salts can only be absorbed actively in the distal gut, and this has significant implications in patients who undergo ileal resection and have inflammatory bowel disease.

Chylomicrons have an inner core that consists of 90% triglycerides, a lesser amount of cholesterol, cholesterol esters, and fat-soluble vitamins, and traces of other lipids. Their outer layer consists of 80% to 90% phospholipid and specialized apolipoproteins. Although they account for only 1% of the mass, the specialized apolipoproteins of chylomicrons are essential for fat absorption. Apoprotein A and apoprotein B are synthesized by the intestinal mucosal cells, are probably found preformed in the tubular system, and are added before the nascent chylomicrons enter the Golgi apparatus. If these proteins are not synthesized or if the Golgi membrane formation is defective, triglycerides accumulate in the vesicles of the smooth endoplasmic reticulum and do not enter the Golgi system. This is the characteristic abnormality in the genetic disorder, congenital abetalipoproteinemia (68). Because chylomicrons are large particles, they cannot cross the intercellular junctions of the capillaries and are, therefore, excluded from the portal blood.

There are some lipolytic products that enter the portal system, including glycerol and medium-chain fatty acids. These compounds are water soluble, are absorbed without incorporation into micelles, are transported directly into the enterocyte, diffuse into the subepithelial space, and enter the capillaries to reach the portal blood. Because of this distinct metabolic virtue, medium-chain fatty acids have been used effectively as nutritional supplements in patients with chronic pancreatitis and pancreatic insufficiency.

Multiple clinical conditions may cause abnormal lipid assimilation that results in fat malabsorption. Gastric disorders that consequently lead to hemigastrectomy may decrease transit time and thus cause fat malabsorption. Patients with exocrine pancreatic insufficiency, chronic pancreatitis, or total pancreatectomy may have fat malabsorption if not supplemented with adequate amounts of the appropriate pancreatic enzymes. However, normal digestion can occur if at least 10% to 15% of endogenous pancreatic enzymes are secreted. Zollinger-Ellison syndrome, characterized in part by hypersecretion of hydrochloric acid, causes the pH of the duodenal contents to be reduced to the point of inhibiting pancreatic lipase. Interruption of the enterohepatic circulation or low intestinal luminal concentrations of bile salts also impairs fat absorption. Finally, pathologic conditions that adversely affect the mucosal cell transport of fatty acids and monoglycerides and the lymphatic transport of chylomicrons may be associated with fat malabsorption and maldigestion. Quantitatively, a diagnosis of fat malabsorption is made if more than 7 g of fat appear in the feces per day.

Enterohepatic Circulation

The enterohepatic circulation involves a cyclic process of bile salt secretion into the intestine, efficient absorption from the ileum, and hepatic reabsorption from the portal blood. The principal constituents of the enterohepatic circulation are bile acids, however, some organic anions, drugs, and hormone metabolites may also be involved. Bile acids are synthesized by the liver and stored in the gallbladder, where they are concentrated interdigestively as bile salts. Their secretion into the intestine is mediated by the hormone cholecystokinin, which is released from mucosal endocrine cells of the duodenum by such dietary components as peptides, essential amino acids, and hydrolyzed lipids. In the circulation, CCK promotes gallbladder contraction (69). Bile

salts serve several important functions during the assimilation of foodstuffs (70). They stimulate bile flow and emulsification of food and facilitate the absorption of lipolytic products through the formation of micelles. They also serve as fluid secretagogues in the intestine.

The major constituents of bile are bile acids (in the form of bile salts), bile pigment (bilirubin diglucuronide), cholesterol, phospholipids, proteins, electrolytes, and water. Although cholesterol, phospholipids, and proteins are present at lower concentrations in the bile than in plasma, the concentrations of bile acids and bile pigment in bile are up to 1000 times greater than those in plasma. During obstructive jaundice, bile acids are responsible for pruritus. Bile pigments are the end products of the catabolism of hemoglobin and, to a lesser extent, myoglobin, by the reticuloendothelial system. The heme portion of the molecule is converted via biliverdin to the yellow pigment, bilirubin, which is transported to the liver for excretion in the bile. When the albumin-bound bilirubin traverses the membrane of the hepatocyte, the protein moiety is cleaved and the bilirubin is conjugated intracellularly to glucuronic acid and, to a lesser extent, to sulfate. This process is accomplished by the enzyme, uridine diphosphoglucuronosyltransferase. Absence of this enzyme is responsible for the genetic disorder, Crigler-Najjar syndrome.

By the time the conjugated bilirubin reaches the colon, it is almost completely changed to urobilinogen, most of which appears in feces. Small amounts may be reabsorbed in the colon and returned to the liver or to the kidneys where urinary excretion occurs.

Bile salts are classified according to the number and molecular distribution of hydroxyl groups in the sterol nucleus and by the nature of their conjugation with amino acids. The functional characteristics of bile acids are determined by the number of hydroxyl groups. The major bile acids are cholic and chenodeoxycholic acids, which are synthesized in the liver from cholesterol. The secondary bile acids, deoxycholic and lithocholic acids, however, are formed by anaerobic bacteria in the intestine and eventually become involved in the enterohepatic circulation. All bile acids secreted into bile by the liver are conjugated either with glycine or taurine. Although one-third of bile acids are conjugated with taurine and two-thirds of bile acids are conjugated with glycine, no major functional differences are apparent between the two. Some bile acids, such as lithocholate, are sulfated in addition to conjugation with glycine and taurine.

Bile acids contain both hydrophilic and hydrophobic functional groups and are, by definition, detergents with characteristic emulsifying properties. Several physical factors, such as the pH of the surrounding milieu and the pKa of bile acids, determine the effectiveness of the bile acids as detergents (71). Furthermore, a critical concentration of conjugated bile acids must be maintained for the optimal absorption of dietary fats to form polymolecular aggregates, called micelles, into which lipolytic products are solubilized.

Primary bile acids excreted in the bile as salts are reabsorbed in the distal small bowel by two different mechanisms. Passive absorption occurs throughout the entire gastrointestinal tract, whereas active absorption is confined to the terminal ileum and is a sodium-dependent process. As the polarity of the bile salts decreases, active transport decreases and passive absorption increases, because unconjugated bile acids, having fewer hydroxyl groups, are more readily absorbed passively.

A bile salt pool of approximately 2 g is recycled through the enterohepatic circulation five to six times a day. With disruption of the enterohepatic circulation, such as occurs in ileal resection or ileal dysfunction (one example of which is Crohn's disease), the amount of bile reaching the colon is increased. This has a potent cathartic effect, resulting in malabsorption and diarrhea. In addition to stimulating colonic motility, the two dihydroxycholic bile acids, deoxycholic and chenodeoxycholic acid, increase net intestinal water secretion. With resection of the terminal ileum, the liver is not able to compensate for the fecal losses of bile salts. This causes a significant decrease in bile salt secretion, contributing to steatorrhea because of insufficient micelle formation. Alterations in the enterohepatic circulation may also be caused by binding resins, such as cholestyramine, bacterial overgrowth, and cholestasis.

Vitamins

Vitamins are organic compounds that cannot be produced by the body but are vital to its metabolism. The relative solubility in water or lipids determines the general mechanism by which vitamins are absorbed.

Vitamins A, D, E, and K have limited solubility in water and depend on bile salt micelles for their absorption, primarily in the jejunum. Vitamin A, or retinol, is ingested and absorbed as β-carotene. Once within the enterocyte, the β-carotene is cleaved into two retinol molecules. Dietary retinol esters are hydrolyzed in the intestinal lumen by pancreatic carboxylesterase and then absorbed. The vitamin A thus absorbed from the lumen is esterified in the mucosa primarily with palmitic acid, transported within the chylomicrons into the lymph, and stored as retinol palmitate in the liver. Esters of dietary vitamins D and E are hydrolyzed by cholesterol ester before being solubilized within micelles. Vitamin D is delivered to the liver in chylomicron remnants where it undergoes 25-hydroxylation. Subsequently, metabolism involves renal synthesis of the 1,25-dihydroxy derivative, a potent regulator of calcium metabolism.

Dietary vitamin K (K_1) is absorbed in the intestine by an active transport system, whereas bacterially derived K_2 is absorbed passively from the lumen. Except for retinol, which is reesterified, the fat-soluble vitamins appear in exocytosed chylomicrons biochemically unchanged by metabolic processes within the enterocyte.

The water-soluble vitamins, which include ascorbic acid (vitamin C), biotin, choline, inositol, nicotinic acid, paraaminobenzoic acid, riboflavin, thiamine, and vitamin B_6, were considered to be predominantly absorbed by passive diffusion. However, their transport is now thought to be more complex and may require several different processes. Vitamin C is absorbed by an active transport process, which is energy dependent, requiring sodium. Whereas biotin absorption requires active transport similar to that of ascorbic acid and sugars, choline is absorbed by facilitated diffusion. Inositol absorption is accomplished by both simple diffusion and a carrier-mediated system. Nicotinic acid, and probably riboflavin, are absorbed in the proximal small intestine by active processes, and riboflavin uptake is enhanced in the presence of bile salts.

The absorption of thiamine occurs in the jejunum by resin diffusion, but at low concentrations, absorption via an active transport system predominates. Vitamin B_6 (pyridoxine) appears to be absorbed rather rapidly by simple diffusion in the proximal intestine. Folate is absorbed primarily in the duodenum and jejunum by two transport mechanisms, one carrier-mediated, the other, by passive transport (72).

Vitamin B_{12} absorption occurs primarily in the terminal ileum (72) and requires intrinsic factor, a glycoprotein secreted by the parietal cells of the gastric mucosa. Binding of this factor to the vitamin protects it from proteolytic digestion. Specific receptors in the terminal ileum take up the B_{12}-intrinsic factor complex. The actual uptake of vitamin B_{12} is by pinocytosis. Vitamin B_{12} enters the portal blood and is transported in the plasma by a β-glycoprotein, transcobalamin (58). Any pathologic condition that interferes with the production or secretion of intrinsic factor or the attachment of the B_{12}-intrinsic factor complex in the ileum leads to vitamin B_{12} malabsorption and deficiency syndrome.

Short Bowel Syndrome

The patient with short bowel syndrome after massive small-intestinal resection represents one of the greatest clinical challenges a general surgeon must face. Maintaining optimal nutritional and metabolic support until maximum bowel adaptation can occur is the first priority of therapy. Short bowel syndrome is not a clinical entity precisely defined by a specific length of residual functioning small intestine, but rather is an aggregation of clinical signs and symptoms characterized primarily by intractable diarrhea, steatorrhea, weight loss, dehydration, malnutrition, and malabsorption of fats, vitamins, and other nutrients. Secondary or more specific subsequent consequences of short bowel syndrome include hypovolemia, hypoalbuminemia, hypokalemia, hypocalcemia, hypomagnesemia, hypozincemia, hypocupricemia, fatty acid and vitamin deficiencies, anemias, hyperoxaluria, and metabolic acidosis (73). The actual presentation of the patient with short bowel syndrome depends on several factors: (a) the extent and site of resection; (b) the presence or absence of the ileocecal valve; (c) the residual function of the remaining small bowel, stomach, pancreas, biliary tree, and colon; (d) the adaptive capacity of the intestinal remnant; (e) the primary disease that precipitated the loss of the small bowel; and (f) the amount and activity of the residual disease in the intestinal remnant (74–78).

The minimum length of small bowel sufficient for adequate absorption is controversial because of the variable residual absorptive capacity of the remaining remnant, the wide variation in the length of the normal small intestine, and the difficulty in obtaining reproducible measurements of the length of the remaining bowel after massive resection. Depending on the state of contraction or relaxation of the intestine, intraoperative estimates of the length of the normal intact small intestine in the adult vary from 260 to 800 cm (approximately 8 to 26 feet) (78). The mean length of normal small intestine during life is 350 cm (11 to 12 feet) and post-mortem is 600 cm (20 feet). The great variability makes it difficult to determine the exact length of the remaining small bowel, and makes it virtually impossible to estimate the percentage of the total length of small bowel that the remaining segment represents. Moreover, many surgeons not only measure the length of the resected small bowel, rather than measuring the length of the remaining intestinal segment, but then they fail to describe accurately the nature and extent of the remaining small bowel in the patient's medical record for future reference. Furthermore, because inflamed bowel shortens after operation, the symptomatic outcome of massive small bowel resection does not correlate well with the intraoperative estimated length of resection (79).

Because of the rather generous functional reserve capacity of the small bowel, resection of the small intestine does not usually result in significant problems with digestion and absorption (80,81). Indeed, resection of as much as 40% of the small intestine is usually well-tolerated, provided that the duodenum, the distal half of the ileum, and the ileocecal valve are spared (82). However, resection of 50% or more of the small intestine usually results initially in significant malabsorption, which can eventually be tolerated without additional nutritional support. However, resection of 75% or more of the small intestine usually leaves the patient with 70 to 100 cm (2 to 3 feet) of remaining intestine, resulting in the short bowel syndrome. This can substantially impair the ability of the patient to maintain normal nutrition and metabolism. This patient will likely require special nutritional care on a long-term or permanent basis, especially with the loss of the terminal ileum and the ileocecal valve.

The severity of symptoms after massive small bowel resection is related both to the extent of the resection and the specific level of the resected small bowel (83). However, the minimal residual small intestinal absorptive surface required to sustain life without permanent parenteral nutritional support appears to vary with each patient (84,85). Development of effective total parenteral nutrition has revolutionized the treatment of the short bowel syndrome by allowing maintenance of adequate nutrition until the remaining bowel can adapt maximally to oral feeding, thus significantly reducing the morbidity and mortality rates (86–91). Prolonged survival has now been achieved in a number of patients having an intact duodenum and 15 cm (6 inches) of residual jejunum, with or without the colon (75,81). In addition to the entire duodenum, if approximately 60 cm (2 feet) of jejunum or ileum remain functional, survival has been the rule rather than the exception. Preservation of the ileocecal valve is of paramount importance during massive small bowel resection. By significantly increasing the intestinal transit time, it appears to increase the absorptive capacity of the remaining small bowel to approximately twice that anticipated for the same length of small bowel without an intact ileocecal valve. Primarily as a result of mucosal hyperplasia and villous hypertrophy, absorption in the residual intestinal segments of patients with short bowel syndrome can increase as much as fourfold. Therefore, in a patient with an intact ileocecal valve, the total absorptive capacity of the remaining bowel can potentially be increased eightfold.

As stated earlier, absorption of fluid, electrolytes, and nutrients depends on the site and extent of the small bowel resection. The intestinal phase of digestion occurs initially within the duodenum, where pancreatic enzymes and bile acids aid digestion of all nutrients and promote fat absorption. It is unusual for the duodenum to be resected together with extensive segments of the small bowel. However, total duodenectomy leads to malabsorption of calcium, folic acid, and iron (74). Proteins, carbohydrates, and fats are absorbed virtually completely in the first 150 cm of the jejunum, so that only small quantities of these macronutrients ever reach the ileum (92).

The small intestine receives and processes about 8 liters of fluid per day, including dietary ingestion and endogenous secretions. Normally, about 80% of the water transported is absorbed in the small bowel, leaving approximately 1.5 liters of fluid to enter the colon. The colon usually absorbs about 1 to 2 liters of fluid with a maximal absorptive capacity of approximately 6 liters of fluid per day (93). Colon absorption is regulated by aldosterone. Large proximal small bowel resections result in little diarrhea because the ileum and colon have a great capacity to reabsorb excess fluid and electrolytes. Conversely, extensive or total ileal resection produces a greater potential for malabsorption and diarrhea. This increases the volume of fluid reaching the colon, and depending on the length of ileal resection, bile salt diarrhea (cholorrhea) or steatorrhea may ensue with significant loss of fat-soluble vitamins. If the ileocecal valve has been resected, transit time may decrease, and bacterial colonization of the small bowel will eventually occur, aggravating both cholorrhea and steatorrhea. As the length of ileal and colonic resection is increased, essential absorptive surface area is lost, resulting in progressive dehydration, hypovolemia, and electrolyte disturbances. If the colon remains in continuity with the residual small bowel after massive resection, malabsorbed bile salts can be deconjugated by colonic bacteria, stimulating colonic secretion and aggravating diarrhea. With extensive ileal resection, an irreversible loss of bile salts occurs even if the colon is in continuity. Although the excess losses stimulate hepatic synthesis of bile salts, a higher incidence of cholelithiasis occurs in these patients. Because the transit time in the ileum is usually slower than in the jejunum (and this remains so after massive intestinal resection), intestinal transit is slowed, and fecal output decreases as the length of residual ileum increases.

After extensive small bowel resection, intestinal lactase activity may be decreased and produce lactose intolerance (94). The unhydrolyzed lactose can cause increased hyperosmolality in the intestinal lumen. Moreover, the fermentation of the lactose by bacteria in the colon can produce a large amount of lactic acid and can further aggravate the osmotic diarrhea (74).

The water-soluble vitamins and minerals (vitamin B complex, vitamin C, calcium, and iron) are absorbed in the proximal small intestine, whereas magnesium diffuses passively throughout the entire small bowel (74). The ileum is the sole site for absorption of vitamin B_{12} and the bile salts. Jejunectomy with preservation of the ileum produces no permanent defects in the absorption of protein, carbohydrate, or electrolytes (95). The ileum can compensate for most of the absorptive functions but not for the secretion of jejunal entero-hormones. After jejunal resection, decreased secretion of cholecystokinin and secretin decrease gallbladder contraction and pancreatic secretion. Furthermore, gastric hypersecretion is greater than after ileal resection. Because of the loss of inhibitory hormones such as GIP and VIP secreted in the jejunum, gastrin levels rise, thus stimulating gastric hypersecretion (96). Significant gastric hypersecretion can be documented within 24 hours postoperatively, and the mucosa distal to the stomach can be injured by the high gastric acid output. Subsequently, the high salt load secreted in the stomach, together with the inactivation of digestive enzymes by the low intraluminal pH, serves to compound the other causes of diarrhea already present in short bowel syndrome.

Normally, the colon functions as a major site of water and electrolyte absorption. As the ileal effluent increases, the colon increases its normal absorptive capacity by 3 to 5 times (97). Furthermore, the colon has a moderate capacity to absorb nutrients, and concomitant colon resection can affect the symptomatic and nutritional courses of patients with massive bowel resection. Malabsorbed carbohydrates that reach the colon are fermented by bacteria to yield short-chain fatty acids, principally acetate, butyrate, and propionate (98,99). Short-chain fatty acids can be absorbed by the colon in quantities up to 500 calories per day and enter the portal circulation to become a fuel source for the body (100,101). Although retention of the colon is highly desirable, its presence is associated with potential complications. In addition to having choleretic diarrhea induced by the bile salts, patients with massive bowel resection and an intact colon have a tendency to form calcium oxalate renal stones. This results from the increased absorption of dietary oxalate, which is normally rendered insoluble by calcium in the intestinal lumen and therefore, ordinarily unabsorbable. However, in patients with short bowel syndrome and steatorrhea, intraluminal intestinal calcium is bound preferentially to unabsorbed fatty acids, leading to decreased binding and increased colonic absorption of oxalate (82).

Finally, preservation of the ileocecal valve during distal small bowel resection is important because the ileocecal valve ordinarily slows intestinal transit and prevents bacterial reflux from the colon into the small bowel. Nutrients that reach the intestinal lumen, especially vitamin B_{12}, become substrates for bacterial metabolism rather than being absorbed from the mucosa (82). Furthermore, bacterial overgrowth in the small bowel in patients with short bowel syndrome receiving total parenteral nutrition appears to increase the incidence of liver dysfunction (102).

Small Intestinal Motility

Small intestinal myoelectric and contractile activity can be divided into two main categories, fed and fasted. The fed state is characterized by irregular groups of contractions that mix the ingesta with digestive enzymes and secretions and propel the contents in the aboral direction. The fasted state is characterized by the periodic occurrence of the MMC. The MMC in the small intestine is a cyclically occurring pattern of electrical and mechanical activity that usually starts in the duodenum and migrates aborally to the distal ileum (39,103). MMC cycling is initiated when nearly all digestible materials have been cleared from the upper gastrointestinal tract. The intense contractions of the MMC propel residual food, secretions, and desquamated cells to the colon. MMC cycles are imitated every 90 to 150 minutes in the human and take approximately 90 minutes to migrate to the distal ileum. In addition to the fed and fasted patterns of activity, other nonspecific types of contractions occur in the small intestine to move intestinal contents rapidly in the oral or aboral direction.

Table 17.12.
Classification of Small Intestine Contractions

1. Individual phasic contractions
2. Organized groups of contractions
   A. Migrating myoelectric (motor) complex
   B. Migrating complex clustered contractions
3. Special propulsive contractions
   A. Giant migrating contractions
   B. Retrograde giant contractions

Because the functions of the small intestine are varied and complex, different types of contraction with specific temporal and spatial organizations exist to accomplish these functions. Small intestinal contractions may be categorized into three groups: individual phasic contractions; organized groups of contractions; and special propulsive contractions (104) (Table 17.12).

Individual Phasic Contractions

Except when special propulsive contractions are present, individual phasic contractions are the basic unit of contractile activity in both the fed and fasted states. The patterns of these contractions are controlled by myogenic, neural, and chemical mechanisms. Myogenic control refers to the electrical activity of the smooth muscle of the small intestine (104). In the small intestine, ECA—rhythmic oscillations in smooth muscle membrane potential—occurs. These electrical oscillations do not result directly in muscle contractions, but their frequency determines the rate at which membrane depolarization can occur. During any ECA depolarization, if the membrane potential reaches a threshold level, ERA—a burst of electrical oscillations—occurs. This results in smooth muscle contraction, the force of which is determined by the intensity of the ERA burst. Because contractions can only occur with ERA bursts and ERA bursts can only occur once during each ECA cycle, the frequency of ECA at any site determines the maximum rate of contractions.

Neural control includes both the extrinsic and intrinsic nerves that innervate the smooth muscle cells. Extrinsic parasympathetic innervation is via the vagus. Extrinsic sympathetic innervation is from thoracic spinal cord, impulses of which travel via the celiac and superior mesenteric ganglia and along the mesenteric vessels to the small intestine. The majority of nerve fibers in the vagus are sensory and respond to both distension and contraction of the small intestine. Vagal efferent fibers synapse on both cholinergic excitatory nerves and nonadrenergic, noncholinergic inhibitory nerves. Postsynaptic, sympathetic nerves inhibit small intestinal contraction by decreasing the release of acetylcholine from cholinergic nerve endings.

Chemical control refers to the effect of various peptides and neurotransmitters on contractile activity. These substances may act at any level to induce changes, including via the CNS, extramural ganglia, the intrinsic nervous system, or directly on the smooth muscle.

Fed State

Within a few minutes of eating a meal, the MMC cycle is replaced with intermittent and irregular contractions. The disruption of MMC cycling by a meal appears to be mediated by both hormonal and neural mechanisms. Fed state contractions mix the intestinal chyme with secretions and expose it to the mucosal surface to facilitate absorption. The rate of propulsion and mixing depends on the content of the meal and the time required for digestion and absorption.

Organized Groups of Contractions

Migrating Myoelectric Complexes

The MMC cycle in the small intestine has four distinct phases of activity (39,104) (Fig. 17.11). Phase I is characterized by minimal or no ERA and, therefore, minimal or no contraction. During phase II, irregular bursts of ERA and contractions occur. During phase III (the activity front), intense bursts of ERA occur during each ECA cycle, resulting in regular, high-amplitude contractions. Phase IV is characterized by a short period of irregular ERA and contraction similar to those in phase II. Phase I occupies 40% to 60% of the MMC cycle time; phase II, 20% to 30%; phase III, 5% to 10%; and phase IV, 0% to 5%. The mean migration velocity of the MMC is 4 to 6 cm/min in the proximal small intestine and 1 to 2 cm/min in the distal intestine.

The duodenal MMC cycle is coordinated with cyclic motor activity in the LES, the stomach, and the gallbladder. During phase III in the stomach, there are increases in LES resting tone and phasic contraction of the LES.

The site of origin of the MMC cycle, the cycle length, and the distance and velocity of migration are normally highly variable. Even in disease states, the MMC cycle is usually present, except for subgroups of patients with selected diseases, including Chagas disease, scleroderma, and small intestinal bacterial overgrowth.

Plasma concentrations of the peptide hormone, motilin, peak in a cyclical manner during phase III of the MMC cycle in the duodenum. Parenteral administration of motilin initiates a premature MMC in the duodenum. From this information, it has been hypothesized that plasma motilin concentrations cycle independently, and, at a given threshold level, this hormone triggers phase III of the MMC in the duodenum. No mechanism for the spontaneous release of motilin has yet been reported. Although an association exists between the initiation of MMCs in the duodenum and a peak in plasma motilin concentration, a direct cause-and-effect relationship between fluctuations in plasma motilin levels and MMC cycling has not been demonstrated. An alternate explanation is that plasma motilin levels cycle as a result

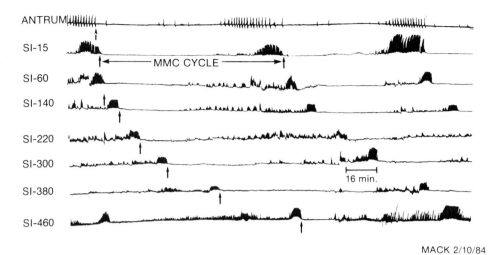

ANTRUM
SI-15
MMC CYCLE
SI-60
SI-140
SI-220
SI-300
SI-380
16 min.
SI-460

MACK 2/10/84

Figure 17.11. Migrating motor complex in the small intestine and cyclic motor activity in the stomach of the dog as recorded by strain gauge force transducers. *Arrows* indicate end of phase III of the MMC cycle at each site. Numbers on the left represent the distance of the small intestine (SI) strain groups from the pylorus. From Sarna SK, Otterson MF. Gastrointestinal motility. Some basic concepts. Pharmacology 1988;36(suppl 1):7–14. Reprinted by permission of S. Karger AG, Basel.

of the MMC cycle and serve to coordinate both MMC cycling and other phenomena related to MMC cycling. This theory postulates that as contractile activity increases during phase III, increasing amounts of motilin from the duodenum and jejunum (where the majority of motilin is stored) are released until a peak is reached during phase III. This release could then coordinate gallbladder emptying, gastric and LES cyclic motor activity, and the release of other hormones. Motilin could also act as a positive feedback mechanism to assist in the initiation of the MMC.

The MMC is a spontaneously cyclical phenomenon without an external stimulus. The basis for many such cyclical phenomena is an autonomous oscillator. MMCs seem to cycle spontaneously because they are not abolished by extrinsic denervation and, although exogenous motilin initiates MMCs, spontaneous MMCs can occur without significant increases in plasma motilin concentrations. The precise location of the MMC relaxation oscillator has not been identified, but a likely possibility is the enteric nervous system.

The intense contractions of phase III of the MMC cycle serve to purge the small intestine of residual food, undigestible solids, secretions, and desquamated cells, and propel them into the colon. Therefore, the function of the MMC cycle may be to keep the stomach and the small intestine cleared of desquamated cells and secretions between meals. This proposal is supported by the observation that disruption of the MMC cycle is associated with bacterial overgrowth in some patients.

Migrating Clustered Contractions

Migrating clustered contractions (MCCs), or discrete clustered contractions or minute rhythms, are groups of small intestinal contractions that last 1 to 2 minutes and migrate aborally over short distances not exceeding 40 cm (104). MCCs occur in both the fed and fasted states. In the fasting state, they occur irregularly during phase II activity, migrate distally at a velocity of 5 to 10 cm/

min, and occur at a rate of 5 to 10/hr. Like MMCs, migrating clustered contractions propel intestinal contents to their forefront and move them over short distances.

The frequency of occurrence of MCCs increases in patients with partial small bowel obstruction and with irritable bowel syndrome. Postprandially, patients with partial small bowel obstruction have a significant increase in MCCs. They are sometimes associated with abdominal cramping. Patients with irritable bowel syndrome have an increase in the incidence of MCCs and higher amplitude contractions during MCCs in the fasted state (105). MCCs may also be associated with abdominal cramping in these patients.

Special Propulsive Contractions

Giant Migrating Contractions

Giant migrating contractions (GMCs), or prolonged propagated contractions or power contractions, occur infrequently and irregularly in the fasted state. They are 1.5 to 2 times larger in amplitude and 4 to 6 times longer in duration than the phasic contractions that occur during MMCs. These contractions normally begin in the distal small intestine and migrate to the terminal ileum at a rate of 1 cm/sec. GMCs are highly propulsive and appear to empty the contents of the distal small intestine rapidly into the proximal colon. The physiologic role of GMCs has not been established, but it may be to either clear the distal small intestine of colonic contents that have refluxed into the terminal ileum or simply to empty the normal contents of the terminal ileum into the colon. This may be necessary because MMCs do not always reach the very terminal ileum. GMCs are initiated by opioids, erythromycin, luminal administration of short-chain fatty acids, and abdominal irradiation, and their incidence is increased during infection with the nematode *Trichinella spiralis*.

Retrograde Giant Contractions

Retrograde giant contractions, like GMCs, are of large amplitude and long duration. They originate in the mid small intestine and migrate in the orad direction to the antrum at a velocity of 8 to 10 cm/sec. They usually precede the expulsion of vomitus.

Colonic Motility

Colonic contraction propels the luminal contents in an aborad direction and expels the fecal material both at rates which permit absorption of water and electrolytes and storage of fecal debris (106,107). There are two principal types of colonic contraction, individual phasic contractions and giant migrating contractions. Individual phasic contractions constitute the major element of motor activity in the colon, as is the case for the remainder of the gastrointestinal tract. These contractions may be organized into clusters. GMCs occur infrequently and result in mass movement of luminal contents (108). Individual phasic contractions of the colon are controlled by myogenic, neural, and chemical mechanisms (108).

Myogenic Control

Myogenic control is via the omnipresent oscillation of the smooth muscle membrane potential known as electrical control activity. ECA controls the timing of phasic contractions but does not cause them. An excitatory neural or chemical stimulation must be present during the ECA cycle for a contraction to occur. When excitatory input is present, a second type of electrical activity is seen, the ERA. A 1:1 relationship exists between ERA and contractions (106,107) (Fig. 17.12).

Occasionally, ERA is continuous over more than one ECA cycle. Under these conditions, a third type of electrical activity is seen, the contractile electrical complex (CEC). CEC has a frequency of 25 to 40 cycles/min and is usually associated with contractions of 30 seconds or longer in duration. CEC is thought to control prolonged contractions, because its duration is about the same as that of the contraction (106).

Neural Control

Neural control refers to the control of contractions by the autonomic and enteric nervous systems. The autonomic nervous system consists of the parasympathetic and sympathetic innervation of the colon.

The parasympathetic innervation of the colon is supplied by the vagus and pelvic nerves (107). These nerves contain both motor and sensory fibers. The motor fibers are mainly excitatory for contractile activity. The vagus nerves are thought to innervate the proximal half of the colon, whereas the pelvic nerves innervate the distal half. However, recent evidence indicates that both the vagus and pelvic nerves may innervate the entire colon, with the number of vagal fibers decreasing in an aborad direction and pelvic fibers decreasing in an orad direction. The preganglionic fibers of the vagus and pelvic nerves synapse on neurons of the enteric ganglia, which then constitute the postganglionic fibers.

Efferent electrical stimulation of the vagus and pelvic nerves results in contractions of colonic smooth muscle (108). The effect of efferent vagal stimulation is completely blocked by atropine, whereas stimulation of the pelvic nerves is only partially blocked by this drug (106,108). These data suggest that preganglionic vagal fibers synapse only on postganglionic cholinergic neurons and pelvic fibers synapse on both cholinergic and noncholinergic postganglionic excitatory neurons in the enteric ganglia.

The sympathetic nerves to the colon also contain both motor and sensory fibers. The motor fibers are mainly inhibitory (106,107). The colon receives sympathetic fibers from thoracic roots 5 through 12 and lumbar roots 2 through 5 of the spinal cord. The preganglionic fibers from the thoracic roots synapse in the superior mesenteric ganglia, whereas the postganglionic fibers innervate the proximal colon. The preganglionic fibers from the lumbar roots synapse in the inferior mesenteric ganglia, with the postganglionic fibers innervating the entire colon.

Efferent electrical stimulation of the sympathetic

Figure 17.12. Myogenic control of phasic contractions, or ERA, of the colon. The *top* tracing is contractile activity recorded with a strain gauge force transducer. The *middle* tracing is the electrical signal recorded from a bipolar electrode, filtered between 0 and 0.3 Hz to bring out the ECA. The *bottom* tracing is from the same electrode filtered between 5 and 10 Hz to bring out the ERA. A 1:1 relationship exists between ERA and phasic contractions. *T*, strain gauge transducer; *E*, bipolar electrode.

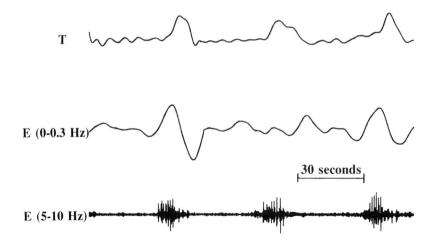

nerves to the colon inhibits both normal contractile activity and that induced by vagal and pelvic nerve stimulation but does not inhibit contractions induced by local intraarterial injection of acetylcholine (106). This evidence suggests that the postganglionic sympathetic nerves synapse on the enteric ganglion where they have their influence on colonic contraction by inhibiting the release of acetylcholine.

The enteric nervous system consists mainly of the myenteric and submucosal plexuses (106,107). These plexuses receive input from extrinsic parasympathetic and sympathetic nerves and mechanoreceptors and chemoreceptors in the gut wall. They also receive input through interneurons from both adjacent ganglia and from ganglia in the corresponding plexus. This information is integrated within the ganglia, and the appropriate contractile response is elicited.

In addition to the postganglionic cholinergic neurons, the enteric nervous system has many peptidergic neurons. The exact physiologic role of these peptide neurotransmitters remains to be ascertained.

Chemical Control

The release of various chemicals from nerve endings as well as endocrine and paracrine cells can also modulate contractile activity in the colon (106,107). As with neural control, these chemicals can have either an excitatory or an inhibitory action on colonic contraction. They may act directly on colonic smooth muscle, at the enteric ganglia, or at sites distant to the gut wall. Many different types of chemicals, including amines, peptides, and eicosanoids, effect colonic smooth muscle.

Contractile Activity of the Colon

Flow of chyme into the colon is regulated by the ileocecal junction, which is thought to act as a sphincter (106,107). The ileocecal junction contains a zone of higher pressure than that recorded in either the ileum or colon. Periodically, the sphincter relaxes, allowing ileal contractions to propel chyme into the colon.

Once the chyme has entered the colon, it is acted on by colonic contractions. For the most part, phasic contractions of the colon are not coordinated at adjacent sites. This type of activity results in a back-and-forth mixing movement of luminal content, which exposes it to the mucosal surface for absorption of water and electrolytes.

Occasionally, phasic contractions at adjacent sites become coordinated over short distances and propagate in either an orad or, more commonly, an aboral direction. This causes propulsion of luminal content in the direction of propagation of these contractions. In addition, clusters of phasic contractions may migrate in either an orad or aboral direction, also resulting in propulsion of luminal content in the direction of migration (106,109).

Phasic contractions recorded from the colon of various species are organized differently. In monkeys, phasic contractions are principally individual and occur randomly. They rarely are organized into clusters of groups of contractions (108,110). Colonic contractile activity in dogs, however, is organized primarily as groups of contractions with periods of complete quiescence between them (109). The organization of human colonic contractile activity tends to be in between that of monkeys and dogs, with randomly occurring contractions interspersed between groups of contractions (111).

Although individual phasic contractions and clusters of contractions result in slow distal propulsion, most aboral movement of luminal content takes place during what is called a mass movement (106,107). The mass movement of luminal content is the result of a giant migrating contraction. GMCs are two to three times greater in amplitude than phasic contractions and have a duration of 20 to 40 seconds in the colon (Fig. 17.13). They usually migrate no more than a third of the distance of the colon, emptying all luminal content from that segment of bowel. GMCs occur infrequently, normally no more than three times a day in healthy humans (106).

Movement of fecal material into the rectum by phasic contractions and GMCs during mass movements causes rectal distension. Distension of the rectum results in the retro sphincter reflex, which causes relaxation of the internal anal sphincter. If this reflex is invoked when it is convenient to defecate, a series of voluntary and involuntary acts take place, resulting in defecation (106,107). A GMC is induced, which supplies the major propulsive force for movement of fecal material from the descending and sigmoid colon (see Fig. 17.13). Along with this, a relaxation of the internal and external anal sphincters occurs, which allows fecal material to pass. These events

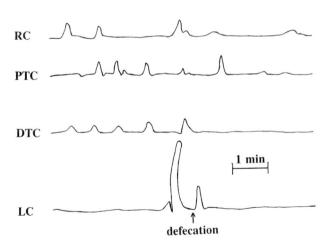

Figure 17.13. Contractile activity recorded from the colon of a nonhuman primate by strain gauge force transducers. A giant migrating contraction in the left colon is followed by a spontaneous defecation. Note the much greater amplitude of the GMC compared with normal phasic contractions of the colon. *RC,* right colon; *PTC,* proximal transverse colon; *DTC,* distal transverse colon; *LC,* left colon.

may also be accompanied by contraction of abdominal muscles and the diaphragm to increase intra-abdominal pressure and lowering of the pelvic floor. This is described in greater detail in the next section.

Defecatory Mechanisms

Planning medical or surgical therapy in disorders of defecation requires a fundamental understanding of its physiologic mechanisms. In this section, the relationships between anorectal sensation, internal anal sphincteric function, external anal sphincteric function, and colorectal motility with respect to defecation will be discussed. In addition, the interaction between diet and output of fecal material will be reviewed.

Anatomical Considerations

Anatomical structures that are important to the mechanics of defecation include the levator ani striated muscle, the anal canal, the circular smooth muscle layer of the colon and rectum, and the enteric nerves. The levator ani muscle forms the floor of the pelvis. Fibers of the levator ani as the puborectalis muscle surround the junction of the anal canal and the rectum. The puborectalis muscle contracts at rest, forming an angle, the anorectal angle, between the anal canal and the rectum (Fig. 17.14). The anal canal itself is from 2.5 to 4 cm long. Within this structure, the internal anal sphincter is a thickening of the terminal circular smooth muscle layer of the rectum which surrounds the proximal anal canal, while the external anal sphincter, which is the distal continuation of the levator ani muscle, surrounds the distal anal canal. The intrinsic enteric nerves form a neural network through the myenteric plexus, beginning at the internal anal sphincter and extending cephalad. In the anal canal, the myenteric plexus adjacent to the internal anal sphincter contains small, compact nerve cell bodies. This neural network abruptly changes at the interface

of the anal canal with the rectum, at which point the plexus contains large, irregular nerve cell bodies (112). An intact network of intrinsic, nonadrenergic inhibitory nerves in the myenteric plexus is required to produce descending relaxation of the internal anal sphincter, which is induced by rectal distension. In contrast, the external anal sphincter is innervated by spinal motoneurons through the inferior rectal nerves. Thus, the levator ani muscle is innervated by nerve fibers that originate extrinsic to the gut.

Sensory Function

Progressive balloon distension of the rectum has been used as a quantitative means of examining sensory function and its relationship to defecation (113). These studies show that balloon distension to an average of 60 mL is required to reach the threshold of stretch receptor perception, distension to 90 mL is required to elicit the urge to defecate, and distension to 190 mL elicits a painful sensation. In addition, there are receptors in the anorectal region that aid in the discrimination between intraluminal gas, fluid, or solid fecal material. The belief that these sensory mechanisms are of physiologic significance in normal defecation is supported by the finding of abnormal sensation in subgroups of patients with fecal incontinence or constipation.

Anal Canal Function

Pressure recordings within the anal canal have demonstrated marked asymmetry of basal, squeeze, and relaxation pressures (114). There appear to be two separate pressure regions in the anal canal. Squeeze pressures are higher posteriorly in the proximal anal canal and are higher anteriorly in the distal anal canal. Balloon insufflation in the rectum shows that the normal reflex relaxation is of higher amplitude in the proximal anal canal compared with the distal anal canal. This gradient in reflex relaxation may allow an individual to remain continent while sensory sampling of rectal contents occurs. Under normal conditions, rectal distension pro-

Figure 17.14. Perineal descent during the Valsalva maneuver. In proctography, the pelvic floor is defined by a line drawn between the symphysis pubis and the tip of the coccyx; to define the anorectal angle, a *dashed line* is drawn through the rectum to a *beaded chain* held by traction in the internal anal canal. In these sagittal sections, the anatomic relationships of the internal anal sphincter (IAS) and the external anal sphincter (EAS) are shown. Note that during the Valsalva maneuver, the anorectal angle (*arrow*) becomes more obtuse and the distance between the pubococcygeal line and the internal anal canal increases by 2 to 4 cm (normal perineal descent).

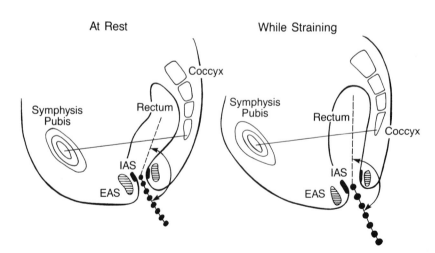

duced by increasing accumulation of fecal material can induce descending relaxation of the internal anal sphincter and voluntary contraction of the external anal sphincter to protect continence. At that time, increasing intra-abdominal pressure by the Valsalva maneuver produces descent of the perineum and permits defecation (115) (see Fig. 17.14). Alternatively, intra-abdominal pressure can be increased by leaning forward during manual application of pressure to the anterior abdominal wall. Some authors have stated that the process of defecation cannot begin until fecal material passes beyond the rectosigmoid junction. In addition, the anorectal angle might function as a flap valve. In this model of defecation, during the Valsalva maneuver, relaxation of the puborectalis muscle produces perineal descent. This could facilitate defecation by making the anorectal angle more obtuse. The physiologic validity of these theories has not been fully determined.

Colorectal Motility

Manometric recordings of the contractile activity of human colon have suggested the presence of two types of contractions. The first type is nonpropagating, low-amplitude phasic contractions that probably do not significantly enhance transit of fecal material. The second type is a high-amplitude, rapidly progressive contraction (Fig. 17.15), which is most likely the manometric equivalent of colonic mass movement (116). Coordinated contractions of the circular smooth muscle are required for movement of material through the colon and rectum. Scintigraphic studies have suggested that dur-

ing normal defecation, a mass movement can propel material from the splenic flexure of the colon through the rectum. Several studies have supported the belief that mass movements involving the sigmoid colon and rectum follow a circadian rhythm because they occur more frequently after awakening in the morning and after meals (117).

Dietary Considerations

Two decades ago, Burkitt and colleagues (118) described a direct relationship between fiber intake and stool output. Dietary fiber in this setting referred only to the undigestible portion of food. By comparing stool weights between people in the United Kingdom and in Africa, they found a higher per day stool weight and decreased intestinal transit time in Africans on a high-fiber diet. As caveats, this study was carried out in young, healthy volunteers, and it is known that a high prevalence of sigmoid volvulus exists in West African countries. Older individuals may, therefore, have increasing difficulty responding to high dietary fiber intake. More recent work by Bannister and associates (119) in the United Kingdom showed that higher intrarectal pressures and increased time during the Valsalva maneuver were needed to expel small, harder materials from the rectum, compared with large, softer materials. These results suggest that dietary fiber might facilitate defecation in normal individuals by producing larger, softer stools.

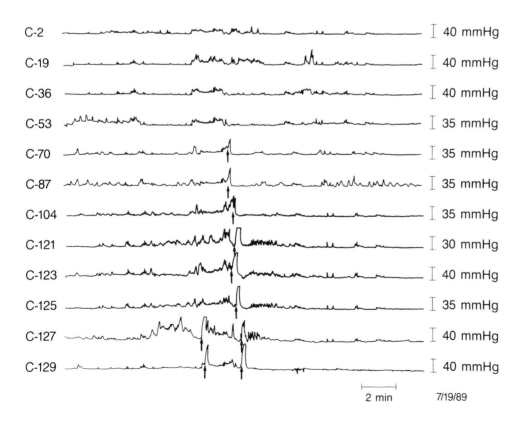

Figure 17.15. Manometric recording of giant migrating contractions in human colon. A perfused catheter was positioned in the ascending colon by colonoscopy. The tracing shows high amplitude contractions that begin in the rectum (*arrows* from recording sites C-127 to C-129) and in the distal transverse colon (*arrows* from recording sites C-70 to C-129) with rapid distal propagation. This colonic motor activity was accompanied by the patient's sensing a need to defecate.

Summary

The process of defecation requires four principal mechanisms: anorectal sensory stimulation causing an urge to defecate in response to rectal distension; reflex relaxation of the internal anal sphincter mediated by intrinsic nonadrenergic inhibitory nerves; colorectal motility, chiefly manifested by rapid, high-amplitude propagating contractions; and an increase in intra-abdominal pressure by the Valsalva maneuver to produce perineal descent. In this proposed model of defecation, propagating colonic contractions propel fecal material into the rectum. Distension of the rectum produced by accumulation of fecal material induces descending relaxation of the internal anal sphincter and voluntary contraction of the external anal sphincter to protect continence. At that time, normal individuals sense the urge to defecate. Increasing their intra-abdominal pressure by the Valsalva maneuver produces perineal descent by relaxing the puborectalis muscle and facilitates passage of fecal material. As an additional feature of defecation, there is a direct relationship in normal individuals between dietary fiber intake and the output of fecal material. Dietary fiber may assist the process of defecation by producing bulkier, softer stools. A fundamental understanding of these physiologic mechanisms is required to plan medical or surgical intervention in disorders of defecation.

REFERENCES

1. Bayliss WM, Starling EH. The mechanisms of pancreatic secretion. J Physiol (Lond) 1902;28:325–353.
2. Pearse AGE. Diffuse neuroendocrine system peptides common to brain and intestine and their relationship to the APUD concept. In: Hughes J, ed. Centrally acting peptides. Baltimore: University Park Press, 1978:49–57.
3. Johnson LR. Regulation of gastrointestinal growth. In: Johnson L, ed. Physiology of the gastrointestinal tract. 2nd ed. New York: Raven, 1987:301–333.
4. Brown JC, Dryburgh JR, Ross SA, Dupre J. Identification and actions of gastric inhibitory polypeptide. Prog Hormone Res 1975;31:487.
5. Schwartz JH. The transport of substances in nerve cells. Sci Am 1980;242:152–171.
6. Alberts B, Bray D, Lewis J, Raff M, Roberts K, Watson JD. Molecular biology of the cell. New York, Garland, 1989.
7. Weisbrodt NW. Motility of the small intestine. In: Johnson LR, ed. Physiology of the gastrointestinal tract. New York: Raven, 1987:631–664.
8. Debas HT. Peripheral regulation of gastric acid secretion. In: Johnson LR, ed. Physiology of the gastrointestinal tract. New York: Raven, 1987:931–946.
9. Johnson LR. Regulation of gastrointestinal growth. In Johnson LR, ed. Physiology of the gastrointestinal tract. New York: Raven, 1987:301–334.
10. Debas HT. Clinical significance of gastrointestinal hormones. Adv Surg 1987;21:157–188.
11. Stern AL, Hansky J, Korman MG, et al. Pancreatic polypeptide release following surgery for duodenal ulcer disease. Dig Dis Sci 1980;25:485–488.
12. Taylor IL. Pancreatic polypeptide release following gastric surgery. Dig Dis Sci 1980;25:481–484.
13. Miller AJ. Deglutition. Physiol Rev 1982;62:129–184.
14. Doty RW, Bosma JF. An electromyographic analysis of reflex deglutition. J Neurophysiol 1956;19:44–60.
15. Kahrilas PJ. Functional anatomy and physiology of the esophagus. In: Castell DO, ed. The esophagus. Boston: Little, Brown & Co., 1992:1–27.
16. Kahrilas PJ, Dodds, WJ, Hogan WJ. The effect of peristaltic dysfunction on esophageal volume clearance. Gastroenterology 1988;94:73–80.
17. Mittal RK, Rochester DF, McCallum RW. Electrical and mechanical activity in the human lower esophageal sphincter during diaphragmatic contraction. J Clin Invest 1988;81:1182–1189.
18. Dent J, Holloway RH, Toouli J, et al. Mechanisms of lower esophageal sphincter incompetence in patients with symptomatic gastroesophageal reflux. Gut 1988;20:1020–1028.
19. Schofield GC, Ito S, Bolander RP. Change in membrane surface areas in mouse parietal cells in relation to high levels of acid secretion. J Anat 1979;128:669–692.
20. Sachs G. The gastric proton pump. The H^+/K^+-ATPase. In: Johnson LR, Christensen J, Jackson MJ, et al, eds. Physiology of the gastrointestinal tract. Vol. 2. 2nd ed. New York: Raven, 1981: 865–882.
21. Soll AH, Wollin A. Histamine and cyclic AMP in isolated canine parietal cells. Am J Physiol 1979;237:E444–E450.
22. Soll AH, Amirian DA, Thomas LP, et al. Gastrin receptors on isolated canine parietal cells. J Clin Invest 1984;73:1434–1447.
23. Debas HT, Mulholland MW. Drug therapy in peptic ulcer disease. Curr Prob Surg 1989;26:26(1):1–56.
24. Feldman M. Gastric secretion. In: Sleisenger MH, Fordtran JS, eds. Gastrointestinal disease. Pathophysiology, diagnosis, management. 3rd ed. Philadelphia: WB Saunders, 1983:541–558.
25. Tache Y. Central nervous system regulation of gastric acid secretion. In: Johnson LR, Christensen J, Jackson MJ, et al, eds. Physiology of the gastrointestinal tract. Vol. 2. 2nd ed. New York: Raven, 1987:911–930.
26. Walsh JH, Grossman M. Gastrin. N Engl J Med 1975;292: 1324–1332.
27. Debas HT. Peripheral regulation of acid secretion. In: Johnson LR, Christensen J, Jackson MJ, et al, eds. Physiology of the gastrointestinal tract. Vol. 2. 2nd ed. New York: Raven, 1987.
28. McGuigan JE. Side effects of histamine-2-receptor and antagonists. Clin Gastroenterol 1931;12:819–838.
29. Fundes JW, Mercer JE. Cimetidine histamine H_2 receptor antagonist occupies androgen receptors. J Clin Endocrinol Metab 1979; 48:189–191.
30. Hammer R, Berrie CP, Birdsall NJY, et al. Pirenzepine distinguished between different subclasses of muscarinic receptors. Nature 1982;2:900–902.
31. Hirschowitz BJ, Fong J, Molina E. Effects of pirenzepine and atropine on vagal and cholinergic gastric secretion and gastrin release and on heart rate in the dog. J Pharmacol Exp Ther 1983;225: 263–268.
32. Maton PN. Omeprazole. N Engl J Med 1991;324:965–975.
33. Haru N. Enterochromaffin-like cell carcinoids of gastric mucosa in rats offer life-long inhibition of gastric secretion. Digestion 1986;35(suppl 1):42–55.
34. Samloff IM, Townes PL. Electrophoretic heterogenicity and relationships of pepsinogens in human urine, serum, and gastric mucosa. Gastroenterology 1970;58:462–469.
35. Donaldson RM. Intrinsic factor and the transport of cobal. In: Johnson LR, Christensen J, Jackson MJ, et al, eds. Physiology of the gastrointestinal tract. Vol. 1, 2nd ed. New York: Raven Press, 1987:959–974.
36. Flemstrom G, Turnberg LA. Gastroduodenal defense mechanisms. Clin Gastroenterol 1984;13:327–354.
37. Meyer JH. The physiology of gastric motility and gastric emptying. In: Yamada T, Alpers DH, Owyang C, et al, eds. Textbook of gastroenterology. Philadelphia: JB Lippincott, 1991:137–157.
38. Malagelada JR, Azpiroz F. Determinants of gastric emptying and transit in the small intestine. In: Wood JD, ed. Handbook of physiology. Section 6, The gastrointestinal system. Vol. I, Motility and circulation. Bethesda, MD: American Physiological Society 1989: 909–937.
39. Sarna SK. Cyclic motor activity; migrating motor complex 1985. Gastroenterology 1985;89:894–913.
40. Read NW, Houghton LA. Physiology of gastric emptying and pathophysiology of gastroparesis. Gastroenterol Clin North Am 1989;18:359–374.
41. Lang IM, Sarna SK. Motor and myoelectric activity associated

with vomiting, regurgitation and nausea. In: Wood JD, ed. Handbook of physiology. Section 6, The gastrointestinal system. Vol. I, Motility and circulation. Bethesda, MD: American Physiological Society, 1989:1179–1198.

42. Lang IM. Digestive tract motor correlates of vomiting and nausea. Can J Physiol Pharmacol 1990;78:242–253.

43. Lang IM, Sarna SK. Neural control of initiation and propagation of the retrograde contraction associated with vomiting. In: Brooks FT, Evers P, ed. Nerves and the gastrointestinal tract. Lancaster, UK: MTP Press 1989:726–731.

44. Gadacz TR, Richter HM III. Physiology of the small intestine. In: Zuidema GD, ed. Shackelford's surgery of the alimentary tract. 3rd ed. Philadelphia: WB Saunders, 1991:237–263.

45. Wright HK, Zucker KA, Ballantyne GH. Gastrointestinal function. In: Davis JH, ed. Clinical surgery. St. Louis: CV Mosby, 1987:235–265.

46. Dempsey DT, Ritchie WP. Anatomy and physiology of the stomach. In: Zuidema GD, ed. Shackelford's surgery of the alimentary tract. 3rd ed. Philadelphia: WB Saunders, 1991:3–14.

47. Castro GA. Digestion and absorption. In: Johnson LR, ed. Gastrointestinal physiology. St. Louis: CV Mosby, 1991:108–130.

48. Guyton AC. Textbook of medical physiology. 8th ed. Philadelphia: WB Saunders, 1991;726–734.

49. West JB. Best and Taylor's physiology of medical practice. 12th ed. Baltimore: Williams & Wilkins, 1991:693–706.

50. Kimmich GA, Randles J. Evidence for an intestinal NA-Sugar transport coupling stoichiometry of 2.0. Biochem Biophys Acta 1980;596:43.

51. Sellin, JH. Physiology of digestion and absorption. In: Miller, TA ed. Physiologic basis of modern surgical care. St. Louis: CV Mosby, 1988:330–346.

52. Adibi SA. Protein assimilation. In: Berk JE, ed. Bockus gastroenterology. 4th ed. Philadelphia: WB Saunders, 1985:3:15:30–37.

53. Sleisenger MH, Kim YS. Protein digestion and absorption. N Engl J Med 1991;300:659.

54. Freeman HJ, Kim YS. Digestion and absorption of protein. Annu Rev Med 1979;2:799.

55. Adibi SA, Kim YS. Peptide absorption and hydrolysis. In: Johnson LR, ed. Physiology of the gastrointestinal tract. New York: Raven, 1981:1073.

56. Fogel MR, Ravitch MM, Adibi SA. Absorptive and digestive function of the jejunum after jejunoileal bypass for treatment of human obesity. Gastroenterology 1976;71:729–33.

57. Waldmann TZ. Protein-losing enteropathies. In: Bockus HL, ed. Gastroenterology. 3rd ed. Philadelphia: WB Saunders, 1976:361–386.

58. Gray GM. Mechanism of digestion and absorption of food. In: Sleisenger MH, Fordtran JS, eds. Gastrointestinal disease—pathophysiology, diagnosis, management. 3rd ed. Philadelphia: WB Saunders, 1983:844–853.

59. Borgstrom B. Fat assimilation. In Bockus HL, ed. Gastroenterology. 4th ed. Philadelphia: WB Saunders, 1985:1510–1519.

60. Hamilton JA, Small DM. Solubilization and localization of triolein in phosphatidylcholine bilayers. A 136 NMR study. Proc Natl Acad Sci U S A 1981;78:6878–6882.

61. Hildebrand H, Borgstrom B, Bekassy A, et al. Isolated co-lipase deficiency in two brothers. Gut 1982;23:243–246.

62. Borgstrom B. Importance of phospholipids, pancreatic phospholipase A₂, and fatty acid for the digestion of dietary fat. Gastroenterology 1980;78:954–962.

63. Hofmann AF. Fat absorption and malabsorption: physiology, diagnosis, and treatment. Viewpoints Dig Dis 1977;9:4.

64. Westergaard H, Dietschy JM. Delineation of dimensions and permeability characteristics of the two major diffusion barriers to passive mucosal uptake in the rabbit intestine. J Clin Invest 1974;54:718.

65. Wilson FA, Dietschy JM. Characterization of bile absorption across the unstirred water layer and brush border of the rat jejunum. J Clin Invest 1972;51:3015.

66. Lack L, Weiner IM. Intestinal absorption of bile salts and some biological implications. Fed Proc 1963;22:1334–1338.

67. Go VLW, Hofmann AF, Summerskill WHJ. Pancreozymin bioassay in man based on pancreatic enzyme secretion potency of specific amino acids and other digestive products. J Clin Invest 1970;49:1558–1564.

68. Meyer JH, Kelly GA. Canine pancreatic responses to intestinally perfused proteins and protein digests. Am J Physiol 1976;231:682–691.

69. Malagelada JR, Go VLW, DiMagno EP, et al. Interactions between intraluminal bile acids and digestive products on pancreatic and gallbladder function. J Clin Invest 1973;52:2160–2165.

70. Javitt, NB. Hepatic bile formation. N Eng J Med 1976;295:1464–1469.

71. Hofmann AF, Small DM. Detergent properties of bile salts. Correlation with physiological function. Annu Rev Med 1967;18:333–376.

72. Alpers DH. Absorption of water-soluble vitamins, folate, minerals and vitamin D. In: Sleisenger MH, Fordtran JS eds. Gastrointestinal disease—pathophysiology, diagnosis, management. 3rd ed. Philadelphia: WB Saunders, 1983:830–843.

73. Dudrick SJ, Latifi R, Fosnocht DE. Management of the short-bowel syndrome. Surg Clin North Am 1991;71:625–643.

74. Allard J, Jeejeebhoy K. Nutritional support and therapy in the short bowel syndrome. Gastroenterol Clin North Am 1989;18:589–601.

75. Deitel M, Wong KH. Short bowel syndrome. In: Deitel M, ed. Nutrition in clinical surgery. Baltimore: Williams & Wilkins, 1980:189–208.

76. Dudrick SJ, Jackson D. The short bowel syndrome and total parenteral nutrition. Heart Lung 1983;12:195–201.

77. Gouttebel M, Saint-Aubert B, Astre C, et al. Total parenteral nutrition needs in different types of short bowel syndrome. Dig Dis Sci 1986;31:718–723.

78. Weser E. Nutritional aspects of malabsorption. Short gut adaptation. Clin Gastroenterol 1983;12:443–461.

79. Tilson MD. Pathophysiology and treatment of short bowel syndrome. Surg Clin North Am 1980;60:1273–1284.

80. Dudrick SJ, Englert DM. Management of the short bowel syndrome. In: Miller TA, Dudrick SJ, eds. The management of difficult surgical problems. Austin: University of Texas Press 1981:225–235.

81. Dudrick SJ, O'Donnel JJ, Englert DM. Ambulatory home parenteral nutrition for short bowel syndrome and other diseases. In Deitel M, ed. Nutrition in clinical surgery. Baltimore: Williams & Wilkins, 1985:276–287.

82. Trier JS. The short bowel syndrome. In: Sleisenger MH, Fordtran JS, eds. Gastrointestinal disease—pathophysiology, diagnosis, management. Philadelphia: WB Saunders, 1973:971–977.

83. Weser E, Fletcher JT, Urban E. Short bowel syndrome. Gastroenterology 1979;77:572–579.

84. Wilmore DW, Dudrick SJ. Effects of nutrition on intestinal adaptation following massive small bowel resection. Surg Forum 1969;20:398–400.

85. Wilmore DW, Holtzapple PG, Dudrick SJ, et al. Transport studies, morphological and histochemical findings in intestinal epithelial cells following massive bowel resection. Surg Forum 1971;22:361–363.

86. Conn HJ, Chavez Cm, Fain WR. The short bowel syndrome. Ann Surg 1972;175:803–814.

87. Dudrick SJ. A clinical review of nutritional support of the patients. Am J Clin Nutr 1981;34:1191–1198.

88. Sheldon GF. Role of parenteral nutrition in patients with short-bowel syndrome. Med J Aust 1979;67:1021–1029.

89. Stewart GR. Home parenteral nutrition for chronic short-bowel syndrome. Med J Aust 1979;2:317–319.

90. Wilmore DW, Johnson DJ. Metabolic effects of small bowel reversal in treatment of the short bowel syndrome. Arch Surg 1968;97:784–791.

91. Wilmore DW, Dudrick SJ, Daly JM, et al. The role of nutrition in the adaptation of the small intestine after massive resection. Surg Gynecol Obstet 1971;132:673–680.

92. Borgstrom B, Dahlquist A, Lundh G, et al. Studies of intestinal digestion and absorption in the human. J Clin Invest 1957;36:1521–1536.

93. Debongnie J, Philips S. Capacity of the human colon to absorb fluid. Gastroenterology 1978;74:698–703.

94. Ricotta J, Zuidema FD, Gadacz RT, et al. Construction of an ileocecal valve and its role in massive resection of the small intestine. Surg Gynecol Obstet 1981;152:310–314.

95. Wright HK, Tilson MD. Short gut syndrome. Pathophysiology and treatment. Curr Probl Surg 1971;8:1–51.

96. Strause E, Gerson E, Yalow RS. Hypersecretion of gastrin associ-

ated with the short bowel syndrome. Gastroenterology 1974;66:175–180.

97. Philips SF, Giller J. The contribution of the colon to electrolyte and water conservation in man. J Lab Clin Med 1973;81:733–746.

98. Bond JH, Levitt MD. Fate of soluble carbohydrate in the colon of rats and humans. J Clin Invest 1976;57:1158–1164.

99. Bond JH, Currier BE, Buchwald H, et al. Colonic conservation of malabsorbed carbohydrates. Gastroenterology 1980;78:444–447.

100. Haverstad T. Studies of short-chain fatty acid absorption in man. Scand J Gastroenterol 1980;21:257–260.

101. Pomare EW, Branch WJ, Cummings JH. Carbohydrate fermentation in the human colon and its relation to blood acetate concentrations in venous blood. J Clin Invest 1985;75:1148–1154.

102. Capron JP, Gineston JL, Herve MA, et al. Metronidazole in prevention of cholestasis associated with total parenteral nutrition. Lancet 1983;1:446–447.

103. Weisbrodt NW. Motility of the small intestine. In: Johnson LR, ed. Physiology of the gastrointestinal tract. Vol. I. New York: Raven 1981:411–443.

104. Sarna SK, Otterson MF. Small intestinal physiology and pathophysiology. Gastroenteral Clin North Am 1989;18:375–404.

105. Sarna SK. Giant migrating contractions and their myoelectric correlates in the small intestine. Am J Physiol 1987;16:G697–G705.

106. Sarna SK. Physiology and pathophysiology of colonic motor activity (Part I). Dig Dis Sci 1991;36:998–1019.

107. Christensen J. Motility of the colon. In: Johnson LR, ed. Physiology of the gastrointestinal tract. New York: Raven, 1981:445–471.

108. Dapoigny M, Cowles VE, Zhu YR, et al. Vagal influence on colonic motor activity in conscious non-human primates. Am J Physiol 1992;25:G231–G236.

109. Sarna SK, Condon RE, Cowles VE. Colonic migrating and nonmigrating motor complexes in dogs. Am J Physiol 1984;9:G335–G360.

110. Frantzides CT, Condon RE, Schulte WJ, et al. Effect of morphine on colonic myoelectric and motor activity. Am J Physiol 1990;21:G247–G252.

111. Condon RE, Frantzides CT, Cowles VE, et al. Resolution of postoperative ileus in humans. Ann Surg 1986;203:574–581.

112. Mebis J, Penninck F, Geboes K, et al. Neuropathology of Hirschsprung's disease. En Face study of microdissected intestine. Hepatogastroenterology 1990;73:596–600.

113. Bielefeldt K, Enck P, Erckenbrecht JF. Sensory and motor function in the maintenance of anal continence. Dis Colon Rectum 1990;33:674–678.

114. Williamson JL, Nelson RL, Orsay C, et al. A comparison of simultaneous longitudinal and radial recordings of anal canal pressures. Dis Colon Rectum 1990;33:201–206.

115. Infantino A, Masin A, Pianon P, et al. Role of proctography in severe constipation. Dis Colon Rectum 1990;33:707–712.

116. Bassotti G, Gaburri M. Manometric investigation of high-amplitude propagated contractile activity of the human colon. Am J Physiol 1988;255:G660–G664.

117. Holdstock DJ, Misiewicz JJ, Smith T, et al. Propulsion (mass movements) in the human colon and its relationship to meals and somatic activity. Gut 1980;11:91–99.

118. Burkitt DP, Walker ARP, Painter NS. Effect of dietary fiber on stools and transit-times, and its role in the causation of disease. Lancet 1972;2:1408–1411.

119. Bannister JJ, Davison P, Timms JM, et al. Effect of stool size and consistency on defecation. Gut 1987;28:1246–1250.

18 Liver, Biliary Tract, and Pancreas

Andrew S. Klein | Keith D. Lillemoe | Charles J. Yeo | Henry A. Pitt

Anatomy

An understanding of the anatomy of the liver, biliary tract and pancreas begins with embryology. At the fourth week in the development of the human embryo, a projection appears in the ventral wall of the primitive midgut. At this 3-mm stage, three buds can be recognized. The cranial bud develops into two lobes of the liver, whereas the caudal bud becomes the gallbladder and extrahepatic biliary tree (Fig. 18.1). The ventral pancreas, which eventually becomes the pancreatic head and uncinate process, also develops from the caudal bud. The third primitive bud develops from the dorsal surface of the midgut to become the anlage of the remainder of the pancreatic head as well as the neck, body, and tail of the pancreas (1).

By the 12-mm stage (see Fig. 18.1), the ventral pancreatic bud has rotated 180° clockwise around the duodenum. This rotation causes fusion of the ventral and dorsal buds to form the complete pancreas by the sixth or seventh week of gestation. Within another week, a completely open lumen has formed in the gallbladder, bile ducts, and pancreatic ducts. By the 12th week of fetal life, the liver begins to secrete bile, and the pancreas secretes fluid that flows via the extrahepatic biliary tree and pancreatic ducts, respectively, into the duodenum.

Liver

The liver occupies the entire area under the right hemidiaphragm, and the left lobe extends beyond the midline into the left upper quadrant. In the adult, the liver ranges in weight from 1200 to 1600 g and is the single largest organ in the body. The average adult liver measures 23 cm transversely, 15 cm anteroposteriorly, and 6 cm vertically. The liver's anterior and superior diaphragmatic surfaces are covered with peritoneum. On either side of the inferior vena cava, but primarily on the right, bare diaphragmatic areas have no serosal covering.

The smooth appearance of the anterior and superior surfaces of the liver is interrupted only by the falciform ligament emanating from the umbilical fissure. Early descriptions of anatomy used the falciform ligament to divide the liver on its superior surface into a large right and small left lobe (Fig. 18.2A). Two additional lobes were also described on the inferior surface (the quadrate lobe) between the umbilical fissure and the gallbladder fossa, and on the caudate lobe wedged between the groove of the inferior vena cava, the transverse hilar fissure, and the umbilical fissure. However, these lobar divisions, based on surface topography of the liver, do not coincide with the course of the intrahepatic vasculature and bile ducts and, therefore, are of little importance when performing an anatomical resection.

The lobar and segmental anatomy of the liver is determined by the sequential branching of the portal vein, hepatic artery, and biliary tree as they enter the parenchyma at the hilum. All three of these structures follow roughly parallel courses and bifurcate just before entering the liver. This major bifurcation divides the liver into left and right lobes. According to Couinaud's classification, the caudate lobe is segment I, segments II to IV are on the left, and segments V to VIII are on the right (see Fig. 18.2B).

The left portal vein, hepatic artery, and hepatic duct run along the surface of the liver for several centimeters before entering the liver parenchyma. After entering the liver on the left, these structures bifurcate with one branch, continuing directly into the lateral segment, Couinard's segment IV. The right portal vein, hepatic artery, and hepatic duct bifurcate into anteromedial and posterolateral branches shortly after entering the parenchyma. In Couinard's classification, segments V and VIII originate from the anteromedial branch, and segments VI and VII arise from the posterolateral branch. Anomalies of the main portal veins are extremely unusual. In comparison, the so-called normal anatomy of the hepatic arteries is present in only 55% to 65% of the popula-

441

Figure 18.1. Development of the liver, biliary tract, and pancreas from the 3-mm to the 12-mm stage. From Lindner HR. Embryology and anatomy of the biliary tract. In: Way LW, Pellegrini CA, eds. Surgery of the gallbladder and bile ducts. Philadelphia: WB Saunders, 1987:4.

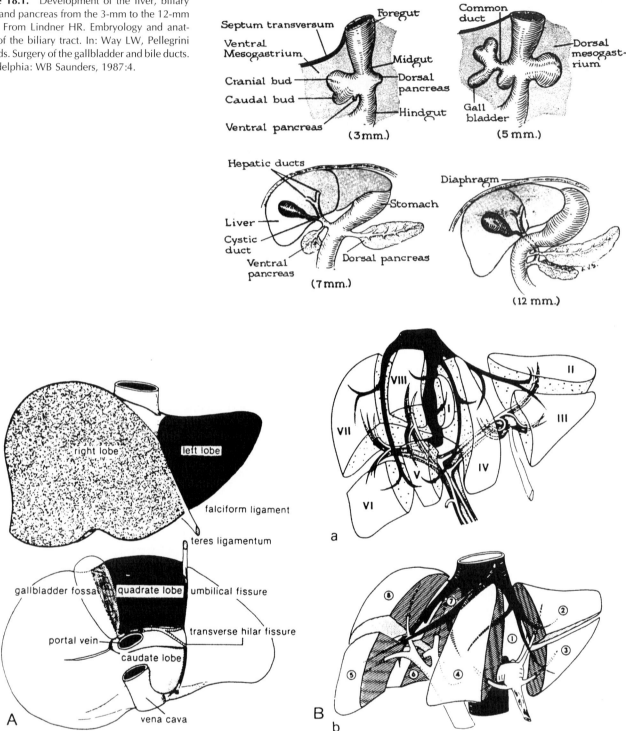

Figure 18.2. **A,** Historical lobar anatomy of the liver. **B,** Functional segments of the liver according to Couinard's classification in the (a) exvivo position and (b) in situ position. From Bismuth H. Surgical anatomy of the liver. In: Bengmark S, Blumgart LH, eds. Liver surgery. New York: Churchill Livingstone, 1986:1, 3.

tion. Generally, the common hepatic artery arises from the celiac axis and gives rise to the right and left hepatic arteries. The two most common arterial anomalies are a replaced right hepatic artery, originating from the superior mesenteric artery, and a left hepatic artery arising from the left gastric artery (2).

Three hepatic veins drain the liver. Unlike the portal veins and hepatic arteries, the hepatic veins do not follow lobar or segmental anatomy (see Fig. 18.2B). The left hepatic vein drains most of the left lobe, the right hepatic vein drains most of the right lobe, and the middle hepatic vein drains both lobes. The three hepatic veins enter the inferior vena cava at the superior aspect of the liver just below the diaphragm. Occasionally, the middle vein will join the right or left vein before entering the vena cava. Multiple smaller veins also enter the vena cava directly from the hepatic parenchyma or via the caudate lobe.

Biliary Tract

The anatomy of the biliary tract can be divided into various segments, including the intrahepatic ducts, the right and left hepatic ducts, the common hepatic duct, the gallbladder, the cystic duct, the common bile duct, and the sphincter of Oddi. The intrahepatic ducts were discussed in the section on the liver. As a rule, these ducts drain the liver segments and are separated into right and left lobar branches (see Fig. 18.2B). Occasional variations do exist; for example, a right segmental branch may drain into the left hepatic duct or vice versa.

Most patients have a bifurcation where the right and left hepatic ducts join to form the common hepatic duct. This junction may occur as a wide or an acute angle, or the two hepatic ducts may run parallel to each other before joining. In some patients, three hepatic ducts will join to form the common hepatic duct. Usually, the hepatic ducts meet just outside of the liver parenchyma, with the cystic duct entering 2 to 3 cm distally. Occasionally, the two hepatic ducts do not unite until after the cystic duct has joined the right hepatic duct.

The cystic duct is generally about 5 cm long but may vary markedly from 0.5 to 8 cm, depending on its mode of junction with the hepatic duct. The cystic duct usually runs dorsally, to the left and inferiorly to join the common hepatic duct (CHD) at an acute angle on its right side. However, the cystic duct may (a) enter the right hepatic duct, (b) join the CHD at a right angle, (c) parallel the CHD, (d) enter the CHD dorsally, (e) enter the CHD on its left side, (f) enter the CHD behind the duodenum, or (g) join the CHD as it enters the duodenal wall (1). The mode of entrance of the cystic duct into the CHD may be spiral as well as angular or parallel. The cystic duct usually has 4 to 10 crescentic folds known as the spiral valves of Heister. The cystic duct, the common hepatic duct, and the hilum of the liver form Calot's triangle.

The gallbladder is a pear-shaped organ that lies on the inferior surface of the liver at the junction of the left and right hepatic lobes between Couinard's segments IV and V (see Fig. 18.2B). The gallbladder varies from 7 to 10 cm in length and from 2.5 to 3.5 cm in width. The gallbladder's volume varies considerably, being large during fasting states and small after eating. A moderately distended gallbladder has a capacity of 50 to 60 ml of bile but may become much larger with certain pathologic states. The gallbladder has been divided into four areas: the fundus, body, infundibulum, and neck. Hartmann's pouch is an asymmetric bulge of the infun-dibulum that lies close to the gallbladder's neck. The neck points in a cephalad and dorsal direction to join the cystic duct.

The common bile duct (CBD) begins at the junction of the cystic duct with the common hepatic duct. The average CBD length is about 7.5 cm, but this figure varies considerably, depending on the site of union of the cystic duct with the common hepatic duct. The CBD diameter is usually less than 1.0cm, but this figure increases with age and increases dramatically in diameter when obstructed. The CBD can be separated into the (a) supraduodenal, (b) retroduodenal, (c) pancreatic, and (d) intraduodenal intramural portions (Fig. 18.3A). The CBD opens into the ampulla of Vater and usually, but not always, unites with the pancreatic duct just within the bowel wall (see Fig. 18.3B). The CBD enters the duodenum near the junction of the second and third portions in nearly 90% of the population (1).

The entire sphincteric system of the distal bile duct and the pancreatic duct is commonly referred to as the sphincter of Oddi. This term is imprecise because the sphincter is subdivided into several sections and contains both circular and longitudinal fibers. The sphincter mechanism functions independently from the surrounding duodenal musculature and has separate sphincters for the distal bile duct, the pancreatic duct, and the ampulla. In more than 90% of the population, the common channel, where the biliary and pancreatic ducts join, is less than 1.0 cm in length and lies within the ampulla. In the rare situation in which the common channel is longer than 1.0 cm or the biliary and pancreatic ducts open separately into the duodenum, pathologic biliary or pancreatic problems are likely to develop.

The common bile duct, the common hepatic artery, and the portal vein lie in the hepatoduodenal ligament. Normally, the CBD is on the right, the common hepatic artery is on the left, and the portal vein is in a dorsal position between the two. The right hepatic artery usually passes dorsal to the common hepatic duct and ventral to the portal vein. When the right hepatic artery is replaced and originates from the superior mesenteric artery, it lies to the right and dorsal to the CBD and to the right and just ventral to the portal vein. The blood supply to the extrahepatic biliary tree arises from the right and left hepatic, common hepatic, gastroduodenal, and pancreatoduodenal arteries. Within the common hepatic duct and common bile duct, longitudinal vessels run in the 3-o'clock and 9-o'clock positions. The cystic artery arises from the right hepatic artery in 95% of the population but may arise from any of the other adjacent arteries (1). The gallbladder and biliary ducts receive nerve fibers from both the sympathetic and parasympathetic nervous systems. These nerves begin at the celiac plexus and travel via the hepatic plexus along the hepatic artery and portal vein. The hepatic plexus contains fibers from the posterior vagus and is joined just inferior to the liver by branches from the anterior vagus. The

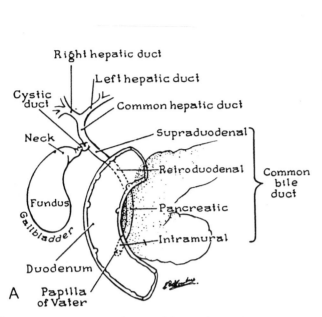

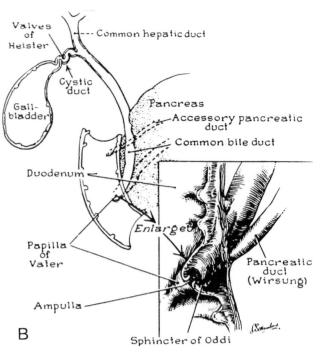

Figure 18.3. **A,** Anatomic division of the extrahepatic biliary tract. **B,** Relationship of the gallbladder and bile ducts to the duodenum. From Gadacz TR. Anatomy, embryology, congenital anomalies, and physiol- ogy of the gallbladder and extrahepatic biliary ducts. In: Zuidema GD, Turcotte JG, eds. Shackelford's surgery of the alimentary tract. 3rd ed. Philadelphia: WB Saunders, 1991;3:139.

lymphatic drainage from the gallbladder may go directly into the liver or toward the cystic duct. Lymph drainage from here and along the common bile duct courses toward the liver and into a deep pancreatic group of nodes, which eventually drain back to the celiac nodes (1, 2).

Pancreas

The pancreas is a retroperitoneal organ extending in an oblique, transverse position from the duodenal C-loop to the hilum of the spleen. The pancreas lies anterior to the right renal vessels, vena cava, portal vein, aorta, superior mesenteric artery, splenic vein, and left renal vessels. The celiac axis, hepatic artery, and splenic artery run along its cephalad edge, and the transverse mesocolon borders the pancreas inferiorly. The stomach and greater omentum cover most of the pancreas anteriorly. The normal pancreas weighs 80 to 90 g and is approximately 20 cm in length. The body of the pancreas measures approximately 4 to 5 cm in width and 1.5 to 2 cm in thickness (3).

The pancreas is divided into five parts: the head, uncinate, neck, body, and tail. The pancreatic head lies adjacent to the second lumbar vertebra and is intimately attached to the duodenum. The distal CBD passes through the pancreatic head (see Fig. 18.3B), although in approximately 15% of people, the CBD remains in a groove on the posterior aspect of the pancreas. The uncinate process lies adjacent to the third and fourth portions of the duodenum and next to the superior mes-

enteric vein (SMV). The uncinate process also extends behind the SMV and portal vein to the right edge of the superior mesenteric artery.

The neck of the pancreas joins the head and the body. The pancreatic neck overlies and is grooved by the junction of the SMV and splenic veins as they become the portal vein. Usually, no anterior venous tributaries of the SMV or portal vein extend from the pancreatic neck. The communication of the gastroduodenal artery with the right gastroepiploic artery lies on the anterior surface of the pancreatic neck (Fig. 18.4). These vessels run between the pancreatic neck and the pylorus, which also covers the pancreatic neck anteriorly.

The body of the pancreas extends to the left of the neck beyond the superior mesenteric vessels. The body usually crosses the vertebral column at the level of the first lumbar vertebra. Superiorly, the pancreatic body lies adjacent to the celiac axis and splenic arteries, whereas the ligament of Treitz and the proximal jejunum are related inferiorly. The splenic vein lies in a groove posteriorly, and multiple small veins enter it from the pancreas. The inferior mesenteric vein also joins the splenic vein to the left of the ligament of Treitz and along the inferior border of the body of the pancreas. No specific landmark defines the merger of the body and tail of the pancreas. Normally, the pancreatic tail extends into the splenic hilum; however, in patients with chronic pancreatitis, the tail of the pancreas may contract away from the spleen.

The pancreas has two ducts draining into the duodenum: the main duct of Wirsung and the accessory duct

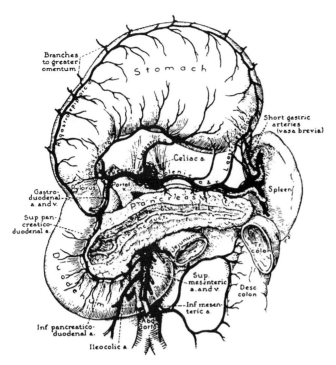

Figure 18.4. Blood supply of the pancreas and duodenum. The stomach is shown reflected upward, and the pancreatic duct is exposed. From Jones T, Shepard WC. A manual of surgical anatomy. Philadelphia: WB Saunders, 1950.

Table 18.1.
Major Functions of the Liver

Energy metabolism
Protein synthesis
Detoxification
Bile production
Reticuloendothelial clearance

of the pancreas. The venous blood from the pancreas drains into the portal system via the superior mesenteric or splenic veins or directly into the portal vein.

The pancreas is innervated by both sympathetic fibers from the splanchnic nerves and parasympathetic fibers from the vagus. The preganglionic efferent fibers of splanchnic nerves pass through the celiac ganglion before reaching the pancreas. Afferent pain fibers have cell bodies in the dorsal root ganglia of T5 to T12. The efferent and afferent parasympathetic fibers also have cell bodies in the brain and pass via the posterior vagus through the celiac ganglion without synapsing before entering the pancreas. Lymphatic drainage extends in all directions but concentrates in pancreatoduodenal and preaortic nodes near the origins of the superior mesenteric artery and the celiac axis.

of Santorini (see Fig. 18.3B). The main pancreatic duct extends from the tail of the pancreas toward the head. In the body of the pancreas, the main duct usually runs midway between the superior and inferior borders and closer to the posterior than to the anterior surface. The main pancreatic duct normally measures 3 to 4.5 mm in diameter. After passing into the neck of the pancreas, the main pancreatic duct extends in a caudal and posterior direction before joining the distal bile duct at the ampulla. The accessory pancreatic duct usually drains the anterior, superior portions of the pancreatic head via a minor papilla, which enters the duodenum approximately 2 cm proximal and slightly anterior to the ampulla of Vater. In 90% of the population, the main and accessory pancreatic ducts join near the junction of the head and neck of the pancreas.

The pancreas derives its blood supply from the gastroduodenal, superior mesenteric, and splenic arteries and sometimes from the celiac and hepatic arteries. The anterior and posterior pancreatoduodenal arcades are the terminal vessels supplying the pancreatic head and duodenum. The superior arteries arise from the gastroduodenal artery and the inferior arteries come from the superior mesenteric artery (see Fig. 18.4). The neck, body, and tail of the pancreas receive blood from superior dorsal and inferior transverse pancreatic arteries. These usually arise from the splenic artery and run within the substance of the gland. When the right hepatic artery arises from the superior mesenteric, it usually runs along with the portal vein posterior to the neck

Hepatic Physiology

The human liver is a complex organ that, in its usual state of health, provides a variety of essential functions. One classification of these major functions is presented in Table 18.1. As a result of its dual blood supply from the portal vein and hepatic artery, the liver is uniquely situated at the interface between the abdominal viscera and the systemic circulation. In this position, both anabolism and catabolism of carbohydrates, lipids, and proteins are coordinated within the liver to satisfy the ever changing availability of substrates and metabolic demands of the body. Detoxification of xenobiotics absorbed through the intestinal tract is handled by hepatic enzyme systems. Bile production, to aid in intestinal absorption and to excrete breakdown products from processed autogenous tissues (i.e., heme from senescent red blood cells), is another major function of the liver. Filtration of pathogens that invade the body through the intestinal tract and enter the portal circulation occurs in the hepatic reticuloendothelial system. This specialized network of cells is primarily responsible for the phagocytosis, killing, and elimination of these organisms.

This section provides an overview of the liver's major functions and a framework for assessment of the liver's integrity in individual patients. The pathophysiologic processes associated with liver derangement will be discussed later in this chapter. A complete exposition of the multitude of other physiologic functions of the liver, including the metabolism of vitamins, hormones, specific drugs, toxins, metals, and porphyrins, is beyond the scope of this chapter. Although limitations of space preclude their discussion in detail, these other liver functions should not be considered less important or critical to survival.

Energy Metabolism

The liver is the central clearinghouse for the generation, conversion, distribution, and storage of energy sources required by the body. Many specialized cells in the body are able to use a limited spectrum of fuels, and the survival of these tissues depends directly on the liver's ability to consistently provide these fuels. Glucose, for instance, is the sole substrate for red blood cells, which lack mitochondria, and is the preferred energy source for the renal medulla and the central nervous system (4). In response to insufficient exogenous glucose, hepatic glycogen is catabolized rapidly to yield glucose by a process called glycogenolysis. The amount of glycogen is limited, and thus for extended periods of glucose deprivation, amino acids, lactate, pyruvate, glycerol, and propionyl-CoA serve as carbon sources for gluconeogenesis in the liver. The glucose produced by these processes is then transported into the bloodstream. Ketones are a second major energy source produced by the liver for use in remote locations. During prolonged fasting, increased levels of fatty acids are generated by lipolysis of adipose tissue. Oxidation of these fatty acids in hepatocyte mitochondria and, possibly peroxisomes, results in the formation of ketone bodies, primarily acetoacetate, which serve as an important secondary fuel for brain and muscle.

In the presence of abundant exogenous nutrients, the liver converts the absorbed fuel into substrates that can be stored locally, such as glycogen, or exported for storage at distant sites, such as fatty acids, glycerol, and lipoproteins. The portasystemic interface at the level of the hepatocyte is essential to the regulation of these complex anabolic and catabolic processes. The intermingling of absorbed fuel from the digestive tract with metabolic products from distant tissues establishes the synthetic or degradative drive for the liver at any point in time. These pathways should not be thought of as mutually exclusive and, indeed, may be catalyzed by distinct enzymes, which explains, in part, how both anabolic and catabolic reactions may proceed and be regulated simultaneously.

Protein Synthesis

A specialized function of the human hepatocyte is the synthesis and secretion of plasma proteins (Table 18.2). Protein synthesis takes place on the polyribosome, a subcellular structure located in the cell cytoplasm. In general, secretory protein synthesis occurs on polyribosomes anchored to the rough endoplasmic reticulum

Table 18.2.
Plasma Proteins Secreted by the Liver

Albumin	Fatty acid-binding protein
α-fetoprotein	Ferritin
α_1-antitrypsin	Haptoglobin
α_2-macroglobulin	Hemopexin
Ceruloplasmin	Serum amyloid A protein
C-reactive protein	Transferrin

Table 18.3.
Coagulation Factors and Inhibitors of Hepatic Origin

Fibrinogen (I)	Factor XI
Prothrombin (II)	Hageman factor (XII)
Proaccelerin (V)	Fibrin-stabilizing factor (XIII)
Proconvertin (VII)	α_2-antiplasmin
Factor IX	Antithrombin (III)
Stuart-Prower factor (X)	C_1 Inhibitor

(RER), and intracellular proteins are translated on free polyribosomes (5). This distinction is thought to be related to the presence of a hydrophobic N-terminus sequence of extra amino acids, a feature common among secretory proteins, which as a group are first synthesized as precursor molecules. The initial N-terminus sequence, which is actually translated on free ribosomes, subsequently facilitates attachment to the RER. The extra amino acids of the precursor are then cleaved from the parent peptide before being secreted from the hepatocyte.

Albumin is the protein produced in largest quantity by the human liver. Albumin is a single polypeptide chain composed of 581 amino acid residues organized into three relatively equal-sized domains. A healthy adult synthesizes approximately 10 g of albumin daily, and the half-life of this protein is roughly 22 days (6). Albumin binds to a variety of other molecules, including bilirubin, thyroid hormone, cortisol, testosterone, metals, and pharmaceutical agents, and plays an important role in the transport of these substances. Other transport or carrier proteins synthesized and secreted by the liver are transferrin, haptoglobin, ferritin, hemopexin, and ceruloplasmin. Fetoprotein, another secretory protein produced by hepatocytes, is thought to be the fetal counterpart of albumin. A striking degree of conservation exists between these two proteins, and a duplication of a common ancestral gene may account for the observed homology (5, 6).

The liver is responsible for the production of a number of proteins essential for hemostasis. Fibrinogen is a large dimeric protein synthesized exclusively by the hepatocyte, which, in the presence of thrombin, gives rise to fibrin monomers, the building blocks of fibrin. Thrombin itself is derived from prothrombin, a glycoprotein also of hepatic origin. These and other coagulation factors synthesized by the liver are listed in Table 18.3.

Table 18.4.
Phase II Detoxification Enzymes

Catechol-*O*-methyltransferase
Glutathione-*S*-transferase
N-acetyltransferase
Sulfotransferase
UDP glucuronosyltransferase

Detoxification

The body is constantly exposed to endogenous and exogenous substances, which, if not processed and eliminated from the circulation, may cause considerable damage. Xenobiotics refer to agents, such as drugs and toxins, that are not employed in normal metabolic pathways to maintain the integrity of a cell or tissue. In some instances, detoxification is a misnomer because the products of xenobiotic metabolism may be more potent or harmful than the parent compound. Detoxification occurs primarily in the liver but can also occur in the kidney, lung, and intestines. The metabolic reactions involved consist primarily of oxidation, reduction, hydrolysis (Phase I reactions) and conjugation (Phase II reactions), depending on the specific substrate. In addition to the generation of a biologically less active compound, many of these reactions tend to promote conversion of a chemical to a more polar and hence more water soluble molecule, which can then be excreted by the kidneys (7).

The Phase I enzyme system in humans, which is most important in xenobiotic metabolism, is the cytochrome P-450 system, which is located on hepatocyte microsomes. The Phase II reactions comprise a heterogeneous group of transferase enzymes that catalyze the combination of the target molecule with an endogenous agent to yield compounds of decreased activity (Table 18.4). The same biochemical reactions that reduce the toxic load from certain xenobiotic agents may actually increase the potency of others with a positive (cyclophosphamide to aldophosphamide) or negative (parathion to paraoxon) therapeutic impact (8).

The detoxification of endogenous substances is also an important function of a healthy liver. Ammonia is the nitrogen-containing waste product of amino acid and nucleic acid catabolism. Substantial amounts of ammonia are also derived from the action of intestinal bacteria upon dietary protein. Within the liver, ammonia is detoxified to urea via enzymes of the urea cycle. Methionine, its metabolite mercaptan, and aminobutyric acid are also products of protein degradation, which, if not processed by the liver, are thought to exert neurotoxic effects.

Bile Production

Hepatocyte Bile Formation

The formation of bile by the hepatocyte serves two functions. Bile represents the route of excretion for cer-

tain organic solids, such as bilirubin and cholesterol, and it facilitates intestinal absorption of lipids and fat-soluble vitamins. Bile secretion results from the active transport of solutes into the canaliculus followed by the passive flow of water. Water constitutes about 85% of the volume of bile.

The major organic solutes in bile are bilirubin, bile salts, phospholipids, and cholesterol. Bilirubin, the breakdown product of spent red blood cells, is conjugated with glucuronic acid by the hepatic enzyme glucuronyl transferase and is excreted actively into the adjacent canaliculus. Normally, a large reserve exists to handle excess bilirubin production, which might exist in hemolytic states. Bile salts are steroid molecules synthesized by the hepatocyte. The primary bile salts in humans, cholic and chenodeoxycholic acid, account for more than 80% of those produced. The primary bile salts, which are then conjugated with either taurine or glycine, can undergo bacterial alteration in the intestine to form the secondary bile salts, deoxycholate and lithocholate. The purpose of bile salts is to solubilize lipids and facilitate their absorption. Phospholipids are synthesized in the liver in conjunction with bile salt synthesis. Lecithin is the primary phospholipid in human bile, constituting over 95% of its total. The final major solute of bile is cholesterol, which is also produced primarily by the liver with little contribution from dietary sources.

The normal volume of bile secreted daily by the liver is 500 to 1000 ml. Bile flow depends on neurogenic, humoral, and chemical control. Vagal stimulation increases bile secretion. Splanchnic stimulation causes vasoconstriction with decreased hepatic blood flow and, thus, diminished bile secretin. Gastrointestinal hormones including secretion, cholecystokinin, gastrin, and glucagon all increase bile flow, primarily by increasing water and electrolyte secretion. This action probably occurs at a site distal to the hepatocyte. Finally, the most important factor in regulating the volume of bile flow is the rate of bile salt synthesis by the hepatocyte. This rate is regulated by the return of bile salts to the liver by the enterohepatic circulation.

Micelle Formation

Cholesterol is highly nonpolar and insoluble in water; thus, it is insoluble in bile. The key to maintaining cholesterol in solution is the formation of micelles, a bile salt-phospholipid-cholesterol complex. Bile salts are amphipathic compounds containing both a hydrophilic and hydrophobic portion. In aqueous solutions, bile salts are oriented with the hydrophilic portion outward. Phospholipids are incorporated into the micellar structure, allowing cholesterol to be added to the hydrophobic central portion of the micelle. In this way, cholesterol can be maintained in solution in an aqueous medium. Recently, the concept of mixed micelles as the only cholesterol carrier has been challenged by the demonstra-

Figure 18.5. Interrelationships of bile salts, lecithin, and cholesterol. The graph is a plan taken from a tetrahedron at 90% water concentration. The tetrahedral plot is used to record the relationships of the four major constituents of bile: water; bile salts; lecithin; and cholesterol. The area enclosed by the triangular coordinates can be divided into four zones, representing the physical state of the solutes in bile: crystals of cholesterol plus liquid (A); cholesterol crystals plus cholesterol liquid crystals plus liquid (B); liquid crystals plus liquid (C); and the micellar zone in which cholesterol is in water solution through the formation of cholesterol-lecithin-bile salt micelles. The solid line is the 10% solute line. From Admirand WH, Small DM. The physiochemical basis of cholesterol gallstone formation in man. J Clin Invest 1968; 47:1043.

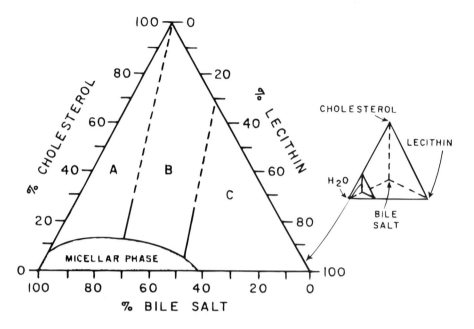

tion that much of the biliary cholesterol exists in a vesicular form. Structurally, these vesicles are made up of lipid bilayers of cholesterol and the phospholipid lecithin. In their simplest and smallest form, the vesicles are unilamellar, but an agreation may take place, leading to multilamellar vesicles. Present theory suggests that in states of excess cholesterol production, these large vesicles may also exceed their capability to transport cholesterol, and crystal precipitation may occur.

Cholesterol solubility depends on the relative concentration of cholesterol, bile salts, and phospholipids (9). By plotting the percentages of each component on triangular coordinates, the micellar zone in which cholesterol is completely soluble can be demonstrated (Fig. 18.5). In a solution composed of 10% solutes similar to bile, the area under the curve represents the concentration at which cholesterol is maintained in solution. In the area above the curve, bile is supersaturated with cholesterol, and precipitation of cholesterol crystals can occur.

A mathematical model of cholesterol solubility has been developed (10); it is influenced by the relative concentrations of lipid components and the total lipid composition. A numerical value, known as the cholesterol saturation (or lithogenic) index, is derived that expresses the relative degrees of cholesterol saturation. When the cholesterol saturation index is greater than 1.0, the solution is supersaturated with cholesterol. Changes in the relative concentrations of bile salts, cholesterol, or phospholipids alter the capacity of micelles, thus changing the solution's cholesterol saturation index.

Enterohepatic Circulation

Bile salts are synthesized and conjugated in the liver, secreted into bile, stored temporarily in the gallbladder, passed from the gallbladder into the duodenum, absorbed throughout the small intestine but especially in

the ileum, and returned to the liver via the portal vein. This cycling of bile acids between the liver and the intestine is referred to as the enterohepatic circulation (Fig. 18.6). The total amount of bile acids in the enterohepatic circulation is defined as the circulating bile pool. In this highly efficient system, nearly 95% of bile salts are reabsorbed. Thus, of the total bile salt pool of 2 to 4 g, which recycles through the enterohepatic cycle 6 to 10 times daily, only about 600 mg of bile salt are actually excreted into the colon. Bacterial action in the colon on the two primary bile salts, cholate and chenodeoxycholate, results in the formation of the secondary bile salts, deoxycholate and lithocholate. Although some deoxycholate is reabsorbed passively by the colon, the remainder is lost in fecal waste.

The enterohepatic circulation provides an important negative feedback system on bile salt synthesis. Should the recirculation be interrupted by resection of the terminal ileum, or by primary ileal disease, abnormally large losses of bile salts can occur. This situation increases bile salt production to maintain a normal bile salt pool. Similarly, if bile salts are lost by an external biliary fistula, increased bile salt synthesis is necessary. However, except for those unusual circumstances in which excessive losses occur, bile salt synthesis matches losses, maintaining a constant bile salt pool size. During fasting, approximately 90% of the bile acid pool is sequestered in the gallbladder.

Bilirubin Metabolism

Heme, released at the time of degradation of senescent erythrocytes by the reticuloendothelial system, is the source of approximately 80% to 85% of the bilirubin produced daily. The remaining 15% to 20% is derived largely from the breakdown of hepatic hemoproteins (11). Both enzymatic and nonenzymatic pathways for

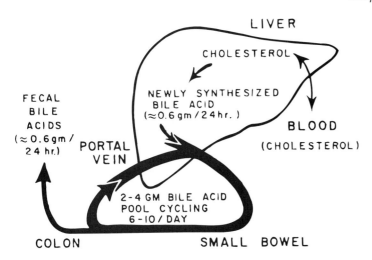

Figure 18.6. Enterohepatic circulation of bile salts. Cholesterol is taken up from plasma by the liver. Bile acids are synthesized at a rate of 0.6 g/24 hr and are excreted through the biliary system into the small bowel. Most of the bile salts are reabsorbed in the terminal ileum and are returned to the liver to be extracted and reexcreted. Modified from Dietschy JM. The biology of bile acids. Arch Intern Med 1972;130:473–474.

the formation of bilirubin have been proposed. Although both may be important physiologically, the microsomal enzyme hemeoxygenase, found in high concentration throughout the liver, spleen, and bone marrow, plays a major role in the initial conversion of heme to biliverdin. Biliverdin is then reduced to bilirubin by the cytosolic enzyme biliverdin reductase in a NADH-dependent reaction before being released into the circulation. In this "unconjugated" form, bilirubin has a very low solubility. Bilirubin is bound avidly to plasma proteins, primarily albumin, before uptake and further processing by the liver. The liver is the sole organ capable of removing the albumin-bilirubin complex from the circulation and esterifying the potentially toxic bilirubin to water-soluble, nontoxic monoconjugated and deconjugated derivatives. Conjugated bilirubin is then excreted into the duodenum.

Reticuloendothelial Function

The reticuloendothelial system (RES) is a group of cells whose function in both health and disease remains incompletely understood. Composed primarily of resident, fixed phagocytes suspected of having a common monocyte-macrophage lineage, the RES is located primarily within the liver, although the spleen and lung also display clinically significant levels of activity. The function initially identified with this group of cells is the clearance of particulate matter from the circulation. The alimentary tract is the main portal of entry for pathogens. Given its direct exposure to both portal and systemic blood, the liver is perfectly positioned to extract and destroy invading bacteria, fungi, and parasites. Although endothelial cells have been shown to possess phagocytic properties, the principal liver cell of the RES is the Kupffer cell. In addition to its ability to phagocytize and destroy infectious agents, the Kupffer cell functions to clear the circulation of old or damaged blood cells, cellular debris, fibrin degradation products, and endotoxin. Recently, the significant role played by Kupffer cells in the elaboration and regulation of prostaglan-

Table 18.5.
Five Categories of Liver Function Tests

Organic ion transport/drug metabolism	Biosynthetic capacity
Serum bilirubin	Prothrombin time
Bromsulphalein excretion	Serum albumin
Indocyanine green excretion	Serum cholesterol
Serum bile acids	Serum fibrinogen
^{14}C breath tests	Serum glucose
Hepatocyte injury/cholestasis	Serum urea
Serum transaminases	Detoxification capacity
Lactate dehydrogenase	Serum ammonia
Alkaline phosphatase	Reticuloendothelial function
γ-glutamyltranspeptidase	Technetium sulfur colloid
5'-nucleotidase	Serum immunoglobulins
Leucine aminopeptidase	Circulating endotoxin

dins, interleukins, oxygen-free radicals, tumor necrosis factor, and other signal molecules has been appreciated.

Liver Function Tests

Liver function tests can be grouped into five broad categories: (a) those that define the liver's capacity to transport organic ions and metabolize drugs; (b) those that identify injury to the hepatocytes; (c) those that reflect the biosynthetic capacity of the liver; (d) those that indicate reduced detoxification capacity; and (e) those that demonstrate the functional status of the RES (Table 18.5). Determination of the patient's bilirubin is the most common means by which we assess the liver's capacity to transport organic anions and metabolize drugs. In the setting of bilirubin elevation, distinction between conjugated and unconjugated levels gives some indication of the cause of the hyperbilirubinemia. Increases in unconjugated bilirubin are often the result of overproduction (hemolysis), decreased conjugation (Gilbert's syndrome and Crigler-Najjar syndrome), or decreased hepatic uptake. Conjugated hyperbilirubinemia is found with parenchymal liver disease, biliary obstruction, and defective excretion (sepsis, pregnancy, drug toxicity, and Dubin-Johnson syndrome).Unfortunately, the bilirubin determination is an insensitive test for hepatic dysfunction.

Dye excretion tests, such as Bromsulphalein and indocyanine green, are more sensitive than bilirubin, but their value in clinical medicine is limited by their non-specificity and their side effects (12). Serum bile acids, which are highly specific indicators of liver dysfunction, may also aid in the diagnosis of certain forms of chronic liver disease. However, as an indicator of acute liver failure, serum bile acids offer no advantage over serum bilirubin. Breath tests are performed by orally administering a ^{14}C-labeled substance (e.g. ^{14}C-aminopyrine) that is metabolized primarily in the liver to carbon dioxide. The ^{14}C-labeled carbon dioxide in the exhaled breath is collected and measured; thus it is possible to determine the degree of hepatic metabolism over time. The ^{14}C breath test is used infrequently because of significant expense and inconvenience.

Hepatic enzyme levels in the serum are the principal means by which hepatocyte damage is identified. Aspartate aminotransferase (AST) and alanine aminotransferase (ALT) are the most sensitive indicators of hepatocyte injury. Both AST and ALT are usually present in low concentrations (less than 40 IU/liter). However, with cellular injury or changes in cell membrane permeability, these enzymes leak into the circulation. Aminotransferases are also found in brain, heart, skeletal muscle, kidney, lung, and leukocytes. Of the two, ALT is the more sensitive and specific test for hepatocyte injury (13). Lactate dehydrogenase (LDH) is a cytoplasmic enzyme found in tissues throughout the body. Even though hepatic LDH isoenzymes can be segregated and isolated, the diagnostic specificity of this test is poor. Alkaline phosphatase is found in the canalicular membrane of the hepatocytes, and thus a rise in the serum level of this enzyme reflects cholestasis. Glutamyl transpeptidase and 5'-nucleotidase are used to confer specificity to an elevated alkaline phosphatase level.

Circulating products of hepatic metabolism are used to estimate the synthetic and catabolic potential of the liver. Decreased serum levels ovalbumin, cholesterol, fibrinogen, glucose, or urea as well as prolongation of the prothrombin time often reflect serious synthetic dysfunction. An elevated ammonia level is associated with decreased detoxification capacity of the liver.

Assessment of the hepatic RES function remains an imprecise art. Technetium sulfur colloid is phagocytosed by Kupffer cells and has been used for years to evaluate the liver anatomically. In the normal patient, about 90% of the radiopharmaceutical will localize intrahepatically, and 10% will be distributed between the spleen and bone marrow. If the Kupffer cells are damaged, diminished liver uptake will occur, but as a measure of RES function, this type of scan is not particularly accurate. Measurement of serum immunoglobulins or circulating endotoxin levels may also be used as indicators of hepatic RES function.

Biliary Physiology

Biliary physiology is less complex than that of either the liver or the pancreas. Nevertheless, the bile ducts can absorb and secrete; the gallbladder has unique absorptive capacities; and the sphincter of Oddi is a complex group of muscles that has multiple functions which impact the physiology of the liver, gallbladder, and pancreas.

Bile Ducts

After leaving the canaliculus, bile enters a series of slightly larger conduits progressing from intralobular to septal to lobar ducts. The right and left hepatic lobar ducts join outside the liver to form the common hepatic duct. During its passage through the collecting system, canalicular bile is modified by the absorption and secretion of electrolytes and water. The gastrointestinal hormone, secretin, increases bile flow primarily by increasing the secretion by the bile ducts and ductules through the active secretion of chloride-rich fluid. Bile ductular secretion is also stimulated by other hormones such as cholecystokinin, gastrin, and cerulean. The bile duct epithelium is also capable of the absorption of water and electrolytes. This role may be of primary importance in the storage of bile during fasting in patients who have previously undergone cholecystectomy.

Gallbladder Function

The main function of the gallbladder is to concentrate and store hepatic bile during the fasting state, thus allowing for its coordinated release in response to a meal. To serve this overall function, the gallbladder has absorptive, secretory, and motor capabilities. The usual capacity of the human gallbladder is only about 40 to 50 ml. Thus, the gallbladder would be filled quickly by the 600 ml of bile produced each day were it not for its remarkable absorptive capacity. The gallbladder's mucosa has the greatest absorptive capacity per unit area of any structure in the body. Bile is usually concentrated 5-fold by the absorption of water and electrolytes. This absorptive process causes a marked change in bile composition during this period of storage (Table 18.6). However, with maximum absorption by the gallbladder epithelium, bile can theoretically be concentrated up to 10-fold.

Absorption

Active Na-Cl transport by the gallbladder epithelium is the driving force for the concentration of bile. Water is passively absorbed in response to the osmotic force generated by solute absorption. The concentration of

Table 18.6.
Composition of Hepatic and Gallbladder Bile

Characteristic	Hepatic	Gallbladder
Na (mEq/liter)	160	270
K	5	10
Cl	90	15
HCO$_3$	45	10
Ca	4	25
Mg	2	—
Bilirubin (mEq/liter)	1.5	15
Protein (mEq/liter)	150	—
Bile Acids (mEq/liter)	50	150
Phospholipids (mEq/liter)	8	40
Cholesterol (mEq/liter)	4	18
Total Solids (mEq/liter)	—	125
pH	7.8	7.2

bile may affect both calcium and cholesterol solubilities. The concentration of calcium in gallbladder bile, which is an important factor in gallstone pathogenesis, is influenced by serum calcium, hepatic bile calcium, gallbladder water absorption, and the concentration of organic substances, such as bile salts in gallbladder bile (13). Although the gallbladder mucosa does absorb calcium, this process is not nearly as efficient as for sodium or water. As the gallbladder bile becomes concentrated, several changes occur in the bile's capacity to solubilize cholesterol. The solubility in the micellar fraction is increased, but the stability of phospholipid-cholesterol vesicles is greatly decreased. Because cholesterol crystal precipitation occurs preferentially by vesicular rather than micellar mechanisms, the net effect of concentrating bile is an increased tendency to nucleate cholesterol (14). Absorption of organic compounds also occurs; lipid solubility is the major determinant of movement across the gallbladder mucosa. However, the absorption of bilirubin, cholesterol, phospholipids, and bile salts is minimal compared with that of water. Thus, these organic compounds are significantly concentrated by the normal absorptive process that occurs in the gallbladder. Unconjugated bile salts are absorbed more readily than conjugated bile salts and may actually damage the gallbladder's mucosa, causing a nonselective increase in absorption of other solutes. Thus, increased absorption of unconjugated bile salts, caused by bacterial deconjugation or mucosal inflammation, may impair cholesterol solubility and, therefore, promote cholesterol gallstone formation.

Secretion

The gallbladder's epithelial cells secrete at least two important products into its lumen: glycoproteins and hydrogen ions. Secretion of mucus glycoproteins occurs primarily from the glands of the gallbladder neck and cystic duct. The resultant mucin gel is believed to constitute an important part of the unstirred layer (diffusion-resistant barrier) that separates the gallbladder cell

membrane from the bulk solution of bile (15). This mucus barrier may be very important in protecting the gallbladder's epithelium from the strong detergent effect of the highly concentrated bile salts found in the gallbladder. Prostaglandins play an important role as stimulants of gallbladder mucin secretion. Furthermore, considerable evidence suggests that mucin glycoproteins play a role as a pronucleating agent for cholesterol crystallization.

The acidification of bile occurs by the transport of hydrogen ions by the gallbladder epithelium, probably through a sodium-exchange mechanism. Acidification of bile promotes calcium solubility, thereby preventing its precipitation as calcium salts. The gallbladder's normal acidification process lowers the pH of gallbladder bile, which normally varies from approximately 7.1 to 7.3. Compared with gallbladder bile, the bile secreted by the liver is slightly alkaline, pH 7.5 to 7.7, so that excess losses of hepatic bile may cause metabolic acidosis.

Motor Function

Gallbladder filling is facilitated by tonic contraction of the ampullary sphincter, which maintains a constant pressure in the common bile duct (10 to 15 mm Hg). The gallbladder does not, however, simply fill passively and continuously during fasting. Rather, periods of filling are punctuated by brief periods of partial emptying of concentrated bile and partial filling of dilute hepatic bile in a bellows-like fashion. This partial emptying and filling process occurs simultaneously with phase III activity of the migrating myoelectric complex (MMC). The release of stored bile from the gallbladder requires a coordinated motor response of gallbladder contraction and sphincter of Oddi relaxation. This activity is mediated by both neural and humoral factors. One of the main stimuli to gallbladder emptying is the hormone cholecystokinin, which is released from the duodenal mucosa in response to a meal. Many other hormonal and neural influences, however, are necessary for coordinated action of the gallbladder and sphincter of Oddi.

When stimulated by a meal, the gallbladder empties 50% to 70% of its contents within 30 to 40 minutes. Gallbladder refilling then occurs gradually over the next 60 to 90 minutes. Vagal stimulation results in gallbladder contraction, and splanchnic sympathetic activity is inhibitory. Between meals, the gallbladder empties approximately 10% to 15% of its volume with each passage through the duodenum of phase III MMC. This process is mediated, at least in part, by the hormone motilin (16). Defects in gallbladder motility, which increase the residence time of bile in the gallbladder, play a central role in the pathogenesis of gallstones.

Sphincter of Oddi Function

The human sphincter of Oddi is a complex structure that is separate from the duodenal musculature. Endo-

Figure 18.7. Sphincter of Oddi (SO) manometric pressure profile obtained by catheter pull through from the common bile duct (CBD) into the duodenum. The CBD pressure and SO basal pressure are both referenced to duodenal pressure. Sphincter of Oddi phasic wave amplitude was measured from basal SO pressure. The CBD to duodenal pressure gradient is indicated by the parallel broken lines. From Geenen JE, Toouli J, Hogan WJ, et al. Endoscopic sphincterotomy: follow-up evaluation of effects on the sphincter of Oddi. Gastroenterology 1984;87:754–758.

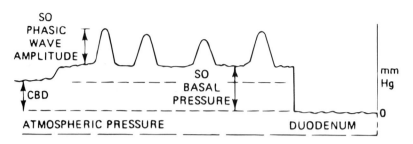

scopic manometric studies have demonstrated that the human sphincter of Oddi creates a high-pressure zone between the bile duct and the duodenum (Fig. 18.7). This sphincter regulates the flow of bile and pancreatic juice and also prevents the regurgitation of duodenal contents. This latter function is achieved by keeping pressure within the bile and pancreatic ducts higher than duodenal pressure (17). The sphincter of Oddi also has very high pressure phasic contractions. The exact functions of these phasic waves in humans is not known, but they may play a role in preventing regurgitation of duodenal contents.

Both neural and hormonal factors influence the sphincter of Oddi. In humans, sphincter of Oddi pressure and phasic wave activity diminishes in response to cholecystokinin. Thus, sphincter pressure relaxes in response to a meal, allowing the passive flow of bile into the duodenum. In some other species, cholecystokinin administration results in an increase in sphincter of Oddi phasic wave activity, suggesting that bile may be pumped actively into the duodenum by the sphincter. During fasting, high-pressure phasic contractions of the sphincter of Oddi persist through all phases of the MMC. Recent animal studies suggest, however, that sphincter of Oddi phasic waves do vary to some degree in concert with the MMC. Thus, sphincter of Oddi activity undoubtedly is coordinated with the partial gallbladder emptying that occurs during phase III of the MMC.

Neurally mediated reflexes link the sphincter of Oddi with the gallbladder and stomach to coordinate the flow of bile and pancreatic juice into the duodenum. The cholecysto-sphincter of Oddi reflex allows the human sphincter to relax as the gallbladder contracts (18). Similarly, antral distension causes both gallbladder contraction and sphincter relaxation (19).

Pancreatic Physiology

Two distinct organ systems exist within the pancreas: the exocrine pancreas and the endocrine pancreas. The exocrine pancreas comprises approximately 85% of the volume of the gland; 10% of the gland is accounted for

by extracellular matrix and 4% by blood vessels and the major ducts, leaving only 2% of the volume for the endocrine pancreas. The acini and ductal systems comprise the exocrine portion of the pancreas. The acinus is the basic subunit of the exocrine pancreas. Each acinus is composed of a single layer of acinar cells assuming a roughly spheroid configuration. Acinar cells (Fig. 18.8) contain abundant zymogen granules in their narrow, centrally located apical portion; they also have a large nucleus, abundant endoplasmic reticulum, and an active Golgi complex. The pancreatic ductal system originates with the centroacinar cells of each individual acinus and incorporates intercalated duct cells along the ductal pathway, terminating in the main excretory duct of the pancreas (Fig. 18.9). Centroacinar cells contain sparse cytoplasm and a small Golgi complex and are devoid of zymogen granules, yet they contain high concentrations of the enzyme carbonic anhydrase, which catalyzes the following reaction:

$$H_2O + CO_2 = H^+ + HCO_3^-$$

The endocrine pancreas is served by the nearly spheroid collections of endocrine cells scattered throughout the pancreatic parenchyma, termed the islets of Langerhans. Up to 1 million islets are located within each gland. Each islet is composed of several distinctive cell types. The centrally located insulin-producing cells make up 70% of the islet population. Glucagon-producing cells make up approximately 20% of each islet, and they are generally located at the periphery of each islet. Also located in the periphery of each islet are the somatostatin-producing cells (5%) and pancreatic polypeptide secreting (PP-secreting) cells (5% to 10%).

Exocrine Function

The final secretory product of the exocrine pancreas derives from the combination of ductal and acinar cell functions. Water and electrolyte secretion originate from the centroacinar and intercalated duct cells. Pancreatic enzymes originate from acinar cells. The final product is a clear isotonic solution with a pH of 8 and a specific gravity that varies between 1.007 and 1.035. Basal secretory rates of the exocrine pancreas average 0.2 to 0.3 ml/min; maximal rates approach 5 ml/min with appropri-

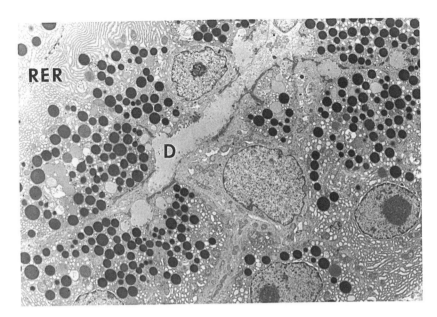

Figure 18.8. Electron micrograph of multiple acinar cells and a section of terminal duct (D). The acinar cells contain extensive rough endoplasmic reticulum (RER) and numerous electron-dense spherical zymogen granules. (Uranyl acetate and lead citrate; 2000.)

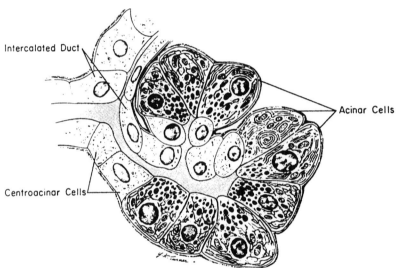

Figure 18.9. Schematic representation of the relationships between acinar cells and the cells of the pancreatic ductal system, including centroacinar cells and intercalated duct cells. From Bloom W, Fawcett DW. A textbook of histology. 10th ed. Philadelphia: WB Saunders, 1975:738.

ate secretagogue stimulation. The anion composition of exocrine pancreatic juice varies with the rate of pancreatic secretion (Fig. 18.10). At low secretory rates, the concentrations of chloride and bicarbonate ions are nearly equivalent to plasma. With neurohumoral stimulation, the bicarbonate component increases in concentration while the chloride concentration falls (20). In contrast, the composition of sodium and potassium in the pancreatic exocrine effluent remains constant; the concentrations of these cations are roughly equivalent to plasma.

Secretin is the principal stimulant of pancreatic water and electrolyte secretion. The term hormone was first used in reference to secretin, a 27 amino acid peptide first extracted from the dog jejunum by Bayliss and Starling in 1902. Secretin is synthesized and stored in the mucosal S cells of the crypts of Lieberkühn of the proximal small bowel, and it is released into the blood in the presence of luminal acid and bile. Secretin stimulates

pancreatic water and electrolyte secretion by binding to pancreatic ductal cell receptors and effecting signal transduction via the adenylate cyclase second messenger system. The result is an increase in intracellular cAMP. Several endogenous inhibitors of pancreatic water and electrolyte secretion have been identified; however, their physiologic roles remain to be defined. In particular, somatostatin, pancreatic polypeptide, and glucagon have all been speculated to play a humoral or paracrine role in the reduction of pancreatic water and electrolyte secretion.

The synthesis and excretion of digestive enzymes from pancreatic acinar cells have been the subject of many sophisticated experimental studies since the early work of Palade (21). Acinar cells are programmed to direct more than 90% of their biosynthetic effort toward the production and storage of a mixture of approximately 20 different digestive enzymes and enzyme precursors. Experiments using radiolabeling techniques

Figure 18.10. Relationship between the rate of secretion and the concentration of electrolytes in pancreatic juice compared with the electrolyte concentration of plasma. From Bro-Rasmussen F, Killmann SA, Thaysen JH. The composition of pancreatic juice as compared to sweat, parotid saliva and tears. Acta Physiol Scand 1956;37:97–113.

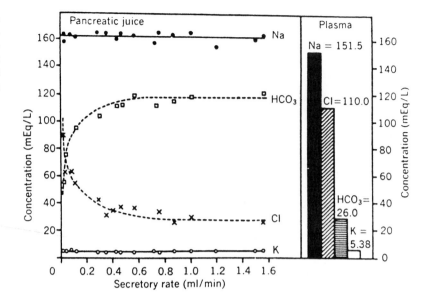

have delineated a stepwise sequence of intracellular events occurring within the acinar cell, leading to the final digestive enzyme products. Within the acinar nucleus, DNA is transcribed to yield mRNA, which travels to the cytoplasm where it is translated on the microsomes of the rough endoplasmic reticulum into proenzymes. These proenzymes subsequently pass to the Golgi apparatus where they are packaged within a glycoprotein vesicular membrane. Zymogen granules formed at the level of the Golgi apparatus contain a full complement of the digestive enzymes. Zymogen granules then migrate to the cell apex where the granule's membranes fuse with the acinar cell membrane (exocytosis), leading to extrusion of the zymogen granule contents into the centroacinar luminal space.

Specific enzymes synthesized and released into the ductal system include the endopeptidases, such as trypsinogen, chymotrypsinogen, and proelastase, as well as exopeptidases, such as procarboxypeptidase A and B. Other enzymes include amylase, lipase, phospholipase, colipase, ribonuclease, and deoxyribonuclease. All peptidases synthesized by acinar cells are released into the pancreatic ductal system in an inactive form. Duodenal mucosal enterokinase serves to activate trypsinogen to the active enzyme trypsin, which further activates the other peptidases.

The control of pancreatic acinar cell secretion is mediated by specific secretogogues acting on acinar cell receptors. Secretogogues, such as cholecystokinin (CCK) and acetylcholine, stimulate acinar cell enzyme secretion via a membrane transduction process involving the receptor-mediated hydrolysis of phosphatidylinositol-4,5-bisphosphate, generating two intracellular messengers: inositol-1,4,5-triphosphate and diacylglycerol (22). The formation of inositol-1,4,5-triphosphate leads to the release of Ca^{2+} from intracellular stores. The generation of diacylglycerol activates protein kinase C, an ubiqui-

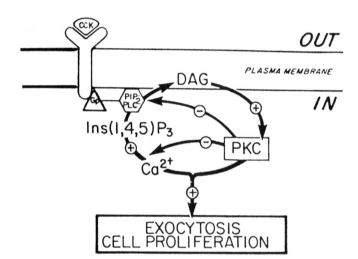

Figure 18.11. Schematic representation of the possible molecular basis of CCK action on a pancreatic acinar cel. A single receptor is coupled, via a G protein (Gp), to an effector mechanism, involving hydrolysis of phosphatidyl-4,5-triphosphate (PIP2) to yield diacylglycerol (DAG) and inositol-1,4,5-triphosphate (Ins (1,4,5)P3). PCL, phospholipase C; PKC, protein kinase C. From Bruzzone R. The molecular basis of enzyme secretion. Gastroenterology 1990;99:1157–1176.

tous calcium- and phospholipid-dependent phosphorylating enzyme, which has been implicated in the mediation of a number of intracellular processes, including exocytotic secretion, changes in ion channel conductance, receptor affinity, and cell proliferation (Fig. 18.11). CCK is the most potent endogenous hormone known to stimulate pancreatic enzyme secretion.

A most important aspect of pancreatic exocrine secretion involves the response of the gland to an ingested meal. The functional reserve of the pancreas is enormous. A total of 80% to 90% of the functional acinar mass must be absent for clinical evidence of malabsorption to appear. Thus, normal digestion is associated with an excess of pancreatic enzymes. In addition to the enzyme products, the exocrine pancreas also secretes water, bicarbonate, and electrolytes, which help to neutralize acidic gastric chyme and to maintain the pH in the optimal range for the activity of most pancreatic enzymes. A key aspect of this neutralizing function is the requirement that pH is maintained above 4.0 at the level of the ampulla of Vater and beyond intraluminal.

The physiologic control of pancreatic secretion lacks a fine-tuning mechanism, is overwhelmingly stimulatory, and is controlled by interacting neurohormonal mechanisms (23). During the cephalic phase of digestion, stimuli activate vagal efferent signals, which follow parasympathetic pathways to stimulate pancreatic exocrine secretion and account for one-fourth to one-third of the maximal pancreatic response. In addition, cephalic phase stimulation of gastric acid secretion, both by direct cholinergic influence on parietal cells and via the release of antral gastrin, leads to duodenal acidification. This acidification releases secretin, which stimulates pancreatic bicarbonate secretion. During the gastric phase of digestion, antral distention and the presence of protein in the antrum stimulate the release of gastrin. Gastrin itself serves as a weak stimulator of pancreatic enzyme secretion because of the sequence homology between gastrin and the C-terminus pentapeptide-amide sequence of CCK. Furthermore, gastrin-stimulated gastric acid secretion contributes to duodenal acidification, secretin release, and resultant bicarbonate secretion.

The intestinal phase of pancreatic exocrine secretion commences when chyme reaches the upper small intestine. This phase is quantitatively the most important, involving both neural and hormonal mechanisms. Duodenal acid and bile cause secretin release, which stimulates pancreatic bicarbonate secretion from duct cells. The presence of fat or protein in the duodenum stimulates CCK release, which causes pancreatic enzyme secretion from acinar cells. Current evidence supports the existence of considerable overlap and potentiating interactions between secretin and CCK in stimulating the pancreatic exocrine response. In addition to these hormonally mediated events, enteropancreatic vagovagal reflexes stimulated by luminal bile salts, fatty acids, and amino acids can serve as an important stimulus for pancreatic exocrine secretion.

Recent evidence has clarified the role of different dietary constituents in postprandial pancreatic enzyme secretion (24). Diets high in carbohydrate (50% to 80%) are associated with the lowest postprandial amylase, lipase, and trypsin outputs, whereas diets high in fat (40%) are associated with the highest postprandial output of these enzymes. The variations in pancreatic enzyme secretion associated with different dietary constituents may have important implications in the pathogenesis and treatment of human diseases of the pancreas. For example, the risk of developing chronic alcoholic pancreatitis has been related to the amount of protein in the diet, and a diet that minimally stimulates pancreatic secretion may be most beneficial in patients convalescing from acute pancreatitis.

Endocrine Pancreas

The principal endocrine function of the pancreas involves maintenance of glucose homeostasis. The association between the pancreas and diabetes mellitus was established in 1888 in a canine model, when near total pancreatectomy produced glucose intolerance. In 1922, Banting and Best isolated a pancreatic extract, containing what is now called insulin, that effectively lowered serum glucose levels in hyperglycemic dogs. Insulin is a two-chain disulfide-linked peptide hormone that is the secretory product of the islet cell. Insulin biosynthesis in humans is confined strictly to the cells in the endocrine pancreas.

Recent work in the field of molecular biology has shown that the human insulin gene is located near the end of the short arm of chromosome 11, in band p15.5. This gene contains three exons separated by two intervening introns. The intron sequences are present in the gene and the primary RNA transcript, and they are removed from the mRNA precursor by splicing before the mRNA moves from the nucleus to the cytoplasm. A critical point of control in insulin gene expression is at the stage of transcription initiation. The effects are mediated through specific DNA sequences located in the 5'-flanking region of the gene and appear to involve recognition of these sequences by protein factors present in cells.

In 1967, the precursor of insulin, proinsulin, was discovered. Both proinsulin synthesis and insulin secretion are stimulated by hyperglycemia. The induction of proinsulin synthesis is achieved mainly by enhancement of the translation efficiency of proinsulin mRNA on the membrane-bound polysomes (translational control). The actual release of insulin from the cell into the portal blood is under a variety of controls, including not only the level of glycemia but also vagal interactions and local concentrations of inhibitory peptides such as somatostatin. In the setting of pancreatic injury, exemplified by both acute and chronic pancreatitis, a circulating insulin deficiency state has been documented (25).

Glucagon

Glucagon was first detected in 1923 in side fractions of insulin extracts. Glucagon is a single-chain peptide with 29 amino acid residues, synthesized and released from islet cells. The hormone is one of a family of homologous peptides that includes secretin, vasoactive intestinal polypeptide (VIP), gastric-inhibitory polypeptide (GIP), and growth hormone releasing factor (GRF). The biologic properties of glucagon can be divided into four categories: *(a) effects on metabolism,* including stimulation of glycogenolysis, gluconeogenesis, and ketogenesis in the liver, stimulation of lipolysis in adipose tissue, and stimulation of insulin secretion; *(b) effects on gastrointesti-*

nal secretion, including inhibition of gastric acid and pancreatic exocrine secretion; *(c) effects on intestinal motility*, including inhibition of intestinal peristaltic activity; and *(d) effects on the cardiovascular system*, including increase in heart rate and in the force of cardiac contraction.

Somatostatin

Initially isolated in 1973 from the hypothalamus, somatostatin is now known to have widespread distribution throughout the body. Somatostatin is acyclic tetradecapeptide synthesized and released from islet cells and many other brain-gut sources. In the pancreas, somatostatin is present mainly in the 14 amino acid form, whereas a 28 amino acid precursor of somatostatin called prosomatostatin predominates in other tissues. Somatostatin receptors have been found on pancreatic acinar cell membranes and on the secretory vesicles of pancreatic islet cells. Somatostatin has a broad spectrum of gastrointestinal activity, including inhibition of gastric acid, pepsin, and pancreatic exocrine secretion; inhibition of gastrointestinal motor activity and ion secretion (26); reduction of gastrointestinal blood flow; and inhibition of pancreatic islet insulin, glucagon, and PP release. The intracellular mechanisms of somatostatin action involve primarily the activation of the inhibitory G protein in the adenylate cyclase system, whereby somatostatin binding inhibits the activation of adenylate cyclase and reduces intracellular cAMP levels. However, all inhibitory actions of somatostatin cannot be explained solely by cAMP-dependent cell activation mechanisms, and some may involve regulation of intracellular Ca^{2+} turnover.

Pancreatic Polypeptide

Pancreatic polypeptide is a 36 amino acid peptide localized exclusively in the islet cells of the pancreas. The PP family of homologous peptides includes PP, neuropeptide Y, and peptide YY. PP cell densities increase from the tail of the gland to the head of the gland; concentrations of PP are five to eight times higher in the pancreatic head than in the tail. In humans, total pancreatectomy results in undetectable levels of PP in both basal and postprandial serum, supporting the notion that the pancreas is the only significant site of PP secretion. The mechanisms of release of PP after a meal are complex and include a characteristic biphasic pattern with an early peak followed by a long plateau. PP release following a meal is stimulated during the cephalic, gastric, and intestinal phases of digestion and appears to depend on both cholinergic and adrenergic modulation. The most likely physiologic role for PP involves inhibition of pancreatic exocrine secretion. Multiple pharmacologic effects of PP have been reported, including modulation of gastric acid secretion, alterations in intestinal motility, and suppression of islet insulin release. In humans, PP has also been used as a marker for pancreatic

endocrine tumors. However, the clinical importance of the identification of elevated PP levels remains to be established convincingly.

Islet-Acinar Interactions

The intimate anatomic relationship between the exocrine and endocrine pancreas is undeniable, as the islets of Langerhans are dispersed throughout the acinar and ductal tissues of the exocrine pancreas. Accumulating structural and functional evidence suggests a close integration of the exocrine and endocrine portions of the pancreas. For example, the presence of specific islet hormone receptors on the plasma membranes of pancreatic acinar cells gives support to the notion of direct regulation of the function of the acinar cells by islet hormones.

Autoradiographic studies have shown that insulin-binding sites in the acinar parenchyma are not distributed evenly. Rather, the acinar cells located around the islets (peri-insular region) show higher densities of receptor labeling than those at a distance from the islets (teleinsular regions). Morphometric studies have demonstrated that the peri-insular acinar cells are twice as large as those found in the teleinsular regions. Determination of volume densities of the different cellular organelles have shown that peri-insular cells contain many more zymogen granules than teleinsular cells. Despite these differences in zymogen granule numbers, the actual content and type of enzymes in the granules of cells from the two regions are similar. However, the pattern of response to secretagogues differs between peri-insular and teleinsular cells. For example, during vagal stimulation, the release of zymogen granules by peri-insular acinar cells is slow, whereas the teleinsular cells are rapidly depleted of zymogen granules.

Further evidence in support of the theory of islet-acinar interaction comes from the existence of an islet-acinar portal blood system (27). The arterial supply of the pancreas originates from the celiac and superior mesenteric arteries. Branches of these vessels travel along the interlobular and intralobular septa and eventually contribute to the arterioles that penetrate the islets, giving rise to an extensive capillary network. After supplying the endocrine tissue, these capillaries radiate from the islet to supply the acinar tissue. Thus, the acinar cells located around the islets of Langerhans may be exposed to very high levels of islet hormones.

Clinical data also lend support to the notion of islet acinar interaction. Multiple studies have shown that pancreatic exocrine function is reduced in many subjects with Type I diabetes, despite insulin treatment. Furthermore, latent or overt diabetes mellitus is seen in 40% to 70% of patients with chronic pancreatitis. In all, ample evidence comes from structural, functional, and clinical sources to substantiate the hypothesis that a close integration exists between pancreatic endocrine and exocrine functions.

Hepatic Pathophysiology

The pathophysiology of the liver is complex, with many diverse problems capable of altering normal hepatic function. For the purposes of this chapter, hepatic pathophysiology has been grouped into four areas: congenital disorders; inflammatory disorders; cirrhosis; and neoplasms.

Congenital Disorders

Congenital hepatic diseases can be divided into those involving the bile ducts and those primarily confined to the hepatic parenchyma. Congenital bile duct problems, such as biliary atresia, choledochal cysts, and Caroli's disease, will be discussed in "Biliary Pathophysiology" (below). Compared with these rare diseases, congenital bile duct hamartomas are encountered commonly at surgery as small fibrotic nodules that masquerade as tiny metastatic lesions. Rarely, congenital hamartomas may be cystic and achieve a large enough size to cause symptoms. When this situation occurs, the cystic hamartoma may be confused with a simple cyst, a cystadenoma, or a cystadenocarcinoma.

Congenital hepatic cysts can be either isolated or multiple simple cysts or a manifestation of polycystic disease. Like bile duct hamartomas, small congenital simple cysts are observed commonly during laparotomy for other disorders. Biopsy or partial or complete excision may be appropriate if a concern exists about metastatic disease, a cystadenoma, or a cystadenocarcinoma. However, most of these lesions, which have the typical appearance of a thin-walled cyst containing clear fluid, do not need to be biopsied or resected.

Simple congenital cysts rarely achieve sufficient size to cause symptoms. When they do cause symptoms, the most common complaints are a steady, dull pain or pressure-related problems such as nausea, vomiting, early satiety, weight loss, or respiratory distress (28). Biliary obstruction occurs only rarely as the result of a simple congenital cyst. When symptomatic, surgical management, as opposed to percutaneous aspiration or drainage, even with sclerosing agents, is indicated because the recurrence and complication rates are high with nonoperative management. Surgical options include partial cyst excision, complete enucleation, hepatic resection, and, if bile is present in the cyst, Roux-en-Y cystojejunostomy. In most cases, laparoscopic partial cyst excision is adequate to relieve symptoms and prevent recurrence.

Polycystic liver disease usually occurs concomitantly

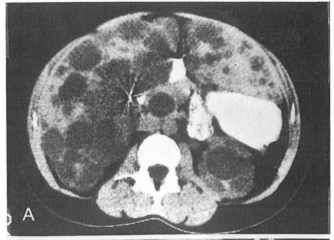
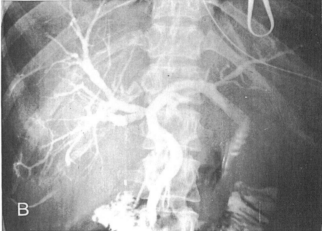

Figure 18.12. **A,** CT scan of a patient with polycystic disease of the liver, kidneys, and pancreas. **B,** Operative cholangiogram, demonstrating a relatively normal biliary tree despite the huge number of intrahepatic cysts. From Doty JE, Pitt HA. Cystic lesions of the liver and biliary tree. In: Moody FG, ed. Surgical treatment of digestive diseases. Chicago: Year Book Medical, 1986;336.

with polycystic renal disease (Fig. 18.12). Cysts are rarely present in the pancreas, spleen, or adrenal glands. Despite apparently massive hepatic involvement, these patients rarely develop biliary obstruction or hepatic failure. In fact, renal failure, with the need for dialysis and renal transplantation, is usually the most serious problem confronting these patients. Occasionally, however, the hepatic cysts may cause sufficient symptoms, analogous to those that occur with massive simple cysts, to warrant surgical intervention. As with simple cysts, percutaneous aspiration, drainage, or sclerosis has been associated with problems and should be avoided. Open surgery with partial resection of cysts with or without adjacent hepatic parenchyma usually relieves symptoms.

The other frequently encountered congenital hepatic disorder is the hemangioma. Small, asymptomatic hepatic hemangiomas are often observed at laparotomy and usually should not be biopsied. Hemangiomas have a typical appearance of a pink-red, soft, "spongy" lesion that refills rapidly after compression. Large hepatic hemangiomas may cause pain, but spontaneous hemorrhage is rare (29). Thus, hepatic resection may be indicated for relief of symptoms, but recent analyses suggest that asymptomatic hemangiomas may be observed safely. A typical appearance on contrast-enhanced CT scan, magnetic resonance imaging, or a tagged red-cell nuclear medicine scan, along with negative tumor markers, justifies long-term observation of asymptomatic hemangiomas.

Inflammatory Disorders

A wide variety of inflammatory problems may affect the liver. This broad category includes infections by bacteria, fungi, parasites, and viruses as well as toxins, chemicals, and drugs that can injure the liver. The bacteria, fungi, and parasites that can produce clinically significant liver disease in humans are presented in Table 18.7. Patients who develop systemic sepsis from a broad spectrum of pathogens may manifest some degree of liver dysfunction. The dominant hepatic pathogen in any given population varies with respect to geographic and socioeconomic factors. Protozoan and helminthic infections, for example, are a serious health hazard in regions with poor sanitation or among people who consume raw meats or fish. These problems are far less common in the United States than in less well-developed parts of the world. Among the long list of infectious hepatic problems, hepatic abscesses and parasitic infections of the liver will be discussed in more detail.

Hepatic Abscess

Liver abscesses secondary to either bacterial or amebic infections have many common features and are a frequent source of diagnostic confusion. Although amebic abscesses are more prevalent worldwide, pyogenic

Table 18.7.
Bacteria, Fungi, and Parasites That Cause Injury to the Liver

Pyogenic abscess	Fungal infections
Enteric aerobes	Actinomycosis
Skin aerobes	Aspergillosis
Enteric anaerobes	Candidiasis
Bacterial infections	Coccidioidomycosis
Brucellosis	Cryptococcosis
Listeriosis	Nocardiasis
Gonococccus	Parasitic infections
Salmonella typhi	Amebiosis
Tuberculosis	Ascariasis
Tularemia	Capillariasis
Miscellaneous infection	Clonorchis
Leptospirosis	Dicrocoeliosis
Syphilis	Echinococcosis
Q fever	Fascioliasis
	Toxocariasis
	Opisthorchiasis
	Schistosomiasis

liver abscesses are encountered more frequently in Western cultures. Within the United States, the incidence of amebic and pyogenic abscesses is nearly equal in the southwestern and south-central states (30). Symptomatic amebiasis is complicated by abscess formation in only 3% to 9% of cases. Patients with amebic abscesses often present with the gradual onset of fever, weakness, malaise, and abdominal discomfort. Jaundice is unusual, and if present, liver function tests are elevated only marginally. A serious complication and source of significant morbidity is rupture of the amebic abscess into neighboring abdominal viscera, the free peritoneal cavity, the pleural space, or the pericardium. Fortunately, most cases of amebic abscess are curable with appropriate medical therapy, including metronidazole. Surgical intervention is rarely necessary.

Patients with bacterial hepatic abscesses often have a more fulminant presentation and may appear toxic early in the course of their disease. The presence of other intra abdominal pathology, such as biliary tract disease, diverticulitis, trauma, extrahepatic malignancy, or remote abdominal infection are predisposing factors for the development of this type of hepatic abscess. Elevations of bilirubin, alkaline phosphatase, and amino transferases are noted in more than 50% of patients. Compared with amebic abscesses, pyogenic abscesses are more likely to be multiple, to require surgical intervention, and to have a fatal outcome. Treatment includes systemic antibiotics, covering both aerobic and anaerobic organisms, and abscess drainage. In carefully selected patients, percutaneous drainage will suffice. Approximately one-third of patients with pyogenic hepatic abscesses will require open surgical drainage.

Parasitic Infections

Many parasites appear capable of causing hepatic infections. Three organisms that have a substantial impact on public health worldwide are schistosomiasis, clonorchis, and echinococcus. Schistosomiasis is an infection caused by flatworms of the Schistosoma mansoni and s. japonicum species. These flatworms are endemic throughout Africa and the Middle East and portions of Japan, China, Indonesia, and the Philippines (31). Aquatic snails are the intermediate host for the schistosomules. When human infection occurs, the parasites gain access by boring through the skin. They disseminate via the lymphatic system and have a tendency to reside within mesenteric veins. The ova of the parasite are released into the portal circulation and become lodged in the hepatic sinusoids, producing presinusoidal portal venous obstruction. Eradication of schistosomes is difficult, but fortunately, effective control can be obtained by simply sterilizing the adult worm. Effective chemotherapy includes the administration of praziquantel, oxamniquine, and hycanthone. Patients with schistosomiasis characteristically have preservation of their liver function and generally do not manifest the clinical signs of chronic liver disease. Medical intervention for complications of chronic infection involves the treatment of portal hypertension, including bleeding varices and hypersplenism.

The liver fluke Clonorchis sinensis was first identified as a human pathogen by McConnell in 1875 (31). Clonorchis is found in many east Asian countries where raw fish and shellfish are commonly eaten. Humans are the primary hosts for Clonorchis. When contaminated fish are ingested, the fluke gains access to the biliary tree through the ampulla of Vater. There, the parasite itself, as well as a number of metabolic products, irritate the biliary epithelium. The chronic inflammation and subsequent bile stasis are thought to be responsible for the increased incidence of choledocholithiasis, cholangitis, and cholangiocarcinoma found with liver fluke infestation. Administration of praziquantel has a 50% cure rate for this parasitic liver infection.

Hydatid disease of the liver is caused most frequently by Echinococcus granulosus, a tapeworm with worldwide distribution. Dogs are the definitive host, and cattle, sheep, and humans are the intermediate hosts. Eggs of the parasite are passed in the stool of an infected dog and inadvertently ingested by the intermediate host. The larva penetrate the intestinal mucosa and become disseminated throughout the body; however, a preference exists for migration to the liver. Many patients remain asymptomatic for years after infection. Diagnosis during a medical workup for unrelated illness or the gradual onset of vague abdominal complaints are common presenting scenarios. Liver function tests are usually normal. Serological tests for echinococcal infection confirm the diagnosis in more than 80% of cases. The Casoni skin test is rarely used now. Computerized tomography often reveals a characteristic multilocular cyst with scoliceal "sand" and calcification of the cyst wall (Fig. 18.13). To date, no medical treatment has been proven effective. Percutaneous needle aspiration should be avoided as a diagnostic or therapeutic maneuver because spillage of the highly antigenic cyst contents into the free peritoneal cavity can be disastrous. Spontaneous rupture of a hydatid liver cyst is associated with major risks of morbidity and mortality. For this reason, surgical management has become the treatment of choice (32).

Viral Hepatitis

A wide variety of viruses are capable of producing acute inflammation of the liver (Table 18.8). Reference to the entity of *viral hepatitis*, however, usually focuses on hepatitis A, hepatitis B, or hepatitis C (previously referred to as non-A, non-B hepatitis). Hepatitis A, at one time referred to as infectious hepatitis because of the recognized fecal-oral route of transmission, is an RNA virus with an incubation period of 2 to 6 weeks. Hepatitis B is a DNA virus spread predominantly by

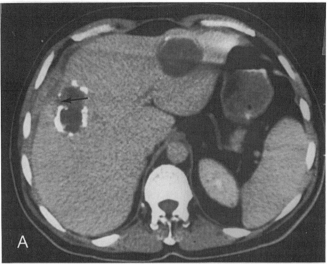

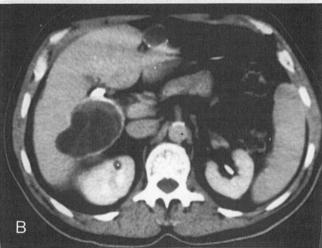

Figure 18.13. **A,** CT scan of a patient with multiple echinococcal cysts. Note the calcification in both the cysts and the transdiaphragmatic rupture (arrow). **B,** CT scan in the same patient, showing two more echinococcal cysts near the gallbladder fossa (with multiple daughter cysts) and on the periphery of segment III. Note the calcification in both cysts. From Pitt HA, Korzelius J, Tompkins RK. Management of hepatic echinococcosis in southern California. Am J Surg 1986;152:110–115.

Table 18.8.
Viral Causes of Hepatitis

Hepatitis A	Enterovirus
Hepatitis B	Epstein-Barr virus
Hepatitis C	Herpes simplex
Hepatitis D	Lassa fever
Adenovirus	Marburg virus
Cytomegalovirus	Rubella
Ebola virus	Yellow fever

the parenteral route or through sexual contact. Many cases of so-called non-A, non-B hepatitis are now believed to be related to infection with hepatitis C, a recently identified RNA flavivirus.

Although hepatitis A tends to produce a more pronounced gastrointestinal disturbance, the clinical course of viral hepatitis is often similar, regardless of the specific virus responsible. A prodrome of weakness, fatigue, headache, nausea, and anorexia heralds the acute phase of the illness (33). In many patients, however, the infection remains clinically inapparent. Jaundice is a variable finding with acute viral hepatitis. Those patients destined to develop an icteric form of the disease often note darkening of their urine and lightening of their stool before overt jaundice becomes apparent. On examination, tender hepatomegaly is characteristic, with splenomegaly and posterior cervical adenopathy often noted. Elevated serum amino transferase levels reflect the hepatocyte necrosis, which accompanies the acute infection. Hypertransaminasemia may predate the development of symptoms by one or more weeks. However, the degree of elevation does not correlate well with severity of illness (34). Mild prolongations of the prothrombin time may occur, but severe synthetic dysfunction is unusual.

Most patients with hepatitis A have a self-limited course of infection, and persistent or chronic forms rarely develop. By comparison, hepatitis B and hepatitis C are associated with a 10% and 50% rate of chronic active hepatitis, respectively. The development of chronic viral infection of the liver increases the risk of cirrhosis, portal hypertension, and hepatoma.

Patients with hepatitis A, B, or C occasionally develop fulminant hepatic failure, which is defined as the development of hepatic encephalopathy within 8 weeks of the onset of an acute illness in a patient without preexisting liver disease. In addition to encephalopathy, these patients manifest a profound coagulopathy, acidosis, and hypoglycemia. Supportive medical therapy alone for patients who have progressed to stage III or IV encephalopathy is associated with a 60% to 85% mortality. Liver transplantation has been effective in the rescue of certain patients with fulminant hepatitis.

Toxic Agents

Because of its primary role in the biotransformation of drugs and xenobiotics, the liver is very susceptible to damage from both primary substrates and various metabolic by-products. Table 18.9 lists some of the compounds known to cause liver injury. Metabolites are

usually more potent toxins than the parent compound. For example, carbon tetrachloride, halothane, isoniazid, and acetaminophen are degraded into substances that, in turn, produce hepatocyte necrosis. Stimulation of the hepatic "detoxification" enzyme pathways by alcohol and barbiturates actually results in greater liver injury from these agents.

Acute hepatic toxicity can occasionally be attributed to dietary components. Botanical hepatotoxins pose a threat to individuals who consume wild picked herbs, fungi, and other plants as part of a "natural" diet. Amanita phalloides, for example, is an innocuous appearing mushroom with no distinctive taste or odor that would otherwise alert the unwary mushroom hunter to the fact that a mere teaspoonful of this fungus contains sufficient anatoxin to cause fatal hepatic necrosis. Ingestion of *bush teas*, prepared from pyrrolizidine alkaloid-containing herbs can cause veno-occlusive disease of the liver, which is fatal in some cases. Alcohol, considered by some individuals to be a significant and sometimes dominant component of their diet, is the food substance most commonly recognized as contributing to hepatic injury. Although alcohol is a relatively weak hepatotoxin, alcohol abuse accounts for the majority of liver disease seen in the United States.

Cirrhosis

In mammals, the liver is uniquely able to respond to parenchymal damage by the process of regeneration. The architecture of such reconstruction is often abnormal because of an increased amount of connective tissue that divides the regenerating liver into nodules. The presence of nodular parenchyma and diffuse fibrosis characterize hepatic cirrhosis. Cirrhotic livers can be subclassified on the basis of their gross appearance. Those with nodules uniformly less than 3 mm in diameter are classified as having micronodular cirrhosis, while those with most nodules measuring greater than 3 mm have macronodular cirrhosis. Mixed cirrhosis indicates an equal representation of both sizes. The nodular pattern may be helpful in identifying the etiology of underlying liver disease (i.e., micronodular cirrhosis and alcohol abuse), but this subclassification is hardly precise.

Cirrhosis is the final common pathway for a broad spectrum of diseases and toxins that damage the liver (Table 18.10). In the United States, alcoholic liver disease

Table 18.9.
Compounds That Cause Liver Injury

Acetaminophen	DDT
Aflatoxin	Halothane
Alcohol	Isoniazid
Anatoxin	Methotrexate
Anabolic steroids	Methyldopa
Arsenic	Oxyphenisatin
Azathioprine	Phenothiazine
Carbon tetrachloride	Rifampicin
Chloroform	Tannic acid
Cimetidine	Vinyl chloride
Copper salts	Yellow phosphorus

Table 18.10.
Diseases Associated with Hepatic Cirrhosis

α_1-antitrypsin deficiency	Hypervitaminosis A
Autoimmune hepatitis	Jejunoileal bypass
Budd-Chiari syndrome	Primary biliary cirrhosis
Chronic active hepatitis	Sclerosing cholangitis
Chronic alcohol abuse	Toxic hepatitis
Cystic fibrosis	Tyrosinemia
Glycogen storage diseases	Wilson's disease
Hemochromatosis	

and chronic active hepatitis are the most common precipitating factors. Regardless of etiology, the clinical picture of a person with severe cirrhosis is dominated by the findings of hepatocellular failure and portal hypertension. The former gives rise to jaundice, steatorrhea, encephalopathy, and endocrine abnormalities. Laboratory examination often reveals low serum albumin and fibrinogen levels, prolonged coagulation times, anemia, and hyperbilirubinemia. Failure of the reticuloendothelial system is reflected by frequent episodes of infection, especially with pathogens of intestinal origin and often in the form of spontaneous bacterial peritonitis.

The overgrowth of connective tissue that characterizes the cirrhotic liver compresses the small hepatic venules, resulting in a functional obstruction of the hepatic venous drainage. The increased resistance of blood flow through the liver produces elevated pressure in the portal venous system (i.e., portal hypertension). As opposed to presinusoidal portal hypertension associated with schistosomiasis infestation, portal hypertension secondary to hepatic cirrhosis is primarily postsinusoidal. Normal portal pressure is approximately 5 to 10 mmHg. Most patients with clinically significant portal hypertension have portal pressures in excess of 18 to 20 mmHg. The pathophysiologic response to this process is dilatation of collateral veins varicies between the portal and systemic circulations or varices. Varices can occur throughout the upper and lower gastrointestinal tract, the retroperitoneum, and the abdominal wall. The sequelae of portal hypertension also include the development of ascites, hypersplenism, and a hyperdynamic cardiac output. Surgical intervention for hepatic cirrhosis focuses on the three major complications of portal hypertension: bleeding esophageal varices; intractable ascites; and hypersplenism.

By virtue of the massive gastrointestinal hemorrhage that can accompany their rupture, esophageal varices are a significant source of morbidity and mortality. Nonsurgical control of variceal hemorrhage begins with administration of pharmacologic agents, such as vasopressin, or the hormone octreotide, which decrease splanchnic blood flow and hence diminish portal venous and esophageal variceal pressure. Sclerotherapy is also effective. This process refers to the infusion of irritants into or around the esophageal varix in an attempt to promote scarring. Surgical procedures for persistent or recurrent bleeding episodes have been designed to either disrupt the portal inflow into the fragile variceal vessels or shunt blood directly from the portal/mesenteric system into the systemic venous system. The so-called portal systemic or mesenteric systemic shunts are effective means of lowering pressure within the variceal vessel, thereby decreasing its propensity to bleed.

Hepatic ascites is an intraperitoneal transudate that forms in response to low intravascular colloidal pressure and sodium retention in the setting of portal hypertension. Although diuretics and sodium restriction control ascites in 95% of patients, massive accumulations can lead to the secondary morbidity of respiratory compromise, abdominal wall herniation, and the development of spontaneous bacterial peritonitis (35). Direct diversion of the ascitic fluid from the peritoneal cavity into the bloodstream with a peritoneal venous shunt is rarely required. In many centers, shunts of both the portal systemic and peritoneal venous variety have been largely abandoned as treatment for patients with portal hypertension and cirrhosis in favor of total liver replacement by orthotopic liver transplantation.

Primary biliary cirrhosis (PBC) is an inflammatory disorder of the intrahepatic bile ducts most commonly identified in middle-aged women. PBC is a cholestatic disease notable for the development of pruritis, jaundice, fatigue, and malaise. As opposed to patients with established hepatic cirrhosis, many patients with PBC tend to have preservation of their hepatocyte function. Their serum biochemical profile typically reveals an elevated alkaline phosphatase level, modest hypertransaminemia, normal or nearly normal coagulation times, and a bilirubin level that increases in the later stages of illness. The diagnosis of PBC is supported by the presence of high titers of antimitochondrial antibody, a liver biopsy with evidence of bile duct inflammation and periportal fibrosis, and a characteristically normal cholangiogram. No specific treatment is available for PBC, although antiinflammatory agents, oral bile acids, and immunosuppressive agents have been used with variable degrees of success. Medical intervention is directed toward the relief of symptoms that, in the case of pruritis, may be disabling. End stage PBC may progress to frank cirrhosis for which liver transplantation may be appropriate treatment.

Neoplasms

Both benign and malignant tumors occur in the liver (Table 18.11). Although advances in surgical technique and postoperative care have significantly reduced the morbidity of liver surgery, an understanding of the natural history of these lesions is essential to providing the most intelligent therapeutic recommendations for each patient.

Benign Tumors

Hemangiomas of the liver occur in approximately 2% of the population. With increasingly sophisticated abdominal scans, clinicians frequently identify them inci-

Table 18.11.
Neoplasms of the Liver

Benign	Malignant
Bile duct adenoma	Cholangiocarcinoma
Focal nodular hyperplasia	Hepatoblastoma
Hemangioma	Hepatoma
Hepatocyte adenoma	Metastatic cancer
Infantile hemangioendothelioma	Sarcoma
Teratoma	

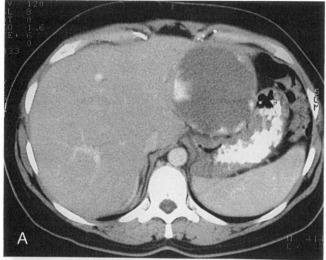

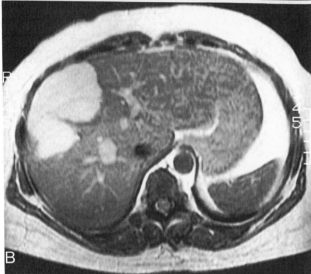

Figure 18.14. **A,** CT scan of the liver, showing an 8-cm hemangioma of the left lobe of the liver. Immediately after administration of intravenous contrast, peripheral enhancement of the lesions is noted. Central scarring is consistent with old hemorrhage and fibrosis. **B,** MRI of the abdomen, showing three hemangiomas of the liver in another patient. All lesions demonstrated characteristic centripetal filling with hypointensity on T1-weighted (not shown) and hyperintensity on T2-weighted (shown) images.

dently during the workup of unrelated disorders. As mentioned in the previous "Congenital Disorders," most hemangiomas less than 5cm are asymptomatic. Larger lesions may be painful or produce a sensation of pressure, but liver function tests usually remain within normal limits. Abdominal CT combined with selective angiography, ^{51}Cr-labeled red cells, and magnetic resonance scans are very accurate in the diagnosis of hemangiomas (Fig. 18.14). Confusion with other hepatic neoplasms rarely occurs. The potential complications of massive hemorrhage or rapid enlargement are rare. Surgical intervention should be limited to severely symptomatic patients with lesions confined to a portion of the liver that can be safely resected (36).

Two benign conditions of the liver that are the source of considerable diagnostic and therapeutic confusion are focal nodular hyperplasia (FNH) and liver cell adenoma. Both are more commonly found in women, are more likely to develop in patients taking oral contraceptives, and may be difficult to distinguish on the basis of noninvasive tests (29). The etiology of FNH remains obscure. Unlike hepatocyte adenomas, which represent actual neoplasia, FNH is thought to be a reactive disorder, perhaps a product of hepatocellular regeneration. Although complications of FNH are unusual, hepatocyte adenomas have a well-recognized incidence of spontaneous rupture, hemorrhage (as high as 30% in one large series), and malignant degeneration. As a rule, hepatocyte adenomas should be surgically removed, and for large unresectable lesions, liver transplantation should be considered.

Malignant Tumors

Malignant tumors of the liver may originate from resident hepatic cells (hepatocellular carcinoma, cholangiocarcinoma, and sarcoma) or, more commonly, from distant sites of primary neoplasia. Hepatocellular carcinoma (HCC), the most frequently diagnosed primary liver tumor in the United States, typically develops in the setting of chronic liver injury. Liver function tests often reflect the underlying liver disease and thus are not particularly useful in identifying patients with HCC. However, fetoprotein levels are elevated in 50% to 75% of patients and should be used regularly to screen high-risk patients. Hepatocellular carcinoma is often referred to as the 30% tumor—30% are surgically explored, 30% are resected, and 30% survive long term (37).Unfortunately, this equation translates into a 10% resectability rate with prolonged survival in only 3% or 4% of patients.

Metastatic liver tumors may occur along with widespread systemic dissemination or may represent a focal site of secondary tumor growth. The latter pattern has a more favorable prognosis but, unfortunately, is noted in less than 5% of all cases. Isolated hepatic metastasis tends to occur in a limited number of diseases, e.g., colon cancer, carcinoid tumors, and gastric leiomyosarcoma. Hepatic resection for selected patients with isolated liver metastases has been associated with prolonged survival and is indicated in selected patients.

Biliary Pathophysiology

The pathophysiology of the biliary tree is also a diverse group of problems, including congenital atresia and cystic disease, gallstone formation, and motility disorders as well as biliary infections, strictures, and tumors. For the purposes of this chapter, biliary pathophysiology has been grouped into five categories: congenital disorders; calculous disease; motility disorders; benign strictures; and neoplasms.

Congenital Disorders

Biliary Atresia

Biliary atresia is the lack of a lumen in part or all of the extrahepatic biliary tract, causing complete obstruction to bile flow. The incidence of biliary atresia is 1 in 10,000 to 13,000 live births, therefore representing the most common condition causing persistent jaundice in the newborn. Two theories are currently proposed to explain the etiology of biliary atresia. The first is based on the embryologic development of the bile ducts. Originally hollow, the hepatic diverticulum becomes a solid mass of cells that later recanalizes to form the bile ducts. Biliary atresia may be a failure of this recanalization process. The other prevailing theory is that biliary atresia is the result of an ongoing inflammatory process, such as a viral infection, that leads to progressive destruction of the extrahepatic bile ducts shortly after birth.

A number of variations of biliary atresia exist with respect to the extent of the ductal obliteration (Fig. 18.15) (38). A correctable variant preserves the intrahepatic and proximal extrahepatic biliary tree, thus allowing biliary reconstruction. Unfortunately, the incidence of this variant is rare and is seen in only 1% to 2% of patients. More than 90% of cases of biliary atresia are considered uncorrectable (Kasai type III), in which the entire biliary tree is obliterated. In approximately 10% of patients, the proximal system is obliterated, but the distal bile duct and gallbladder are patent. The pioneering work by Kasai and colleagues in the late 1950s has led to the recognition that intrahepatic ducts may be patent at birth with subsequent destruction during the first 2 to 3 weeks of life (39). This realization led to the development of the Kasai procedure or the hepatic portoenterostomy. In this operation, a transection of hepatic parenchyma is made above the fibrous cone of obliterated proximal bile ducts. A loop of small bowel is then anastomosed to the exposed area of the liver surface.

Although the procedure was originally met with skepticism, the Kasai procedure and its subsequent modifications are now the initial treatment of choice for most patients with biliary atresia. In recent reports, 66% to 80% of patients with biliary atresia can be managed successfully if an adequate corrective operation is carried out within the first 60 days of life. Postoperative prevention of cholangitis is imperative to obtain these results. Unfortunately, in many cases, reestablishment of bile flow does not equate with cure. The availability of hepatic transplantation provides definitive therapy for those patients in whom hepatic portoenterostomy has failed. Current 1-year survival for pediatric liver transplant patients is approximately 70% to 80%. Recently, the use of living, related donors has provided suitable liver parenchyma for transplantation, thereby decreasing the high mortality rates of infants on transplantation waiting lists.

Choledochal Cysts

Choledochal cysts are the other common congenital anomaly of the biliary system. The cystic dilatation can involve either the extrahepatic biliary tree alone or may have associated intrahepatic cystic dilatation (30% of cases). Choledochal cysts occur more often in females and may present either during childhood or as an adult. Although choledochal cysts are often called congenital lesions, it is probably more appropriate to say that patients are born with the propensity for the development of cysts. Most evidence now suggests that an alteration in the arrangement of the choledochopancreatic duct junction leads to a mixing of pancreatic juice and bile with resultant destruction of the wall of the biliary tree, leading to cystic dilatation (Fig. 18.16) (40). This theory explains why some choledochal cysts do not present until adulthood. Moreover, chronic irritation of the ductal mucosa and bile stasis probably explains why these cysts are potentially premalignant abnormalities.

The clinical manifestations of choledochal cysts are variable. Epigastric pain is the most common symptom. Fever and jaundice may also occur, especially in patients with choledochal cysts and intrahepatic ductal dilatations. Complications include biliary obstruction, stone formation, and cholangitis. Cholangiocarcinoma may

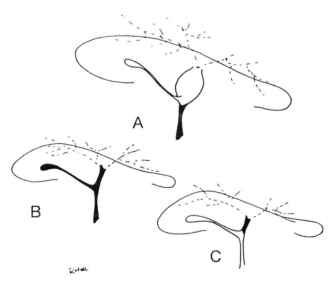

Figure 18.15. Three variants of biliary atresia. **A,** Correctable atresia. Proximal patency is often misleading because the hilar bilepseudocysts are lined only by granulation tissue and covered by fibrous tissue. **B,** Noncorrectable atresia. This is the most common type; the entire extrahepatic ductal system is obliterated. **C,** Similar to noncorrectable atresia, the proximal ducts are obliterated in this type, but patency of the gallbladder, cystic duct, and common bile duct is preserved. In all types, intrahepatic ducts are hypoplastic. From Karrer FM, Hall RJ, Stewart BA, et al. Congenital biliary tract disease. In: Pitt HA, ed. Biliary tract surgery. Surg Clin North Am 1990;70:1405.

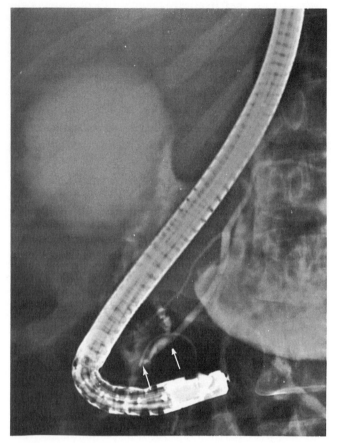

Figure 18.16. Endoscopic retrograde cholangiopancreatogram, demonstrating a large choledochal cyst. Note the abnormal choledochopancreatic duct junction with a long common channel (arrows). From Doty JE, Pitt HA. Cystic lesions of the liver and biliary tree. In: Moody FG, ed. Surgical treatment of digestive diseases. Chicago: Year Book Medical, 1986;334–351.

also develop, and the incidence of this abnormality increases with the age of the patient at presentation. Surgical treatment is recommended for choledochal cysts, and the procedure of choice is excision of the cyst and reconstruction of the biliary tree with a Roux-en-Y choledochojejunostomy.

Calculous Disease

Gallstones represent a failure to maintain certain biliary solutes, primarily cholesterol and calcium salts, in a solubilized state. Gallstone disease is a substantial international health care problem. In the United States, the overall incidence of gallstones is reported to be 10% to 12%, which translates to 25 to 30 million people. The incidence is increased in both women and in the elderly. Gallstones are classified by their cholesterol content as either cholesterol or pigment stones. Pigment stones are further classified as either black or brown. Pure cholesterol gallstones are uncommon (10%) with most cholesterol stones containing calcium salts in their center, or nidus. Pigment stones are also composed of calcium salts of one or more of four primary anions: bilirubinate;

carbonate; phosphate; and long-chain fatty acids, primarily palmitate. Black pigment stones occur more frequently in the setting of hemolysis and are the type of pigment stones found most commonly in Western populations. Brown pigment stones are earthy, are often associated with chronic biliary infection, and are the type of pigment stones found most often in the Orient. In most American populations, 70% to 80% of gallstones are cholesterol, and pigment stones account for the remaining 20% to 30%.

An important biliary precipitate in gallstone pathogenesis is biliary "sludge," which refers to a mixture of cholesterol crystals, calcium bilirubinate granules, and a mucin gel matrix. Biliary sludge has been observed clinically in prolonged fasting states or with the use of long-term total parenteral nutrition (TPN). Both of these conditions are also associated with gallstone formation. Prospective studies in humans indicate that biliary sludge may be a precursor of gallstones (41). The finding of macromolecular complexes of mucin and bilirubin, similar to biliary sludge in the central core of most cholesterol gallstones, suggests that the sludge may serve as the nidus for gallstone growth.

Cholesterol Gallstone Pathogenesis

The pathogenesis of cholesterol gallstones is clearly multifactorial but essentially involves three stages: (a) cholesterol saturation; (b) nucleation; and (c) stone growth. For years after the classic studies of Small (42) and colleagues, gallstones were thought to result primarily from a defect in the hepatic secretion of biliary lipids and were primarily a liver disease. Yet this view ignored the fact that almost all gallstones form in the gallbladder. In recent years, it has become increasingly clear that gallbladder mucosal and motor function also play key roles in gallstone formation. The entire body of research and clinical information on the pathogenesis of cholesterol gallstones is far beyond the scope of this chapter, but the three stages of gallstone formation will be addressed.

Cholesterol Saturation. As discussed previously, cholesterol is an organic molecule that is virtually insoluble in an aqueous medium such as bile. The transport of cholesterol in bile occurs primarily in mixed micelles and cholesterol-phospholipid vesicles. Excess cholesterol secretion is known to surpass the ability of these carriers to maintain cholesterol in solution, resulting in cholesterol supersaturation. This situation creates the thermodynamic state that allows cholesterol precipitation. However, cholesterol supersaturation has been demonstrated to be present in many normal humans without gallstones. Furthermore, significant overlap exists in cholesterol saturation index in patients with and without gallstones. Thus cholesterol supersaturation results in a metastable state in which cholesterol precipitation may or may not take place. Additional factors in bile must be present, therefore, to either enhance or inhibit the nucleation of cholesterol leading to the next stage in gallstone formation.

Nucleation. Nucleation refers to the process in which solid cholesterol monohydrate crystals form and conglomerate. Numerous investigators have demonstrated that nucleation occurs more rapidly in gallbladder bile of patients with cholesterol stones than in individuals with cholesterol saturated bile without stones. The gallbladder is the site of the major kinetic events associated with cholesterol nucleation. One important event occurring in the gallbladder is the concentration of bile. The concentration of bile leads to a net transfer of phospholipids and cholesterol from vesicles to micelles (Fig. 18.17). The phospholipids are transformed more efficiently than cholesterol, leading to cholesterol enrichment of the remaining vesicles. These cholesterol-rich vesicles aggregate to form large multilamellar liquid vesicles that then precipitates cholesterol monohydrate crystals.

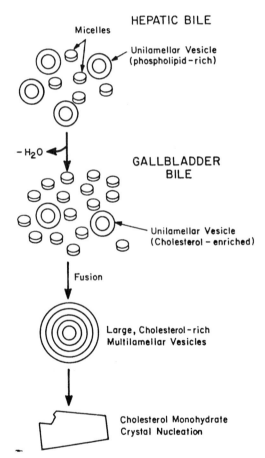

Figure 18.17. Concentration of bile leads to net transfer of phospholipid and cholesterol from vesicles to micelles. Phospholipids are transferred more efficiently than cholesterol, leading to cholesterol enrichment of the remaining (remodeled) vesicles. Aggregation of these cholesterol-rich vesicles to form multilamellar liquid crystals may be followed by precipitation of excess cholesterol as solid crystals of cholesterol monohydrate. From Vessey DA. Metabolism of drugs and toxins by the human liver. In: Zakin D, Boyer TD, eds. Hepatology: a textbook of liver disease. 2nd ed. Philadelphia: WB Saunders, 1990:1492.

Another factor promoting vesicle aggregation is the presence of pronucleating factors in gallbladder bile. Because cholesterol nucleation occurs in the mucin gel layer in various animal models and in human sludge, mucin glycoproteins produced by the gallbladder may serve as a nucleating agent. Mucin glycoproteins have been found to accelerate cholesterol nucleation in model bile systems and in human bile. Furthermore, increased mucus secretion has been reported as an early event in animal models with experimentally induced cholesterol gallstones. More recently, nonmucinglycoproteins in bile, including immunoglobulins, have been implicated as pronucleating agents and antinucleating agents. In addition, calcium salts may serve as a nidus for cholesterol crystallization. Current theory also suggests that the gallbladder's mucus gel serves as a large matrix, or scaffold, of protein in which the nucleation reaction may occur (43). Similar events are recognized to occur in other biomineralization processes, such as in bone and dental formation.

Stone Growth. For gallstones to cause clinical symptoms, they must obtain a size sufficient to produce mechanical injury to the gallbladder or obstruction of the biliary tree. Growth of stones may occur in two ways: *(a)* progressive enlargement of individual crystals or stones by deposition of additional insoluble precipitate at the bile-stone interface; or *(b)* fusion of individual crystals or stones to form a larger conglomerate. Current evidence suggests that both patterns of growth contribute to the enlargement of stones. The gallbladder is again key in this stage as increased residence time in the gallbladder likely contributes to gallstone growth. This hypothesis is supported by a number of experimental and clinical observations. First, in numerous animal models, a defect in gallbladder motility has been recognized before gallstone formation. Second, gallbladder emptying induced with cholecystokinin can reduce the incidence of gallstone formation. Finally, gallbladder muscle contractility in animal models is decreased before the development of stones. Gallstone formation also occurs in clinical states with gallbladder stasis, as seen with prolonged fasting, the use of long-term TPN, and in patients with somatostatin-producing tumors or those receiving long-term somatostatin therapy.

Pigment Gallstone Pathogenesis

With the current recognition that calcium salts are present in most, if not all, cholesterol gallstones, renewed interest has developed in the events leading to the precipitation of calcium salts. The solubility of calcium salts, like that of cholesterol, is a critical factor in gallstone pathogenesis. Calcium precipitation occurs only if the solubility product (K) of one or more of the four calcium salts is exceeded (44). Thus, increases in the biliary concentration of calcium or in the anions, bilirubin, carbonate, phosphate, or palmitate may all result in calcium salt precipitation. Calcium enters bile by passive connection with water in response to the concentration of bile salts as dictated by the Gibbs-Donnan equilibrium. Thus, factors that increase the bile salt concentration in the bile, such as gallbladder concentration, increased time bile remains in the gallbladder, or stasis, will increase free calcium in the bile. The calcium may then precipitate as an insoluble calcium salt and serve as a nidus for stone formation.

Increased plasma calcium, as in hyperparathyroidism, will also increase biliary calcium. Increases in biliary anions can occur in a variety of clinical states. Unconjugated bilirubin increases if the bilirubin load increases, as in hemolytic states, or if excessive deconjugation occurs, as when certain bacteria are present in the biliary tree. Calcium phosphate and calcium salts of long-chain fatty acids such as palmitate may result from excessive hydrolysis of biliary lecithins by bacterial phospholipases. Increased biliary carbonate occurs with defective acidification of bile. All of these circumstances predispose to the formation of pigment gallstones.

As previously stated, pigment gallstones are classified as either black or brown pigment stones. Black pigment stones are typically tarry and are associated frequently with hemolytic conditions or cirrhosis. These stones are usually not associated with infected bile and are located almost exclusively in the gallbladder. In contrast, brown stones are earthy in texture and are typically found in the bile ducts, especially in Oriental populations. Brown stones often contain more cholesterol and calcium palmitate (Fig. 18.18) and occur as primary common duct stones in Western patients with disorders of biliary motility and associated bacterial infection (45). In these settings, bacteria containing the enzyme -glucuronidase cause enzymatic hydrolysis of soluble conjugated bilirubin glucuronide to form free bilirubin. This water-insoluble component then combines with calcium to produce the calcium bilirubinate matrix for stone formation.

Gallstone Treatment

Symptomatic gallstone disease accounts for substantial morbidity, mortality, and economic losses. Although gallstones do not invariably cause disease, more than 600,000 biliary tract operations are performed annually in the United States for symptoms or complications of cholelithiasis. The management of asymptomatic gallstones has been controversial, but most experts recommend that these patients should be observed and not treated. Data from large population studies suggest that in truly asymptomatic patients, the likelihood of the development of symptoms is only approximately 1% to 2% per year. Furthermore, serious complications rarely occur without the development of symptoms before the acute problem.

A number of symptoms are associated with gallstone disease. The most common is biliary colic, which is a right upper quadrant ormidepigastric pain that is generally characterized by rapid increase in intensity with a plateau of discomfort lasting for several hours, usually followed by gradual decrease of intensity. The pain seldom lasts more than 8 hours and in most cases is caused by cystic duct impaction or passage of a stone. The usual onset of biliary colic following a meal suggests a role of postprandial gallbladder contraction in the development of this symptom. Other nonspecific symptoms of biliary tract disease include dyspepsia without pain, increased flatulence, or fatty food intolerance. Recent studies suggest that in patients with biliary colic, symptomatic improvement following cholecystectomy can be expected in more than 90% of patients, whereas in those with more nonspecific symptoms, only 75% of the pa-

Figure 18.18. Percent of black (n = 17) and brown (n = 5) stones containing individual calcium salts and cholesterol. Statistical analysis compares black and brown pigment stone groups. From Kaufman HS, Magnuson TH, Lillemoe KD, et al. The role of bacteria in gallbladder and common duct stone formation. Ann Surg 1989;205:584–592.

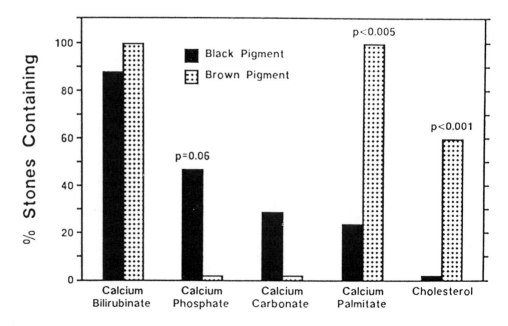

tients experience long-term relief of symptoms following removal of the gallbladder (46).

The treatment of symptomatic gallstones has changed tremendously in the last decade. For over a century, traditional open cholecystectomy had been used for the treatment of calculous biliary tract disease with excellent result in the elective setting. In recent years, the development of laparoscopic cholecystectomy has revolutionized gallbladder surgery. Currently, laparoscopic cholecystectomy is equally effective as open cholecystectomy and has tremendous advantages in terms of patient comfort and minimizing of time away from productive activity. Although the incidence of bile duct injury following the laparoscopic procedure is higher than with open cholecystectomy (0.4% to 0.6% versus 0.1 % to 0.2 %), much of this difference has been associated with the learning curve with this procedure. Nonoperative management of gallstones includes dissolution with oral bile acids, extracorporeal shockwave lithotripsy, and percutaneous extraction or dissolution with organic solvents. All of these techniques, however, have disadvantages, including limited application to subsets of patients, relatively low initial efficacy, and high recurrence rates. As a result, these nonoperative options are not very cost effective and, with the advent of laparoscopic cholecystectomy, have fallen out of fashion.

Acute Cholecystitis

Acute cholecystitis complicates the course of symptomatic gallstones in 10% to 20% of patients. In most cases, the initial event is obstruction of the cystic duct by a gallstone. However, the progression of events during acute cholecystitis after the obstruction of the cystic duct is not entirely clear. Obstruction of the cystic duct does not progress to cholecystitis in all patients. A presumed sequence of events suggests that cystic duct occlusion in the presence of saturated bile activates inflammatory mediators, including prostaglandins, which are present in high concentrations in the wall of the gallbladder. Prostaglandins stimulate the mucosa of the gallbladder to secrete and not absorb water, thereby exacerbating gallbladder distension. As the gallbladder distends with mucus, luminal pressure increases and gallbladder perfusion is impaired with resultant necrosis or perforation. High concentrations of bile acids have also been implicated as initiators of the inflammatory response because these substances increase transepithelial transport of water. Another possible mediator of inflammation in acute cholecystitis is lysolecithin, a product of the action of phospholipase A on lecithin.

Edema of the gallbladder wall from venous and lymphatic obstruction develops early in acute cholecystitis. If the cystic duct stone dislodges, the attack may be brief and self-limited, but if the gallbladder remains obstructed, the subsequent development of ischemia or secondary infection will determine the severity of the disease. Bacterial infection appears to play a secondary role in the pathogenesis of acute cholecystitis. Aerobic bacteria can be cultured from gallbladder bile in about half of the patients with acute cholecystitis. Although infection is not an important factor in the development of cholecystitis, suppurative complications may produce much of the morbidity and mortality as the disease progresses. Anaerobes are not commonly isolated from patients with acute cholecystitis, except for the small percentage of patients with empyema or gangrene of the gallbladder. In these rare situations, Clostridia perfringens may be present and require high-dose penicillin therapy.

Choledocholithiasis

Common duct stones are classified as either primary (those that form in the common duct) or secondary (those that form in the gallbladder and pass into the common bile duct). Approximately 15% of patients with gallbladder stones will have stones in their common bile duct, whereas 95% of the patients with common bile duct stones have gallbladder stones. Most secondary gallstones represent a complication of long-standing gallbladder stone disease and are associated with factors such as multiple small stones, a large cystic duct, and a low entrance of the cystic duct. In most cases, primary common bile duct stones are associated with bile stasis and infection. Primary common bile duct stones are brown pigment in nature and are described as earthy or mud-like. They often crumble easily when manipulated. Bile stasis, as a result of abnormalities of sphincter of Oddimotor activity, results in the overgrowth of bacteria with an associated increase in the bacterial enzyme -glucuronidase. This situation facilitates deconjugation of bilirubin with subsequent calcium salt precipitation. The differentiation of primary from secondary common bile duct stones is important, as their clinical management may differ. In patients with secondary stones, cholecystectomy and choledocholithotomy are almost always adequate therapy. In patients with primary common bile duct stones, further drainage of the common bile duct may be necessary to prevent continued bile stasis and further stone formation.

Acute Cholangitis

Cholangitis is an acute bacterial infection of the biliary tree. Charcot was the first to recognize cholangitis. His original report described the triad of fever, jaundice, and right upper quadrant pain. He postulated that the condition was caused by "stagnant bile," usually associated with an obstructed bile duct. In the century since Charcot's initial description, it has been recognized that the pathophysiology of cholangitis requires a combination of two factors: bacterial contamination of the bile

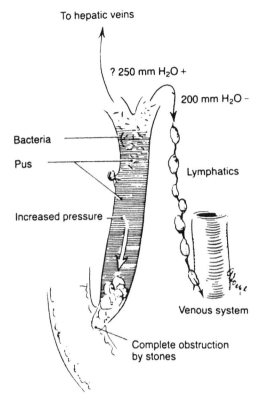

To hepatic veins

? 250 mm H$_2$O +

200 mm H$_2$O −

Bacteria

Pus

Lymphatics

Increased pressure

Venous system

Complete obstruction
by stones

Figure 18.19. Cholangitis is caused by the combination of biliary obstruction, often attributable to distally impacted stones and bactibilia. Bacteria then reflux into the hepatic veins and perihepatic lymphatics, resulting in systemic bacteremia. From Pitt HA, Longmire WP Jr. Suppurative cholangitis. In: Hardy JM, ed. Critical surgical illness. 2nd ed. Philadelphia: WB Saunders, 1980:380.

and increased biliary pressure (Fig. 18.19). The resultant increased intraductal pressure causes the reflux of bacteria into the hepatic veins and perihepatic lymphatics, resulting in bacteremia. Biliary obstruction contributes to both aspects by increasing bacterial concentrations as a result of stagnation and by increasing biliary pressure.

Common bile duct stones are the most common cause of biliary obstruction, resulting in cholangitis. Malignant biliary obstruction rarely presents with cholangitis. The advances in invasive biliary tract procedures, however, have changed the spectrum of this disease. Manipulations of the biliary tract, either percutaneously or transampullary, can be associated with both the introduction of bacteria and sudden increases in biliary tract pressure, which may result in cholangitis.

Although the bile is normally sterile, positive cultures are found in up to 90% of patients with choledocholithiasis and in virtually all patients with acute cholangitis. Blood cultures are also positive in 40% to 50% of patients with cholangitis. The most common organisms associated with acute cholangitis are Gram-negative coliforms, including Escherichiacoli and Klebsiella pneumoniae. Enterococcus is the third most common organism in most series. Anaerobic bacteria, particularly Bacteroides fragilis, are also important pathogens, espe-

cially in elderly patients with choledocholithiasis and patients with indwelling biliary stents. In recent years, a change in the spectrum of bacterial infection has occurred as more and more cases of cholangitis are seen following biliary tract manipulations (47). In such cases, previously uncommon Gram-negative rods such as Pseudomonas spp. and Enterobacter spp. and yeast are now being isolated.

The spectrum of disease of acute cholangitis can range from a mild self-limited illness to a life-threatening condition with septic shock. The therapy for cholangitis must, therefore, be individualized on the basis of the severity of the disease. Virtually all patients require rehydration and prompt institution of broad-spectrum antibiotic. Historically, the combination of a penicillin, an aminoglycoside, and an agent effective against anaerobic bacteria has been recommended to provide empiric coverage for the potential infecting organisms. Recently, synthetic penicillins have become available that provide a similar broad-spectrum of coverage against Gram-negative aerobes, enterococcus, and anaerobes. These agents may provide excellent single-agent coverage without the potential nephrotoxicity of the aminoglycoside. The vast majority of patients with cholangitis will respond to antibiotics and intravenous fluids without the need for urgent biliary decompression. However, emergency biliary decompression may be necessary in the small subset of patients with septic shock. Currently, the preferred route of biliary decompression depends on the likely cause of obstruction and available expertise in percutaneous biliary drainage and endoscopic sphincterotomy.

Motility Disorders

Abnormalities of biliary motility may affect both the gallbladder and sphincter of Oddi. As mentioned above, a defect in gallbladder motility is thought to be an early event in the pathogenesis of gallstones. As a result, some patients who have not yet developed macroscopic gallstones may present with typical biliary symptoms. If an extensive workup reveals no other source for the symptoms and if some objective evidence of abnormal gallbladder emptying or early gallstone disease has been demonstrated, cholecystectomy may be justified and often results in relief of symptoms. Among the multiple diagnostic tests to confirm symptomatic a calculous cholecystitis, quantitative nuclear medicine gallbladder function studies and duodenal drainage with a search for cholesterol crystals or calcium bilirubinate granules have been used most frequently.

An abnormality in the function of the sphincter of Oddi has long been suspected as the source of abdominal pain in patients with biliary symptoms and no common duct stones after cholecystectomy. However, this problem has been difficult to diagnose. Current diagnostic modalities include specialized nuclear medicine studies, focusing on bile duct to duodenal delivery time; ultrasound measurement of bile duct diameter in response to a fatty meal or intravenous cholecystokinin; and transendoscopic measurement of the sphincter of Oddi and biliary baseline pressure and phasic wave activity.

Endoscopic manometric observations in the biliary tree are often open to considerable interpretive errors and have the disadvantage of requiring invasive technology. They require an endoscopist with specific expertise and have been associated with a high incidence of pancreatitis if the manometry catheter is in the pancreatic sphincter. Recent studies using radionuclide scanning to determine emptying rates of the common bile duct may provide a noninvasive quantitative method of providing repeated observation in such patients.

Biliary manometric studies of symptomatic postcholecystectomy patients have demonstrated a number of abnormalities. First, a group of patients has been identified with elevation of baseline sphincter of Oddi pressure above 40 mmHg. This group of patients with sphincter stenosis may benefit by the performance of an endoscopic or surgical sphincterotomy (48). The etiology of the stenosis in these patients is presumed secondary to scarring from recurrent passage of common bile duct stones or biliary debris. Other patients with postcholecystectomy symptoms who only have an altered response of the sphincter to intravenous cholecystokinin or abnormally rapid phasic waves are less likely to have a favorable response to sphincterotomy.

The decision to perform a sphincterotomy for biliary pain attributed to sphincter dysfunction is made best in a patient with frequent or severe symptoms in whom objective support for the diagnosis has been obtained. Enthusiasm for the procedure must be tempered because the procedure is associated with a low, but real, risk of morbidity and mortality. Moreover, if sphincter of Oddi dysfunction is being considered, a trial of a calcium channel blocker to reduce sphincter pressure may be indicated before sphincterotomy.

Benign Strictures

Benign strictures of the bile duct are rare problems that cause considerable patient morbidity. Sclerosing cholangitis and iatrogenic strictures are the most common benign strictures.

Primary Sclerosing Cholangitis

Primary sclerosing cholangitis is an idiopathic disease characterized by inflammatory, fibrous strictures of the intrahepatic and extrahepatic bileducts that cannot be attributed to other causes, such as operative trauma, choledocholithiasis, or cholangiocarcinoma. The cause of primary sclerosing cholangitis is unknown. Several etiologic theories have been proposed, including

Table 18.12.
Possible Etiologies of Sclerosing Cholangitis

Autoimmune	Association with other autoimmune disease; circulating immune complexes; frequency of HLA-BB
Bacterial	Cases occuring after suppurative cholangitis; portal bacteremia with ulcerative colitis
Viral	Reovirus-induced murine biliary atresia; reovirus titers in children with biliary atresia; reovirus titers in patients; association with AIDS
Congenital	Cases involving only common bile duct; reports in siblings; report of long common channel
Copper	Serum and hepatic copper levels
Drug-induced	Formalin treatment of hepatic echinococcosis; hepatic arterial fluorodeoxyuridine (FUDR)
Histiocytosis X	Reports of three cases

autoimmune responses, bacterial and viral infections, and congenital lesions (Table 18.12). In recent reports, more than half of the cases of sclerosing cholangitis have been associated with inflammatory bowel disease, primarily ulcerative colitis.

The clinical course of patients with primary sclerosing cholangitis is variable. Some patients are identified because of mild liver function abnormalities detected during an evaluation for ulcerative colitis. These patients may be asymptomatic for years, whereas other patients may have rapidly worsening course and die from progressive liver failure. Patients often have exacerbations and remissions. Because of the variable clinical course and the infrequency of the disease, the response to treatment has been difficult to evaluate. The most common symptoms of sclerosing cholangitis are persistent jaundice and pruritus. Despite the name, acute cholangitis is an unusual finding. The diagnosis is usually made by endoscopic retrograde cholangiopancreatography. Findings reveal diffusely distributed strictures, often producing a beaded appearance to the bileducts. Both intrahepatic and extrahepatic ductal involvement are present in most patients.

No medical therapy has been proven to alter patient survival, although recent trials suggest that ursodeoxycholic acid can improve liver function tests. Proctocolectomy in patients with ulcerative colitis has not proven to improve the outcome or delay the progression of the biliary tract disease. Biliary reconstruction has been recommended in patients with a dominant stricture. Such strictures are found frequently at the hepatic bifurcation. Cameron and associates have reported improvement of jaundice after resection of the hepatic bifurcation, bilateral dilatation, stenting the hepatic ducts, and hepaticojejunostomy (49). In addition, an improvement in survival has been seen in patients without preexisting cirrhosis. With the advent of liver transplantation, a trend exists toward the avoidance of hepaticobiliary surgical procedures that might make subsequent hepatic transplantation difficult. The role of balloon dilatation in these patients has yet to be clearly established. Liver transplantation has become the procedure of choice for patients with sclerosing cholangitis, established cirrhosis, and liver failure. However, bile duct resection and reconstruction may be indicated in selected patients with extrahepatic obstruction as well as those in whom a secondary cholangiocarcinoma is suspected.

Benign Bile Duct Stricture

The vast majority of bile duct strictures occur after injury to the bile duct during cholecystectomy or other upper abdominal operations. The exact incidence of iatrogenic bile duct injury is unknown; however, recent studies suggest that the incidence of bile duct injury during open cholecystectomy is 1 to 2 in 1000 cases (50). Large surveys suggest that laparoscopic cholecystectomy is associated with an increased incidence of bile duct injury in the range of 3 to 5 per 1000 cases (51,52). A number of factors are associated with bile duct injury during either open or laparoscopic cholecystectomy, including inadequate exposure and lighting, inexperience, and failure to identify structures before clamping, ligating, or dividing them. Failure to recognize congenital anomalies of the bile duct, such as insertion of the right hepatic duct into the cystic duct or a long common wall between the cystic duct and common bile duct, may also lead to injury. Factors increasing the risk of injury during laparoscopic cholecystectomy include (a) the visual perception through the laparoscope, (b) excessive cephalad displacement of the gallbladder fundus and infundibulum creating an alignment of the cystic duct and the common bile duct, and (c) tinting of the common bile duct due to retraction of a short cystic duct.

In recent years, the importance of ischemia of the bile duct in the formation of postoperative strictures has been emphasized. Unnecessary dissection around the bile duct during cholecystectomy or bile ductanastomosis may divide or injure major arteries of the bile duct. These run in the 3- and 9-o'clock positions (Fig. 18.20). Division of these arteries may result in ischemia, which may contribute to fibrosis and stricture formation. Finally, a tremendous local inflammatory reaction can develop in adjacent tissues to respond to a bile leak or surgical clips. This reaction may be intensified if infection is present. Finally, the development of a neuroma has been identified as a cause for late bile duct strictures.

The clinical presentation of postoperative bile duct strictures is variable. In the era of open cholecystectomy, nearly 80% of strictures were identified within the first year after the initial operation (53). However, in the remaining patients, the presentation may be delayed for years after the initial operative procedure. After open cholecystectomy, the most common early presentation of bile duct strictures is the development of jaundice with or without cholangitis. This mode of presentation is associated with a progressive increase in liver function tests, particularly total bilirubin and alkaline phospha-

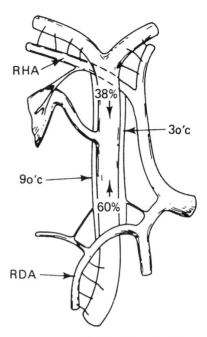

Figure 18.20.   Anterior view of the blood supply of the human bile duct. The blood supply to the bile ducts in the hilum of the liver (above) and the retropancreatic bile duct (below) from adjacent arteries is profuse. The supraduodenal bile duct blood supply is axial and tenuous, with 60% from below and 38% from above. The small main axial vessels (3 and 9 o'clock arteries) are vulnerable and damage easily. RHA, right hepatic artery; RDA, retroduodenal artery; 9o'c, nine o'clock; 3o'c, three o'clock. From Terblanche J, Allison HF, Northover JMA. An ischemic basis for biliary strictures. Surgery 1983;94:52.

tase. These changes can often be seen as early as the second or third postoperative day. As with open cholecystectomy, bile duct injury during laparoscopic cholecystectomy is usually not recognized at the time of operation. In most patients, the injury during laparoscopic cholecystectomy involves transection of the bile duct. Leakage of bile via a trochar site or the accumulation of bile in the abdomen (bile ascites/peritonitis) is the mode of presentation seen most commonly. Serum bilirubin will be elevated modestly in this setting because of reabsorption of bile from the peritoneal cavity. Patients presenting with postoperative bile duct strictures months to years after cholecystectomy frequently have episodes of cholangitis. These episodes are often mild and respond to antibiotic therapy.

The gold standard for the evaluation of patients with a presumed bile duct stricture is cholangiography. Either endoscopic retrograde cholangiography (ERC) or percutaneous transhepatic cholangiography (PTC) is useful in defining biliary anatomy. In most cases, however, PTC is more valuable because it defines the anatomy of the proximal biliary tree, which may be used in the reconstruction. Moreover, during PTC, transhepatic catheters can be placed, which can be useful in providing decompression of the biliary tract.

The management of bile duct strictures has changed substantially since the introduction of either percutaneous or endoscopic techniques for dilatation of strictures. The operative management of bile duct strictures in most cases involves resection of the stricture with reconstruction as a hepaticojejunostomy or choledochojejunostomy with or without a transanastomotic stent. In general, success rates after the surgical management of benign bile duct strictures approach 85% to 90%. Initial success rates with transhepatic or endoscopic balloon dilatation of bile duct strictures have approached that of surgical reconstruction. However, long-term follow-up is not available in many reports.

In a retrospective study from the Johns Hopkins Hospital that compared patients managed at the same institution by both operative reconstruction and percutaneous dilatation, surgical reconstruction was associated with an 88% success rate with a mean follow-up of 57 months (52). Percutaneous dilatation alone was successful in only 55% of patients with a similar follow-up. The total length of stay, hospital costs, morbidity, and mortality were similar. A similar report comparing endoscopic dilatation and surgery showed that surgical reconstruction was successful in 83% of patients, whereas endoscopic dilation was successful in 75% with similar mean follow up at 46 to 50 months (55). Unfortunately, because complete bile duct transection occurs in most patients with laparoscopic injuries, neither percutaneous nor endoscopic techniques are applicable.

Neoplasms

Gallbladder Cancer

Primary gallbladder cancer, although the most common malignant lesion of the biliary tract, is an uncommon abdominal malignancy. The cause of gallbladder cancer remains unknown. However, several factors have been associated with this disease. Gallstones are present in up to three-fourths of the patients with carcinoma of the gallbladder, suggesting that they may play a role in the pathogenesis. Because the vast majority of gallbladder cancers are adenocarcinoma, benign neoplasms of the gallbladder, such as adenomatous polyps, may also have a predilection for malignancy. Thus, a sequence of epithelial metaplasia to carcinoma may be important in the genesis of gallbladder cancer, especially in patients with gallstones.

Unfortunately, symptomatic gallbladder carcinoma is rarely curable. Gallbladder carcinoma is most likely to be successfully treated surgically only when a small carcinoma is found incidentally during cholecystectomy for symptomatic cholelithiasis. Gallbladder cancers are locally aggressive and typically invade the liver and surrounding portal structures and the duodenum. Attempts to palliate surgically are often difficult because of extensive involvement of the portal hepatic structures. In those rare cases for which tumor is recognized and felt to be resectable, a resection of surrounding hepatic parenchyma and regional lymph node dissection might be appropriate. Adjuvant radiation may improve survival in patients with gallbladder cancer, but the overall prognosis for stage III and IV patients has been poor.

Cholangiocarcinoma

Malignant neoplasms of the extrahepatic biliary tree are also uncommon. The most frequent location for cholangiocarcinoma is in the perihilar area, although these neoplasms can be found throughout the biliary tree (56). The etiology of cholangiocarcinoma remains unknown. In humans, cholangiocarcinoma has been linked to a number of etiologic factors. Strong associations have been found between cholangiocarcinoma and sclerosing cholangitis, ulcerative colitis, cystic disease of the bile duct, and liver fluke (Clonorchis sinensis) infestation. Bile stasis, chronic inflammation, and reflux of pancreatic exocrine secretions are associated with many of the conditions and lead to malignant transformation of the bile duct epithelium.

The majority of patients with cholangiocarcinoma have jaundice at initial examination. Unfortunately, jaundice does not develop until complete obstruction of either the common hepatic duct, common bile duct, or both right and left hepatic ducts has occurred. Therefore, the tumor is often far advanced before it becomes symptomatic. Fever and pain are unusual symptoms, unless bile duct manipulations have been performed. Once the presence of biliary obstruction has been established, the anatomic site and the nature of the obstruction can be obtained by PTC or ERC. PTC is the preferred diagnostic approach when imaging studies suggest a proximal lesion. Studies from above are more likely to determine the proximal extent of the obstruction, information that is essential for surgical planning.

The management of cholangiocarcinomas is dictated by the site and the size of the lesion. Purely intrahepatic lesions may be managed with hepatic resection. For tumors arising at the bifurcation of the hepatic ducts, resection of the bifurcation and biliary reconstruction with a Roux-en-Y hepaticojejunostomy is preferred by many experts. Whether hilar resection should include a hepatic resection and/or the use of long-term transhepatic stents remains debatable. Lesions arising more distally in the common hepatic duct should be resected and continuity of the biliary tract reestablished by a hepaticojejunostomy. Distal tumors are often difficult to distinguish from other periampullary malignancies. The treatment for tumors in this location should be a pancreatoduodenectomy.

Unfortunately, long-term survival rates for patients with cholangiocarcinoma are poor. In most surgical reports of perihilar cholangiocarcinoma, peritoneal or liver metastases are identified at laparotomy in 15% to 25% of cases. Resection rates vary widely from 10% to 75%, depending on the aggressiveness of the surgeon.

More radical operations are associated with a higher operative mortality and a better long-term survival. Debate continues regarding the relative merits of various surgical palliative procedures and percutaneously or endoscopically placed stents. The best long-term survivals, of 30% to 40%, have been achieved with pancreatoduodenectomy for the most distal lesions.

Pancreatic Pathophysiology

The pathophysiology of the pancreas also represents an interesting mix of congenital problems, acute and chronic inflammatory disorders, and a diverse group of benign and malignant exocrine and endocrine tumors.

Congenital Disorders

Three important congenital abnormalities of the pancreas include annular pancreas, heterotopic pancreas, and pancreas divisum. *Annular pancreas* is a rare condition thought to arise from failure of the normal clockwise rotation of the ventral pancreatic primordium to join the dorsal pancreatic primordium. Here, histologically normal pancreatic tissue partially or completely encircles the second portion of the duodenum. Varying degrees of duodenal obstruction have been associated with annular pancreas. Although most individuals have signs of this abnormality in childhood, in some patients symptoms will not occur until later in life. Surgical management of obstructive symptomatology is accomplished by bypass surgery in the form of duodenojejunostomy. Resection or division of the annular pancreatic tissue is not recommended because of the risk of duodenal or pancreatic fistula formation.

The development of pancreatic tissue outside of the pancreas, most commonly in the stomach, duodenum, or small bowel, is referred to as *heterotopic pancreas*. This heterotopic tissue usually resides in a submucosal location and may vary histologically from entirely normal pancreas to rudimentary pancreatic structures. Complications such as intestinal obstruction, ulceration, and hemorrhage may arise. When intestinal obstruction occurs, it is often caused by intussusception, with the ectopic pancreatic tissue serving as the intussusceptum.

Pancreas divisum is a congenital abnormality resulting from failure of fusion of the two primordial pancreatic ductal systems. In patients with pancreas divisum, the larger, dorsal portion of the pancreas is drained via the duct of Santorini into the duodenum through the minor duodenal papilla (Fig. 18.21). The major duodenal papilla usually communicates with a small duct of Wirsung, which drains the inferior portion of the head and uncinate process of the pancreas. The significance of pancreas divisum remains controversial. A small percentage of patients (less than 10%) undergoing endoscopic retrograde cholangiopancreatography (ERCP) for presumed pancreatic pathology have pancreas divisum. In patients with pancreas divisum associated with idiopathic pancreatitis, the pathophysiology has been hypothesized to involve relative stenosis of the minor duodenal papilla. Papilloplasty of the minor papilla has been successful in treating recurrent attacks of pancreatitis in selected patients with pancreas divisum, if the pancreas is free of fixed fibrotic parenchymal changes.

Inflammatory Disorders

Acute Pancreatitis

Acute pancreatitis involves a wide spectrum of illness (54). The majority of patients experience mild to moder-

Figure 18.21. **A,** Normal pancreas with absence of the duct of Santorini. **B,** Normal pancreas with the duct of Santorini. **C,** Pancreas divisum with small duct of Wirsung. **D,** Pancreas divisum with no absence of the duct of Wirsung. From Rattner DW, Warchaw AL. Surgical approach to the patient with biliary symptoms but no biliary calculi. In: Sawyers JL, Williams LF, eds. Difficult problems in general surgery. Chicago: Year Book Medical, 1989:217.

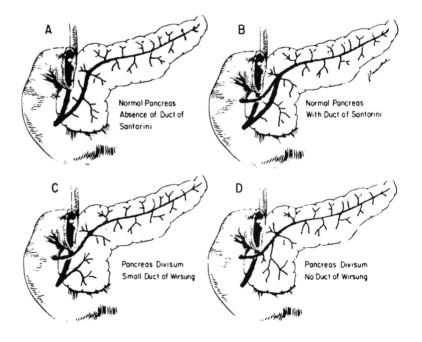

Table 18.13.
Causes of Acute Pancreatitis

Afferent limb syndrome	Idiopathic
Alcohol	Ischemia
Biliary tract disease	Pancreatic cancer
Drugs	Penetrating duodenal ulcer
Duodenal obstruction	Trauma
Familial	Scorpion venom
Hypercalcemia	Sphincter of Oddi dysfunction
Hyperlipidemia	Viral infection

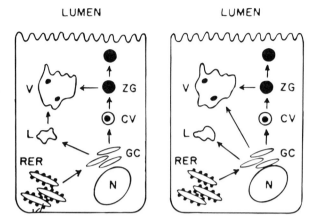

Figure 18.22. **Left,** The changes induced in mice fed the CDE diet, which blocks exocytosis and causes zymogen granules (ZG) to fuse with lysosomes (L) to form large vacuoles (V) that contain both lysosomal hydrolases and digestive zymogens. **Right,** In rats given supramaximal doses of cerulein, impaired separation of lysosomal hydrolases and digestive zymogens results in the formation of large vacuoles that contain both types of enzyme. N, nucleus, RER, rough endoplasmic reticulum, GC, Golgi complex, CV, condensing vacuole. From Steer ML, Meldolessi J. The cell biology of experimental pancreatitis. N Engl J Med 1987;316: 144–150.

Table 18.14.
Ranson's Prognostic Signs of Acute Pancreatitis

At Admission	During Initial 48 hr
Age over 55 years	Hematocrit fall >10%
WBC >16,000 cells/mm³	BUN elevation >5 mg/dL
Glucose >200 mg/dl	Ca^{2+} fall to <8 mg/dL
LDH >350 IU/L	Arterial pO_2 <60 mm Hg
SGOT >250 IU/dL	Base deficit >4 mEq/L
	Fluid sequestration >6 liters

ate symptoms and show gross pathologic changes of mild parenchymal edema. Less than 10% of patients develop a severe life-threatening illness associated with severe hemorrhagic destruction of the pancreas. Multiple causes of acute pancreatitis exist (Table 18.13). In the United States, alcohol-related pancreatitis and gallstone pancreatitis account for more than 90% of all cases. The predominant clinical feature of acute pancreatitis is midepigastric abdominal pain, frequently associated with nausea and vomiting. Fever, tachycardia, epigastric tenderness, and abdominal distension typically are found on physical examination. Hypotension, hypovolemia, hypoperfusion, and cerebral abnormalities can also be seen in patients with severe pancreatitis.

A number of animal models have been developed to study acute pancreatitis on a cellular and molecular level (57). Two have been particularly well-studied. In one model, mice are fed a choline-deficient diet supplemented by 0.5% ethionine (CDE diet). In the second, intravenous infusion of supramaximal doses of the CCK agonist cerulein is administered to rats. Results of such experimental work suggest that some pancreatitis-inducing stimuli prevent the extrusion of zymogen granules from individual acinar cells. This situation leads to fusion of the zymogen granules with intracellular lysosomes, activation of the zymogen proenzyme trypsinogen, and generation of active intracellular trypsin, which is capable of cellular autodigestion (Fig. 18.22). Although this mechanism is supported by several other models of acute pancreatitis, it is not applicable to all.

The diagnosis of acute pancreatitis is suspected by clinical criteria and supported by laboratory and radiographic findings. The measurement of serum amylase and, in some institutions, amylase isoenzymes and lipase, are the most commonly used laboratory tests. Although abdominal sonography may be useful in assessing cholelithiasis in patients suspected of having gallstone-associated pancreatitis, sonography is not ideal for evaluation of the common duct or pancreatic parenchyma. Currently, CT is the most widely accepted radiographic method used to confirm the diagnosis of acute pancreatitis. A correlation appears to exist between the degree of CT abnormality and the patient's clinical course.

The severity and prognosis of an attack of acute pancreatitis can be predicted using routinely available clini-

cal and laboratory parameters termed Ranson's prognostic signs (Table 18.14). Patients with two or fewer prognostic signs generally require simple supportive care, whereas patients with three or more prognostic signs have a stepwise increase in morbidity and mortality rates (58). The initial management of patients with acute pancreatitis should be nonoperative. Standard therapy includes intravenous fluid and electrolyte replacement, control of abdominal pain, and prohibition of oral intake. Although it is common practice to treat patients with three or more of Ranson's prognostic signs with broad-spectrum intravenous antibiotics and nasogastric decompression, only one randomized trial has shown that antibiotics (imipenem) improves clinical outcome (59). Operative intervention is indicated in four specific circumstances: *(a)* uncertainty of clinical diagnosis; *(b)* treatment of pancreatic sepsis; *(c)* correction of associated biliary tract disease; and *(d)* deterioration of clinical status. With the widespread availability of abdominal CT scanning, the need to perform an exploratory laparotomy to exclude a surgically correctable disease has become uncommon. Pancreatic sepsis occurs in up to 5% of all patients with pancreatitis, and the frequency is directly proportional to the severity of the disease. The diagnosis of pancreatic sepsis is suspected by clinical criteria, strengthened by positive laboratory and CT findings, and may be supported further by CT-guided percutaneous aspiration of peripancreatic fluid collections. The treatment of infected pancreatic or peripancreatic necrosis combines antibiotic therapy with prompt surgical debridement and drainage. The two accepted alternatives for achieving drainage are the liberal use of suction drains and open packing of the abscess cavity (60).

Definitive biliary tract surgery during the index admission with pancreatitis is now favored in the majority of patients with gallstone-associated pancreatitis. In most circumstances, laparoscopic cholecystectomy serves as the most appropriate biliary procedure. The most controversial indication for operative therapy in acute pancreatitis is that of deterioration of the clinical status. Proponents of early intervention recommend operative procedures ranging from local debridement to formal total pancreatectomy. However, most authorities reserve pancreatic resection for patients with documented infected necrosis.

Chronic Pancreatitis

Chronic pancreatitis is marked pathologically by irreversible parenchymal destruction. This is usually associated with recurrent or persistent abdominal pain of pancreatic origin combined with evidence of endocrine and/or exocrine insufficiency. Chronic pancreatitis may be caused by alcohol abuse, hyperparathyroidism, congenital abnormalities of the pancreatic duct, pancreatic trauma, and hyperlipidemia. Familial and idiopathic varieties also exist. The diagnosis of chronic pancreatitis is usually suspected by the clinical setting. Routine laboratory tests are not often helpful. Plain abdominal films may reveal pancreatic calcifications. Abdominal CT scanning is used to evaluate the size and texture of the gland, to inspect for pancreatic nodularity or parenchymal calcifications, and to assess for pancreatic ductal enlargement. Endoscopic retrograde pancreatography is useful to document ductal abnormalities.

Nonoperative management of chronic pancreatitis encompasses treatment of endocrine and exocrine insufficiency and control of abdominal pain. Diabetes may require cautious insulin administration. Exocrine insufficiency is treated with exogenous pancreatic enzyme supplementation. Pain relief may be obtained in some patients by complete abstinence from alcohol. Persistent pain may require analgesics. Patients who undergo unsuccessful nonoperative management are considered for surgical treatment.

Surgical treatment falls into three groups: ampullary procedures; ductal drainage procedures; and ablative procedures. The choice of surgical procedure depends on the findings on pancreatic imaging by CT and pancreatic ductal anatomy by ERCP, and the surgeon must consider the results of previous operative procedures. Ampullary procedures currently have limited application. The ductal drainage procedure most commonly used involves a side-to-side pancreaticojejunostomy (Puestow procedure). Determinants of success for the side-to-side pancreaticojejunostomy include a pancreatic duct greater than 1cm in diameter, the presence of pancreatic calcifications, and a pancreatic-jejunal anastomosis longer than 6 cm. Ductal drainage does not improve established pancreatic exocrine or endocrine dysfunction, although it may delay the rate of progressive impairment. Ablative procedures are generally reserved for patients who are not candidates for or have undergone unsuccessful ductal drainage procedures. In rare patients with disease limited to the body and tail of the gland, distal pancreatectomy may be applicable. When the parenchymal disease primarily affects the head of the gland, pylorus-preserving pancreatoduodenectomy has been successful in certain patients. Newer duodenum-sparing procedures involving partial resection of the head of the gland, combined with pancreatic ductal drainage via a pancreaticojejunostomy, have been popularized by Frey (61) and Beger (62).

Pancreatic Duct Disruptions

Pancreatic duct disruptions include internal pancreatic fistulae such as pancreatic pseudocysts, pancreatic ascites, and pancreatic pleural effusion and external pancreatic fistulae. These entities most commonly occur in the settings of alcoholic pancreatitis, pancreatic trauma, and operative misadventures.

Pancreatic pseudocysts are localized collections of pancreatic secretions that lack an epithelial lining. They occur as the result of surrounding tissues walling off a pancreatic duct disruption. Up to 10% of patients develop pancreatic pseudocysts after an episode of acute alcoholic pancreatitis. Clinical findings include upper abdominal pain, nausea, vomiting, and epigastric tenderness. The majority of patients have elevations of the serum amylase. Definitive diagnosis is made by CT or ultrasound. Recent evidence suggests that strict size criteria alone are not sufficient to determine the need for operative intervention. Up to 50% of pseudocysts can be managed nonoperatively without complication (62–64). For pseudocysts that require operative intervention, preoperative endoscopic pancreatography may be useful. Options for the management of pseudocysts include internal drainage via cystojejunostomy, cystogastrostomy, or cystoduodenostomy; excision; external drainage; and percutaneous or endoscopic drainage techniques.

Pancreatic ascites occurs when exocrine secretions extravasate from the pancreatic duct and drain freely into the peritoneal cavity (65). Pancreatic pleural effusion results when similar extravasation occurs into the retroperitoneum, tracking cephalad through the diaphragm into the thorax. Both these entities may occur in the absence of a history of clinical pancreatitis. Painless massive ascites is the hallmark of pancreatic ascites. Primary pulmonary symptoms, such as dyspnea, chest pain, and cough, suggest a pancreatic pleural effusion. Analysis of the ascitic or pleural fluid reveals high levels of amylase and protein. In both entities, nonoperative treatment is initially indicated for a 2 to 3-week period. For inpatients not cured by nonoperative management, operative intervention will be necessary. Delineation of pancreatic duct anatomy by ERCP is crucial in operative management. In most of these patients, Roux-en-Y pancreatojejunostomy or distal pancreatectomy is indicated.

An external pancreatic fistula is present when pancreatic exocrine secretions drain through a drain site or wound for more than 7 days. Contrast injection of the sinus tract and CT should be used to delineate the anatomy of the fistula tract. Total parenteral nutrition is often used to avoid pancreatic stimulation by oral intake and to maximize tissue anabolism. Somatostatin analogue (octreotide) usually decreases pancreatic output and, therefore, may accelerate fistula closure when proximal pancreatic duct obstruction is not present. The majority of external pancreatic fistulas close nonoperatively.

Neoplasms

Benign Exocrine Tumors

Benign neoplasms of the exocrine pancreas are uncommon. Cystadenomas comprise less than 10% of all cystic pancreatic lesions. These tumors may be difficult to differentiate from malignant cystic neoplasms or pancreatic pseudocysts. They can be cured by appropriate resection. Solid and papillary neoplasms of the pancreas are rare tumors, typically found in young women in the body or tail of the gland. On gross examination, these neoplasms appear as large rounded masses often containing hemorrhagic and macrocytic areas. These tumors are generally curable by appropriate resection.

Malignant Exocrine Tumors

In the United States, approximately 28,000 new cases of cancer of the exocrine pancreas are diagnosed each year, and more than 25,000 deaths occur annually, making it the fifth most common cause of cancer death. These tumors are more common in blacks, cigarette smokers, and males and may be linked to the presence of diabetes and alcohol use. Recently, the molecular genetics of pancreatic cancer have been unraveled, with common findings being oncogene mutations of K-ras and losses of tumor suppressor genes, such as p53, MTS1 (p16), and DCC (66). Adenocarcinoma of the head of the pancreas is the most common of the four malignant neoplasms classified as periampullary neoplasms;

this class also includes carcinomas of the ampulla, duodenum, and distal common bile duct. The typical clinical features are jaundice, weight loss, and abdominal pain. The majority of patients have abnormalities of the liver function tests. Currently available serologic tests, such as carcinoembryonic antigen (CEA), CA19-9, and others, are not accurate enough for diagnosis or screening. CT scan is used to determine the size of the primary neoplasm and to screen for hepatic metastases. The site of the biliary obstruction is defined by cholangiography, using either the percutaneous transhepatic or the endoscopic retrograde route. An algorithm for the diagnosis and management of these patients is presented in Figure 10.23. In patients with localized tumors, angiography with portal venography can be used to stage for resectability and to determine the vascular anatomy (67). Alternatively, vascular anatomy can be defined by dynamic, contrast-enhanced, thin-section CT scanning, obviating the need for angiography.

Many patients with periampullary carcinoma are candidates for operative therapy. Palliative surgery is performed in patients with unresectable or metastatic disease discovered at the time of laparotomy or in patients whose symptoms are managed poorly nonoperatively. Palliative surgery seeks to alleviate biliary obstruction, gastric or duodenal obstruction, and tumor-associated pain (68).

In patients who are candidates for resection, the standard resection for periampullary carcinoma involves a pancreatoduodenectomy (Whipple's operation). Recently, the pylorus-preserving modification of Whipple's resection has gained popularity. Accumulated data indicate no compromise in survival in patients undergoing pylorus preservation. The overall 5-year survival rate for patients with resected carcinoma of the head of the pancreas exceeds 20% in some centers (69–72). Based on a recent analysis of 201 patients who underwent pancreaticoduodenal resection for adenocarcinoma of the head of the pancreas, the parameters found to be the most important determinants of prognosis include tumor size, resected nodal status, margin status, and tumor DNA content.

In patients with advanced unresectable disease, neither chemotherapy nor radiotherapy alone has been associated with consistent improvements in survival. However, the combination of radiation and chemotherapy has prolonged survival after potentially curative pancreatoduodenectomy (73). Results of treatment of unresectable cancer of the head of the pancreas using either external beam or intraoperative radiation therapy have shown some variable improvement in local tumor control, variable improvement in control of abdominal and back pain, but only minimal improvement in long-term survival.

Carcinoma of the body and tail of the pancreas accounts for up to 25% of all cases of pancreatic cancer. At initial examination, patients generally report weight

ALGORITHM FOR THE EVALUATION OF JAUNDICE

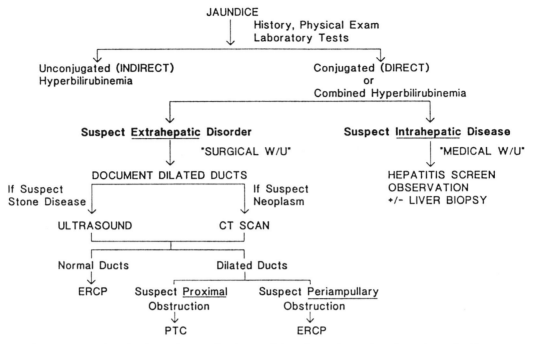

Figure 18.23. Algorithm for evaluation of patients with jaundice. W/U, workup. From Lipsett PA, Pitt HA. Jaundice: mechanisms and differential diagnosis. In: Toouli J, ed. Surgery of the biliary tract. London: Churchill Livingstone, in press.

Table 18.15.
Classification of Functional Pancreatic Islet Cell Tumors

Tumor Name	Major Hormone(s)	Cell Type	Syndrome	Malignancy Rate	Extrapancreatic Location
Insulinoma	Insulin	β-cell	Hypoglycemia	<15%	Rare
Gastrinoma (Zollinger-Ellison syndrome)	Gastrin	non-β-cell	Peptic ulcer, diarrhea	<50%	Frequently in duodenum
Vipoma (Verner-Morrison syndrome)	VIP, prostaglandins, PHI[a]	non-β-cell	Watery diarrhea, hypokalemia, achlorhydria	Majority	10%
Glucagonoma	Glucagon	α-cell	Hyperglycemia, dermatitis	Majority	Rare
Somatostatinoma	Somatostatin	δ-cell	Hyperglycemia, steatorrhea, gallstones	Majority	Rare

[a] Peptide histidine isoleucine.

loss and abdominal pain, without jaundice. Abdominal CT is the best initial radiographic study. ERCP may document a pancreatic duct cutoff. Visceral arteriography may be useful to define the extent of major vessel involvement. Good-risk patients without evidence of metastatic disease and with favorable arteriographic findings may be best served by abdominal exploration and resection. Overall, the resectability rate is less than 10%, and the prognosis is poor (73).

Endocrine Tumors

Pancreatic endocrine tumors are rare, with a clinical frequency of 5 per 1 million per year. These tumors are divided into functional and nonfunctional varieties. Functional endocrine tumors are conventionally named according to the major hormonal product of the tumor (Table 18.15). The general principles applicable to the

management of patients with suspected functional tumors include the following: recognition of the abnormal physiology or characteristic syndrome; detection of hormone elevations in serum; and the localization and staging of the tumor. Standard radiographic techniques available for tumor localization include CT with intravenous and oral contrast, visceral angiography, endoscopic ultrasonography, transhepatic portal venous sampling, and intraoperative ultrasonography.

Insulinoma is the most common endocrine tumor of the pancreas. Patients typically present with neuro glycopenic symptoms and catecholamine-surge symptoms. The most reliable method for diagnosis involves a monitored fast of up to 72 hours with documentation of hypoglycemia and elevated insulin levels. Supportive tests include documentation of elevations in serum C-peptide and proinsulin levels, absence of sulfonylureas on toxicologic screening, and absence of anti-insulin antibodies. After biochemical diagnosis and appropriate localization studies, the treatment of insulinoma is surgical resection. Up to 90% of patients have benign solitary pancreatic adenomas (76).

Gastrinoma (Zollinger-Ellison syndrome) is the second most common functional endocrine tumor. Clinical manifestations include peptic ulcer disease, abdominal pain, reflux esophagitis, and diarrhea. The fasting serum gastrin is almost always elevated above normal. The diagnosis of gastrinoma is supported by measurement of gastric acid secretion, with a basal acid output (BAO) in excess of 15 mEq/hr and a BAO: maximal acid output (BAO:MAO) ratio in excess of 0.6. In patients with hyperchlorhydria and a fasting serum gastrin level of less than 1000 pg/mL, it is appropriate to perform a secretin stimulation test. After an intravenous infusion of secretin, a 200pg/mL or greater increment in circulating serum gastrin is diagnostic of gastrinoma.

After confirmation of the diagnosis, patient management first involves control of gastric acid hypersecretion. Hypersecretion should be controlled using proton pump blockade with either omeprazole or lansoprazole. Next, patients with gastrinoma should undergo radiographic localization studies to attempt to localize the primary tumor and to assess for metastatic disease. In the absence of documented unresectable disease, all patients with sporadic gastrinoma should undergo exploration with curative intent. Improvements in early diagnosis, preoperative localization, and intraoperative assessment have yielded surgical cure rates approaching 35% (74,75). Late recurrence in up to 60% of patients thought to have been cured have recently been reported.

Vipoma (Verner-Morrison syndrome, pancreatic cholera, WDHA syndrome) is associated with watery diarrhea, hypokalemia, and either achlorhydria or hypochlorhydria. Preoperative preparation must include correction of fluid and electrolyte deficits and appropriate localization studies. More than one-half of the reported cases have been malignant, most commonly associated with widespread hepatic metastases. Octreotide (somatostatin analogue) may be useful in reducing circulating vasoactive intestinal polypeptide (VIP) levels and controlling the diarrhea.

The glucagonoma syndrome is marked by mild diabetes and severe dermatitis (necrolytic migratory erythema). Patients may also demonstrate malnutrition, anemia, glossitis, and venous thrombosis. Serum glucagon levels are usually well in excess of 120 pg/mL. Preoperative management includes treatment of hyperglycemia and attention to the malnutrition that is typical of patients with glucagon excess. The majority of patients have metastatic disease precluding the possibility of complete tumor resection.

The somatostatinoma syndrome is associated with gallstones, diabetes, and steatorrhea. Because these clinical findings are nonspecific, this rare pancreatic endocrine tumor is difficult to diagnose. Management encompasses preoperative treatment of hyperglycemia and malnutrition combined with standard radiographic localization and staging studies. Like vipomas and glucagonomas, the majority of reported somatostatinomas have been malignant.

REFERENCES

1. Linder HR. Embryology and anatomy of the biliary tree. In: Way LW, Pellegrini CA, eds. Surgery of the gallbladder and bile ducts. Philadelphia: WB Saunders, 1987:322.
2. Ratych RE, Smith GW. Anatomy and physiology of the liver. In: Zuidema GD, Turcotte JG, eds. Shackelford's surgery of the alimentary tract. 3rd ed. Philadelphia: WB Saunders, 1991;3:273–286.
3. Quinlan RM. Anatomy and embryology of the pancreas. In: Zuidema GD, Turcotte JG, eds. Shackelford's surgery of the alimentary tract. 3rd ed. Philadelphia: WB Saunders, 1991;3:318.
4. Alberti KGMM, Johnston DG, Taylor R. Carbohydrate metabolism in liver disease. In: Wright R, Millward-Sadler GH, Alberti KGMM, et al, eds. Liver and biliary disease. 2nd ed. East Sussex, UK: Bailliere Tindall,1985:45–64.
5. Tavill AS. Hepatic protein metabolism: Basic and applied biochemical and clinical aspects. In: Arias IM, Frenkel M, Wilson JHP, eds. The liver annual. 3rd ed. Amsterdam: Elsevier Science Publishers, 1983:50–87.
6. Tavill AS. Protein metabolism and the liver. In: Wright R, Millward-Sadler GH, Alberti KGMM, et al, eds. Liver and biliary disease. 2nd ed. East Sussex, UK: Bailliere Tindall, 1985:87–117.
7. Vessey DA. Hepatic metabolism of drugs and toxins. In: Zakin D, Boyer TD, eds. Hepatology: a textbook of liver disease. 2nd ed. Philadelphia: WB Saunders, 1990:197–230.
8. Alvares AP. Oxidative biotransformation of drugs. In: Arias IM, Popper H, Schachter D, et al, eds. The liver biology and pathology. New York: Raven, 1982:265–280.
9. Admirand WH, Small DM. The physiochemical basis of cholesterol gallstone formation in man. J Clin Invest 1968;47:10–43.
10. Carey MD. Critical tables for calculating the cholesterol saturation of native bile. J Lipid Res 1978;19:945.
11. Blanckaert N, Schmid R. Physiology and pathophysiology of bilirubin metabolism. In: Zakmin D, Boyer TD, eds. Hepatology: a textbook of liver disease. 2nd ed. Philadelphia: WB Saunders, 1990: 246–296.
12. Sherlock S. Viral hepatitis. In: Sherlock S, ed. Diseases of the liver and biliary system. 7th ed. London: Blackwell Scientific, 1985: 251–279.
13. Moore EW. Biliary calcium and gallstone formation. Hepatology 1990;12:206S–218S.
14. Holzbach RT. Recent progress in understanding cholesterol crystal nucleations as a precursor to human gallstone formation. Hepatology 1986;6:1403–1410.
15. Smithson KW, Miller DB, Jacobs LR, et al. Intestinal diffusion barrier: unstirred water layer or membrane surface mucous coat? Science 1981;214:1241–1244.
16. Itoh Z, Takahashi I. Periodic contractions of the canine gallbladder during interdigestive state. Am J Physiol 1981;240:G183–G188.
17. Geenen JE, Hogan WJ, Dodds WJ, et al. Intraluminal pressure recording from the human sphincter of Oddi. Gastroenterology 1980;78:317–323.
18. Webb TH, Lillemoe KD, Pitt HA. Gastro-sphincter of Oddi reflex. Am J Surg 1988;155:193–198.
19. Wyatt AP. The relationship of the sphincter of Oddi to the stomach, duodenum, and gallbladder. J Physiol London 1967;193: 225–243.
20. Bro-Rasmussen F, Killmann SA, Thaysen JH. The composition of pancreatic juice as compared to sweat, parotid saliva and tears. Acta Physiol Scand 1956;37:97–113.
21. Palade GE. Intracellular aspects of the process of protein secretion. Science 1975;189:347–358.
22. Bruzzone R. The molecular basis of enzyme secretion. Gastroenterology 1990;99:1157–1176.
23. Malagelada JR. Gastric, pancreatic, and biliary responses to a meal. In: Johnson LR, ed. Physiology of the gastrointestinal tract. New York: Raven, 1981;893–924.

24. Boivin M, Lanspa SJ, Zinsmeister AR, et al. Are diets associated with different rates of human interdigestive and postprandial pancreatic enzyme secretion? Gastroenterology 1990;99:1763–1771.

25. Yeo CJ, Bastidas JA, Schmieg RE Jr., et al. Pancreatic structure and glucose tolerance in a longitudinal study of experimental pancreatitis-induced diabetes. Ann Surg 1989;210:150–159.

26. Anthone GJ, Bastidas JA, Orandle MS, et al. Direct proabsorptive effect of octreotide on ionic transport in the small intestine. Surgery 1990;108:1136–1142.

27. Bonner-Weir S, Orci L. New perspectives on the microvasculature of the islets of Langerhans in the rat. Diabetes 1982;31:883–889.

28. Doty JE, Pitt HA. Cystic lesions of the liver and biliary tree. In: Moody FG, ed. Surgical treatment of digestive diseases. Chicago: Year Book Medical, 1986;334–351.

29. Jones RS. Hemangioma. In: Cameron JL, ed. Current surgical therapy. 3rd ed. Toronto: BC Decker, 1989;212–216.

30. Conter RL, Pitt HA, Tompkins RK, et al. Differentiation of pyogenic from amebic hepatic abscesses. Surg Gynecol Obstet 1986; 162:114–118.

31. Ong GB. Helminthic diseases of the liver and biliary tract. In: Wright R, Millward-Sadler GH, Alberti KGMM, et al, eds. Liver and biliary diseases. 2nd ed. East Sussex, UK: Bailliere Tindall, 1985;1523–1559.

32. Pitt HA, Korzelius J, Tompkins RK. Management of hepatic echinococcosis in southern California. Am J Surg 1986;152:110–115.

33. Sherlock S. Assessment of liver function. In: Sherlock S, ed. Diseases of the liver and biliary system. 7th ed. London: Blackwell Scientific, 1985;15–27.

34. Wallnofer H, Schmidt E, Schmidt FW, et al. Acute viral hepatitis. In: Diagnosis of liver disease. Stuttgart: George Thieme, 1977; 33–65.

35. Conn HO, Atterbury CE. Cirrhosis. In: Schiff L, Schiff E, eds. Disease of the liver. 6th ed. Philadelphia: JB Lippincott, 1987;725–864.

36. Cady B. Liver tumors. In: Cameron JL, ed. Current surgical therapy. 3rd ed. Philadelphia: BC Decker, 1989;212–216.

37. Sugarbaker PH. Hepatic neoplasia. In: Bayless TM, ed. Current therapy in gastroenterology and liver disease. Philadelphia: BC Decker, 1986;412–417.

38. Kasai M. Treatment of biliary atresia with special reference to hepatic portoenterostomy and its modifications. In: Bill A, Kasai M, eds. Biliary atresia and choledochal cyst. Progress in pediatric surgery. Munich: Urban & Schwarzenburg, 1974;6:5–52.

39. Kasai M, Suzuki S. A new operation for "non-correctable" biliary atresia: hepatic portoenterostomy. Shujitsu 1959;13:733–738.

40. Babbitt DP. Congenital choledochal cysts. New etiological concept based on anomalous relationships of the common bile duct and pancreatic bulb. Ann Radiol 1969;12:231–234.

41. Carey MC, Cahalane MJ. Whither biliary sludge? Gastroenterology 1988;95:508–518.

42. Small DM. The formation of gallstones. Adv Intern Med 1970;16: 243–260.

43. Lee SP, Lim TH, Scott AJ. Carbohydrate moieties of glycoproteins in human hepatic and gallbladder bile, gallbladder mucosa and gallstones. Clin Sci Mol Med 1979;56:533–539.

44. Moore EW. The role of calcium in the pathogenesis of gallstones: Ca^{++} electrode studies of model bile salt solutions and other biologic systems. Hepatology 1984;4:228S–234S.

45. Trotman BW, Soloway RD. Pigment gallstone disease: summary of the National Institutes of Health-international workshop. Hepatology 1982;2:879–890.

46. Gilliland TM, Traverso W. Modern standards for comparison of cholecystectomy with alternative treatments for symptomatic cholelithiasis with emphasis on long-term relief of symptoms. Surg Gynecol Obset 1990;170:329–344.

47. Lipsett PA, Pitt HA. Acute cholangitis. Surg Clin North Am 1990; 70:1297–1312.

48. Geenen JE, Toouli J, Hogan WJ, et al. Endoscopic sphincterotomy: follow-up evaluation of effects on the sphincter of Oddi. Gastroenterology 1984;87:754–758.

49. Cameron JL, Pitt HA, Zinner MJ, et al. Resection of hepatic duct bifurcation and transhepatic stenting for sclerosing cholangitis. Ann Surg 1988;207:614–622.

50. Andren-Sandberg A, Alinder G, Bengmark S. Accidental lesions of the common bile duct at cholecystectomy: pre- and perioperative factors of importance. Ann Surg 1985;201:328–332.

51. Orlando R, Russell JC, Lynch J, et al. Laparoscopic cholecystectomy: a statewide experience. Arch Surg 1993; 128:494–499.

52. Deziel DJ, Milikan KW, Economou SG, et al. Complications of laparoscopic cholecystectomy: a natural survey of 4292 hospitals and an analysis of 77,604 cases. Am J Surg 1993;165:9–14.

53. Pitt HA, Miyamoto T, Parapatis SK, et al. Factors influencing outcome inpatients with postoperative biliary strictures. Am J Surg 1982;144:14–21.

54. Pitt HA, Kaufman HS, Coleman J, et al. Benign postoperative biliary strictures: operate or dilate? Ann Surg 1989;210:417–427.

55. Davids PHP, Tanka AKF, Rauws EAJ, et al. Benign biliary strictures: surgery of endoscopy? Ann Surg 1993; 217:237–243.

56. Broe PJ, Cameron JL. The management of proximal biliary tract tumors. Adv Surg 1981;15:47–76.

57. Yeo CJ, Cameron JL. Acute pancreatitis. In: Zuidema GD, Turcotte JG, eds. Shackelford's surgery of the alimentary tract. 3rd ed. Philadelphia: WB Saunders, 1991;3:19–36.

58. Steer ML, Meldolessi J. The cell biology of experimental pancreatitis. N Engl J Med 1987;316:144–150.

59. Ranson JHC, Rifkind KM, Roses DF, et al. Prognostic signs and the role of operative management in acute pancreatitis. Surg Gynecol Obstet 1974;139:69–81.

60. Pederzoli P, Bassi C, Vesentini S, et al. A randomized multicenter clinical trial of antibiotic prophylaxis of septic complications in acute necrotizing pancreatitis with imipenem. Surg Gynecol Obstet 1993;176:480–483.

61. Frey CF, Smith GJ. Description and rationale of a new operation for chronic pancreatitis. Pancreas 1987; 2:701–707.

62. Beger HG, Buchler M, Bittner R, et al. Duodenum-preserving resection of the head of the pancreas in severe chronic pancreatitis. Ann Surg 1989;209:273–278.

63. Yeo CJ, Bastidas JA, Lynch-Nyhan A, et al. The natural history of pancreatic pseudocysts documented by computed tomography. Surg Gynecol Obstet 1990;170:411–417.

64. Vitas GJ, Sarr MG. Selected management of pancreatic pseudocysts: operative versus expectant management. Surgery 1992;3: 123–130.

65. Williams KJ, Fabian TC. Pancreatic pseudocyst: recommendations for operative and nonoperative management. Am Surg 1992;58: 199–205.

66. DiGuiseppe JA, Hruban RH. Pathobiology of cancer of the pancreas. Semin Surg Onc 1995; 11:87–96.

67. Dooley WC, Cameron JL, Pitt HA, et al. Is preoperative angiography useful in patients with periampullary tumors? Ann Surg 1990; 211:649–655.

68. Cameron JL. Chronic pancreatic ascites and pancreatic pleural effusions. Gastroenterology 1978;74:134–140.

69. Lillemoe KD, Sauter PK, Pitt HA, et al. Current status of surgical palliation of periampullary carcinoma. Surg Gynecol Obstet 1993; 176:1–10.

70. Yeo CJ, Cameron JL, Lillemoe KD, et al. Pancreaticoduodenectomy for cancer of the head of the pancreas: 201 patients. Ann Surg 1995; 221:721–733.

71. Geer RJ, Brennan MF. Prognostic indicators for survival after resection of pancreatic adenocarcinoma. Am J Surg 1993;165:68–73.

72. Trede M, Schwall G, Saeger H. Survival after pancreaticoduodenectomy. Ann Surg 1990; 211:447–458.

73. Nordback IH, Hruban RH, Boitnott JK, et al. Carcinoma of the body and tail of the pancreas. Am J Surg 1992;164:26–31.

74. Kalser MH, Ellenberg SS. Pancreatic cancer. Adjuvant combined radiation and hemotherapy following curative resection. Arch Surg 1985;120:899–903.

75. Yeo CJ. ZES: Current approaches. Contemp Gastroenterol 1990;3: 1729–1776.

76. Andersen DK. Current diagnosis and management of Zollinger-Ellison syndrome. Ann Surg 1989; 210:685–703.

19 Hematology

Carol E. H. Scott-Conner | Edward E. Rigdon | William A. Rock, Jr. | Anne T. Mancino

Overview of Hemostasis

Performance of even the most minor surgical procedure depends on a complex, interdependent set of events resulting in the formation of a stable clot. The vascular endothelium, platelets, and circulating substances are all contributing factors (1–3).

When a vessel is cut, the initiation phase begins as platelets attach to the exposed subendothelial collagen (Fig. 19.1). Von Willebrand factor, synthesized and released by endothelial cells, assists in platelet attachment to collagen. Adherent platelets spread out and release substances from cytoplasmic granules that cause local vasoconstriction and stimulate platelet aggregation, thus recruiting more platelets. In addition, platelets synthesize and release vasoactive amines. Circulating factors of the coagulation cascade are activated.

The next phase of coagulation is termed the "amplification phase," as an amplifying series of reactions generates the local accumulation of thrombin, culminating in the conversion of fibrinogen to fibrin. Thrombin is itself a powerful stimulus for platelet aggregation, and more platelets accumulate in the growing thrombus during the propagation phase.

Primary hemostasis denotes the events leading to the formation of the initial hemostatic plug (a mass of adherent platelets). As fibrin accumulates, the platelet plug stabilizes and a fibrin clot forms through the mechanism of secondary hemostasis. The clot is composed of fibrin, platelets, and erythrocytes. Cross-linking of fibrin further stabilizes the clot, which contracts as a result of the activity of the contained platelets.

Contraction of smooth muscle fibers within the vessel wall causes local vasoconstriction and is potentiated by neural and humoral factors. Platelets synthesize and release thromboxane A_2, a potent vasoconstrictor. Endothelial cells synthesize prostacyclin, a vasodilator and inhibitor of platelet aggregation, as well as endothelial-derived relaxing factor.

Propagation of thrombus beyond the site of injury is limited by several major regulatory mechanisms (Table 19.1). Initiation of coagulation is moderated by tissue factor pathway inhibitor (TFPI) (1,2). Excess local thrombin complexes with thrombomodulin on the endothelial cell surface. Thrombin thus bound to thrombomodulin is no longer able to participate in the clotting cascade and no longer causes platelet aggregation. Moreover, the thrombin-thrombomodulin complex activates protein C, which, with its cofactor protein S, inactivates factors Va and VIIa of the clotting cascade. Thrombin is also inactivated by circulating antithrombin III. The activity of this factor is accelerated by heparin sulfate on cell surfaces of endothelial cells (or by exogenous heparin).

Substances such as platelet-derived growth factor are released by degranulating platelets and stimulate vascular repair. Other platelet-released substances are chemotactic for phagocytic leukocytes that are thus stimulated to accumulate in the region of injury to clean up the debris.

Finally, when healing and restoration of endothelial continuity has occurred, the fibrinolytic system is activated and the occluding thrombus is lysed. Plasminogen bound to fibrin within clot produces local accumulation of plasmin, where it is protected from circulating inactivators and where its activity is localized to the region of need.

Primary hemostasis, the formation of the initial platelet plug, requires the presence of adequate numbers of normally functioning platelets as well as substances synthesized by endothelial cells (collagen and von Willebrand factor) and products of the coagulation cascade (thrombin and fibrinogen). Deficits of primary hemostasis are recognized in the operating room when normal avascular planes continue to ooze as numerous small capillaries continue to bleed, despite the application of pressure and the passage of time (3).

Secondary hemostasis requires the participation of

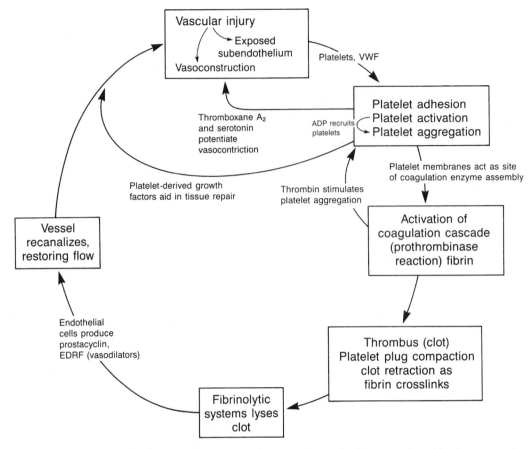

Figure 19.1. Overview of the hemostatic system. Vascular injury triggers platelet aggregation with subsequent activation of the coagulation cascade and formation of a clot composed of platelets, erythrocytes, and fibrin. Plasminogen is bound to fibrin within the clot; the active form, plasmin, initiates clot lysis when healing has occurred.

Table 19.1.
Regulatory Mechanisms that Control Procoagulant Pathways and Limit Clot Formation

Phase of Coagulation	Control Mechanism
Initiation	Tissue Factor Pathway Inhibitor (TFPI) inhibits tissue thromboplastin-induced coagulation by inhibiting the interaction of Factors VIIa, Xa, and tissue factor complex on a cell membrane
Amplification	Protein C pathway, activated by complex of thrombomodulin and thrombin on an endothelial cell surface
Propagation	Antithrombin III

the coagulation cascade to form a stable clot. Platelet phospholipid and other substances are critical for the initiation and amplification phases of coagulation. The endothelial cell participates by down regulating an amplifying system that would otherwise culminate in massive intravascular coagulation.

Abnormalities in the endothelial cell may cause excessive or pathologic bleeding or, more commonly, inappropriate thrombosis. When the fibrinolytic system is activated prematurely, clots form normally only to lyse prematurely. The result is delayed rebleeding after initial satisfactory hemostasis.

Hemostasis thus may be thought of as a tightly regulated system of interdependent factors. Platelets, the coagulation cascade, endothelial cells, and the fibrinolytic system all interact. In the sections that follow, each of the major elements will be considered separately. Congenital and acquired defects of each element will be considered as examples of deranged physiology, and the effects of pharmacologic interventions will be detailed. Complex disorders of hemostasis will be discussed last.

The Platelet and Formation of the Primary Hemostatic Plug

Platelets are disc-shaped elements of the blood, averaging 1.5 to 3.5 μm in length. They lack DNA but contain all of the other major cellular components. Platelets consist of three primary functional elements: secretory granules, an intrinsic contractile system, and a specialized surface membrane with a thick proteoglycan coat that contains specific receptors.

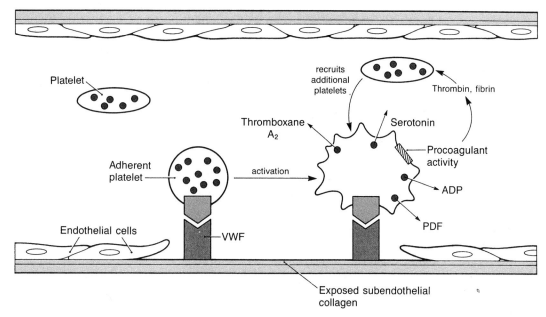

Figure 19.2. The three phases of platelet function are adherence, activation, and aggregation.[1] Platelets adhere to the exposed subendothelium with the aid of von Willebrand's factor (vWF), synthesized and released by endothelial cells. Adherent platelets become activated, changing shape and releasing the contents of their granules. This recruits more platelets into the growing thrombus (platelet aggregation). Thrombin activation of platelets exposes binding sites for Xase and the prothrombinase complex (procoagulant effect). Thus, the growing platelet thrombus acts as a site for assembly of enzymes of the coagulation reaction as well as a scaffold upon which the fibrin clot forms[1].

Platelets are responsible for primary hemostasis (the formation of a platelet plug) at sites of endothelial damage. As shown in Figure 19.2, three steps must occur in sequence: platelet adherence, activation, and aggregation (1–6). Platelet activation occurs when platelets adhere to a site of vascular injury, change shape, and degranulate. Platelet membranes provide a surface for activation and assembly of coagulation enzyme complexes, culminating in the generation of fibrin. Platelets also secrete growth and chemotactic factors important for tissue repair (4).

Platelet Production and Destruction

Platelets are fragments of megakaryocyte cytoplasm, and most of the contents of platelets are derived from megakaryocytes. Megakaryocytes, the precursor cells of platelets, are the largest cells in normal bone marrow. They are commonly multinucleate. Two steps have been identified in platelet production. Megakaryocyte-colony-stimulating factor and granulocyte-macrophage-colony-stimulating factor cause pluripotent marrow stem cells to differentiate into the megakaryocyte cell line. Thrombopoietin, a substance isolated from the plasma of thrombocytopenic patients and from embryonal kidneys, stimulates the final maturation and release of platelets. Megakaryocytes extrude cytoplasmic projections called proplatelets into the sinusoids of the bone marrow. These are released as a string of platelet fields that further fragment into individual platelets in the circulation. In addition, some megakaryocytes enter the circulation from the bone marrow sinusoids and break up into platelets in the pulmonary circulation.

The number of circulating platelets in a given individual remains remarkably constant, suggesting that a finely tuned mechanism regulates platelet release. Platelet production can be increased up to sixfold in response to increased platelet destruction. In states of rapid platelet release, platelets vary in size, and a preponderance of relatively large platelets may be noted. These large platelets actually correspond to several platelet fields and would, under normal circumstances, have been further subdivided into several normal-size platelets.

The average life span of a platelet is 8 to 12 days. Platelets are removed from the circulation by several mechanisms. Senescent platelets are destroyed primarily in the bone marrow and secondarily in the spleen and liver. Platelets contribute to normal vascular integrity. Capillary permeability to plasma and particulate substances is increased in thrombocytopenic states. A fixed loss of 7 to 10×10^9 platelets per day may reflect this function. In the circulation, platelets form aggregates that are reversible in the absence of fibrin stabilization. Formation of these reversible aggregates does not decrease the life span of the involved platelets. Approximately 33% of the platelet pool is sequestered in the spleen. The adhesive properties of platelets slow transit through the splenic sinusoids, where large numbers of platelets can be demonstrated adhering to reticular and endothelial cells. These sequestered platelets are freely exchangeable with those in the blood and are released in large numbers in response to epinephrine (which de-

Table 19.2.
Causes of Thrombocytopenia

Spurious
Underproduction
  Drugs and toxins
  Infiltrative disease of the bone marrow
  Aplastic marrow
  Paroxysmal nocturnal hemoglobinuria
Over-destruction
  Immunologically mediated
    ITP
    Posttransfusion purpura
    Heparin-induced thrombocytopenia
  TTP
  DIC
  Hypersplenism

Table 19.3.
Causes of Reactive Thrombocytosis

Chronic inflammatory disorders
  Most of the so-called rheumatoid disorders
  Crohn's disease
  Chronic ulcerative colitis
Recovery from acute infection
Acute hemorrhage
Hemolytic anemia
Iron deficiency anemia
Malignancy
Post-splenectomy
Response to drugs
  Vincristine
  Epinephrine
Rebound phenomenon
  After discontinuation of myelosuppressive agents
  Alcohol withdrawal

creases splenic blood flow and causes an increase of 25% to 50% in the platelet count) and exercise. In hypersplenism states, increased splenic sequestration of platelets may result in thrombocytopenia. After splenectomy, the entire platelet pool is contained within the circulation. Thrombocytosis occurs immediately after splenectomy and persists to a varying extent thereafter, and the platelet count no longer rises in response to epinephrine or exercise (5).

Disorders of Platelet Number

Thrombocytopenia may result from underproduction or abnormal destruction of platelets (Table 19.2). As a screening test, examination of a properly prepared blood smear should demonstrate 6 to 10 platelets per high-power field. Platelets may vary in size or clump in the presence of EDTA anticoagulant. Automated cell counters will not detect these changes and may yield spurious results. For this reason, an abnormal platelet count should always be confirmed by visual inspection of a blood smear. Examination of the smear also provides important information on platelet size and may reveal additional evidence, such as the characteristic red cell fragmentation of microangiopathic hemolytic anemia (seen in disseminated intravascular coagulation or thrombotic thrombocytopenic purpura).

Thrombocytopenia caused by decreased production occurs with replacement of functioning marrow by tumor, leukemic cells, or fibrosis and in response to myelosuppressive drugs and radiation. Several drugs and toxins exhibit a selective and generally temporary effect on platelet production. Chronic alcohol ingestion causes thrombocytopenia in some patients, apparently by a direct toxic effect on megakaryocytes. A rebound thrombocytosis may accompany alcohol withdrawal. Other drugs that can cause thrombocytopenia include thiazide, diuretics, estrogens such as DES, and interferon. Paroxysmal nocturnal hemoglobinuria is a stem cell disease for which platelet production is reduced and platelets are consumed by inappropriate thrombus formation, resulting in profound thrombocytopenia (7–9).

Bone marrow examination will reveal a normal or increased number of megakaryocytes when thrombocytopenia is the result of increased platelet destruction. Immunologically mediated platelet destruction, usually caused by an IgG-type antibody, occurs in idiopathic thrombocytopenic purpura, posttransfusion purpura, and heparin-induced thrombocytopenia (10–14).

Thrombocytosis, an excess of circulating platelets, occurs in reaction to a number of stimuli (Table 19.3). Primary thrombocytosis is a myeloproliferative disorder sometimes occurring in association with polycythemia vera or other myeloproliferative disorders. Despite an increased number of platelets, hemostasis is impaired, either because the platelets are qualitatively abnormal or because of abnormal binding of von Willebrand factor. Thrombotic complications also can occur, especially in older patients. Thus, these patients are aptly described as being in double jeopardy. Clinical manifestations include focal mucocutaneous bleeding, thrombosis, headaches, neurologic symptoms and transient ischemic attacks, digital ischemia, hepatic and portal vein thrombosis, and recurrent abortions. It is extremely important to recognize the increased surgical risk that patients with this disorder present, particularly when the platelet count is greater than $1,500,000/mm^3$. Reduction of the platelet count by platelet apheresis or by myelosuppressive therapy is effective treatment and is mandatory before any elective surgery. Aspirin is used only when the thrombotic complications dominate, and its use may result in catastrophic hemorrhage (15,16).

Hemostatic abnormalities rarely occur in secondary or reactive thrombocytosis (in contrast to primary thrombocytosis). Reactive thrombocytosis in surgical patients is most commonly seen after splenectomy. Because of fear of thrombosis, many clinicians treat platelet counts greater than $1,000,000/mm^3$ with antiplatelet drugs. These complications are rare, however, except in patients with hemolytic anemia; and even there, the incidence of thrombosis correlates poorly with the platelet count (17).

Table 19.4.
Contents of Platelet Alpha Granules

Platelet specific proteins (indicate platelet activation when measured in the serum)
    Platelet factor 4 (chemotactic for neutrophils, physiologic function not known, high affinity for heparin)
    Beta-thromboglobulin (biologic function not known)
    Basic protein
Coagulation factors
    Fibrinogen
    Factor X
    Factor VIII
    von Willebrand's factor
Glycoproteins
    Thrombospondin (an adhesive glycoprotein)
    Fibronectin
    Albumin
Growth factors
    Platelet-derived growth factor (PDGF)
    Transforming growth factor-β (TGF-β)
    Connective tissue activating peptide
Other substances
    Immunoglobulin G
    Osteonectin

Platelet Granules

On both light and electron microscopy, abundant cytoplasmic granules are a prominent feature, making up approximately 20% of platelet volume. Currently, these are subdivided into two main types: α-granules and dense granules (or dense bodies). α-Granules contain platelet-specific proteins, coagulation factors, and other proteins (Table 19.4). α-Granule contents are released during platelet activation. Dense granules contain ATP, ADP, GTP, GDP, pyrophosphate, orthophosphate, calcium, and serotonin. Although most of the contents of platelet granules are derived from megakaryocytes, serotonin is absorbed by platelets from the enterochromaffin cells of the gut and stored in dense granules. Several of the constituents of α-granules are synthesized within platelets (18).

Activated platelets degranulate, releasing the contents of α-granules and dense bodies. Platelet-specific proteins are substances released only by platelets (primarily α-granule contents). Detection of one of these substances in the serum is presumptive evidence for platelet activation. The mechanism of release is complex and probably involves a complex canalicular system continuous with the extracellular milieu rather than simple exocytosis.

ADP, released from dense granules, stimulates platelet shape change and aggregation. It requires the ability of the platelet to synthesize prostaglandins and hence is inhibited by aspirin. The significance of platelet serotonin release during normal hemostasis is unknown. Platelet derived serotonin may be significant in migraine and may contribute to the pulmonary vasoconstriction accompanying pulmonary embolism.

Thrombin is physiologically the most important platelet agonist. It stimulates degranulation and activates phospholipase A_2, which stimulates synthesis and release of thromboxane A_2 and its precursors.

Growth factors released by platelets include platelet-derived growth factor (PDGF), transforming growth factor-β (TGF-β), and connective tissue-activating peptide (CTAP-III). In cell cultures, TGF-β produces loss of contact inhibition and induces formation of colonies when another growth factor (such as epidermal growth factor) is present. TGF-β may be particularly important in bone development and healing. CTAP-III stimulates metabolic activity in connective tissue (18).

Lysosomal enzymes (acid hydrolases) are found within small vesicles and are generally lumped with α-granules on morphologic grounds. Acid hydrolases are released in high concentrations into the surrounding milieu during platelet activation. The significance of this is unknown at present, and although platelets can be demonstrated to engulf foreign particles in vitro, no significant phagocytic or bacteriocidal function is believed to exist. Other structures formerly designated as granules by light microscopy have now been identified as organelles, such as mitochondria. Only α-granules and dense bodies are currently believed to be important and unique contributors to platelet function (18).

Storage pool deficiency disorders, in which α-granules or dense bodies are absent or decreased, may be congenital or acquired. These are associated with a mild to moderate hemostatic defect. Dense granule defects correlate best with decreased ADP, attesting to the importance of this substance in platelet function. Although these disorders are clinically rare, study of involved individuals has provided important insights into the function of platelet granules in normal hemostasis (19).

In addition to release of preformed substances stored in α-granules and dense bodies, activated platelets synthesize and release prostaglandins, the most important of which is thromboxane A_2. Arachidonic acid is produced in activated platelets by the action of phospholipase C and phospholipase A_2 on membrane-bound phospholipids. Cyclooxygenase converts arachidonic acid to thromboxane A_2 via intermediate prostaglandins G_2 (PGG$_2$) and H_2 (PGH$_2$). Thromboxane A_2, PGG$_2$ and PGH$_2$ are secreted and function as vasoconstrictors and strong stimulants of platelet aggregation. Other arachidonic acid metabolites are strong chemotaxis substances for neutrophils (20,21).

Aspirin irreversibly inhibits cyclooxygenase, thus blocking platelet conversion of arachidonic acid to thromboxane A_2. The aspirin effect lasts for the life span of the platelet. Because thromboxane A_2, PGG$_2$, and PGH$_2$ are important stimulants for platelet aggregation, formation of the initial hemostatic plug is impaired. The bleeding time is prolonged, and platelet aggregation studies demonstrate a consistent abnormality. Other nonsteroidal antiinflammatory agents show similar but

Table 19.5.
Drugs that Affect Platelet Function

Cyclooxygenase inhibitors
  Aspirin
  Nonsteroidal anti-inflammatory agents
Antibiotics
  Penicillins
    Carbenicillin
    Penicillin G
    Ticarcillin
    Nafcillin
  Cephalosporins
    Moxalactam
    Cefotaxime
  Nitrofurantoin
Dextran

Table 19.6.
Platelet Receptors

Glycoprotein
  Ia - Collagen
  Ib - Thrombin
  Ib/IX - von Willebrand factor
  IIb/IIIa - Fibrinogen, fibronectin, von Willebrand factor, vitronectin
  IV - Thrombospondin (released from alpha granules)

less pronounced effects (Table 19.5). Because cyclooxygenase is also responsible for the production of PGI_2 by endothelial cells, the release of this substance is altered as well. The differential sensitivity of these systems is the basis for current low-dose aspirin therapy (22–24).

Intrinsic Contractile System

Rapid and characteristic changes in platelet shape occur with platelet activation. The normally disc-shaped platelet extends pseudopods, becoming more like a spiny sphere. Proteins of the cytoskeleton, organized into microtubules, microfilaments, and intermediary filaments, are responsible for the maintenance of platelet structural stability and the conformational changes accompanying platelet activation. These proteins include actin, myosin, actomyosin, tubulin, a number of regulatory proteins that control actin polymerization, and proteins that anchor filaments to the cell membrane (25).

Actin is the most abundant protein in platelets. Myosin is also present in platelets, and the existence of actomyosin (initially termed thrombosthenin) was demonstrated in platelets as the first extra-skeletal muscle site. The ratio of actin to myosin (100:1) heavily favors actin. When actin is complexed with myosin in actomyosin, the same actin:myosin ratio (7:1) is seen as in skeletal muscle, although the typical thick and thin skeletal muscle filaments are not noted in platelets. The contractile activity of actomyosin is probably the factor responsible for clot retraction (18).

Cross-polymerization of actin, anchored to the cell membrane and organized in a system of microfilaments, may be responsible for some of the conformational changes associated with platelet activation.

Actin is maintained in microfilaments of F-actin by a continuous, energy-requiring process termed the actin treadmill. In the actin treadmill, actin depolymerizes at one end, and an actin monomer is added at the other end in an ATP-requiring process, which uses 40% of the resting platelet's ATP consumption (18). A system of microtubules surrounds the periphery of the resting platelet and helps maintain the discoid shape. Platelet

secretion requires the presence of microtubules, which move to the center of the platelet, disappear, and then reappear (repolymerize) within pseudopods.

Platelet Membrane Receptors

Receptors on platelet membranes form a critical part of the hemostatic mechanism. A platelet agonist, such as thrombin, binds to a specific receptor on the surface of a platelet. A second messenger is generated on the cytoplasmic side of the membrane, thus transmitting the message to the inside of the platelet. The final effect for many stimulatory platelet agonists appears to be an increase of intracellular calcium. Receptor agonists that inhibit platelet function all stimulate adenylate cyclase, resulting in an increase in platelet cAMP (25,26).

Most identified receptors are glycoproteins (Table 19.6). Specific receptors have been recognized for thrombin, ADP, epinephrine, serotonin, vasopressin, and prostanoids—PGG_2, PGH_2, and thromboxane A_2 (which stimulate platelet activation) and prostacyclin, PGE_1, and PGD_2 (which, by stimulation of adenylate cyclase, cause platelet inhibition). Additional receptors bind fibrinogen, von Willebrand factor, calcium, thrombospondin, and fibronectin. These contribute to platelet adhesion to surfaces and stabilization of the platelet thrombus by fibrinogen. von Willebrand factor acts as a bridge between glycoprotein Ib and IIb/IIIa sites on platelets and binding sites on collagen in the subendothelium, thus producing adhesion of platelets to the site of injury (26,27).

Membrane receptors for fibrinogen are critically important for platelet aggregation and the formation of a stable clot. The identification of a "platelet-type" bleeding diathesis in patients with abnormal fibrinogen or congenital hypofibrinogenemia or afibrinogenemia underscores the importance of this mechanism. More than 50,000 of the glycoprotein IIb/IIIa receptor complexes that bind fibrinogen are present on the surface of unstimulated platelets. These are not capable of fibrinogen binding until the receptor site is exposed by a steric change in the local receptor environment. Exposure of the receptor site occurs after platelet activation and appears to require prior binding of ADP, perhaps to an adjacent receptor. Chymotrypsin treatment of platelets also exposes fibrinogen receptors, which then bind normally. Over a period of 10 to 30 minutes, the initially reversibly bound fibrinogen becomes irreversibly bound. The requirement that platelet activation occurs before fibrinogen receptor activation provides an obvious protective mechanism against spontaneous formation of platelet aggregates. The IIb/IIIa receptor is also involved in the phenomenon of clot retraction observed in vitro. Ends of fibrin strands bind to the receptor, and contractile elements in the platelet cytoskeleton produce the force that compacts the clot. Factor XIIIa is needed to stabilize the clot by promoting fibrin cross-linkage. In the absence of XIIIa, clot retraction is poor, and a loose clot forms. Abnormal wound healing is noted as well.

Platelet membranes provide a surface on which elements of the coagulation cascade form enzyme complexes that culminate in the formation of thrombin. In addition, α-granules release significant amounts of some clotting factors, including factor V. Approximately 20% of factor V is located within platelet α-granules. Factor Va derived from α-granules may be more significant for hemostasis than serum factor Va (as evidenced by studies of individuals deficient in one or the other). Patients lacking in serum factor V, but having adequate platelet factor V, have minimal bleeding problems. Factor V is secreted from α-granules and activated by thrombin or by a platelet protease. Activated factor V binds to specific platelet membrane receptors, becoming a binding site for factor Xa and forming, with calcium, the prothrombinase complex that catalyzes the conversion of prothrombin to thrombin.

Platelet Membrane Receptor Defects

Defects in platelet membrane receptors have been identified and produce predictable alterations in hemostasis. Analysis of these rare disorders as experiments of nature have provided important insights into normal platelet function and, for that reason, are briefly mentioned here (19,28).

In Glanzmann's thrombasthenia, platelet glycoprotein IIb/IIIa is deficient or abnormal. Platelet aggregation with and binding to fibrinogen during clot formation is, therefore, impaired. Characteristically, these patients have a prolonged bleeding time, absent clot retraction, and no demonstrable platelet aggregation in response to any agonist.

Bernard-Soulier syndrome platelets have a deficiency in glycoprotein Ib, V, and IX. Because glycoprotein Ib binds platelets to the subendothelium via von Willebrand factor, platelet adhesion is impaired. Platelets are large, and moderate thrombocytopenia is often present. Ristocetin-induced platelet agglutination is decreased (similar to the defect observed in von Willebrand disease) and this cannot be corrected by addition of von Willebrand factor. This rare autosomal recessive disorder may cause severe, even fatal, mucocutaneous bleeding (19,28).

von Willebrand disease was originally named *vascular hemophilia* and was thought to be a vascular disease; it should be suspected in any individual with an increased bleeding time despite a normal platelet count and normal clot retraction. The more common form of this heterogeneous group of relatively common disorders is characterized by insufficient production of von Willebrand factor (vWF) by endothelial cells. Because vWF is important for initial attachments of platelets to subendothelial collagen in regions of high shear, a platelet type of bleeding diathesis results (29–36). von Willebrand factor is synthesized by endothelial cells and stored intracellularly in Weibel-Palade bodies. It is released and circulates as a heterogeneous family of multimers, ranging tremendously in molecular weight. Because the larger multimers have more binding sites, they are more important for platelet attachment (35,36).

Most of the common forms of von Willebrand disease are inherited as autosomal dominants. Because many individuals are only mildly affected, the true incidence in the population is unknown. Ristocetin, an antibiotic that was withdrawn from clinical use because it produced thrombocytopenia, causes platelet agglutination via enhanced binding of plasma vWF to platelet receptors. The ability of ristocetin to induce platelet agglutination is used as a test for von Willebrand disease. The test depends on the concentration of ristocetin, and results and interpretation vary with different forms of von Willebrand disease. It has been largely superseded by the availability of direct testing for von Willebrand factor antigen and multimers.

Desmopressin (DDAVP) is a vasopressin analogue that causes release of vWF from endothelial cells. It is useful in mild forms of von Willebrand disease (37–39). An uncommon syndrome, pseudo-von Willebrand disease, has been identified in several families. Platelets contain either an increased number of binding sites for vWF or receptors with a greater affinity for vWF. Abnormal binding of normally produced vWF to platelets produces a relative defect in circulating vWF, particularly the larger multimers (29).

Assessment of Platelet Function

The bleeding time is the standard method for assessing primary hemostasis. A blood pressure cuff is placed on the upper arm and inflated to 40 mm Hg. Small wounds are made in a standardized fashion on the forearm. The blood is pulled away by capillary action with a piece of filter paper (by gently touching the edge of the blood pool at the wound site) at 20 second intervals, and the time to cessation of bleeding is measured. Protocols vary and standardization of the test is important. In most laboratories, a normal bleeding time is 2 to 9 minutes. Thrombocytopenia, drugs such as aspirin, or platelet dysfunction from any cause will prolong the bleeding time. Even with careful standardization, the variability of the bleeding time to risk of bleeding has come under question. This variability is especially pronounced between individual patients. Hence the value of the bleeding time as a screening test is doubtful. Be-

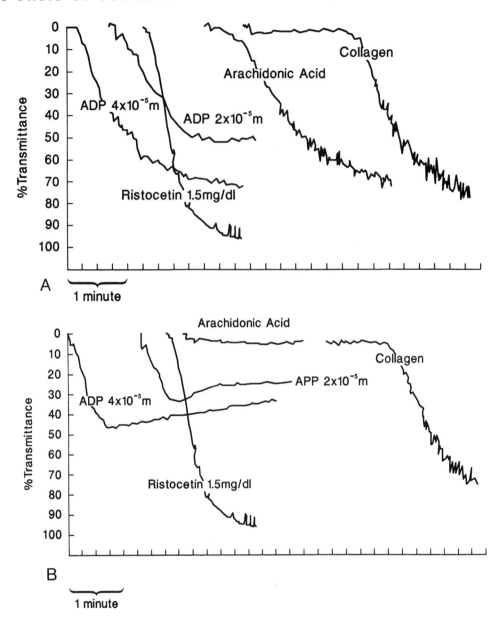

Figure 19.3. Platelet aggregometer tracings. The response of normal platelets is shown in the top tracing. Aspirin significantly impairs the response to all aggregating agents with the exception of Ristocetin (bottom tracing). The aspirin effect is irreversible and lasts for the lifetime of the platelet.

cause the bleeding time is relatively nonspecific, platelet aggregation studies are used when a specific platelet disorder is suspected (e.g., a congenital platelet disorder or drug effect) (40–42).

Platelet aggregation studies are done by measuring the light transmitted through a suspension of stirred platelets. Changes in platelet shape during activation and clumping of platelets during platelet aggregation increases the amount of light transmitted. When an agonist such as thrombin is added, a small initial drop in light transmission typically occurs as platelets change shape from discs to spheres. As platelet aggregation occurs, light transmission increases. Two waves of aggregation can be identified with the proper concentration of some agonists such as epinephrine (Fig. 19.3). The first wave occurs in direct response to the agonist and consists of formation of reversible aggregates. Platelet secretion of ADP causes the second wave, which is char-

acterized by the formation of large permanent aggregates. When a high concentration of a strong agonist such as thrombin is used, the first and second waves merge. Routine platelet aggregation uses a battery of agonists. These are usually ADP, weak ADP, collagen, ristocetin, and arachidonic acid. Epinephrine is generally not used because it does not induce aggregation in 50% of normal subjects. Arachidonic acid is specific and very sensitive to medication effects. The remainder of the agonists are useful in screening for congenital platelet defects (43).

The Coagulation Cascade and Formation of the Fibrin Clot

The fragile platelet plug must be stabilized by fibrin to form a strong, stable clot in which erythrocytes, plate-

Table 19.7.
Names Associated with Coagulation Enzymes and Cofactors

Factor	Name
V	Proaccelerin
VII	Proconvertin
VIII	Anti-hemophiliac factor (AHF)
IX	Christmas factor
X	Stuart-Power factor
XI	Plasma thromboplastin antecedent
XII	Hageman factor
XIII	Fibrin-stabilizing factor

Table 19.8.
Vitamin K Dependent Coagulation Factors

II (Prothrombin)
VII
IX
X
Protein C
Protein S

lets, and elements of the clotting and fibrinolytic system are trapped within a meshwork of cross-linked fibrin strands.

Enzymes and Cofactors of the Coagulation Cascade

Originally conceived as a sequential, amplifying cascade or series of reactions in which activation of one enzyme results in activation of the next enzyme, the coagulation system is now thought of as one central reaction (1,2,44). In this reaction, a serine protease and a nonenzymatically active protein cofactor assemble on cell membranes in the presence of calcium ions. The resulting enzyme complexes increase the speed of reactions critical for clot formation by a factor of 10^4 to 10^5. Three major reactions will be considered here: the final prothrombinase reaction, and both the intrinsic and extrinsic Xase pathways that produce activated factor X needed by prothrombinase. The classical intrinsic and extrinsic pathways were derived from observations of blood clotting in vitro. These are discussed at the end of this section and are related to two commonly used laboratory measures of blood coagulation: the prothrombin time (PT) and partial thromboplastin time (PTT). The enzymes and cofactors of the coagulation system are numbered with Roman numerals in order of discovery; thus, the numbers assigned do not relate to the order in which they appear in the reaction. Fibrinogen is factor I, prothrombin is factor II, tissue factor is factor III, and ionized calcium is factor IV. These four factors are generally referred to by name rather than by number. Factors V to XIII are commonly referred to by Roman numerals, and the activated forms are designated with an *a*; thus, activated factor V is denoted factor Va. There is no factor VI. Eponyms and descriptive terms associated with factors V to XIII are encountered occasionally and are listed in Table 19.7. In addition to the numbered elements of the cascade, von Willebrand factor, prekallikrein, and high molecular weight kininogen (HMWK) are important components.

Most of the enzymes and factors essential for coagulation are synthesized in the liver. Hepatic synthesis has been confirmed for fibrinogen, factor V, and a group of factors that requires vitamin K for synthesis (Table 19.8). Factor XIII, important for fibrinogen cross-linkage, is synthesized partially in megakaryocytes and partially in the liver. Levels of factor XIII are depressed in severe liver disease. Factor VIII is probably made in several sites, including the liver. Although liver transplant has corrected factor VIII deficiency in patients with hemophilia A, factor VIII levels may be increased (rather than decreased) in severe liver disease, possibly as an acute phase response, but also suggesting that alternate sites of production are important (45).

All vitamin K-dependent factors contain N-terminus γ-carboxyglutamate amino acid residues, which are essential for binding to membrane surfaces in the presence of calcium (46). Vitamin K is a necessary cofactor for the enzyme vitamin K dependent carboxylase, responsible for posttranslational carboxylation. Although some vitamin K is synthesized by gastrointestinal flora, an additional dietary intake of 1 to 3 μg/kg/day is required. A normal person will develop vitamin K deficiency 1 to 2 weeks after cessation of oral vitamin K intake. In the absence of vitamin K, the final carboxylation of the vitamin K dependent factors does not occur and the resulting factors are functionally inert. The PT is elevated, and the PTT may be elevated with severe vitamin K deficiency or with a low normal initial factor IX. Within 12 to 24 hours after administration of intravenous vitamin K, complete correction occurs. Two of the vitamin K dependent factors, protein C and protein S, form part of a critical anticoagulant system that limits the formation of thrombosis. These factors are discussed in "Endothelial Cells and the Regulation of Coagulation" later in this chapter.

Sodium warfarin interferes with vitamin K reductase and vitamin K epoxide reductase, enzymes that produce and recycle the reduced form of vitamin K needed for carboxylation. This produces a state of vitamin K deficiency with impaired synthesis of the vitamin K dependent factors. Although a direct relationship exists between the dose of coumarin and the anticoagulant effect produced in an individual patient, there are tremendous differences between patients. Dietary vitamin K intake, drug ingestion, hereditary resistance to vitamin K, liver function, and patient compliance all affect the response. Drug interaction with coumarin is so common that any drug should be considered to have the potential for interaction, and a patient on coumarin should have frequent PT checks during initiation or change in concomitant medications. Because coumarin interferes with the synthesis of protein C and protein S as well as coagulation proteins, thrombotic complications occasionally occur. These are discussed in more detail in "Down Regulation of Coagulation by Endothelial Cells" later in this chapter (47,48).

Fibrinogen is produced in large quantities by the liver; serum levels average 300 mg/dL, and fibrinogen has a serum half-life of 3 days. Hepatic output of fibrinogen is increased up to eightfold in response to inflammatory stimuli, including a number of monokines, and thus is one of the so-called acute phase reactants. Fibrinogen is the stable precursor of fibrin, the monomer from which fibrin clots are built.

Coagulation In Vivo

Thrombin is the critical enzyme that cleaves fibrinogen, the precursor of fibrin, into fibrin monomers, which then polymerize into long strands and are stabilized by factor XIII. Circulating enzymes and cofactors of the coagulation cascade provide a mechanism for controlled generation of thrombin via the prothrombinase reaction. Because generation of thrombin to cleave fibrinogen is the final goal of the coagulation cascade, the prothrombinase reaction will be taken as the starting point of this discussion.

The Prothrombinase Reaction

The prothrombinase complex is composed of factor Xa (an enzyme) and factor Va (a nonenzymatic cofactor), assembled on a suitable membrane surface in the presence of calcium ions (Fig. 19.4). It speeds the enzymatic conversion of prothrombin to thrombin by 280,000

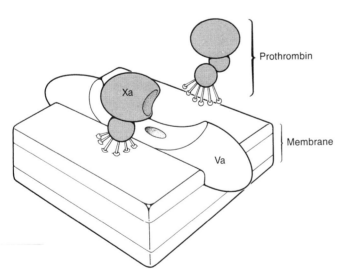

Figure 19.4. The prothrombinase complex consists of factors Xa and Va on a suitable phospholipid membrane surface in the presence of calcium ions. Platelet activation by thrombin results in exposure or steric change in membrane receptors, which act as binding sites for Xase and the prothrombinase complex[1].

times. As stated by Tracy (49), "the prothrombinase complex catalyzes in 2 minutes what free factor Xa would catalyze in 1 year." Factor Xa is activated by either the intrinsic Xase or extrinsic Xase mechanism (discussed below). Specialized prothrombinase receptors are present on platelets, monocytes, lymphocytes, neutrophils, and vascular endothelium. Platelets probably form the most important site of prothrombinase assembly during in vivo clotting. Prothrombin binds to phospholipids and hence accumulates on membrane surfaces in the vicinity of the prothrombinase complex. Factor Va increases the reaction speed by 10,000 times and thus is a necessary cofactor. Thrombin accelerates the conversion of factor V, the circulating and relatively inactive form, to factor Va. Initial activation of Va before generation of significant amounts of thrombin through the prothrombinase complex probably occurs by direct activation of membrane-bound factor V by factor Xa.

The activity of the prothrombinase complex is modulated by three principal mechanisms: the abundance of thrombin generated by the initial production of thrombin by TF-VIIa (after TFPI neutralization) which activates cofactor V and VIII; inactivation of factor Va by activated protein C; and inhibition by the antithrombin III system (the site of action of heparin) (49–57).

Activation of Factor X

Factor IXa (a protease) associates with its cofactor VIIIa (activated by thrombin) on a membrane surface in the presence of calcium ions to catalyze the conversion of factor X to Xa. This complex increases the activation of factor X by a rate of 10,000 times over that produced by factor IXa alone. Factor VIII circulates in low concentrations in noncovalent linkage with its carrier protein, von Willebrand factor. Factor VIII is stabilized by von Willebrand factor in the circulation, and when it dissociates from factor VIII, VIIIa is formed. Factor VIII is activated by Xa and thrombin. Activated factor VIII binds to membranes and can be inactivated proteolytically by activated protein C. Factor VIIIa is unstable in the circulation and must be bound to factor IXa in the activating complex to be stabilized (49–56).

The primary activator of blood coagulation is a complex of tissue factor (TF) and activated factor VII complex (TF-VIIa). Tissue factor pathway inhibitor (TFPI) rapidly neutralizes the TF-VIIa complex as it is generated. However, sufficient factor Xa is left to generate thrombin. The small amount of thrombin left over is sufficient to activate cofactors V and VIII. The activation of VIII with factor IX proceeds to convert factor X to factor Xa and to continue the generation of thrombin and eventually the fibrin for the fibrin clot. This modification of the previous cascade explains why factor XII, prekallikrein, and high molecular weight kininogen deficiencies are not associated with clinical bleeding but will prolong the aPTT (49–56).

Thrombin

Thrombin not only produces fibrin monomers by enzymatically cleaving fibrinogen, it also down regulates the coagulation cascade by binding to thrombomodulin on the endothelial cell surface. It is a potent platelet agonist, stimulating platelet aggregation, and it acts as a chemoattractant and mitogen for monocytes. By binding to monocytes, thrombin induces the release of interleukin-1, causing a number of substances (including plasminogen-activator inhibitor I, which depresses activity of the fibrinolytic system) to be synthesized (49).

As fibrin polymerization progresses, thrombin binds to fibrin. Although less than one thrombin molecule is bound per fibrin monomer, a significant amount of thrombin is incorporated within the growing clot. The binding of proteolytically active thrombin may serve to limit the spread of thrombin outside the region of thrombus formation but also may yield a burst of procoagulant material when clot lysis occurs (56,57).

Factor XIIIa stimulates cross-linkage of fibrin to produce a mechanically stable clot. In the absence of factor XIIIa, the clot is weak and wound healing is impaired. Fibrin enhances the rate of activation of factor XIII.

Hirudin is a natural anticoagulant found in the saliva of the medicinal leech Hirudo medicinalis. This 65 amino acid peptide binds competitively to thrombin, neutralizing many of its actions and interfering with its enzymatic activity in vivo and in vitro. Known for over a century but overshadowed by the discovery of heparin, hirudin is under investigation as an anticoagulant that may have some clinical applications (58–62).

Assessment of Coagulation In Vitro

Two measures of in vitro coagulation, the prothrombin time and partial thromboplastin time, are used as screening tests for disorders of the coagulation cascade and to monitor anticoagulant therapy (Fig. 19.5). These tests are relatively crude and generally are not prolonged until factor levels fall below 30% of normal.

Prothrombin Time

In the one-step prothrombin time test, a mixture of calcium and thromboplastin is added to citrated blood and the time to clot formation is measured. This provides a measure of the so-called extrinsic pathway of coagulation (because tissue thromboplastin, a factor extrinsic to blood, must be added). The PT is prolonged by deficiencies in factors VII (activated by tissue factor on a phospholipid surface in the presence of calcium), X (converted to Xa by VIIa), Factor V, prothrombin, and fibrinogen. It is used clinically to monitor oral anticoagulation with coumarin-type drugs. Tissue thromboplastin is a mixture of tissue factor, a necessary cofactor in the extrinsic Xase system, and phospholipid membrane fragments on which the system assembles. Tissue

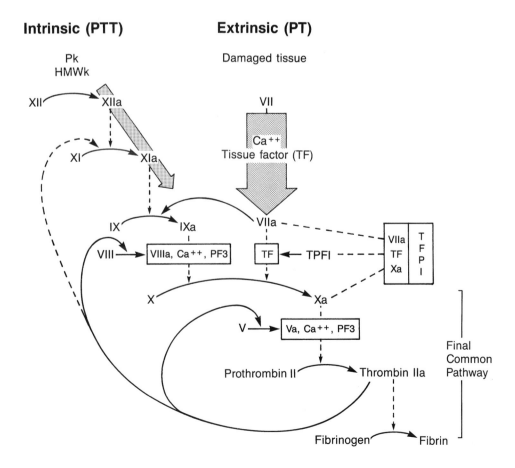

Intrinsic (PTT) **Extrinsic (PT)**

Figure 19.5. Overview of the coagulation cascade, showing components assessed by the PT and PTT. The path of primary *in vivo* significance is the so-called "Extrinsic" pathway, initiated by tissue damage. Components along this pathway are assessed using the Prothrombin time (PT). Components along the "intrinsic" pathway are assessed using the Partial thromboplastin time (PTT). Thrombin exerts feedback effects at various points in the cascade as shown by the loops. Tissue factor pathway inhibitor (TFPI) has an inhibitory effect which modulates the response[1,2,14].

thromboplastins vary in their composition, and difficulties in standardization of this test and in comparability of results from one laboratory to another are common. Significant differences in oral anticoagulant regimens described in the American and British literature underscored this problem recently. Depending on the laboratory, normal PT averages 12 ± 2 sec (48).

Partial Thromboplastin Time

The partial thromboplastin time measures the slower intrinsic pathway. In vitro, activation of the intrinsic pathway requires all of the clotting factors with the exception of factor VII. Normal levels of Hageman factor (factor XII), prekallikrein, and high molecular weight kininogen are required for a normal PTT. However, they do not appear to be important in vivo because individuals lacking these factors do not bleed abnormally. The PTT is used commonly to monitor anticoagulation with heparin.

The lupus anticoagulant is an acquired anticardiolipin antibody that prolongs the PTT by inhibiting the activity of the phospholipid used in the test. Clinical bleeding is rare. The antibody was described initially in patients with systemic lupus erythematosus. It has subsequently been identified in a wide variety of autoimmune disorders, in association with drugs, in acute infections, and in patients with neoplasia. Despite the elevated PTT, an increased risk of venous thrombosis or spontaneous abortions may be seen in some patients (70,71).

Thrombin Time

The thrombin time (TT) measures the thrombin-induced conversion of fibrinogen to fibrin and is prolonged in states of decreased fibrinogen or by the presence of an abnormal form of fibrinogen, or circulating anticoagulants, including fibrin degradation products (FDP). This test is a useful screen for hypofibrinogenemia when a quantitative fibrinogen is not available. Its marked sensitivity to heparin rules out this test for most hospitalized patients with keep-open arterial lines (72).

Disorders of the Coagulation Cascade

Congenital disorders of coagulation are a heterogeneous group of disorders for which clotting factors are produced in decreased numbers or in abnormal forms. These are conventionally grouped according to the factor that is diminished or abnormal (for example, factor VIII in hemophilia A). Factor levels must be significantly below normal before screening tests such as the PT and PTT are prolonged. Affected individuals vary in the severity of bleeding problems, depending on how much of the factor is present or how abnormal it is. For example, in hemophilia A, the PTT remains normal until factor VIII falls below 30% of normal levels. A personal or

family history of spontaneous bleeding, especially bleeding into joints, soft tissues, or body cavities, or a history of abnormal bleeding after surgery or trauma are important clues.

When surgery is necessary in individuals with coagulation disorders, replacement therapy is guided by serum factor levels. In Hemophilia A and most disorders, factor levels should be brought to 100% before elective surgery and held at 40% of normal until all drains and sutures are out. However, patients with hemophilia B will develop thrombotic complications at >50% and should not be brought above this level. This underscores the importance of knowing the appropriate factor level target for each disorder and following factor levels. Additional factor replacement at the time of suture removal may be required. In some disorders, wound healing is delayed. This should be anticipated and sutures should be left in for a longer period than usual (4,17,74–77). Topical hemostatic agents and fibrin glue may be useful but cannot replace meticulous hemostasis (78).

Hemophilia A

Classic hemophilia (factor VIII deficiency) is a sex-linked recessive genetic disorder that is carried by the female members of a kindred and that affects males almost exclusively. It is by far the most commonly inherited coagulation disorder, occurring in approximately 1 of 10,000 male births and accounting for 80% of all congenital factor deficiencies. Clinical manifestations correlate with factor VIII levels, which vary from less than 1% in severely affected individuals to as high as 40% in those with mild hemophilia. The degree of severity varies between kindreds but tends to be similar among affected males within a kindred. Patients with factor VIII levels greater than 5% rarely bleed spontaneously but will have bleeding problems after surgery or trauma. Most carriers of hemophilia A have factor VIII levels that are >50% and have no difficulty with spontaneous bleeding or with abnormal bleeding after surgery (79).

Fresh frozen plasma (FFP) and cryoprecipitate both contain factor VIII in relatively low concentrations (1 unit/ml of FFP, 5 to 10 units/ml of cryoprecipitate). The preferred replacement source is factor VIII concentrate, a pooled plasma product that is now treated to inactivate HIV and hepatitis viruses (79–85). Sterilized factor VIII concentrates were not available until 1984, and at present, approximately 90% of severely affected multiple transfused hemophiliacs have chronic active or chronic persistent hepatitis. The same percentage is HIV positive (83).

Antifactor VIII antibodies (factor VIII inhibitors) develop in 10% to 15% of severely affected hemophiliacs, usually in response to prior factor VIII infusion. Most of these patients have extremely low factor VIII levels. Their management is complicated, and patients with hemophilia A should be screened for factor VIII inhibitors before surgery so that appropriate treatment can be used (80). Factor VIII inhibitors occasionally occur in nonhemophiliac patients and can cause a clinical bleeding diathesis with prolonged PTT and decreased factor VIII levels clinically similar to classic hemophilia (71–80). Factor VIII levels are also decreased in patients with von Willebrand disease because vWF acts as a carrier molecule for factor VIII (71–80).

Hemophilia B

Christmas disease (factor IX deficiency) was identified when it was observed that blood from one hemophiliac corrected the prolonged clotting time of another patient with hemophilia. The pattern of inheritance and clinical manifestations are similar. Generally, the PT is normal and the PTT is prolonged; however, factor IX activity must be less than 30% of normal for prolongation to occur. Heat-treated, concentrated preparations of factor IX are available. Calculation of dosage is complicated by loss of 50% of infused factor IX (perhaps by binding to endothelial cells or movement into intravascular space). Factor IX infusion has been complicated by venous and arterial thromboses when levels greater than 50% were attained; for this reason, treatment generally aims at producing factor IX levels of approximately 50% normal (75–78).

Other Inherited Factor Deficiencies

Hereditary deficiencies of factor V (parahemophilia), factor VII, factor X (Stuart-Prower factor), and factor XI occur. All are extremely rare. Most are inherited as autosomal recessives, and a great deal of heterogeneity exists within each disorder.

Hageman factor (factor XII) deficiency highlights the difference between coagulation in vivo and in vitro. Decreased factor XII levels prolong the PTT, but even complete absence of factor XII does not cause abnormal bleeding. Patients deficient in Hageman factor are asymptomatic and generally are identified on screening PTT. The diagnosis is confirmed by specific factor XII assays. No treatment is indicated, as abnormal bleeding does not occur after surgery. Hageman factor is also a component of the intrinsic system for the conversion of plasminogen to plasmin, which causes clot lysis. Whether deficiency of factor XII predisposes to thrombosis is uncertain. The index patient (Hageman) died of pulmonary embolism after a pelvic fracture, and thrombotic complications have been reported in other patients with this deficiency.

Prekallikrein (Fletcher factor) deficiency and deficiency in HMWK produce clinical syndromes similar to Hageman factor deficiency. The PTT is prolonged, but abnormal bleeding does not occur. Prekallikrein and HMWK are also components of the intrinsic plasminogen activation system.

Several forms of combined factor deficiency syndromes have been identified in kindreds. Some of these are caused by deficient enzymes in the vitamin K dependent carboxylation system. The mechanisms of the other syndromes are unknown.

Patients with amyloidosis, the nephrotic syndrome, and Gaucher disease may develop an acquired coagulation disorder owing to increased clearance of coagulation factors. In the case of amyloidosis, factor X is bound with high affinity to amyloid fibrils, resulting in an acquired factor X deficiency despite normal production. Replacement therapy is difficult because infused factors also bind readily (83).

Endothelial Cells and the Regulation of Coagulation

Endothelial cells form a continuous barrier that contains and maintains the fluidity of blood. In a 70-kg adult, the total endothelial cell surface area exceeds 1000 m^2. Forming a nonleaking closed circuit, endothelial cells are far more than a simple passive lining of vascular conduits. Endothelial cells actively participate in and modulate the hemostatic response to vessel injury by several mechanisms (86–89).

Blood flow in normal vessels is laminar, with the fastest flow in the center of the channel. Erythrocytes and larger formed elements tend to channel in the center. Platelets are found in the slower-moving layers immediately adjacent to the endothelium. In the microcirculation, endothelial cell:platelet ratios may exceed 1:1, and significant inhibition of platelet function by PGI$_2$ and other substances secreted by endothelial cells occurs. Stasis, the first element of Virchow's triad, occurs more commonly in larger vessels such as the deep veins of the calf. Here, platelet aggregates may form and transient activation of coagulation enzymes may occur. Reestablishment of blood flow rapidly disperses these aggregates. Regions of abnormal blood flow, such as bifurcations and stenoses, produce turbulence that may contribute to endothelial cell damage and thrombosis (88,89).

Endothelial cells lie on a subendothelial matrix, which they secrete. Healthy endothelium forms a functionally seamless coating, resistant to platelet aggregation, over the thrombogenic sub-endothelium. Endothelial cells are joined by intercellular adhesion molecules (ICAMS) which form tight junctions and limit the permeability of the endothelium to plasma and cells. Cells that normally pass through the capillary wall, such as neutrophils, monocytes, basophils, and eosinophils, first adhere to endothelial cell adhesion molecules (ELAMS) by specialized receptors and then pass between endothelial cells. Platelets probably play an important role in the maintenance of capillary integrity. Thrombocytopenia is associated with increased capillary fragility and a measurable increase in permeability to erythrocytes and carbon particles. The subendothelial matrix is composed of collagen, elastin, fibronectin, thrombospondin, vitronectin, mucopolysaccharides (heparan sulfate, dermatan sulfate, and chondroitin sulfate), laminin, von Willebrand factor, and other substances. These provide mechanical stability and contribute to adhesion of endothelial cells to the basement membrane. Endothelial cells and their basement membrane (subendothelium) constitute the intima of large vessels. The subendothelium provides an additional mechanical barrier against blood loss after injury and acts as a potent stimulus for platelet aggregation. The importance of the subendothelium in maintenance of capillary integrity is emphasized by vitamin C deficiency in which an abnormal collagen is formed in the subendothelium and petechial bleeding results despite normal platelet function (89).

Intact endothelial cells are nonthrombogenic and, especially in the microcirculation where the endothelial cell surface area:blood volume ratio is high, secrete substances that inhibit and may deactivate platelets. Probably the most important platelet-inactivating substance is prostacyclin (PGI_2). At low concentrations, prostacyclin binds to specific platelet receptors and stimulates adenylate cyclase, increasing platelet cAMP and inhibiting many platelet functions. PGI_2 synthesis requires the enzyme cyclooxygenase (which is blocked by aspirin). Despite initial concerns, this aspirin effect does not appear to be clinically significant and is overshadowed by the therapeutic effect on thromboxane A_2 synthesis. The effect of PGI_2 on platelets is most pronounced in regions of high shear stress, such as the microvasculature. Thrombin induces synthesis and release of PGI_2. Endothelial cells also inactivate ADP, a potent platelet agonist (89).

When the endothelium is damaged, exposed subendothelium acts as a potent stimulus for platelet adhesion. Platelet adhesion to the subendothelium in regions of high flow requires von Willebrand factor, which is secreted into the subendothelium by the endothelial cells. Adherent platelets spread out, change shape, and degranulate, releasing substances such as thromboxane A_2 and serotonin, which attract more platelets and cause vasoconstriction (88,89).

Vasoconstriction is an immediate response to injury and may temporarily halt bleeding from small vessels that are completely transected. This is caused by contraction of vascular smooth muscle and by elastin in the subendothelium. The response is most pronounced in arteries and negligible in the great veins. In the operating room, this is noted as the tendency for small bleeders to retract and bleed later, when vasoconstriction relaxes. Regional closure of precapillary sphincters decreases blood flow to the area of injury. This vasoconstriction is mediated neurogenically and humorally, involving α-adrenergic agonists, thromboxane A_2 (synthesized and released by platelets), serotonin released by platelets, and endothelium. Local vasoconstriction is mediated by prostacyclin and endothelial cell-derived relaxing factor, both synthesized by the endothelial cell (90).

Platelets release growth factors, including platelet-derived growth factor (mitogenic and chemotactic for smooth muscle cells and fibroblasts), that probably contribute to vascular repair by stimulating fibroblasts and smooth muscle cells. The endothelium is repaired by initial migration of adjacent endothelial cells. Although endothelial cells synthesize a protein that is similar to PDGF, they lack receptors for and do not appear to respond to PDGF (34,86,90–93).

Down Regulation of Coagulation by Endothelial Cells

Endothelial cells have an extremely important role in modulating the coagulation system. Two primary mechanisms have been identified: (a) the presence of cell-surface molecules similar to heparin that bind antithrombin III, inactivating coagulation enzymes; and (b) thrombomodulin on endothelial cell surfaces binds thrombin, inactivating it and forming a powerful activator of protein C. In addition, endothelial cells secrete tissue-type plasminogen activator that converts fibrin-bound plasminogen to plasmin, initiating clot lysis (94).

Antithrombin III is made by the liver. It neutralizes thrombin by forming a complex with it. Activation of antithrombin III increases the rate of complex formation 1,000-fold. Physiologic activation occurs when antithrombin III binds to proteoglycans (heparan sulfate) on endothelial cell surfaces and in the subendothelial matrix. Activated antithrombin III is a major inhibitor of thrombin and factor Xa, with some inhibition of factors IX, XI, and XII. Antithrombin III is a necessary cofactor for the pharmacologic agent heparin, which binds to antithrombin III and increases its activity 1,000 to 10,000 times (95–103).

Both congenital and acquired states of antithrombin III deficiency occur. The congenital form is inherited as an autosomal dominant. Affected individuals have 40% to 60% of normal levels and have an increased incidence of venous thrombosis. Antithrombin III levels are decreased in patients with cirrhosis of the liver and the nephrotic syndrome. Approximately 2% of patients with idiopathic venous thrombosis have been found to have decreased antithrombin III. Specific replacement therapy is available (98,102–107).

Thrombomodulin is located in high concentration (approximately 50,000 sites per cell) on endothelial cells of all organs except the brain. When bound to thrombomodulin, thrombin loses its procoagulant properties, including fibrinogen cleavage, factor V activation, and platelet activation. Thrombomodulin provides a means for localizing thrombin effect to the site of injury and

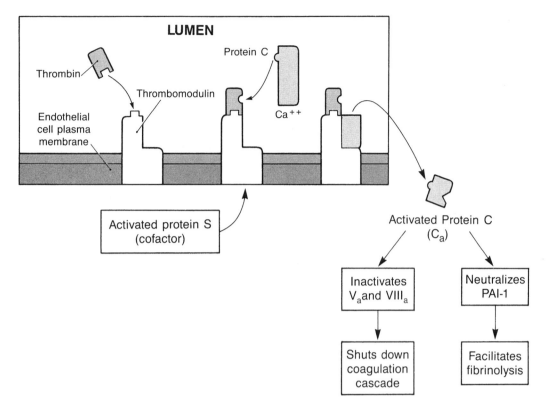

Figure 19.6. Thrombomodulin-protein C system. The system is activated when thrombomodulin and thrombin form a complex on the endothelial cell plasma membrane. In addition to shutting down the coagulation cascade, the system contributes to the initiation of fibrinolysis by neutralizing PAI-1[1,15].

limits its effect in proximity to intact endothelial cells. Thrombin bound to thrombomodulin is endocytosed gradually by the endothelial cell, providing a means for removing excess thrombin (108–117).

Protein C and protein S are synthesized in the liver and require vitamin K for carboxylation. Thrombin activates protein C slowly. The rate of activation is increased 1000 times by the binding of thrombin to thrombomodulin on endothelial cell surfaces (Fig. 19.6). Protein S is a necessary cofactor. Activated protein C is a potent inactivator of factors Va and VIIIa (critical enzymes of the coagulation cascade) and also neutralizes plasminogen-activator inhibitor I (facilitating fibrinolysis). The protein C pathway provides a link to inflammatory mediators and is important in host defense (110–116,118).

A total of 10% to 15% of patients with unexplained venous thrombosis have been identified as having either protein C or protein S deficiency. Several kindreds with protein C or protein S deficiency and pronounced thrombotic diatheses have been identified. However, screening of large numbers of blood donors has demonstrated that asymptomatic protein C deficiency is relatively common in the general population, suggesting that an additional factor may be necessary to produce thrombosis. Thrombotic complications (e.g., warfarin-induced skin necrosis) sometimes occur early in the course of oral anticoagulation with vitamin K antagonists. This may be more likely in patients deficient in protein C or protein S (119–127).

Disorders of the Endothelial Cell

Endothelium exposed to endotoxin, interleukin-1, or tumor necrosis factor loses thrombomodulin function. The resulting loss of down regulatory function may contribute to the development of widespread intravascular thrombosis characteristic of disseminated intravascular coagulation (DIC) (128). DIC is part of a spectrum of consumptive thrombohemorrhagic disorders in which inappropriate uncontrolled activation of the hemostatic mechanism occurs, with deposition of thrombus in areas where no local injury exists, resulting in widespread areas of local ischemia, tissue dysfunction, and possibly cellular death. DIC is discussed in more detail with other complex disorders of coagulation.

Thrombotic Thrombocytopenic Purpura

Widespread occlusion of the microvasculature with hyaline thrombi accounts for the diverse clinical manifestations of the uncommon disorder thrombotic thrombocytopenic purpura. Fluctuating neurologic signs, thrombocytopenia, and microangiopathic hemolytic anemia form the characteristic triad; renal dysfunction and fever are often present as well. The primary laboratory hemostatic abnormality is thrombocytopenia. Endothelial cell abnormalities have been identified, including abnormal prostacyclin synthesis and decreased tissue plasminogen activator (perhaps related to inappropriate release of plasminogen-activator inhibitor I by endothelial cells). Unusually large circulating vWF multimers, possibly released by damaged endothelial cells, have been found in the serum and may stimulate platelet activation. Unusually high serum levels of vWF and the presence of vWF multimers in the serum of patients in remission from TTP have been documented, whereas a decrease in these levels during acute exacerbation suggests consumption during formation of microthrombi (129).

Plasmapheresis is the most effective treatment and probably acts by removing toxic substances and replacing an inhibitor by infused FFP. Despite thrombocytopenia, platelet transfusion is not indicated, as this may worsen formation of microthrombi.

Hemolytic-uremic syndrome is a closely related disorder of infancy and childhood and is occasionally seen in adults. Renal symptoms predominate and neurologic dysfunction is rare. A genetic predisposition seems to exist, but as with TTP, the inciting factor appears to be endothelial cell damage (129).

The Fibrinolytic System and Healing

The fibrinolytic system allows remodeling and removal of thrombus to occur as wound healing proceeds (Fig. 19.7). A complex system of activators and inhibitors regulate the conversion of plasminogen to plasmin, the enzyme that cleaves fibrin and causes the clot to dissolve (130–132).

Plasminogen and Plasmin

Plasminogen, the inactive form of plasmin, is synthesized in the liver and circulates in the blood. Cleavage of a single peptide bond converts plasminogen to plasmin, an active enzyme that is capable of degrading both fibrin and fibrinogen. During clot formation, 4% to 10% of the locally available plasminogen binds to fibrin through lysine-binding sites and is incorporated into the growing thrombus, modulated by α_2-antiplasmin.

Both congenital dysplasminogenemias (disorders in

which an abnormal form of plasminogen exists) and hypoplasminogenemias (normal plasminogen formed in decreased amounts) occur rarely and are manifested clinically by thrombotic diatheses (133,134).

ϵ-aminocaproic acid (EACA) inhibits fibrinolysis by competitively binding to the lysine binding sites of plasminogen. This prevents plasminogen (and plasmin) from binding to fibrin substrate. A similar synthetic agent, tranexamic acid (AMCA) has less renal excretion and is effective at lower concentrations (135).

Plasminogen Activators

Two major classes of plasminogen activators have been identified. Tissue-type plasminogen activator (tPA) and urokinase-type plasminogen activator (uPA) both cleave plasminogen, generating plasmin.

Tissue-type plasminogen activator is produced by endothelial cells and released into the circulation. It is cleared rapidly by the liver (half-life approximately 5 min). High local concentrations of thrombin and conditions of venous stasis stimulate tPA release. tPA binds avidly to fibrin, bringing it into close proximity to fibrin-bound plasminogen. In addition, the enzymatic activity of tPA is greater when fibrin-bound. Thus, tPA produces plasmin within the thrombus, with little activation of circulating plasminogen (57).

The highly clot-specific property of tPA appears to enhance its dose-predictable activity when administered as a therapeutic agent, but it does not enhance its efficacy or safety compared with urokinase or streptokinase. In addition, it does not prevent the potential bleeding complications associated with all thrombolytic agents. Fibrin-bound tPA will initiate thrombolysis with equal efficacy in undesirable locations where hemostasis is essential (e.g., arterial puncture sites and spontaneous internal hemorrhages) and in desirable, or therapeutic, locations (e.g., coronary arteries and vascular grafts). tPA is also the most expensive currently available thrombolytic agent (136–143).

Urokinase-type plasminogen activators are found in limited amounts in the blood. Urokinase is a uPA that is responsible for the fibrinolytic activity of urine. uPAs lack the fibrin affinity of tPA and do not exhibit a greater enzymatic activity for plasminogen in the presence of

Figure 19.7. Overview of fibrinolytic system. The fibrinolytic system is activated when plasminogen is converted to plasmin. Substances that facilitate this conversion (shown above the arrow) such as tPA and uPA are termed "activators." Inhibitors of the fibrinolytic system are shown below the arrow and include α_2-antiplasmin, PAI-1, and PAI-2. Links between the coagulation and fibrinolytic systems have been demonstrated in vitro but not in vivo. In vitro, XIIa, XIa, or kallikrein can convert plasminogen to plasmin, hence activating the fibrinolytic system[130].

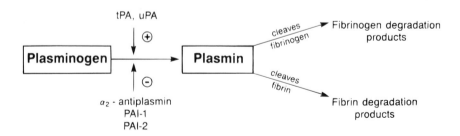

fibrin. Urokinase is extremely effective and dose predictable as a thrombolytic agent, has no immunologic side effects, and is intermediate in cost. Urokinase is the most widely used thrombolytic agent for intra-arterial infusion into the peripheral arterial system and grafts (136–139,144,145).

Streptokinase, a glycoprotein produced by β-hemolytic streptococci, is not a proteolytic enzyme and does not convert plasminogen to plasmin. Instead, it complexes with plasminogen, and this complex is then capable of activating other plasminogen molecules. The affinity of streptokinase for fibrin is low, and like uPA, streptokinase is not selective for fibrin-bound plasminogen. Because streptokinase is a nonhuman protein, it may elicit profound allergic (febrile) responses, which limits its clinical utility. Preformed antibodies to streptokinase also may bind and inactivate it, but in clinically administered doses this effect is usually overwhelmed and a thrombolytic state is achieved easily. Some dose-response unpredictability may occur because the streptokinase-plasminogen complex resists inactivation by α-antiplasmin and because degradation products are multiple and maintain variable activity. Streptokinase can be effective and is the least expensive thrombolytic agent available (136–139,142,144–147).

Although tPA activates only fibrin-bound plasminogen, it can directly lyse circulating fibrinogen without activating plasmin. The resulting hypofibrinogenemia, activation of the complement system, and the production of thrombocytopenia in some patients (mechanisms unknown) can cause significant systemic coagulopathy after its administration. Urokinase and streptokinase also cause a decrease in circulating plasma fibrinogen by activating circulating plasminogen. All of these agents also reduce circulating plasminogen, possibly even to the point of depletion and spontaneous thrombosis. The resulting hypofibrinogenemia and plasminogenemia are greatest in the first few hours after initiating an effective thrombolytic infusion, and thereafter the levels of fibrinogen gradually increase and fibrinogen degradation products stimulate hepatic fibrinogen synthesis. Although hypofibrinogenemia is generally greatest with streptokinase and least with tPA, the occurrence of hemorrhagic complications is actually greatest with tPA because of its multiple effects on the coagulation system (142).

No significant difference in therapeutic effectiveness of thrombolysis exists between these agents when used at sufficient doses to achieve a thrombolytic state. The rapid effect of tPA has some hypothetical appeal in its application to acute coronary artery thrombosis, but there is conflicting evidence that it results in a lower mortality rate, and in fact it is associated with the highest incidence of rethrombosis (142).

The intrinsic plasminogen activating system is initiated by contact of Hageman factor (factor XII) with a surface. Factor XIIa converts prekallikrein to kallikrein, which enhances the activity of uPA. Thus, activation of the intrinsic coagulation system in vivo also activates fibrinolysis. Plasmin activates factor XII, producing an amplifying system.

Inhibitors of Fibrinolysis

The two major physiologic inhibitors of fibrinolysis are α2-antiplasmin and plasminogen-activator inhibitor I (PAI-I). α2-antiplasmin binds avidly to circulating plasmin and irreversibly inactivates it, preventing a generalized fibrinolytic state. Within a thrombus, the situation is more complex. During clot formation, small amounts of α2-antiplasmin are incorporated within the fibrin mesh and bound covalently to fibrin as factor XIIIa stimulates fibrin cross-linkage. Mature clots in which fibrin cross-linkage has occurred are much more resistant to plasmin than fresh thrombi for this reason. When plasmin is subsequently generated within the thrombus, it must saturate the binding sites of this inhibitor before clot lysis occurs. This prevents premature clot lysis. Plasmin bound to fibrin is relatively resistant to inactivation by α2-antiplasmin, however, and once the small amount of inhibitor bound within the fibrin is saturated, additional plasmin generated within the thrombus is protected from the effects of circulating inhibitor. Congenital α2-antiplasmin deficiency causes pathologic hyperfibrinolysis with premature clot dissolution (130).

Plasminogen-activator inhibitor I is synthesized by endothelial cells and released into the blood and extracellular matrix. It is one of the interleukin-1 mediated acute phase reactants; thus, the synthesis and release of PAI-I can occur in response to a variety of stimuli, including bacterial endotoxin. PAI-I binds to and inhibits tPA, preventing cleavage of plasminogen to plasmin and inhibiting fibrinolysis. PAI-I is elevated in patients with acute myocardial infarction, and elevation of PAI-I may represent the most common abnormality of the hemostatic system that predisposes to thrombosis (148,149).

Plasminogen-activator inhibitor II (PAI-II) can be isolated from the trophoblastic epithelium of the placenta during pregnancy and occurs in increasing amounts in maternal plasma. A corresponding decrease in fibrinolytic activity occurs, which peaks at the time of separation of the placenta and then rapidly returns to normal. This protective mechanism helps prevent exsanguinating hemorrhage from the raw surface of the uterus, but it accounts in part for the increased incidence of venous thromboembolism and may contribute to the pathophysiology of eclampsia (148–150).

Hyperfibrinolysis

Pathologic activation of the fibrinolytic mechanism occurs in response to severe stress, heat stroke, and in association with certain neoplasms. Currently, it occurs most often as a side effect of fibrinolytic therapy (148,151).

Current Use and Assessment of Fibrinolysis

In current vascular surgical practice, thrombolytic agents are increasingly used for both therapeutic and diagnostic applications. In some situations, lysis of thrombus in native arteries or grafts may be the only acute therapy needed to revascularize severely ischemic organs; however, in most cases, it is a temporary remedy that is of greatest benefit in allowing accurate radiographic diagnosis of underlying pathology for appropriate treatment (140,144–146).

The euglobulin lysis time is used to evaluate systemic fibrinolysis and is believed to reflect primarily the level of plasminogen activators. Acidified, diluted plasma (the euglobulin fraction) is relatively free of inhibitors of fibrinolysis. The euglobulin fraction is allowed to form a fibrin clot, and the time to subsequent clot lysis (90 minutes to 6 hours) is measured. A more rapid lysis (less than 1 hour) implies that circulating activators are present.

Measurement of the TT is more useful in monitoring the systemic fibrinolytic state achieved during fibrinolytic therapy because it is quicker and more widely available. A satisfactory fibrinolytic state is achieved when the TT is two times normal (147,152).

Plasminogen, fibrinogen, and fibrinogen/fibrin degradation products can be measured directly. Most bleeding complications related to fibrinolytic therapy occur when fibrinogen levels have diminished to less than 50 to 100 mg/dL. The thrombolytic infusion rate should be reduced by 50% if the fibrinogen level is <150 mg/dL, discontinued if the fibrinogen level is <100 mg/dL, and FFP should be administered prophylactically to replenish fibrinogen if the level is <80 mg/dL (143,145–147,152,153).

An increased risk of hemorrhagic complications has also been correlated with fibrin degradation products (FDPs) greater than 100 U/dL, but this has been more variable, and a quantitative assay for FDPs is not readily available in many laboratories (142).

A practical protocol for monitoring the systemic administration of fibrinolytic agents is to measure the TT every 6 hours until a lytic state is achieved and thereafter to measure the TT and fibrinogen level every 12 hours. Blood samples must be placed in ice immediately after withdrawal to prevent continued in vitro activity (142, 143, 145–147). However, no method of monitoring has been found to eliminate the potential risks associated with fibrinolytic therapy. Indeed, the use of monitoring tests is considered futile by some, like those who monitor effective dose administered by clinical response and who feel bleeding complications are reduced to the minimum possible by limiting doses to quantities determined safest by empirical clinical experience.

During administration of fibrinolytic agents via intra-arterial catheters, it is also necessary systemically to anticoagulate the patient with heparin to reduce the potential complications related to formation of thrombus along the catheter. Anticoagulation should be monitored by PTT in a standard fashion (140,144,146).

The risks of bleeding during the use of systemic fibrinolytic therapy may be reduced by avoiding invasive procedures (including i.m. injections, nasogastric tube insertion, and urethral catheterization), limiting venipunctures to only essential circumstances and holding pressure at least 10 minutes afterward, and prescribing strict bed rest to avoid even minor trauma (142,147).

Relative contraindications to the use of systemic fibrinolytic agents are circumstances with moderate risk of hemorrhage or thromboembolism, such as recent operation or arterial puncture, recent peptic ulceration, intracardiac or valvular vegetations, etc. Use of fibrinolytic agents is absolutely contraindicated when significant risk of producing fatal hemorrhagic complications exists, such as after recent intracranial hemorrhage or trauma, pregnancy, or recent liver or spleen injury (140,147).

Complex Disorders of Hemostasis and Thrombosis

In complex disorders, an abnormality of more than one component of the hemostatic mechanism exists. Disseminated intravascular coagulation and the bleeding diatheses associated with uremia, liver disease, and multiple transfusions are all encountered commonly in surgical practice. Each of these representative disorders was mentioned briefly above. They are now discussed individually in greater detail and used to relate the various components of the hemostatic and fibrinolytic systems (1–4,17,154,155).

Disseminated Intravascular Coagulation

Disseminated intravascular coagulation (DIC) is the manifestation of an underlying disease process and may be classified as acute or chronic. The clinical picture may be dominated primarily by bleeding or by thrombosis. A number of conditions have been identified that cause or contribute to DIC (Table 19.9).

Chronic DIC accompanies a number of disorders, including malignancy, aortic aneurysms, liver disease, and peritoneovenous shunting. Chronic low-grade DIC has been estimated to occur in as much as 10% of patients with abdominal aortic aneurysms—exacerbations may occur with impending rupture as blood dissects through tissue planes and local consumption of clotting factors occurs. Occasional acute DIC with bleeding after repair has been reported. Coagulation abnormalities

Table 19.9.
Causes of Diffuse Intravascular Coagulopathy (DIC)

Sepsis
  Gram-negative bacteria
  Gram-positive bacteria
  Viruses
Hemolysis (massive)
  Transfusion of incompatible blood
Ischemia
Hypotension
Hypoperfusion
Brain injury
Obstetrical emergencies
Snake bite
Localized DIC
  Aneurysms
  Hemangiomas
  Allograft rejection
  Glomerulonephritis
Malignancy, especially prostatic cancer

Table 19.10.
Laboratory Abnormalities in Diffuse Intravascular Coagulopathy

Decreased platelets
Decreased fibrinogen
Decreased prothrombin
Decreased levels of factors V, VIII, XIII
Increased fibrin degradation products

consistent with DIC also occur with dissecting aneurysms. Classic causes of acute DIC, usually with hemorrhagic manifestations, include obstetrical emergencies (abruptio placentae and amniotic fluid embolism) and massive brain trauma (156–162). Localized deposition of fibrin with laboratory evidence of DIC may occur in allograft rejection and proliferative glomerulonephritis.

Acute DIC in surgical patients is heralded frequently by bleeding, with oozing from all tubes, wounds, and vascular access sites. Shock, ischemia, and infection are the most common precipitating factors. Severe acidosis and multiple blood transfusions often complicate the picture.

The thrombotic manifestations of DIC are uncommon and consistent with thrombosis in the microcirculation, including focal dermal ischemia, renal failure, focal neurologic signs, delirium and coma, and gastrointestinal ulcerations. These are more commonly seen in patients with the chronic forms of DIC. Patients with malignancy may develop a characteristic migratory thrombophlebitis (particularly associated with mucinous adenocarcinoma, but also seen with acute leukemias).

Infection with gram-negative bacteria is the single most frequent etiology of DIC. Endotoxin-induced damage to endothelial cells, with loss of thrombomodulin, may be a factor. Endotoxin also damages platelets, causing release of platelet factors, and activates the fibrinolytic system (128,162,163).

The laboratory abnormalities and clinical manifestations in DIC reflect consumption of clotting elements and enhanced fibrinolysis (Table 19.10). Therapy must be directed at correcting the underlying condition while supporting the patient with transfusion of specific hemostatic elements. Generally, a vigorous search for sepsis is undertaken in the surgical patient. Treatment with heparin may be appropriate for the occasional patient with chronic DIC and primarily thrombotic manifestations. It is rarely applicable in surgical patients, in whom

hemorrhagic symptoms dominate. Supportive care with replacement of platelets and clotting factors is appropriate in the bleeding patient, and concern that this will "fuel the fire" of DIC associated thrombosis seems to be unwarranted. Even when fibrinolysis is a prominent component, treatment with inhibitors of the fibrinolytic system is fraught with hazard. It may cause widespread deposition of thrombus throughout the microcirculation. For this reason, antifibrinolytic agents such as ϵ-aminocaproic acid should not be given alone but always accompanied by the administration of heparin (3,4,17,154).

Uremia

Uremia may cause a complex bleeding diathesis that is characterized by abnormal platelet function and improved by dialysis. In some patients, thrombocytopenia is present and contributes to the problem. However, transfused platelets are ineffective and are rapidly becoming abnormal. Platelet adherence to subendothelial collagen is impaired. Although the total amount of circulating von Willebrand factor may be normal, the largest von Willebrand factor multimers (which may be most important for platelet adhesion) are decreased. Platelet synthesis of thromboxane A_2 is decreased, and uremic platelets have lower than normal concentrations of serotonin, ADP, and von Willebrand factor. An increased amount of cAMP and intracellular calcium is also present. An additional defect is seen in the endothelial cell. Endothelial prostacyclin production increases and, paradoxically, levels of endothelially derived von Willebrand factors increase (164,165). Fibrinogen and several of the clotting factors may be decreased. Antithrombin III and protein C are decreased, and the fibrinolytic system is impaired, probably the result of circulating inhibitors.

The main treatment for uremic bleeding is adequate dialysis and elevation of the hematocrit. The effects of dialysis last 2 to 3 days. Cryoprecipitate infusion also may correct the bleeding problem, as does desmopressin, a synthetic analogue of vasopressin (DDAVP). Conjugated estrogens shorten the bleeding time in uremia by an unknown mechanism. They have been most useful in patients with gastrointestinal bleeding and telangiectasias (166–171).

Liver Disease

Severe liver disease produces a coagulopathy by several mechanisms. Synthesis of all coagulation factors, with the exception of factor VIII, is decreased. Vitamin K deficiency may result from decreased oral intake, malabsorption, or biliary obstruction, resulting in deficiency of the vitamin K dependent procoagulant and anticoagulant factors. Fibrinogen synthesis is decreased in severe liver failure, and an abnormal fibrinogen may be produced. This hypofibrinogenemia may also adversely affect platelet function. Thrombocytopenia is common in patients with portal hypertension and secondary hypersplenism (172,173).

Hepatic clearance of particulate substances, including macroaggregates, from the bloodstream is decreased. Endotoxin absorbed from the gut is poorly cleared from the portal circulation and may spill over into the systemic circulation. A chronic low-grade disseminated intravascular coagulation may result. Poor hepatic clearance of plasminogen activators results in a state of systemic fibrinolysis (173).

Peritoneovenous shunting for ascites (LeVeen or Denver shunt) causes direct infusion of procoagulant material into the venous circulation, again triggering DIC (174). Treatment of these multifactorial abnormalities involves replacement of clotting factors with FFP, cryoprecipitate, and vitamin K as needed (173).

Multiple Transfusion

Massive transfusion is defined as the transfusion of one or more blood volumes (5000 ml in a 70-kg adult) within 24 hours. Transfused blood is deficient in platelets as well as coagulation factors (175–186).

Diffuse bleeding during massive transfusion generally is caused by thrombocytopenia. Platelet dysfunction results from even moderate hypothermia (common in patients receiving massive transfusion), compounding the problem (187,188). The physiologic response to a hemorrhage includes an increase in circulating platelets, which include a high percentage of large young platelets freshly released from the bone marrow, which are extremely effective hemostatically. Rapid bleeding overwhelms this mechanism. Platelet counts should be obtained during massive transfusion, and platelet transfusion may be necessary after 6 to 10 units of packed red cells have been given, particularly if the patient has been taking aspirin. Evidence of defective primary hemostasis (oozing from raw surfaces, including avascular planes) is an indication for platelet transfusion. Routine platelet transfusion after infusion of a certain number of units of packed cells has not been shown to be beneficial (189,190).

Transfused blood is deficient in factors V and VIII as well as in platelets; however, in the absence of preexisting disease, an isolated decrease in these factors during transfusion is rarely sufficient to cause a coagulopathy. Fresh frozen plasma supplies all coagulation factors and should be given when clinical observation or laboratory tests suggest that the coagulation cascade is defective.

Prophylactic administration of FFP or administration by formula (for example, giving two units of FFP for every six units of packed red blood cells) has not been shown to be effective and subjects the patient to significant unnecessary risk of transmission of infectious diseases (191).

Platelet concentrates contain significant amounts of fibrinogen in addition to platelets (190,191). Cryoprecipitate is the primary source of fibrinogen and factor VIII replacement and is also used to enhance platelet function in acquired platelet defects such as in uremia.

Hematopoiesis

The observation that mixed colonies of cells arose from a single clone of bone marrow cells injected into lethally irradiated mice provided the evidence for the presence of stem cells (192,193). A relatively small number of long-lived stem cells form the basic pool from which all other cells are derived. The different formed elements of the blood (erythrocytes, granulocytes, lymphocytes, and platelets) are derived from pluripotent stem cells, which are morphologically indistinguishable. These stem cells are able to replicate themselves and to produce more differentiated cells. In a process that has been termed *death by differentiation,* the offspring of these stem cells become progressively more differentiated and lose proliferative ability with each cell division until the mature form, incapable of replication, is produced and released into the circulation. Stem cells first undergo an initial differentiation into lymphopoietic or hematopoietic progenitor cells. Lymphopoietic progenitor cells are the origin of both T and B lymphocytes. Lymphopoiesis is a complex process, involving the initial formation of T and B lymphocyte progenitor cells within the thymus and marrow, with subsequent processing of lymphocytes within aggregates of lymphoid tissue, such as lymph nodes. This is discussed in more detail in Chapter 7. It is conventional to use the term *hematopoiesis* to cover the genesis of all nonlymphocyte blood cell lines, and this is the process that will be discussed here. Hematopoietic progenitor cells undergo further differentiation into progenitor cells of granulocyte (neutrophil, basophil, and eosinophil), erythrocyte, or megakaryocyte lineage (Fig. 19.8).

Initial production of blood cells occurs in the yolk sac of the growing embryo. By the second month of fetal life, the liver has become an important hematopoietic organ, joined during later fetal development by the spleen. Hematopoietic cells first appear in the bone marrow at about the fifth month of gestation, and the center of hematopoietic activity gradually shifts until, at birth, the marrow is active and hematopoiesis has virtually ceased in extramedullary (outside of the bone marrow) locations. However, for the next several years, the volume required by the hematopoietic cell mass nearly approximates the volume available within the marrow

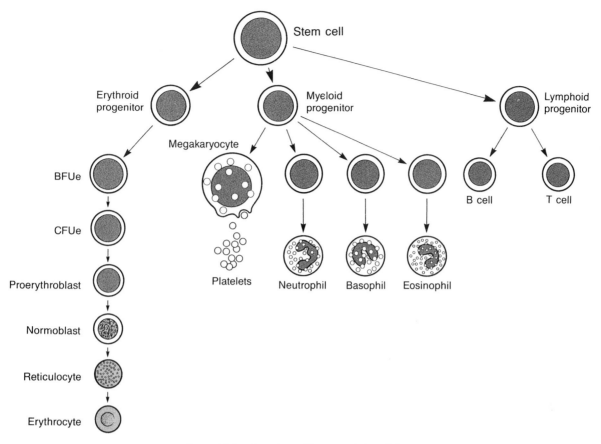

Figure 19.8. Overview of hematopoietic cell lines.

cavities. Hence, under conditions of stress, extramedullary hematopoiesis may again occur in the liver and spleen in normal children. By age 4, fat has begun to appear in the marrow, indicating that there is excess room. The hematopoietic cells gradually recede and become localized within the central marrow locations of the vertebrae, skull, ribs, and pelvis. The predilection of these cells for central marrow is illustrated by the selective repopulation of these areas by intravenously administered marrow cells during marrow transplantation. Fat cells occupy the remaining space in the long bones of the extremities (194).

In the adult, hematopoietic activity normally occurs only within the marrow. A nutrient artery supplies blood to the marrow sinusoids, which are lined by a continuous monolayer of endothelial cells. Nests of hematopoietic cells corresponding to different cell lines occupy the extravascular spaces, tending to cluster in characteristic locations. Megakaryocytes, the progenitor cells of platelets, lie closely adjacent to the sinusoid wall, as do the erythroblastic islands in which reticulocytes are formed. Myeloid stem cells that differentiate into granulocyte cell lines generally are located deep within the extravascular space. The marrow cavity forms a complex environment in which endothelial cells, fibroblasts, macrophages, and other stromal cells interact with hematopoietic cells. Mature cells exit the marrow by pushing through endothelial cells into the marrow sinusoids (194–196).

Growth Factors

Hematopoietic growth factors (originally called colony-stimulating and burst-stimulating factors) are glycoproteins that function as trophic hormones for stem and progenitor cells. Most growth factors are stimulatory for more than one cell line but have predominant activity for one. In the absence of specific growth factors, progenitor cells not only fail to differentiate but die (197–199).

These growth factors form part of a tightly controlled system that maintains cell counts within relatively small tolerances and adapts to changing needs. The bone marrow of the average adult generates 2.4 million erythrocytes per second and twice as many platelets (197). Bleeding, stress, and infection are stimuli for an increase of up to 6 to 10 times in output of the appropriate cell line, which is promptly shut off when the abnormal demand ceases.

Inhibitors of hematopoiesis include steroids, interferons, TGF-β, tumor-necrosis factor, lactoferrin, transferrin, ferritin, and arachidonic acid metabolites (197).

Potential clinical applications for growth factors include measurement of fetal umbilical cord erythropoietin levels as an indicator of in utero hypoxia and the administration of growth factors to ameliorate chemotherapy and/or radiation therapy induced myelosuppression. Growth factors also might be used to enhance platelet and blood donation, improve host defense, and enhance dose intensity in responsive neoplasms (199). Uses in cancer have been tempered by reports of leukemic transformation in preleukemic states and the observation that some tumors possess receptors for growth factors (199). The use of erythropoietin to ameliorate the anemia of chronic renal failure is an encouraging first step.

Erythropoiesis

Erythropoiesis provides an illustration of this process and is of central interest to surgeons. Erythropoiesis occurs within well-defined erythroblastic islands next to the vascular wall. Each erythroblastic island consists of one or two central macrophages. Maturing erythroid cells surround the macrophage and are engulfed by projections of the macrophage's cytoplasm. This architecture is lost in the typical diagnostic bone marrow aspirate, but may be appreciated in a marrow biopsy specimen (194,200).

The differentiating cells of the erythroid line are collectively referred to as the *erythron*. Three functional compartments are recognized: early progenitor cells (recognizable only by their capacity to give rise to erythroid colonies in vitro); erythroid precursors (proerythroblasts and marrow reticulocytes); and reticulocytes/erythrocytes. As differentiation progresses, cells become recognizable as erythroid precursors and gain sensitivity to their specific growth factor, erythropoietin. Erythropoietin stimulates transformation to proerythroblasts, which subsequently multiply and mature (200).

Reticulocytes lose their nucleus within the bone marrow and exit the marrow by passing through the endothelial cells. This appears to require a pressure gradient from within the marrow and considerable deformation of the reticulocyte. The reticulocyte continues its maturation within the bloodstream.

Erythropoietin

Erythropoietin is a glycoprotein hematopoietic growth factor that primarily stimulates erythroid precursors but has secondary effects on megakaryocytes. In the fetus, the liver is the major source of production of erythropoietin. After birth, over 90% of erythropoietin is produced in the kidney, and only about 10% is made in the liver. Anemia of prematurity may be related to failure to switch from hepatic to renal production of erythropoietin. Hepatic production of erythropoietin becomes important in anephric patients and is abolished experimentally by hepatectomy (198–201).

Erythropoietin production is increased by tissue hypoxia caused by anemia, hypoxemia, ischemia, and ab-

normal hemoglobin (increased affinity for oxygen, hence less delivery of oxygen at the tissue level) (Fig. 19.9). Carbon monoxide blocks this response, suggesting that the renal oxygen sensor may be a heme protein (H5). The site of synthesis lies within cells adjacent to the proximal renal tubules. Hypoxia stimulates the release of erythropoietin with a 5 to 6-hour delay. In the bone marrow, erythropoietin binds to specific receptors on erythroid progenitor cells; each cell has approximately 1000 receptors for erythropoietin. In the absence of erythropoietin stimulation, these cells die (198–201).

Normal levels of erythropoietin average 10 to 20 U/liter (or approximately 2 pmol). This amount is sufficient for normal replacement of worn-out erythrocytes. The level of erythropoietin increases as the hematocrit decreases, reaching 100 times normal at a hematocrit of 20% (200). This increased erythropoietin stimulates progenitor cells and accelerates the marrow transit time, resulting in the release of large, immature "stress" reticulocytes (200,202). A brief dose of erythropoietin results in an increase in circulating reticulocytes 4 to 5 days later.

Some cerebellar tumors produce polycythemia and may, by some unknown (probably neurohumoral) mechanism, stimulate erythropoietin release (200). A particular human hepatoma cell line is a rich source of erythropoietin and has provided a useful model (201). It is uncertain whether another substance shuts off erythropoietin production during polycythemia.

Clinical Uses of Erythropoietin

The anemia of chronic renal failure is multifactorial. Decreased or absent renal production of erythropoietin, hemolysis, small but obligate blood loss during hemodialysis, and nutritional factors all contribute. The administration of recombinant erythropoietin in doses ranging from 25 to 500 U/kg 3 times a week causes a dose-dependent rise in hematocrit and a significant improvement in well-being (202–205). Many of the nonspecific symptoms associated with chronic renal failure, such as fatigue, ameliorate as the anemia is corrected. Often a coexisting iron deficiency is unmasked and must be corrected as well.

Administration of erythropoietin allows more frequent blood donation and facilitates more frequent phlebotomy in patients with iron overload syndromes (202). The use of erythropoietin in other kinds of anemia (sickle-cell disease and anemia occurring after surgery) has had varied results (201–203). Anemias caused by rheumatoid arthritis, cancer, multiple myeloma, and the anemia of chronic disease are associated with low levels of endogenous erythropoietin and respond better to exogenous administration (202).

Anemia and Blood Transfusion

Acute blood loss does not immediately lower the hematocrit and results in anemia only after transcapil-

Kidney   **Blood**   **Marrow**

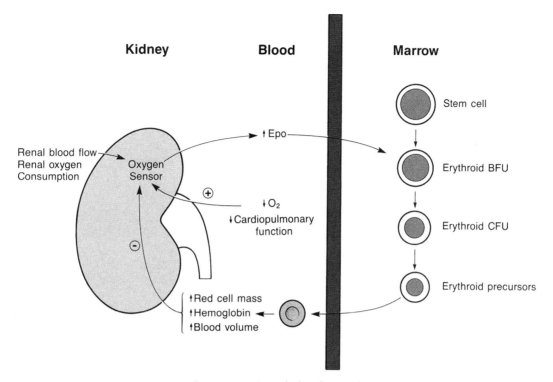

Figure 19.9. Control of erythropoiesis.

lary refill or intravenous infusion of crystalloid or colloid restores the circulating blood volume. Within several hours, erythropoietin output is increased and the process of erythropoiesis is accelerated. Several weeks later, red cell mass is reestablished. Excessive blood loss requires transfusion of donor red cells. Packed red blood cells are obtained when the approximately 200 to 250 ml of plasma are removed from a unit of whole blood. A small amount of preservative solution is added, and the resulting suspension has a volume of between 200 and 250 ml and a hematocrit of 50% to 80%. Packed red cells also contain leukocytes and platelets that, although not functional, are antigenic and may cause febrile transfusion reactions (206). Leukocyte reduction filters, when used in processing donor blood or at the bedside, significantly reduce febrile events and HLA sensitization. The indications for the use of various allogeneic blood products are summarized in Table 19.11.

Red Cell Surface Antigens

On their surface, red cells carry antigens from more than 30 different systems. Leukocytes carry HLA antigens, and platelets carry both HLA and platelet-associated antigens. Because the leukocytes and platelets that are incidentally infused with packed red blood cells are normally well-tolerated, blood is typed and cross-matched only for red cell antigens. Although any of the red cell surface antigens are capable of producing reactions in a susceptible recipient, the two important systems are the ABH (ABO) and Rh systems (212–214).

Table 19.11.
Indications for Allogeneic Blood or Blood Component Transfusion (208)

Product	Indications
Packed RBCs	Hematocrit <21–24%
Washed RBCs	Allergic Reactions
Leukocyte-reduced PRBCs	Febrile reactions, delay alloimmunication to HLA antigen
Irradiated PRBCs	Prevent graft vs host disease by terminating lymphocyte function in donor blood
Fresh frozen plasma	PT >18 sec, aPTT >55–60sec
Cryoprecipitate, pooled donors	Fibrinogen <100 mg/dl, source of vWF and Factor VII
Cryoprecipitate, single donor	Fibrin glue at wound site combined with bovine thrombin
Platelet concentrate	Platelet deficiency, <50,000/mm³ and platelet dysfunction

The ABH System. Antigens of the ABH system share common features with many naturally occurring proteins. Possibly for this reason, individuals who lack the A or B antigen on the surface of their erythrocytes possess strong IgM antibodies to these antigens (even in the absence of prior transfusion) and will have an immediate reaction if transfused with cells containing either of these antigens. Because IgM antibodies fix complement, transfusion of ABH incompatible blood causes immediate intravascular hemolysis of the transfused cells and/or cardiovascular collapse, and may be fatal.

Two genes determine the ABH genotype; there are six possible genotypes but only four phenotypes. The most common of these is blood type O (corresponding to the H antigen), occurring in 47% of the general population in the United States. Individuals of blood type O have antibodies to A and B and will react to blood from A or B (or AB) donors. Because H is antigenically weak, most people (regardless of their blood type) can accept blood from an O donor. Type A is almost as common, occurring in 41% of the U.S. population. The genotype may be either AA or AH. These individuals possess antibodies to B. Types B (genotype BB or BH) and AB are rare, occurring in 9% and 3% of the population, respectively.

A separate gene, the secretor gene, determines whether these antigens are water soluble and hence are found in secretions such as saliva. Approximately 80% of Western Europeans carry this gene and are termed *secretors* (212,213).

The Rh System. Individuals who lack antigens of the Rh system do not generally possess strong preformed antibodies. Prior exposure (by transfusion or during pregnancy) is necessary to sensitize the individual. There are six common antigens in this system, but the D antigen (Rh positive) is the most common (occurring in 85% to 95% of the population that is positive) (214).

Transfusion Reactions

Between 2% to 5% of patients who receive blood will experience an adverse reaction. The majority of these reactions are febrile allergic reactions to antigens or pyrogens (significantly reduced by leucocyte reduction filtration). The most serious reactions are hemolytic transfusion reactions with the most severe of these resulting from transfusion of ABO incompatible blood. When incompatible red cells are infused, recipient anti-A or anti-B antibodies bind to the red cells, causing activation of complement and lysis of the donor cells. When massive, the intravascular hemolysis causes activation of the coagulation cascade, resulting in the release of vasoactive substances. Vascular collapse, shock, and renal failure may result. The majority of these ABO mismatches arise from clerical or system error outside of the blood bank. The severity of the reaction is related to the type of incompatibility and the total amount of blood transfused. When DIC results, abnormal bleeding may be the first sign of a transfusion reaction. This is especially true when the event occurs while the patient is anesthetized.

Fever may be the first sign of a serious hemolytic transfusion reaction, and for this reason, when a fever is documented the transfusion should be stopped. However, most febrile reactions are the result of antibodies to leukocytes. Packed red blood cells may be leukocyte reduced (preferred) or washed to remove leukocytes. This is necessary in patients with a history of febrile reactions. Allergic reactions to plasma proteins are associated with urticaria and hives and may be mild or se-

vere. The severe form may cause laryngeal edema and death. Milder forms may be treated successfully with antihistamines. Washing the packed red cells will reduce the allergic response significantly and may be required with repeated allergic episodes.

Delayed hemolytic reactions occur when antibodies against the infused red blood cells are produced rapidly after infusion. In many instances, prior transfusions have sensitized the recipient. Typically, the antibody level was low before transfusion and hence not detected on routine screening. Transfusion of red cells results in an anamnestic response with rapid increase in antibody levels and hemolysis several days after transfusion.

Adverse effects of blood transfusion are not limited to potential transfusion reactions, but include suppression of the immune system, possible transmission of disease, and depression of the normal erythropoietin rise after hemorrhage. For all of these reasons, blood should be transfused only when needed and not according to a formula (206–215).

Acknowledgment

The assistance and critical review of the manuscript by Robert S. Rhodes, M.D., and Francis S. Morrison, M.D., are gratefully acknowledged.

REFERENCES

1. Roberts HR, Lozier JN. New perspectives on the coagulation cascade. Hospital Practice 1992;97–112.
2. Furie B, Furie BC. Molecular and cellular biology of blood coagulation. New Engl J Med 1992;326:800–805.
3. Clagett GP. Unexpected coagulopathies during surgery. Problems in General Surgery 1984;1:200–215.
4. Dykes C, Sobel M. The management of coagulation problems in the surgical patient. Adv Surg 1991;24:229–257.
5. Paulus J-M, Aster RH. Production, distribution, life-span and fate of platelets. In: Williams WJ, Beutler E, Erslev AJ, et al, eds. Hematology. 4th ed. New York: McGraw-Hill, 1990:1251–1260.
6. Bennett JS. Mechanisms of platelet adhesion and aggregation: An update. Hospital Practice 1992;124–140.
7. Birgens HS, Hancke S, Rosenklint A, et al. Ultrasonic demonstration of clinical and subclinical hepatic venous thrombosis in paroxysmal nocturnal haemoglobinuria. Br J Haematol 1986;64:737–743.
8. Devine DV, Siegel RS, Rosse WF. Interactions of the platelets in paroxysmal nocturnal hemoglobinuria with complement. Relationship to defects in the regulation of complement and to platelet survival in vivo. J Clin Invest 1987;79:131–137.
9. Doukas MA, DiLorenzo PE, Mohler DN. Intestinal infarction caused by paroxysmal nocturnal hemoglobinuria. Am J Hematol 1984;16:75–81.
10. Morrison FS, Mollison PL. Post transfusion purpura. New Engl J Med 1966;275:243–248.
11. King DJ, Kelton JG. Heparin-associated thrombocytopenia. Ann Int Med 1984;100:535–540.
12. Warkentin TE, Kelton JG. Heparin-induced thrombocytopenia. Prog Hemost Thromb 1991;10:1–34.
13. Warketin TE, Kelton JG. Heparin and platelets. Hematol Oncol Clin North Am 1990;4:243–264.
14. Rice L, Huffman DM, Levine ML, et al. Heparin-induced thrombocytopenia/thrombosis syndromes. Blood 1986;68S:339a.
15. McIntyre KJ, Hoagland HC, Silverstein MN, et al. Essential thrombocythemia in young adults. Mayo Clin Proc 1991;66:149–154.

16. Schafer AI. Essential thrombocythemia. Prog Hemost Thromb 1991;10:69–96.

17. Silver D. Complications of coagulation and splenectomy. In: Greenfield L, ed. Complications in surgery and trauma. 2nd ed. Philadelphia: JB Lippincott, 1990:193–202.

18. Holmsen H. Composition of platelets. In: Williams WJ, Beutler E, Erslev AJ, et al, eds. Hematology. 4th ed. New York: McGraw-Hill, 1990:1182–1200.

19. Rao AK. Congenital disorders of platelet function. Hematol Oncol Clin North Am 1990;4:65–86.

20. Hectman HB, Huval WV, Mathieson MA, et al. Prostaglandin and thromboxane mediation of cardiopulmonary failure. Surg Clin North Am 1983;63:263–283.

21. Prescott SM, McIntyre TM, Zimmerman GA. The role of platelet-activating factor in endothelial cells. Thromb Haemost 1990;64:899–903.

22. Webster MWI, Chesebro JH, Fuster V. Platelet inhibitor therapy: agents and clinical implications. Hematol Oncol Clin North Am 1990;4:265–289.

23. FitzGerald GA. Dipyridamole. N Engl J Med 1987;316:1247–1257.

24. Goodnight SH. Mechanism of the anti-thrombotic effects of fish oil. Bailliere's Clin Haematol 1990;3:601–623.

25. Ashby B, Daniel JL, Smith JB. Mechanism of platelet activation and inhibition. Hematol Oncol Clin North Am 1990;4:1–26.

26. Colman RW. Platelet receptors. Hematol Oncol Clin North Am 1990;4:27–42.

27. McEver RP. The clinical significance of platelet membrane glycoproteins. Hematol Oncol Clin North Am 1990;4:87–105.

28. George JN, Nurden AT, Phillips DR. Molecular defects in interaction of platelets with the vessel wall. N Engl J Med 1984;311:1084–1098.

29. Ginsburg D. The von Willebrand factor gene and genetics of von Willebrand disease. Mayo Clin Proc 1991;66:506–515.

30. Gralnick HR, Williams SB, McKeown LP, et al. Platelet von Willebrand factor. Mayo Clin Proc 1991;66:634–640.

31. Meyer D, Pietu G, Fressinaud E, et al. von Willebrand factor: structure and function. Mayo Clin Proc 1991;66:516–523.

32. Miller JL. von Willebrand disease. Hematol Oncol Clin North Am 1990;4:107–128.

33. Weiss HJ. Von Willebrand factor and platelet function. Ann N Y Acad Sci 1991;614:125–137.

34. Jaffe EA. Cell biology of endothelial cells. Hum Pathol 1987;18:234–239.

35. Mayadas TN, Wagner DD. Von Willebrand factor biosynthesis and processing. Ann N Y Acad Sci 1991;614:153–166.

36. Sixma JJ, deGroot PG. Von Willebrand factor and the blood vessel wall. Mayo Clin Proc 1991;66:628–633.

37. Cattaneo M, Moia M, Delle Valle P, et al. DDAVP shortens the prolonged bleeding times of patients with severe von Willebrand disease treated with cryoprecipitate. Evidence for a mechanism of action independent of released von Willebrand factor. Blood 1989;74:1972–1975.

38. DiMichele DM, Hathaway WE. Use of DDAVP in inherited and acquired platelet dysfunction. Am J Hematol 1990;33:39–45.

39. Mannucci PM. Desmopressin: A nontransfusional hemostatic agent. Annu Rev Med 1990;41:55–64.

40. Lackner H, Karpatkin S. On the "easy bruising" syndrome with normal platelet count: a study of 75 patients. Ann Intern Med 1975;83:190–196.

41. Rodgers RP, Levin J. A critical reappraisal of the bleeding time. Semin Thromb Hemost 1990;16:1–20.

42. Lind S. The bleeding time does not predict surgical bleeding. Blood 1991;77:2547–2552.

43. Bennett JS, Shattil SJ. Platelet function. In: Williams WJ, Beutler E, Erslev AJ, et al, eds. Hematology. 4th ed. New York: McGraw-Hill, 1990:233–1250.

44. Roberts HR, Tabarea AH. Overview of the coagulation reaction. In: High KA, Roberts HR, eds. Molecular basis of thrombosis and hemostasis. New York, Marcel Decker, Inc., 1995:35–50.

45. Bontempo FA, Lewis JH, Gorene TJ, et al. Liver transplantation in hemophilia A. Blood 1987;69:1721–1724.

46. Corriveau DM, Fritsma GA, eds. Hemostasis and thrombosis in the clinical laboratory. Philadelphia: JB Lippincott, 1988.

47. Bovill EG, Malhotra OP, Mann KG. Mechanisms of vitamin K antagonism. Bailliere's Clin Haematol 1990;3:555–581.

48. Hirsh J. Oral anticoagulant drugs. N Engl J Med 1991;324:1865–1875.

49. Tracy PB. Regulation of thrombin generation at cell surfaces. Semin Thromb Hemost 1988;14:227–233.

50. Wun T. Tissue factor pathway inhibitor. In: High KA, Roberts HR, eds. Molecular basis of thrombosis and hemostasis. New York: Marcel Decker, Inc., 1995;331–353.

51. Malar RA, Kless AJ, Griffin JH. An alternative extrinsic pathway of human blood coagulation. Blood 1982;60:1353–1358.

52. Nordfang O, Valentin S, Bec TC, et al. Inhibition of extrinsic pathway inhibitor shortens the coagulation time of normal plasma and of hemophiliac plasma. Thromb Haemost 1991;66:464–467.

53. Carson SD, Brozna JP. The role of tissue factor in the production of thrombin. Blood Coagulation and Fibrinolysis 1993;4:281–291.

54. Mann KG, Jenny RJ, Krishnaswamy S. Cofactor proteins in the assembly and expression of blood clotting enzyme complexes. Ann Rev Biochem 1988;57:915–956.

55. Fenton JW. Regulation of thrombin generation and functions. Sem Thromb Hemost 1988;14:234–240.

56. Abbate R, Gori AM, Modesti PA, et al. Heparin, monocytes, and procoagulant activity. Haemostasis 1990;20(Suppl 1):98–100.

57. Mosesson MW. Fibrin polymerization and its regulatory role in hemostasis. J Lab Clin Med 1990;116:8–17.

58. Jakubowski JA, Maraganore JM. Inhibition of coagulation and thrombin-induced platelet activities by a synthetic docopeptide modeled on the carboxy-terminus of hirudin. Blood 1990;75:399–406.

59. Adams SL. The medicinal leech: historical perspectives. Sem Thromb Hemost 1989;15:261–264.

60. Hoffmann H, Siebeck M, Spannagl M, et al. Effect of recombinant hirudin, a specific inhibitor of thrombin, on endotoxin-induced intravascular coagulation and acute lung injury in pigs. Am Rev Respir Dis 1990;142:782–788.

61. Markwardt F. Development of hirudin as an antithrombotic agent. Sem Thromb Hemost 1989;15:269–282.

62. Fenton JW. Thrombin interactions with hirudin. Sem Thromb Hemost 1989;15:265–268.

63. Mueh JR, Herbest KW, Rapaport S. Thrombosis in patients with the "lupus"-type circulating anticoagulant. Ann Intern Med 1980;92:156–159.

64. Greisman SG, Thayaparan R-S, Godwin TA, et al. Occlusive vasculopathy in systemic lupus erythematosus. Association with anticardiolipin antibody. Arch Intern Med 1991;151:389–392.

65. White GC, Marder VJ, Colman RW, et al. Approach to the bleeding patient. In: Colman RW, Hirsh J, Marder VJ, et al, eds. Hemostasis and thrombosis: basic principles and clinical practice. Philadelphia: JB Lippincott, 1994:1134–1147.

66. Krieger JN, Hilgartner MW, Redo SF. Surgery in patients with congenital disorders of blood coagulation. Ann Surg 1977;185:290–294.

67. Blomback M, Johansson G, Johnsson H, et al. Surgery in patients with von Willebrand's disease. Br J Surg 1989;76:398–400.

68. Hilgartner MW. Factor replacement therapy. In: Hilgartner M, Pochedly C, eds. Hemophilia in the child and adult. New York: Raven Press, 1989:1–26.

69. Morgan CH, Penner JA. Bleeding complications during surgery: part I. Defects of primary hemostasis and congenital coagulation. Lab Med 1986;17:207–212.

70. Kram HB, Nathan RC, Stafford FJ, et al. Fibrin glue achieves hemostasis in patients with coagulation disorders. Arch Surg 1989;124:385–387.

71. Thompson AR. Molecular biology of the hemophilias. Prog Hemost Thromb 1991;10:175–214.

72. Repke D, Gemmell CH, Guha A, et al. Hemophilia as a defect of the tissue factor pathway of blood coagulation: effect of factors VIII and IX on factor X activation of a continuous-flow reactor. Proc Natl Acad Sci U S A 1990;87:7623–7627.

73. Broze GJ. Why do hemophiliacs bleed? Hospital Practice 1992;71–86.

74. Berry EW. Use of DDAVP and cryoprecipitate in mild to moderate hemophilia A and von Willebrand's disease. Prog Clin Biol Res 1990;324:269–278.

75. Pisciott PT, ed. Factor VIII concentrate. In: Blood transfusion therapy—a physician's handbook. Arlington, VA: American Association of Blood Banks, 1989:27–29.

76. Pisciott PT, ed. Factor IX concentrate. In: Blood transfusion ther-

apy—a physician's handbook. Arlingtion, VA: American Association of Blood Banks, 1989:30–31.

77. Lollar P. The association of factor VIII with von Willebrand factor. Mayo Clin Proc 1991;66:524–534.

78. Roberts HR, Jones MR. Hemophilia and related conditions—congenital deficiencies of prothrombin (factor II), factor V, and factors VII to XII. In: Williams WJ, Beutler E, Erslev AJ, et al, eds. Hematology. 4th ed. New York: McGraw-Hill, 1990:1453–1473.

79. Rose EH, Aledort LM. Nasal spray desmopressin (DDAVP) for mild hemophilia and von Willebrand disease. Ann Intern Med 1991;114:563–568.

80. Kasper CK. Treatment of factor VIII inhibitors. Prog Hemost Thromb 1989;9:57–86.

81. Preissner KT. Anticoagulant potential of endothelial cell membrane components. Haemostasis 1988;18:271–300.

82. Tomasini BR, Mosher DF. Vitronectin. Prog Hemost Thromb 1991;10:269–305.

83. Owen J, Kvam D, Nossel HL, et al. Thrombin and plasmin activity and platelet activation in the development of venous thrombosis. Blood 1983;61:476–482.

84. Jaffe EA. Vascular function in hemostasis. In: Williams WJ, Beutler E, Erslev AJ, et al, eds. Hematology. 4th ed. New York: McGraw-Hill, 1990:1322–1337.

85. Wu KR. Endothelial cells in hemostasis, thrombosis and inflammation. Hospital Practice 1992;145–166.

86. Vanhoutte PM, Luscher TF, Graser T. Endothelium-dependent contractions. Blood Vessels 1991;28:74–83.

87. Marcum JA, Rosenberg RD. Role of endothelial cell surface heparin-like polysaccharides. Ann N Y Acad Sci 1989;556:81–94.

88. van Hinsbergh WWM. Regulation of the synthesis and secretion of plasminogen activators by endothelial cells. Haemostasis 1988;18:307–327.

89. Brenner BM, Troy JL, Ballermann BJ. Endothelium-dependent vascular responses: mediators and mechanisms. J Clin Invest 1989;84:1373–1378.

90. Stern DM, Kaiser E, Nawroth PP. Regulation of the coagulation system by vascular endothelial cells. Haemostasis 1988;18:202–214.

91. Bauer KA, Rosenberg RD. Role of antithrombin III as a regulator of in vivo coagulation. Semin Hematol 1991;28:10–18.

92. Beresford CH, Owen MC. Antithrombin III. Int J Biochem 1990;22:121–128.

93. Hathaway WE. Clinical aspects of antithrombin III deficiency. Semin Hematol 1991;28:19–23.

94. Jackson CM. Mechanism of heparin action. Baillieres Clin Haematol 1990;3:483–504.

95. Conrad HE. Structure of heparan sulfate and dermatan sulfate. Ann N Y Acad Sci 1989;556:18–28.

96. Levine MN, Hirsh J. Clinical potential of low molecular weight heparins. Bailliere's Clin Haematol 1990;3:545–554.

97. Menache D. Antithrombin III: An introduction. Semin Hematol 1991;28:1–2.

98. Menache D. Replacement therapy in patients with hereditary antithrombin III deficiency. Semin Hematol 1991;28:31–38.

99. Rosenberg RD. Actions and interactions of antithrombin and heparin. N Engl J Med 1975;292:146–151.

100. Salzman EW. Heparin for prophylaxis of venous thromboembolism. Ann N Y Acad Sci 1989;556:371–385.

101. Tollefsen DM, Sugimori T, Maimone MM. Effect of low molecular weight heparin preparations on the inhibition of thrombin by heparin cofactor II. Semin Thromb Hemost 1990;16:66–70.

102. Bauer KA, Rosenberg RD. Congenital antithrombin III deficiency: insights into the pathogenesis of the hypercoagulable state and its management using markers of hemostatic system activation. Am J Med 1989;87:39S–43S.

103. Buller HR, ten Cate JW. Acquired antithrombin III deficiency: laboratory diagnosis, incidence, clinical implications, and treatment with antithrombin III concentrate. Am J Med 1989;87:44S–48S.

104. Mannucci PM, Tripodi A. Laboratory screening of inherited thrombotic syndromes. Thromb Haemost 1987;57:247–251.

105. Blaisdell FW. Acquired and congenital clotting syndromes. World J Surg 1990;14:664–669.

106. Felez J. Biochemical aspects of the pathogenesis of venous thrombosis. Acta Chir Scand Suppl 1990;556:9–17.

107. Joist JH. Hypercoagulability: Introduction and perspective. Sem Thromb Hemost 1990;16:151–157.

108. Dittmann WA, Majerus PW. Structure and function of thrombomodulin: a natural anticoagulant. Blood 1990;75:329–336.

109. Carlson TH. Clearance of thrombin in vivo: significance of alternative pathways. Mol Cell Biochem 1986;71:97–105.

110. Esmon CT, Johnson AE, Esmon NL. Initiation of the protein C pathway. Ann N Y Acad Sci 1991;614:30–43.

111. Esmon CT. The regulation of natural anticoagulant pathways. Science 1987;235:1348–1352.

112. Esmon CT. The roles of protein C and thrombomodulin in the regulation of blood coagulation. J Biol Chem 1989;264:4743–4746.

113. Esmon CT, Owen WG. Identification of an endothelial cell cofactor for thrombin-catalyzed activation of protein C. Proc Natl Acad Sci U S A 1981;78:2249–2252.

114. Esmon NL. Thrombomodulin. Prog Hemost Thromb 1989;9:29–55.

115. Esmon NL. Thrombomodulin. Semin Thromb Hemost 1987;13:454–463.

116. Esmon NL, Esmon CT. Protein C and the endothelium. Semin Thromb Hemost 1988;14:210–215.

117. Thompson EA, Salem HH. The role of thrombomodulin in the regulation of hemostatic interactions. Progress in Hematology 1987;15:51–70.

118. Clouse LH, Comp PC. The regulation of hemostasis—the protein C system. N Engl J Med 1986;314:1298–1304.

119. Allaart CF, Aronson DC, Ruys T, et al. Hereditary protein S deficiency in young adults with arterial occlusive disease. Thromb Haemost 1990;64:206–210.

120. Comp PC, Elrod JP, Karzenski S. Warfarin-induced skin necrosis. Semin Thromb Hemost 1990;16:293–298.

121. Comp PC. Overview of the hypercoagulable states. Semin Thromb Hemost 1990;16:158–161.

122. Miletich J, Sherman L, Broze G. Absence of thrombosis in subjects with heterozygous protein C deficiency. N Engl J Med 1987;317:991–996.

123. Schafer AI. The hypercoagulable states. Ann Int Med 1985;102:814–828.

124. Thomas JH. Edgar J Poth lecture. Pathogenesis, diagnosis, thrombosis. Am J Surg 1990;160:547–551.

125. Thomas JH, Pierce GE, Delcore R, et al. Primary hypercoagulable states in general and vascular surgery. Am J Surg 1989;158:491–494.

126. Rosenberg RD, Bauer KA. Thrombosis in inherited deficiencies of antithrombin, protein C, and protein S. Hum Pathol 1987;18:253–262.

127. Clark DA, Williams WL, Marlar RA. Mesenteric vein thrombosis associated with a familial deficiency of free protein S. Arch Pathol Lab Med 1991;115:617–619.

128. Moore KL, Andreoli SP, Esmon NL, et al. Endotoxin enhances tissue factor and suppresses thrombomodulin expression of human vascular endothelium in vitro. J Clin Invest 1987;79:124–130.

129. Remuzzi G, Garella S. Hemolytic uremic syndrome and TTP: Variable expression of a single entity. Kidney Int 1987;32:282.

130. Francis CW, Marder VJ. Physiologic regulation and pathologic disorders of fibrinolysis. Hum Pathol 1985;18:263–275.

131. Bennett CR, Mueller S, Anderson HV, et al. Thrombolytic therapy: A state of the art review. Hospital Practice 1992;61–72.

132. Loskutoff DJ, Curriden SA. The fibrinolytic system of the vessel wall and its role in the control of thrombosis. Ann N Y Acad Sci 1990;598:238–247.

133. Robbins KC. Classification of abnormal plasminogens: dysplasminogenemias. Semin Thromb Hemost 1990;16:217–220.

134. Leebeek FW, Knot EA, ten Cate JW, et al. Severe thrombotic tendency associated with a type I plasminogen deficiency. Am J Hematol 1989;30:32–35.

135. Nilsson IM. Clinical pharmacology of aminocaproic and tranexamic acids. J Clin Pathol 1980;33(Suppl 14):41.

136. Collen D, Lijnen HR. Thrombolytic therapy. Ann N Y Acad Sci 1991;614:259–269.

137. Marder VJ, Sherry S. Thrombolytic therapy: Current status. Part I. N Engl J Med 1988;318:1512–1520.

138. Marder VJ, Sherry S. Thrombolytic therapy: Current status. Part II. N Engl J Med 1988;318:1585–1595.

139. Weitz JI. Mechanism of action of the thrombolytic agents. Balliere's Clin Haematol 1990;3:583–599.

140. Meyerovitz MF, Goldhaber SZ, Reagan K, et al. Recombinant tissue-type plasminogen activator versus urokinase in peripheral arterial and graft occlusions: a randomized trial. Radiology 1990; 175:75–78.

141. Francis CW, Marder VJ. Concepts of clot lysis. Annu Rev Med 1986;37:187–204.

142. Rao AK, Pratt C, Berke A, et al. Thrombolysis in myocardial infarction (TIMI) trial—phase I: hemorrhagic manifestations and changes in plasma fibrinogen and the fibrinolytic system in patients treated with recombinant tissue plasminogen activator and streptokinase. J Am Coll Cardiol 1988;11:1–11.

143. Marder VJ. The use of thrombolytic agents: choice of patient, drug administration, laboratory monitoring. Ann Intern Med 1979;90: 802–808.

144. Belkin M, Belkin B, Bucknam CA, et al. Intra-arterial fibrinolytic therapy. Efficacy of streptokinase versus urokinase. Arch Surg 1986;121:769–773.

145. Comerota AJ, Rubin RN, Tyson RR, et al. Intra-arterial thrombolytic therapy in peripheral vascular disease. Surg Gynecol Obstet 1987;165:1–8.

146. Earnshaw JJ, Gregson RH, Makin GS, et al. Early results of low dose intra-arterial streptokinase therapy in acute and subacute lower limb arterial ischemia. Br J Surg 1987;74:504–507.

147. Conrad J, Samama M. Theoretic and practical considerations on laboratory monitoring of thrombolytic therapy. Semin Thromb Hemost 1987;13:212–222.

148. Stump DC, Taylor FB Jr, Nesheim ME, et al. Pathologic fibrinolysis as a cause of clinical bleeding. Semin Thromb Hemost 1990; 16:260–273.

149. Wiman B, Hamsten A. The fibrinolytic enzyme system and its role in the etiology of thromboembolic disease. Semin Thromb Hemost 1990;16:207–216.

150. Bonnar J, Daly L, Sheppard BL. Changes in the fibrinolytic system during pregnancy. Semin Thromb Hemost 1990;16:221–229.

151. Kwaan HC, Keer HN. Fibrinolysis and cancer. Semin Thromb Hemost 1990;16:230–235.

152. Totty WG, Gilula LA, McClennan BL, et al. Low-dose intravascular fibrinolytic therapy. Diagnostic Radiology 1982;143:59–69.

153. Verhaeghe R, Wilms G, Vermylen J. Local low-dose thrombolysis in arterial disease of the limbs. Simin Thromb Hemost 1987;13: 206–211.

154. Addonizio VP, Stahl RF. Bleeding. In: Wimore DL, Brennan MF, Harken AH, et al, eds. American College of Surgeons care of the surgical patient. Vol. I. Critical care. New York: Scientific American, 1992:1–13.

155. Morgan CH, Penner JA. Bleeding complications during surgery: part II. Acquired hemorrhagic disorders. Laboratory Medicine 1986;17:262–266.

156. Mulcare RJ, Royster TS, Weiss HJ, et al. Disseminated intravascular coagulation as a complication of abdominal aortic aneurysm repair. Ann Surg 1974;180:343–349.

157. Nand S, Messmore H. Hemostasis in malignancy. Am J Hematol 1990;35:45–55.

158. Saldeen T. Clotting, microembolism, and inhibition of fibrinolysis in adult respiratory distress. Surg Clin North Am 1983;63: 285–304.

159. Siebert WT, Natelson EA. Chronic consumption coagulopathy accompanying abdominal aortic aneurysm. Arch Surg 1976;111: 539–541.

160. Sherman LA. DIC in massive transfusion. Prog Clin Biol Res 1982; 108:171–189.

161. Ten Cate JW, Timmers H, Becker AE. Coagulopathy in ruptured or dissecting abdominal aortic aneurysm. Am J Med 1975;59: 171–176.

162. Schafer AI. Bleeding and thrombosis in the myeloproliferative disorders. Blood 1984;64:1–12.

163. Suffredini AF, Harpel PC, Parrillo JE. Promotion and subsequent inhibition of plasminogen activation after administration of intravenous endotoxin to normal subjects. N Engl J Med 1989;320: 1165–1172.

164. Carvalho AC. Acquired platelet dysfunction in patients with uremia. Hematol Oncol Clin North Am 1990;4:129–143.

165. Castillo R, Lozano T, Escolar G, et al. Defective platelet adhesion on vessel subendothelium in uremic patients. Blood 1986;68: 337–342.

166. Bronner MH, Pate MB, Cunningham JT. Estrogen-progesterone therapy for bleeding of gastrointestinal telangiectasias in chronic renal failure. Ann Int Med 1986;105:371–374.

167. Janson PA, Jubelier SJ, Weinstein MJ, et al. Treatment of the bleeding tendency in uremia with cryoprecipitate. N Engl J Med 1980; 303:1318–1322.

168. Lethagen S, Rugarn P, Aberg M, et al. Effects of desmopressin acetate (DDAVP) and dextran on hemostatic and thromboprophylactic mechanisms. Acta Chirurgica Scandinavia 1990;156: 597–602.

169. Soslau G, Schwartz AB, Putatunda B, et al. Desmopressin-induced improvement in bleeding times in chronic renal failure patients correlates with platelet serotonin uptake and ADP release. Am J Med Sci 1990;300:372–379.

170. Triulzi DJ, Blumberg N. Variability in response to cryoprecipitate treatment for hemostatic defects in uremia. Yale J Biol Med 1990; 63:1–7.

171. Mannucci PM, Remuzzi G, Pusinerif F, et al. Deamino-8D-agrinine vasopressin shortens the bleeding time in uremia. N Engl J Med 1983;308:8–12.

172. Krauss JS, Jonah MH. Platelet dysfunction (thrombocytopathy) in extrahepatic biliary obstruction. South Med J 1982;75:506–507.

173. Rock WA. Laboratory assessment of coagulation disorders in liver disease. Clin Lab Med 1984;4:419–442.

174. Addonizio VP Jr, Fisher CA, Strauss JF III, et al. Preliminary characterization of the procoagulant material in human ascites. Surgery 1987;101:753–762.

175. Collins JA. Recent developments in the area of massive transfusion. World J Surg 1987;11:75–81.

176. Harrigan C, Lucas CE, Ledgerwood AM, et al. Primary hemostasis after massive transfusion for injury. Am Surg 1982;48:393–396.

177. Hewson JR, Neame PB, Kumar N, et al. Coagulopathy related to dilution and hypotension during massive transfusion. Crit Care Med 1985;13:387–391.

178. Patterson A. Massive transfusion. Int Anesthesiol Clin 1987;25: 61–74.

179. Phillips TF, Soulier G, Wilson RF. Outcome of massive transfusion exceeding two blood volumes in trauma and emergency surgery. J Trauma 1987;27:903–910.

180. Riska EF, Bostman O, von Bonsdorff H, et al. Outcome of closed injuries exceeding 20 unit blood transfusion need. Injury 1988; 19:273.

181. Rudolph R, Boyd CR. Massive transfusion: complications and their management. South Med J 1990;83:1065–1070.

182. Rutledge R, Sheldon GF, Collins ML. Massive transfusion. Crit Care Clin 1986;2:791–780.

183. Sawyer PR, Harrison CR. Massive transfusion in adults. Diagnoses, survival and blood bank support. Vox Sang 1990;58: 199–203.

184. Wilson RF, Dulchavsky SA, Soullier G, et al. Problems with twenty or more blood transfusions in 24 hours. Am Surg 1987; 53:410–417.

185. Edmunds LH, Addonizio VP. Massive transfusion. In: Colman RW, Hirsh J, Marder VJ, et al, eds. Hemostasis and thrombosis: basic principles and clinical practice. Philadelphia: JB Lippincott, 1987:913–919.

186. Wudel JH, Morris JA Jr, Yates K, et al. Massive transfusion: outcome in blunt trauma patients. J Trauma 1991;31:1–7.

187. Ferrara A, MacArthur JD, Wright HK, et al. Hypothermia and acidosis worsen coagulopathy in the patient requiring massive transfusion. Am J Surg 1990;160:515–518.

188. Valeri CR, Feingold H, Cassidy G, et al. Hypothermia-induced reversible platelet dysfunction. Ann Surg 1987;205:175–181.

189. Reed RL II, Heimbach DM, Counts RB, et al. Prophylactic platelet administration during massive transfusion: A prospective, randomized, double-blind clinical study. Ann Surg 1986;203:40–48.

190. Slichter SJ. Platelet transfusion therapy. Hematol Oncol Clin North Am 1990;4:291–311.

191. Pisciott, PT, ed. Massive transfusion. In: Blood transfusion therapy—a physician's handbook. Arlington, VA: American Association of Blood Banks, 1989:52–53.

192. Till JE, McCulloch EA. A direct measurement of the radiation sensitivity of the normal mouse bone marrow. Radiat Res 1961; 14:213–218.

193. Becker AG, McCulloch EA, Till JA. Cytological demonstration of the clonal nature of spleen colonies derived from transplanted mouse marrow cells. Nature 1963;197:452–454.

194. Erslev AJ, Lichtman MA. Structure and function of the marrow. In: Williams WJ, Beutler E, Erslev AJ, Lichtman MA, eds. Hematology. 4th ed. New York: McGraw-Hill, 1990:37–47.

195. Quesenberry PJ, McNiece IK, Robinson BE, et al. Stromal regulation of lymphoid and myeloid differentiation. Blood Cells 1987; 13:137–146.

196. Torok-Storb B. Cellular interactions. Blood 1988;72:373–385.

197. Robinson BE, Quesenberry PJ. Review: Hematopoietic growth factors: overview and clinical applications. Part I. Am J Med Sci 1990;300:163–170.

198. Robinson BE, Quesenberry PJ. Review: Hematopoietic growth factors: overview and clinical applications. Part II. Am J Med Sci 1990;300:237–244.

199. Robinson BE, Quesenberry PJ. Review: Hematopoietic growth factors: overview and clinical applications. Part III. Am J Med Sci 1990;300:311–321.

200. Erslev AJ. Production of erythrocytes. In: Williams WJ, Beutler E, Erslev AJ, et al, eds. Hematology. 4th ed. New York: McGraw-Hill, 1990:389–398.

201. Bunn HF. Erythropoietin: current status. Yale J Biol Med 1990; 63:381–386.

202. Erslev AJ. Erythropoietin. N Engl J Med 1991;324:1339–1344.

203. Krantz SB. Erythropoietin. Blood 1991;77:419–434.

204. Eschbach JW, Kelly MR, Haley NR, et al. Treatment of the anemia of progressive renal failure with recombinant human erythropoietin. N Engl J Med 1989;321:158–163.

205. Eschbach JW, Abdulhadi MH, Browne JK, et al. Recombinant human erythropoietin in anemic patients with end-stage renal disease: results of a phase III multicenter clinical trial. Ann Intern Med 1989;111:992–1000.

206. Greenburg AG. Indications for transfusion. In: Wilmore DL, Brennan MF, Harken AH, et al, eds. American College of Surgeons care of the surgical patient. Vol. I. Critical care. New York: Scientific American, 1989:1–19.

207. Hebert PC, Wells G, Marshall J, et al. Transfusion requirements in critical care: A pilot study. JAMA 1995;273:1439–1444.

208. Rock WA Jr, Boral LI. Blood product replacement in obstetrics and gynecology. In: Rock JA, Faro S, Gant NF, et al, eds. Advances in obstetrics and gynecology. Mosby-Year Book 1995;2:71–90.

209. Welch HG, Meehan KR, Goodnough LT. Prudent strategies for elective red blood cell transfusion. Ann Inter Med 1992;116: 323–332.

210. Dodd RY. The risk of transfusion-transmitted infection. New Engl J Med 1994;327:419–420.

211. College of American Pathologists. Practice parameters for the use of fresh frozen plasma, cryoprecipitate, and platelets. JAMA 1994; 271:777–781.

212. Harmening-Pittiglio D, Flynn JC. The ABO blood group system. In: Harmening D, ed. Modern blood banking and transfusion practices. 2nd ed. Philadelphia: FA Davis, 1989:78–104.

213. Silberstein L, Spitalnik SL. Blood group antigens and antibodies. In: Rossi EC, Simon TL, Moss GS, eds. Principles of transfusion medicine. Baltimore: Williams & Wilkins, 1990:63–78.

214. O'Connor KL. The Rh blood group system. In: Harmening D, ed. Modern blood banking and transfusion practices. 2nd ed. Philadelphia: FA Davis, 1989:105–119.

215. Pisciotto, PT, ed. Transfusion reactions. In: Blood transfusion therapy—a physician's handbook. Arlington, VA: American Association of Blood Banks, 1989:77–86.

20 The Musculoskeletal System

Keith C. Donatto

Introduction

Bone, together with cartilage, ligaments, and tendons, is referred to collectively as the connective tissues. Their main function is mechanical: they provide support, movement, and protection for the body. Unlike the parenchymal organs (e.g., the liver and kidneys), which are composed of cellular elements, the connective tissues are composed of mostly extracellular substances that are appropriate for the mechanical functions of these tissues.

Bone is well-suited to the special needs of vertebrates. An upright posture places substantial load on the skeleton. Given the fact that a 1-in.^{3} block of bone can support a load of 2 tons, its comprehensive strength is more than adequate. Its tensile strength approximates that of a cast iron, yet it is 3 times lighter and 10 times more flexible (1). These impressive mechanical properties depend on bone's matrix structure. Separate from this is the biologic behavior of bone, which depends on the composition of the bone matrix and the activities of the living bone cells.

In a cursory view of orthopedics as a field, bone could appear to be treated as an inert material similar to plastic or metal. However, bone is composed of dynamic living cells that perform specific biologic functions in addition to acting as structural material. Like most of the tissues in the body, bone is innervated, supplied by blood vessels and lymphatics, and consists of both an intracellular and extracellular matrix. It is different, however, from these other tissues in that the matrix to cell ratio is much higher. Bone is composed of a heterogenous population of cells. Each of these cells has a specialized function, such as bone formation, bone remodeling, bone repair, and mineral homeostasis. The large, extracellular organic matrix of bone is formed primarily by collagen. This organic matrix of bone mineralizes to produce the unique integration of organic and inorganic matrices

that give bone its great strength. During life, the matrix is dynamic. The living cells within the matrix continually alter their environment and, consequently, the properties of the bone. Because of this, traumatic injuries may be repaired and bone restored to its original strength and form without scar formation (1). The durability of this matrix is seen after cellular functions within the bone cease. Even after death, bone retains most of its strength owing to its mineralization.

Bone Formation

There are two mechanisms of bone formation: enchondral ossification and intramembranous ossification (1–6). Although some bones, such as the vertebral column and most of the appendicular skeleton, form through enchondral ossification, others, such as the bones in the face, form by intramembranous ossification. Some bones are formed by both mechanisms (e.g., the clavicle). These bones have their primary formation through intramembranous ossification, but there is a secondary center of ossification and a growth plate that forms through enchondral ossification. These mechanisms, although different, do not alter the ultimate structure of mature bone.

Enchondral Ossification

Bones formed by enchondral ossification begin with an aggregation of undifferentiated mesenchymal cells. These cells first form a mesenchymal model of the bone that they are to become. They then differentiate into chondrocytes, which form a hyaline cartilage model of bone. Chondrocyte hypertrophy occurs and is associated with vascular invasion, which leads to matrix mineralization. The vascular buds are accompanied by osteoprogenitor cells, which are pluripotent at that time. They eventually differentiate into osteoblasts, forming a bone matrix on the mineralized cartilage. Osteoclasts

then resorb the trabeculae of bone and calcified cartilage. Osteoblasts replace the mixed calcified cartilage
and immature bone with mature lamellar bone (1,5,6).
This process is responsible for formation of all long
bones other than the clavicle. The short bones and the
epiphyseal centers of ossification are also formed by enchondral ossification. This process continues in the
growth plate until skeletal maturity is reached. This
same process participates in the healing of certain fractures throughout the life of the bone.

Intramembranous Ossification

Intramembranous bone formation is initiated by aggregation of common mesenchymal cells into condensed layers. Within these layers, a loose collagenous
matrix of vessels, osteoprogenitor cells, fibroblasts, and
common mesenchymal cells are synthesized (1). As in
enchondral ossification, the osteoprogenitor cells differentiate into osteoblasts. They begin to deposit a bone
matrix and, subsequently, become mature osteocytes. In
contrast to enchondral ossification, no cartilaginous
model of the bone is formed. Most of the bones formed
by intramembranous ossification are flat bones. This
process occurs during embryonic development. Subsequently, bones that are formed by intramembranous ossification grow by periosteal new bone formation. This
process also increases the diameter of bones that originally were formed by enchondral ossification. The periosteum forms new bone directly without a preceding
cartilaginous model. Therefore, it is often considered a
form of intramembranous ossification.

The Growth Plate

The growth plate, or epiphysis, is the area in which
enchondral ossification takes place. It is responsible for
the increase in length of maturing bones. The growth
plate has been divided into separate zones, according
to cell morphology and function (Fig. 20.1). It begins at
the top of the reserve zone and ends at the last intact
transverse septum of the hypertrophic zone. The reserve
zone begins immediately beneath the secondary bony
epiphysis. It is followed by the proliferative zone and
then the hypertrophic zone. The hypertrophic zone is
subdivided into the zone of maturation, the zone of degradation, and the zone of provisional calcification.

Proliferative Zone

The proliferative zone is within the epiphyseal plate.
It is located directly beneath the bony epiphysis and
consists of sparsely distributed round to spherical cells
that exist singly or in pairs. The cells are separated
widely by a cartilaginous matrix. These cells contain
more lipid bodies and vacuoles than do cells in any other
zones (7). In contrast, the chondrocytes in the proliferative zone are more flattened and are arranged in longitudinal columns separated by a long, longitudinal cartilage septa. The matrix in this zone constitutes
approximately 75% of the volume; the cells account for
the remaining 25% (7). Cells in this area show a high
rate of metabolic activity and rapidly proliferate. They
are primarily responsible for the longitudinal growth of
long bones and providing cells for the rest of the growth
plate. Although the central cells divide and synthesize
matrix, the cells on the periphery of the proliferative
zone produce appositional growth.

Hypertrophic Zone

Histologic examination of the hypertrophic zone
shows more spherical and greatly enlarged cells. A great

Figure 20.1. Zonal division of the
cartilaginous portion of a growth plate.

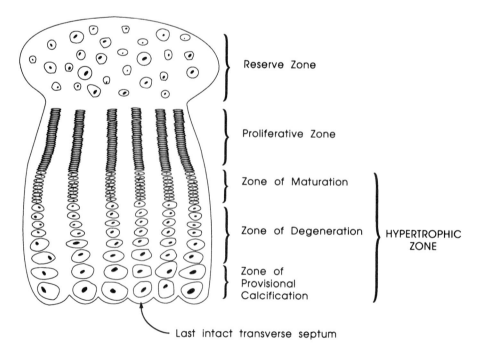

change of the ratio of relative volumes of matrix to cells also occurs. Here, the matrix constitutes only about 40% of the volume, and the cells account for the remaining 60% (7). Based on changes in the cells and the matrix, the hypertrophic zone can be divided into three separate zones: the zone of maturation, the zone of degeneration, and the zone of provisional calcification. The arrangement in the hypertrophic zone resembles that of the proliferative zone. Chondrocytes are arranged in columns that are separated by cartilaginous septa. As each cell passes through the entire hypertrophic zone, they enlarge to fivefold the size they were in the proliferative zone. As they progress downward, they undergo degenerative changes that end in degeneration and cell death at the base of the cell column. In this area of cell death is the zone of provisional calcification. Here, the longitudinal cartilage septa calcify, whereas the transverse septa, joining adjacent longitudinal septa, do not. An abrupt change from uncalcified to calcified matrix occurs. This mineralization does not extend beyond the region of provisional calcification.

Once calcification occurs, the sequence of events that replaces calcified cartilage with mature lamellar bone is initiated.

Bone Structure

Bones are classified into three groups according to their shape: long bones, short bones, and flat bones (3). Long bones (the femur and tibia) are composed of a thick-walled tubular mid-section called the diaphysis. Each end of a tubular bone is characterized by an expansion of the structure. The cortical wall of bone at each end is much thinner. This area of bone is called the metaphysis. Farther toward the end of the bone is the epiphysis. This area is covered with articular cartilage and constitutes one portion of a synovial joint. Short bones have the same composition as long bones but are approximately the same length in all directions. Examples include the carpal bones of wrist and the tarsal bones of the foot. Most of these bones have relatively thin cortices on their external surfaces. Flat bones are characterized by a large discrepancy in dimensions. Their length usually is much larger than their width; examples include the scapula and the wing of the ilium.

Bone is also divided into cortical and cancellous components. Cortical bone is commonly known as compact bone, whereas cancellous bone is known as trabecular bone. Cortical bone, the predominant form in the skeleton (constituting approximately 80% of total body bone volume), is found primarily in the diaphysis of long bones (3). Trabecular bone is found primarily in the vertebral bodies, flat bones of the pelvis, and the metaphysis of long bones. Each individual bone is composed of both a cortical and cancellous component.

Both types of bone are dynamic. Hence, the structure is modified in response to load, hormonal influence, and the stress of mobilization. However, the responses to these influences differ in both manner and rate for the two different types of bone. Cancellous (trabecular) bone is characterized by large surface area per unit volume. Its cell population lies primarily between lamellae and the surface of the trabeculae. In contrast, cortical bone is much more dense. It has approximately 5% of the surface area per unit volume of cancellous bone (3,8). Most of its cell population lies between lamellae and is surrounded completely by a mature bony matrix. Another difference between these two forms of bone is found in their nourishment. Blood vessels rarely penetrate cancellous bone, and hence the cells receive nourishment by diffusion from marrow vessels. In contrast, diaphysial cortical bone relies primarily on a complex intraosseous circulatory system.

Remodeling occurs through different means as well. In cortical bone, osteoclasts must tunnel through dense compact bone to allow remodeling. Cancellous bone is remodeled by cells lying on the abundant trabecular surfaces. Because of this organization, cancellous bone usually has a higher rate of metabolic activity and remodeling. Therefore, it responds more rapidly to changes in mechanical loads and metabolic disease.

Given all these differences in the structure of cancellous and cortical bone, the material properties of these two forms are surprisingly similar. To eliminate the structural differences, discrepancies in density and orientation must be compensated for during testing. Thick, stiff, tubular cortical bone provides maximum resistance to torsion and bending, whereas the more flexible trabecular bone more evenly distributes suddenly applied loads. As may be inferred, both of these properties are desirable and each has its importance in resisting injury to the structural integrity of the bone.

Mineralized Bone

Mineralized bone exists in two forms: woven (immature) and lamellar (mature). Woven bone may be viewed as the template of mature lamellar bone. It forms the embryonic skeleton and normally is replaced by mature bone as the skeleton develops. This type of bone forms on the calcified cartilage model during enchondral ossification. Osteoclasts and chondroclasts resorb woven bone in calcified cartilage, which is then replaced with mature lamellar bone. Woven bone is rarely found in the normal human skeleton after the age of 5 years. However, it may appear in healing fractures, certain metabolic diseases, neoplastic processes, or in response to inflammation.

Distinct biologic and mechanical differences exist between these two forms of bone. This results from the manner in which the bone is formed by osteoblasts. The

Figure 20.2. Schematic view of the cortical portion of the shaft of a long bone. It is composed of osteons, or haversian systems, with inner and outer circumferential lamellae. A complete osteon is composed of a central haversian canal, cement line, concentric lamellae, canaliculi, and lacunae. Interstitial lamellae lie between completed haversian systems. Volkmann's canals establish cross-connections between osteons.

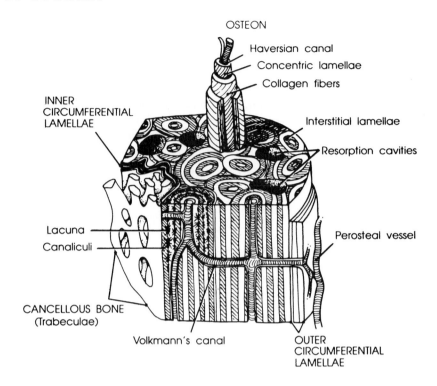

matrix of woven bone has a high deposition rate and turnover compared with lamellar bone. Woven bone also has a more random pattern of collagen fibrils. These fibrils contain approximately four times as many osteocytes per unit volume as does lamellar bone (3,8). This explains the difference in turnover rates. In addition, the osteocytes of woven bone are not homogenous. They are of different size, orientation, and distribution compared with those found in lamellar bone. Given the lack of orientation of collagen fibrils, the mineralization of woven bone follows an irregular pattern. Deposits vary in size and relationship to the fibril. The combination of a high cell and water content, irregular mineralization, and lack of collagen fibril orientation leads to a more flexible and easily deformed type of bone.

The collagen fibrils of lamellar bone are more uniform in diameter and are tightly organized into parallel sheets. There are distinct lamellae 4 to 12 μm thick with a more even distribution of mineralization of the matrix. This microscopic structure gives lamellar bone its strength and rigidity (Fig. 20.2).

Each lamella consists of densely packed collagen fibrils that are oriented in the same direction. Fibrils and adjacent lamellae run in different directions. This alternating pattern is responsible for the strength of the bone. The collagen fibrils interconnect within a single lamella and between lamellae.

The bulk of the diaphyseal cortical bone of the mature skeleton is formed by osteons (3,8,9). These structures consist of a centrally placed neurovascular canal surrounded by concentric interconnected lamellae (see Fig. 20.2). Cement lines, or reversal lines, mark sites where bone resorption has ceased and new bone formation be-

gins. These lines also define the outer boundary of an osteon. The osteons spiral around the diaphysis having the same orientation as the long axis of the bone. The central canal of an osteon, the Haversian canal, contains blood vessels and lymphatics. Occasionally, nerves may also be found within the canal. The living osteocytes must have a constant blood supply to perform their functions. Because diffusion of nutrients through mineralized bone matrix is limited, the cells depend primarily on small connections between the central canal and the osteocytes. Regulation of bone metabolism depends on the connection between the central canal to the osteocytes as well as a connection from osteocyte to osteocyte. This is accomplished by canaliculi, which contain the cell processes of the osteocytes. The canaliculi extend in a radial pattern from the central canal, similar to spokes of a bicycle wheel.

The osteons branch and anastomose, as do the canaliculi. They also join obliquely oriented vascular canals, referred to as Volkmann's canal. These intraosseous vascular canals run both in the longitudinal direction of the bone and toward the periosteal and endosteal surfaces. For this reason, woven bone must be replaced by mature lamellar bone to meet the demands of the strength and structural integrity placed on the mature skeleton.

Blood Supply

Diaphyseal and metaphyseal bone have essentially the same pattern of blood supply and can be divided

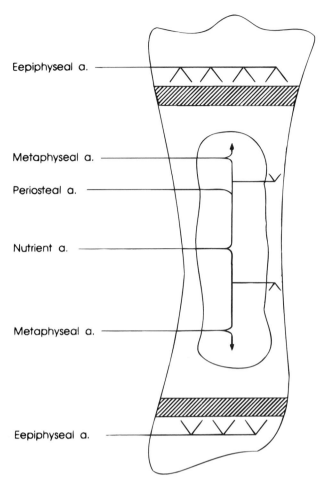

Eepiphyseal a.

Metaphyseal a.

Periosteal a.

Nutrient a.

Metaphyseal a.

Eepiphyseal a.

Figure 20.3. Schematic diagram of the blood supply to a typical long bone. The nutrient artery branches proximally and distally after entering the medullary canal. Periosteal vessels give diaphyseal and metaphyseal bone a dual blood supply by joining the medullary system. The metaphyseal arteries also anastomose with the medullary system. The epiphysis receives a direct blood supply. At maturation with physeal closure, an anastomosis forms between the medullary vascular system and the epiphyseal system.

seus anastomosis develops between the penetrating epiphyseal arteries and the medullary arteries. Although this anastomosis may be extensive, the epiphyseal penetrating vessels still provide an important contribution.

The vascular supply of periosteum is also complex. The fine vessels that overlie the surface of the periosteum anastomose with vessels within the skeletal muscle and with vessels in the cambium layer. An intraosseous connection is achieved via penetration of cambium vessels into the cortical bone. Similar to the fate of the epiphyseal vessels, periosteal vessels eventually diminish and their contribution to the total blood supply of bone becomes less important. Although they are no longer substantial contributors to the total blood supply of bone, these periosteal vessels do remain active and constitute a portion of the bone circulation throughout life (3).

Because of the anastomosis between the periosteal system and the medullary vascular system, the diaphysis has a dual blood supply. This suggests that the diaphysis can receive the majority of its necessary blood supply from either the periosteal or medullary system. As such, damage to one or the other of these systems will not necessarily lead to death of the bone.

Periosteum

The periosteum is a tough connective tissue membrane covering the external surface of bone and consisting of an outer fibrous layer and an inner, more vascular layer. The inner layer contains cells that are capable of becoming osteoblasts and is thus referred to as the cambium or the osteogenic layer. The cells of this layer can also form hyaline cartilage under appropriate circumstances. During bone growth, these cells secrete the organic matrix that enlarges the diameter of the bone. The dense outer layer has fewer cells and much more collagen and is, therefore, much stronger than the inner layer. With age, the periosteum becomes thinner and the inner cambium layer loses its osteogenic capacity. At skeletal maturity, the cambium layer has disappeared almost completely, and the more superficial fibrous layer has become thin and atrophic. Although these metabolic and structural changes occur at skeletal maturity, the periosteum is still capable of forming bone throughout life.

The Cellular Component of Bone

Bone is a dynamic living entity. As such, bone has several different types of cells that perform specific functions necessary for growth and maturation. These cells

into three sources: nutrient arteries, metaphyseal penetrating arteries, and periosteal arteries (Fig. 20.3). The nutrient artery is the main supplier of diaphyseal and metaphyseal bone (3,6,10). It enters the diaphysis and branches to run longitudinally in the bone. There are multiple anastomoses between the terminal ends of the proximal and distal branches of the nutrient artery and the fine branches from the periosteal and metaphyseal arteries. This configuration of interconnected arteries forms the medullary arterial system. Normally, this system supplies the majority of periosteum covered cortical bone. This pattern changes where muscle or ligaments insert onto the bone. In these areas where dense fascial tissue is connected, periosteal vessels supply the outer third of the cortex.

In bone with open physes, the epiphysis depends primarily on its penetrating vessels for its blood supply. Rarely do the medullary vessels cross the open physeal plate. At maturity, with closure of the physis, an interos-

include osteoprogenitor cells, osteoblasts, osteocytes, and osteoclasts.

The osteoprogenitor or undifferentiated cells reside in several areas. They are usually found in the bone canal, the endosteum, or the periosteum (3,6). These cells are small and are irregularly shaped. They are mononuclear and contain relatively few organelles. Until stimulated by specific mechanical and histochemical signals, they remain in this immature undifferentiated state. Once stimulated, they proliferate and differentiate into more mature osteoblasts.

In contrast to undifferentiated osteoprogenitor cells, osteoblasts line bone surfaces, and their physical form differs according to their metabolic activity. If the osteoblasts have been stimulated to synthesize osteoid, they assume a round to oval or even polyhedral shape (3,6,11). They become separated from the bone on which they lay because of the deposition of osteoid. Metabolically active osteoblasts contain an abundant endoplasmic reticulum, multiple mitochondria, and large Golgi membranes. These organelles are responsible for powering the cell as well as for production of the numerous proteins found in osteoid. Just as mature osteocytes have complex interconnections among themselves, the immature osteoblasts are also connected to osteocytes deep within the mineralized matrix. These specialized contacts may help to coordinate both the deposition and maturation of the newly deposited osteoid (6,11).

Active osteoblasts have differing fates. If the cell remains on the bone surface, the synthetic activity is reduced and the cell becomes flatter, with a significant decrease in its organelle component. If the osteoblast surrounds itself with matrix, it becomes an osteocyte. Again, this cell has less cytoplasm and fewer organelles than active osteoblasts. Osteoblasts, although extremely active metabolically, rarely divide.

Osteocytes are the predominant cell found in mature bone. They remain mononuclear, as do their osteoblast precursors. Similarly, organelle content and cytoplasm varies with metabolic activity. These cells maintain a dynamic interconnection among themselves via long cytoplasmic processes. The metabolic activities are well-coordinated via this contact with other mature and immature cells within the bone matrix. Because of this extensive structural arrangement and interconnection in bone, osteocytes can govern the function of a large amount of mineralized bone matrix surface area. This is important in cell-mediated exchange between bone fluid and blood.

Although osteocytes are thought of primarily as the cells that are responsible for maintenance of bone, evidence exists that these cells may also participate in bone resorption. They may also exhibit some hypertrophy and contribute to some new bone synthesis. They do participate in the hypercalcemic response to parathyroid hormone by removing mineral from the surrounding bone matrix (3).

Unlike the previously mentioned cells, the osteoclast is primarily a cell of bone resorption. Its structure, which is well-suited to its role in extensive bone remodeling, is characterized by multiple nuclei and a large irregular form. Its organelle content is much more substantial than both the osteoblast and osteocyte. The distinguishing feature of these cells is their ruffled, or brush border. It is a complex folding of the cytoplasmic membrane that is designed specifically for bone matrix resorption. The complex involutions of the cytoplasmic membrane increase the surface area of the cell relative to the bony surface. There is also a region—the clear zone—within the cell that is free of organelles. The clear zone surrounds the brush border and may in fact allow unobstructed movement of this structure. Deep to the ruffled border is a region containing membrane-bound vesicles and vacuoles. These structures may be separate and distinct from the brush border or be a continuation of that membrane. They appear to contain the collagen and mineral that has been resorbed from mature bone and brought into the cell.

Osteoclasts are found in both cancellous and dense cortical bone. The method of bone resorption differs between these two types of bone. In cancellous bone, osteoclasts' cells create a clear zone around them, known as a Howship's lacuna. This clear zone is formed by direct resorption of the surrounding porous bone. In contrast, the osteoclasts of dense cortical bone lead to osteonal cutting cones that remodel the bone (3,6,8,9). Osteoclasts may vary in their metabolic activity. They are mobile and may gain or lose nuclei and organelles according to bone-mediated mineral metabolism (3).

Although the three cell lines (osteoblasts, osteocytes, and osteoclasts) are connected, the osteoclast's origin is uncertain. The pluripotent osteoprogenitor cells clearly have the capacity to differentiate into osteoblasts, if the appropriate stimulation is received. These osteoblasts may mature to become osteocytes. Most bone biologists agree that the osteoblast and osteoclast come from different cell lines. Experiments have shown that blood-borne monocytes form osteoclasts (3). The differentiation of a monocyte and osteoclast may be mediated by contact between the monocyte precursor cell and the mineralized bone matrix. If this is the case, the monocyte is somehow attracted to the bone matrix, and its differentiation into an osteoclast depends on a specific component within the matrix. The life span of the osteoclast is unknown.

Bone Matrix

Bone has mechanical properties that are a function of its extracellular matrix. The combination of an inorganic and organic component leads to a strong, yet dynamic construct. The inorganic component of bone constitutes 70% to 80% of bones' net weight. This corresponds to an organic component of 10% to 20%; water makes up the remainder of the weight (3). The excellent tensile strength of bone is primarily the result of collagen (8). Collagen's orientation and function as scaffolding for mineralization gives bone its final shape. Compressive forces are resisted primarily by the rigid mineral component of the matrix. An imbalance in the ratio of either component will lead either to a soft, pliable structure that is not resistive to compressive forces, or to a brittle and rigid structure that can be fractured easily. Inspection of the makeup of the organic matrix of bone reveals more than 90% Type I collagen; the remaining 10% is a complex of noncollagenous proteins, glycoproteins, and proteoglycans (3,11). Type I and Type II are the primary collagens found in the body. Type I collagen differs from other collagen at both the molecular and macroscopic levels. Its relatively large diameter fibrils make it ideal for tissues subjected to large tensile loads.

Osteoblasts are responsible for deposition of the immature organic matrix (3,6,11). The matrix first appears as osteoid, which contains a large amount of water and noncollagenous matrix macromolecules. Although the materials within the osteoid do not change, the relative composition of the organic matrix is dynamic. As mineralization of the matrix occurs, the large amount of water and noncollagenous matrix molecules are lost. An apparent deposition of more insoluble mineral molecules also occurs. The collagen precursor remains constant in its absolute amount, although its form changes. Once the process of mineralization is complete, the new mature organic matrix remains relatively unchanged until resorption. Any abnormality in the makeup of the organic component results in bone that is less resistant to mechanical forces than is normal bone.

Although the mechanisms of matrix mineralization remain controversial, this deposition radically changes the material properties of the immature bone. Although varying postulations exist as to how matrix mineralization is controlled, most theories agree that osteoblasts are responsible for both deposition of immature osteoid and have some control over its subsequent mineralization (3). Osteoid (bone matrix) contains molecules that combine both organic and inorganic components. The organic collagen has bonding sites that can catalyze mineral nucleation as well as maturation of mineral crystals. This mineralization process seems to be controlled by osteoblasts that not only induce the process but also produce inhibitors that may govern the rate of inorganic ion transfer. This is done primarily through the regulation of calcium and phosphates progression from a soluble ion state to a relatively insoluble crystalline state. Calcium may also be sequestered intracellularly and released at the appropriate time to stimulate mineralization.

In newly mineralized bone, calcium and phosphate bind in an array of patterns. Some of the calcium phosphate is relatively soluble, whereas more mature calcium phosphate crystallizes into hydroxyapatite particles. The greater the maturity of the bone, the more insoluble hydroxyapatite it contains. Other elements and compounds may also be present. These include sodium, magnesium, citrate, and fluoride. The crystalline form of these minerals is found usually within the structure of the collagen fibrils of mature bone. Once the process of mineralization begins, it proceeds over a prolonged period of time, gradually increasing the amount of mineral content, thus leading to an increase in bone density.

Calcium Metabolism

The levels of intracellular and extracellular calcium are tightly regulated. At the macroscopic level, calcium balance is maintained by three organ systems: intestine, bone, and kidney (11). In all these systems, hormones are used to modulate organ function with respect to calcium metabolism.

Calcium is absorbed actively from the duodenum. This is accomplished by a calcium-binding protein located in the duodenal wall. In low-calcium diets, the majority of dietary calcium is taken up by this active absorption process. Farther along in the small intestine, the jejunum allows passive diffusion of calcium. In diets replete with calcium, the majority of calcium is absorbed via the passive transport system. This is the result of the limitation of active transport by the amount of available calcium-binding protein, the intestinal pH level, and the transit time in the duodenum. The dietary requirement for calcium changes throughout life. Early and late in life, there is an increased need for calcium. During maturation, skeletal mineralization makes great demands on the body's stores of calcium. Similarly, later in life, there is an increased need for dietary calcium to counteract the net loss of calcium from the body caused by increased bone resorption. During these periods of increased stress, the recommended intake is approximately 1500 mg of elemental calcium per day (11). Given an adequate dietary intake, the average adult absorbs approximately 300 to 400 mg of elemental calcium per day (11). Between 33% and 50% of this is secreted back into the intestinal lumen, resulting in a net intake of approximately 200 mg/day. The normal blood level of calcium is 9 to 10 mg/dl; approximately 50% of this is bound to plasma protein (primarily albumin), and 45% is in the form of free ion. The remaining fraction may be bound tightly to phosphate or citrate (11).

The delicate balance of intracellular and extracellular calcium is modulated closely by hormones secreted from several different endocrine organs. The important endocrine and other elements include the parathyroid glands, skin, liver, kidneys, gonads, adrenal tissues, and the thyroid.

Parathyroid Hormone

Parathyroid hormone is synthesized as a larger prehormone in the parathyroid glands. This large precursor is cleaved rapidly into the metabolically active, 84 amino acid, single-chain peptide (11). The rate of its synthesis and release is inversely related to the amount of extracellular ionized calcium available. Transcription of this hormone does not appear to depend on the cytosolic calcium ion concentration.

The principal target tissues for parathyroid are bone and kidney. First and second messenger systems are activated via specific membrane receptors within tissue of the bone and kidney. In bone, specific receptors for parathyroid hormone have been found on osteoblasts and osteoblast precursors but not on osteoclasts. This may imply that it is the osteoblast that regulates proliferation and activation of the osteoclast in response to a parathyroid hormone challenge. Osteocytes also appear to have parathyroid hormone receptors. When stimulated, they rapidly mobilize the calcium salts immediately surrounding them. In the kidney, parathyroid hormone decreases phosphorus reabsorption in the proximal tubule. This is mediated through activation of adenyl cyclase. In the distal tubule, parathyroid hormone increases the reabsorption of calcium.

Vitamin D

Vitamin D is a hormone that may regulate calcium homeostasis via two mechanisms. Vitamin D_3 (cholecalciferol) can be formed when ultraviolet light contacts the skin. Its precursor is endogenously synthesized 7-dehydrocholesterol. The other major source is vitamin D_2 (ergocalciferol) (12). This form of vitamin D is found primarily in cod liver oil and in fortified milk.

Vitamin D from the skin undergoes C-25 hydroxylation in the liver to produce the major circulating prohormone, calcifediol. Calcitriol, the physiologically active form of the vitamin, is produced in the kidney (Fig. 20.4). The enzyme for this C-1 hydroxylation is activated by parathyroid hormone. In the presence of a low level of parathyroid hormone, the C-24 site is hydroxylated instead of the C-1 site. This yields the inactive metabolite 24,25-dihydroxycholecalciferol ($24,25(OH)_2$-D_3) (12). Calcitriol, the active metabolite of vitamin D, has the intestine and bone as its principal target tissues. In the intestine, it induces production of a calcium-binding protein, which is responsible for active calcium transport. In the bone, its function is less well understood, but it is thought to promote the differentiation of osteoclasts and to modify their activity and number.

Fracture Healing

The fracture of a bone initiates a predictable sequence of events, resulting in the ultimate restoration of the injured bone towards its original state. This sequence begins with inflammation, followed by repair, and finally remodeling (4,13). Energy requirements for fracture healing are highest during the repair phase when the cells and the fracture callus are undergoing mitosis and synthesizing large volumes of a new matrix.

Inflammation

The trauma that is required to fracture a bone damages not only the bone matrix itself but also the periosteum, muscle, and surrounding soft tissues. Immediately after fracture, a hematoma accumulates between the fracture ends, within the medullary canal, and beneath the elevated periosteum. The damage to the vascular supply of the bone causes death of osteocytes as far back as the first junction of collateral channels (4). Hence, the immediate ends of the fracture have no living

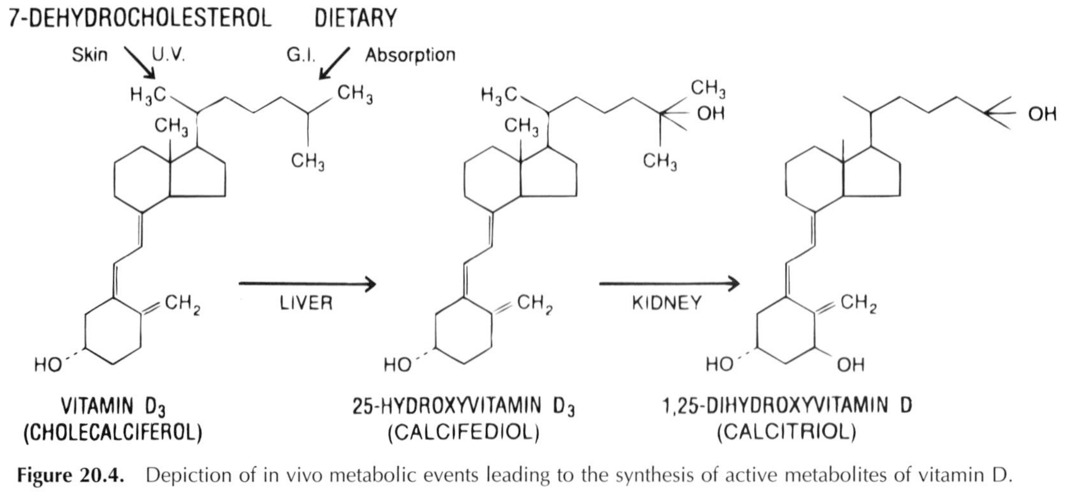

Figure 20.4. Depiction of in vivo metabolic events leading to the synthesis of active metabolites of vitamin D.

cells. Periosteum that has been stripped and torn may also be devitalized.

The injured and dying cells, along with platelets and other cells, release inflammatory mediators. These chemicals cause blood vessels in the area of the fracture to dilate and their basement membranes to become more permeable. Exudation of plasma occurs, leading to the acute edema seen in the region of a recent fracture. Inflammatory cells, including polymorphonuclear leukocytes, macrophages, and lymphocytes, migrate to the region. The polymorphonuclear leukocytes are the first to respond. As the acute inflammatory response subsides, necrotic tissue is resorbed and the area is replaced by fibroblasts, which start producing a new fibrous matrix.

Repair

The disruption of bone tissue and the surrounding blood vessels leads to exposure of bone matrix proteins. This, combined with release of chemotactic factors during the inflammatory phase, stimulates fracture repair (4,13,14). Evidence also indicates that electrical stimuli may play a role in healing fresh fractures (4,13,14). Such studies suggest that the electronegativity found in the region of a fresh fracture may be a factor in new bone formation. The amount of electronegativity depends on cell viability. As the fracture heals, the degree of electronegativity and its importance decreases.

Organization of the fracture hematoma is recognized as the first step in fracture repair. Migration of repair cells to the area is aided by the hematoma, which provides a fibrous scaffold that facilitates migration and attachment. Cells within the hematoma produce growth factors and other proteins that serve to induce initial events required for fracture repair. These include cell migration, proliferation, and synthesis of a new tissue matrix. At the time of cell migration, the microenvironment is acidic. The pH gradually returns to neutral and then becomes slightly alkaline as healing progresses. The alkaline pH promotes mineralization of the fracture callus.

Blood supply during fracture healing is extremely important. Under ordinary circumstances, it is the periosteal vessels that contribute the majority of capillary buds early in the healing phase. The reconstituted nutrient artery becomes more important in the latter stages of the healing process. The exact stimuli responsible for angiogenesis has not been defined.

The stimulus for necrotic bone resorption also remains unidentified. Prostaglandins do not seem to have a significant influence in this process (4). They have been found in large amounts in the region of fresh fractures in experimental animals. The cells responsible for resorption of necrotic bone are the osteoclasts. Prostaglandins have been shown to increase osteoclast activity and cause recruitment of new osteoclasts.

The majority of cells that are responsible for osteogenesis during early fracture healing appear in the fracture site with the granulation tissue. These cells seem to be associated with the invasion of capillary loops, but their precise source remains unknown. Other cells responsible for a portion of bone formation are the pluripotential mesenchymal cells. They initially form fibrous tissue and cartilage, which eventually becomes bone. Some of these cells also arrive at the fracture site via migration at the time of the onset of angiogenesis. Other cells originate from the local injured tissues. The cellular, or cambium, layer of the periosteum is responsible for formation of the earliest bone. Cells within the cambium are highly active. Osteoblasts from the exposed endosteal surfaces also participate in bone formation. Viable osteocytes near the fracture site do not appear to form repair tissue.

Fracture callus consist of fibrous tissue, cartilage, and woven bone. These tissues are derived from the proliferation and differentiation of mesenchymal cells in the area. The original fibrin clot is eventually replaced with a loose fibrous matrix. Contained within the matrix are Types I and III collagen, glycosaminoglycans, and proteoglycans. Consequently, the soft callus becomes a more dense fibrocartilage or hyaline-like cartilage. During the resultant enchondral ossification and intramembranous bone formation, the concentration of Type I collagen increases until matrix mineralization occurs. The newly formed woven bone eventually remodels to lamellar bone, and the content of collagen and other proteins returns to normal levels.

For mineralization of fracture callus to occur, the fibrocartilaginous callus matrix must be removed, and chondrocytes and osteoblasts must release calcium phosphate complexes into the new matrix. This matrix is different from the soft callus in that a high concentration of Type I collagen fibrils exist. Spaces within these collagen fibrils are the site for deposition of calcium hydroxyapatite crystals.

The new bone that arises in the regions of low oxygen tension near the center of the inflammatory action is primarily cartilage and is called the soft callus. Bone formed at the periphery of the inflammatory response is through the process of intramembranous ossification. This is called the hard callus. Cartilage within the callus is replaced gradually by maturing bone through the process of enchondral ossification. This enlarges the hard callus, thus increasing the stability of the fracture fragments. The process of new bone formation continues until the fracture site has been bridged, thus restoring continuity between the cortical bone fragments.

As mineralization continues, a fusiform mass of callus gradually envelopes the bone ends. This large callus contains a preponderance of woven bone. The increasing mineral content directly correlates with increasing hardness of the callus. With the increase in maturation of both internal and external callus, union progresses.

However, healing is still not complete. The callus is still immature and is weaker than normal bone. It will only gain full strength during remodeling.

Remodeling

Fracture remodeling continues years beyond radiographically apparent union. During the final stages of repair, woven bone is replaced by lamellar bone. The previously fusiform callus is reduced in size so that the fracture site more closely resembles uninjured bone. After all woven bone has been replaced, osteoclastic resorption continues so that poorly placed trabecula are also removed and new struts are laid down along the lines of force. At the completion of callus remodeling, the new bone has been altered to perform the function demanded of it.

The above mechanism of fracture healing characterizes only fractures that are not rigidly stabilized. If rigid stabilization is used and bone surfaces are in contact, formation of a callus is minimized (4). Healing occurs in a primary fashion. If a direct contact occurs between the ends of cortical bone with a minimum of motion, lamellar bone forms directly across the fracture site. This is accomplished in a fashion parallel to the long axis of the bone and is accomplished by direct extension of osteons.

Osteoporosis

Osteoporosis is a condition of reduced bone mass that impairs skeletal function. The National Institutes of Health Consensus Conference (15) has defined primary osteoporosis as an age-related disorder characterized by decreased bone mass in absence of other recognizable causes of bone loss and an increased susceptibility to fractures. Approximately 15 to 20 million people in the United States suffer from osteoporosis (15), the consequences of which are severe. At least 1.2 million fractures each year occur in patients with osteoporosis (538,000 vertebral bodies, 227,000 hips, 172,000 distal forearms, and 283,000 other limb sites) (16). Approximately 33% of all women over 65 will sustain vertebral fractures during their lifetime (17). Of patients who live to be 90 years old, 32% of women and 17% of men will also sustain a hip fracture (15). Hip fractures are associated with higher mortality rate, disability, and medical costs than all other osteoporotic fractures combined. The mortality rate for patients sustaining hip fractures increases 12% to 20% over that for individuals of the same age without hip fractures (11). Of those patients who survive, 50% will require long-term nursing home care and fewer than 30% will return to their prefracture lifestyle (18). The annual cost of acute and long-term care

for hip fractures alone has been estimated to exceed $7 billion in the United States.

All adults suffer decreases in bone stock after the fourth decade of life, but certain individuals are at increased risk. These patients at the highest risk are slim, white, postmenopausal female of Northwestern European decent. Factors that add to an increased risk in this patient profile are cigarette smoking, excessive ethanol use, poor calcium intake, and a sedentary life-style (11,17,18). A major risk factor appears to be early or surgically induced menopause.

Cigarette smokers have significantly more bone loss and an increased incidence of both vertebral and hip fractures. Tobacco may enhance the degradation of estrogen. Patients with heavy ethanol intake have a decreased bone density of the vertebral bodies and femoral necks (18). Ethanol has been shown to depress osteoblast function directly (11).

Declining bone mass is now thought to be a universal phenomenon of aging. Peak bone mass is achieved between the third and fourth decades of life in both sexes. It is affected by gender, nutrition, race, exercise, and overall health. Peak bone mass is approximately 30% higher in men than in women, and 10% higher in blacks than in whites (15). A slow phase of bone loss commences at about the age of 35 years. This continues for both sexes at the rate of 0.3% to 0.5% per year (11) and is directly related to continuous negative calcium balance. After surgical or natural menopause, an accelerated phase of bone loss begins at the rate of 2% to 3% per year and lasts for 6 to 10 years, after which bone loss returns to its basal slow phase of 0.3% to 0.5% per year (17).

Bone contains both trabecular and cortical components. Cortical bone has a high volume and low surface area, whereas trabecular bone has a low volume and high surface area. Because remodeling of bone takes place on the surface, trabecular bone, with its higher surface area and metabolic activity, is the first area to be resorbed during times of net skeletal loss. Consequently, the incidence of Colles and vertebral fractures rises soon after menopause. These two fractures occur at sites that contain large amounts of trabecular bone. Conversely, the proximal femur is composed primarily of cortical bone and, therefore, lags 10 to 15 years behind the vertebral body with respect to patient age at time of fracture (11).

Riggs and Melton (17) have subclassified involutional osteoporosis based on these two patterns of fracture and bone loss. Type 1, or postmenopausal osteoporosis, occurs in females 51 to 65 years old, involves areas of predominately trabecular bone, and is characterized by vertebral and Colles fractures. Decreased estrogen levels play a primary role in Type 1 osteoporosis. In contrast, Type 2, or senile osteoporosis, occurs in both men and women, usually after 75 years. It involves both cortical bone and trabecular bone and is characterized by fractures of the hip, pelvis, proximal humerus, and proximal tibia. The bone loss in Type 2 osteoporosis is related to aging and long-term calcium deficiency. The calcium deficiency is possibly secondary to decreased vitamin D activity and increased parathyroid hormone activity.

Basic Cartilage Biology

Cartilage is another specialized form of connective tissue that is composed of cells and a complex matrix. Unlike bone, cartilage has a low metabolic rate, is relatively avascular, and has a high compressive strength coupled with elasticity. Its properties are the result of the large amount of fibrous macromolecules and ground substance contained within the matrix. This matrix is synthesized by mature cartilage cells called chondrocytes. They encase themselves within cavities in the matrix called lacunae.

There are three types of mature cartilage tissue: hyaline, fibrous, and elastic. All three types contain mature chondrocytes within a matrix and fibers embedded in a ground substance. The difference in properties of these types of cartilage are caused by the distribution, structure, and number of fibers and chondrocytes.

Hyaline Cartilage

Hyaline cartilage is the most prevalent form of cartilage in the body. It is found on the bone surfaces of joints (articular cartilage) and on the ventral ends of ribs. In the immature skeleton, it is also found at the growing ends of long bones. This dynamic cartilaginous model serves as a precursor for the final structure of mature cortical and cancellous bone.

All cartilage develops from mesenchymal tissue. Cells within the mesenchyme differentiate and transform into chondroblasts. This aggregation of cells and surrounding matrix is called precartilage. As the chondroblasts become more active, they synthesize and secrete matrix into the extracellular space. This in turn entraps them within a lacuna. With the continuation of matrix production, the space between individual cells gets larger. Cells that are completely surrounded by maturing extracellular matrix are called chondrocytes.

The newly formed precartilage model is surrounded by a fibrous covering, called the perichondrium. It is composed of two layers. The outer fibrous layer, which consists of dense connective tissue, surrounds an inner layer that is adjacent to the precartilage. The inner region contains a layer of flattened cells, which have the potential to differentiate into active chondrocytes.

Growth

Maturing cartilage grows in two ways: interstitial and appositional. Interstitial growth is characterized by an individual mature chondrocyte that divides within its own lacuna. The aggregate group of new cells within one lacuna is called the cell nest. Each of these maturing chondrocytes continues to secrete matrix that eventually separates the cells from each other. The resulting expansion of the cartilage from within is known as interstitial growth.

The matrix does exert some limitation on this expansion. As it ages, interstitial growth declines rapidly. Further growth is then achieved by the addition of cartilage to the outer surface. Undifferentiated cells of the inner chondrogenic layer of the perichondrium proliferate and differentiate into chondroblasts. These active chondroblasts deposit matrix around themselves in a process that is identical to those within the lacunae. This particular type of cartilage formation is termed appositional growth.

These two types of growth should not be considered separate. During the early part of embryonic development, both types of growth occur simultaneously. It is only during the later aspect of growth, when the matrix has expanded to its limitation, that growth is primarily appositional. Eventually, the chondrogenic activity of the perichondrium and the interstitium becomes dormant.

Chondrocytes

The appearance of chondrocytes differs with respect to the cells' age. Young cells are usually flattened or elliptical, with their long axis oriented parallel to the surface of the underlying cartilage. In contrast, older cells are round or hypertrophied. The organelles within the cytoplasm are similar to those found in fibroblasts. There is a large endoplasmic reticulum and a prominent Golgi zone. Whereas younger cells tend to have a high concentration of organelles, the older chondrocytes tend to have fewer organelles associated with matrix synthesis. They are characterized more by an abundant amount of cytoplasmic glycogen.

Matrix

All types of cartilage contain similar types of chondrocytes and chondroblasts; however, the matrix of hyaline cartilage differs greatly from fibrocartilage or elastic cartilage. The physical and chemical properties of hyaline cartilage are a result of the components within the matrix. Hyaline cartilage contains collagen and proteoglycans. Estimates of the collagen content of the cartilage matrix range from about 50% to 70% of the dry weight (6). The proteoglycans have a protein core with covalently bound chondroitin sulfate and keratin sulfate side chains. The proteoglycans play an important role in the transport of water and electrolytes within the matrix. They also bind to collagen fibers and fibrils, forming a network that contributes to the gel-like qualities of the ground substance. This heavy molecular weight substance acts as a barrier to limit free movement of large macromolecules.

Cartilage is unique in that it contains only Type II collagen. Chondroblasts and chondrocytes secrete collagen as tropocollagen molecules consisting of triple helixes of three α_1-proteins. Within the extracellular fluid, the tropocollagen is linked enzymatically into stable collagen fibers.

Fibrocartilage differs dramatically from hyaline cartilage. Instead of having an abundant ground substance, its ground substance is sparse. Numerous collagenous fibers are visible as large irregular bundles associated with groups of chondrocytes. Although these chondrocytes may be aligned in rows parallel to the collagen bundles, more often they are distributed individually or in pairs.

Fibrocartilage has a structure that is intermediate between dense connective tissue and hyaline cartilage. It never occurs alone but usually merges with neighboring tendons, ligaments, or hyaline cartilage. It arises initially as ordinary connective tissue in which a transformation of fibroblasts into chondroblasts occurs. These chondroblasts then secrete a thin layer of matrix around themselves. Because of the small amount of matrix synthesized, the abundant collagenous bundles do not become infiltrated by the sparse matrix. No perichondrium is found in fibrocartilage.

Fibrocartilage occurs where both support and tensile strength are necessary. Examples include the pubic symphysis, attachments of tendons and ligaments, and the intervertebral disks. The type of cartilage that is formed after an injury to an articular surface has a firm fibrous texture which macroscopically resembles dense connective tissue.

Elastic cartilage is similar to hyaline cartilage, but its chondrocytes can produce elastic fibers as well as collagen fibrils and nonfibrous intercellular substance. With the addition of the elastic fibers, this cartilage provides a flexible form of support. It is typically found in the auricle of the ear, the epiglottis, and parts of the larynx.

Similar to hyaline cartilage, elastic cartilage forms a perichondrium at its periphery. The elastic fibers are less dense near the perichondrium and gradually blend into the fibrous layer. The growth of elastic cartilage is essentially the same as that of hyaline cartilage.

Nutrition

Owing to its avascularity, cartilage has a slow turnover and inherent stability to compressive forces. Although early embryonic cartilage is filled with blood vessels, mature cartilage receives its nutrients and rids waste products via diffusion. The large amount of fluid within the matrix permits nutrients, waste products, and dissolved gases to diffuse readily to and from capillaries located outside the perichondrium. This structure of cartilage leads to a slightly anaerobic environment. Conse-

quently, chondrocytes function predominately by a glycolytic metabolism and have an extremely high lactate content. If the cartilage becomes too thick, efficient diffusion ceases and the chondrocytes die.

Regeneration

Because of its avascularity and limited diffusion potential, hyaline cartilage has only a small capacity to regenerate. When cartilage is damaged in adults, the injured region usually becomes necrotic. This necrotic area is then resorbed and slowly filled with newly formed connective tissue from the surrounding perichondrium and nearby fascia. Some of this connective tissue may differentiate into cartilage cells that lay down fibrocartilage. However, no hyaline cartilage is produced, and the majority of the tissue remains as a scar of dense connective tissue.

Articular Cartilage

Articular cartilage is found at the end of bones that are joined by a capsule. In most respects, it is typical of hyaline cartilage. However, articular cartilage lacks a perichondrium and has a unique collagen organization. Three zones compose this structural modification: a tangential zone with the fibers oriented parallel to the surface of the joint; a deep radical zone with fibers at right angles to the surface of the joint; and a transitional area uniting these two zones. This network closely resembles numerous overlapping arches, which are called Benninghof arcades. This orientation creates a densely packed network of collagen located immediately beneath the articular surface. This is the ideal structure for sustaining the constantly changing stresses on the joint.

Proteoglycans, in association with a large amount of water and cartilage cells, are found within the collagenous framework. The chondrocytes are divided into zones. At the surface is a narrow layer of flattened chondrocytes called the gliding layer, or tangential zone. Beneath this is the transitional zone in which more ovoid to rounded chondrocytes are distributed randomly. Underneath lies the radial zone, which marks the boundary between the cartilage above and the zone of calcified cartilage below. Between the radial zone and the zone of calcified cartilage lies the tidemark. This area represents the superficial edge of the layer of calcified cartilage. Last, the layer of calcified cartilage fuses with subchondral bone, a mature type of cortical bone with haversian systems. During the growth of the epiphysis of the long bones, the chondrocytes in the deeper layers undergo the same sequence of proliferation, maturation, hypertrophy, and calcification as those of the growth plate. After epiphyseal growth is complete, the lower zones of chondrocytes are converted into compact bone, whereas the more superficial layers remain as articular coverage.

The cartilage in articular surfaces receives its nutrition as previously described. When a load is placed on the surface, the fluid is extruded from the cartilage into the joint space, thus lubricating the surfaces of bone. Reciprocally, removing the load results in reabsorption of the fluid by the matrix. This sponge-like effect functions as the transport mechanism of nutrients and waste through the avascular articular cartilage.

Joints

The skeleton is formed by the interconnection of bones by articulations, which are called joints. Bones within these joints are connected to each other by a wide variety of connective tissues that permit varying amounts of movement between adjacent bones. Connections with little to no bone movement are called synarthroses, slightly movable joints are called amphiarthroses, and those that contain a fluid-filled cavity and are freely movable are referred to as diarthroses. The amphiarthroses and diarthroses bear most of the skeletal load.

Synarthroses

Synarthrotic joints are either immobile or show limited movement. They are grouped into three subclasses by the type tissue involved in the connection between the bones. If the articulation is via connective tissue only, it is termed a syndesmotic joint; if the linkage is through cartilage, it is a synchondrotic joint; and if the connection is bone, it is a synostotic joint.

Syndesmotic Joints

The numerous sutures of the cranial bones constitute syndesmotic joints. These are remnants of mesenchymal tissue that form the adjacent bones. During growth and development, the undifferentiated connective tissue between the bones contain osteogenic precursors that can subsequently add new bone to the free edges by appositional means. This results in enlargement of bones such as those found in the cranial cavity. At maturity, the skull stops growing, and these connective tissue sutures may slowly be replaced by bone. At this point, the syndesmotic joint is transformed into a synostosis.

Synchondrotic Joints

In synchondroses, bones are joined by hyaline cartilage. Usually, these joints are present only during development and show limited mobility. An example is the junction of the ribs and sternum. The growth plate in growing mammals is also a synchondrotic joint. It connects the epiphysis and metaphysis of a long bone. Its major function, similar to that of syndesmotic joints, is to permit continued bone growth and expansion. This is accomplished by the process of enchondral ossification.

These joints are also frequently converted to a synostosis at bony maturity.

Synostotic Joints

Synostotic joints are formed from bone arising from within either connective tissue or cartilaginous joints. Most of these joints occur in adults and are believed to function in stabilizing parts of the skeleton after the bones have stopped growing.

Amphiarthroses

A prime example of an amphiarthrotic articulation is the intervertebral disc situated between the vertebral bodies. Each disc is constructed like an automobile tire in its radial assignment of outer fibers with a soft gelatinous inner tube or core known as the nucleus pulposus. The fibrous outer casing is called the annulus fibrosus. The annulus is composed of concentrically arranged fibrocartilage encased within a sheet of dense connective tissue. This entire outer tissue component is derived from mesenchymal precursors. In contrast, the nucleus arises from the notochord and is composed of only a few round mesenchymal cells embedded in a semifluid gel. Functionally, it is the more liquid nucleus that dissipates the forces in the spine. Unfortunately, the nucleus undergoes chondroid metaplasia, making it brittle and inelastic with age (6). The annulus becomes less absorbent because of an increase in collagen fiber content associated with a loss of moisture and sulfated glycosaminoglycans.

Diarthroses

The diarthrodial joint is characterized by articular cartilage within a capsule connecting the ends of bones (Fig. 20.5). This capsule is lined with a synovial membrane and encloses a fluid-filled cavity. These joints are

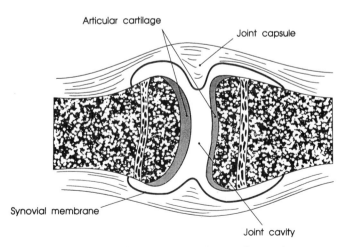

Figure 20.5. Schematic diagram of a typical synovial joint. The opposing articular surfaces are covered by articular cartilage. The joint is enclosed by a synovial membrane.

the most mobile of all joints and consequently are subject to a large amount of friction between the hyaline cartilage coverings of the apposing articular surfaces. The synovial fluid is critical in reducing this friction.

The joint capsule consists of an outer layer of dense fibrous tissue lined by an inner, loosely constructed synovial membrane. The capsule is continuous with the outer layer of adjacent periosteum and is attached to the margins of the articular cartilage. It contributes to the stability of the joint secondary to its relative inelasticity. Regions of the capsule are thickened to form ligaments. Occasionally, gaps may be found within the capsule. These gaps allow synovial membrane outpouchings to develop, called bursae. Bursae serve to separate the main body of the joint from the muscle or tendon to which it is attached, thereby reducing the friction on these structures.

The inner synovial membrane is a loosely textured sheet of vascular connective tissue, which is similar to pericardium. It lines the joint capsule but not the articular cartilage surfaces. A one to three-cell layer faces the joint cavity. Two cell types line this synovial. Some cells resemble macrophages and are collectively called type A histocytic cells. The second cell type resembles a fibroblast and is characterized by a smoother cell surface and an abundance of granular endoplasmic reticulum. This classification is not rigid, as the two cell types may represent different functional stages of the same cell. Functionally, these cells secrete the synovial mucin and are phagocytic.

A loosely textured fibrous connective tissue layer lies under the synovial layer. This layer contains numerous capillary vessels, which merge into a deeper portion of the connective tissue adjacent to the capsule. No basement membrane exists in the synovial membrane, thereby eliminating any barrier between capillary walls and the joint cavity. Thus, the joint cavity can be considered an intercellular space. This structure of the joint cavity is important for understanding the process of exudate formation and inflammatory joint diseases.

Synovial Fluid

The fluid found within diarthrodial joints is produced from the combination of the ultrafiltrate from the synovial capillaries with the mucin produced by the type B synovial cells. Compared with blood serum, the synovial fluid consists of a fluid with 33% of the protein concentration. These proteins are principally albumin, although enzymatic proteins and complement system proteins are also present. Viscosity of the synovial fluid is attributed to the mucin secreted by the type B synovial cells. It consists of hyaluronic acid and covalently bound proteins. Hyaluronic acid is highly polymerized and is responsible for the viscous properties of the synovial fluid. However, the lubricating properties of the fluid are probably derived from a glycoprotein constituent.

Normal synovial samples contain fewer than 300 leukocytes per millimeter, and no more than 25% of them are polymorphonuclear leukocytes.

Articular Cartilage Repair

Because of its avascular nature and limited diffusion capacity, articular cartilage is not repaired easily. In fact, reparative mechanisms are limited to the periphery of the joint. In these regions, cartilage is immediately adjacent to the synovial membrane. The lining cells of the membrane are able to proliferate and produce a form of fibrocartilage rather than normal hyaline or articular cartilage. The fibrocartilage is not ideal for the types of forces seen in the articulation of joint surfaces. It is not as resistant to either sheer or comprehensive forces as is normal articular cartilage. Although the formation remains certain, its long-term survivability and usefulness have yet to be determined.

Because of the inability of mature cartilage cells to mitose, cells damaged outside of the immediate periphery of the joint die without the benefit of any reparative mechanisms.

Osteoarthritis

Osteoarthritis is the most prevalent form of articular cartilage degeneration. It may result from childhood developmental abnormalities such as Legg-Calvé-Perthes disease and congenital hip dysplasia (19). Traumatic changes may also cause an incongruity of joint surfaces that predispose the joints to articular cartilage damage. In cases for which etiologies are known, osteoarthritis is sometimes described as secondary. Idiopathic osteoarthritis is described as primary.

The etiology of osteoarthritis has yet to be completely determined. Theories can be grouped into two basic categories: excessive force in normal tissue and insufficient chondrocyte response to normal forces. The excessive forces may occur from developmental abnormalities, leading to incongruity of joint surfaces. This leads to a change in normal joint biomechanics that may produce excessive sheer forces at the surfaces of articular cartilage. Excessive stress can also occur from direct trauma. In both cases, enzymes synthesized by the chondrocytes themselves may be the early mediators in the breakdown of the articular cartilage (19). Simple aging has a deleterious effect on the fatigue strength of articular cartilage.

Nonsteroidal antiinflammatory agents have been the mainstay in symptomatic relief of arthritic symptoms. These drugs are similar in their pharmacologic properties, and no one agent has been proven to be consistently better than the others. There is a wide range of patient response to a particular nonsteroidal agent, and one drug may be more beneficial in an individual case. The most common side effect associated with the use of non-steroidal agents has been the development of symptomatic peptic ulcers.

REFERENCES

1. Buckwalter JA. Proteoglycan structure in calcifying cartilage. Clin Orthop 1983;172:207–232.
2. Boskey AL. Current concepts of the physiology and biochemistry of calcification. Clin Orthop 1981;157:225–257.
3. Buckwalter JA, Cooper RR. Bone structure and function. In: Griffing PP, ed. Instructional course lectures. St. Louis: CV Mosby, 1987:27–48.
4. Buckwalter JA, Cruess RL. Healing of the musculoskeletal tissues. In: Rockwood CA, Green DP, eds. Fractures in adults. Philadelphia: JP Lippincott, 1991:181–211.
5. Reddi AH. Cell biology and biochemistry of endochondral bone development. Coll Research 1981;1:209–226.
6. Jee WSS. The skeletal tissues. In: Weiss L, ed. Histology: cell and tissue biology. New York: Elsevier Science, 1977:200–255.
7. Brighton CT. Longitudinal bone growth: the growth plate and its dysfunctions. In: Griffing PP, ed. Instructional course lectures. St. Louis: CV Mosby, 1987:3–25.
8. Carter DR, Spengler DM. Mechanical properties and composition of cortical bone. Clin Orthop 1978;135:192–217.
9. Cooper RR, Milgram JW, Robinson RA. Morphology of the osteon. J Bone Joint Surg Am 1966;48A:1239–1271.
10. Trueta J. The role of the vessels in osteogenesis. J Bone Joint Surg Am 1963;45B:402–418.
11. Lane JM, Bockman RS, Buss DD. Bone metabolism and metabolic bone disease. In: Poss R, ed. Orthopaedic knowledge update 3. Park Ridge, IL: American Academy of Orthopaedic Surgeons, 1990:29–46.
12. Audran M, Kumar R. The physiology and pathophysiology of vitamin D. Mayo Clin Proc 1985;60:851–866.
13. Brand RA, Rubin CT. Fracture healing. In: Evarts, ed. Surgery of the musculoskeletal system. New York: Churchill, Livingstone, 1990:93–114.
14. Kuhlman RE, Bakowski MJ. The biochemical activity of fracture callus in relation to bone production. Clin Orthop 1975;107:258–265.
15. National Institutes of Health. Consensus development conference statement on osteoporosis. JAMA 1984;252:794–799.
16. Kelsey JF. Osteoporosis: prevalence and incidence. In: Osteoporosis: program and abstracts. NIH Consensus Development Conference, April 2–4, 1984:25–28.
17. Riggs L, Melton LJ. Involutional osteoporosis. N Engl J Med 1986;314:1676–1686.
18. Barth RW, Lane JM. Osteoporosis. Orthop Clin North Am 1988;19(4):845–858.
19. Goldberg VM. Arthritis. In: Fitzgerald R, ed. Orthopaedic knowledge update 2. Park Ridge, IL: American Academy of Orthopaedic Surgeons, 1987:35–47.

CHAPTER

21 Basic Neuroscience

Roger D. Smith / *Robert L. Tiel* / *Robert J. Johnson*

The past 20 years have witnessed a virtual explosion of new information in the neurosciences. In fact, the 1990s have been declared the "Decade of the Brain" by the President of the United States. An understanding of basic principles of neuroscience will benefit all those practicing surgery, as the nervous system integrates so many bodily functions and organ systems. This chapter will outline fundamental aspects of neuroanatomy, neurophysiology, and neuropathology and will introduce some of the newer discoveries in the neurosciences that may prove applicable to a wide variety of surgical disciplines.

Cellular Anatomy and Physiology

The central nervous system (CNS) contains more than 30 billion cells. These are divided morphologically and functionally into three major groups: the neurons, the neuroglial cells, and the microglia that represent the reticuloendothelial system in the brain and spinal cord. The neurons and the glia maintain a complex relationship that allows for the orderly passage of information in the nervous system.

Cellular Morphology

The Neuron

The neuron is the functional unit of the nervous system. Depolarization of the neuronal membrane propagates an electrochemical impulse that is transferred to other neurons through specialized junctions called synapses. In this way, information is continually processed in the nervous system. The neuron is divided into the cell body or soma and the cell processes—the axon and the dendrites. The morphology of these processes allows classification of neurons into unipolar, bipolar, and multipolar neurons. Unipolar neurons have a single process arising from the soma that gives rise to both the dendrite and the axon. The dorsal root ganglion cell, which brings somatic sensation to the CNS, is the prototype of this neuronal type. Bipolar neurons with a single dendrite and an axon are found in special sensory systems such as the retina and vestibule. By far the largest group is the multipolar type. Elaboration of the dendritic tree allows for a greatly increased surface area for synaptic contact. A single Purkinje cell in the cerebellum may receive 150,000 synapses, allowing for extremely fine modulation of the cell activity.

The axon is the neuronal process along which the electrochemical impulse is propagated to communicate with subsequent neurons. The axon may be long, extending 3 m from the brain or spinal cord, yet arising from a 20-μ to 40-μ soma. This is a complex structure containing microtubules and filaments that transport the axoplasm, containing neurotransmitters and other chemicals, over great distances to and from the soma. The origin of the axon, the axon hillock, is the most electrically excitable portion of the neuron and generally gives rise to the nerve action potential.

The Glia

Glial cells include astrocytes, oligodendrocytes, ependymal cells, and microglia. Astrocytes are found throughout the CNS. They are characterized by extensive processes that completely encase the neurons, isolating them from each other except at synapses and also separating the neuron from direct contact with the capillary by special astrocytic foot processes. Although the astrocytes are polarized to -90 mV internally, they are not electrically excitable and cannot propagate an action potential. Astrocytes may play a role in regulating the extracellular ionic environment, especially potassium that is liberated during neuronal depolarization. Astrocytes respond to ischemia and injury, initially with swelling, and subsequently with proliferation to form scarring in the brain. They give rise to the majority of primary brain tumors.

Oligodendrocytes are smaller than astrocytes and are more concentrated in white matter. These cells form the

522

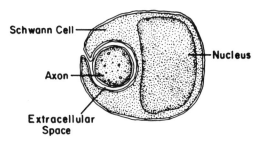

Figure 21.1. Concentric layers of the Schwann cell membrane encase a peripheral nerve axon as myelin. From Morrell P. Myelin. In: Adelman G, ed. Encyclopedia of neuroscience. Vol. 2. Boston: Birkhauser, 1987: 729.

myelin that electrically insulates the axons and greatly increases the rate of nerve impulse propagation. In the peripheral nervous system, this function is carried out by the Schwann cell. In both cases, the myelin is formed by concentric layers of the lipid-rich cell membrane of the glial cell (Fig. 21.1). There are varying degrees of myelination of different axons and tracts. Axonal conduction velocities are directly proportional to the degree of myelination. Unmyelinated nerve fibers indent the oligodendrocyte or Schwann cell but are not surrounded by the concentric lamellae of myelin.

Ependymal cells line the cerebral ventricles, and over the vascular choroid plexus, they are specialized so that they can produce cerebrospinal fluid. The ependyma is a single layer of cuboidal epithelial cells that exhibits secretory and absorptive functions and provides a cellular layer between the cerebrospinal fluid in the ventricle and the extracellular space of the brain. Ependymal cells lining the ventricle are relatively permeable to solutes, although those of the choroidal epithelium show tight junctions controlling the passage of solutes from the capillaries of the choroid plexus into the cerebrospinal fluid.

Microglia represent the reticuloendothelial cells of the CNS and are derived from outside the brain and spinal cord. Microglial proliferation occurs in response to infectious processes, although blood-derived lymphocytes and neutrophils represent a major part of an inflammatory response in the CNS. Whether microglial cells are truly resident in the brain tissue or derived only from blood elements is still unclear.

Other Cell Types

The capillaries of the CNS are characterized by a special penta laminar interdigitation referred to as a tight junction. This inhibits the passage of molecules from the bloodstream into the CNS, forming a blood-brain barrier.

The meninges are mesenchymal tissues that completely envelop the brain and spinal cord. The dura mater is approximated to the skull but is more separated in the spine. It functions as a bone-forming tissue in the skull during development and provides a relatively competent barrier to encroachment of infection or tumor into the nervous system. The thin trabeculated arachnoid contains the cerebrospinal fluid. It is approximated loosely to the spinal cord and forms cisterns at the base of the brain. Over the brain surface there is closer approximation to the Pia. The Pia mater is approximated tightly to the surface of the brain and spinal cord. The leptomeninges (the arachnoid and the Pia) follow the blood vessels into the brain parenchyma for some distance as the Virchow-Robin spaces.

Synapses and Receptors

Contact between neurons occurs at a synapse, a specialized structure composed of a presynaptic axonal terminal bouton containing neurotransmitter and a postsynaptic membrane-bound protein designated a receptor. The discovery of new neurotransmitters and the elucidation of the complex role of receptors has been one of the most exciting developments in current neuroscience.

As the action potential arrives at the axon terminal, the presynaptic membrane is depolarized, opening protein channels in the membrane that are permeable to calcium. Neurotransmitter molecules are packaged into discrete quanta by membranes. The entry of calcium into the cytoplasm causes these membranes to fuse with the presynaptic membrane and release the neurotransmitter into the synaptic cleft. There is a 200-A distance from the presynaptic membrane to the receptor membrane. Neurotransmitter molecules migrate to the receptor proteins and bind with them, causing conformational changes that increase or decrease the permeability of the adjacent membrane channels to various ions, including potassium, sodium, and chloride. This may depolarize or hyperpolarize the postsynaptic membrane, thus facilitating or inhibiting the propagation of further nerve impulses. Muscle cells have similar post-synaptic receptors in a specialized area of the membrane called the motor end plate. Nerve action potentials are translated into muscle contraction across these synapses.

The action of the neurotransmitter at the synapses must be reversed quickly to allow a new signal to arrive. Synapses may have enzymes that destroy the neurotransmitter, or reuptake of the neurotransmitter into the axon may occur for reuse. The pharmacologic effect of many agents are to (*a*) mimic the neurotransmitter substance, (*b*) block its action at the receptor or prevent its release from the presynaptic membrane, (*c*) prevent its enzymatic degradation or prevent its reuptake.

Different receptors may respond to a given neurotransmitter with different physiologic consequences. For most of the better evaluated neurotransmitters, such as the vasoactive amines and acetylcholine, several subsets of receptors have been identified. Thus, a neurotransmitter may be inhibitory at a given synapse but excitatory at another.

A second and extremely important concept in the function of receptors is that, rather than changing ion conductance as the primary response to the neurotransmitter-receptor interaction, biologic information may be conveyed by the release of so-called second messengers by the cell membrane. Second messengers, such as cAMP, phosphoinositides, and calcium, may catalyze the phosphorylation of proteins concerned with cellular metabolic processes, the increase (up-regulation) or decrease (down-regulation) of other membrane receptors, or even gene expression of factors such as cell growth or differentiation. Intermediate between a receptor and a second messenger are membrane-associated proteins such as the G protein that, when activated by the neurotransmitter-receptor complex, binds GTP and protein kinase C, which catalyzes phosphorylation of the phosphoinositide system. As with ion permeability changes, the same neurotransmitter may be excitatory or inhibitory to the associated membrane protein catalyzing the formation of the second messenger. For example, norepinephrine stimulates adenyl cyclase to form cAMP at β-adrenergic receptors, inhibits the same enzyme at α_2-receptors, and activates phospholipase C at α_1-adrenergic receptors. A more thorough understanding of these mechanisms should open new avenues to pharmacologic therapy.

Nerve Action Potential

Selective permeability of the neuronal membrane to different ion species creates an electrical potential across the membrane that is negative on the inside of the membrane and positive on the outside. Proteins in the cell membrane act as channels to the passage of ions across the membrane, and there are specific channels for potassium, sodium, chloride, and calcium. The membrane is much more permeable to potassium than to sodium. This allows a concentration gradient to be maintained for sodium and potassium across the cell membrane. The presence of negatively charged protein molecules within the cytoplasm that cannot cross the membrane creates an opposing force to the migration of potassium ions out of the cell. Although the concentration gradients of all ionic species contribute to the resting potential of the cell membrane, the equilibrium potential of potassium contributes most to this potential. Thus, the resting potential (EMF in mV) is approximated by the Nernst equation for potassium concentration inside and outside the neuron: EMF $= -61 \times \log$ conc K^+ in/conc K^+ out. This varies from -50 to -90 mV, depending on the type of neuron. A more complete mathematical description, the Goldmann equation, accounts for the concentrations of all relevant ions (1).

The nerve impulse is generated by depolarization of the membrane that is then propagated along the axon to the synapse. Depolarization of sensory receptors or nerve endings occurs through a variety of sensory stimuli—mechanical, temperature, light, chemical, etc. Depolarization within the nervous system is caused by the binding of neurotransmitters to receptors across synapses. The depolarization of hundreds or thousands of synapses on dendrites, soma, and even the axon is summated over time until a threshold depolarizing potential is reached in the region of the axon hillock. This is generally about -45 mV. When threshold is reached, a self-propagating depolarization along the axon occurs—the so-called all-or-none response—which conveys the action potential along the entire length of the axon to the synapse. Although the propagation of an impulse may occur in either direction along a cell membrane, a period of refractivity after depolarization directs propagation toward the synapse.

Depolarization occurs when molecular changes in the postsynaptic membrane allow opening of the previously gated sodium channels. Increased permeability to sodium allows an influx of sodium ions along the concentration gradient toward its equilibrium potential of $+40$ mV. The sodium channel gate quickly closes to allow the return of negativity to the inside of the membrane. An increased permeability to potassium creates a temporary period of relative refractoriness to depolarization that gradually returns toward baseline. This series of molecular exchanges is recorded as an action potential. The action potential depolarizes the adjacent membrane to propagate the impulse along the axon. Myelinated nerve fibers are insulated, except at small regular bare spots called the nodes of Ranvier where sodium channels are clustered. Depolarization jumps from one node to the next, markedly accelerating the process and increasing axonal conduction velocity. This is termed saltatory conduction (Fig. 21.2). Sodium accumulated within the axon during depolarization is expelled by an energy-consuming protein exchange transfer mechanism called the sodium-potassium pump.

A neurotransmitter may depolarize or hyperpolarize the postsynaptic membrane. These voltage changes are called excitatory postsynaptic potentials (EPSP) and inhibitory postsynaptic potentials (IPSP), respectively. Hyperpolarization may result from increased conductance of potassium ion or chloride ion that will increase the interior negativity of the cell. Depolarization is primarily a function of sodium conductance. Increasing or decreasing the number of various receptors at the synapse is a mechanism to increase or decrease its sensitivity to incoming neural connections and may form the basis for such functions as learning and accommodation.

Neuroanatomy

The nervous system is classically divided into the CNS, the peripheral nervous system (PNS), and the autonomic nervous system (ANS). The CNS is enclosed within the bone of the skull and spine and covered by

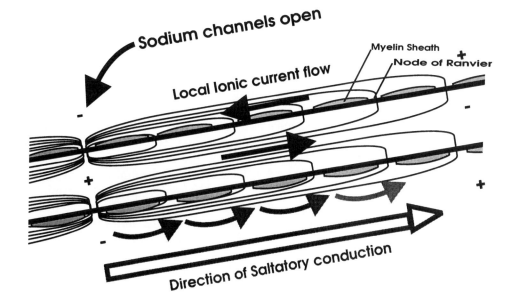

Figure 21.2. Saltatory conduction. Currents generated at node of Ranvier are propagated to the next node, bypassing the insulated portion of the axon and thus accelerating nerve conduction velocity. Note that the current generated can trigger 4-5 nodes ahead of the active site.

the meninges: the dura mater, arachnoid, and Pia. The PNS and ANS are also ensheathed in investing layers of mesenchymal tissue.

Gross Anatomy of the CNS

The Skull, Spine, and Meninges

The skull is formed of multiple plates that fuse after birth through sutures to form the calvarium and the skull base. The paired frontal, parietal, and temporal bones and the occipital bone are membranous bones that form the calvarium. Portions of the frontal bones, temporal bones, occipital bone, and the sphenoid bone are endochondral bone formed from cartilage and comprise the skull base. Small areas of the ethmoid and zygomatic bones are also in contact with the dura. Three fossae are recognized in the skull base. The anterior fossa is formed by the orbital roofs, cribriform plate, and planum sphenoidale. The middle fossa is formed by the greater wing of the sphenoid and petrous portion of the temporal bone on each side, and the posterior fossa by the clivus of the sphenoid and occipital bones and the petrous portions of the temporal bones. The tentorium cerebelli, a dural fold extending from the clinoid processes of the sella turcica and the petrous ridges of the temporal bones to the occipital bone, separates the posterior fossa or infratentorial compartment from the supratentorial compartment. The tentorial hiatus or notch separates the two sides of the middle fossa and allows passage of the brainstem from the supra- to the infratentorial compartment. A sickle-shaped fold of dura, the falx cerebri, extends from the crista galli of the cribriform plate to the tentorium and separates the cerebral hemispheres. The opening at the base of the clivus and occipital bone, the foramen magnum, allows the brainstem to pass through to the spinal cord. Displacements or herniations of brain tissue through these dural and bony apertures are char-

acteristic of mass brain lesions and have important physiologic consequences.

The spine is composed of segmental vertebrae and includes 7 cervical vertebrae, 12 thoracic (rib-bearing) vertebrae, 5 lumbar vertebrae, a sacrum of 5 fused sacral vertebrae, and a coccyx of 2 to 5 vertebrae. A common variation is attachment of the fifth lumbar vertebra to the sacrum (sacralization) or nonattachment of the first sacral vertebra to the sacrum (lumbarilization). The first cervical vertebra (atlas) forms a ring to support the cranium and allow rotation. The second cervical vertebra (axis) incorporates the body of C1 as the odontoid process or dens through the ring of the atlas. The remainder of the cervical, thoracic, and lumbar vertebrae are composed of a body anteriorly and a dorsal arch attached to the body by pedicles and formed by the facet joints (articulating processes), laminae, and spinous processes. The sacral bones are fused into a single triangular-shaped bone but maintain foramina for the exit of sacral nerve roots. Anterior and posterior longitudinal ligaments run the length of the spine, and the intersegmental ligamenta flavum between the lamina and interspinous ligaments between the spinous processes add additional strength to the spinal column. Cartilaginous intervertebral discs from C2 to L5 allow flexibility to the spine and dissipate forces applied to the spinal column. The disc is composed of a fibrous annulus and a softer central nucleus pulposus. Degeneration of the nucleus pulposus through aging, trauma, and weakening of the annulus may lead to disc herniation into the spinal canal, a substantial cause of neurologic morbidity.

With growth of the individual prenatally through adolescence, a relative ascendancy of the spinal cord occurs in relation to the bony spine. Thus, in adulthood, the tip of the spinal cord, the conus medullaris, ends at about the L1–L2 disc space. The nerve roots continue caudally as the cauda equina and exit at their appropriate segmental bony level. The Pia arachnoid continues to about S2 as the filum terminale, and the dura attaches to the coccyx. A lesion at the C7 vertebra may be associated with a T1 spinal cord lesion, and a lesion at the T11 vertebra may be associated with an L3 lesion. As the C1 nerve root exits above the atlas, there are eight cervical spinal segments but only seven cervical vertebrae. Below C8, the nerve roots exit below the pedicles of the corresponding vertebra. Thickened arachnoid bands, the dentate or denticulate ligaments, attach the spinal cord to the dura at each segmental level. These ligaments serve as a landmark for the midpoint of the spinal cord in the A-P direction.

The Brain

The brain weighs about 1400 to 1600 g in the adult (about 2% of body weight). It can be divided grossly into the cerebral hemispheres, the brainstem—diencephalon, midbrain (mesencephalon), pons, medulla—and the cerebellum. The cerebral hemispheres occupy the supratentorial compartment, the brainstem passes through the tentorial notch and lies behind the clivus as it courses down to the foramen magnum, where it becomes spinal cord. The cerebellum occupies the infratentorial compartment behind and lateral to the brainstem. The cerebellum and brainstem account for about 15% to 20% of the brain's mass.

The cerebral hemispheres are essentially symmetrical, with their surfaces characterized by convolutions (gyri) and fissures (sulci). The neuronal cell bodies are on the surface of the brain (gray matter), and the myelinated axons project internally (white matter). Deep gray nuclei are found subcortically. The cerebral hemispheres are connected by broad white matter tracts—the corpus

callosum, anterior, posterior, and hippocampal commissures. The cerebral hemispheres are divided into four lobes: frontal, temporal, parietal, and occipital, although these do not show distinct anatomical boundaries (Fig. 21.3). The frontal lobe is the portion of the cerebral hemisphere that is anterior to the central sulcus of Rolando and superior and medial to the Sylvian fissure. The basal ganglia, nucleus basalis, and insula of Reil are contained within the frontal lobe. The cortex of the frontal lobe is subdivided further into the precentral gyrus (primary motor cortex) just anterior to the central sulcus and premotor cortex, including the area for conjugate eye movements just anterior to this. More frontally are the transversely oriented superior, middle, and inferior frontal gyri. The inferior gyrus, usually on the left side, contains the primary motor speech area. The orbital surface of the frontal lobe is divided by the olfactory sulcus into the gyrus rectus medially and the orbital gyri laterally. Deep to the Sylvian fissure is the insular cortex covering the basal ganglia. The edges of cortex around the Sylvian fissure are called operculae.

The temporal lobe lies inferior to the Sylvian fissure. It is separated from the parietal lobe by a line running from the posterior edge of the Sylvian fissure inferiorly to the preoccipital notch and on its inferomedial surface by a line from the splenium of the corpus callosum to the preoccipital notch. The mesial gyri, the uncus, contain the hippocampus. Superior, middle, and inferior temporal gyri are recognized on the surface of the temporal lobe. The transverse gyri of Heschl are contained in the temporal opercula and represent the primary auditory cortex.

The parietal lobe extends from just behind the central sulcus, which separates it from the frontal lobe, to the

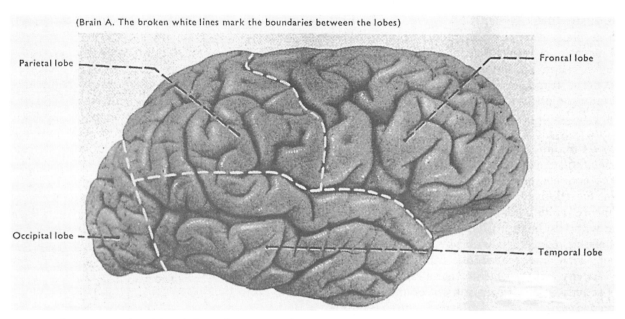

(Brain A. The broken white lines mark the boundaries between the lobes)

Parietal lobe

Frontal lobe

Occipital lobe

Temporal lobe

Figure 21.3.   Lobes of the right hemisphere. From Zuckerman S. A new system of anatomy. London: Oxford University Press, 1961:498.

parieto occipital sulcus on the mesial cerebral hemisphere, separating it from the occipital lobe. A line from the parieto occipital sulcus to the posterior Sylvian fissure to the preoccipital notch divides the parietal lobe from the temporal and occipital lobes on the surface of the hemisphere. The postcentral gyrus immediately behind the central sulcus is the primary sensory cortex. A mixture of sensory and motor functions exist in the pre- and postcentral gyri; these are sometimes termed the sensorimotor cortex. More posteriorly, the parietal lobe is divided into superior and inferior parietal lobules by the interparietal sulcus. The inferior parietal lobule contains the supramarginal and angular gyri, which on the left side are usually concerned with speech reception, reading, writing, and calculation. Body organization and spatial relationships are important right-sided parietal lobe functions. The occipital lobe is that cortex posterior to the parietal and occipital lobes. The cortex faces primarily mesially. The deep horizontal calcarine fissure separates the cuneate gyrus superiorly from the lingual gyrus inferiorly. These form the primary visual cortex, with the central (macular) visual cortex close to the occipital pole.

On the mesial surface of the cerebral hemispheres, the hippocampus, the fornix, and the cingulate gyrus above the corpus callosum run in close proximity to the ventricular system. These, in association with the anterior subcallosal area, the amygdala of the temporal lobe, and parts of the diencephalon, subserve arousal and emotion and are sometimes termed the limbic lobe.

White matter tracts are divided into: *(a)* association fibers that connect cortical neurons within the same hemisphere; *(b)* commissural fibers that connect corresponding areas of cortex in opposite hemispheres; *(c)* and projection fibers that run from the cerebral hemispheres to the brainstem and spinal cord. Important association fiber bundles include the arcuate fasciculus from the temporal to the frontal lobe and the optic radiations from the thalamus to the occipital cortex. The main portions of the two cerebral hemispheres are connected through the corpus callosum, the primary cerebral commissure. The anterior commissure connects the temporal lobes, and the hippocampal commissure connects the hippocampal cortex bilaterally. The posterior commissure is in the diencephalon and connects pretectal nuclei concerned with eye movements. Projection fibers include the long tracts, such as the corticospinal and extrapyramidal pathways. The white matter of the cerebral hemisphere is called the centrum semiovale above the basal ganglia and the internal capsule as it passes through the basal ganglia and thalamus to the brainstem.

The deep nuclei of the cerebral hemispheres include the basal ganglia—caudate, putamen, and globus pallidus—that are believed to modulate motor function but also seem to be concerned with behavior, affect, and ideation. Functionally, these are related closely to the thalamus and brainstem nuclei. The nucleus basalis of Meynert is located caudal to the basal ganglia and may play a role in cognitive function.

The diencephalon includes the paired thalami, the hypothalamus, the pineal gland, the habenular nuclei, and the subthalamus. Except for olfaction, all sensory information coming into the cerebral hemispheres is relayed through the thalamus. The thalamus maintains reciprocal connections with all areas of cerebral cortex and has been considered the key to understanding brain function. The thalami abut the ventricular system, forming the floor of the lateral ventricles and the medial walls of the third ventricle. The hypothalamus sits beneath the third ventricle and is continuous with the pituitary stalk. It has extensive hormonal and visceral functions. The pineal gland is in the roof of the third ventricle, and the subthalamus is continuous with the mesencephalon. The subthalamic area is functionally related to the basal ganglia and is sometimes included in this term.

The mesencephalon (midbrain) is characterized by the quadrigeminal plate (the superior and inferior colliculi) dorsally and the cerebral peduncles (the corticospinal and corticopontine tracts) ventrally. The cerebral aqueduct (of Sylvius) in the mesencephalic tegmentum connects the third and fourth ventricles. The tegmentum contains the nuclei of cranial nerves III and IV; the red nuclei; the substantia nigra; the ascending long tracts, including the decussation of the superior cerebellar peduncles; and the reticular formation. Cranial nerves III and IV exit from the mesencephalon ventrally and dorsally, respectively.

A pontomedullary sulcus ventrally divides the mesencephalon from the pons. The cerebral peduncles pass through the base of the pons and are dispersed into bundles of nerve fibers. Corticospinal and corticobulbar fibers continue caudally. Corticopontine fibers synapse with pontine nuclei and project to the cerebellum as the middle cerebellar peduncles. The tegmentum of the pons contains the nuclei of cranial nerve V with its associated spinal nucleus and tract, the nuclei of cranial nerves VI and VII, the long ascending tracts, and the reticular formation. Cranial nerve V exits the pons, and cranial nerve VI exits the pontomedullary sulcus at the caudal end of the pons. Cranial nerve VII exits laterally at the pontomedullary sulcus. The fourth ventricle separates the pons from the cerebellum.

The medulla is separated from the pons by the pontomedullary sulcus. The corticospinal tracts form the pyramids on the base of the medulla, and these decussate at this level before entering the spinal cord. The medullary tegmentum contains the nuclei for cranial nerves VIII through XII, the decussation of the posterior columns, the olivary nuclei, the long ascending tracts, and the reticular formation. The fourth ventricle ends dorsal to the medulla at the obex through a midline opening, the foramen of Magendie. The lateral openings,

Figure 21.4. Drawing of the brainstem with the cerebral and cerebellar peduncles cut. From Carpenter MB, Sutin J, eds. Human neuroanatomy. 8th ed. Baltimore: Williams & Wilkins, 1983:49.

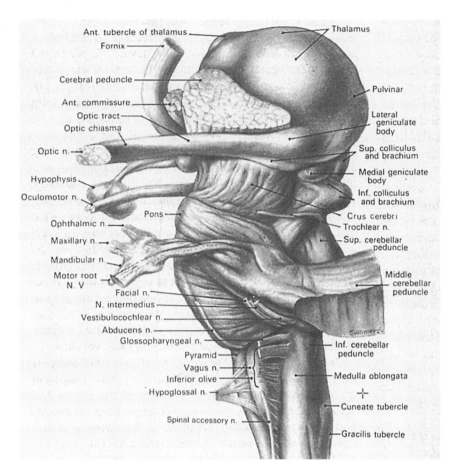

the foramina of Luschka, are located above the pontomedullary sulci (Fig. 21.4).

The cerebellum lies dorsal to the brainstem and is attached to it through three peduncles: the superior (brachium conjunctivum) to the mesencephalon; the middle (brachium pontis) to the pons; and the inferior (restiform body) to the medulla. The cerebellum is composed of a midline vermis and two hemispheres. Anatomically, there are multiple lobes of the cerebellum based on connections between the hemispheres and the vermis. Functionally, the cerebellum may be divided into the flocculonodular lobe (archicerebellum), concerned with vestibular function; the anterior lobe (paleocerebellum), concerned with spinal reflexes; and the posterior lobe (neocerebellum), concerned with fine-motor activity. The cerebellum functions to coordinate motor activity at an unconscious level and to set postural muscles to allow coordinated voluntary movements. The output of the cerebellum is through the superior cerebellar peduncles to the thalamus and brainstem nuclei.

The Spinal Cord

The spinal cord runs from the cervicomedullary junction to the inferior body of the L1 vertebra. It is a segmental structure composed of central gray matter surrounded by ascending and descending white matter tracts. Small rootlets are given off ventrally and dorsally, and these combine at each segmental level to give a ventral motor root and a dorsal sensory root that exit the spine. The cell bodies of the dorsal root are in the dorsal root ganglion outside the spinal cord, whereas those of the motor root are in the ventral column of gray matter cells. Autonomic fibers also contribute to the ventral root. Sensory fibers may be contained in the ventral root to explain the failure of dorsal rhizotomy in relieving pain.

The spinal cord diameter gradually reduces from rostral to caudal as motor tracts synapse and sensory input is added. Cervical and lumbar enlargements of the spinal cord signify neural output to the extremities. Spinal cord tracts are divided into three columns: the posterior columns, conveying vibration, touch, and joint position; the lateral columns, containing the corticospinal (motor) and lateral spinothalamic (pain and temperature) tracts; and the anterior columns, conveying touch sensation. Many other ascending and descending tracts share these three columns (Fig. 21.5).

Intrinsic Architecture of the CNS

Reflex Arcs

The nervous system operates through a hierarchy of reflexes from the most basic monosynaptic stretch reflex through segmental, suprasegmental, autonomic, on up

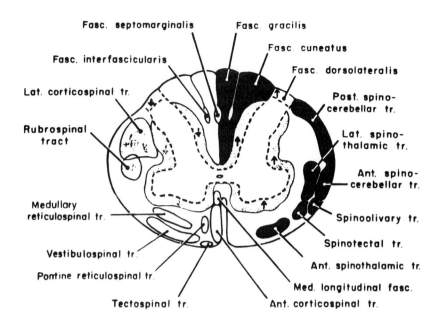

Figure 21.5. Diagram of the ascending and descending tracts of the spinal cord. From Carpenter MB, Sutin J, eds. Human neuroanatomy. 8th ed. Baltimore: Williams & Wilkins, 1983:302.

to complex behavioral reflexes. The term *reflex* implies a stereotyped and unconscious or involuntary response to a sensory input. The prototype monosynaptic stretch reflex involves a specialized sensory receptor in the muscle, the muscle spindle, which, when activated by lengthening, transmits an afferent impulse over a large myelinated (Ia) fiber to an excitatory synapse on the α-motor neuron supplying that muscle. This results in contraction of the skeletal muscle fiber to restore the length of the muscle spindle. The resting length or tension in the muscle spindle is influenced by a τ-motor neuron that in turn receives input from segmental and suprasegmental interneurons. The same afferent fiber that excites the α-motor neuron of the stretched muscle inhibits the motor neurons of antagonistic muscles through interposed inhibitory neurons.

Increasingly complex responses, such as withdrawal of a limb in response to pain, setting of proximal muscles to allow fine movements of distal muscles, locomotion, visceral responses, and so forth, can be considered extensions of this concept, with progressively larger numbers of excitatory and inhibitory interneurons involved in the reflex. Many reflexes are genetically coded into the architecture of the nervous system, although others can be learned, modified, and forgotten over the lifetime of an individual. Understanding how responses are elicited and how they can be modified by experience is a key goal of the neurosciences.

Ascending Sensory Systems

Sensation below the head is conveyed into the spinal cord through neurons located in the dorsal root ganglia. These unipolar neurons carry information received from specialized nerve endings sensitive to a variety of external stimuli into the dorsal horn of the central gray matter of the spinal cord. The central gray matter has been sub-

divided into 10 laminae (I to X) by Rexed based on cell type and functional considerations (2). Laminae I to VII are in the dorsal horn and intermediate area, laminae VIII to X in the ventral horn, and lamina X in the area of the central canal. A functional division of sensory information occurs at a spinal cord level, with pathways for conscious position sense, pain and temperature, touch, and unconscious position sense ascending in discrete nerve bundle tracts.

Posterior Columns. The large myelinated nerve fibers subserving pressure, vibration, and joint position (proprioception) pass through the dorsal root entry zone without synapse and ascend as the posterior (dorsal) columns. These remain ipsilateral in the spinal cord. As the upper thoracic area is reached, two ipsilateral fasciculi are recognized: the fasciculus gracilis, medially serving the lower portion of the body, and the fasciculus cuneatus, laterally carrying information from the upper extremities. These ascend to the lower medulla where they synapse on their respective nuclei, the gracilis and cuneatus. The axons of these second-order neurons decussate at the lower medullary level as the internal arcuate fibers and ascend contralaterally in the brainstem as the medial lemnisci. The medial lemnisci terminate in the ventral posterolateral nucleus of the thalamus, and the third-order neuron reaches the postcentral gyrus—the primary somatosensory cortex. Thus, these modalities of sensation become conscious at the synapse of the third-order neuron.

Pain Pathways

Lateral Spinothalamic Tract. Smaller nerve fibers that carry the sensations of pain and temperature (nociception) enter the spinal cord through the dorsal root and ascend or descend one or two segments as Lissauer's tract. These synapse primarily on neurons in laminae I, II, and V. Lamina II, the substantia gelatinosa, is composed primarily of interneurons, whereas laminae I and V are the primary projection neurons for ascending pain pathways. The nociceptive neurotransmitter, substance P, is found in high concentration in these gray matter laminae. A complex interaction between excitatory and inhibitory interneurons in the substantia gelatinosa has been suggested to modulate pain pathway transmission (gate theory), but the exact mechanisms of this remain unclear.

The projection axons from laminae I and V cross just in front of the central canal of the spinal cord as the anterior commissure and ascend contralaterally in the anterior portion of the lateral column as the lateral spinothalamic tract. As destruction of this tract does not completely abolish pain sensation contralaterally, other ascending pathways have been postulated. The lateral spinothalamic tract ascends through the brainstem to reach the thalamus, but many of the fibers synapse with the brainstem reticular formation so that the number of fibers projecting directly to the thalamus is reduced considerably. The lateral portion of the spinothalamic tract projects to the ventral posterior thalamic nuclei and is concerned with more acute, localized pain. The medial portion projects to the medial and intralaminar thalamic nuclei, as do those fibers synapsing through the reticular formation. These may convey less localized, more chronic pain. Ventroposterior thalamic neurons project to the somatosensory cortex, although the medial and intralaminar nuclei have extensive connections with the limbic system and frontal lobes.

Although pain perception results from afferent transmission from pain-sensitive nerve endings, considerable modulation of pain pathways by other neuronal groups exist at both the spinal cord and the brainstem levels. Areas of the brainstem concerned with pain modulation include the periaqueductal gray matter, the hypothalamic periventricular gray matter, the dorsal pontine tegmentum, and the ventral medullary reticular formation. These pathways converge in the ventral medulla and travel in the spinal cord in the dorsal part of the lateral column to synapse on cells of laminae I, II, and V in the spinal gray matter dorsal horn. One system uses the amine neurotransmitters norepinephrine and serotonin from the pons and medulla, respectively, to inhibit spinal nociceptive neurons and to interconnect brainstem pain-modulating centers. Another system uses the endogenous opioid peptide neurotransmitters enkephalin, β-endorphin, and dynorphin. These peptides and their receptors are located in the periaqueductal gray matter, hypothalamus, ventral medulla, and dorsal horn of the spinal cord. The precise interconnections of these pain pathways remain to be elucidated.

Spinocerebellar Tracts. Information from muscle and joint stretch and pressure receptors, including muscle spindles and Golgi tendon organs, is conveyed through the spinal cord to the cerebellum by the spinoc-

erebellar tracts. These transmit unconscious proprioception and are thought to function in coordinating fine-motor movements and setting postural and antagonistic muscles.

Afferent fibers from the dorsal root ganglion enter the spinal cord and may ascend or descend several segments in the posterior Lamina VII (Clark's nucleus). The second-order neurons ascend on the dorsal margin of the lateral column as the posterior spinocerebellar tract. In the medulla, these join with the inferior cerebellar peduncle to terminate in the cerebellar vermis.

Neurons that give rise to the anterior spinocerebellar tract are localized less discretely in the spinal gray matter and are concentrated in the base of the dorsal and ventral horns. They receive afferents from ipsilateral and contralateral joint receptors in the lower extremities and pass with the superior cerebellar peduncle to the anterior lobe of the cerebellum. Inherited ataxias may selectively affect the spinocerebellar tracts and their connections.

Anterior Spinothalamic Tract. The sensation of light touch is conveyed through tactile receptors (Meissner's corpuscles) to the dorsal root ganglion and into the dorsal horn, where synapses occur in laminae I, IV, and V. Second-order axons cross in the anterior commissure to the contralateral anterior column, where they ascend as the anterior spinothalamic tract. Itching and tickling may be sensations subserved by this tract.

Descending Motor Systems

Spinal Motor Neurons. Muscular contraction is initiated by the firing of motor neurons in the spinal cord and brainstem. These motor neurons are the only connection of the CNS to muscles and thus represent the final common pathway of the excitatory and inhibitory motor pathways within the CNS. Two types of motor neurons are recognized: the larger α- and the smaller γ-motor neurons. The α-motor neuron innervates the skeletal muscle fibers through a specialized synaptic connection, the motor end plate, using acetylcholine as a neurotransmitter. One motor neuron innervates a few hundred to several thousand muscle fibers. This is termed a motor unit. The γ-motor neuron innervates the muscle spindle, a specialized receptor that sets muscle tone and monitors stretch and contraction.

Spinal motor neurons are arranged in columns in the ventral horn of spinal gray matter in laminae VIII and IX. The α-motor neurons (anterior horn cells) are arranged into medial and lateral groups, with the medial group supplying muscles attached to the axial skeleton and the lateral group supplying the muscles of the trunk and extremities. The lateral group is organized somatotopically so that the more medial neurons supply proximal muscles and the more lateral neurons, the more distal muscles. In addition, neurons supplying flexor muscles are dorsal to those supplying extensor muscles.

The α-motor neuron is termed the lower motor neuron. All descending neurons that modulate the activity of the lower motor neuron are called upper motor neurons. The lower motor neuron synapses directly to the muscle, and its loss results in atrophy of the muscle, loss of tone and stretch reflexes, and spontaneous contractions of muscle, such as fasciculations. Upper motor neuron lesions cause hypertonia, increased stretch reflexes, release of spinal reflexes, and spasticity. Spasticity refers to tonic contraction of antigravity muscles that will suddenly release with stretching of the muscle. The concept of upper and lower motor neuron lesions is extremely important in localizing a neurologic lesion.

Corticospinal Tracts. The corticospinal tracts include those nerve fibers that originate in the cerebral cortex and connect with motor neurons in the brainstem and spinal cord. Each corticospinal tract contains about 1 million axons located in the precentral and postcentral gyri and the premotor area of the frontal lobe. The large pyramidal cells of Betz account for about 40,000 axons in each corticospinal tract. The corticospinal tract passes through the subcortical white matter (corona radiata) and the internal capsule at the level of the basal ganglia and thalamus to form the cerebral peduncle with the corticopontine fibers. The tract courses through the basis pontis to form the medullary pyramids. The corticospinal tract is also termed the pyramidal tract because of this formation. Fibers given to the brainstem motor nuclei are called corticobulbar fibers, and those that pass into the spinal cord are corticospinal fibers. About 90% of the corticospinal fibers cross in the pyramidal decussation and travel in the dorsal half of the lateral column as the lateral corticospinal tract. The remaining 10% of fibers descend ipsilaterally in the anterior column as the anterior corticospinal tract that ends at upper thoracic cord levels. These latter fibers cross in the anterior commissure to supply contralateral anterior horn cells. The corticospinal tract is responsible for volitional movement, especially of the upper extremities, and interruption of the tract leads to paralysis.

Extrapyramidal Descending Motor Tracts. The remaining descending motor tracts originate in the brainstem and course to spinal levels. These tracts are more concerned with coordination of movements, postures, and muscle tone. Many descending motor tracts are recognized. Most important are the rubrospinal, vestibulospinal, and reticulospinal tracts.

Fibers from the red nucleus descend in the spinal cord as the rubrospinal tract to synapse upon the motor neurons supplying flexor muscles. The vestibulospinal tract originates from the lateral vestibular nucleus and synapses primarily upon extensor motor neurons. Thus, an antagonistic role exists between the rubrospinal and vestibulospinal tracts in control of posture and tone. The reticulospinal tract descends from the lower brainstem to the spinal cord. The reticulospinal tract is involved in respiration, cardiopressor responses, bladder function, and pain modulation.

Brainstem Nuclei and Tracts

Motor Nuclei and Cranial Nerves. Muscles controlling eye movements, facial and masticatory movements, and movement of the tongue and pharyngeal muscles are subserved by motor neurons in the brainstem. These in turn are under reflex and voluntary control from cortical, brainstem, and spinal cord influences.

Cranial nerves controlling ocular movements and pupillary reflexes are the oculomotor, (CN III), trochlear (CN IV), and the abducens (CN VI). These exit the brain stem, traverse the cavernous sinus, and enter the orbit through the superior orbital fissure. The abducens nerve supplies the lateral rectus muscle to abduct the eye, and the trochlear nerve innervates the superior oblique muscle to depress and intort the eye. All other ocular muscles, including lid elevators and pupillary sphincters, are supplied by the oculomotor nerve.

Eye movements are coordinated by multiple controlling influences. The median longitudinal fasciculus (MLF) interconnects the nuclei of CN III, IV, and VI and connects these with the vestibular system and ascending and descending axons in the reticular formation. The tract extends from the cervical spinal cord to the upper mesencephalon. Damage to the MLF gives dysconjugate gaze difficulties, particularly medial rectus dysfunction on attempted lateral gaze and nystagmus. This is termed internuclear ophthalmoplegia. Conjugate gaze is controlled by two "gaze centers," one in the pons and one in the frontal lobe. Damage to the pontine gaze center causes the patient to look away from the side of the lesion. The gaze center in the posterior frontal lobe projects through the superior colliculus to the oculomotor complex. Damage to one cerebral hemisphere causes the patient to look toward the side of the lesion. The superior colliculi are responsible for allowing an object of interest to be brought into the center of the visual field. The pretectal area just rostral to the superior colliculi mediates the pupillary light reflex and subserves upward gaze.

The facial nerve (CN VII) is a complex nerve supplying the muscles of facial expression. It also carries parasympathetic fibers and afferent axons conveying taste and somatic sensation. The facial nerve nucleus is just beneath the floor of the fourth ventricle in the caudal pons. The fibers of the nerve course over the abducens nucleus, turn laterally, and exit the lateral pontomedullary junction just beneath the foramen of Luschka. The nerve passes with CN VIII into the internal auditory canal, runs through the temporal bone to exit the stylomastoid foramen, and branches in the parotid gland to supply facial muscles. Corticobulbar fibers cross in the pons to supply the facial nerve nucleus. The upper one-third of the face has more bilateral representation, so that upper motor neuron lesions tend to affect the lower two-thirds of the face primarily. These are distinguished from lower motor neuron lesions, where all ipsilateral facial muscles are weak.

The autonomic portion (nervus intermedius) passes into the internal auditory canal with the motor facial nerve but diverges in the temporal bone to send parasympathetic fibers to the pterygopalatine ganglion (lacrimal and nasal glands), via the superficial petrosal nerve, and to the submandibular ganglion (submandibular and sublingual glands), via the chorda tympani connection to the trigeminal nerve. The chorda tympani carries the afferent fibers for taste on the anterior tongue back to the geniculate ganglion in the temporal bone and with the facial nerve back to the solitary (gustatory) nucleus in the medulla.

The muscles of mastication—the masseters, pterygoids, and temporalis—are supplied by the motor division of the trigeminal nerve (CN V). This nerve exits the foramen ovale and runs with the mandibular branch of the trigeminal nerve.

The muscles of the pharynx and larynx receive innervation from the glossopharyngeal (CN IX), vagus (CN X), and spinal accessory (CN XI) nerves whose cell bodies lie in the nucleus ambiguus adjacent to the medullary reticular formation. The glossopharyngeal nerve is primarily a sensory nerve but also supplies the stylopharyngeal muscles. The cranial portion of CN XI supplies the vocal cords through the recurrent laryngeal nerve. The spinal portion of CN XI originates from cells in the upper cervical spinal cord and supplies the trapezius and sternocleidomastoid muscles. The remainder of the palatal and pharyngeal muscles are supplied by the vagus nerve. The extensive autonomic functions of these cranial nerves will be discussed with the ANS. These three nerves exit the jugular foramen to pass to the pharynx and neck. The glossopharyngeal nerve (CN IX) courses over the internal carotid artery and beneath the styloid process and external carotid artery. It reaches the posterior tongue and pharynx beneath the hyoglossus muscle. The vagus nerve is joined by the cranial portion of the accessory nerve and first courses between and then behind the internal carotid artery and jugular vein in the carotid sheath. The spinal accessory nerve diverges from the vagus nerve in the carotid sheath, passes through the sternocleidomastoid muscle, and posteriorly enters the trapezius muscle.

The hypoglossal nerve (CN XII) innervates the muscles of the tongue. The nerve arises from cells near the midline in the lower medulla and emerges as rootlets between the pyramid and olive to coalesce into a single nerve that exits the hypoglossal foramen on the skull base. There is usually prominent bilateral corticobulbar supply, so weakness is more apparent with lower motor neuron lesions. The strongest muscle, the genioglossus, protrudes the tongue, so with weakness deviation exists to the ipsilateral side. After exiting the hypoglossal

canal, the nerve passes between the internal carotid artery and jugular vein and anterior to the external carotid and lingual arteries. It gives off the descendens hypoglossi (ansa cervicalis) nerve, passes deep to the digastric muscle, and enters the muscles of the tongue.

Sensory Nuclei and Cranial Nerves.   Sensation on the face, nasal cavity, teeth, mouth, and part of the skull base is conveyed by the trigeminal nerve (CN V). The three peripheral divisions of this nerve—the ophthalmic, maxillary, and mandibular—pass through the superior orbital fissure, foramen rotundum, and foramen ovale, respectively, to their cell bodies in the trigeminal (Gasserian) ganglion, located in a trough in the temporal bone (Meckel's cave). Fibers from the trigeminal ganglion carrying pain sensation enter the brainstem and descend as the spinal trigeminal tract, which continues into the cervical spinal cord. These synapse on the adjacent spinal trigeminal nucleus, which is continuous with the substantia gelatinosa of the spinal cord. Secondary axons cross the brainstem and ascend to the ventral posteromedial thalamus as the trigeminothalamic tract. Fibers conveying pain and general sensation around the ear, tonsil, and pharynx are also carried with the facial, glossopharyngeal, and vagus nerves and enter the spinal trigeminal nucleus.

Taste sensation enters the medulla from the facial nerve (anterior tongue), glossopharyngeal nerve (posterior tongue and pharynx), and a few fibers of the vagus nerve (epiglottis) to enter the lateral portion of the nucleus solitarius in the medulla. General sensation from the tongue, pharynx, larynx, and thoracic and abdominal viscera is conveyed via the glossopharyngeal and vagus nerves to the medial portion of the nucleus solitarius. Second-order neurons ascend to the ventral posteromedial nucleus of the thalamus and reticular formation. Cranial nerves I (olfactory) and II (optic) represent brain tracts and will be discussed with the thalamus.

The vestibulocochlear nerve (CN VIII) has two anatomical and functional components: the cochlear, carrying hearing, and the vestibular, carrying the sense of equilibrium and orientation in space. Both components of the nerve arise from receptors in the temporal bone: the cochlear nerve from the cochlea, and the vestibular nerve from the labyrinth.

Sound waves are transmitted from the tympanic membrane through the middle ear ossicles to the oval window of the inner ear. The inner ear (organ of Corti) consists of a tectorial and a basilar membrane suspended in fluid (perilymph). Sound waves oscillate the basilar membrane, distorting hair cells and propagating an impulse. These bipolar cells have cell bodies in the spiral ganglion within the cochlea. The afferent axons form the cochlear nerve and course to the medulla to synapse on the cochlear nuclei lateral to the inferior cerebellar peduncle. Axons from the cochlear nuclei form the acoustic striae that both cross and ascend uncrossed as the lateral lemnisci. The lateral lemniscus synapses primarily in the ipsilateral inferior colliculus in the midbrain, with some fibers crossing to the opposite inferior colliculus and others coursing directly to the medial geniculate body of the thalamus. All fibers eventually reach the medial geniculate body. Geniculocortical fibers project to the temporal operculum (transverse gyri of Heschl), the primary auditory cortex. Loss of the cochlear nerve or nucleus causes complete unilateral deafness. Lesions of the brainstem and cortex do not cause complete deafness but may affect localization of sound and perhaps discrimination.

Receptors in the labyrinth—the utricle, saccule, and semicircular canals—transmit impulses through the vestibular ganglion (Scarpa's) along the superior and inferior vestibular nerves to the vestibular ganglia in the medulla. Vestibular connections are widespread, but particularly important connections include the flocculonodular lobe of the cerebellum, the median longitudinal fasciculus (see above), and the vestibulospinal tract to motor neurons in the spinal cord. Vestibular stimulation results in vertigo (a sense of whirling and nausea) and nystagmus (rhythmic oscillations of the eyes). Vestibular tracts are concerned with oculocephalic and tonic neck reflexes and subserve decerebrate rigidity after brainstem injury.

Brainstem Reticular Formation. The central core of polysynaptic neurons in the brainstem is called the reticular formation. The reticular formation extends from the lower medulla to the upper mesencephalon. Descending and ascending projections arise from cells in the larger medial reticular formation. Descending reticulospinal fibers primarily facilitate deep tendon reflexes and extensor motor tone. This is effected through the τ-efferent motor neuron system. The medullary reticular formation contains the respiratory and vasomotor centers.

An ascending central reticular polysynaptic pathway, independent of the ascending lemniscal sensory systems, is responsible for generalized cortical arousal and is termed the ascending reticular activating system (ARAS). This system receives collaterals from all ascending sensory systems but does not convey a specific sensory modality. It is responsible for the waking pattern on EEG and is believed to be the basis for consciousness.

Cerebellum

The cerebellum is responsible for coordination of muscle movements and tone. Information delivered to the cerebellum does not enter consciousness but allows the setting of postural and associated muscles, allowing smooth voluntary movement. Afferent impulses from muscle spindles, joint receptors, and tendon organs are carried to the cerebellum via the spinocerebellar tracts. These combine with the corticopontine tracts to influence cerebellar efferent neurons.

The cerebellar cortex is thrown into folds (folia) and consists of three layers: the superficial molecular layers, the Purkinje cell layer, and the granular layer (Fig. 21.6). Ascending sensory fibers entering the cerebellar cortex are modulated by neurons in the deeper granular layer

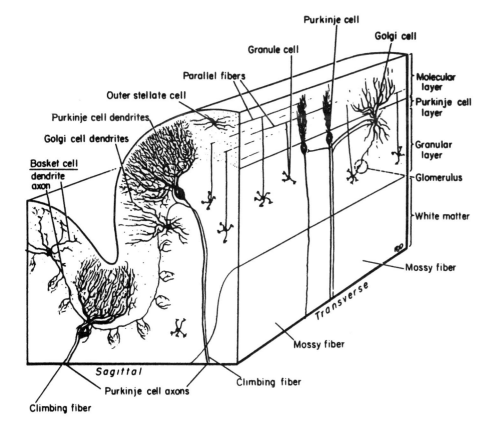

Figure 21.6. Diagram of the cerebellar cortex. From Carpenter MB, Sutin J. Human neuroanatomy. 8th ed. Baltimore: Williams & Wilkins, 1983:458.

before ascending to the molecular layer to synapse with Purkinje cell dendrites. Axons of the Purkinje cells course in the cerebellar white matter to the deep cerebellar nuclei and the vestibular nucleus. They use GABA as an inhibitory neurotransmitter.

The deep cerebellar nuclei—the fastigial, globose, emboliform, and dentate—are located within the white matter close to the fourth ventricle and project as the superior cerebellar peduncle to the ventrolateral nucleus of the contralateral thalamus. The thalamocortical fibers mainly synapse on primary motor cortical areas.

Functionally, there are three cerebellar zones: a vermal (midline) cerebellar cortex, which projects the fastigial nucleus and secondarily to the vestibular nuclei, regulating extensor (postural) tone; a paravermal zone, projecting to the globose and emboliform nuclei and then to the red nucleus, facilitating flexor tone; and a lateral zone, projecting to the dentate nucleus, to the ventral lateral nucleus of the thalamus, and finally to the sensorimotor cerebral cortex to coordinate pyramidal tract function. Lesions involving the vernal and paravermal zones produce gait disturbance and imbalance (ataxia) and often cause nystagmus and speech dysfunction. Lesions involving the lateral zone (cerebellar hemisphere) include hypotonia, tremor, dysmetria, dysdiadochokinesia, and other types of muscle coordination asynergia.

Thalamus

The paired thalami, separated by the third ventricle, are large nuclear masses responsible for the integration of sensory information. All sensation except olfaction is processed in the thalamus before arriving at a cortical level. The thalamic nuclei project to all areas of the cerebral cortex and, in turn, receive input from corresponding cortical areas. Because the specific ascending sensory pathways and the ascending reticular-activating system converge in the thalamus, the thalamus is considered to bring sensory information into awareness.

The thalamus contains multiple nuclear groups with complex relationships. The ventral nuclei convey sensation of pain, touch, vibration, position and temperature to the primary sensory cortex (post central gyrus) in a topographical manner. The ventral nuclei also modulate motor activity. The lateral and medial geniculate bodies subserve vision and hearing respectively. Anterior and dorsal nuclei are related to the limbic system concerned with the emotional and affective processing of information. The intralaminar nuclei are thought to be involved in general arousal responses and central control of pain.

Hypothalamus

The hypothalamus forms the walls of the third ventricle below the hypothalamic sulcus and is connected to the pituitary gland through the infundibulum and pituitary stalk. This small area of brain is vitally important for control of autonomic, endocrine, and behavioral functions. The hypothalamus has afferent and efferent connections to multiple areas of the nervous system, including the brainstem, spinal cord, pituitary gland, and limbic system.

The hypothalamus functions as the brain center for autonomic function. Both sympathetic and parasympathetic activity are coordinated in the hypothalamus. In general, the anteromedial area of the hypothalamus is responsible for parasympathetic functions, and the posterolateral area regulates sympathetic activity. Osmoreceptors in the anterior hypothalamus constitute a thirst center and are related to the supraoptic nucleus, where the antidiuretic hormone (ADH) vasopressin is formed. The lateral area of the hypothalamus seems concerned with hunger, and the ventromedial area with satiety. The anterior hypothalamus also controls temperature regulation by its connections with other hypothalamic areas.

Another important function of the hypothalamus is hormonal regulation. The neuropeptides vasopressin (ADH) and oxytocin are secreted directly from axons in the posterior lobe of the pituitary, with their cell bodies in the supraoptic and paraventricular nuclei. The hormones of the anterior lobe of the pituitary are regulated by releasing factors from the hypothalamus that are brought to the pituitary gland through the hypophyseal portal system rather than through direct neural connections. These releasing factors regulate growth hormone, adrenocorticotropic hormone, thyroid-stimulating hormone, luteinizing hormone, follicle-stimulating hormone, prolactin, and their target organs through a complicated feedback mechanism. These factors are, in turn, acted on by afferent fibers to the hypothalamus from other brain centers.

Finally, the hypothalamus acts as a center for behavior and emotional expression. Attentiveness, somnolence, and the visceral components of rage, fear, aggressiveness, and pleasure are produced by electrical stimulation of areas of the hypothalamus in animals. The neuroanatomical connections of these complex behaviors in humans are unclear.

Basal Ganglia

The basal ganglia are located in the deep frontal lobe and diencephalon and are concerned with motor function. They consist of the corpus striatum (caudate, putamen, and globus pallidus), the claustrum, the subthalamic nuclei, and the substantia nigra. The caudate and putamen are termed neostriatum and seem to be a unified nucleus anatomically divided by the internal capsule. The globus pallidus is medial to the putamen and separated from the thalamus by the posterior limb of the internal capsule. The subthalamic nucleus lies just caudally in the diencephalon, and the substantia nigra lies farther caudally in the midbrain tegmentum. These nuclei form circuits that modulate and connect the motor cortex, thalamus, and descending motor pathways.

Afferents to the striatum include cerebral cortex, thalamus, and substantia nigra. All areas of the cortex project to the caudate and putamen, but the sensorimotor cortex and premotor areas are better represented. The striatum receives bilateral projections from the cortex. An important afferent input to the striatum is the substantia nigra. Melanin-containing cells in the substantia nigra convey the neurotransmitter dopamine to the putamen and caudate. Degeneration of these nigral cells is associated with Parkinsonism. A reciprocal striatonigral pathway uses GABA and substance P as neurotransmitters, which are inhibitory and excitatory, respectively. Finally, there is a serotonin-transmitted pathway from the dorsal brainstem to the striatum that has been implicated in behavioral disturbances.

The primary output of the caudate and putamen (striatum) is to the globus pallidus. The globus pallidus does not receive fibers directly from the cerebral cortex, thalamus, or substantia nigra. Striatopallidal fibers use GABA as a neurotransmitter.

Lesions of the basal ganglia are associated with alterations in tone and involuntary movements. Muscular rigidity and slowness in initiating movements as well as tremor are characteristic of Parkinsonism, for which the primary lesion is loss of dopamine-producing cells in the substantia nigra. Chorea (quick involuntary movements), athetosis (writhing movements), and dystonia (fixed postural movements) are found in Huntington's disease and other genetic disorders and are associated with neuronal atrophy and loss of GABA in the neostriatum. Ballism (violent movements of the extremities) occurs with lesions in the contralateral subthalamic nucleus. The efferent fibers of the basal ganglia course to the thalamus and, subsequently, to the cerebral cortex but not to the lower brainstem or spinal cord. Thus, the modulation of motor activity from the basal ganglia is thought to be mediated through the corticospinal tract.

Visual System

The visual system is concerned with the processing of visual information (light) and voluntary and reflex movements of the eyes that fix the visual image to be processed. Eye movements and tracking were discussed under brainstem nuclei. The visual world seen by each eye is termed the visual field. The visual fields generally are divided into superior and inferior, nasal, and temporal quadrants. The lens inverts and transposes the visual field onto the retina so that the temporal fields are on the nasal retina, the superior fields on the inferior retina, etc. The photosensitive cells, or the rods (low illumination) and cones (high illumination and color), are connected by bipolar cells to the retinal ganglion cells whose axons form the optic nerves. The optic nerves pass from the orbit through the optic foramina to the subarachnoid chiasmatic cistern, where they partially decussate as the optic chiasm. Only the fibers from the nasal retina that represent the temporal visual fields cross. Posterior to the chiasm, the fibers are called the optic tracts, with each tract carrying the contralateral hemivisual field. The tracts encircle the hypothalamus and synapse in the lateral geniculate body of the thalamus. Those fibers concerned with eye movements and pupillary reactions go directly to the area of the superior colliculus without entering the lateral geniculate body.

The visual fibers coursing from the thalamus to the occipital cortex are termed the geniculocalcarine tract or optic radiations. Superior fibers carrying the inferior visual field course adjacent to the ventricle to reach the occipital lobe superior to the calcarine fissure. Inferior fibers carrying the superior visual field course forward into the temporal lobe and follow the temporal horn of the ventricle posteriorly to end in the occipital lobe inferior to the calcarine fissure (Fig. 21.7). Thus, temporal lesions give a homonymous (both eyes) superior quadrantanopsia, and parietal lesions give an inferior quadrantanopsia. Occipital lesions are associated with homonymous hemianopsia. The more posterior the lesion, the more similar (congruous) the field loss in each eye. Macular fibers end in the occipital pole, and peripheral retinal fibers end more rostrally.

Processing of visual information occurs at all levels of the visual system. In the retina, one ganglion cell receives several rods and cones. The receptive area for each ganglion cell is circular and has an excitatory center and inhibitory margin or an inhibitory center and excitatory margin. Neurons in the lateral geniculate body have a similar anatomical mechanism to enhance discrimination. Occipital (striate) cortex has a columnar arrangement of neurons; the columns are stimulated by edges of light/dark in various orientations, and the columns of cells respond more to images in one or the other eye. Interconnections between these columns of cells allow patterns to be formed and provide binocular vision. Adjacent association cortex connects these patterns to memory and recognition.

Olfactory System

Olfactory sensory cells are found in a specialized epithelium in the nasal mucosa. These are bipolar neurons that project their axons through the cribriform plate of the ethmoid bone to the olfactory bulb, where they synapse on mitral cells. Axons of mitral cells form the olfactory tract that courses posteriorly in the olfactory sulcus between the gyrus rectus and the orbital gyri and divides into medial and lateral stria. The smaller medial stria runs to the subcallosal (septal) area, although the larger lateral stria synapses in the prepiriform area of the temporal lobe. This cortex then projects to the parahippocampal gyrus (uncus and entorhinal areas) and

Figure 21.7.   Diagram of the visual pathways showing the optic chiasm and optic radiations. From Carpenter MB, Sutin J. Human neuroanatomy. 8th ed. Baltimore: Williams & Wilkins, 1983:541.

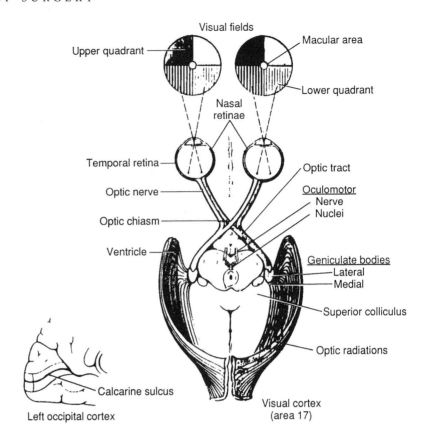

the amygdala. Olfaction is the only sensation not processed by the thalamus.

Cerebral Cortex and Higher Cortical Functions

Cortical Architecture.   The cerebral cortex is characterized by alternating layers of larger pyramidal and smaller granule cells. Typically, the adult cerebral cortex contains six layers: I, consisting mainly of dendrites; II, an external granular layer; III, an external pyramidal layer; IV, an internal granular layer; V, an internal pyramidal layer; and VI, a layer of fusiform cells. Areas of the hippocampus contain only three layers: a molecular layer, a pyramidal or granular layer, and a polymorphic layer. Six-layered cortex is called neocortex, and three-layered cortex is called allocortex. Development of these layers varies in different areas of the cortex. Efferent axons of cortical neurons are termed association fibers if they synapse within the same hemisphere, commissural fibers if they connect to corresponding regions of the opposite hemisphere, and projection fibers if they course to subcortical destinations. Association and commissural fibers arise mainly from cells in layers II and III, and projection fibers primarily from pyramidal cells in layer V. Cells in layer VI project to the thalamus. In addition to the horizontal layers of cells, the cortex is arranged into vertical columns that extend through all six layers and form functional physiologic units. This organization is particularly apparent in visual and sensory cortex.

Motor Areas.   The precentral gyrus contains mainly pyramidal neurons, including the giant Betz cells, and is considered the primary motor area, although it accounts for only about 30% of axons in the corticospinal tract (Fig. 21.8). The largest nerve fibers in the corticospinal tract originate from this area. Stimulation of this gyrus results in discrete movements of the contralateral face and limbs; the face area is closest to the Sylvian fissure, the arm area is located more superiorly on the frontal lobe, and the lower extremity is on the mesial aspect of the hemisphere (Fig. 21.9). Destruction of the gyrus causes contralateral paralysis that is initially flaccid but later shows some return of tone. Spasticity is not characteristic.

Adjacent rostrally to the primary motor area is the premotor area. Stimulation of cortex closest to the primary motor area results in similar movements but requires a greater stimulus, while stimulation more rostrally on the superior frontal gyrus causes aversive head and eye movements and posturing of the trunk and extremities. Bilateral movements of the face and pharyngeal muscles can be elicited. The cortex on the medial surface of the superior frontal gyrus is called the supplementary motor area, and stimulation results in posturing and bilateral movements. Ablation of the premotor area does not cause paralysis, but removal of the primary motor and premotor areas gives paralysis for which spasticity is a prominent feature. Almost 40% of axons in the corticospinal tract come from neurons in the postcentral gyrus (parietal lobe), and sensations are

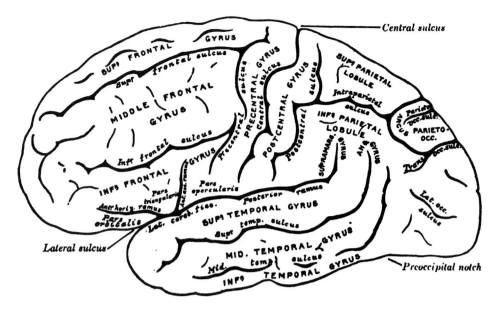

Figure 21.8. Lateral view of the cerebral hemisphere, showing the precentral and postcentral gyri in relation to other areas of cortex. From Goss CM. Gray's anatomy. 28th ed. Philadelphia: Lea & Febiger, 1970:842.

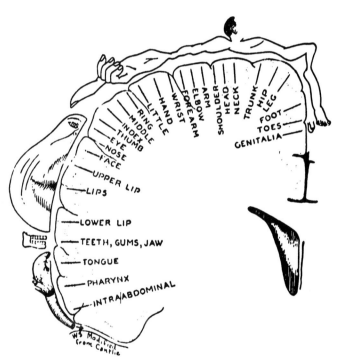

Figure 21.9. Motor homunculus, showing motor representation in the precentral gyrus. From Goss CM. Gray's anatomy. 28th ed. Philadelphia: Lea & Febiger, 1970:849.

Figure 21.10. Sensory homunculus, showing tactile sensory representation in the postcentral gyrus. From Goss CM. Gray's anatomy. 28th ed. Philadelphia: Lea & Febiger, 1970:850.

described with stimulation of the precentral gyrus. Therefore, the precentral and postcentral gyri have overlapping functions and are together called sensorimotor cortex.

Sensory Areas. The postcentral gyrus represents the primary cortical sensory area. Granule cells predominate (granular cortex). The edge of the gyrus closest to the central sulcus receives the major output of the ventral posterior thalamic nuclei, and this area responds most readily to cutaneous stimuli (Fig. 21.10). The posterior edge of the gyrus receives finer fibers and responds

to joint movement and deep pressure. A secondary somatic sensory area is described along the parietal operculum of the Sylvian fissure.

Visual cortex is located in the occipital lobe above and below the calcarine fissure and was discussed under the visual system. Auditory cortex is composed of two transverse gyri on the superior temporal lobe buried in the Sylvian fissure. The anterior gyrus is the primary auditory area and the posterior auditory association cortex. The auditory cortex receives its primary input from the medial geniculate body of the thalamus. Each ear has bilateral cortical representation, so destruction of the auditory cortex on one side does not significantly decrease hearing but does affect spatial localization of sound. Taste is represented in the parietal operculum near the somatic tongue area. Vestibular function is found on the posterior edge of the postcentral gyrus near the end of the interparietal sulcus.

Association Areas.   Areas of cortex not concerned directly with primary motor and sensory functions are termed association cortex. This cortex integrates the primary sensory modalities with memory and experience and allows symbolic interpretation and expression of events such as language, calculation, and spatial construction. Speech function resides in the left hemisphere of most people, including left-handed individuals. Speech comprehension depends on the temporoparietal cortex at the posterior end of the Sylvian fissure (Wernicke's area), and, to some degree, speech production depends on cortex of the posteroinferior frontal lobe (Broca's area). These areas are connected by white matter association fibers, the arcuate fasciculus. Inability to understand and form language is termed aphasia and is divided into receptive (fluent) aphasia, when comprehension is lost, and expressive (nonfluent) aphasia, when production is lost. Most patients with aphasia show elements of both. Characteristics of aphasia include inability to form words, word deletions, inability to name objects, repetitive use of a word (perseveration), and inability to follow spoken commands.

Inability to recognize sensory information and assign meaning to it is called an agnosia. With visual agnosia, an object is seen but not recognized. Inability to read is termed alexia and is a type of visual agnosia. Lesions of the left hemisphere cortex between the primary visual areas and the inferior parietal lobe (angular gyrus) create visual agnosias. Similarly, auditory agnosias, for which sound is heard but not interpreted, occur with lesions of the left posterior temporal lobe and connections to the inferior parietal lobe. Receptive aphasia is basically a high-level auditory agnosia. Tactile agnosia or astereognosis is the inability to recognize objects by touch and is associated with lesions of the left supramarginal gyrus (parietal lobe). These specific agnosias involve the formulation of language, reading, and writing. They result from left hemisphere lesions, although contralateral astereognosis is present with lesions of either hemisphere. The parietal cortex of the right hemisphere seems to be concerned with spatial and constructional relationships. Damage to right parietal cortex results in the inability to draw figures and recognize spatial relationships. Nonrecognition and neglect of the opposite side of the body are associated with more severe damage. Nevertheless, right-left disorientation and inability to recognize fingers, in association with writing and calculation difficulties, form a specific syndrome (Gerstmann's) related to damage to the left angular gyrus. Finally, some agnosias result from an inability to transfer information from the right to the left hemisphere caused by lesions in the corpus callosum. They are termed disconnection syndromes. Damage to the dominant supramarginal gyrus and adjacent parietal lobe can impair the execution of learned motor skills in the absence of paresis. This condition is termed apraxia. A patient understands what is being requested but is unable to carry out the task. The impairment involves all extremities. Lesions in the frontal lobe anterior to the primary motor areas may also cause difficulty in execution of movements in the absence of paresis, but this is more of a clumsiness or difficulty in initiation of movement. Gait apraxia would be an example.

Hippocampal and Limbic Structures.   The hippocampus is found in the posterior mesial temporal lobe adjacent to the temporal horn of the lateral ventricle and lies in the choroidal fissure. It is composed of three-layered cortex (allocortex). Axons of the hippocampal pyramidal cells form the fornix, the efferent projection of the hippocampus. Partial decussation of the fornices (hippocampal commissure) occurs as they course beneath the corpus callosum and on top of the thalamus. The fornix splits over the anterior commissure near the foramina of Monro into precommissural fibers, which reach the septal area and anterior hypothalamus, and more numerous postcommissural fibers, which synapse in the mammillary bodies of the posterior hypothalamus. The mammillothalamic tract projects to the anterior and intralaminar nuclei of the thalamus, which themselves project to the cingulate gyrus. This loop from cingulate gyrus to entorhinal cortex to hippocampus to mammillary bodies via the fornix to thalamus and back to cingulate gyrus is termed the Papez circuit. Bilateral damage to any component of this circuit causes severe impairment of short term memory. Other components of the limbic system include the amygdala, prefrontal and orbitofrontal cortex, the septal area, and nucleus basalis (Meynert).

Limbic structures are concerned with memory, affect, emotion, and behavior. The hippocampus seems important in short-term memory and learning. Bilateral destruction results in loss of acquisition of new memories but spares long-standing memories and experiences. Damage to the mammillary bodies may cause a similar syndrome (Korsakoff's). The hippocampus possibly influences the expression of emotion by connecting the cortex to the hypothalamus and brainstem through the Papez circuit. However, experimentally, stimulation of the amygdala is more consistent in producing autonomic and psychic concomitants of strong emotional states. Bilateral destruction of the amygdala seems to lessen aggressive behavior. Disconnection of the prefrontal area (prefrontal lobotomy) results in lessening of anxiety but also decreased concentration and attention span, lessening of drive and initiative, and impaired social behavior. Bilateral cingulum lesions decrease the affective components of pain without as profound an effect on attentiveness.

The Peripheral Nervous System

General Considerations

The peripheral nervous system (PNS) consists of 31 pairs of segmental spinal nerves and the cranial nerves that were discussed under brainstem, above. The spinal nerves contain motor, sensory, and visceral elements. Motor (ventral) and sensory (dorsal) roots form the spinal nerve at each level. Visceral fibers travel with the ventral root and will be discussed in the next section. In the cervical and lumbar areas, the spinal nerves form plexuses, where redistribution of axons takes place to form the peripheral nerves.

The peripheral nerves are invested in a connective tissue sheath, the epineurium. Within the nerve the axons are arranged in fascicles bound by perineurium. The perineurium is the first level of a blood-nerve barrier. A regrouping of axons into different fascicles occurs along the course of a nerve such that when a segment of nerve is removed, the fascicles no longer precisely match. Connective tissue within the fascicle invests each axon as the endoneurium. Finally, the axon is surrounded by myelin, the concentric laminations of the cell membranes of Schwann cells, which increases the rate of conduction of the nerve impulse in relation to its thickness. Even unmyelinated axons are believed to be in contact with, but not invested by, Schwann cells.

Peripheral nerve fibers are classified by size in an ABC system. Size depends on the diameter of the axon and, more important, the thickness of the myelin sheath. Myelinated fibers are designated group A and may be subdivided α through δ. Diameters range from 2 μ to 20 μ, and nerve conduction velocities (NCVs) range from 20 m/sec to 120 m/sec. B fibers are myelinated preganglionic autonomic fibers, 2 to 5 μ in diameter, and C fibers are unmyelinated fibers, 1 μ to 2 μ in diameter with NCVs less than 2 m/sec. Larger A sensory fibers subserve joint and tendon receptors, muscle spindles, and pressure receptors. Smaller A_δ and C fibers carry pain (nociceptive) impulses. Motor neurons to skeletal muscle are A_α and those to muscle spindles are A_γ. A similar classification system uses Roman numerals I to IV for large to small fibers.

Each motor neuron synapses with many muscle fibers. The axon and its associated muscle fibers are termed a motor unit. Muscle contraction represents the simultaneous firing of many motor units within the given peripheral nerve.

When a nerve is severed, the distal portion of the nerve undergoes a progressive degeneration (Wallerian) that may take several days, depending on the length of the nerve. Schwann cells form tubules to allow regrowth of the nerve, but scar tissue inhibits this process. The axon also dies back a few millimeters, and the endoplasmic reticulum of the cell shows dispersion of RNA (chromatolysis). The neuromuscular synapse dissipates, and the entire muscle fiber becomes sensitized and may spontaneously contract (fibrillation). This process is usually evident by 3 weeks after a nerve injury and forms the basis of an electromyographic examination (EMG) for nerve injury.

Anatomy of the PNS

The 31 spinal nerves are divided into 8 cervical, 12 thoracic, 5 lumbar, 5 sacral, and 1 coccygeal. Shortly after exiting the intervertebral foramina, the spinal nerves divide into dorsal and ventral rami. The dorsal rami supply motor innervation to the long extensors of the back and sensation over the spine.

The cervical plexus is formed from the first four cervical segments. C2, with its dorsal ramus, supplies the occipitalis muscle and the skin of the scalp as the occipital nerves. C2–C4 supply the hyoid muscles, via the ansa cervicalis, and the diaphragm, via the phrenic nerve. The phrenic nerve is supplied primarily by C4. It runs on the lateral border of the anterior scalene muscle, passes anterior to the subclavian artery, and lies in the mediastinum in close relation to the vagus nerve. It supplies the diaphragm from its inferior surface.

The brachial plexus is formed by the spinal nerves (roots) of C5 through T1. These form upper (C5, C6), middle (C7), and lower (C8, T1) trunks (Fig. 21.11). The trunks form anterior and posterior divisions that give rise to three cords named for their relation to the axillary artery. The lateral cord is formed by the anterior divisions of the upper and middle trunks (C5–C7), the medial cord by the anterior division of the lower trunk (C8, T1), and the posterior cord from the posterior divisions of all three trunks (C5–C8). The cords then give rise to the major peripheral nerves, although nerves are given off the plexus all along their course. From the cervical spine, the plexus runs beneath the clavicle, in front of the scapula, and over the first rib. It is covered by the scalene muscles and courses behind the pectoralis minor muscle. It is intimately related to the subclavian and axillary artery and vein.

Nerves to the scalene muscles, rhomboids (dorsal scapular nerve C5), and serratus anterior (long thoracic nerve C5–C7) are the most proximal branches of the plexus and exit at a root to trunk level. The upper trunk gives the suprascapular nerve (C5, C6) to the supraspinatus and infraspinatus muscles. At the cord level, the lateral cord gives the lateral pectoral nerve (C5–C7), the medial cord, the medial pectoral nerve (C8, T1), and the medial cutaneous nerve of the arm and forearm; the posterior cord provides the nerves to the latissimus dorsi (C6–C8) and subscapular muscles (C5–C7). The posterior cord gives rise to the axillary nerve (C5) to the deltoid muscle and becomes the radial nerve. The lateral cord divides into the musculocutaneous and lateral half of the median nerves, and the medial cord divides into the ulnar and medial half of the median nerves.

The musculocutaneous nerve (C5–C7) runs through

Figure 21.11. Diagrammatic drawing of the brachial plexus. From Goss CM. Gray's anatomy. 28th ed. Philadelphia: Lea & Febiger, 1970:965.

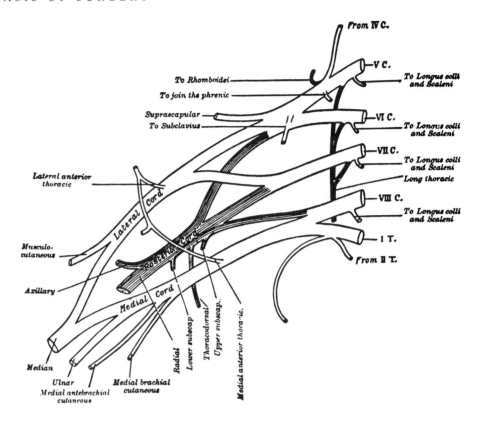

the coracobrachialis muscle and between the biceps and brachialis muscles, which it supplies. It emerges as the lateral cutaneous nerve of the forearm on the radial side of the forearm. The median nerve (C6–T1) runs with the brachial artery on the medial side of the upper arm; passes between the heads of the pronator teres in the antecubital fossa; gives off the anterior interosseous branch, which supplies forearm muscles; and passes beneath the carpal tunnel to supply the thenar muscles and sensation to the thumb, index finger, middle finger, and median half of the ring finger. Muscles supplied by the median nerve, in order, are pronator teres; palmaris longus; flexor carpi radialis; flexor digitorum superficialis, as anterior interosseous nerve-flexor pollicis longus, flexor digitorum profundus (half), and pronator quadratus; in the hand, abductor pollicis brevis, opponens pollicis, and flexor pollicis brevis; and the first two lumbricales.

The ulnar nerve (C8, T1) initially runs with the brachial artery but passes posteriorly between the medial epicondyle and the olecranon, courses through the flexor carpi ulnaris muscle, and runs with the ulnar artery to enter the hand, where it provides sensation to the small finger and ulnar half of the ring finger. Muscles supplied by the ulnar nerve, in order, are flexor carpi ulnaris, flexor digitorum profundus (half), palmaris brevis, hypothenar, adductor pollicis, lumbricales, and interossei. The radial nerve (C5–C8) is the continuation of the posterior cord as it passes between the heads of the triceps muscle. It winds around the humerus in the spiral groove giving off the posterior cutaneous nerve of

the forearm. Coursing alongside the brachioradialis muscle, it divides near the elbow into a superficial sensory branch and a deep branch to the extensor muscles of the forearm, called the posterior interosseous nerve. Innervation of the extensor carpi radialis occurs before this division. The superficial sensory branch supplies the dorsum of the radial side of the hand and fingers. Muscles supplied by the radial nerve, in order, are triceps, anconeus, brachioradialis, extensor carpi radialis, extensor digitorum, extensor carpi ulnaris, extensor pollicis longus, abductor pollicis longus, extensor indicis, and extensor pollicis brevis.

The 12 thoracic segments give intercostal nerves at each level. T1 is mainly part of the brachial plexus, and T2 gives some sensory innervation to the upper inner arm. The intercostal nerves run between the pleura and the intercostal muscles on the inferior edge of the rib. On the abdominal wall, the nerves run between the internal oblique and transversus abdominis muscles and come through the posterior rectus sheath. These nerves innervate the intercostal and abdominal wall musculature and give lateral and anterior cutaneous branches to the skin of the chest and abdomen.

The first three and the upper portion of the fourth lumbar nerves form the lumbar plexus (Fig. 21.12). Anterior divisions of the lumbar plexus give rise to the iliohypogastric (L1), ilioinguinal (L1), genitofemoral (L1, L2), and obturator (L2–L4) nerves. The first three nerves are primarily sensory nerves. The iliohypogastric and ilioinguinal nerves run from the lateral border of the psoas muscle on the quadratus lumborum muscle and behind

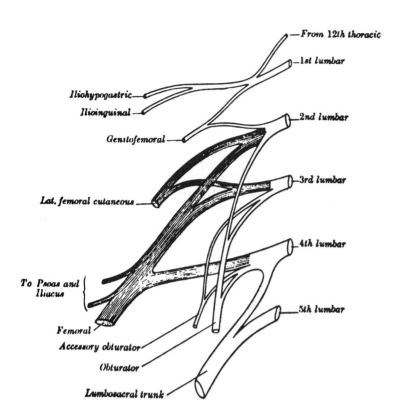

From 12th thoracic

1st lumbar

Iliohypogastric

Ilioinguinal

2nd lumbar

Genitofemoral

3rd lumbar

Lat. femoral cutaneous

4th lumbar

To Psoas and
Iliacus

5th lumbar

Femoral

Accessory obturator

Obturator

Lumbosacral trunk

Figure 21.12. Diagrammatic drawing of the lumbar plexus. From Goss CM. Gray's anatomy. 28th ed. Philadelphia: Lea & Febiger, 1970:988.

the kidney. They course in close relation to the inguinal canal and supply the pubis and scrotum or labia, respectively. The genitofemoral nerve passes through the psoas muscle beneath the ureter and runs with the spermatic cord or round ligament to supply the scrotum or labia. The nerve supplies the cremaster muscle. The obturator nerve enters the pelvis from the medial edge of the psoas muscle and supplies the obturator, gracilis, and adductor thigh muscles as well as sensation to the medial thigh.

The posterior divisions of the lumbar plexus form the iliopsoas (L2, L3), femoral (L2–L4), and lateral femoral cutaneous (L2, L3) nerves. The iliopsoas nerves arise primarily from spinal nerves L2 and L3 before dividing to supply the psoas muscle. The femoral nerve leaves the lateral edge of the psoas muscle and passes beneath the inguinal ligament with the femoral artery and vein and supplies the quadriceps femoris and sartorius muscles. It ends as the cutaneous sensory saphenous nerve, which courses all the way to the medial foot. The lateral femoral cutaneous nerve passes beneath the inguinal ligament close to the anterior superior iliac spine to supply the lateral thigh to the knee. Entrapment results in a common painful syndrome, meralgia paresthetica.

The lumbosacral plexus (sacral plexus) arises from spinal nerves L4 to S3 (Fig. 21.13). The principal nerves formed by this plexus are the sciatic (L4-S3), the gluteals (L4-S1), and the pudendal (S2–S4). The sciatic nerve is a composite nerve of two divisions, the peroneal and the tibial, which generally diverge at a midthigh level but may split much higher. The anterior division of the plexus forms the tibial nerve and the posterior division

forms the peroneal. The sciatic nerve exits the pelvis through the greater sciatic foramen (sciatic notch) below the piriformis and gluteal muscles and runs between the biceps femoris and semimembranosus muscles in the thigh. The peroneal nerve passes laterally under the head of the fibula and supplies the extensor muscles of the lower leg and sensation to the dorsum of the foot. The tibial nerve runs through the popliteal fossa, continues distally between the soleus and gastrocnemius muscles, and passes around the medial malleolus to supply the sole of the foot as the plantar nerves. The peroneal division of the sciatic supplies the following muscles, in order: biceps femoris (short head), peroneus longus, tibialis anterior, extensor digitorum longus, extensor hallucis longus, peroneus tertius, peroneus brevis, and extensor digitorum brevis. Muscles supplied by the tibial division, in order, are biceps femoris (long head), semimembranosus, semitendinosus, adductor magnus (part), gastrocnemius, soleus, flexor hallucis longus, flexor digitorum longus, tibialis posterior, and intrinsic foot.

The superior gluteal nerve supplies the gluteus medius and minimus muscles, and the inferior gluteal nerve supplies the gluteus maximus muscle. They exit the pelvis above and below the piriformis muscle, respectively. The pudendal nerve passes into the ischiorectal fossa through the lesser sciatic foramen, where it gives rectal and perineal nerves. The inferior rectal nerve supplies the external rectal sphincter, although the perineal nerve goes to the external bladder sphincter and to the genitalia.

Figure 21.13. Diagrammatic drawing of the sacral plexus. From Goss CM. Gray's anatomy. 28th ed. Philadelphia: Lea & Febiger, 1970:998.

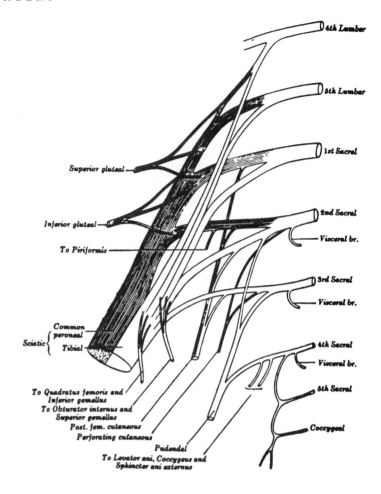

The Autonomic Nervous System

General Considerations

The autonomic nervous system (ANS) refers to that part of the CNS and PNS concerned with visceral functions as opposed to somatic, by which is generally meant the innervation of blood vessels, glands, skin appendages, heart, viscera, and pupils. The central portion of the system includes the hypothalamus and reticular formation in the brain and the intermediolateral cell column in the spinal cord. The peripheral portion of the system is characterized by a two-neuron system with an interposed autonomic ganglion. The ANS is divided into two parts: a sympathetic and a parasympathetic system (Fig. 21.14). These systems generally have opposing actions on the target organ. Although central control for both systems arises in the hypothalamus and reticular formation, preganglionic nerves of the sympathetic system are found only in the thoracolumbar spinal cord, and preganglionic nerves of the parasympathetic system are found in the brainstem and sacral spinal cord. Sympathetic ganglia are generally close to the spinal cord, whereas parasympathetic ganglia tend to be close to or within the organ supplied. Both sympathetic and parasympathetic preganglionic neurons use acetylcholine (ACh) as their neurotransmitter. ACh is also the neurotransmitter for postganglionic parasympathetic neurons

and for postganglionic sympathetic neurons (sudomotor) to sweat glands, but the receptor for the neurotransmitter is different. Autonomic ganglia primarily have nicotinic receptors, which are blocked by hexamethonium, whereas smooth muscle receptors are muscarinic and are blocked by atropine. The enzyme acetylcholinesterase destroys released ACh in the synapse. The remainder of postganglionic sympathetic nerve fibers are adrenergic and use norepinephrine at synapses. Adrenal and other chromaffin tissue release epinephrine into the circulation after stimulation. Two general categories of receptors exist at adrenergic synapses, α and β, although subcategories are recognized. In general, α-receptors are excitatory and β-receptors are inhibitory, although the heart and viscera are exceptions. Norepinephrine is catalyzed by the enzymes monoamine oxidase (MAO) and catechol-o-methyl-transferase (COMT), although reuptake by the nerve terminal is the most potent regulatory mechanism.

The Sympathetic System

Preganglionic cell bodies lie in the intermediolateral cell column of the spinal cord between T1 and L2. Postganglionic cell bodies are found in either the sympathetic trunks (chains) or the prevertebral ganglia. The sympathetic trunks are formed by ganglia that are inter-

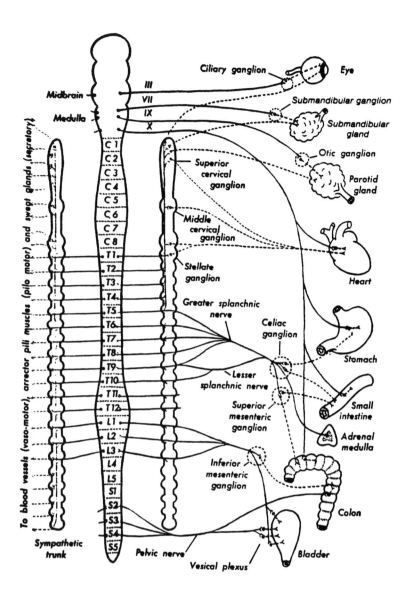

Figure 21.14. Diagram of the ANS. From Carpenter MB, Sutin J. Human neuroanatomy. 8th ed. Baltimore: Williams & Wilkins, 1983:211.

connected but not strictly segmental and run from C1 to the coccyx. The trunks lie on the anterior surface of the lateral masses in the cervical spine and transverse processes in the thoracolumbar spine and cross in front of the sacral promontory to fuse at the coccyx. There are three cervical ganglia: the superior, middle, and inferior (stellate). The nerve fibers from the spinal cord are myelinated (B fibers) as they enter the sympathetic trunks and are called white rami communicantes. Postganglionic nerve fibers returning to the spinal nerve are unmyelinated (C fibers) and are called gray rami communicantes. The preganglionic fibers run up and down in the sympathetic trunk and some synapse with postganglionic neurons within the trunk. Others pass through to reach the prevertebral ganglia. The prevertebral ganglia are related to the abdominal aorta and its branches and are embedded in extensive plexuses, including cardiac, pulmonary, celiac, superior and inferior mesenteric, renal, and hypogastric (pelvic) plexuses. Three nerves, composed of white rami communicantes, course from the thoracic sympathetic chain as the greater, lesser, and

least splanchnic nerves. The first two go to the celiac plexus and the last go to the renal plexus, where they synapse on postganglionic neurons. Postganglionic nerve fibers reach their target organ by traveling with cranial or spinal nerves, by coursing in the adventitia of arteries, or via a combination of both.

The Parasympathetic System

Four parasympathetic ganglia are recognized in the head. The ciliary ganglion receives preganglionic fibers from the Edinger-Westphal nucleus (oculomotor) in the midbrain, via the oculomotor nerve, and sends postganglionic fibers to the pupil. It is located within the orbit. The pterygopalatine ganglion is in close relation to the maxillary division of the trigeminal nerve near the foramen rotundum. It receives preganglionic fibers from the superior salivatory nucleus in the pons, via the intermedius portion of the facial nerve, and supplies the lacrimal and intranasal glands. The submandibular ganglion at the base of the tongue receives similar input via the facial nerve and chorda tympani and supplies the submandibular and sublingual glands. Finally, the otic ganglion that is adjacent to the mandibular division of the trigeminal nerve near the foramen ovale receives preganglionic fibers from the inferior salivatory nucleus in the medulla, via the glossopharyngeal nerve, and supplies the parotid gland.

Preganglionic cell bodies in the dorsal motor nucleus of the vagus nerve distribute their fibers to widespread synapses in the viscera. The vagus nerve exits the skull through the jugular foramen and lies behind the carotid artery and jugular vein in the neck. The right vagus nerve passes in front of the right subclavian artery and in front of the aortic arch on the left. The right nerve is applied to the trachea more closely. The nerves run in the mediastinum behind the root of the lung, giving off recurrent laryngeal nerves that run in the tracheoesophageal groove and fibers that enter the cardiac and pulmonary plexuses. The vagus nerves form a plexus around the esophagus from which emerge an anterior and a posterior trunk, with contributions from both nerves. The anterior trunk supplies the anterior stomach, liver, and biliary system. The posterior trunk joins the abdominal autonomic plexus and is distributed to all the viscera, including the intestine as far as the transverse colon. Some recent evidence suggests that vagal innervation may go all the way to the rectum. In the intestinal wall, the vagal fibers synapse with cells in the submucosal (Meissner) and myenteric (Auerbach) plexuses.

Sacral preganglionic parasympathetic fibers travel with S2–S4 to the hypogastric plexus between the iliac arteries, where pelvic splanchnic nerves emerge to supply the descending colon and rectum, bladder, and genital organs.

Visceral Afferents

Visceral afferent fibers that originate from sensory receptors in the viscera course with the sympathetic and parasympathetic nerves. Sympathetic afferents travel with splanchnic and other sympathetic nerves to the sympathetic trunks and pass into the white rami communicantes to their cell bodies in the dorsal root ganglia. Although all afferent cell bodies are in the dorsal root ganglia, it is estimated that 20% of ventral root fibers represent visceral afferents and another 10% represent somatic afferents. These enter the spinal cord with the ventral root and are distributed to spinal gray matter. Parasympathetic afferents travel with the facial, glossopharyngeal, and vagus nerves with cell bodies in the geniculate, inferior glossopharyngeal (petrosal), and inferior vagal (nodose) ganglia, respectively. Sacral visceral afferents pass with the pelvic nerves to the dorsal root ganglia of S2–S4 and enter the conus medullaris.

Visceral Reflexes

The simplest autonomic reflex arc involves afferent input from a visceral or somatic afferent fiber, with its cell body in the dorsal root ganglion. This synapses on an interneuron in the spinal cord gray matter, which in turn connects to a preganglionic autonomic neuron in the intermediolateral column of the cord. The preganglionic cell synapses on a postganglionic cell in an autonomic ganglion, which is the final effector cell. Thus, three synapses are involved, unlike the monosynaptic arc of a deep tendon reflex. Segmental reflexes from the abdominal viscera include reddening of the skin and contraction of the abdominal musculature (guarding) from distension, inflammation, and cramping of the intestine and inhibition of intestinal motility (ileus) from peri-intestinal inflammation.

Reflexes concerning cardiac rate, cardiac contractility, and systemic arterial blood pressure (SAP) are mediated through the reticular formation in the medulla in what is considered a cardiovascular autonomic center. Heart rate is affected both by vagal fibers and sympathetic afferents through the cardiac nerves (T1–T5), which converge in the superficial and deep cardiac plexuses in front and behind the aortic arch, respectively, and the cardiac ganglia near the sinoatrial and atrioventricular nodes. Sympathetic input is β-adrenergic and increases heart rate. Parasympathetic input decreases heart rate through a muscarinic type receptor. β-adrenergic sympathetic nerves also synapse directly on cardiac muscle cells, increasing contractility and, consequently, stroke volume and cardiac output. There is no direct parasympathetic effect on cardiac contractility. Cardiac visceral afferents travel with the vagus nerve to the medulla and with the sympathetic nerves to the cervicothoracic spinal cord both to monitor reflex activity and to convey cardiac pain.

Arterial blood pressure depends on the rate and contractility of the heart but more so on vasoconstriction of the arterioles, which is mediated through α-adrenergic sympathetic receptors. There is no direct parasympathetic supply to the arterioles of the skin and muscles, but parasympathetic input to the coronary vessels and some viscera (especially the kidney) have been demonstrated. Baroreceptors in the aortic arch (vagal) and carotid sinus (glossopharyngeal) provide afferents to the nucleus solitarius in the medulla to maintain arterial blood pressure. A constant secretion of epinephrine from the adrenal medulla also helps to maintain blood pressure. When blood pressure drops, there is reflex vasoconstriction of the arterioles to the skin and abdominal viscera and constriction of the venous system. This is associated with dilatation of the arterioles of the brain and the coronary arteries and an increase in heart rate. With muscular activity, there is a marked dilatation of blood vessels to muscle that is sympathetic but cholinergically mediated, probably through a nicotinic-type receptor. Cardiac output is increased, and there is vasoconstriction of the blood vessels to the skin and abdominal viscera. The afferent signaling of these responses is not well understood.

There is thought to be a respiratory center in the medullary reticular formation that can be divided into inspiratory and expiratory areas. These are under the control of a pontine respiratory center that, in turn, is influenced by hypothalamic, limbic, and cortical centers. Visceral and somatic afferents have their sensory endings in the epithelium of the respiratory tract from the trachea and major bronchi to the alveoli. In addition to touch, stretch, and pain receptors, some endings respond to carbon dioxide tension (chemoreceptors). Cell bodies for these fibers are in the nodose ganglion of the vagus nerve. These synapse through the medullary respirator center with motor nerves to the diaphragm and accessory muscles of respiration in the spinal cord to mediate respiratory and cough reflexes. Chemoreceptors are also found in the carotid and aortic bodies, which respond to carbon dioxide and, to a lesser extent, oxygen tension in the blood. These fibers accompany the carotid sinus nerve (glossopharyngeal) and vagus nerve, respectively.

Swallowing reflexes involve sensory (glossopharyngeal) and motor (vagal) inputs. Although the pharynx and upper esophagus are supplied by the vagus nerve, they are striated muscle and thus are not considered autonomic. The esophagus gradually becomes autonomic innervated smooth muscle. The presence of food initiates the swallowing reflex and a wave of esophageal contraction. Overstimulation of the posterior pharynx causes the gag reflex. Vagal stimulation increases peristalsis in the gastrointestinal tract, relaxes sphincters, and increases secretion of hydrochloric acid and pepsin in the stomach. Sympathetic stimulation has the opposite effects and causes vasoconstriction in the intestinal vasculature. Visceral pain is conducted through the sympathetic visceral afferents. Gallbladder, biliary, and pancreatic ducts are contracted and sphincters are relaxed by parasympathetic stimulation. Sympathetic stimulation inhibits contraction of the ducts and closes the sphincters. Rectal and anal reflexes are mediated through the sacral parasympathetic system.

Parasympathetic supply to the kidney is through the vagus nerve, and sympathetic supply is through the celiac ganglion and splanchnic nerves to the renal plexus. Parasympathetic stimulation increases and sympathetic stimulation decreases renal blood flow; hence urinary output. The ureter receives parasympathetic input from both the vagus nerve and the sacral segments and sympathetic input from the lower splanchnic nerves. Stimulation of either system has little effect on ureter function, and the kidney and ureter can be denervated as in transplantation without any functional impairment. Micturition is mediated through the parasympathetic system. Stretch receptors in the bladder wall stimulate visceral afferents that travel with the pelvic nerves to spinal cord levels S2–S4. Parasympathetic efferents over the same nerves cause contraction of the detrusor muscle and relaxation of the sphincters. These neurons are influenced by a micturition center in the pontine reticular forma-

tion, which in turn is under cortical control. Sympathetic input mildly inhibits bladder contraction but may be responsible for preventing reflux into the ureters. Erection is caused by parasympathetically (S2–S4) induced vascular engorgement of the penis. Emission of semen is a sympathetic function, and ejaculation is a combination of autonomic and somatic activities.

The Cerebral Circulation

Cerebrovascular Anatomy

The arterial blood supply to the brain arises from the aortic arch. The right common carotid and subclavian arteries are the primary branches of the innominate artery. The left common carotid artery usually arises directly from the aortic arch. The vertebral arteries are proximal branches of the subclavian arteries. The common carotid arteries bifurcate at about the C3–C4 level into internal carotid arteries (ICA), carrying blood to the brain, and external carotid arteries, carrying blood to the neck, face, mouth, jaw, scalp, and meninges. Potential anastomoses between the two systems exist, especially around the orbit and upper face, which become important with carotid artery stenosis or occlusion.

Small branches of the intracavernous ICA supply the pituitary gland and meninges and have surgical importance in cases of carotid-cavernous fistula. Intracranial branches of the ICA, in order, are the ophthalmic, which courses with the optic nerve to the orbit; the posterior communicating, which crosses the oculomotor nerve and connects to the posterior cerebral artery; the anterior choroidal, which runs between the uncus and the cerebral peduncle before entering the choroidal fissure; the small superior hypophyseal branches, which run along the pituitary stalk; and the terminal branches of the anterior and middle cerebral arteries.

The two ICA systems are interconnected through the anterior communicating artery, a channel of considerable variability. The posterior communicating artery connects each ICA to the basilar artery through the posterior cerebral arteries. This system of junctions is called the circle of Willis. In 10% to 15% of cases, the posterior cerebral artery will be supplied primarily by the ICA. Variability of size of these arterial segments is common and has relevance to the ability of diseased carotid arteries to sustain the cerebral circulation.

The anterior communicating artery courses horizontally to the skull base between the frontal lobe and optic chiasm, giving medial striate branches to the basal ganglia, cortical branches to the orbital frontal lobe, and with the anterior communicating artery, branches to the optic chiasm and hypothalamus. Distal to the anterior communicating artery, paired anterior cerebral (pericallosal) arteries ascend over the genu of the corpus callosum and remain in the callosal cistern to anastomose with smaller pericallosal branches of the posterior cerebral arteries. Cortical branches, including fronto-orbital, frontopolar, callosomarginal, and cuneal, supply the mesial cerebral hemisphere. Disorders of consciousness, affect, and hypothalamic function occur with ischemia in the proximal anterior cerebral artery distribution. More distal ischemia affects the legs more than the arms because of the mesial hemisphere cortical representation. Bilateral ischemia in this distribution can cause leg weakness, gait disturbance, and bladder dysfunction, suggestive of spinal cord disease.

The middle cerebral artery (MCA) is the primary continuation of the ICA, coursing in the Sylvian fissure between the frontal and temporal lobes and over the insula of Reil. Lateral striate or "lenticulostriate" branches arise before the primary bifurcation of the artery and perforate the basal frontal lobe to supply the basal ganglia and internal capsule. Because the corticospinal fibers are concentrated at the genu and posterior limb of the capsule, occlusion of a small lenticulostriate branch can cause a profound contralateral hemiplegia, often in the absence of sensory findings. At the edge of the insula, the MCA bifurcates and turns posteriorly. In general, the superior trunk supplies the frontal lobe back to the central sulcus and the inferior trunk supplies the parietal and temporal lobes, but considerable variation exists in the patterns of branching. Viewed in a sagittal plane, the middle cerebral artery supplies the lateral two-thirds of the cerebral hemisphere and the basal ganglia, and the anterior cerebral and posterior cerebral artery supply the medial one-third of the hemisphere anteriorly and posteriorly, respectively. The anterior choroidal artery divides to supply the uncal area of the temporal lobe and continues between the temporal lobe and brainstem, supplying the lower diencephalon and posterior internal capsule before entering the choroidal fissure in the temporal horn of the ventricle to supply the choroid plexus.

The vertebral arteries arise from the subclavian artery on each side and ascend through the foramina transversaria of the cervical vertebrae from C6 to C2. They exit at C2, cross behind the atlas, and enter the foramen magnum anterior to the hypoglossal nerve rootlets. The vertebral arteries join at the pontomedullary junction to form the basilar artery, which continues anterior to the pons and mesencephalon and divides between the cerebral peduncles into the posterior cerebral arteries. Connection of these arteries to the ICA through the posterior communicating arteries completes the circle of Willis.

Three pair of cerebellar arteries arise from the vertebral and basilar arteries in the posterior fossa. The posterior inferior cerebellar artery (PICA) is a branch of the vertebral artery, usually at the level of the medulla. It courses underneath cranial nerves IX, X, and XI, supplying the lateral medulla; courses around the cerebellar tonsil; gives branches to the choroid plexus of the fourth ventricle; and divides into inferior vermian and hem-

ispheral branches. The anterior inferior cerebellar artery is usually the smallest of the cerebellar arteries. It arises from the basilar artery at the lower pons in close relation to the origin of cranial nerve VI. It then follows CN VII and VIII into the cerebellopontine angle, supplying the lateral pons; loops laterally; and courses on the inferior surface of the cerebellum. The superior cerebellar artery (SCA) arises near the basilar artery bifurcation, courses around the midbrain and pons between CN III and V, and divides into hemispheral and superior vermian branches. A reciprocal size relationship generally exists among the cerebellar arteries.

The posterior cerebral artery (PCA) is the terminal branch of the basilar artery. It courses around the midbrain anterior to CN III and supplies the thalamus and midbrain. Over the quadrigeminal plate, the artery gives branches to the hippocampal (posterior temporal) area and divides into a calcarine branch, supplying the visual cortex, and a parieto occipital branch, going to visual and parietal association areas.

Paramedian branches of the basilar artery supply the medial brainstem. More inferiorly, the anterior spinal artery, a common branch of the vertebral arteries, supplies the medial medulla and continues caudally to supply the spinal cord. Perforating branches to the thalamus are termed anterior if they arise from the posterior communicating artery and posterior if they arise from the posterior cerebral artery. The posterior cerebral arteries also give off medial and lateral posterior choroidal arteries, which supply the diencephalon and choroid plexus. In the spinal cord, the anterior spinal artery is reconstituted by segmental arteries, including the large lumbar radicular artery of Adamkiewicz, which serves the cord below about T10 and is important in operations on the abdominal aorta. The anterior spinal artery supplies the anterior two-thirds of the cord, and the paired posterior spinal arteries supply the dorsal one-third.

Cerebral veins can be divided into superficial and deep systems. The superficial system drains superiorly and inferiorly from the superficial middle cerebral veins of the Sylvian fissure. Superiorly running veins drain into the superior sagittal sinus. The largest of these is called the vein of Trolard. Inferiorly running veins drain into the sphenoparietal, petrosal, and transverse (lateral) sinuses. The largest of these is termed the vein of Labbe. The veins are considered anastomotic because blood can drain through them in either direction. Veins from the mesial hemisphere drain into the falx and the inferior and superior sagittal sinuses.

The deep venous system includes the deep anterior and middle cerebral veins that form the basal vein of Rosenthal. This vein courses around the brainstem in close relation to the posterior cerebral artery and enters the vein of Galen in the quadrigeminal area. Subependymal veins in the ventricles drain the deep hemisphere. Septal and caudate veins join to form the internal cerebral vein. The thalamostriate vein runs on top of the thalamus in the floor of the lateral ventricle. It joins the internal cerebral vein near the foramen of Monro (venous angle), and the paired internal cerebral veins continue posteriorly in the roof of the third ventricle to drain into the vein of Galen. Posterior fossa veins drain from the cerebellum and around the brainstem toward midline to form the precentral cerebellar veins, which in turn drain into the vein of Galen. Other posterior fossa veins empty directly into the petrosal, transverse, and cavernous sinuses. Pericallosal veins from the splenium of the corpus callosum also enter the vein of Galen. The vein of Galen is thus formed by the paired internal cerebral, basal, precentral cerebellar, and pericallosal veins. It lies dorsal to the quadrigeminal (collicular) plate and drains into the straight sinus at the junction of the falx and tentorium.

The superior sagittal and straight sinuses converge at the torcula (torcular Herophili) and continue as the paired transverse (lateral) sinuses. These are joined by the superior petrosal sinuses behind the mastoid processes and descend as the sigmoid sinuses, which form the jugular bulbs at the jugular foramen, and continue into the neck as the internal jugular veins. Connections between the sigmoid, petrosal, and cavernous sinuses and the pterygoid plexus allow for collateral drainage when the internal jugular veins are blocked. The torcula may be incomplete, most often with the superior sagittal sinus and superficial system running to the right transverse sinus and the straight sinus and deep system draining to the left. This can preclude elective ligation of a major sinus.

The basal subarachnoid space is divided into a system of well-defined cisterns. These compartments allow a convenient road map for understanding vascular and cranial nerve anatomy. Especially well developed is a sheet of arachnoid, Lilliequist's membrane, extending across the tentorial notch between the unci of the temporal lobes and surrounding the pituitary stalk, effectively dividing the supratentorial and infratentorial compartments ventrally. Cisterns above this membrane include: the carotid cistern with the ICA and its branches; the chiasmatic cistern with the optic nerves and ophthalmic arteries; the Sylvian cistern with the middle cerebral artery and its branches; the crural cistern with the anterior choroidal artery and basal vein of Rosenthal; the lamina terminalis cistern with the anterior cerebral and anterior communicating and recurrent arteries; and the callosal cistern with the pericallosal arteries. Cisterns around the upper brainstem include: the interpeduncular cistern with the basilar bifurcation, posterior cerebral and posterior communicating arteries, and CN III; the ambient cistern with the posterior cerebral, superior cerebellar, and posterior choroidal arteries; the quadrigeminal cistern with the vein of Galen, pineal gland, and CN IV; and the velum interpositum cistern with the posterior medial choroidal artery and the internal cerebral veins. Posterior fossa cisterns in-

clude: the prepontine cistern with the basilar artery, origins of the AICA, and CN VI; the cerebellopontine cistern with AICA, CN V, VII, and VIII, and the foramen of Luschka; the premedullary cistern with the anterior spinal artery and CN XII; the cerebellomedullary cistern with the vertebral arteries, PICA, and CN IX, X, and XI; and the cisterna magna with the distal PICA and the foramen of Magendie. These relationships form the basis of a microsurgical anatomy for basal tumors and intracranial vascular surgery.

Cerebrovascular Physiology

The brain has a mass of about 1500 g (2% body weight) and has a total brain blood flow of about 750 mL/min (15% of cardiac output). Each carotid artery carries about 300 mL/min, and the vertebrobasilar system carries 150 mL/min. Thus, average CBF is about 50 mL/100 g/min. Separate gray and white matter compartments are recognized with CBF of 75 to 80 mL and 20 to 25 mL/100 g/min, respectively. Capillary density in gray matter is also about four times that of white matter. The metabolic rate of oxygen ($CMRO_2$) in the brain under resting conditions is about 3.0 to 3.5 mL/100 gm/min (20% of total body oxygen consumption), and the metabolic rate of glucose (CMRGlu) is 25 to 30 mol (3.5 to 5.0 mg)/100 g/min. The brain depends on a continuous supply of oxygen and glucose, and with total global ischemia, unconsciousness ensues in about 10 seconds and irreversible damage occurs in 4 to 5 minutes.

CBF remains constant over a range of systemic arterial blood pressures (ABP) generally between about 60 and 170 torr mean ABP. This is termed autoregulation (Fig. 21.15). The range of autoregulation will be elevated in chronic hypertension. Autoregulation is based on the underlying vascular caliber. This caliber and therefore

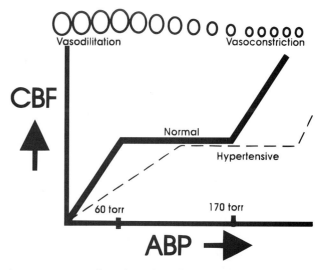

Figure 21.15. Graphic relationship of CBF to ABP with progressive vasoconstriction being responsible for the flat portion of the curve (autoregulation). Note that the curve is shifted to the right in hypertension.

CBF depends greatly on the arterial tension of carbon dioxide ($PaCO_2$) increasing or decreasing about 2.5% for each 1 torr change in $PaCO_2$ between 30 and 60 torr.

Poiseuille's Law

$$CBF = \frac{\{\pi(P_1 - P_2)R^4\}}{\{8\eta L\}}$$

describing Newtonian flow through a cylinder gives particular insight into mechanisms controlling CBF. The dependance on pressure (P_1-P_2) shows a direct relationship to CBF. The dependance on vessel caliber shows a fourth power relationship to vessel radius and illustrates how even minor vessel dilatation may cause significant increases in CBF. The symbol for viscosity (η) shows an inverse relationship. Agents such as mannitol, which decrease viscosity as well as hemodilution, will increase CBF.

Activation of brain areas causes a focal increase in CBF, $CMRO_2$, and CMRGlu. This is called coupling of CBF to metabolism. The precise regulatory mechanism is not clear, but adenosine is believed to be an important signal, whereas H^+, K^+, and CO_2 seem less important.

Cerebrospinal Fluid (CSF)

CSF is contained in the ventricles and the cerebral and spinal subarachnoid spaces and is continuous with the brain extracellular space through the ependyma and pia mater. These spaces contain about 150 mL CSF in the young adult, of which 25 mL is in the ventricles, 50 mL is in the spinal subarachnoid space, and 75 mL is in the cerebral subarachnoid space and cisterns. There are two C-shaped lateral ventricles composed of an atrium in the central portion and frontal, temporal, and occipital horns in these lobes, respectively. Each communicates through a foramen of Monro at the anterior end of the thalamus with the third ventricle, which lies between the thalami and has recesses into the hypothalamus and pineal areas. The aqueduct of Sylvius in the midbrain connects the third ventricle to the fourth ventricle, which lies between the pons and medulla ventrally and the cerebellum dorsally. Two lateral openings (the foramina of Luschka) and one midline opening (the foramen of Magendie) communicate the ventricles to the subarachnoid space. Around the spinal cord and base of the brain, the subarachnoid space is large and forms cisterns, described in more detail previously. On the cortical surface, the arachnoid is more closely applied to the pia and extends into the sulci and white matter around the blood vessels as the Virchow-Robin spaces.

CSF is produced in the choroid plexus, a special vascularized epithelium that extends from the choroidal fissure in the temporal horn, where it receives the anterior and lateral posterior choroidal arteries, through the atrium to the foramen of Monro and into the roof of the third ventricle, where it receives the medial posterior choroidal artery. There is no choroid plexus in the frontal or occipital horns. Choroid plexus is also found in the roof of the fourth ventricle, where it is supplied by choroidal branches of the PICA.

About 70% of CSF is generated by the choroid plexus, the other 30% from brain capillaries and metabolic water. CSF production is 0.35 mL/min, or about 500 mL/day. Thus, the entire CSF volume turns over three to four times each 24 hours. Generation of CSF results from hydrostatic forces and through an active Na^+ transport system that depends on Na^+/K^+/ATPase. The role of carbonic anhydrase in the Na^+ transport is unclear, but acetazolamide, a carbonic anhydrase inhibitor, decreases production of CSF. CSF production is selective with increased Mg^{2+} and Cl^-; decreased glucose, K^+, Ca^{2+}; and negligible protein secreted compared with plasma levels. CSF is absorbed at the arachnoid villi, clusters of arachnoid cells that project into the dural sinuses. These act as one-way valves, requiring a pressure of about 3 torr to open, and preventing reflux of blood and plasma into the CSF. The villi have the capacity to absorb about five times normal CSF production. Resting pressure of the CSF is between 60 and 180 mm H_2O (5 to 13 torr).

Inflammation within the meninges causes an increase in protein, appearance of white blood cells, and sometimes lowering of glucose in CSF. Subarachnoid hemorrhage is associated with ruptured cerebral aneurysms, vascular malformations, and trauma. Neoplastic cells may be seen in cases of CNS malignancy. Lumbar puncture (LP) is used to obtain CSF for diagnostic tests, measure intracranial pressure (ICP), and deliver therapeutic agents into the CSF (intrathecally).

Generally, the lumbar subarachnoid space is in communication with the cerebral subarachnoid space. When this is not the case, a pressure gradient may exist. Under these circumstances, LP will lower spinal pressure and may cause brain or spinal cord displacement (herniation), often with disastrous consequences. A focal neurologic deficit should always be viewed as a relative contraindication for LP until more precise information (CT/MR) is available. Markedly elevated protein on LP (Froin's syndrome) may be an indicator of a spinal block and a precursor to an impending spinal herniation.

An imbalance in the production or absorption of CSF causes ventricular enlargement (hydrocephalus). Hydrocephalus is categorized as obstructive, meaning the ventricular system is blocked, or communicating, meaning the subarachnoid pathways or arachnoid villi are obstructed. In most cases of obstructive and acute communicating hydrocephalus, intracranial pressure is increased, resulting in headache, vomiting, visual disturbance, and decreased level of consciousness. Congenital stenoses, brain tumors, acute hemorrhage, and inflammation are common etiologic factors. In cases of chronic communicating hydrocephalus, the intracranial pressure (ICP) may be normal because of a compensated ventriculomegaly. Typical symptoms in this setting are dementia, gait apraxia, and urinary incontinence. The etiology is often obscure. Sometimes, a prior history of meningitis or subarachnoid hemorrhage may be obtained, whereas in other cases it is idiopathic (normal pressure hydrocephalus).

Blood-Brain Barrier

The brain extracellular space constitutes about 15% of brain volume. Although relatively free passage of solutes exists between the CSF in the ventricles, subarachnoid spaces, and the extracellular space, molecules in the blood are selectively allowed passage into the extracellular space and CSF. This is termed the blood-brain barrier (BBB) and is based on special connections between capillary endothelial cells (tight junctions). The BBB continues out into the peripheral nerve at the level of the perineurial capillaries to continue as the blood nerve barrier. The BBB serves both to control the chemical environment of the neurons and glial cells and to protect the brain from potentially harmful substances. In general, lipid-soluble compounds pass easily through the capillary endothelium, and ionic compounds pass with difficulty. Water and diffusible gases such as oxygen and carbon dioxide are not restricted. To allow entry of important nutrients such as glucose and amino acids, specific transport systems are used. These enzymatic groups are stereospecific, saturable, and competitively inhibited. A similar process is used for returning small ionic molecules from the CSF to the bloodstream. The circumventricular organs (area postrema, median eminence, etc.) are areas where the BBB is not present and allow receptors in the brain to sense molecules in the blood.

Delivery of drugs into the CSF depends on their lipid solubility and use of carrier mechanisms. In pathologic states, the capillary endothelium can be damaged or tight junctions can be destroyed, rendering the BBB inoperable. This contributes to vasogenic edema and may allow circulating toxins to pass into the brain. However, loss of the BBB allows intravascular contrast media to enhance abnormal areas of the brain on imaging studies and allows chemotherapeutic agents and antibiotics to pass in the brain and CSF more easily. Intravenous mannitol will temporarily open the BBB and has been used to improve delivery of antineoplastic drugs.

Cerebral Electrical Activity

Electroencephalography

All neurons exhibit continuous generation of electrical impulses. Excitation and inhibition can be considered alterations in the rate of neuron firing. When groups of neurons, firing simultaneously, are large enough, change in potential can be recorded through the scalp as an electroencephalogram. Cortical cells, especially pyramidal cells, are oriented perpendicular to the surface and arranged in columns. Electrically, these create dipoles. Their dendritic potentials summate to create waves of depolarization and repolarization. The EEG records the differences in potential between bipolar electrodes or a unipolar electrode and a reference, amplifies the microvolt potentials, and records them on an oscilloscope or chart paper for analysis. Usually, 16 electrodes are used, and a given array of electrodes is termed a montage.

EEG activity is categorized by frequency. α-waves (8 to 13 Hz) predominate in the occipital areas at rest. They are synchronous between the two hemispheres and are believed to be generated from thalamic and brainstem sources. β-activity (14 to 30 Hz) results from arousal, eye opening, and some drugs. It predominates in the frontal and central areas. It is of lower voltage than α-activity and nonsynchronous. θ-waves (4 to 7 Hz) and δ-waves (1 to 3 Hz) are considered pathologic in an awake adult and, when localized, suggest a structural brain lesion. Sharp voltage activity (spikes); high-frequency, high-voltage discharges; distinctive spike; and special wave patterns are associated with seizure disorders. Diffuse encephalopathies show loss of normal patterns and generalized slowing. Triphasic waves are associated with hepatic encephalopathy.

The use of EEG monitoring during carotid endarterectomy is based on the correlation of CBF with EEG. An EEG record will show slowing with ischemia and will become isoelectric with a reduction of CBF below 20 mL/100g/min. EEG monitoring can be used to asses the need for intraoperative vascular shunting.

Evoked Potentials

Evoked potentials refer to the electrical responses obtained in cortex, brainstem, or spinal cord after stimulation elsewhere in the nervous system. Typically, responses are averaged over many repetitions to enhance the desired response and to average out background activity. Evoked potentials demonstrate continuity in the pathways being evaluated and, when altered, suggest dysfunction specific to these pathways.

Somatosensory evoked potentials (SSEPs) use stimulation of the median or tibial nerves and record over the somatosensory cortex (postcentral gyrus). They primarily record conduction in the posterior columns, medial lemniscus, thalamus, and cortex. The principal cortical response has a latency of about 19 msec. Visual evoked responses (VERs) record potential changes in the occipital cortex in response to flashing lights or checkerboard patterns and evaluate transmission through the retina, optic nerves, optic tracts, lateral geniculate body, optic radiations, and occipital cortex. Brainstem auditory evoked responses (BAERs) are obtained by stimulating with repetitive clicks in the ear and recording over the auditory cortex. Depolarizing waves are demonstrated in the cochlea, auditory nerve, and brainstem structures in addition to the cortex. These are termed far-field potentials. BAER are used primarily to demonstrate brainstem abnormalities. Methods under investigation to record motor evoked potentials include electrical and magnetic stimulation of the motor cortex and spinal corticospinal tracts.

Evoked potentials have proven useful for intraoperative monitoring and diagnostic evaluations. SSEPs are used in spinal operations and operations on the abdominal aorta to monitor spinal cord function. They can be used to evaluate cerebral function in carotid surgery and in cases of subarachnoid hemorrhage. Motor evoked potentials may be more predictive of outcome in these settings. BAERs are used in operations in the posterior fossa and VERs in pituitary and other operations around the optic nerves and chiasm.

Sleep

The sleep-wake cycle is one example of circadian rhythms that seem to be genetically encoded and are found in all animals. The inherent sleep-wake cycle in humans is closer to 25 to 26 hours but is modified by environmental factors to create a 24-hour periodicity. Five stages of sleep are described based on EEG and observation. The resting individual shows α-rhythm in the occipital areas. As sleep comes, the EEG shows progressive slowing through θ to δ-wave activity. Specific wave complexes—sleep spindles and K complexes—appear in deeper sleep. This process then reverses itself and returns to lighter sleep patterns; the cycle is repeated three or four times a night. During the earlier stages of sleep, there is a loss of muscle tone associated with rapid eye movements (REMs). REM sleep is correlated with dreaming and seems to be a necessary component of sleep. The brainstem basis for non-REM sleep is postulated to be serotonergic neurons in the raphe nuclei; for REM sleep, it is thought to be noradrenergic neurons in the locus ceruleus. Sleep is independent of coma, and destruction of the ascending reticular activating system (ARAS) does not abolish sleep cycles.

Pathologic Conditions

Decreased Levels of Consciousness

Consciousness is appreciated instinctively but not defined easily. Clinically, a person is considered fully conscious when he or she is attentive and responsive, demonstrating spontaneous purposeful activity and using coherent thought patterns. Affective abnormalities such as anxiety, fear, and depression generally are not considered disordered levels of consciousness, whereas agitation, sluggishness, or incoherence may be the earliest findings in a patient lapsing into coma. Similarly, patients with dementia and psychosis are considered to retain consciousness, although they might be immobile and unresponsive. Decreased levels of consciousness include: lethargy, where a person is drowsy, needs to be stimulated to respond and often does so incompletely, but is verbal and will follow command; stupor or obtundation, where there is minimal verbalization and limited response to command but there is semipurposeful to purposeful response to pain; semicoma, where there is no verbalization and stereotyped or reflex responses to pain; and coma, where the patient is unresponsive to pain or command. These classifications form a continuum, and full description is preferred in medical communication (Table 21.1). The Glasgow coma scale is commonly used to grade levels of consciousness in head-injured patients and gives a score from 15 (fully awake) to 3 (comatose) based on best verbal response, best motor response, and eye opening.

The physiologic basis of consciousness is considered to be the ascending reticular activating system (ARAS) in the upper pons and midbrain and its projections through the nonspecific thalamic nuclei and hypothalamus to the limbic and prefrontal cortex and ultimately to the cerebral hemispheres, especially the left hemisphere. Isolated lesions of one hemisphere do not impair consciousness, although they may depress affect. Therefore, a patient must have either widespread damage to both hemispheres or a lesion affecting the ARAS to experience a decrease in level of consciousness.

Table 21.1.
Glasgow Coma Scale. The GCS is the sum total of responses in each category. Scores range between 3 and 15

Eye Opening	
4	Spontaneous
3	To Sound
2	To Pain
1	None

Motor Response	
6	Follows Commands
5	Localizes stimulus
4	Withdraws
3	Flexion posturing
2	Extension posturing
1	No Movements

Verbal Response	
5	Oriented
4	Confused
3	Words
2	Sounds
1	None

As the brain exquisitely depends on oxygen and glucose for function, any deprivation of these—such as through anoxia, decreased CBF with hypotension, insulin overdosage, or carbon monoxide or cyanide poisoning—will lead to decreased consciousness. Similarly, a variety of metabolic and toxic alterations can lead to coma, including hyponatremia, hypocalcemia, myxedema, meningitis, uremia, hyperammonianemia, and a host of anesthetic and sedative drugs. Some of these affect the entire brain; others act more specifically on pathways concerned with consciousness.

Structural lesions in the brain cause coma if they involve the ARAS and its projections. Thus, lesions in the upper brainstem may be associated primarily with coma. Hemispheral lesions produce coma by secondary effects on the upper brainstem, as is discussed in "Herniation Syndromes."

Cerebral Ischemia

Cerebral ischemia is a common denominator of many pathologic processes, including arterial occlusion, hypotension, subarachnoid hemorrhage, head injury, local and generalized increases in brain pressure, and brain herniation syndromes. Resting CBF for the whole brain is about 50 mL/100 g/min. This can be lowered acutely to about 20 mL/100 g/min without change in function. Below this level, EEG changes are appreciated, suggesting that ischemia first affects synaptic transmission. Between 8 and 10 mL/100 g/min, there is a precipitous rise in extracellular potassium; this has been thought to signify cell death. CBF of less than 20 mL/100 g/min over a 30-minute period is often associated with cerebral infarction.

The relationships between CBF, the metabolic rate of oxygen ($CMRO_2$), and the metabolic rate of glucose (CMRGlu) with ischemia are becoming clarified by positron emission tomographic (PET) scanning. Cerebral metabolism normally regulates CBF. With a decrease in CBF, $CMRO_2$ and CMRGlu are maintained initially by increased extraction of oxygen and glucose from the blood. This is termed misery perfusion. When CBF is inadequate to maintain metabolism, $CMRO_2$ and CMRGlu decline and infarction occurs. The area surrounding the area of infarction shows increased CBF (luxury perfusion) and, for a time, an increase in CMRGlu. Areas functionally connected but remote from the site of infarction show a decline in both CBF and $CMRO_2$. Those cases showing preservation of metabolism and reduced blood flow (misery perfusion) may represent an indication for revascularization, whereas those showing absence of metabolism and luxury perfusion would not be expected to benefit.

One clinical method that gives insight into CBF is measurement of the difference between arterial and venous oxygen saturation. This is measured by arterial O_2 sampling at a peripheral site and sampling of venous

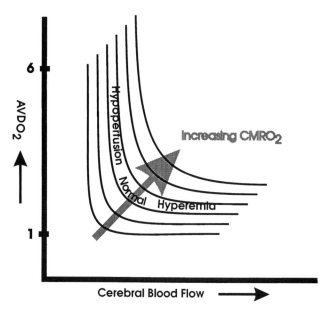

Figure 21.16. Graphic representation of the relationship between $AVDO_2$ and CBF at different levels of $CMRO_2$.

blood from the jugular bulb. The latter assumes complete mixing of venous blood from both hemispheres. A fixed relationship exists between $AVDO_2$ and CBF at any given $CMRO_2$ (Figure 21.16). High values of 5 or 6 $CMRO_2$ suggest ischemia, whereas low values of 1 suggest relative hyperemia.

Mechanisms leading to ischemic cell death have undergone intensive investigation (3). One of the early biochemical changes in ischemia is the release of arachidonic acid from the cell membrane. This occurs before depletion of ATP stores and is, therefore, believed to be an active phenomenon. Arachidonic acid is metabolized further in the presence of oxygen to prostaglandins and leukotrienes, which are involved in vasoactive and inflammatory processes that may propagate tissue damage. Ischemia changes are seen first at synapses with the release of excitatory neurotransmitters, especially glutamate. Depolarization of the postsynaptic membrane allows influx of calcium, and when this is excessive, it can activate phospholipases. These attack the cell membrane to release arachidonic acid. Glutamate receptors, especially the *N*-methyl-*d*-aspartate (NMDA) receptor, have been implicated in this process, and selective receptor blockers have been suggested to protect against cerebral ischemia (4).

An important component of these destructive chemical reactions seems to be the generation of oxygen-derived ionic radicals, termed free radicals. Oxygen in tissue can undergo several reductions to form superoxide anion. In addition, hydrogen peroxide and its reduced form, the hydroxyl radical, can also be produced. These intermediate radicals are extremely reactive and initiate chemical reactions that are destructive to proteins and phospholipid membranes. Sources for generation of free radicals of oxygen include xanthine oxidase, catecholamine oxidation, mitochondrial electron transport, metabolism of prostaglandins and leukotrienes, peroxidation of lipid membranes, and phagocytosis. Lipid peroxidation is associated with the oxidation of ferrous iron, which in turn oxidizes the double bonds of fatty acids in the membranes of the cell and its organelles. This perpetuates a cycle of free radical generation. Possible protective compounds include corticosteroids, amino steroids, vitamin E, vitamin C, mannitol, xanthine oxidase inhibitors, DMSO, and the enzyme superoxide dismutase. Another important component of cell membrane damage is the increased entry of calcium into the cell cytoplasm that catalyzes untoward lipid and protein reactions. Calcium channel blockers such as nimodipine may attenuate this effect. Acidosis occurs in ischemic tissue as the metabolism of glucose is converted to anaerobic glycolysis, which results in the production of lactic acid. This effect is potentiated by hypercapnia. This would suggest that glucose and lactate containing intravenous fluids may be harmful in cerebral ischemia and emphasizes the importance of preventing hypoxia, hypercapnia, and acidosis in the arterial blood.

In addition to neuronal damage, ischemia also injures the cerebral microcirculation. Reduced blood flow occurs through areas of ischemia after reopening of the circulation (no-reflow phenomenon), which is attributed to endothelial swelling. A few hours after ischemia, the capillaries become permeable to macromolecules, signifying breakdown of the BBB. Associated with this is cerebral edema, which at first involves the glial cells (cytotoxic) and subsequently the extracellular space (vasogenic). The microcirculation either undergoes necrosis or recovers so that after a few weeks the BBB is restored. Damage to the microcirculation may represent a limiting factor to attempted CBF restoration in the clinical setting.

Cerebral Edema

Cerebral edema, or an increase in brain tissue water content, results from a variety of insults: ischemic, traumatic, neoplastic, and others. Increased water in the brain ultimately derives from the vascular system and is, therefore, related to capillary integrity, the BBB, and the ionic environment of the tissue itself. When pathologic conditions within the tissue increase the ionic or oncotic (protein) osmotic pressure of the extracellular fluid, water moves into the extracellular space and subsequently into glial cells. This is termed cytotoxic edema. With damage to the capillary endothelium (ischemia or trauma) or difference in capillary endothelial structure (abscesses or neoplastic processes), solutes and proteins are lost into the extracellular space osmotically carrying water with them. This is termed vasogenic edema. Edema fluid moves through the brain by bulk flow and is eventually transferred into the subarachnoid space

and ventricles. White matter shows more compliance than gray matter, and edema, therefore, tends to accumulate there.

A variety of biologically active compounds has been implicated in production of cerebral edema. The prostaglandins, leukotrienes, and oxygen-derived free radicals cause cerebral edema when injected directly into brain tissue. Bradykinin and other peptides within the kallikrein-kinin system also have been associated with production of brain edema. Ischemic brain edema shows increased levels of histamine and serotonin in the tissue. A variety of toxins are used experimentally to produce brain edema, but they may act through the above mechanisms.

Cerebral edema is important clinically because it raises intracranial pressure and induces brain shifts and herniation syndromes. Local compression of the microvasculature has been suggested but is unproven. Also unclear is whether cerebral edema per se affects neurologic function by changing the local environment. Experimental studies of controlled focal edema have shown no alteration in neurologic function.

Raised Intracranial Pressure

Pressure-Volume Relationships

Mathematical models to describe intracranial pressure (ICP) assume the skull to be an essentially inelastic container with several volume compartments (Monro-Kellie hypothesis): the brain tissue itself (1500 mL), which is considered incompressible, although it can be distorted or shifted; the cerebral blood volume (CBV; 200 mL), which relates to CBF and vascular diameter; and the cerebrospinal fluid (CSF 100 mL), which may be displaced out of the cranium into the spinal canal and cranial nerve foramina or resorbed into the venous circulation. Of the CBV, only about 50 mL (3.5% of brain volume) is intraparenchymal; the rest is in the larger arteries, veins, and sinuses. CBV, rather than CBF, is a determinant of ICP. ICP varies with uncompensated changes in one or more of these volume compartments.

The pressure volume relationship describes a curve that is relatively flat to pressure increases over additions of volume until a point at which the curve rapidly steepens to become almost vertical (Figure 21.17). The flat area of the curve is presumed to demonstrate compensatory mechanisms such as movement of blood or CSF out of the cranial cavity, and the steep portion represents exhaustion of these compensatory mechanisms. The ability of the intracranial space to accommodate increases in volume is termed compliance (dV/dP), and the resistance to increases in volume is termed elastance (dP/dV). The actual curve generated by addition of volume depends on the compliance and elastance of the system and, therefore, varies between patients and pathologic processes. The important consequences of these pressure-volume relationships are that, depending

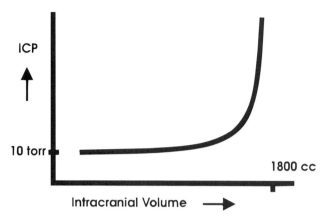

Figure 21.17. Relationship between intracranial volume and ICP.

where a given ICP is on the curve, small increases in volume may give precipitous rises in ICP or be well compensated, and small decreases in volume may dramatically lower ICP, as on the steep portion of the curve. Clinically, these curves must be generated by addition of known volumes of fluid to the intracranial space. ICP is distributed fairly evenly throughout the intracranial cavity and from tissue to ventricular pressure, although tentorial herniation may create a pressure gradient between the supratentorial and infratentorial compartments. Nevertheless, the presence of focal masses results in brain shifts away from the mass with severe physiologic consequences.

Clinically, ICP can be measured by pressure transducers coupled to intraventricular cannulae, subarachnoid cannulae (Richmond bolt), epidural fiber optic sensors, and miniature strain gauge pressure transducers. ICP of more than 15 torr is considered elevated. In addition to static pressure measurements, three types of pressure waves (Lundberg) are recognized. A waves (plateau waves) are intermittent elevations of ICP from 50 to 100 torr, lasting several minutes and probably related to vasodilatation. These are associated with elevated ICP and herald clinical deterioration. B waves are 1/min rhythmic fluctuations to 50 torr associated with period respirations and a decreased level of consciousness. C waves are 4 to 8/min waves to 20 torr related to periodic fluctuations in arterial blood pressure (Traube-Hering-Meyer) waves. Fourrier waveform analysis has shown that the component frequencies of an ICP waveform shift towards higher frequencies with reduced compliance, but this observation also depends on heart rate and venous outflow resistance. ICP monitoring is used so that physicians may initiate treatment for raised ICP before clinical deterioration ensues.

CBF and ICP

To quantify a relationship between CBF and ICP, an equation similar to Ohm's law can be used with cerebral perfusion pressure (CPP)—the difference between systemic arterial pressure (SAP) and ICP—representing the

potential or voltage, the CBF representing the current flow, and their quotient representing the resistance. CPP = CBF × CVR, where CPP is expressed in torr, CBF in mL/100 g/min, and CVR in torr/mL/100 g/min. With generalized increase in ICP, CBF is maintained until CPP drops below 50 torr. However, CBF is better maintained at the same CPP reached by elevation of ICP than by lowering of SAP. After a period of reduced CPP, lowering ICP to improve CPP causes hyperemia associated with decreased CVR (vasodilatation).

Finally, with repeated lowering of CPP, CBF eventually begins to decline even when CPP is restored, suggesting an increase in CVR consistent with capillary endothelial swelling or microcirculatory sludging. With a focal lateralized mass, CBF decreases at the site of the lesion, and with herniations, there are widespread areas of ischemia not directly correlated to elevation of ICP and decrease in CPP. These do not occur with decreases in CPP caused by cisternal infusion when lateralized mass effect is not present. Thus, the relationship between ICP and CBF is complex, with CBF in individual areas of the brain dependent not only on a given ICP (CPP) but on anatomical location, vascular anatomy, preservation of autoregulation, rapidity of ICP increase, neuronal metabolism, and a host of other factors.

Herniation Syndromes

The most important consequence of increased ICP, especially in relation to lateralized mass effect, is brain herniation. Two dural folds, the falx cerebri and the tentorium cerebelli, divide the intracranial space into compartments. The falx separates the two hemispheres as deep as the corpus callosum, and the tentorium separates the cerebrum from the cerebellum with an opening, the tentorial notch or hiatus, to allow the brainstem to pass through. At the foramen magnum, the medulla passes through to spinal cord. Because these structures are essentially unyielding, pressure effects will cause the brain to move through these openings, creating pressure and vascular effects on vital structures.

With a supratentorial mass, especially frontal, subfalcial herniation occurs with the cingulate gyrus and anterior cerebral arteries herniated beneath the falx to the opposite side. More important is herniation of the uncus of the temporal lobe through the tentorial notch. This causes downward displacement of the upper brainstem with associated pressure effects. Two syndromes are recognized, which differ in their earliest presentation. However, both exhibit a rostrocaudal pattern of neurologic deterioration with recognizable brainstem levels of dysfunction. The central type with bilateral temporal lobe herniation begins as agitation, decreasing level of consciousness, small reactive pupils, bilateral increased tone and Babinski sign, and Cheyne-Stokes respirations. The lateral type begins with decreased level of consciousness, ipsilateral oculomotor paresis generally beginning with a dilated nonreactive pupil and later involving lid elevation and extraocular movements, contralateral hemiparesis, and a sustained hyperventilation. Frequently, an initial hemiparesis ipsilateral to the lesion occurs, explained by compression of the opposite cerebral peduncle against the tentorial edge (Kernohan's notch syndrome). Both syndromes progress to decreased responsiveness, decorticate posturing (arm flexed, leg extended) to decerebrate posturing (all extremities extended), midrange nonreactive pupils, loss of oculocephalic and oculovestibular reflexes, loss of corneal reflexes, and ataxic breathing patterns. Progression leads to herniation of the cerebellar tonsils through the foramen magnum with medullary compression, resulting in loss of motor tone, loss of gag and cough reflexes, apnea, and eventually cardiovascular collapse and death. Early signs of tentorial herniation may evolve over minutes, although full progression to death generally takes hours to days, especially if respiration is supported. If herniation cannot be reversed rapidly, hemorrhages appear in the brainstem, leading to a poor prognosis, even if pressure is subsequently relieved.

Increased ICP is managed by head elevation, which improves venous return to the heart; hyperventilation, which causes cerebral vasoconstriction and reduces CBV; mannitol, an osmotic diuretic, which decreases the brain tissue compartment by shrinking the extracellular and perhaps the intracellular space; and in some situations, barbiturates, which decrease $CMRO_2$ and consequently CBF and CBV. Corticosteroids have a beneficial effect with tumors, abscess, and inflammatory diseases and are thought to improve vasogenic edema, although a reduction in ICP is difficult to demonstrate. In many situations, removing a mass lesion or damaged brain is necessary, especially in the frontal and temporal lobes, to control ICP.

Brain Tumors

Brain tumors generally are categorized as: (a) primary, meaning tumors originating from neuroglial tissues, the meninges, reticuloendothelial cells, and vascular cells intrinsic to the brain; and (b) secondary, or metastatic from tumors elsewhere in the body. Intrinsic brain tumors arise most commonly from glial cells. Astrocytomas, ependymomas, and oligodendrogliomas are seen in decreasing order of frequency and commonly show characteristics of more than one glial type. Poorly differentiated glial tumors—glioblastoma multiforme—are the most common glial tumors in adults. Brain tumors are the second most common form of neoplasia in children and are usually malignant, whereas some cystic astrocytomas in the cerebellum are compatible with decades of survival. Primitive embryonic cells give rise to a variety of tumors—medulloblastoma, germinoma, neuroblastoma, and others in this age group. Protein markers, especially nerve growth factor (NGF)

and glial fibrillary acidic protein (GFAP), have been better used to classify these tumors types. In children, tumors arise most commonly in the posterior fossa and around the ventricular system, although in adults they are more common in the cerebral hemispheres, basal ganglia, and thalamus.

Extrinsic brain tumors arise most often from the coverings of the brain (meningioma, acoustic neuroma, and epidermoid) and are usually not invasive into brain tissue. Pituitary adenomas are usually included in this group because they grow into the intracranial cavity. Despite the histologically benign nature of these extraaxial tumors, their typical locations at the base of the skull, around the brainstem, from cranial nerves, and along the dural sinuses can pose considerable problems for complete removal.

Malignant tumors outside the nervous system commonly metastasize to the brain, both the supratentorial and infratentorial compartments. Lung and breast tumors are the most common metastatic lesions, followed by kidney, melanoma, and gastrointestinal malignancies. Lesions commonly present at the gray-white matter junction, a site were there is a significant reduction in the arteriolar density. Metastatic tumors can be associated with considerable edema of the surrounding brain. Although multiplicity is common, solitary metastases occur and may be the first presenting symptoms of the disease.

The terms benign and malignant are applied less easily to brain tumors. Primary brain tumors, even histologically poorly differentiated, rarely metastasize outside the nervous system, and death is caused by progressive brain involvement. However, histologically well-differentiated tumors are frequently not resectable, and if they are intrinsic to the brain, they generally lead to death. Pathologic criteria for increased aggressiveness in gliomas include hypercellularity, mitoses, pleomorphism, necrosis surrounded by pseudo palisading cells, and hypervascularity. Necrosis seems best correlated to prognosis.

Kinetic studies of tumor growth rates has been proposed to define malignancy better and to aid in prognosis. The cell cycle time, the time between successive mitoses, has been divided into four phases: a mitotic (M) phase during which the cell is dividing; a postmitotic phase (G_1) of RNA synthesis; a phase of DNA synthesis (S); and a premitotic (G_2) phase before cell division. Cells not actively proliferating are considered to be in the G_0 phase. The proportion of proliferating cells to the total cell population is termed the growth fraction (GF). Growth fraction is approximated by the number of cells in S phase that can be labeled. The growth fraction has been measured by autoradiography with [3H]thymidine, DNA flow cytometry, and monoclonal antibody directed against bromodeoxy-uridine-labeled nuclei or against the nuclear antigen Ki-67. Not surprisingly, glioblastoma and medulloblastoma show a much

Table 21.2.
Tumor Syndromes Associated with Neural Involvement and Chromosome Location

Tumor Syndrome	Typical Tumor Types	Chromosome Location
Hereditary cutaneous malignant melanoma/dysplastic nevus syndrome	Dysplastic nevi, melanoma	1p
Von Hippel-Lindau Syndrome	Hemangioblastoma, pheochromocytoma, renal cell carcinoma	3p
Multiple endocrine neoplasia Type I	Pituitary tumor, parathyroid adenoma, endocrine pancreatic tumors	11p
Multiple endocrine neoplasia Type 2	Pheochromocytoma, medullary thyroid carcinoma	10
Familial retinoblastoma	Retinoblastoma, osteosarcoma	13q
Neurofibromatosis (NF-1)	Neurofibroma, optic glioma, neurofibrosarcoma	17q
Neurofibromatosis (NF-2)	Vestibular schwannoma, meningioma, spinal nerve root neurofibroma	22q
Tuberous sclerosis	Subependymal giant cell astrocytomas hamartomas	16q

higher GF than astrocytoma and meningioma, and some subgroups of biologic activity are beginning to emerge.

Neurofibromatosis, an autosomal dominantly inherited disease, is associated with a marked increase in the incidence of several of the most common brain tumors—gliomas, schwannomas, and meningiomas. Sixteen percent of patients with primary brain tumors have a family history of cancer. With glioblastoma multiform, primary CNS lymphoma, and neuroblastoma, the figure nearly doubles. Many hereditary disorders are associated with neural tumors (Table 21.2). Current theory postulates the presence of tumor-promoting genes (oncogenes) and tumor-suppressing genes (antioncogenes). Genetic abnormalities in this condition may be acquired environmentally, accounting for spontaneously occurring brain tumors. Nitrosourea compounds are especially effective in inducing gliomas experimentally. Epidermal growth factor and platelet-derived growth factor have been considered oncogenic expressions in malignant gliomas. Heterozygosity or nonsymmetrical alleles have been demonstrated in glioblastoma on chromosomes 7, 10, and 22. Meningiomas show an estrogen or progesterone receptor in about half of cases, and abnormalities on chromosomes of 22 have been noted.

The failure of surgery and, for the most part, radiation therapy to alter significantly the course of intrinsic brain tumors has prompted increased investigation into molecular biologic and immunologic areas.

Neurotrauma

Head Injury

Brain trauma includes a spectrum of pathophysiologic consequences: synaptic impairment, neuronal disruption, ischemia, increased intracranial pressure, edema, bleeding, and herniation syndromes. With cerebral concussion, there is transient loss of consciousness attributed to traction on the upper brainstem and reversible synaptic impairment in the reticular-activating system. Persistent mild impairment of higher cortical functions has been recognized in more severe cases of cerebral concussion. Boxers subjected to repeated concussion may later show a degenerative-type dementia.

With more severe closed head injury, prolonged unconscious may occur, and amnesia, both retrograde and posttraumatic (antegrade), is common. Immediately after injury, there is a marked increase in CBF attributed to vasoparalysis, which is not blocked by sympathectomy or vagotomy and is believed to be brainstem mediated. Afterward, there is a period of decreased CBF owing either to reduced metabolic demand or to vasospasm. Both decreases in $CMRO_2$ and angiographic vasospasm have been demonstrated after head injury.

Cerebral contusions commonly result from head injury. A contusion may develop beneath the site of impact (coup contusion) but more commonly develops where the brain has struck the internal aspect of the skull on the contralateral side (contrecoup contusion). The irregular surface of the skull base over the orbits and at the sphenoid and petrous ridges make frontal and temporal lobe contusions more common. Brain contusions initially show small ecchymoses often at the crowns of the gyri. Edema develops around the areas of contusion and, although it is maximal between 48 and 96 hours, it may persist for weeks. In some cases, sizable intracerebral hematomas occur at the time of injury, and in still others, small areas of contusion coalesce over a few days into sizable clots (delayed traumatic intracerebral hematoma).

Extra-axial hematomas are well recognized complications of head injury. Epidural hematoma usually is associated with skull fracture and bleeding from the meningeal arteries or sinuses. Such hematomas are typically temporoparietal but may occur anywhere, including the posterior fossa. Subdural hematoma results from shearing of bridging veins to the sinuses and from brain lacerations. They are often holoconvex, extending from front to occiput. Skull fractures are present in about 50% of subdural hematomas and are often on the contralateral side. If not fatal, a subdural membrane can envelop the clot, and a chronic subdural hematoma may form, which may gradually increase in size. Subdural hematomas present as a variety of neurologic syndromes.

Untreated brain mass lesions, whether contusions or hematomas, may progress rapidly to brain herniations as described previously. Early diagnosis and treatment are mandatory to preserve neurologic function in these cases. Some patients with severe closed head injury will show no abnormalities on imaging studies and are considered to have diffuse axonal shearing injuries. Some of these patients make remarkable recoveries, but others are left in a permanent vegetative state.

Spinal Cord Injury

Trauma to the spinal cord may occur biomechanically, with or without spinal column fracture, or by penetrating injuries. Except for penetrating injuries, most spinal cord injuries are contusive in nature, and complete severance of the spinal cord is uncommon. Experimentally, the earliest finding in a contusive cord lesion is hemorrhage of the gray matter, with subsequent necrosis of the white matter. This occurs within days. Nevertheless, functional impairment is often complete from the time of injury, and strategies to prevent delayed necrosis of the white matter pharmacologically are controversial. At present, only one randomized controlled study has shown that the administration of methylprednisolone within 8 hours of spinal cord injury results in improved recovery (5).

About half of spinal injuries are cervical and half are thoracolumbar. Also, about half of spinal cord injuries are complete and half are incomplete. Clinical syndromes depend on the level of injury—cervical, thoracolumbar, conus, cauda equina—but syndromes relating to the cross-sectional anatomy of the cord are recognized. Hemisection of the cord (Brown-Sequard syndrome) causes ipsilateral paralysis and position/vibration sense loss, and contralateral pain and temperature loss. Ipsilateral segmental sensory loss completes the syndrome. Anterior cord syndrome describes loss of motor, pain, and temperature sensation bilaterally with preservation of position and vibration sense (posterior column function). This syndrome may have a vascular basis. Central cord syndrome describes an injury for which weakness in the arms, especially distally, is out of proportion to leg weakness, and sensory functions are preserved partially or completely. It is the most common incomplete injury and is associated with preexisting cervical spondylosis. Finally, a central cyst (syringomyelia) can cause loss of pain and temperature sensation, with preservation of other sensory modalities in the upper extremities before motor involvement that is of the central cord type. Most incomplete spinal cord injuries represent a mixture of the above syndromes, but one type often predominates.

In the initial phase of a complete spinal cord injury, the muscles below the injury are flaccid, reflexes are absent, and the autonomics are impaired. This is termed spinal shock, which does not denote decreased blood pressure, although mild hypotension is common. Over a period of weeks, tone and reflexes return and eventually become hyperactive with associated pathologic reflexes.

The mechanisms underlying spinal shock and subsequent development of spasticity are unknown. Perhaps a mechanism similar to Wallerian degeneration in peripheral nerves occurs in descending corticospinal inhibitory pathways with initial release of excessive neurotransmitter, then gradual degeneration of the axon and disinhibition of local reflex arcs. During spinal shock, the bladder is atonic, ileus is common, and the skin is prone to pressure necrosis, all requiring immediate attention in the injured patient.

Peripheral Nerve Injury

Peripheral nerve injury can be graded according to the type of injury a nerve fiber has sustained (Seddon) or from the injury a peripheral nerve has sustained (Sunderland). Both systems are useful conceptually and clinically.

In the Seddon system, neuropraxia is the mildest injury a fiber can receive and is associated physiologically with loss of conduction. The axon is in continuity but is focally demyelinated at the injury site. The endoneurium or connective tissue sheath is intact, and restoration of function occurs with remyelination usually within weeks to months. This type of injury is seen in positioning palsies or after prolonged periods of immobilization. Axonotmesis is a more severe injury in which axonal continuity is lost in addition to demyelination, but the connective tissue sheath is intact. Recovery will depend on axonal regeneration. The fidelity of regeneration is expected to be excellent. Neurotmesis adds to axonotmesis the disruption of the connective tissue support of the axon. This type of injury can range from internal disruption of the connective tissue to nerve transection. With axonotmetic and neurotmetic injuries, Wallerian degeneration occurs. The axon degenerates toward the motor end plate, and Schwann cells form tubules to receive regenerating axons.

Many nerve injuries leave the nerve in gross continuity with varying degrees of intraneural damage. The Sunderland grading method is based on the anatomical structure of the nerve, with progressive grades reflecting more severe damage.

Grade 1 is disruption of the myelin sheath, which manifests as a Conduction block.

Grade 2 is the loss of axon continuity with preservation of all layers of connective tissue framework. The endoneurial, perineurial and epineurial layers all remain intact.

Grade 3 is loss of axon continuity with loss of endoneurial integrity. In this setting, internal endoneurial scarring can prevent re-innervation, and disruption of the endoneurial sheath may allow mismatched re-innervation as regenerating axons stray from their proper endoneurial sheaths.

Grade 4 is loss of perineural integrity and thus disruption of the fascicle. This is associated with more intraneural scarring and consequently less effective nerve regeneration. As in grade 3 injuries, the connective tissue disruption will allow mismatch to occur with regeneration, potentially degrading functional recovery.

Grade 5 is loss of epineural continuity and thus transection of the nerve.

Most clinical nerve injuries result from of four basic types of trauma: laceration, compression, stretch, and high velocity missile injury.

Laceration to nerve may be caused by knife wounds, shattered glass, or by more blunt mechanisms such as chain saws, propeller blades, auto metal, and animal bites. Up to 20% of suspected transection injuries actually leave the nerve in continuity, and some of these may recover without surgery. However, most laceration injuries are Sunderland grade 4 or 5 and consequently will require surgical intervention. Direct end-to-end repair, with proper fascicular alignment using either epineurial or fascicular suture, is the mainstay of treatment.

Acute compression injuries are identified by a characteristic history of prolonged immobility. In patients previously well, this immobility usually is associated with extreme fatigue, alcohol intoxication, drug-abuse, or general anesthesia. The type of injury is usually neuropraxic and/or axonotmetic, but on occasion, endoneurial damage does occur. The recovery time will be the major indicator of degree of injury, as these injuries usually do not require surgical intervention. Motor fibers are the most susceptible to compression. They are the first to fail, the last to recover, and, in mild injuries, may be the only ones to suffer.

As a nerve is stretched more than 6% to 20% of its length, nerve function starts to fail, cross sectional area decreases, and intraneural pressure increase. Nerve injury proceeds, starting at Sunderland grade 1 and progressing grade by grade until the upper 30% limit is reached. At this point, the perineurium and then the epineurium give way and the nerve ruptures. In mixed motor sensory nerves, stretching may affect all function, or sensation alone, but seldom affects motor disability without sensory impairment. Given the lengths over which the stretching forces may take place, the damage tends to be spread over a length of nerve rather that at a precise point. Consequently, surgical repair often requires the use of grafts. As the perineurium provides significant strength to peripheral nerve, the absence of this layer at the spinal rootlet level contributes significantly to the propensity for nerve root avulsion from the spinal cord.

High velocity missiles generate forces which take the form of shock waves, with high pressure regions in front of and lateral to the moving body and pressure associated with the formation of a temporary explosive cavity in the track of the missile. Consequently, structures adjacent to and also distant from the missile path may be stretched abruptly and deformed. Nerves directly in the path may be severed or torn, but most are injured secondarily due to sudden stretch, with all grades of injury being observed afterwards.

Nerve recovery passes through several stages. After an initial period of retrograde demyelination of the axon and chromatolysis of the cell nucleus, wherein new RNA is manufactured, the axons begin sprouting and will grow into the distal nerve sheath unless inhibited by distance or scar. Once neurotization of the distal stump is achieved, the nerve fibers grow toward the motor endplates and sensory terminals. A period of time is required for these connections to be reestablished. This process continues until the active fiber pool is numerous enough to elicit muscle activity or provide sensation. This process takes months to years to complete. The presence of regenerating unmyelinated fibers may be ascertained by tapping over the course of a nerve. Elicited paresthesias (Tinel's sign) are indicative of the forward advance of these axons but are no guarantee of useful functional return.

A useful clinical approximation for recovery of motor function is an overall growth rate of 1 inch per month. The regenerative rate for axons is faster in the proximal limb than in the distal limb. When an axon is lacerated, the time for retrograde degeneration, sprouting, and spanning the injury reduces the expected rate of recovery. This delay may be 2 weeks with axonotmetic injuries and up to 4 weeks with sutured neurotmetic injuries. In stretch injuries, the growth rate is slower.

The time course of nerve recovery will ultimately indicate the degree of injury. Lack of clinical recovery 16 weeks after nerve injury usually indicates a grade 3 or higher injury. The functional potential of nerve recovery decreases with the passage of time. Although variation exists in the intrinsic recoverability of nerves and in the percentage of strength necessary for useful function in associated muscles, most muscles are subject to a 24 month limit of denervation, after which no useful motor recovery is expected from reconnection. The exceptions to this rule are large proximal muscles such as biceps, gastrocnemius-soleus, quadriceps, and, surprisingly, the facial muscle. When sensory function is considered, the period of effective repair may be increased by several years.

Electromyography may further clarify the pattern of neuronal injury and recovery. By 3 weeks after axonotmetic or neurotmetic injury, denervational changes of increased insertional activity, fibrillation potentials, and positive sharp waves may be identified. Later with reinnervation of at least 200 to 400 fibers, motor units under volitional control may be identified.

At least three to four thousand myelinated fibers must be present for significant reinnervation to occur. This forms the basis for direct operative evaluation of injured nerve with Nerve Action Potential (NAP) recordings in those patients with proximal injuries which show no spontaneous recovery in the initial months after nerve injury. The absence of a NAP after adequate time for axonal regrowth to have crossed the damaged segment is an indication that no useful recovery can be anticipated. In such a case, the damaged area is resected and grafts from sensory nerves, such as the sural, can be used as substitute conduit for regenerating axons.

Seizures and Epilepsy

Seizures result from excessive and/or hypersynchronous, usually self-limited abnormal activity of neurons predominately located in the cerebral cortex. A seizure may occur in the normal human brain from a variety of noxious stimuli depending on individual thresholds. In some, mild sleep deprivation, alcohol withdrawal, and in children, fever, can provoke a seizure. In contradistinction, epilepsy is a condition wherein the disturbance of the brain, either microscopic or macroscopic, is responsible for the seizure endures and is responsible for repetitive events. Seizures result in a variety of symptoms, depending upon the area of brain involved. Seizures occurring in childhood and adolescence often have no radiologic abnormalities and may have a genetic basis, whereas seizures in adults are more likely to have an associated structural abnormalities.

Seizures are classified as generalized when a loss of consciousness occurs and partial when consciousness is preserved. Complex partial seizures have some alteration in consciousness and are associated with foci in the temporal and frontal lobes. Partial seizures may become generalized. Generalized seizures include tonic-clonic (grand mal) and absence (petit mal) and are believed to be generated with participation of the brainstem reticular formation and thalamic nuclei because of the observed symmetrical electrocortical activity. Partial seizures are associated more commonly with a focal brain lesion. Simple partial seizures may be motor (Jacksonian) where progressive involvement of one side of the body, sensory or other, exists. Complex partial seizures (temporal lobe seizures) frequently have automatism and visceral components.

The spike and wave discharge is the EEG signature of a seizure; this reflects abnormal depolarization and hyperpolarization events occurring synchronously in the abnormal region. The spike of the EEG is formed by the summation of the excitatory depolarization, whereas the wave represents the summation of the inhibitory after hyperpolarizing potentials.

Seizures tend to be self limited but are often repetitive and at times continuous (status epilepticus). CRMO$_2$ and CBF increases considerably in the involved areas, often with CBF unable to meet metabolic demand, creating a relative ischemia. Interictally metabolism and CBF may be reduced significantly in 70% to 80% of patients. This finding has been used in Positron Emission Tomography (PET) to localize seizure foci.

Ion channel physiology is important in understanding the mechanisms by which anticonvulsant medica-

Table 21.3.
Sites of Action of Seizure Medications

	Use-Dependant Inhibition of Sodium Channels	Enhanced GABA Receptor Chloride Current	Inhibition of T-Type Calcium Current
Phenytoin	+ +	–	–
Carbamazepine	+ +	–	–
Valproate	+ +	+/?	–
Ethosuximide	–	–	+ +
Barbiturates	+	+ +	–
Primidone	+	–	–
Benzodiazepines	+	+ +	–

tions work (Table 21.3). Drugs such as phenytoin, carbamazepine, and valproate bind to activated sodium channels from the inside the cell membrane and maintain the channel in an inactive form temporarily. Its short duration of blockage will therefore minimally affect the normal functioning of the sodium channels but will greatly impede the rapid repetitive firing of neurons characteristic of a seizure.

The chloride channel complex is regulated by GABA a major inhibitory neurotransmitter of the brain. Opening of the chloride channel by GABA allows chloride ions to enter the neuron and hyperpolarize the cell, thereby making the neuron more difficult to fire. GABA is synthesized in gabaergic nerve terminals by the enzyme glutamic acid decarboxylase (GAD). After its release, it is taken up into neurons and glia by specific transporters (GAT). GABA is metabolized by GABA transaminase as part of the GABA shunt. The GABA receptor is divided into two types: A and B. The A receptor is formed from five peptide subunits which surround a channel permeable to CL-.

Chloride channel activity can be enhanced by three mechanisms: (a) by prolonging the channel's opening time; (b) by increasing its opening frequency; and (c) by increasing the channel's conductance. Benzodiazepines act by increasing the frequency of channel openings and barbiturates act by prolonging the channel's opening time. New anti-epileptic drugs (AED) have been developed to exploit the understanding of GABA functioning. Tigabine (TGB) binds to GAT inhibiting neuronal reuptake of GABA in the synaptic cleft and has shown efficacy in the treatment of partial complex seizures. Vigabatrin is an irreversible inhibitor of GABA transaminase and has been shown to increase CSF GABA content and reduce seizure frequency in AED resistant CPS.

Calcium channel physiology is also important in seizure understanding. Ethosuximide, an anticonvulsant effective only in absence seizures, has been shown to block a voltage dependant calcium channel in thalamocortical relay neurons.

Another focus of AED control is the excitatory amino acids. Glutamate coupled with glycine is the major excitatory neurotransmitter of the cortex. Substantial evidence points to the role of abnormal expression or enhanced function in various acquired forms of epilepsy. Three receptor types are recognized currently: the AMPA receptor, the kainic acid receptor, and the NMDA receptor. The NMDA receptor, when activated, allows flow of CA++ and sodium ions. It has multiple regulatory sites and is a main focus for AED development. The ion channel is affected by magnesium and the dissociative anesthetics such as ketamine. The sedative effects of drugs developed to block this receptor may limit their usefulness in epilepsy, but the potentially toxic effects of EAAs in trauma and stroke suggests that this class of drugs may have neuro protective functions.

Seizures are terminated by an active inhibitory process. Adenosine is thought to be involved with seizure termination and explains why toxic levels of aminophylline may induce seizures which are extremely difficult to control. Second messengers, such as cyclic nucleotides, calcium, and G-proteins, offer potential sites of pharmacologic manipulation.

After a seizure, a period of drowsiness and confusion (postictal state) occurs that clears over a few hours. With partial and generalized seizures, a postictal neurologic deficit, such as hemiparesis, commonly occurs and clears over 24 to 48 hours (Todd's paralysis).

Surgical excision of the seizure focus is being considered more often in chronic seizure disorders that have not responded favorably to AED therapy. Accurate localization of the seizure focus can be obtained with depth electrodes; continuous recordings, including video monitoring to correlate seizures to EEG events; and PET/MRI scanning.

Brain Death

The advent of artificial ventilation has created medical conditions wherein the brain may be completely and irreversibly damaged and the cardiac function maintained. As a consequence, the concept of brain death has been developed to apply to these situations in which the prior standard of death, i.e., the cessation of heartbeat, is not a useful criterion of an organism's ability to recover. Understanding the criteria for brain death is important because the increased availability of organs for transplantation has been allowed by the general acceptance of this concept. The definition of brain death involves legal, ethical, and clinical considerations. Universal criteria for brain death and the acceptance of brain death as equivalent to cardiorespiratory arrest do not exist for every state and country. In making the determination of brain death, therefore, it is important to be familiar with hospital, community, and state guidelines regarding this important question.

The most commonly applied criteria in the United States use the guidelines of the President's Commission, which considers a patient to have died when cerebral and brainstem functions are absent and when the situa-

Table 21.4.
Modification of Brain Death Criteria for Children and Infants Less than 5 Years Old

Infants 7 Days to Two Months
Two examinations and two confirmatory EEGs separated by at least 48 hours

Infants 2 Months to 1 Year
Two examinations and EEGs separated by at least 24 hours unless CBG studies document no cerebral perfusion

Children 1 to 5 Years
When an irreversible cause exists, a 12 hour time interval between examinations is recommended. In cases of hypoxiaischemia, a 24 hour interval is recommended. If an EEG shows electrical silence or a CBF study demonstrates no cerebral perfusion, the time interval between examinations may be reduced.

tion is deemed irreversible based on a known cause for brain dysfunction, no known therapy that will promote recovery, and an adequate period of observation.

Brain death determination rests primarily on the clinical examination. The patient is unresponsive to command or pain and shows no spontaneous movements. Limited limb withdrawal is considered a spinal reflex and not relevant. Brainstem reflexes are not elicitable, including pupillary reaction, oculocephalic reflexes (doll's eyes), oculovestibular reflexes (cold calorics), and corneal, gag, and cough reflexes. The patient is apneic with endotracheal oxygen, and the Pa_{CO_2} is allowed to rise above 60 torr. The clinical examination is conducted in the absence of sedative drugs, with the temperature higher than 95°C and the systolic blood pressure above 95 torr. Ancillary tests include an isoelectric (flat) EEG and absence of CBF on angiography or radioisotope scan. When ancillary testing is used as an adjunct to clinical examination, brain death may not be declared until the adjunctive test fully supports the clinical diagnosis. Appropriate periods of observation between two examinations range from 6 to 24 hours, and some hospitals require examinations by two independent examiners, especially in cases of transplantation.

The declaration of brain death in children poses additional challenges. The report of the President's Commission outlines criteria valid in children over 5 years of age. The supposition of increased resistance to injury in the child's brain is controversial and lacks good clinical support. As a consequence, a task force of pediatricians and neurologists developed guidelines to deal with the problem of pediatric brain death (Table 21.4).

The time of death is generally considered when cardiac arrest occurs in cases for which life support is withdrawn. Time of death is at the time of brain death determination in cases of transplantation.

Future Directions

Despite the wealth of information that has contributed to the understanding of the nervous system, many of the most fundamental questions remain unanswered or are understood at only a superficial level: How does the nervous system develop? What are the underlying mechanisms for learning and memory? Can the nervous system regenerate, and if so, how? Can neuronal cell death in trauma and ischemia be prevented? Why does the nervous system age and degenerate? Are the genetic changes in neoplasia reversible or preventable? Why do patients with stroke show gradual recovery over months? Can consciousness and behavior be understood completely in electrochemical terms? Many additional basic questions could be posed.

A major area of research effort in the neurosciences is presently in the fields of molecular biology and genetics. The search for neurotransmitters, the structure of their receptors, and the genes regulating them dominates much of the neuroscience literature. The discovery of nerve growth factors has raised hope for promoting regeneration in the nervous system and perhaps elucidating mechanisms underlying neoplasia. Ischemic cell death is considered to be, at least partially, a receptor-mediated phenomenon. Learning and memory may relate to the up-regulation of receptors in given neuronal circuits in response to repeated sensory experiences and input. In general, emphasis has shifted from the "hard-wiring" of the nervous system to chemical neurotransmitter relationships. Both are essential to proper function of the nervous system, but the neurochemical relationships might lend themselves more easily to therapeutic manipulation.

Recent years have seen the introduction of imaging modalities such as MRI and PET and SPECT scanning that create both physiologic and anatomical maps of the nervous system and help clarify the interrelationship of various brain areas in normal and abnormal functional activities. Nervous tissue is being transplanted in degenerative diseases and spinal cord injuries, and in-dwelling pumps and slow-release polymer capsules containing neurotransmitters are being evaluated. Genetic abnormalities associated with brain tumors have been described, and the role of oncogenes and suppressor genes in neoplasia is being elucidated. Plasticity within the nervous system to recover lost functions is under intense scrutiny. Familiarity with the basic concepts of neuroscience will benefit all physicians in understanding developments relevant to their own specialties and keeping abreast of advances in this important area.

REFERENCES

1. Hodgkin AL, Huxley AF. Quantitative description of membrane current and its application to conduction excitation in nerve. J Physiol 1952;117:500.
2. Rexed B. The cytoarchitectonic organization of the spinal cord in the cat. J Comp Neurol 1952;96:415.
3. Nordstrom CH, Rehncrona S, Siesjo BK. Cerebral metabolism. In: Youmans JR, ed. Neurological surgery. Philadelphia: WB Saunders, 1990:623–661.
4. Meldrum BS, ed. Frontiers in pharmacology and therapeutics: excitatory amino acid antagonists. Oxford, UK: Blackwell Scientific, 1991.
5. Bracken MB et al. A randomized, controlled trial of methylprednisolone or naloxone in the treatment of acute spinal cord injury. New Engl J Med 1990;322:1405–1411.

SUGGESTED READINGS

Carpenter MB, Sutin J. Human neuroanatomy. 8th ed. Baltimore: Williams & Wilkins, 1983.
Kandel ER, Schwartz JH. Principles of neuroscience. 3rd ed. New York: Elsevier, 1992.
Salcman M, ed. Neurobiology of brain tumors. Concepts in neurosurgery. Baltimore: Williams & Wilkins, 1991.
Schmidt RF, ed. Fundamentals of neurophysiology. 3rd ed. New York: Springer-Verlag, 1985.
Yasargil MG. Microneurosurgery. Vols. 1–2. Stuttgart: Georg Thieme, 1984.
Youmans JR, ed. Neurological surgery. Vols. 1–6. Philadelphia: WB Saunders, 1990.
Kline DG and Hudson AR. Nerve Injuries. Philadelphia: WB Saunders, 1995.

22 Skin and Subcutaneous Tissue Review In General Surgery

Edwin G. Wilkins | Kevin C. Chung | Riley S. Rees | Martin C. Robson |
David J. Smith, Jr.

Anatomy and Physiology

The skin is a highly specialized bilaminate structure that serves as an organ of protection. It controls the invasion of microorganisms, regulates fluid loss or gain, monitors temperature, protects against injury from radiation and electricity, and provides immunologic surveillance. Each function directly reflects a cell or area within the skin (1). The skin is generally 1.2-mm thick but varies from 0.5 to 6 mm. The outer, highly cellular epidermal layer measures 0.06 to 0.8 mm in thickness and is in contact with the dermis through irregular interpapillary ridges and grooves (2).

The outermost stratum corneum is the most important layer and is composed of nonviable, relatively dry keratinized cells. It not only provides protection but also prevents water, electrolyte, and plasma protein loss. Water moves from the strongly hydrated viable dermis through the stratum corneum and then evaporates. The stratum corneum also structurally protects against bacterial invasion. There are two types of skin bacteria: resident and transient flora. Although resident organisms exist in relative equilibrium on the skin, the skin protects against transient bacterial invasion. Exposure to streptococci, staphylococci, and enteric bacteria is frequent, and random cultures may recover any of these. Sebum, the secretion of the sebaceous gland, contains high levels of fatty acids, particularly oleic acid. In addition to lubricating the skin surface, sebum actively destroys streptococci and, to a lesser extent, staphylococci. Any break in the skin or any cutaneous inflammation causes serum accumulation that inactivates sebum. In this situation, streptococci may rapidly colonize the skin. In reality, the stratum corneum is the rate-limiting barrier for most substances.

In most areas of the body, the stratum corneum is only 10 to 15 cell layers, or 10- to 20-μ thick; exceptions are the palms and soles. These layers are strongly inter-digitated, accounting for the high tensile strength of skin. The stratum corneum also resists stretch because of its flexibility. However, the dermis, with its high collagen content, resists and cushions direct trauma. Melanin, the best absorber of ultraviolet light, is primarily in the basal layer of the epidermis but is also present in the stratum corneum.

The inner most layer of epidermis, the stratum germinativum, or basal layer, contains melanocytes and cells destined for keratin production. These are the only proliferating epidermal cells. Melanocytes are confined to the basal layer but can transfer melanin, in melanosomes, to the keratinocytes. Between the outer stratum corneum and the inner stratum germinativum, keratinocytes lie in various stages of differentiation.

The stratum spinosum, or spinous layers, contain most of the viable cells producing keratin and precursor proteins for the granular layer cells. The stratum granulosum primarily produces proteins related to the fully keratinized cells. After migrating into the epidermis, melanocytes, Langerhans cells, and Merkel cells become associated with certain keratinocytes. The melanocytes provide melanin, which absorbs and scatters ultraviolet radiation as well as trapping photochemically active free radicals. Langerhans cells help identify antigens for immunocompetent cells and are particularly important in contact hypersensitivity. Merkel cells are thought to be sensory receptors, acting as mechanoreceptors. Groups of basal cells in the epidermis also form appendages (nails, pilosebaceous apparatuses, eccrine, and apocrine sweat glands) during embryogenesis. No new appendages are added postnatally (3).

The skin also provides a mechanism for temperature regulation, one of the few protective functions not controlled by the stratum corneum. The rate at which heat is lost by radiation is a function of temperature of the cutaneous surface, and in turn, this temperature is a function primarily of blood flow through the skin. Adipose tissue is a good heat insulator, and heat is poorly conducted below the cutaneous surface.

The dermal-epidermal junction undulates in most

areas of the body, increasing surface contact between the two layers to provide resistance of normal skin to shearing. The dermal-epidermal junction, called the basement membrane, functions as a filter to inhibit or prevent passage of molecules >40 kDa (4). Inflammatory cells and neoplastic cells, circulating pemphigus, pemphigoid autoantibodies, immigrant cells, and neurites can penetrate the basement membrane zone. Therefore, these cells must possess some mechanism for disruption of this barrier. The basement membrane zone is frequently the site of immune complex deposition (4).

The dermis, or deeper layer of skin, is 20 to 30 times thicker than the epidermis. It contains the nervous, vascular, lymphatic, and supporting structures for the epidermis and harbors the epidermal appendages. The regions of the dermis respond differently because of differences in structural organization and biochemistry, and each responds uniquely to systemic disease, genetic disease, and environmental assault. The papillary and reticular dermis comprise the two main dermal zones.

The dermis contains fibrous and nonfibrous matrix molecules. The fibrous proteins impart bulk, density, and tensile properties to skin and also allow for compliance and elasticity. Fibrous glycoproteins in the dermis function in cell-matrix attachment. The nonfibrous matrix molecules form the ground substance that influences the osmotic properties of skin; permits cellular migration in a more fluid milieu; and serves as an integrative, continuous medium for all of the other structural elements (5). Fibrous elements of the dermis consist mainly of collagen fibrils and elastic fibers. The collagen in the skin is primarily Type I (85%) and Type III (15%) (6). Type IV collagen is the major component of the basal lamina zone. The elastic fibers contain two components: aligned bundles of microfibrils and a dense elastin matrix. The microfibrils are believed to serve as a template for the elastin matrix.

The nonfibrous portion of the dermis consists of glycosaminoglycans (GAGs) and glycoproteins of the amorphous ground substance. GAGs in the skin include hyaluronic acid, dermatan sulfate, and chondroitin 4- and 6-sulfate. GAGs play a role in cutaneous permeability, allow cellular migration, and influence the polymerization of such fibrous matrix proteins as collagen. GAGs are synthesized by fibroblasts and are turned over in phagocytic vacuoles by macrophages (5).

The papillary dermis is only slightly thicker than the overlying epidermis. Generally, it is separated from the underlying reticular dermis by a horizontal plexus of vessels that provides the overlying papillary dermis with a rich blood supply. The papillary dermis is altered more commonly in environmentally induced skin lesions (actinic damage) than in systemic inherited diseases of connective tissue metabolism. The majority of dermis is reticular dermis. Epidermal appendages either terminate in the lower levels of the reticular dermis or penetrate even deeper into the subcutaneous tissue. Vessels pierce the dermis, supplying blood to the hair follicles and sweat glands.

The human epidermal appendages include nails, hair, sebaceous glands (pilosebaceous apparatus), and eccrine and apocrine sweat glands. Few structures of the skin have as much variability as the pilosebaceous structures. The type of hair, density, and rate of growth all depend on the body region, sex, age, and race of the individual. The eccrine sweat glands are important in thermoregulation. Eccrine and apocrine glands each have unique characteristics. Both have granule-containing secretory cells, myoepithelial cells, modifications of the cells lining the glandular and ductile segments, and a thick connective tissue capsule. Apocrine glands are usually fewer in number, more restrictive in distribution, generally larger in size, and located deeper in the dermis (3).

Trauma

Care of Acute Wounds

Lacerations are the classic skin wound and are managed with débridement of devitalized tissue followed by atraumatic suture closure. Crush injuries are often accompanied by loss of more tissue than would have been suspected initially. The extent of injury may be evaluated with intravenous fluorescein, which diffuses into the interstitial tissue from patent capillaries in the area. Fluorescence under an ultraviolet lamp will indicate blood flow in the region and predicts survival of the tissue. Abrasion injuries involve superficial loss of epithelial elements. Most of the dermis and deeper structures are left intact. Usually, only cleansing of the wound is required, as the remaining epithelial cells will regenerate and migrate to close the wound. Careful cleansing is critical to prevent traumatic tattoos.

Almost all nonmilitary wounds can be closed primarily. The wounded area is cleaned with an antibacterial solution. Local anesthesia is generally adequate for smaller wounds. Agents containing epinephrine should be used with caution. Chemical vasoconstriction is often helpful in tissue with a rich blood supply but may produce detrimental ischemia in other areas, e.g., digital blocks of fingers or toes. The best way to cleanse the wound is sharp débridement to remove clot, debris, and necrotic tissue, followed by irrigation with a physiologic saline solution. Hematoma should be evacuated and all active bleeding controlled. Closure of the wound is undertaken in layers, with absorbable sutures placed in those layers that provide the greatest strength, i.e., dermis and fascia. The epithelium is approximated with superficial placement of nonabsorbable, monofilament suture to seal the wound. Closure of "dead space" is usually not necessary, given proper closure of the skin and fascia. Subcutaneous sutures only serve to necrose fat and introduce an unnecessary foreign body that promotes infection (7).

Great emphasis is often placed on the suture material used for closure, but it is less important than attention to adequate débridement and hemostasis. Newer absorbable sutures include synthetic material of polyglycolic acid, which is absorbed by hydrolysis and is useful for reapproximation of tissue below the epidermis. Nylon is an excellent example of synthetic suture material. It is usually monofilament but may be woven or braided. This material is biologically inert; therefore, it cannot be broken down or absorbed. Suture material, size, and type should be chosen based on the type of reapproximation. Usually, absorbable synthetic suture is preferred for closure of the deep layers. Muscle is friable and holds sutures poorly; therefore, the fascial covering is generally used for approximation. Subdermal tissue is closed, then the skin. For simple lacerations, wound drains are not required. The need for drainage usually suggests the need for better hemostasis. Sutures should be tight enough to approximate, not strangulate, the tissue. Swelling of the tissue will occur over a 24 to 48-hour period and tighten the suture. Excessive tension produces ischemia and additional inflammation. This exaggerates the suture marks across the wound and the "railroad track" appearance of the scar. Although cosmesis is the last element to consider in wound closure, avoidance of excessive tension produces a more desirable result. A dressing is usually placed over the closed wound. To be maximally functional, the dressing should protect the wound, immobilize the area, evenly compress the area, absorb secretions, and be aesthetically acceptable (8).

All wounds are contaminated with bacteria to a greater or lesser extent. Even the wounds considered clean have a bacterial inoculum. Proper wound care with débridement and adequate lavage can markedly diminish the inoculum and result in successful primary wound healing. Exceptions to the primary closure of contaminated wounds include those wounds with a high bacterial inoculum (e.g., human bite), long-time lapse from time of initial injury, or severe crush. In these instances, delayed closure is preferred (9).

The number of bacteria that can be found in a wound and still allow primary wound closure is the most precise definition of an infected wound. This level of contamination is approximately 10^5 organisms per gram of tissue in the otherwise uncompromised wound and host. The proper management of the infected wound should decrease the bacterial count to fewer than 10^5 organisms per gram tissue before wound closure. Débridement is the most important technique to decrease the bacterial count. Frequent dressing changes (q. 4h.) can also decrease the bacterial count. Systemic antibiotics are of little use in local bacterial control because they do not penetrate a granulating wound bed. However,

topical antibacterials, such as mafenide acetate or silver sulfadiazine, are effective. Biologic dressings such as allograft and amniotic membrane also decrease the bacterial level. Successful adherence of a biologic dressing indicates an acceptable bacterial count and will predict success accurately with either wound closure or autograft (9).

To ensure uncomplicated healing of a surgical wound, one needs to understand the stages of wound healing as outlined in Chapter 6. An open wound undergoes a predictable sequence to achieve final wound closure. These stages are inflammation, epithelialization, collagen synthesis, contraction, and remodeling (10). A wound will not heal if this sequence is disrupted. An infected wound prolongs the inflammatory phase and retards epithelialization. Poor nutrition reduces the substrates (Vitamin C and Zinc) needed for collagen synthesis. Steroids directly impede wound contraction. All these adverse conditions must be controlled to minimize complications and maximize both the rate and strength of wound healing.

Burns

Thermal Injury. Human skin can be injured by heat in two ways. One is an immediate direct cellular injury that is followed by a delayed injury caused by progressive dermal ischemia. Skin can tolerate temperatures up to 40°C for relatively long periods of time, but beyond this level, tissue destruction increases logarithmically (11). Tissue destruction is related to both time of exposure and temperature. Direct cell damage results from protein denaturation. Many of these changes may be reversible. The response of cells to heat is neither uniform nor static. The blood supply and the local environment of the wound greatly influence the ultimate cellular response (3).

The classic description by Jackson (12) of three concentric zones of thermal injury in the burn wound provides a practical basis for discussing the local burn injury. The central area of the burn wound, closest to the heat source, is characterized by coagulation of cells (zone of coagulation). Extending concentrically from the central zone of coagulation lies a labile zone of injured cells, which, under the most ideal circumstances, have the potential to survive (zone of stasis). Finally, the zone of hyperemia that has sustained only minimal injury lies peripheral to the zone of stasis. Cells in this zone will normally recover over a period of 7 to 10 days, unless they are subjected to some additional insult (3).

The initial cytologic evidence of thermal injury is a redistribution of the fluid and solid components of the cell nuclei. Imbibition of fluid causes nuclear swelling, membrane rupture, and pyknosis. Cell cytoplasm first becomes granular and then homogeneously coagulated. Progressive denaturation of cell protein occurs as temperatures rise. Thermolabile enzyme systems are blocked at approximately the same temperatures that effect protein denaturation (13). The metabolic response of an individual cell is variable, even within a homogeneous cell population. However, the decrease in enzyme activity less than 50% of normal results in cell death (3).

The idea that the progressive changes in the burn wound may be related to inflammation suggests a possible role of inflammatory mediators, specifically prostaglandin (PG). Inasmuch as thromboxane is a potent platelet aggregator and vasoconstrictor counteracting the action of PGI_2, it was postulated that PGE_2 and PGF_{2a} were present in exudates and tissue fluids of burns in a steady-state relationship because of their bidirectional activity. It was also postulated that this relationship was essential to the preservation and integrity of the cell (14). When the thromboxane response was prevented pharmacologically, platelet adherence was reduced, leukocytes and erythrocytes were prevented from sticking to vessel walls, and vasoconstriction was prevented (15). Thromboxane synthetase inhibition with imidazole, dipyridamole, and methimazole clearly preserved the integrity of the dermal microcirculation.

Vasoactive amines such as histamine are also found in increased concentrations after thermal injury. Histamine is released either as a direct result of heat or by stimulation of mast cells. It is associated with vasodilation and increased microvascular permeability (16). This causes both increased edema immediately and a delayed accumulation of edema in distant unburned areas (17). Prevention of histamine release by H_2-blocking agents such as cimetidine can decrease these effects (18).

Oxygen-free radicals may actually initiate the progressive damage phase of the burn injury. However, their short half-life makes them difficult to study in humans. Free radicals are produced whenever the energy charge of a cell drops below a critical level, limiting the oxygen availability necessary to produce ATP. They are also produced as part of the leukocyte respiratory burst to help prevent bacterial invasion when skin integrity is broached. Both of these stimuli occur at the moment of thermal injury. Ward (19) has shown that free radical scavengers such as catalase or superoxide dismutase can decrease the amount of postburn edema if given before injury. This suggests that free radicals are involved in the pathophysiology of the burn wound. Because oxygen-free radicals can also release arachidonic acid, it is difficult to determine whether they are involved directly in mediating damage or only indirectly involved by increasing the production of PG, thromboxanes, and leukotrienes (16).

Ward (20) summarized the stages of thermolability in burn patients. In acute burns, the complement system is activated by an undefined mechanism. Among the activated products in the complement cascade, C5a appears to be the initiating factor in the inflammatory response. C5a activates intravascular neutrophils' secretion of histamine. Additionally, C5a catalyzes the conversion of xanthine dehydrogenase into xanthine ox-

idase by interacting with the endothelial cells. Elevated level of xanthine oxidase leads to the production of oxygen free radicals (O_2, H_2O_2, HO) which causes increased vascular permeability and intravascular hemolysis. Furthermore, C5a may be a cofactor in the production of cytokines such as TNF-alpha which are active in the inflammatory reaction in burn patients (21).

The multisystemic responses of the burn patient, and the patient's death or survival, are closely related to the successful management of the burn wound. The first response to evaluate is the vascular response. There is both a local and generalized microvascular fluid flux, a generalized impairment in cell membrane function, and an increase in burn tissue osmotic pressure (22). These all lead to edema which, depending on the size of the burn, can be localized to the injured area or become a generalized systemic response.

After burns, the evaporative loss of fluid from the lack of skin coverage can cause marked hypovolemia. Concomitantly, the inflammatory effects of the burn injury cause increased systemic capillary permeability and loss of intravascular volume into the interstitium (23). This massive fluid shift in burns causes severe hypovolemia. If the intravascular volume is not restored, perfusion to all organs will be compromised, and cell death occurs. To assure adequate fluid resuscitation in burn patients, several formulas can be used to assess fluid requirement. The most commonly used formula is the Parkland formula (Table 22.1) (24). Total fluid requirement for the first 24 hours is estimated by multiplying the percent of body surface area burn by the weight of the patient in kilograms and a constant (4ml/kg/ %burn).

$$\text{Volume} = \text{weight (kg)} \times \% \text{ burn} \times 4$$

Lactated ringer is the fluid of choice for the first 24 hours. The percent of body surface area burn is estimated from the Lund and Browder chart (Figure 22.1) (25) which divides the body into regions, with each region consisting of 9% body surface area. Half of the calculated fluid is given during the first 8 hours, and the remaining half is infused in the remaining 16 hours. One must be cautioned that these calculations are only estimates of fluid requirements. Precise intravascular replacement must be based on the urine output which reflects perfusion of vital organs. If the urine output is low despite having given the estimated fluid replacement, additional information can be obtained by measuring the filling pressure of the heart using the Swan-Ganz catheter. Adequate tissue perfusion is usually assured if urine output is 0.5 cc/ kg/hour in an adult or 1 cc/kg/hour in an infant.

Renal function is altered in the burn patient, similar to that seen in any trauma patient. The normal stress response occurs along with the addition of marked loss of extracellular fluid volume (3). The posterior pituitary releases ADH, causing maximal reabsorption of water in the renal tubules. Simultaneously, maximal sodium reabsorption occurs because of aldosterone release from

Table 22.1.

Formula	Electrolyte	Colloid	Glucose in Water
First 24 hours			
Burn budget of FD Moore	Lactated Ringer's, 1000–4000 ml 0.5 N saline, 1200 ml	7.5% of body weight	1500–5000 ml
Evans	Normal saline, 1.0 ml/kg/% burn	1.0ml/kg/% burn	2000 ml
Brooke	Lactated Ringer's, 1.5 ml/kg/% burn	0.5 ml/kg/% burn	2000 ml
Parkland	Lactated Ringer's, 4 ml/kg/% burn		
Hypertonic sodium solution	Volume to maintain urine output at 30 ml/hr (fluid contains 250 mEq Na/L)		
Modified Brooke	Lactated Ringer's 2 ml/kg/% burn		
Second 24 hours			
Burn budget of FD Moore	Lactated Ringer's, 1000–4000 ml 0.5 N saline, 1200 ml	2.5% of body weight	1500–5000 ml
Evans ¹/₂ of 1st 24-hr requirement	¹/₂ of 1st 24-hr requirement ¹/₂ to ³/₄ of 1st 24-hr requirement	¹/₂ of 1st 24-hr requirement	2000 ml
Brooke		¹/₂ to ³/₄ of 1st 24-hr requirement	2000 ml
Parkland		20%–60% of calculated plasma volume	To maintain adequate urine output
Hypertonic sodium solution	¹/₃ Isotonic salt solution orally up to 3500 ml limit		
Modified Brooke		0.3–0.5 ml/kg/% burn	To maintain adequate urine output

0.5N, Halp normal; *Na,* sodium
From Ruitt BA. Fluid resuscitation for extensively burned patients, J Trauma 21 (suppl):690, © by Williams & Wilkins, 1981.

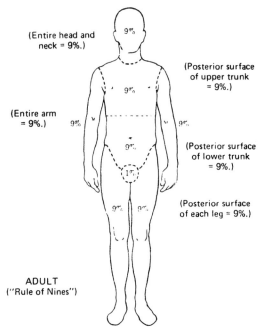

(Entire head and neck = 9%.)

9%

(Posterior surface of upper trunk = 9%.)

(Entire arm = 9%.) 9% 9% 9%

9%

(Posterior surface of lower trunk = 9%.)

1%

(Posterior surface of each leg = 9%.)

9% 9%

ADULT
("Rule of Nines")

Figure 22.1. Estimation of body surface area in burns. Reprinted from Shroeder SA, Krupp MA, Tierney LM Jr., McPhee SJ. Current medical diagnosis and treatment. Norwalk, CT: Appleton & Lange, 1990.

Although the trachea and bronchi dissipate heat rapidly, the upper airway may be burned. This causes edema, obstruction, and further hypoxia. The hypoxia causes a release of mediators that cause constriction in the bronchioles. Combined with edema, this decreased clearance of secretion and decreased cardiac output can lead to a ventilation-perfusion imbalance. The consequences are inadequate peripheral perfusion, lactic acidosis, and further cellular injury. As resuscitation occurs, the products of the peripheral ischemia are recirculated and must be cleared by already damaged lungs (3).

Originally, the lung was thought to be compromised further as resuscitation was begun because of an increase in total body capillary permeability; however, the lung actually may be spared this added insult (3). The normal respiratory response to burning is hyperventilation. Ventilation is about twice normal with minute volumes of up to 14 liters at a ventilatory rate of 20/min (27). This is caused by the increased oxygen needs and the ventilation-perfusion imbalance. In patients with burns over 40% of their total body surface area, a restrictive process with a decreased lung volume, decreased vital capacity, and an increase in pulmonary resistance can be seen (28).

Thermal injury also alters gastrointestinal tract function. The initial response is severe splanchnic vasoconstriction associated with an ileus. If unrecognized, acute gastric dilation can occur, leading to regurgitation and aspiration. Gastroduodenal ulceration, a frequent occurrence in a burn patient, is not always clinically evident and is not a result of an absolute hyperacidity (29). However, patients developing gastroduodenal injury within 72 hours of the burn do have higher basal acid outputs

the adrenals. Under this influence, the kidney will excrete only the amount of urine necessary to handle the solute load. The result is a small amount of concentrated urine with a decreased urine sodium concentration (26).

The pulmonary response to burning is the result of both direct injury and material circulating to the lung from the distant burned area. The lungs may be exposed to decreased oxygen secondary to combustion, and this may be further compromised if smoke inhalation occurs.

than those without gastrointestinal injury (30). Gastrin levels are not increased in thermal trauma and no correlation exists between serum gastrin levels and gastric acid output in burn patients. Therefore, the pathophysiology appears to be a relative hyperacidity combined with either increased mucosal barrier permeability or primary cytotoxicity (3).

Thermal trauma can also alter the hepatobiliary system. These changes may be the result of hypovolemia, hypoxia, or circulating factors requiring clearance. Liver biopsies have shown cloudy swelling as early as 3 hours postburn (3). This progresses to hepatocellular necrosis, vacuolization, and fatty degeneration (2). However, repair occurs with time. In addition, liver function tests all show some abnormalities during the course of a severe burn (31). Biliary tract stasis also occurs, as do changes in the normal bile salt ratios (3). Frequently, sludge forms in the gallbladder (3).

Numerous metabolic and neuroendocrine changes occur throughout the course of injury and recovery. Some of these are due primarily to hypovolemia. However, others occur when perfusion and tissue oxygenation are adequate (32). Hypermetabolism develops with increased oxygen consumption above the basal predicted level in burn patients. This increase in oxygen consumption is linear in patients with up to 40% burns and can reach a heat production of twice normal levels in burns between 50% to 100% (33). Although the exact cause of this hypermetabolism is not fully elucidated, the metabolic rate gradually falls toward normal with wound healing or burn wound closure (3).

The fluid-holding lipid in the skin is destroyed by burning so that up to four times the amount of body fluids can be lost through burned skin (34). Increased evaporative water loss causes cooling of the body, shivering, and additional heat expenditure. Increasing the environmental temperature and humidity can decrease the energy loss caused by evaporation and shivering. The critical temperature appears to be 32° to 34°C (3,35).

The hypermetabolic state after thermal trauma causes protein catabolism, hyperglycemia, decreased glucagon: insulin ratios, and extreme intracellular cation alterations. Intracellular sodium concentrations can rise dramatically and will remain elevated unless daily caloric intake is adequate (36). The negative nitrogen balance accompanying hypermetabolism can cause a nitrogen requirement of up to 20 g/m^2/body surface area (BSA) burn per day during the first month postburn. This nitrogen need is a result of both increased catabolism and decreased protein synthesis (32).

Counter regulatory hormones, glucagon, cortisol, and catecholamines are elevated in burn patients and are thought to play a major role in mediating the catabolic response to injury (32). It appears that these endocrine mediators, working with various inflammatory mediators, are in large part responsible for the various metabolic responses seen after a major burn (3).

Another series of systemic responses to the burn injury involve the immune system. If one artificially divides the immune system into the first barrier of defense (the skin), nonspecific immune factors, and specific host immunity, each is dramatically altered (37). The skin's dryness and keratin layer provide the first barrier to bacterial invasion. Its normal secretion of sebum further provides bactericidal properties. Burning removes the outer layer, and the local inflammatory response leads to an increase in PGE$_2$ and fluid into the wound. Although the fluid fibrin and thrombin help to localize the bacteria, the fluid also tends to neutralize the bacterial properties of sebum (3,38,39).

The nonspecific host response involves inflammation and chemotaxis. The chemotaxis is stimulated by mediators such as complement, opsonins, kinins, and PG. Altered leukocyte chemotaxis has been demonstrated after thermal injury (40,41). Circulating complement is depleted by 50%, and more important, C3a that is essential for both the classic and alternate complement pathways is decreased (37).

Thermal injury alters the natural barrier of the body to invasion by microorganisms. The susceptibility to infection in burn patients relates to the local and systemic defects. Robson stated that burn wound sepsis is a quantitative disturbance between the host's resistance and the bacterial load (42). Locally, thermal injury destroys the skin and alters the balance between endogenous flora and the protective mechanism of the skin. The endogenous flora consist of streptococci, staphylococci, and coliform bacteria (43). These organisms reside in the hair follicles and the orifices of sebaceous glands in the concentration of 10^3 bacteria per gram of tissue (42). In spite of these bacterial concentrations, the skin possesses antibacterial properties which prevent invasion. The sebaceous glands contain sebum which is effective in destroying streptococci and, to a lesser extent, staphylococci. In addition, the high concentration of fatty acids acts as a lubricant for the skin. After thermal injury, the destruction of the sebaceous glands eliminates this natural bactericidal compound and allows unchecked early proliferation of streptococci, and later, infection by other types of bacteria. Furthermore, the accumulation of serum and edema in a burn wound neutralizes any bactericidal properties that might remain, thus promoting bacterial growth.

As the bacteria count reaches a concentration of 10^5 bacteria per gram of tissue, invasion can occur into the dermal-subcutaneous junction. Deeper incursion into the vascular structures leads to thrombosis of the vessels and destruction of surrounding viable tissues. As a consequence, burn wound infection may convert a partial thickness burn into full thickness burn by virtue of ischemia and bacterial autolysis (42).

Prior to the discovery of penicillin, a 30% of total body surface burn had a mortality rate of 50%, with streptococcal infection responsible for most of the deaths (43).

Penicillin use reduced the mortality from streptococcal infection. During the antibiotic era, the bacterial flora in burn wounds changed. In 1964, Moncrief estimated that burn wound sepsis accounted for 70% of all hospital burn deaths, and pseudomonas aeruginosa was the dominant organism (44). Although the incidence of burn wound sepsis from pseudomonas has decreased dramatically because of topical antimicrobials, colonization of the wound with high concentrations of pseudomonas ($>10^5$) can be lethal. The circulation of byproducts or endotoxin from the high pseudomonas concentration can produce gram negative sepsis with septic shock and death. Another organism of interest is clostridium tetani. Because tetanus can occur even in superficial burns, coverage and prophylaxis with tetanus immunoglobulin or tetanus toxoid needs to be instituted based on the patient's immunization history.

Other than the local effects of the burn, systemic effects center on the immunologic deficit which predisposes to infection. Heggars et al. (45) divided the immune deficits into nonspecific and specific immunity. In nonspecific immunity defect, circulating complement is depleted by 50% (45). Total protein level, such as albumin and globulin, will be as low as 50% of normal for the first week after injury (42). In addition, leukocytes in burn patients show impaired phagocytosis and decreased intracellular killing of bacteria (46). Specific immunity deficits are manifested by impaired B cell mediated humoral response and T cell-mediated cellular response. Suppression of the B cell humoral response is evident by the decreased IgA, IgG and IgM. Impaired cellular immunity in burn patients is suggested by lymphocytopenia, delayed rejection of allografts, and a delayed response to normal hypersensitivity antigens (42). In summary, the generalized immunosuppression in burn patients may result from a combination of deficient production of immune system components and overproduction of suppressive toxins and factors (42).

The host's specific immune mechanisms can be divided into T cell-mediated cellular response and B cell-mediated humoral response. Both are altered severely in the burn patient. Impaired cellular immunity in burned patients is suggested by lymphocytopenia, delayed rejection of allografts, and a delayed response to normal hypersensitivity antigens (2). The decreased number of lymphocytes is altered further by a decreased responsiveness of peripheral blood lymphocytes to T cell mitogens (47). There is also an increase in a nonspecific immunosuppressive substances in burn sera that participate in the generation of suppressor T cells (3). The activation of B cell is hindered by an increase in suppressor activity, and the production of antibodies through the humoral response pathway are altered severely (3,48).

Electrical Injury

An electrical injury is a unique form of thermal trauma. Electrical injuries are divided arbitrarily into high-tension (;>1000 V) and low-tension (;<1000 V) injuries (3). The tissue destruction caused by contact with high-voltage electricity is basically a thermal injury. Passage of electric current through a solid conductor causes conversion of electric energy into heat (Joule effect) (49). The amount of heat can be determined by Ohm's law and the Joule effect. The extent of injury depends on the type of current, the pathway of flow, the local tissue resistance, and the duration of contact (50–54).

Several theories to explain the pathologic changes seen after electrical injury have been postulated. The first emphasizes the differences in tissue resistance to current flow. Tissue resistance progressively increases from nerve to blood vessels, muscle, skin, fat, and finally to bone (55–57). Bone, which has the greatest resistance, generates the most heat and would cause greater necrosis in the deep perosseous tissues (3,58–60).

Another theory contests the existence of progressive muscle necrosis. Hunt et al. (50) found that the internal body acts like a volume conductor of a single resistance and not as though it were composed of tissues of varying resistances (50). With the onset of current, flow, amperage, and temperature rose in parallel throughout the limb. By the time of current arcing, both muscle and bone temperature were equal. However, Hunt et al. (50) observed that it took bone longer to dissipate the heat and thought that this prolonged elevation in temperature accounted for the periosseous "core" of necrotic muscle seen clinically. This study proposed that involved muscle and vessels sustain irreversible damage at the time of current passage with immediate microscopic muscular coagulation necrosis and small nutrient artery thrombosis (3). Several studies support this concept (61,62).

A third theory postulates that inflammatory mediators are responsible for the progressive necrosis after electrical injury. Using a rat model, increasing levels of arachidonic acid metabolites, chiefly thromboxane, have been shown in the deep periosseous tissue beneath what appeared to be uninjured skin. With time, the thromboxane increased progressively toward the limb surface until apparently uninjured skin necrosed, just as in the clinical situation (3,49).

The first step in managing the victim of an electrical injury is to choose among the planning options (3). As stated, controversy exists whether the hidden damage of tissue beneath apparently uninjured skin is a slow manifestation of irreversible muscle damage secondary to the original insult or whether it is actually progressive ischemic necrosis secondary to ongoing vascular compromise. The question has important clinical implications. Proponents of the pathophysiologic scheme of immediate irreversible necrosis advise early aggressive débridement to decrease the septic risk of unexcised nonviable muscle. Proponents of the progressive ischemic necrosis accept the inability to discern the full extent of the injury initially and advise cautious initial débridement followed by periodic débridement as demarcation proceeds. Premature closure over partially necrotic tissue is thereby avoided. If the progressive necrosis is because of cellular injury secondary to mediators released by the heat generated, then possible pharmacologic means to block or inhibit these mediators may become useful (52,62,63).

Chemical Injury

Although chemical burns account for only 3% of all burns, they account for 30% of burn deaths (64). Chemical agents burn by oxidation, reduction, corrosion, protoplasmic poisoning, or the ischemic concomitants of vesicant activity (65).

Oxidizing agents usually cause damage because they become oxidized on contact with body tissue. Often the reaction and its by-products account for further toxicity with continued absorption. Commonly encountered oxidizing agents are chromic acid, sodium hypochlorite (Chlorox), and potassium permanganate.

Reducing agents act somewhat similarly and produce protein denaturation by binding free electrons in tissue proteins. Examples of reducing agents are alkyl mercuric agents, hydrochloric acid, and nitric acid.

Corrosive agents act in a variety of ways and are so termed because of the degree of denaturation exerted on tissue protein. Their net effect is eschar formation and a shallow, indolent ulcer. Corrosive agents include phenols and cresols, white phosphorus, dichromate salts, sodium metals, and the lyes.

Protoplasmic poisons produce their effect by forming salts with proteins or by binding or inhibiting calcium or other inorganic ions necessary for tissue viability and function. Examples of such agents include "alkaloidal" acids; acetic acid; formic acid; and metabolic competitors/inhibitors, including oxalic and hydrofluoric acids.

Vesicant agents produce ischemia with anoxic necrosis at the site of contact. Examples are cantharides (Spanish Fly), dimethyl sulfoxide (DMSO), mustard gas, and lewisite. There is also a subgroup of agents that are desiccants and produce their deleterious effects by causing dehydration damage by creating excessive heat in the tissue. Examples of this group are sulfuric acid and muriatic acid (3).

Chemical burns can also be classified as acid or alkali. However, this is not as accurate as classifying the agents by the mechanisms by which they coagulate proteins. Although the mechanism of action of individual acids or alkalis may differ, the wounds they produce share enough similarities to warrant consideration as two separate groups (64). A strong acid has a pH of less than 2. A better predictor than pH alone is the amount of alkali needed to raise the pH of an acid to neutrality (66). Alkalis capable of producing tissue damage usually have pH of 11.5 or more (64). On a volume-to-volume basis, alkaline material usually can cause more tissue damage than acids. This is because acids tend to cause coagulation necrosis with precipitation of protein, whereas alkalis tend to produce liquefaction necrosis, allowing more diffusion of the alkali deeper into the tissue (3,64).

Although there are many similarities in the evaluation of chemical and thermal burns, there are also certain peculiarities in the evaluation of chemical injuries. The agent involved must first be identified. This is crucial not only for treatment of the specific injury but also for associated problems such as systemic toxicity. The severity of a chemical injury is determined by five components: (a) strength; (b) quantity of the agent; (c) manner and duration of skin contact (progression); (d) penetration; and (e) mechanism of action (3,64).

Whatever the chemical agent, first aid consists of removing saturated clothing and irrigating with massive amounts of water. The volume of water dissipates the heat generated by dilution of the agent. In addition, copious irrigation or hydrotherapy will effectively cleanse the wound of unreacted surface chemicals, dilute the chemical already in contact with the tissue, and may restore tissue water lost to the hygroscopic effect of certain agents (3). Water constitutes immediate first aid and should continue at the scene for 20 to 30 minutes and thereafter from anywhere from 2 to 12 hours. Up to 48 hours of continuous irrigation may be necessary for burns involving the eye. No agent has been found superior to water (67).

In general, although a reference book will be useful to elucidate the potential toxicity, agents should not be neutralized because the neutralization process produces heat and furthers tissue necrosis. The one exception to this is hydrofluoric acid (3). The course and results of a chemical injury are determined by the size and depth of the injury. However, the importance of early and copious irrigation cannot be overemphasized (68).

Cold Injury

Human skin may be injured by cold, either by direct cellular injury or by indirect cellular effects. The indirect effects are from microvascular changes that lead to thrombosis and ischemia (3). Some of the recognized and documented changes from direct cellular injury include (a) development of extracellular ice formation, (b) development of intracellular ice formation, (c) cell dehydration with cell shrinkage, (d) abnormal concentration of electrolytes within the cell, (e) thermal shock, and (f) denaturation of lipid-protein complexes (69).

The rate of freezing is crucial to the location of ice crystal formation. Slow cooling causes extracellular ice crystal formation, although rapid freezing causes the more lethal intracellular ice crystal formation. It is unlikely that the clinical cold injury forms intracellular ice crystals; however, extracellular crystals are not totally innocuous. They cause withdrawal of water across the cell membrane that contributes to cell dehydration and ultimate death. In addition, the entire volume of water within a cell is not freezable, and as much as 8% to 10% of the water content is held in the protein complex within the cell (69). This "bound water" always remains in a liquid state. Although the mechanical theory of ice crystals actually disrupting the cell is attractive, minimal laboratory support exists for the concept (3).

A variant of cold injury is the phenomenon of thermal shock, which is a profound and sudden temperature change that is theorized to be incompatible with life (69). The severity of this phenomenon in clinical situations is poorly understood, and whether it affects the cold injury per se is open to debate. Another poorly understood concept is the manner in which sub-zero temperatures will produce denaturation of lipid-protein complexes. Part of the lipid membrane breakup may be caused by the solvent action of the toxic electrolyte concentration within the cell that has resulted from the cellular dehydration (3).

Indirect cellular damage appears to result from progressive microvascular insult and is usually more severe than the direct cellular effects. This is emphasized by the fact that skin subjected to a standard freezing and thawing injury that consistently produced necrosis can survive as a full-thickness skin graft when transplanted to an uninjured recipient site (70). Conversely, uninjured full-thickness skin did not survive when transferred to a recipient bed pretreated with the same freezing injury. Thus the direct skin injury appears reversible, and the progressive nature of the injury is most likely caused by microvascular changes (3).

The primary site of injury appears to be to the vascular endothelium. By 72 hours post-injury and thawing, there is a loss of vascular endothelium in the capillary walls and substantial fibrin deposition. The endothelium may be totally destroyed and the fibrin may saturate the arteriole walls (69). Interestingly, however, the injury appears greatest in the venules where the circulation is slower. Spasm of the arterioles and venules is not enough to explain decreased flow (71). Inasmuch as the changes in cold injury had been shown to be similar to changes seen in other inflammatory states, it was postulated that the progressive dermal ischemia seen in frostbite might be due to the same inflammatory mediators responsible for progressive dermal ischemia in the burn wound. Blister fluids were evaluated from cases of hand frostbite, and levels of PGE_2, PGF_{2a}, and thromboxane B_2 were sampled. The vasoconstricting, platelet-aggregating, and leukocyte-sticking prostanoids (PGF_{2a} and thromboxane B_2) were elevated significantly (72,73). It was postulated that the edema formation seen in frostbite was either due to leakage of proteins caused by release of these factors or secondarily due to white blood cells sticking in the capillaries and increased hydrostatic pressure. The frostbite rabbit ear model was used to test the hypothesis (74). Increased tissue survival was shown when the arachidonic acid cascade was blocked at all

levels. The most marked tissue salvage resulted when specific thromboxane-blocking agents were used (3).

Frostbite occurs rapidly after exposure to freezing temperatures. Clinically, this temperature is 20°F (-6.5°C) or less for 1 or more hour (75). The skin becomes blanched, and a stinging sensation is noted. The part eventually becomes numb with a sensation of clumsiness. The most common system of classifying frostbite injuries is based on the acute physical findings after cold exposure and rewarming. The injuries are classified according to "degree of injury." First-degree injury is characterized by a white or yellowish, firm plaque in the area of injury, sometimes surrounded by erythema and edema (76). Tissue necrosis or loss does not usually occur. However, a causalgia-like pain frequently develops, indicating that some element of nerve damage has been produced. Second-degree injury consists of superficial blisters, containing clear or milky fluid. Erythema and edema frequently surround the blisters. These injuries usually heal spontaneously unless the initial level of injury was deep enough to progress to tissue loss. Injury to the blister may cause desiccation of the underlying tissue and necrosis. Third-degree injury consists of deeper blisters, containing red or purple fluid or areas of darkly discolored skin without blisters. Prognosis for these injuries has been poor, with tissue necrosis common. Partial-thickness injury is associated more commonly with areas of blister formation, although deeply discolored areas usually represent full-thickness injury. Fourth-degree injury in this classification consists of deep cyanosis of the injured part without vesicle formation or local edema. In these injuries, gangrene is often evident within hours of injury (3).

Treatment of frostbite is aimed at blocking direct cellular damage, preventing microvascular thrombosis and tissue loss, or correcting the residual defect. It is important to avoid refreezing after the part has been thawed. Direct cellular damage is minimized by thawing rapidly with immersion in water warmed to between 104° and 108°F (40° and 42°C) (76). The narrow temperature range should be observed closely, because rewarming at lower temperatures is less beneficial for tissue survival, although higher temperatures may produce a burn injury and compound the injury (77,78). McCauley et al. (79) have designed a successful protocol based on the pathophysiology of progressive dermal ischemia (3).

Bites and Stings

Spider Bites

There are 30,000 known species of spiders worldwide and all but two contain venom glands. Most spiders are venomous, and there have been 50 species of spiders that have caused bites requiring medical attention. However, only two species in the United States are a public health problem. These are the brown recluse and the black widow spiders. The biggest problem with the management of spider bites is that it is unusual for patients to recognize what type of spider bit them. Therefore, it is difficult to develop a treatment plan because there is a multitude of products present in venoms.

Loxoscelism. Loxoscelism is a reaction to envenomation of the species of the brown spiders in the genus *Loxosceles*. The spider is found throughout the Midwestern and southern United States. These spiders live in old homes and abandoned barns and houses, are responsible for skin necrosis, and produce difficult wound-healing problems. Systemic symptoms include hemolysis, hemoglobinuria, disseminated intravascular coagulation, renal failure, and death. These spiders are medium size, with a body length between 8 and 15 mm and a leg length between 18 and 30 mm. Typically, they have a small, brown cephalo thorax, and the abdominal color can vary from fawn to dark brown depending on the habitat. The *Loxosceles* species contains a violin-shaped figure on the anterior surface of the cephalo thorax. This feature gives the brown recluse spider the name of "fiddle back" (80). Magnification is required to identify the fiddle, and therefore patients cannot use this feature as an identifying marker on casual observation.

Clinical loxoscelism can present with a broad spectrum of cutaneous reactions and various systemic symptoms. Sometimes this bite is no more than a transient skin irritation and follows a benign course, and sometimes severe local cutaneous skin necrosis results, requiring débridement and skin grafts.

In a typical case, a red cutaneous lesion develops with a central area of necrosis 24 hours after envenomization. The pain is intense, localized, and associated with itching or blistering. The wound can be edematous, mottled, and violaceous, with irregular borders surrounded by a large area of erythema. It usually has a dependant, gravitational spread when it is on the lower extremities.

Histologic biopsies of these skin lesions demonstrate an intense neutrophil vasculitis that is the hallmark of the lesion. Vasculitis persists until the wound is healed. Current treatment includes the neutrophil inhibitor, Dapsone; antibiotics; ice; and elevation (81). No therapy is necessary unless skin necrosis occurs. Immediate surgical excision of these skin lesions, although touted in the past to be effective, is dangerous and can lead to chronic, nonhealing wounds.

Black Widow. The black widow spider of the genus *Latrodectus* is the most notorious spider in North America. The most common species in the United States is *L. mactans*. Typically, the female, or black widow, has a shiny black sepia with an underlying red marking that looks like an hourglass in the mature spider.

These spiders are found in undisturbed areas; under stones, logs and pieces of bark; and around vegetation, barns, privies, outbuildings, stone walls, and trash heaps. The location where the bite occurred must be documented so that a positive identification of the spider can be made.

The bite of the black widow occurs when the web is disturbed, and it is painless without a cutaneous lesion. After a period of time (1 to 6 hours), the patient develops intense pain accompanied with anxiety. Paresthesias, described as a burning sensation, may affect the whole body. The patient's pain is often most intense on the soles of the feet. Often, associated symptoms include a thready pulse, diaphoresis, slurred speech, headache, dizziness, dysphagia, nausea, vomiting, edema, ptosis, and fever. Severe and uncontrolled hypertension with seizures is a dreaded complication of black widow bites.

Treatment begins with local cleansing of the wound site, application of ice, and sedation of the patient. Muscle spasms, headache, vomiting, and paresthesias may be treated with a solution of 10% calcium gluconate. This may need to be repeated every 2 to 4 hours. Intravenous diazepam or narcotics are helpful for muscle spasm. Usually the symptoms are self-limited; but the neurotoxin is virulent, and therefore, envenomization must be treated aggressively.

Tick Bites

Tick bites are common in the spring and summer when people spend a significant amount of time outdoors. The most clinically important tick bites produce a local reaction with an erythematous papule that can develop into a nodular pruritic area. This may be exacerbated by removing the tick and leaving the hypostome and capitulum in the patient. Residual tick parts in the skin may be responsible for post bite nodules.

The major concern of tick bites in the United States is from *Ixodes dammini*, which may be infected by a spirochete responsible for Lyme disease. In this illness, there is chronic migratory arthritis associated with the formation of erythematous halo patches that can be multiple over the patient's body. Patients develop nausea, delirium, fever, and must be treated to prevent persistent arthritis. Before treating the patient with tetracycline, sera should be drawn to confirm the diagnosis. In addition to Lyme disease, Colorado tick fever and Rocky Mountain spotted fever can occur after tick bites. Colorado tick fever is an acute viral illness that produces fever, malaise, and headache and is caused by the tick *Dermacentor andersoni*, or the dog tick. It is common throughout the western United States, and the illness is self-limited. Rocky Mountain spotted fever is caused by a spirochete and can produce erythematous multiple spots over the body. It can be fatal if not treated with appropriate antibiotics. The surgeon may be called on to remove the tick parts, and therefore, it is important for him or her to recognize these illnesses.

Malignant Tumors of the Skin

Basal Cell and Squamous Cell Carcinomas

Basal cell carcinoma and squamous cell carcinoma are the most common skin malignancies and are derived from the basilar keratinocytes. These tumors are in contrast to adnexal carcinoma, which arises in the adnexal structures in the skin. Inasmuch as basal cell and squamous cell carcinomas are common, the surgeon must distinguish them from benign lesions of the skin. Skin biopsy is critical in securing a definitive diagnosis so that appropriate management can be instituted. Either punch biopsy or shave biopsy is acceptable.

Basal cell and squamous cell carcinomas occur at a rate of 600,000 new cases a year. They are most common in the head and neck, followed by the trunk, upper extremities, and lower extremities (82). They occur because of persistent exposure to ultraviolet light and are, therefore, more common in the Sunbelt regions of the United States. Skin cancer is a significant occupational hazard for postal workers, farmers, construction workers, and leisure-time sports enthusiasts. Skin cancer is more common in people with a fair complexion and is seen rarely in blacks, except in certain types of genetic syndromes. The skin melanin, formed from melanocytes, appears to be protective, because albino blacks have a higher incidence of skin cancer than nonalbino blacks.

The most common putative agent for basal cell carcinoma is solar ultraviolet light-type B (UV-B). This is a significant problem in the United States, where tanning beds and sun worshiping have increasingly become part of our culture. The time lag between the appearance of skin cancer and exposure to the sunburn is between 20 and 40 years. Most patients have received most of their sun exposure by the end of adolescence. Efforts to control sun exposure with hats and sun-screens are only marginally effective after adolescence because the majority of patients have approximated their threshold of UV-B radiation by the age of 18 years.

Basal cell carcinoma may also arise in scars from burns, chronic osteomyelitis, nevus sebaceous skin lesions, and chronic sinuses. Basal cell carcinomas do not appear to be more biologically aggressive when they occur in chronic wounds. A third causative agent for basal cell carcinoma is ionizing radiation from the sun. Patients who received prior radiation for tinea capitis or chronic acne are at great risk because the radiation therapy dose was controlled poorly when treating these conditions. DNA damage to the basal keratinocyte is thought to be the putative mechanism.

Multiple basal cell carcinomas may occur in patients who have had arsenical exposure. This is a common chemical component, which was previously used in welding flux or foundries. A compound called Fowler's solution also contains arsenic and may be associated with this type of arsenical carcinoma. This type of skin cancer is associated with visceral malignancies, most commonly, lung cancer. Typically, these patients get multiple tumors that are plaque-like, red, and scaly.

There are three types of genodermatosis that are associated with basal cell carcinoma. The most common is xeroderma pigmentosum. In these patients, there is a defect in DNA replication from ionizing radiation, so that thymidine dimers are formed that cannot be repaired enzymatically. These patients do well until late childhood when they develop ichthyotic skin, and the appearance of basal cell carcinomas, squamous cell carcinomas, or melanomas. This genetic defect is usually fatal in the mid-20s because of metastatic melanoma.

A second genodermatosis is albinism, which is an autosomal recessive trait that prevents melanin formation. These patients are photosensitive and develop multiple focal basal carcinomas and multiple recurrent skin cancers.

Basal cell nevus syndrome is an autosomal dominant genodermatosis that is associated with jaw cysts, palmer pits, and multifocal basal cell carcinoma in situ. These patients develop recurring basal cell carcinomas, requiring multiple surgical procedures. Patients have also been treated with retinoid compounds with some improvement.

The most common phenotype expression of basal cell carcinoma is the nodular type that arises at the interface between the dermis and epidermis. These lesions are characterized by peripheral palisading, stromal retraction, and dermal fibrosis. Another type is the aggressive growth phase basal cell carcinomas. These are the sclerosing or fibrosing type, sometimes called morphea basal cell carcinoma. These tumors have collagenase enzymes that allow the tumor to spread along peripheral nerves or embryonic fusion planes. These tumors frequently have dermal skip areas that make simple circular excisions difficult because of the great potential for recurrence.

The aggressive biologic potential for basal cell carcinoma depends on the surgeon's ability to resect local disease, because regional metastases rarely occur. These tumors grow slowly and destroy tissue through expansion and infiltration of surrounding tissues. Frequently, tumors infiltrate deeply until they encounter a fascial plane and then shelf or skate along the lateral edge of the obstruction. This classically occurs at the interface between skin and muscle. The scalp is a good example of this process because tumors only rarely invade the bone, but they do extend along the galea. These tumors have aggressive growth patterns and spread along vessels or nerves to infiltrate the skull base, orbit, or nose.

Clinically, basal cell carcinomas are asymptomatic, unless they itch, bleed, or produce an open sore. Patients with a history of basal cell carcinoma must be followed regularly because 20% to 40% of those patients develop a second primary carcinoma within 2 years.

The clinical appearance of basal cell carcinoma is typified by the nodular variety that presents with a rodent ulcer and a keratin plug in the center of the lesion. Inasmuch as the nodular basal cell carcinoma contains large amounts of mucin, they appear as pearly white in clinical appearance. A second type of basal cell carcinoma is a superficial spreading variety that forms in large, scaly plaques in the skin. These lesions are frequently confused with psoriasis and may be treated for long periods with steroids to reduce the inflammation before they are biopsied. One of the most difficult basal cell carcinomas to treat is called the morphea type. These tumors have a waxy, yellow, plaque-like appearance and are deeply invasive with aggressive growth patterns. The clinical extent of the tumors are difficult to determine from gross examination.

Pigmented basal cell carcinomas are nodular tumors that are often confused with melanomas because of their dark color. Pigmented basal cell carcinomas are more symmetrical than melanomas and have uniform color distribution and a prolonged history of this tumor.

Another unusual type of basal cell carcinoma is the fibroepithelioma, a pink papule that occurs in nonsun-exposed areas. These lesions can be waxy and plaque-like, and surgical excision is adequate treatment.

The risk factors for basal cell carcinoma recurrence include radiation failure, and tumor location, e.g., the medial canthus, alar base, the preauricular and postauricular areas, and scalp. A large tumor size has a greater potential for morbidity, particularly if an aggressive growth pattern exists. Moh's surgical treatment for primary or recurrent tumors improves the prognosis because it lowers the local recurrence rate.

Squamous cell is the second most common skin cancer and is important because it is more aggressive. It spreads by local extension and direct invasion and through the regional lymphatics. It can cause death. These tumors can be graded as either well, moderately, or poorly differentiated and phenotypically show an ulcerative, infiltrative, or exophytic appearance. Their biologic aggressiveness is directly related to the size of the tumor. Those tumors less than 2 cm in diameter have a recurrence rate of 5%, with a 7% incidence of metastases, although tumors that are more than 2 cm have double the incidence of local recurrence and three times the incidence of regional lymphatic spread. Squamous cell carcinomas are activated by sun exposure and are related to genetic sensitivity to the sun. Other factors that increase the incidence of squamous cell carcinoma are chemical carcinogens, previous radiation therapy, and chronic inflammation.

Presumably, squamous cell carcinoma arises as a result of the two-hit hypothesis. Tumors are thought to be initiated and promoted by repeated exposure to the offending carcinogen. For example, in mice, benzoquinone is the initiator and will bind to keratinocyte DNA to produce strain breaks. Thereafter, repeated exposures to the promoting agents such as dihydroxybiphenomol will promote the formation of a squamous papilloma. This biologic mechanism may be the cause of squamous cell carcinoma arising in pressure sores, burn scars, chronic osteomyelitis, lupus, or scalp perifolliculitis. Squamous cell carcinoma can be promoted by administration of psoralens for the treatment of psoriasis. There

is an increased incidence in patients who are immunosuppressed, and in patients who are photosensitized, such as with those who have had photodynamic therapy. Squamous cell carcinoma can present as a premalignant lesion from leukoplakia of the lower lip, an erythroplakic patch, such as that associated with arsenic, or in actinic keratosis, or cutaneous horn. There are certain nonaggressive subtypes of squamous cell carcinoma, including verrucous carcinoma, which arises in a condyloma or a keratoacanthoma. These are both common after transplantation. Squamous cell carcinoma in situ, Bowen's disease, and an unusual variant called erythroplasia of Queyrat are indolent variants of squamous cell carcinoma. In addition to well-differentiated squamous cell variant, this carcinoma can present as a spindle cell tumor that resembles soft tissue sarcomas. This histologic variant may require a positive vitronectin antibody for the diagnosis. This tumor is thought to be more biologically aggressive than squamous cell carcinoma, and is uncommon.

In the treatment of squamous cell carcinoma, spread to the regional node becomes important in the development of a treatment algorithm. Patients who present with squamous cell carcinoma of the nose, ear, or temple area should have their parotid examined for a regional lymphatic spread. When the tumor extends into the neck, modified radical neck dissection should be performed. Squamous cell carcinomas may arise in the lower extremities and are usually associated with chronic wounds. Because these tumors are biologically more aggressive than other squamous cell carcinomas, regional lymphadenectomy should be strongly considered. If there is regional lymphatic spread of squamous cell carcinoma, adjunctive radiotherapy should be considered. Local recurrence rates are high in patients with positive clinical nodes, and treatment failures occur without the addition of radiotherapy.

Melanoma

Melanoma, first described in 1787, is the fastest-growing skin malignancy and accounts for 3% of all newly diagnosed skin cancers. Although basal cell and squamous carcinomas represent the vast majority of the malignancies diagnosed annually, cutaneous melanoma accounts for approximately 65% of all skin cancer deaths. Because the skin is readily available for examination, the diagnosis is made easily with biopsy and should be distinguished from junctional nevi, pigmented basal cell carcinomas, and hyperpigmented compound nevi. However, more than 50% of melanomas are not clinically suspected before biopsy.

Certain risk factors make the patient more susceptible for the formation of a melanoma. Melanoma may arise in a giant hairy nevus, which is a congenital nevus that is present at birth and darkens after puberty (83). About 60% arising in a congenital nevus occur in childhood, with the remainder occurring in adult life. Obviously, excision of the congenital nevus is preferred to avoid the formation of a melanoma.

Patients who have one primary melanoma have a 20-fold increased chance of developing a second primary melanoma during their lifetimes compared with the general population. A second subset of patients with an increased chance of developing a second primary melanoma consists of those with dysplastic nevus syndrome. Although a sporadic form exists, there is a familial form with a family history of melanoma, formally called BK nevus syndrome. It is now termed dysplastic nevus syndrome and is inherited as an autosomal dominant. These patients must be followed closely after their first melanoma, as there is a significantly increased chance of having a second primary melanoma in their lifetimes. Multiple dysplastic nevi can be the first presenting sign of AIDS.

In the exceedingly rare congenital syndrome, xeroderma pigmentosa, patients develop multiple skin cancers and frequently die from the melanoma. Melanoma is difficult to recognize in these patients because of the ichthyotic (fish-like) skin. Patients who have melanotic skin lesions and show atypical junctional melanocytic hyperplasia (AJMH) on biopsy must have the lesion completely excised, as this is a prodrome to the development of an invasive melanoma.

With regard to genetic predisposition to melanoma, approximately 10% of melanoma arise in a familial setting (84). However, identification of a melanoma gene is difficult because melanomas in these susceptible patients do not follow a simple Mendelian mode of inheritance (85). Intense research efforts have indicated that chromosome 1 and 9 may be the responsible loci for the melanoma genes (86,87).

Melanomas can be divided into different types based on their growth patterns. The most common is superficial spreading melanoma, which has variations in color and is flat in appearance. Superficial spreading melanoma may arise in a preexisting nevus and may develop nodular components within the lesion.

The second variety of melanoma is lentigo malignant melanoma, which may occur on the face or hands and has the appearance of a brownish, reddish patch that can degenerate into invasive melanoma. The incidence of superficial spreading melanoma is 15% among all patients with melanoma.

Nodular melanomas occur in 15% of patients with melanoma. They are blue-black in appearance and occur in the absence of a preexisting mole. These tumors typically ulcerate and frequently have a worse prognosis because of their depth of invasion.

An unusual variant of melanoma is the acrolentiginous lesion that occurs on the palms of the hands, soles of the feet, and in the subungual regions of the nail bed (88). These lesions are diagnosed late in the course of the disease, and may occur in blacks or Hispanics for whom other phenotypic types of melanoma are rare. These tumors rapidly invade deeply and frequently present with regional lymphatic metastases. Because melanoma micro staging is unimportant in these lesions, there is no need to obtain a deep biopsy.

Micro Staging of Melanoma

A biopsy of melanoma is important because it secures the diagnosis of the disease and connotes prognosis, but it is subject to sampling error if not performed correctly. The preferred biopsy technique used in melanoma is to excise the lesion completely. If a shave biopsy is performed, the level of invasion cannot be assessed accurately from the specimen. Moreover, in larger lesions in which there are areas of atypical junctional melanocytic hyperplasia, invasive melanoma cannot be identified because of sampling error. In circumstances in which lesions are large, multiple punch biopsies can be used to sample the lesion.

The micro staging system used to determine diagnosis and prognosis in melanoma has been outlined by Breslow. Previous staging systems using levels of invasion are obsolete because of the great disparity between levels of invasion and the depth of the invasion of the tumor. Using the Breslow classification, micro staging the tumor can be achieved using an ocular micrometer on the microscope and measurements from the top of the granule layer to the tumor depth.

Using depth of invasion as the primary criterion, the overall survival of the patient can be implied. Deep tumors (thick melanoma) have a poor prognosis, and superficial tumors (thin melanoma) have an excellent prognosis. Surgical therapy is based on the level of invasion and the presence or absence of clinically positive lymph nodes. Other factors that the pathologist considers when reviewing the melanoma biopsy is the host lymphatic response. Although lymphatic response matched for depth of invasion shows poor correlation, people with active lymphocytic response have thinner lesions. Recent data suggest that the prognosis of the melanoma can be correlated with the descriptive pattern of invasion. If the melanoma has a radial growth phase, it is considered to have a favorable prognosis, whereas if it has a vertical growth phase, then the prognosis becomes much worse. Ulceration of the tumor connotes a poor prognosis and correlates with depth of invasion.

Clinical Staging

Once the diagnosis of melanoma has been secured by biopsy, it can be staged to determine the prognosis. A clinical staging system that uses stages I, II, and III has been outlined by the American College of Surgeons and is divided based on the presence of regional or systemic metastasis. In Stage I, the tumor is limited to the biopsy site, whereas in Stage II, it is limited to regional nodes, or in transient lymphatic metastasis. In Stage III, there is generalized disease. Unfortunately, one of the short-falls of the staging system is that the vast majority of the patients (85%) falls within the Stage I category, and this limits the selectivity of the staging system. The importance of the staging of the tumor is in the treatment of Stage III disease for which multimodality chemotherapy or experimental protocols are available. To date, chemotherapy protocols and radiotherapy have had limited success in this disease.

Surgical Treatment of Melanoma

The treatment of melanoma depends on the stage of the disease, micro staging of the tumor, histologic description, and the location of the lesion (89). For example, in lesions for which the diagnosis is atypical junctional melanocytic hyperplasia, 0.5-cm margins surrounding the tumor in the surgical specimen are sufficient. A fluorescent light may be used to highlight the white areas and to avoid incomplete excision. In AJMH, the tumors can have occult dysplastic nevus cells that extend beyond the margin of the pigmented areas and will recur if not completely excised. Locally invasive melanomas that are biopsied but incompletely treated have a 60% incidence of local recurrence with a increased risk of regional lymphatic spread. Even after appropriate surgical excision for deep melanomas, the incidence of recurrence is 7%. Therefore, appropriate surgical treatment of the local lesions underpins the success of melanoma treatment.

The primary therapy for invasive melanoma is wide local excision, but the definition of *wide* remains controversial. Excision of more than 3 cm of tissue surrounding the melanoma is probably unnecessary. Although local recurrence connotes a unfavorable prognosis, excision of more than 3 cm of tissue will not eliminate satellitosis caused by "intransigent" dermal metastases. Evidence now suggests that melanomas that are thin (< 1 mm) in depth of invasion and that have a radial growth pattern do not recur after limited resection (< 1 cm). Moreover, World Health Organization studies suggest that the disease-free interval and survival are unaffected by excisions that exceed 1 cm. Therefore, extensive resections should be reserved for tumors that have high-risk factors for local recurrence, such as ulcerated lesions, acrolentigineous lesions, deeply invasive lesions, and stage II disease. In patients for whom the resection of the melanoma with wide margins would cause mutilation, consideration of aesthetic value must be considered because massive surgical excisions do not improve the prognosis in the disease.

Regional Lymphadenectomy

Enormous controversy exists regarding the management of the regional lymph nodes in melanoma. Inasmuch as the majority of the patients are in the Stage I category, disease stage is not helpful in distinguishing the need for lymph node dissection. Many surgeons advocate regional lymphadenectomy to remove micro-metastasis in the absence of clinical disease because it may improve the overall prognosis. There are two types of lymph node dissections for melanoma. In the first, a therapeutic lymph node dissection is performed in the patient who has clinically positive lymph nodes. This therapy is required to remove known disease.

In the second, a prophylactic lymph node dissection has been proposed when prognostic features of the tumor suggest that lymph node dissection would eliminate micrometastatic disease. In studies by Balch et al. (90), tumors that have deep invasion (1.5–4.0 mm) are likely to have micrometastatic disease, and elective lymph node dissection may be of therapeutic value. This study suggested that there was an increased survival in the subgroup of patients with deep extremity melanomas and melanomas of the head and neck when regional lymphatic node dissection was performed. More recent perspective data from the World Health Organization and Mayo Clinic studies showed no difference in survival between high-risk patients undergoing elective lymph node dissection and patients undergoing therapeutic lymph node dissection. The decision to do an elective lymph node dissection requires patient participation and frequently comes after advice from the hospital tumor board or reflects the institution's consensus of opinion.

Specific Sites of Regional Lymphatic Spread—Head and Neck

The complex anatomy of the head and neck and their rich lymphatic drainage makes appropriate management of melanoma in this area difficult. The data from Balch's study suggest that regional lymphadenectomy should be performed in patients with melanomas that have between 1.5 and 4 mm of invasion. Most surgeons prefer "functional" node dissection, preserving the jugular vein, sternocleidomastoid muscle, and the spinal accessory nerve. If the tumor lies above the plane of the parotid gland and involves the temple, the ear, or eyelid, superficial parotidectomy is required in addition to removing the regional lymphatics. Some surgeons would favor superficial parotidectomy and biopsy of a Stage II node as an alternative to a modified neck dissection. Tumors that arise in the scalp may require posterior lymph node dissection in addition to parotidectomy.

Preoperative Workup

The preoperative workup for patients with melanoma should include chest radiograph and liver function studies. The use of CT and MRI scans should be avoided unless specific evidence of metastatic disease exists. After surgical resection, patients with AJC stage I can be followed every 6 months for 5 years with yearly chest radiographs and liver function studies. Patients with AJC stage II or III should be followed clinically every 3 months with yearly chest radiographs and liver function studies. All patients require routine history and physical examinations, and specific questions should be asked regarding the central nervous system and gastrointestinal tract symptoms, because metastatic disease is common in these areas.

Adjunctive Therapy

Adjunctive therapy for melanoma has not been effective. Treatment of patients with 5-(3,3-dimethyl-1-triazenyl)-1*H*-imidazole-4-carboxamide (DTIC) or other nitrosoal have had disappointing success, with response rates between 10% and 20%. Rarely does a patient have complete response rate to chemotherapy. Experimental protocols with IFN-a and adoptive immunotherapy show promise in treatment trials but are not approved for clinical use.

The treatment of melanoma with radiotherapy should be limited to patients who have isolated cutaneous disease and soft tissue recurrences for which surgical resection is not feasible. It has no place in the primary treatment of melanoma. The surgical resection of isolated metastasis to the brain or soft tissue areas may be valuable for palliation but does little to affect prognosis. Overall, adjuvant therapy has been unsuccessful in improving survival in patients with this disease.

Pressure Sores

In 1873, Paget wrote that "bed sores may be defined as the sloughing and the mortification or death of a part produced by pressure." This insightful comment forms the basis for treatment of all pressure sores. They commonly occur in patients with disrupted sensory input from the area. Therapeutic interventions for the treatment of pressure sores were initiated during World War II when increasing reports of excision and closure were reported in young veterans. Treatment of this disorder with pedicle flaps and improved nutrition have complemented the advent of modern bacterial therapy to improve the prognosis.

Pressure sores are often erroneously referred to as decubitus ulcers. Although a majority of pressure sores may occur in the lying down or, in Latin, "decumbere" position, pressure sores can occur from the top of the head to the bottom of the foot corresponding to the bony prominences (91). In patients with paraplegia, the most common location of pressure sores is the ischium, followed by the sacrum and the femoral trochanter. Ulceration over the heel and malleolus are less likely (92). Approximately two-thirds of pressure sores are treated in acute care hospitals. Approximately 60% of these pressure sores are hospital acquired, and 70% of these occur during the first 2 weeks of hospitalization.

The reasons for pressure sores to occur are pressure, shearing forces, friction, and moisture. Of all these rea-

sons, the single most important factor is pressure on the skin, subcutaneous fat, and muscle. In healthy tissue, the normal capillary arteriolar limb pressure is 32 mm Hg and the normal venous limb pressure is 12 mm Hg (93). In an experimental model, constant pressure of 70 mm Hg was applied. Blood flow to the tissue ceased and irreversible tissue damage occurred in 2 hours (94). As the pressure was increased, less time was needed to cause tissue necrosis. Other than pressure, shearing forces were implicated in causing pressure sores. In patients with the head raised, the deeper tissues such as muscle and bone tend to slide down while the skin and subcutaneous tissues remain adherent to the bed. These two opposing forces can disrupt the blood vessels between the two planes, causing ischemia of the overlying skin. The shearing forces coupled with the constant friction of the skin on the sheets may cause skin breakdown. In patients who are incontinent, the moisture and the increased bacterial colonization over the ulcerated skin exacerbate the ulceration. People who are most susceptible to these insults are patients whose underlying diseases affect their sensory perception or their level of consciousness. Spinal cord injury, cerebral vascular accident, and central nervous system diseases are often associated with a high incidence of developing pressure sores.

Pressure sores can be classified into 4 stages (95). Stage I is injury limited to the epidermis with superficial induration and erythema. Stage II is ulceration extending through the dermis but not to the underlying fat. Stage I and II are reversible injuries with good chance for spontaneous healing. Stage III is ulceration extending into the subcutaneous fat and the muscle. Stage IV is ulceration penetrating into underlying bone or into the joint. The appearance of the ulcer may be deceptive and often a small ulceration may mask a large undermined crater below. These conical configurations of the ulcers often exemplify stage III and stage IV pressure sores.

In the treatment of pressure sores, a multidisciplinary approach is mandatory. Since development of pressure sores occurs through a complex interplay between the patient's underlying disease and various mechanical insults, inputs from the surgical, medical, psychiatric, and rehabilitation teams are essential in the management. The best treatment for pressure sore is prevention. All efforts must be made to identify the high risk patients so that appropriate preventive measures can be undertaken. Standardized measures involve placing the patient on a well padded bed and rotating the patient side to side every hour to avoid prolonged pressure in one position. Shearing forces can be minimized by not tilting the head of the bed. Friction can be avoided by lifting the patient instead of dragging the sheets under the patient. Finally, the patient must be maintained in a clean and dry environment. These preventive measures are much more cost effective than the treatment of an established pressure sore which can extend hospital stay by 25 weeks at a cost of over $40,000 (96).

Sheep skin overlying the sheets has been an effective method to reduce sheer force against patient's skin. These are dry, absorb moisture, and are capable of dispersing pressure over a large body surface area. Unfortunately, clinical effectiveness has not been achieved in controlled clinical studies. Alternating pressure devices, with a mattress and air cells, have been designed to inflate and deflate, thereby reducing the pressure on pressure points, have been used extensively, but they are noisy, expensive, and bulky.

Preoperative Management

Many pressure sores may heal without a surgical procedure, because of meticulous wound care, intense nursing efforts, and improved nutrition of the patient. Nonsurgical conservative therapy may be the preferred treatment if the patient's outcome is poor. In initial management of pressure sore patients, wound infections, and sepsis require appropriate attention. Bacteremia has been documented in approximately 50% of patients with pressure sores. About 50% of these cultures are anaerobes. A localized infected bursa requires drainage and necrotic tissue débridement. The most common site of sepsis in pressure sore patients is the urinary tract.

The preoperative management of patients should include correcting the preoperative anemia nutrition deficiency, identification of osteomyelitis, and assessment of joint infections.

Surgery of the Pressure Sore

Before proceeding with an operation, preoperative preparations are necessary. Nutritional status should be optimum along with a hemoglobin of 12 mg/100 mL. The wound should be clean. The bony skeleton in the area should be evaluated for signs of infection. Urinary drainage should be provided by an indwelling catheter. A mechanical bowel cleansing should be accomplished. Oral diazepam or dantrolene sodium is useful in controlling muscle spasms.

Anesthesia may be unnecessary in the smaller ulcers but is preferred for débridement and closure of larger pressure sores. In patients with loss of muscle mass, care must be taken to avoid a second pressure sore.

Total excision of the ulcerated bursa and underlying bony prominence may be required. Staining with methylene blue will outline the full extent of the bursa. Hemostasis should be complete, especially in patients with paralysis. Closure should be obtained with large skin/muscle flaps and the wounds drained with suction catheters.

Occipital ulcerations occur in unconscious or paralyzed patients. These may involve the periosteum, and therefore, a scalp flap is preferable. Scapular and dorsal spine ulcerations may occur in patients with excessive weight loss. These are best handled by excision of the ulcer, bony prominence, and primary closure. Elbow defects can be closed with a local flap from the lateral forearm or with an abdominal flap. However, the abdominal flaps are not recommended in the bedridden patient. Posteriorly based chest flaps can be used to cover the olecranon when the arm is extended. Antero-superior iliac spine ulcers are unusual and can be treated easily with excision of the ulcer, bony prominence, and primary closure.

When the knees are unprotected, they may ulcerate, particularly if the patient is kept in the prone position or has adductor spasms. Usually, these may be covered with split-thickness skin grafts. Local skin flaps are not helpful. If the joint is exposed, closure with muscle flaps or skin grafts are performed.

Sacral ulcers should be excised with removal of the bursa-like lining. Bony prominent spines as well as the posterior iliac spine and sacral ligaments should be removed. The first option and preferred method is a skin rotation flap. Based inferiorly, this flap maintains a good blood supply from the perforating gluteal vessels. It avoids suture lines over the weight-bearing surface of the ischium. The second option is an island gluteus maximus muscle skin flap. Care must be exercised to preserve the gluteal vessels that enter the medial portion of the muscle. Another approach is a rotation gluteus musculocutaneous flap that also has application in closure of ischial defects. A transverse back flap is a safe method. Dissection is at the fascial level and the secondary defect is covered with a STSG.

Ischial ulcers may have an area of involvement that resembles an inverted cone. There may be a small skin ulcer but a much larger area of involvement in the underlying tissues. The ulcer should be excised circumferentially down to the ischium, and then either partial or total ischiectomy should be performed. Complications of total ischiectomy include hematoma, dehiscence, abscess, and perineal ulceration as a late complication. For partial ischiectomy, a curved osteotome can be used to remove 2 cm of bone below the ulcer, care should be taken to avoid fracture of the pelvis or urethral transection. The deep cavity that results can be filled with a V—Y of biceps femoris, semimembranosus, or semitendinosus musculocutaneous unit. The ischiectomy cavity can also be filled with a gluteal musculocutaneous flap.

Greater trochanter ulcers are relatively easy to excise. The greater trochanter can be débrided with an osteotome. Closure can be obtained with an anteriorly based thigh flap or a superiorly based musculocutaneous tensor fascia lata flap.

Ulcerations of the foot and ankle occur in several locations, which include the medial malleolus, lateral malleolus, Achilles tendon, and lateral aspect of the foot. Trophic ulcerations of the heel are seen in ambulatory patients but rarely in paraplegics. The abductor hallucis brevis muscle can be used to cover the medial malleolus and occasionally the Achilles tendon. The abductor digiti quinti muscle can be used occasionally to cover small lateral malleolus ulcers. Partial excision of the Achilles tendon with immediate STSG is favored by some authors. If the Achilles tendon is left uncovered, it will desiccate. Ulcerations on the weight-bearing surface of the heel can be covered by a turnover flap of flexor digitorum brevis or a medial plantar flap. These flaps should cover the entire calcaneus and occasionally the distal portion of the Achilles tendon. Skin grafts are the first choice in ulcers of the foot and ankle, however, they often fail. Flaps are a second choice. Local flaps have not been reliable in this area and should not used in paralyzed patients.

Extensive Pressure Ulcers

The surgical techniques used in the treatment of decubitus ulcers have improved in the past two decades. However, there are some patients with severe ulcers that are not amenable to conventional procedures. Large trochanteric ulcers with pyarthrosis of the hip, osteomyelitis of the pelvis, and flexion contractures have been treated by amputation, hip disarticulation, or resection of the proximal femur. For extensive pressure sores of the sacrum and ischium, high thigh amputations and fillet leg flaps are effective. This technique is superior to bilateral hip disarticulation and provides four points of pressure instead of two, as in hip disarticulation.

A total thigh flap and hip disarticulation can be used for treatment of trochanteric ulcers. These patients often have osteomyelitis of the femur and pyarthrosis of the hip. The disadvantage of this procedure is that acetabulum provides a ready made dead space. Moreover, postoperative stability is possible if the proximal one-third of the femur can be saved.

Postoperative Treatment

Routine postoperative care includes wound suction, urinary drainage and avoidance of fecal soiling. Proper positioning of the patient in the prone position is important. If healing of the flap is complete, then the patient is allowed out of bed by the 3rd week. Air fluidized beds reduce the chances of a second pressure sore.

Complications

Because hematoma is the most frequent complication, prevention of surgical dead spaces is important. Wound separation usually reflects poor planning or persistent spasms. Flap necrosis is disastrous because it causes recurrence of the ulcer. Other complications include infections, pneumonia, thrombophlebitis, and pulmonary embolism.

REFERENCES

1. Holbrook KA. Structure and function of developing human skin. In: Goldsmith LA, ed. Biochemistry and physiology of skin. New York: Oxford University Press, 1983:64–101.
2. Robson MC, Krizek TJ, Wray RC. Care of the thermally injured patient. In: Zuidema GD, Rutherford RB, Ballinger A, eds. Management of trauma. Philadelphia: WB Saunders, 1979:666–736.
3. Robson MC, Smith DJ, Jr. Management of thermal injuries. In: Jurkiewicz MJ, Krizek TJ, eds. Plastic surgery: principles and practice, Vol. 2. St. Louis: CV Mosby, 1990:1355–1420.
4. Briggaman RA. The epidermal-dermal junction and genetic disorders of this area. In: Goldsmith LA, ed. Biochemistry and physiology of skin. New York: Oxford Universtiy Press, 1983:1001–1024.
5. Silbert JE. Proteoglycans and glycosaminoglycans. In: Goldsmith LA, ed. Biochemistry and physiology of skin. New York: Oxford University Press, 1983:448–461.
6. Odland GF. Structure of skin. In: Goldsmith LA, ed. Biochemistry and physiology of skin. New York: Oxford University Press, 1983:3–63.
7. Robson MC, Raine TJ, Smith DJ, Jr. Wounds and wound healing. In: Lawrence P, ed. Essentials of general surgery. Baltimore: Williams & Wilkins, 1988:111.
8. Robson MC, Raine TJ, Smith DJ, Jr. Wounds and wound healing. In: Lawrence P, ed. Essentials of general surgery. Baltimore: Williams & Wilkins, 1988:112.
9. Robson MC, Raine TJ, Smith DJ, Jr. Wounds and wound healing. In: Lawrence P, ed. Essentials of general surgery. Baltimore: Williams & Wilkins, 1988:107–114.
10. Stevenson, T.R., Mathes, S.J. Wound healing. In: Miller, T.A., ed. Physiologic basis of modern surgical care. St. Louis: VC Mosby, 1988:1011.
11. Moritz AR, Henrique FC, Jr. Studies of thermal injury: the relative importance of time and surface temperature in the causation of cutaneous burns. Am J Pathol 1947;23:695.
12. Jackson DM. The diagnosis of the depth of burning. Br J Surg 1953;40:388.
13. Larrey DJ. Memoirs of military surgery. Vol. 2. Baltimore: Joseph Cushing, 1814:156–164.
14. Arturson G. Arachidonic acid metabolism and prostaglandin activity following burn injury. In Ninnemann JL, ed. Traumatic injury: infection and other immunologic sequelae. Baltimore: University Park Press, 1983:57.
15. Raine TJ, Heggers JP, Robson MC, et al. Cooling the burn wound to maintain microcirculation. J Trauma 1981;21:394.
16. Robson MC, Smith DJ, Heggers JP. Innovations in burn wound management. Adv Plast Reconstr Surg 1987;4:149.
17. Boykin JV, Eriksson E, Shelley MM, et al. Histamine mediated delayed permeability response after scald burn inhibited by cimetidine or cold water treatment. Science 1980;209:815.
18. Blank IH. What are the functions of skin lost in burn injury that affect short- and long-term recovery? J Trauma 1984;24(suppl):S10.
19. Ward PA. How does the local inflammatory response affect the wound healing process? J Trauma 1984:24(suppl):S18.
20. Ward PA, Till GO. Pathophysiologic events related to thermal injury of skin. J Trauma 1990;30(12):75–79.
21. Solomkin JS. Neutrophil disorders in burn injury: complement, cytokines, and organ injury. J Trauma 1990;30(12):80–85.
22. Demling RH. Fluid resuscitation. In Boswick JA, ed. The art and science of burn care. Rockville, MD: Aspen, 1987:196.
23. Chung KC, Smith DJ, Jr. Management of thermal, electrical, radiation, and chemical injuries of the hand. In Peimer CA, ed. Surgery of the hand and upper extremity. New York: McGraw-Hill, 1996.
24. Schwartz SI, et al. Principles in surgery, 4th ed. New York: McGraw-Hill, 1984.
25. Schroeder SA, et al. Current medical diagnoses & treatment. Appleton & Lange, California, 1990.
26. Wright HK, Gann DS, Drucker WR. Current concept of therapy for derangements of extracellular fluid. In: Davis JH, ed. Current concepts in surgery. New York: McGraw-Hill, 1965:295–320.
27. Robson MC. Treatment of burns victim. In: Cushieri A, Giles GR, Moossa AR, eds. Essential surgical practice. 2nd ed. London: John Wright, 1988:312–327.

28. Robson MC, Parsons RW. Respiratory problems in thermal injury. In: Rattenborg CC, Via-Regue E, eds. Clinical use of mechanical ventilation. Chicago: Year Book Medical, 1981:156–164.

29. O'Niell JA, Jr. The influence of thermal burns on gastric acid secretion. Surgery 1970;67:267.

30. Rosenthal A, Czaja AJ, Pruitt BA. Gastrin levels and gastric acidity in the pathogenesis of acute gastroduodenal disease after burns. Surg Gynecol Obstet 1977;144:232.

31. Stenberg T, Hogeman KE. Experimental and clinical investigations on liver functions in burns. In: Artz CP, ed. Research in burns. Philadelphia: FA Davis, 1962:171.

32. Wilmore DW. Metabolic changes after thermal injury. In: Boswick JA, ed. The art and science of burn care. Rockville, MD: Aspen, 1987:137–144.

33. Wilmore DW, Long JA, Mason AD, et al. Catecholamines: mediator of the hypermetabolic response to thermal injury. Ann Surg 1974;180:653.

34. Jelenko C III, Ginsburg JM. Water holding lipid and water transmission through homeothermic and poikilothermic skin. Proc Soc Exp Biol Med 1971;136:1059.

35. Arturson G. Evaporation and fluid replacement: research in burns. In: Matter P, Barclay TL, Konickova Z, eds. Transactions of the third international congress on research in burns. Berne: Hans Huber, 1971:520.

36. Curreri PW. Metabolic and nutritional aspects of thermal injury. Burns 1976;2:16.

37. Heggers JP, Heggers R, Robson MC. The immunological deficit encountered in thermal injury. J Am Med Technol 1982;44:99.

38. McCutcheon M. Inflammation, In: Anderson WAD, ed. Pathology. St. Louis: CV Mosby, 1948:14–66.

39. Ricketts LR, Squire JR, Topley E, et al. Human skin lipids with particular reference to the self-sterilizing power of the skin. Clin Sci Mol Med 1951;10:89.

40. Robson MC, Samburg JL, Krizek TJ. Quantitative comparison of biological dressings. J Surg Res 1973;14:431.

41. Warner GF, Dobson EL. Disturbances in the reticuloendothelial system following thermal injury. Am J Physiol 1954;179:93.

42. Robson MC, Smith DJ, Jr. Burned hand. In Jurkiewicz MJ, Krizek TJ, Mathes SJ, et al, eds. Plastic surgery, principles and practice. 1st ed. St. Louis, CV Mosby, 1990;781–802.

43. Krizek TJ. Topical therapy of burns—problems in wound healing, J Trauma 1968;8:276.

44. Moncrief JA, Teplitz C. Changing concepts in burn sepsis. J Trauma 1964;4:233.

45. Heggers JP, Heggers R, Robson MC. The immunological defect encountered in thermal injury. J Am Med Technol 44:99, 1982.

46. Alexander JW, Nixon D. Neutrophil dysfunction of polymorphonuclear leukocytes in patients with burns and other trauma. Surg Gynecol Obstet 1970;130:431.

47. Warden GD. Immunologic response to burn injury. In: Boswick JA, ed. The art and science of burn care. Rockville, MD: Aspen, 1987:118.

48. Arturson G, Johansson SGD, Hogman CF, et al. Changes in immunoglobulin levels in severely burned patients. Lancet 1969;1:546.

49. Robson MC, Murphy RC, Heggers JP. A new explanation for the progressive tissue loss in electrical injuries. Plast Reconst Surg 1984;73:431.

50. Hunt JL, Mason AD, Masterson TS, et al. Pathophysiology of acute electrical injuries. J Trauma 1976;16:335.

51. Sances A, Larson, SJ, Myklebust J, et al. Electrical injuries. Surg Gynecol Obstet 1979;149:97.

52. Esses SI, Peters WJ. Electrical burns: pathophysiology and complications. Can J Surg 1981;24:11.

53. Jaffe RH. Electropathology: a review of pathologic changes produced by electric currents. Arch Pathol 1928;5:837.

54. Sances A, Myklebust JB, Larson SJ, et al. Experimental electrical injury studies. J Trauma 1981;21:589.

55. Mann RJ, Wallquist JM. Early decompression fasciotomy in the treatment of high voltage electrical injury of the extremities. South Med J 1975;68:1103.

56. Solem L, Fischer RP, Strate RG. Natural history of electrical injury. J Trauma 1977;17:487.

57. Sturim HS. The treatment of electrical injuries. J Trauma 1971;11:959.

58. Baxter CR. Present concepts in the management of major electrical injuries. Surg Clin North Am 1970;50:1401.

59. Ponten B, Erickson U, Johansson SH, et al. New observations on tissue changes along the pathway of the current in an electrical injury. Scand J Plast Reconstr Surg 1970;4:75.

60. Skoog T. Electrical injuries. J Trauma 1970;10:816.

61. Hunt JL, McManus WF, Haney WP, et al. Vascular lesions in acute electrical injuries. J Trauma 1974;14:461.

62. Hunt JL, Sato RM, Baxter CR. Acute electric burns. Arch Surg 1980;115:434.

63. Quinby WC, Burke JF, Trelstad RL, et al. The use of microscopy as a guide to primary excision of electrical burns. J Trauma 1978;18:423.

64. Luterman A, Curreri PW. Chemical burn injury. In: Jurkiewcz MJ, Krizek TJ, Mathes SJ, et al, eds. Plastic surgery: principles and practice. St. Louis: CV Mosby, 1990:1355–1440.

65. Jelenko C. Chemicals that "burn." J Trauma 1974;14:65.

66. Moriarty RW. Corrosive chemicals: acids and alkalis. Drug Therapy. 1979;3:89.

67. Stone HH, Martin JD. Pulmonary injury associated with thermal burns. Surg Gynecol Obstet 1969;129:1242.

68. Leonard LG, Scheulen JJ, Munster AM. Chemical burns: effect of prompt first aid. J Trauma 1982;22:420.

69. Zacarian SA. Cryogenics: the cryolesion and the pathogenesis of cryonecrosis. In: Zacarian SA, ed. Cryosurgery for skin and cutaneous disorders. St. Louis: CV Mosby, 1985:1–30.

70. Weatherly-White RCA, Sjostrom B, Paton BC. Experimental studies in cold injury. J Surg Res 1964;4:17.

71. Bellman S, Adams-Ray J. Vascular reactions after experimental cold injury. Angiology 1956;7:339.

72. Cohnheim J. Local disturbances of the circulation. In: Lectures on general pathology. London: New Sydenham Society, 1989:109–171.

73. Robson MC, Heggers JP. Evaluation of hand frostbite blister fluid as a clue to pathogenesis. J Hand Surg 1981;6:43.

74. Raine TJ, London MD, Goluch L, et al. Antiprostaglandins and antithromboxanes for treatment of frostbite. Surg Forum 1980;31:557.

75. Knize DM, Weatherly-White RC, Paton BC, et al. Prognostic factors in the management of frostbite. J Trauma 1969;9:749.

76. Knize DM. Cold injury. In: Converse JM, ed. Reconstructive plastic surgery. Vol. 1. Philadelphia: WB Saunders, 1977:516–530.

77. Fuhrman FA, Crissman JM. Studies of gangrene following cold injury. VII, Treatment of cold injury by immediate rapid rewarming. J Clin Invest 1947;26:476.

78. Mills WJ, Whaley R, Fish W. Frostbite: experience with rapid rewarming and ultrasonic therapy. Alaska Med 1962;3:28.

79. McCauley RL, Hing DN, Robson MC, et al. Frostbite injuries: a rational approach based on the pathophysiology. J Trauma 1983;23:143.

80. Williams HE, Breene RG, Rees R. The brown recluse spider. Knoxville: University of Tennessee Institute of Agriculture PB1191, University of Tennessee Press, 1988.

81. King LE, Rees RS. Dapsone treatment of a brown recluse spider bite. JAMA 1983;250:648.

82. Koplan L, Zaran HA. Recurrent basal cell carcinoma: A review concerning the incidence, behavior, and management of recurrent basal cell carcinoma, with emphasis on the incompletely excised lesion. Plast Reconstr Surg 1980;65:656.

83. Kaplan EK. The risk of malignancy in large congenital nevi. Plast Reconstr Surg 1974;53:421.

84. Greene MH, Fraumeni JF, Jr. The hereditary variant of malignant melanoma. In: Clark WH Jr, Goldman LI, Mastrangelo MJ, eds. Human malignant melanoma. New York: Grune and Stratton, 1979.

85. Skolnick MH, Cannon-Albright LA, Kamb A. Genetic predisposition to melanoma. Eur J Cancer 1994;30(13):1995–2001.

86. Bale SJ, Dracopoli NC, Tucker MA, et al. Mapping the gene for hereditary cutaneous malignant melanoma-dysplastic nevus to chromosome 1P. N Engl J Med 1989;320:1367–1372.

87. Cannon-Albright LA, Goldgar DE, Meyer LJ, etal. Assignment of a locus for familial melanoma MLM, to chromosome 9p13-22. Science 1992;258:1148–1152.

88. Krementz ET, Reed RJ, Coleman WP, et. al. Acral lentiginous melanoma. Ann Surg 195:632–645, 1982.

89. Balch CM, Seng-Jaw S, Milton GW, et al. A comparison of prognostic factors and surgical causes in 1,786 patients with localized

(Stage 1) melanoma treated in Alabama, US, and New South Wales, Australia. Ann Surg 1982;196:677.

90. Balch CM, Murad TM, Soong SJ, et al. A multifactorial analysis of melanoma: prognostic histopathological features comparing Clark's and Breslow's staging methods. Ann Surg 1978;88: 732–742.

91. Rees R, Reilley A, Nanney LB, et al. Sacral pressure sores: treatment with gluteus maximus musculocutaneous flaps. South Med J 1985;78:1147.

92. Colen RS. Pressure sores. In: McCarthy JG, ed. Plastic surgery. Philadelphia: WB Saunders Co., 1990;6:3806–3807.

93. Landis EM. Micro-injection studies of capillary blood pressure in human skin. Heart 1930;15:209.

94. Dinsdal SM. Decubitus ulcers: role of pressure and friction in causation. Arch Phys Med Rehabil 1974;55:147.

95. Shea JD. Pressure sores—classification and management. Clin Orthop 1975:112:89–100.

96. Young JB, Dobrzanski S. Pressure sores: epidemiology and current management concepts. Drugs Aging 1992;2:42–57.

SUGGESTED READINGS

Bauer BS, Kernahan DA, Hugo DE. Lymphangioma circumscriptum—a clinicopathological review. Ann Plast Surg 1981;7:318.

Bowers RE, Graham EA, Tomlinson KM. The natural history of the strawberry nevus. Arch Dermatol 1960;82:667.

Burns AJ, Rohrick RJ. Vascular anomalies and lymphedema. Selected readings. Plast Surg 1988;5:1.

Caro WA, Bronstein BR. Tumors of the skin. In: Moschella SL, Hurley HS, eds. Dermatology. Philadelphia: WB Saunders, 1985:1533–1628.

Garden JM, Polla LL, Tan OT. The treatment of port-wine stains by the pulsed dye laser. Analysis of pulse duration and long-term therapy. Arch Dermatol 1988;124:889.

Ghadially FN, Barton BW, Kerridge DF. Etiology of keratoacanthoma. Cancer 1963;16:603.

Kaban LB, Mulliken JB. Vascular anomalies of the maxillofacial region. J Oral Maxillofac Surg 1986;44:203.

Mulliken JB, Glowacki J. Hemangiomas and vascular malformations in infants and children: a classification based on endothelial characteristics. Plast Reconstr Surg 1982;69:412.

Persky MS. Congenital vascular lesions of the head and neck. Laryngoscope 1986;96:1002.

Schonfeld A, Schattner A, Crespi M, et al. Intramuscular human interferon-beta injections in the treatment of condyloma acuminata. Lancet 1984;1:1038–1045.

WHO. Expert committee on leprosy: 5th report. WHO Tech Rept Ser 607, 1977: 1.

WHO. Report of study group: chemotherapy of leprosy for control programmes. WHO Tech Rept Ser 675,1982:1.

23 Urology/Urinary System

Gerald H. Jordan | Thomas V. Whelan | William G. Horstman | William V. Tynes II | Edwin L. Robey | Greg R. Eure | John F. Stecker, Jr. | Boyd H. Winslow | Scott Fabozzi | Paul F. Schellhammer | Donald F. Lynch

Embryology

The kidneys and gonads are derived from a mesodermal structure, the müllerian ridge. The ridge develops into the metanephros, which matures into the adult renal parenchymal tissues. The müllerian and mesonephric (Wolffian) ducts differentiate, via different stimuli, into portions of the internal genitalia and the urinary tract. The ureteral bud emanates from the distal Wolffian duct, becomes a tubular structure, and migrates rostrally to impact the metanephros. On impacting the metanephros, it stimulates definitive nephrogenic development, causing the metanephros to divide to form the structures of the renal pelvis, infundibula, and calyces. In the female, the Wolffian duct eventually involutes, and its vestiges are termed Gartner's duct cysts. In the male, the Wolffian duct persists and becomes the vas deferens. Agenesis of the Wolffian duct in the male causes aplasia of the vas deferens. Other abnormal conditions in renal development often associated with ureteral genetic anomalies include the multicystic dysplasia constellation.

In the female, the müllerian ducts persist to form the fallopian tubes, uterus, and proximal third of the vagina. Aplasia of the müllerian system in the female leads to the Meyer-Rokitansky Kuster complex, manifested by the lack of fallopian tubes and/or lack of proximal vagina, uterus, and fallopian tubes. In the male, the müllerian duct regresses under the influence of the müllerian inhibition factor. The vestiges become the prostatic utricle (termed müllerian cysts when enlarged) and the appendage testis.

The bladder and proximal urethra are derived from the urogenital sinus, of endodermal origin. After the urogenital sinus arises from the cloaca, it is divided by the transverse rectal folds and becomes the anorectal canal and the anterior urogenital sinus. The urogenital sinus then divides proximally into the bladder, and caudally into the posterior urethra in the male and the entire urethra in the female. Abnormalities of the development of the urogenital sinus and/or cloaca lead to cloacal malformations, cloacal exstrophy, or the classic exstrophy/epispadias complex.

The anterior urethra is derived from mesodermal structures associated with the genital tubercle. The mesoderm develops into the corpus spongiosum and urethral epithelium via a process of proximal tubularization. Failure of the proper progression of anterior urethral development leads to hypospadias and is also a part of the epispadias complex.

In the male, the gonadal ridge differentiates into a testis under the influence of the Y chromosome. In the absence of a Y chromosome, the gonadal ridge differentiates into the ovary. In those anomalies in which abnormal development of the second X chromosome (XO conditions) occurs, ovarian differentiation frequently leads to a streak gonad.

Renal Physiology & Anatomy for Surgeons

The kidney's primary function is regulation of fluid volume. Other crucial homeostatic mechanisms carried out by the kidneys include insulin degradation, erythropoietin production, vitamin D synthesis and activation, secretion of organic ions, ammonia genesis, and bicarbonate reabsorption.

The human kidney is composed of approximately one million functional units termed nephrons. The nephron consists of the corpuscle (glomerulus), the proximal convoluted tubule, the thin loop of Henle, the distal tubule, and the collecting duct (Figure 23.1).

Initial ultra filtration occurs at the level of the renal corpuscle. This filtration is affected by many factors, including: renal blood flow; vascular and tubular oncotic

581

Figure 23.1. Illustration of renal corpuscle. AA: Afferent arteriole. IMC: Intraglomerular mesangial cell. CEC: Capillary endothelial cell. CBM: Capillary basement membrane. VE: Visceral epithelium. PE: Parietal epithelium. GBM: Glomerular basement membrane.

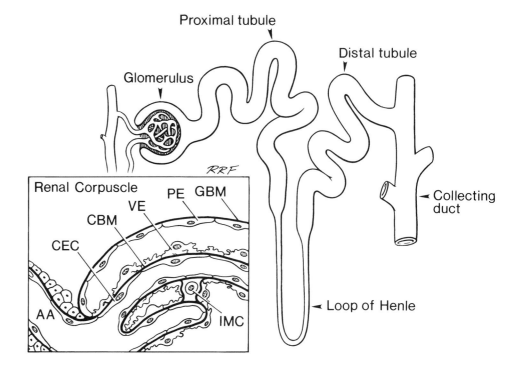

Figure 23.2. Forces responsible for filtration of fluid from the glomerular capillaries and reabsorption of fluid into the peritubular capillaries. The values are considered representative of forces in humans. Pg = glomerular capillary pressure; PB = Bowman's space pressure; πg = Plasma colloid osmotic pressure; πB = Colloid osmotic pressure of filtrate; Kf = Glomerular filtration coefficient; EFP = Effective filtration pressure; Ra = Afferent arteriole resistance; Re = Efferent arteriole resistance; πi = Interstitial colloid osmotic pressure; Pi = Interstitial space hydrostatic pressure; Pc = Capillary hydrostatic pressure; πc = Capillary colloid osmotic pressure; PCU = Peritubular capillary uptake; Kr = Reabsorption coefficient; ERP = Effective reabsorption pressure; Rv = Venous resistance. From: Arends, Horst WJ, Navar LG. Renal circulation and hemodynamics. In Schrier RW, Gottschalk CW, eds. Diseases of the kidney, 4th ed. Boston: Little Brown and Co., 1988.

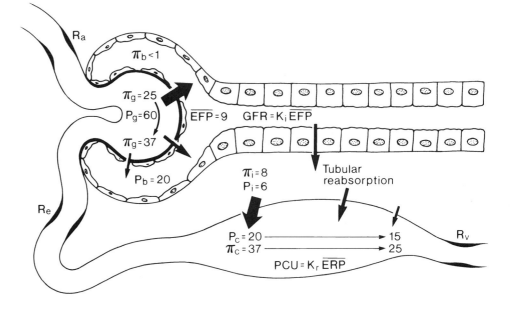

and hydrostatic pressure; size, shape, and electric charge of molecular substances; and mechanical forces associated with the capillary wall (Fig. 23.2). Filtration fluid progresses from the glomerular capillary, into Bowman's space, and into the proximal tubular lumen. Most of the filtered solute is reabsorbed in the proximal tubule. About 25% to 40% of the reabsorption of filtered sodium occurs in the thin limb of the loop of Henle. In man, some nephrons have a long loop of Henle, whereas others have a short one. The quantity of each determines the concentrating ability of the kidney. Because of the relative impermeability to water, the filtrate is diluted in the thin limb of the loop of Henle. Approximately 10% of filtered sodium is reabsorbed in the distal tubule.

Potassium and acid balances are regulated primarily in the collecting duct under the influence of aldosterone.

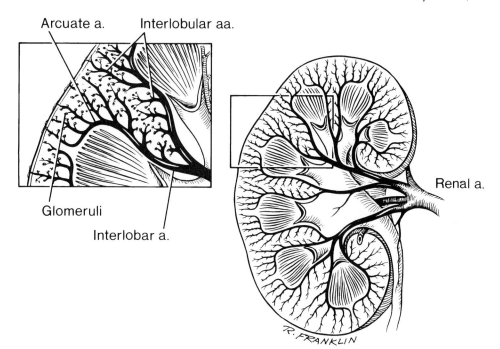

Arcuate a. Interlobular aa.

Glomeruli

Interlobar a.

Renal a.

R. FRANKLIN

Figure 23.3. The macroarterial renal circulation. From: Pitts RF. Physiology of the kidney and body fluids, 3rd ed. Chicago: Year Book Medical Publishers, Inc., 1994: 1–9.

Antidiuretic hormone (vasopressin) also exerts its action at the collecting duct, rendering the duct more permeable to water transport, and further concentrating urine.

The juxtaglomerular apparatus plays a pivotal role in the tubuloglomerular feedback apparatus by contributing to renal blood flow auto regulation. It consists of an intricate complex of cells and blood vessels that are responsible for monitoring a decline in extracellular fluid volume and releasing renin, which converts renin substrate (angiotensinogen) to angiotensin I.

The kidneys receive about 20% of cardiac output, a disproportionately high percentage compared to other organs. Regulation of renal blood flow is critical to maintaining normal glomerular filtration rate over a wide range of systemic pressures. Most individuals require a mean arterial pressure of more than 60 mm Hg to maintain a normal glomerular filtration rate.

Although many congenital variants exist, in most individuals, the renovascular network consists of a single renal artery and vein. In the renal hilum, the artery divides into an anterior division and a posterior division each with five branches. These branches become the interlobar arteries, with the sequence of blood flow as follows: Quillain arcuate arteries to interlobular arteries; interlobular arteries to afferent arcuate arteries; afferent arcuate arterioles to glomerular capillaries; glomerular capillaries to the efferent arterioles; efferent arterioles to the vasa rectae; and vasa rectae to the venous return (Figure 23.3).

Nephrology for Surgeons

The pathophysiology of most renal parenchymal disease is explained through our understanding of the structure and function of the nephron unit. In general, glomerular diseases lead to a loss of protein in the form of either albumin or larger protein molecules.

Nephrosis is characterized by significant proteinuria and scant, if any, cellular sediment. Nephrotic syndrome is defined as more than 3.5 grams per day of proteinuria, systemic edema, hypoalbuminemia, and hyperlipidemia. The pathologic findings for nephrosis include minimal change disease, focal segmental glomerulosclerosis, membranous glomerulopathy, diabetic renal disease, and amyloidosis.

Nephritis is associated with varying degrees of proteinuria, edema, hematuria, and hypertension. The pathologic findings in nephritis include acute poststreptococcal glomerulonephritis, mesangioproliferative glomerulonephritis, membranoproliferative glomerulonephritis, systemic lupus erythematosus, Wegener's granulomatosis, Goodpasture's syndrome, polyarthritis nodosa, and other vascular diseases.

Tubulointerstitial disease states affect solute, water, acid-base, and electrolyte abnormalities. Examples of tubulointerstitial diseases include infectious, toxic, and systemic processes, such as Fanconi's syndrome, lithium nephrotoxicity, and cyclosporine nephrotoxicity.

Vascular insult typically presents as acute tubular necrosis, and is seen in the setting of ischemia. Examples of other diseases affecting the renal vasculature include vasculitis, atheroembolic disease, abnormal renal blood flow associated with dissecting aneurysm, systemic embolization, and renal vein thrombosis.

Renal cystic disease can be either genetic or acquired. Acquired cystic disease develops in patients who are on renal replacement therapy for the treatment of end stage renal disease. Although infrequent, there is a possibility that these cysts will develop into renal cell adenocarcinoma. Imaging has demonstrated that simple cysts are found in a large percentage of the population and are not generally associated with clinical pathology.

The three categories of genetic renal cystic disease all represent a genetic mutation leading to impaired connective tissue formation, and they are determined by the size of the affected kidney. Nephronophthisis (cystic renal medulla complex) is seen in small kidneys; medullary sponge kidney disease is found in normal sized kidneys; and either autosomal dominant or autosomal recessive polycystic kidney disease is noted in large kidneys.

Other hereditary renal diseases are a heterogeneous group of disorders. The most well known is Alport's syndrome. There are six types of Alport's syndrome, all of which manifest as microscopic hematuria and progressive azotemia, and most, but not all, are associated with deafness.

Nephrolithiasis, or renal stone disease, is the third most common affliction of the urinary tract. A number of situations can precipitate crystal formation in the urine, but most are related to an imbalance of the physiochemical state of the urine. This imbalance can be the result of any one, or a combination, of the following: supersaturation, pH abnormalities, a lack of inhibitory substances (i.e., chelators such as citrate), matrix production, infection, or heterogeneous nucleation.

Many disorders are associated with nephrolithiasis; however, the majority of patients have idiopathic hypercalciuria. Secondary causes of stone formation include renal tubular acidosis, hyperparathyroidism, gout, and recurrent urinary tract infections. In patients who have renal tubular acidosis, chronic acidemia induces bone resorption, leading to hypercalciuria and the formation of calcium oxalate stones. Crohn's disease/colitis patients form calcium oxalate stones caused by impaired binding of oxalate in the gut, which leads to hyperoxaluria. Hyperparathyroidism also causes patients to form calcium oxalate stones. Gout can lead to uric acid nephrolithiasis. Finally, recurrent urinary tract infections, especially those with urease production, cause an alkaline urine and infection matrix that leads to formation of triple phosphate stones.

Radiographic Imaging for Genitourinary Diseases

A variety of imaging modalities can be used to investigate the genitourinary tract with the appropriate choice dictated by the clinical situation. Many uroradiologic studies require the injection of intravenous contrast material that can be associated with a number of adverse reactions. Uroradiologic studies should therefore only be ordered after careful consideration of the indications and clinical need for the information provided by the study.

Urolithiasis

The intravenous urogram (IVU) is sill the most often used test to evaluate the genitourinary system. The most common indication for IVU is to evaluate patients with symptoms thought to be caused by urolithiasis. A precontrast view (KUB) of the abdomen is critical if radio-opaque calculi are to be visualized, as it allows visualization of the number, size, and position of such stones. Fifteen percent of calculi are radiolucent, however, and radio-opaque stones can often be obscured by overlying bowel gas and contents.

The IVU detects most stones, including almost all symptomatic ones. After contrast administration, the first sign is delayed contrast excretion on the affected side. Eventually, contrast fills the urinary tract to the level of the obstruction, termed columning. When contrasting columns to a radio-opacity that was first noted on KUB, a definite diagnosis of an obstructing calculus can be made. Because the time it takes for contrast to column to an obstruction offers a rough estimate of the degree of obstruction, delayed films are important in the determination of location and nature of the obstruction. Occasionally, there will be columning of contrast when no definite stone is seen. These patients may require further evaluation with cystoscopy with retrograde pyelography.

Computed tomography (CT) and ultrasonography have been used by some investigators to evaluate patients suspected of having urolithiasis. Non-contrast CT has been used recently to evaluate patients with suspected stones. All stones are radio-opaque on CT, even those not visible on plain radiography, affording non-contrast CT the advantage of allowing a diagnosis without the use of intravenous contrast. Non-contrast CT may therefore prove to be a reliable alternative for the diagnosis of symptomatic ureterolithiasis in patients who cannot receive intravenous contrast.

The most common use of ultrasonography is to determine the presence or absence of hydronephrosis. In some patients with early obstruction, hydronephrosis may not have had time to develop and may lead to a false negative study. Ultrasound is not specific, and many dilations of the collecting systems result from causes other than obstruction. Ultrasound does provide adequate visualization of intrarenal stones. However, because symptomatic stones are located in the ureters, which are obscured in most cases by the bowel, ultrasound is not useful for symptomatic stones.

Trauma

Because CT has proven to be more sensitive and specific, IVU is currently only used in specific settings for evaluation of trauma patients. After injecting intravenous contrast material, a one shot IVU can be done in the emergency department to demonstrate whether both kidneys are present and functioning. An IVU can also be used to demonstrate contrast extravasation in patients with penetrating trauma. However, the IVU is not sensitive for detecting bladder or urethral injuries. A CT is the test of choice for the evaluation of most trauma patients.

Trauma patients who have pelvic fractures must undergo urethral evaluation with retrograde urethrography. Cystography is also useful for the evaluation of patients suspected of having bladder injuries. After the urethra is evaluated adequately, any trauma patient with a pelvic fracture and hematuria should be evaluated with a cystogram.

Masses

IVU is useful in the evaluation of patients with hematuria. An IVU visualizing the entire upper urinary tract is the only non-invasive study that can exclude a mucosal lesion or other filling defect above the bladder. When combined with tomography, an IVU allows visualization of most renal parenchymal masses, and while a specific diagnosis usually cannot be made with IVU, the most common masses noted are benign cysts.

All mass lesions noted on IVU warrant further evaluation with CT, ultrasound, or magnetic resonance imaging (MRI). Magnetic resonance imaging or ultrasound can be used in lieu of CT in patients who cannot receive contrast material.

Ultrasound is the most operator-dependent investigational procedure used in the genitourinary tract. Ultrasound detects almost all renal masses larger than 3-4 cm. It is also the examination of choice in most cases of scrotal pathology and is 100% sensitive in the detection of intraparenchymal testicular lesions. Furthermore, the development of color Doppler has added blood flow information to the ultrasound evaluation, expanding its applications in scrotal evaluation.

CT scan is the most sensitive and specific imaging modality for evaluation of renal masses and has a 95% to 98% sensitivity for detecting renal parenchymal masses. All patients with high clinical suspicion of a renal mass should have CT, even if IVU or ultrasound was negative, since both tests can miss a small percentage of solid renal lesions. CT should also be used in patients in whom a diagnosis remains unclear, despite the performance of IVU and/or ultrasound. However, CT scan is technique-dependent, the nature of the renal lesion being evaluated must be made clear to the radiologist performing the study, as non-contrast images with thin sections may be needed for optimal renal evaluation.

MRI that has been demonstrated to be useful in the evaluation of adrenal lesions may not be as helpful in the genitourinary tract. In general, MRI contributes the same information as a well-performed CT scan. The intravenous contrast for MRI is gadolinium because in the kidney, the signal intensity of many solid renal mass lesions closely matches that of normal renal tissue. MRI can be used to evaluate patients who are allergic to the intravenous contrast material used in IVU and CT scan.

Other

Renal scintigraphy, done with several different radio pharmaceutical agents, allows an estimate of the percentage of renal function coming from each kidney. The most common use of renal scintigraphy is to evaluate renal blood flow and function in patients with renal failure. Another important function of renal scintigraphy is to determine the functional significance of apparent renal obstruction. Renal transplant patients are evaluated routinely with renal scintigraphy, as it allows both evaluation of blood flow to the renal allograft and the function of the allograft.

Physiology of Voiding/Voiding Dysfunction

Voiding Physiology

For complete understanding of voiding dysfunction, it is important to review key aspects of the anatomy and physiology of the bladder as they pertain to voiding. Voiding can be divided into two distinct phases: storage of urine and emptying of urine. The lower urinary tract is composed of the bladder, urethra, striated muscle, and fascial layers. The coordination and integration of the lower urinary tract necessary to accomplish these functions is complex. Storage requires the accommodation of increasing volumes of urine while maintaining low intravesical pressures and the ability to sense fullness. During this phase, the bladder outlet is closed while adjusting for increasing intra-abdominal pressure, and no involuntary bladder contractions result. During emptying, bladder contraction coordinates with relaxation of the sphincter. This involves the concomitant decreases in the resistance of the involuntary (passive) and voluntary (active) sphincters, which allows the bladder outlet to open.

The muscle layers of the bladder wall are composed of detrusor smooth muscle fibers with the ability to exert maximal effective tension over a wide range of fiber lengths. With contraction, the bladder is able to empty continuously and forcefully throughout the voiding phase.

Based on formation of the smooth muscle fibers, the bladder is divided into different regions. The body of the bladder is composed of a mass of muscle fibers that allows the bladder to expand and contract. In the trigone (the base of the bladder), the muscle fibers separate into three distinct muscle layers: inner longitudinal, middle circular, and outer longitudinal. These layers form the internal meatus of the bladder neck and act as a passive sphincter. The passive sphincter is also known as the proximal sphincter mechanism. In males, the prostate assists this mechanism. The outer longitudinal layer extends the entire length of the female urethra, whereas it ends near the membranous urethra in males. These fibers are oriented in a circular fashion, allowing variations in urethral resistance, and are called the intrinsic portion of the distal sphincter mechanism. The bladder neck and distal sphincter mechanisms provide involuntary (passive) mechanisms for continence and are not true anatomic sphincters.

The voluntary or external sphincters are composed of striated muscle fibers and compose the extrinsic portion of the distal sphincteric mechanism. In the female, these fibers form a sphincter around the middle third of the urethra. In males, the external sphincter has fibers surrounding the distal portion of the prostate and the membranous urethra. The external sphincter is also composed of striated muscles of the pelvic floor, including the levator ani and pubococcygeus muscles. The proximal or distal sphincteric mechanisms can provide passive continence in the male, even if one or the other is dysfunctional.

The function of the lower urinary tract requires the activation and coordination of multiple structures to control storage and emptying of urine. The three controlling mechanisms are central, spinal, and peripheral. The central mechanism allows for voluntary control of the bladder and acts as a sphincter mechanism. Central nervous control is divided further into cortical, basal ganglia, and brain stem. Cortical influences are primarily inhibitory to the micturition reflex. The basal ganglia appears to be altered in voiding dysfunction of Parkinson's disease and other neurologic diseases. The brain stem micturition center coordinates filling and emptying of the bladder by influencing the peripheral innervation of the lower urinary tract via the spinal cord.

Although interactions with the spinal cord are not completely understood, there are some purely spinal reflexes that control the lower urinary tract. The spinal cord has two specialized areas involved in micturition: 1) a concentration of sympathetic neurons at the level of T_{11} through L_2; and 2) the parasympathetic (autonomic) and pudendal (somatic) influence located at level S_2 through S_4. The proximal sphincteric mechanism and the intrinsic portion of the distal sphincteric mechanism receives its innervation from sympathetic neurons of the thoracolumbar outflow at T_{11} and L_2, whereas the extrinsic components of the distal sphincteric mechanism receive motor innervation from the spinal cord via the pudendal nerve at the level of S_2 to S_4. Pelvic floor (levator) muscles receive motor innervation between the same area.

The peripheral innervation of the detrusor muscle is part of the parasympathetic nervous system that innervates the bladder through the sacral and pelvic nerves, also called the pelvic plexus. In addition, sympathetic innervation to the detrusor also occurs through the pelvic plexus. Sensory neurons from the bladder are divided into pain, temperature, and proprioceptive sensation. The sensory neurons of the bladder neck and trigone return via the sympathetic trunk. The sensory innervation of the external sphincter returns by way of the pudendal nerve.

Larger volumes of urine are stored to allow quality of life and infrequent voiding. To prevent damage to the upper urinary tract, urine is stored at an intravesical pressure of less than 40 cm of water. To remain continent, the urethral pressure must remain greater than the intravesical pressure at all times. Intravesical pressure during storage is typically 10–20 cm of water. The point at which intravesical pressure exceeds urethral resistance pressure is called the "leak point pressure." "Leak point pressure" has been used to evaluate women with stress urinary incontinence and children with neurogenic bladder disorder.

During storage, as a result of the vesico elastic properties of the bladder wall, the intravesical pressure changes minimally despite increases in volume. However, as the bladder volume reaches capacity, the intravesical pressure gradually increases, provoking an increase in somatic motor activity, and increases the activity of the pelvic floor. Sympathetic activity produces a decrease in bladder contractile activity, inhibition of the parasympathetic ganglia, and stimulation of the beta adrenoreceptors in the bladder. This reflex, known as the "guarding reflex," also closes the bladder outlet through simulation of the alpha adrenergic receptors at the bladder neck and urethra, resulting in maintenance of a ratio between urethral resistance pressure and intravesical pressure. The guarding reflex compensates for sudden increases in intravesical pressure and increases in intra-abdominal pressure through the somatic reflex and voluntary sphincter.

Micturition involves coordinating bladder contraction and a decrease in bladder outlet resistance. The primary control is the sensation of fullness of the bladder, acknowledged in the cortical center, resulting in the voluntary release of controlling mechanisms. The sympathetic reflex is blocked, allowing the bladder neck and urethra to relax and open the outlet while the parasympathetic micturition reflex contracts the distended bladder. Stimulation of voluntary sphincters is also inhibited. Once the bladder is empty, it returns to the storage phase.

Evaluation of Voiding Dysfunction

The evaluation of voiding dysfunction begins with a voiding history, including a history of irritative symptoms (urgency, frequency, and incontinence) and obstructive symptoms (hesitancy and failure to empty). In addition, a complete history of medical problems, neurologic disorders, surgical and obstetrical procedures, and trauma may be important. In most cases, a voiding diary should be included in the initial evaluation.

Physical examination consists of an examination of the neurologic and genitourinary systems. Anal sphincter tone reflects the state of the perineal striated musculature. Deep tendon reflex evaluation provides an indication of segmental and suprasegmental spinal cord function. The bulbocavernosal (BC) reflex provides specific information about the S_2 to S_4 region of the spinal cord. It is elicited in a female by gently pulling on a Foley catheter or by gently stroking the labia majora with a cotton tip applicator while monitoring for perineal muscle contraction. In the male, it is elicited by squeezing the glans penis. Because infection is the most common cause of changes in voiding function, a urine culture should be included in the initial evaluation.

Evaluation of the lower urinary tract begins with cystoscopy, which has become much easier with the advent of the flexible cystoscope. If upper tract pathology is suspected, it should also be examined. Urodynamic studies reproduce clinical symptoms while yielding objective data. The goals of urodynamic study are to evaluate capacity, accommodation, intravesical pressure during storage, intravesical pressure during voiding, the presence and quality of detrusor contraction, the presence of uninhibited contractions, the perception of fullness, the ability to inhibit or initiate voiding, and the presence of residual urine.

As a minimum requirement, the initial evaluation should include flow cystometry and quantification of emptying with a post void residual urine. Normal flow rates are 20–25 mL/second in males, and 20–30 ml/second in females. Normal post void residual urines are minimal. Other normal parameters include a bladder capacity of 400–500 cc, a storage bladder pressure of < 15 cm H_2O pressure (the point of voiding), a first sensation of fullness at approximately 150–250 cc of urine, and a voiding pressure of < 30 cc H_2O pressure.

Voiding Dysfunction

The sources of voiding dysfunction can be separated into three groups: failure to store, failure to empty, and disease processes that affect both.

Failure to Store. Failure to store implies an inappropriate loss of urine or incontinence. The incidence of incontinence in females is much higher than in males because the female urethra is much shorter, lacks the external support of the male urethra, and lacks the resistance forces of the prostate. A healthy urethral mucosa maintains closure that helps to resist leaking; this is an important factor in maintaining continence in the fe-

male. Estrogen plays a key role in supporting a healthy female urethral mucosa.

Incontinence can be the result of either bladder or sphincter pathology. If the bladder is the culprit, the pathology is primarily related to involuntary bladder contractions during the storage phase. This is most commonly associated with infection and inflammation. Incontinence is also associated with benign prostatic hypertrophy. It can also be seen in patients without obstruction (idiopathic detrusor instability).

Detrusor instability is the term used to describe bladder contractions occurring during filling that are not related to neurogenic pathology. Its symptoms include urgency and frequency. Urine leaks occur if the bladder contraction raises intravesical pressure to the point that it exceeds urethral pressure, a phenomenon referred to as urge incontinence. The patient may also note an urgency to void without an uninhibited detrusor contraction, referred to as sensory instability.

The primary treatments for detrusor instability are removal of the underlying cause or the use of anticholinergic drugs. In females, behavior modification, exercises to strengthen the pelvic floor musculature, and postmenopausal estrogen replacement therapy can be helpful. Surgical intervention for detrusor instability includes hydrodilation, bladder augmentation, and, in rare cases, diversion.

Detrusor hyperreflexia is an involuntary bladder contraction of neurogenic origin that occurs during the storage phase. Treatment of detrusor hyperreflexia involves monitoring of intravesical pressure and the use of anticholinergic agents. Lesions above the brain stem—caused by cerebrovascular accidents, dementia, closed head injuries, brain tumor, cerebellar ataxia, normal pressure hydrocephalus, cerebral palsy, and Parkinson's disease—produce a spastic neuropathy resulting in a decrease in bladder capacity, uninhibited bladder contractions, increased intravesical pressure, and hypertrophy of the bladder wall. Such lesions usually cause involuntary bladder contractions while maintaining synergy with the smooth and striated sphincter.

Injuries to the spinal cord cause spasticity of the pelvic striated muscle, with lack of coordinated voiding. Commonly seen in multiple sclerosis, spinal cord injury, tethered cord syndrome, and myelomeningocele, this syndrome is seen occasionally in sacral agenesis. Complete spinal cord injuries above the S_2 level usually result in involuntary bladder contractions, with smooth muscle synergy and striated muscle dyssynergy.

A complicating factor in detrusor hyperreflexia is autonomic dysreflexia, involving an excessive sacral afferent feedback which initiates an uncontrolled sympathetic response. Autonomic dysreflexia classically occurs in patients with spastic lesions (complete spinal cord injuries) above level T_6. The symptoms include a significant increase in blood pressure, headache, and sweating. The treatment is to reverse the initiating cause.

In the urinary tract, the syndrome typically is caused by either a distended bladder, urinary tract infection, or high pressure voiding. Prophylaxis of dysreflexia can include sublingual procardia (10–20 mg). Short term blockage of the response can also be accomplished through the use of the nonselective alpha blocker, phenoxybenzamine. External appliances to collect the urine are used only as a last resort.

Another cause of failure to store urine is low compliance of the bladder wall. In this circumstance, the bladder's ability to store urine at low, constant pressures decreases. Incontinence is the result of overflow caused by the intravesical pressure exceeding the outlet resistance pressure. Anatomic causes of low bladder wall compliance include detrusor hypertrophy secondary to outlet obstruction, bladder wall fibrosis secondary to irradiation, tuberculosis, recurrent infections, chronic catheterization, and multiple bladder procedures. Injury to the pelvic plexus caused by pelvic trauma or surgery also may result in a bladder wall with low compliance.

Stress incontinence is the loss of urine resulting from increased abdominal pressure and is not due to a detrusor contraction. It is the result of the failure of the urethral resistance to compensate for transient increases in intra-abdominal pressure, and can occur because of urethral hypermobility and/or loss of mucosal coaptation. In females, laxity of the pelvic floor muscles, in conjunction with weakening of the pelvic ligaments, causes loss of the normal urethral position in the pelvis and leads to stress incontinence.

Intrinsic sphincter dysfunction is another source of failure to store urine and is the result of a well-supported but poorly functioning urethra. This can result in continuous loss of urine, and it usually occurs in females after a pelvic operation or radiation. In males, failure to store urine because of sphincter dysfunction is most often caused by prostatic surgery.

Although a tendency exists to categorize incontinence by urge versus stress, both can co-exist in the same patient. In addition, some of the surgical procedures that prevent stress incontinence, induce detrusor instability. After radical prostatectomy, continence is maintained by the distal sphincteric mechanism (membranous urethra). If the sphincter is damaged, its function was less than optimal prior to surgery, or its functional length is foreshortened to a degree that the urethral leak point pressure is inadequate; therefore, the patient will have stress incontinence.

The treatment for sphincter deficiency varies depending on the severity of the problem. The use of procedures that potentially obstruct the bladder outlet to prevent incontinence can result in conversion of the problem from failure to store to failure to empty. In females, sphincter incompetence can be treated by a number of procedures with relatively the same rates of success (80%–85%). Depending on severity, anticholinergic medication, collagen injections, or artificial bulbar urethral sphincters may be required. With the advent of clean intermittent catheterization, patients rarely require diversion. In men, surgical intervention after radical prostatectomy is usually delayed for a year to allow for a period of time for continence to be regained. In patients with small contracted bladders, the use of bladder augmentation is used to increase the volume and improve continence.

Failure to Empty. Failure to empty urine can also be divided into bladder and sphincter pathology. Bladder pathology associated with chronic retention can result from outlet obstruction that causes decompensation of the bladder wall and decreased bladder contractile force. After removal of the obstruction, the bladder may not recover completely and continue to fail to empty. Sensory neuropathic disorders, such as diabetes mellitus, tabes dorsalis, and pernicious anemia, can result in decreased sensation of fullness and retention. Genital herpes can produce transient urinary retention that will resolve in weeks to months. Lower motor neuron lesions caused by pelvic surgery or trauma can leave a weak or a contractile bladder. With the inability to effectively empty, overflow incontinence can arise once the intravesical pressure exceeds the leak point pressure. The treatment for these conditions is clean intermittent catheterization. Although cholinergic agonists (i.e., Urecholine) were used in the past, the results have been inconsistent, and these drugs are no longer considered a primary treatment modality for failure to empty...Postoperative retention is usually the result of inhibition of the bladder reflex by opioid mediated mechanisms. Transient over-distension of the bladder while under anesthesia or analgesic medications can also cause postoperative retention. In these situations, the bladder becomes stretched past normal capacity because of a lack of sensation, and the detrusor muscle contractile force is diminished temporarily. The primary treatment is bladder rest with an indwelling catheter or the initiation of a clean intermittent catheterization protocol. In some cases, bladder outlet obstruction will co-exist and have to be corrected as well.

The most common sphincter pathology associated with failure to empty in the adult male is bladder outlet obstruction secondary to benign prostatic hypertrophy (BPH). The pathophysiology and treatment of BPH are discussed later in this chapter. Bladder outlet obstruction is uncommon in females and primarily results from surgery to correct incontinence.

Failure to Store and Failure to Empty. Overflow incontinence is a classic example of a condition characterized by both failure to store and failure to empty. In detrusor sphincter dyssynergy, bladder contraction is not synchronized with relaxation of the sphincter mechanism. This results in a bladder that contracts against a closed outlet, with either reduced flow or complete obstruction. The bladder is therefore unable to empty effectively and slowly becomes distended. Once the bladder's maximum capacity has been reached, the intravesical pressure achieved is greater than the outflow resistance, and the patient has overflow incontinence.

In older patients, detrusor hyperactivity with impaired contractility can result in a similar clinical picture. These patients have elevated residual urines and still have urgency incontinence. Treatment of these conditions should be individualized for each patient.

Adult Urinary Tract Infections

Accounting for more than five million office visits annually in the United States alone, adult urinary tract infection (UTI) is one of the most prevalent infectious diseases seen in modern medical practice. Although they occasionally result from viral or fungal infections, the majority are caused by bacteria, and UTIs represent the most common cause of nosocomial bacterial infections.

The prevalence of UTI varies with age and sex. Approximately 1% of males will acquire a UTI during infancy, often associated with a significantly redundant preputial skin related to phimosis. Beyond that peak, infection in the male is uncommon until the sixth decade of life, at which time about 50% of males are affected with benign prostatic enlargement. The incidence of UTI is far greater in females than in males. In females, the incidence also increases with advancing age; with school age girls experiencing an incidence of 1%–5%, and sexually active post-menopausal women experiencing an incidence of 20%–30%. In the elderly population, a relationship exists between the place of residence and the prevalence of infection. Approximately 20% of elderly women and 10% of elderly men living at home have bacteriuria. These figures increase to 25%–30% of elderly people who reside in a nursing home environment. Furthermore, the figures continue to rise for these patients when hospitalized. There is a direct relationship with the length of hospitalization.

Bacteriuria is defined as the presence of bacteria in the urine. Often this bacterial colonization warrants no treatment. However, when such patients undergo instrumentation or catheter manipulation, they should be treated with antibiotic prophylaxis. At times, colonization of the urine can progress to microbial invasion of the tissues, which is defined as a true infection. The majority of UTIs are caused by an ascending route (reaching the bladder via the urethra), although hematogenous spread is seen occasionally. UTIs are typically caused by intestinal flora. Escherichia coli is the most common causative agent.

Catheter associated UTIs are the most common type of hospital acquired infection. Bacteria easily migrate to the bladder in both men and women in the presence of a catheter. A single transient catheterization produces an infection in approximately 1% of a healthy population, with an increased risk of 10%–20% in the compromised hospital patient. Despite sterile placement and meticulous care, bacterial colonization often occurs within 48 to 72 hours of placement of an indwelling catheter.

UTIs can involve all parts of the urinary tract, either individually or in combination. Clinical symptoms are useful in distinguishing the site of involvement, and diagnosis is confirmed by urine culture.

Lower Urinary Tract Infection

Lower tract infection involves the urethra, bladder, and/or the prostate or epididymis in males. Infection of the urethra, termed urethritis, is seen most often in males. Symptoms include dysuria, or difficulty voiding, and a purulent urethral discharge. Urethritis is often sexually transmitted. "Cystitis" describes an infection of the urinary bladder. It is suspected in the presence of urinary frequency, urgency, suprapubic discomfort, and dysuria.

Infection of the prostate, termed prostatitis, can be either acute or chronic. Acute bacterial prostatitis is often associated with a more dramatic presentation, which may include dysuria, difficulty voiding, urgency, fever, and perineal or lower back discomfort. Chronic prostatitis is thought to be the result of incomplete treatment of the acute condition.

Epididymitis usually results from bacterial migrations through the vas deferens, termed urethrovasal reflux, and has been associated with long-term urethral catheterization. Epididymitis is suspected in the presence of scrotal pain, swelling, and tenderness. In the young male, the diagnosis of epididymitis must be separated from the diagnosis of torsion of the spermatic cord, often a difficult distinction, and one that may involve scrotal exploration. Epididymitis is often sexually transmitted in men under the age of 35, and in the older population is associated with gram negative organisms. Left untreated, epididymitis can involve the testicle, a condition termed epididymo-orchitis.

Upper Urinary Tract Infection

Upper urinary tract infection refers to the involvement of the kidney or collecting system. Termed pyelonephritis, it is usually accompanied by fever, chills, and flank pain. Nausea, vomiting, and flank tenderness may also be present. In the young population, the association of pyelonephritis with vesicoureteral reflux is well established. Patients who do not show a prompt initial response to antibiotic therapy when suspected of having pyelonephritis should be suspected of having an upper urinary tract obstruction. Left untreated, this condition can lead to urosepsis and be fatal.

Evaluation

Collection of a urine specimen is critical to diagnosis of UTIs. In males, collection of urine specimens is accomplished easily by cleaning the glans and retracting the preputial skin. In infants and children, urinary collection is sometimes accomplished by placing a bag over the genitalia. Although this method may be convenient and may often be a matter of necessity, in many ways it suffers from the potential for contamination. In young infants, urine for a sterile sample can be collected by a suprapubic needle tap.

To collect sterile urine specimens in prepubertal girls, catheterization can be accomplished with a 5 or 8 Fr. feeding tube. Because of the potential for vaginal contamination, catheterization is thought to be the only method of obtaining a true sterile specimen in females of childbearing age. Often, clean voided specimens of females show pyuria that are attributed to UTI. However, if the patient is otherwise asymptomatic, treatment should not be initiated solely on the appearance of white cells in a "clean catch specimen."

UTIs during pregnancy pose additional risks and warrant special considerations. Hormonal changes in pregnancy lead to decreased bladder tone, diminished uretero peristalsis, and dilation of the collecting system, all increasing the risk of upper urinary tract infection. Pyelonephritis is the most common bacterial infection complicating pregnancy. Untreated bacteriuria in pregnancy leads to pyelonephritis in about a fourth of cases, and is associated with spontaneous abortion. Patients who do not show a prompt response to antibiotic therapy or who have evidence of sepsis need to be evaluated for obstruction, which in many cases involves exposure of the fetus to small amounts of radiation.

Urolithiasis

In industrialized countries, urolithiasis occurs in 1-5% of the population. The highest incidence is in middle-aged white males. It is estimated that 50% of patients will have recurrent symptoms during the eight years following the initial diagnosis. An understanding of the physiology of stone formation is necessary to prevent such recurrence.

Seventy-five percent of kidney and ureteral calculi are composed of calcium oxalate and/or phosphate. The remaining 25% are either uric acid, struvite (infectious calculi), or cystine calculi. Calcium oxalate stones are more common than calcium phosphate stones.

Calcium Calculi

Risk factors for calcium oxalate lithiasis include low urine output (<1500 cc/day), hypercalciuria, elevated sodium or oxalate excretion, increased protein intake, and low urinary citrate excretion. Maintaining a urine volume of >2 liters/day is an important prevention for all forms of urinary tract calculi, but particularly for calcium oxalate lithiasis. Hypercalciuria is related to either increased absorption of calcium from the bowel, or increased renal excretion of calcium. Increased renal excretion can be related to primary tubular defects or hypercalcemia. Increased sodium intake and excretion increases the amount of calcium excreted in the urine, causing hypercalciuria. Hyperoxaluria usually occurs in short gut syndrome and is characterized by increased oxalate absorption from the colon. It can also be seen in patients who have had a jejunoileal bypass, that has excluded the majority of the small intestine. In these cases, an intact colon is required for hyperoxaluria to occur.

Citrate inhibits most stone formation, especially calcium stone formation. Low urinary citrate usually occurs in the setting of distal renal tubular acidosis, where calcium phosphate stones are most commonly seen.

The factors that identify an individual at risk for development of urinary calculi are detected by measurement of serum chemistries and a 24 hour urine collection that quantitates volumes, calcium, oxalate, citrate, and sodium. The foundation of treatment to reverse these factors that place the patient at risk include increasing fluid intake, particularly water, and avoiding excessive intake of calcium and oxalate. In some patients, the addition of thiazide diuretics decreases calcium excretion, and the addition of citrate containing alkalinizing medications may further decrease the likelihood of stone formation.

Infectious Calculi

Infectious stones typically are composed of struvite or magnesium ammonium phosphate. The pathophysiology is initiated by the enzyme urease, which converts urea to ammonia. Ammonia irritates the epithelium of the collecting system. Proteinaceous material and glycosaminoglycans are secreted in response to mucosal irritation, which creates a substance called matrix. This substance hardens capturing crystals of magnesium ammonium phosphate and calcium, forming struvite. In some patients, these stones fill the entire collecting system and are then referred to as staghorn calculi.

Prevention of infectious calculi involves eradication of chronic urinary tract infections. Treatment of these stones requires removal of all stone material, followed by diligent efforts to maintain a sterile urine. A 24-hour urine collection for measurement of calcium, citrate, oxalate, and uric acid is therefore essential to guide management of these patients.

Uric Acid Calculi

Uric acid calculi occur in approximately 5% of patients with nephrolithiasis. Increased uric acid excretion is related to increased intake or turnover of protein. With an increased intake of protein, there is an increased breakdown of amino acids to uric acid via the enzyme xanthine oxidase. Increased protein excretion is associated with some chemotherapy, especially that used for treatment of lymphoproliferative disease.

Hyperuricemia from gout or other inherited disorders of uric acid metabolism can also result in hyperuricuria and uric acid stone formation. Because uric acid is soluble at a urinary pH of >6.5, once these patients are identified, their stones generally can be prevented by hydration (>2 liters output per day) and by increased urinary alkalization with alkalinizing agents. In patients with hyperuricemia (if renal function is normal) or if the urinary excretion of uric acid is >800 mg daily, allopurinol can be given at a dose of 150–300 mg daily.

Male Infertility

The testes are responsible for spermatogenesis and the secretion of hormones (primarily testosterone). Both functions are controlled by feedback via the hypothalamic-pituitary axis. The initiation of sperm production at puberty requires the presence of both normal luteinizing hormone (LH) and follicle stimulating hormone (FSH) (Fig. 23.4). Luteinizing hormone-releasing hormone (or releasing factor) from the hypothalamus stimulates secretion of LH and FSH from the pituitary. LH then stimulates the Leydig cells of the testicle to produce testosterone. Serum testosterone reduces the secretion of pituitary LH via negative feedback. FSH acts on the Sertoli cells of the seminiferous tubules to produce proteins necessary for spermatogenesis. In combination with other factors, a polypeptide secreted by the Sertoli cell, inhibin, may also influence FSH secretion in a complicated feedback system. The measurement of FSH and LH, as well as testosterone and prolactin, helps to define the etiology of low (oligo) or absent (azo) spermia in the semen analysis.

Factors that result in male infertility are divided into pre-testicular, testicular, and post-testicular. Assignment to one of these groups is made on the basis of history, physical exam, semen analysis, and hormone evaluation.

Pre-testicular infertility is usually the result of abnormal hormone production adversely affecting spermatogenesis. Isolated gonadotropin deficiency or increased production of prolactin can result in abnormal spermatogenesis.

Testicular causes of infertility account for the bulk of male infertility patients. About 40% of this category have a varicocele, and surgical correction may increase sperm production. For another 25% of these patients, cause for the infertility will not be obvious. Their condition is described as idiopathic. These patients often respond to hormonal manipulation (clomiphene citrate [Clomid, Marion Merrell Dow, Kansas City, MO]). The most frequent causes of "testicular infertility" for which a cause can be identified include orchitis, undescended testicles, and toxic effects from such agents as chemotherapy, radiation therapy, or environmental agents.

Post-testicular causes of infertility include problems with delivery of the sperm. They are commonly related to obstructive phenomena. Such patients have vasal agenesis, ejaculatory duct obstruction, prior surgery that has injured the vas, and bilateral epididymitis that has resulted in scarring of the epididymal tubule. These patients are often severely oligospermic or azoospermic. If their testicles exhibit active spermatogenesis, sperm can be retrieved by microaspiration of the epididymis or testicular biopsy and used in association with an in vitro fertilization program.

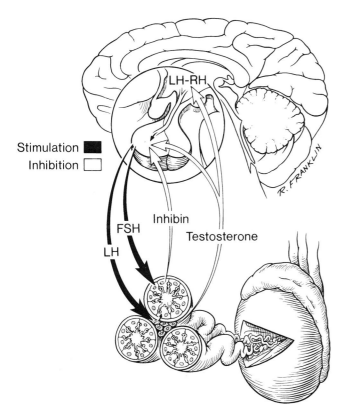

Figure 23.4. The pituitary gonadal axis.

Erectile Dysfunction

Recent advances in the ability to diagnose the pathophysiology of erectile dysfunction have expanded patient options. Detailed evaluation of patients with erectile dysfunction, coupled with individualized treatment, has allowed the majority of patients with organic impotence to return to a satisfactory level of sexual activity.

Testosterone

In patients with demonstrated reduced serum testosterone, exogenous testosterone therapy is warranted, but only when other endocrinopathies associated with reduced testosterone have been excluded. Testosterone enanthate is administered via deep intramuscular injection, in titrated doses. A reasonable beginning dose is 300 mg every 3 weeks.

Pharmacologic Erection Protocols

Pharmacologic erection protocols have won widespread acceptance by patients with erectile dysfunction. Agents that have been used commonly for this purpose without FDA approval include papaverine, regitine, phenoxybenzamine, and prostaglandin E-1. A preparation of prostaglandin E-1 has now been approved for use in intracavernosal injection protocols.

Vacuum Assisted Devices

For some patients with erectile dysfunction, vacuum assisted devices have been effective. Most of these devices consist of plastic cylinders that are fitted over the penis and connected to a pump apparatus that produces a vacuum in the cylinder. The inherent intracorporal pressure converts to tumescence, and a rubber band is placed at the base of the penis to maintain tumescence and whatever rigidity is achieved. Some vascular dilation also appears to be associated with dilation of the corporal bodies. The use of intracorporal injections in association with vacuum assisted devices has been helpful in some cases.

Surgery

In the past, the surgical treatment of terminal erectile dysfunction essentially involved choosing a prosthesis to be implanted. Today, however, other surgical approaches are available, such as revascularization of the penis and surgery for corporal veno-occlusive dysfunction.

Pediatric Urology

Antenatal sonographic imaging has greatly changed management of the fetus with urinary tract abnormalities, and many infants are now born with an already-formulated treatment plan. The developing urinary tract is well visualized by modern sonographic surveillance from approximately 12 weeks of gestation.

Masses

Masses involving the kidney in newborns include Wilms' tumor and congenital mesoblastic nephroma. After appropriate evaluation, both masses should be managed with surgical resection.

Urinary Tract Obstruction and Vesicoureteral Reflux

Because the developing kidney has little to no capacity for concentration of urine, large volumes of dilute urine are produced by the fetal kidney, and many early sonographic images of the urinary tract in gestation raise the question of hydronephrosis or obstruction. However, as gestation proceeds, the physiologic dilation of the urinary tract often diminishes, and antenatal intervention for the fetal urinary tract that is clearly thought to be obstructed remains controversial. If fetal demise is threatened by the absence of amniotic fluid, and there is a picture consistent with bilateral obstruction, usually occurring as a consequence of posterior urethral valves in males, then fetal intervention with a vesicoamniotic shunt may be a reasonable consideration. In most other circumstances, fetal intervention has not proven to be the solution it was once hoped to be. In the child with a suggested urinary tract abnormality, studies should be accomplished in the immediate postnatal period that include another ultrasound and a voiding cystourethrogram. Radionuclide studies to assess obstruction can also be selectively added but offer little information in the immediate postnatal period.

After a particularly stressful delivery, a neonate occasionally experiences transient urinary retention. Greater than 90% of neonates void within the first 24 hours. Those who do not should be evaluated with ultrasound and possibly with a voiding cystourethrogram. In males, high grade infravesical obstruction is the greatest threat to the urinary tract, and immediate attention is necessary to protect neonatal renal function.

Posterior urethral valves generally are managed with neonatal cystoscopy and transurethral ablation of valves. Because of the continued occurrence of urethral stricture associated with neonatal valve ablation, a number of centers continue to advocate immediate treatment with vesicostomy and valve ablation after the child's urinary tract has matured.

The neonatal management of vesicoureteral reflux usually consists of an assessment of renal function with radionuclide imaging and selection of an appropriate course of prophylactic antibiotics. Prevention of an infection allows time for observation of the patient. The indications for surgical management of vesicoureteral reflux are the inability to keep the urinary tract sterile (i.e., breakthrough infections) and/or high volume reflux associated with a bladder with docile storage characteristics.

Recent studies show that the greatest predictor of vesicoureteral reflux resolution is the grade at discovery. Grading of reflux is generally after the Dwoskin/Perlmutter classification. Grade I is low volume reflux that only goes into the ureter. Grade II is reflux of a higher volume, with contrast outlining the entire urinary tract without dilation. Grade III reflux is associated with Grade II findings plus some clubbing of the calyces. Grade IV reflux clearly demonstrates hydronephrosis. In Grade V reflux, the ureters are markedly tortuous and the architecture of the upper tracts is virtually destroyed. The majority of children with Grade III or less at the time of discovery will resolve their reflux in slightly greater than 3 years. Vesicoureteral reflux of a higher grade may ultimately cause renal failure. In Grades IV and V, reflux resolution is far less predictable.

Imaging studies are now sufficiently refined to not only allow for grading of reflux based on the appearance on voiding cystourethrogram, but also on the basis of actual volume refluxed into the upper collecting systems. Short serial studies assessing reflux by both imaging and nuclide analysis help the surgeon when antireflux surgery is necessary. Obstruction of the ureter, either at the ureteropelvic or ureterovesical junction, are assessed by serial ultrasound and radionuclide renography with furosemide. In most of these patients, a voiding cystourethrogram will exclude dilation secondary to reflux. In infants with high grade obstruction, increasing hydronephrosis and declining renal function surgery to protect renal function is indicated.

Spinal Dysraphism

Spinal dysraphism with neurogenic bladder can be diagnosed on antenatal studies. These infants require immediate assessment with ultrasound and a voiding cystourethrogram, which should be scheduled in cooperation with the closure of the myelomeningocele. An important concern in the management of spinal dysraphism is the constantly changing neurologic status. A child who has no hydronephrosis or evidence of reflux at birth can rapidly become a child with marked hydronephrosis, severe neurogenic bladder, and secondary vesicoureteral reflux. If the initial voiding cystourethrogram demonstrates reflux, with or without poor bladder emptying, it may be necessary to initiate intermittent catheterization. These children should also be maintained on prophylactic antibiotics.

In children with spina bifida, regular studies should be done to assess bladder emptying, renal growth, and to monitor the development of hydronephrosis (ultrasound and/or radionuclide scan). Voiding cystourethrogram should also be done to assess reflux.

Embryologic Abnormalities

The development of the male genitalia is a complex embryologic phenomena, and failures of the sequence can cause a variety of abnormalities. The most common lesion encountered is a significantly redundant foreskin and phimosis. If the phimosis does not resolve with gentle retraction of the foreskin during the first years of life, the condition should be treated by circumcision. The first step of the well done neonatal circumcision consists of the takedown of the glanular preputial adhesions, dilation of the preputial skin, and retraction of the skin so that the glans and meatus are visualized completely and examined. If no suspected abnormalities exist, one can proceed with the circumcision.

Circumcision should not be done if any structural abnormality of the penis appears to exist, such as hypospadias or chordee. Hypospadias results from the failure of ventral fusion of the preputial skin, a foreshortened ventrum of the corpora cavernosa, and displacement of the urethral meatus on the ventrum of the penis, proximal to the tip of the glans. Incomplete ventral fusion of the preputial skin is a manifestation of hypospadias; however, the foreskin can be fused ventrally, and lesions of the urethra, including urethral diverticulum, megameatus, or ventral foreshortening of chordee, can exist. The abnormality occurs between the tenth and sixteenth week of gestation. Most theories suggest that it is the result of androgen unresponsiveness during development. The goal of surgery to correct hypospadias is to achieve a straight penis with a durable urethra exiting at the tip of the glans.

Maldescent of the testicles may also be noted at birth. This may affect one or both of the testicles. Premature infants tend to have a higher incidence of testicular maldescent. Testicular descent continues well into the third trimester, and undescended testicles will descend naturally in a number of children early within the first year of life. Therefore, in general, boys born with undescended testicles should be observed for 8 to 9 months with orchiopexy scheduled soon thereafter. However, if bilateral testicular maldescent occurs in concert with an abnormality of the penis, the child should immediately undergo an intersex evaluation. Intersex evaluation includes a karyotype evaluation, an evaluation of the cholesterol to androgen biochemical cascade, and in some cases, imaging studies and/or laparotomy or laparoscopy with gonadal biopsy.

The undescended testicle that fails to reach the scrotum by twelve months of age should be treated surgically. If the testicle is in the canal, inguinal exploration with orchidopexy can be accomplished. No imaging test has been shown to provide consistent localizing information of impalpable, undescended testicles. If examination fails to demonstrate the testis in the canal, it will be necessary to operate on the patient. For both the purpose of localization and for orchiectomy or orchidopexy (in appropriate patients), laparoscopy has proven to be a valuable tool.

The most common cause of gender ambiguity is the adrenogenital syndrome in girls, and possibly in boys as well. Via a number of enzymatic steps, cholesterol becomes both mineral corticoids and glucocorticoids. In the female infant, when the enzymatic blockade alters the synthesis of cortisol and associated hormones, the cascade is swayed towards the production of androgen hormones, leading to virilization. In the male infant, enzymatic blockade interrupts the androgen production, thus leading to inadequate virilization. The initial approach to the infant suspected of adrenogenital syndrome, or any of its variants, is an assessment of the enzymatic cascade, with definition of the enzymatic deficiency and appropriate replacement therapy. This usually includes medications to avoid hypertension, lethal electrolyte disturbances, and inappropriate production of cortisol. The assignment of gender in the child with ambiguous genitalia is a social, and at times a medical, emergency and should be addressed with appropriate exigency.

A second dramatic condition is the exstrophy complex, or cloacal exstrophy. The presentation of classic exstrophy, occurring in 1:30,000 infants, is alarming to physicians as well as parents. The embryology of exstrophy is complex and results from failure of the midline fusion of the myotomes. The etiology of the malfusion is controversial. The exstrophy child is usually otherwise healthy, and an early surgical approach is imperative.

In the classic exstrophy complex, the initial surgical management consists of bladder closure. In the cloacal exstrophy child, the gastrointestinal tract is usually managed by ileostomy, and at a later date, but early in life, the bladder patches are closed as if the classic exstrophy condition existed. After the initial closure, the bladder is intentionally left incontinent. Closure of the bladder is associated with closure of the pelvic bony ring. At later stages, reconstruction is undertaken to treat the epispadiac abnormality of the male penis, bladder neck, and vesicoureteral reflux, which are invariably associated with the exstrophy complex. These procedures are followed with a continuing sequence of operations to improve continence and increase bladder capacity.

Urinary Tract Infection

All anomalies of the urinary tract are heralded by urinary tract infections. Therefore, when a male or nonsexually active female child presents with a urinary tract infection, he or she by definition should be evaluated for other abnormalities. Early intervention unquestionably preserves renal function.

Genitourinary Trauma

Renal injuries are the most common of all urologic injuries. They can be the result of either penetrating or blunt trauma, and they occur in approximately 10% of all blunt injuries to the abdomen. Laceration injuries of the kidney resulting from blunt trauma are usually associated with lower rib fractures or fractures of the lumbar transverse processes. Although the kidney's retroperitoneal location protects it in most circumstances, deceleration injuries can produce enough motion to stretch or even avulse the main renal vessels. Stretching injuries cause disruption of the vascular intima, with subsequent subintimal dissection and secondary thrombosis in the renal artery. Penetrating injuries cause a wide range of injuries of varying severity.

Renal injuries have been divided into four classifications. Grade I is a renal contusion or bruise, Grade II is minor laceration limited to the cortex, Grade III involves a major laceration through the corticomedullary junction, with or without collecting system involvement, and Grade IV involves vascular injuries.

This staging system relies on a complete evaluation of the urinary tract, consisting of a three-tiered approach: clinical evaluation, imaging evaluation, and (when indicated) surgical evaluation and management. For most patients, imaging should be done as the clinical examination alone is unsatisfactory for staging of the injury. The imaging modalities used most often in this situation are the CT scan and/or intravenous urogram. Arteriography and ultrasound are used much less frequently.

The indications for radiographic assessment include gross hematuria, microscopic hematuria associated with shock, clinical suspicion of injury (i.e. fracture of the transverse processes of lumbar vertebra and/or fractures of T_{11} or T_{12} rib), splenic injury, and penetrating injuries with any degree of hematuria. In the pediatric population, the parameters are less well defined, as the child differs in two important ways: the kidneys are larger and more mobile; and the coexistence of a renal anomaly can make the kidney more easily traumatized.

The treatment of renal injuries is mediated by the stage. Grade I and Grade II injuries are self limiting and resolve without treatment. Grade III injuries can follow a more variable course, although certain patients with urinary extravasation have resolved their injuries without the need for surgical intervention. There is increasing enthusiasm for observing these patients. Exceptions would include injuries associated with concomitant injuries requiring exploration, or injuries demonstrated on CT scan to be associated with a large area of devitalized renal tissue.

Ureteral injuries account for approximately 1% of genitourinary trauma, and most are the result of penetrating trauma. Blunt trauma is rarely the cause of ureteral injury, and when it does occur, it is usually in the form of traumatic disruption of the ureteropelvic junction. Traumatic disruption of the ureteropelvic junction is seen far more often in the pediatric population than in the adult population.

Ureteral injuries are often missed, resulting in significant morbidity. No single radiographic assessment is reliable in the assessment of ureteral injuries, and the best evaluation is provided by direct examination of the course of the ureter while the patient is being explored for other purposes. Intravenous urogram and computed tomography will often, but not always, show extravasation. Retrograde pyelography provides excellent visualization, but it is frequently impractical in patients with penetrating trauma and other associated injuries. If the patient has no other reason for exploration, cystoscopy with retrograde pyelography is the imaging modality of choice.

Bladder injuries can occur as a result of either penetrating or blunt trauma. Bladder injuries are classified as extraperitoneal (60%), intraperitoneal (30%), or both (10%). Eighty-five percent of bladder injuries are associated with pelvic fracture, and 10% of pelvic fractures are associated with bladder injury. Therefore, bladder injuries should be suspected in all patients with pelvic fracture, all patients with hematuria, or any patient with a mechanism of injury that suggests the potential for bladder or urethral injury.

The diagnostic study of choice for evaluation of bladder injury is the trauma cystogram. A trauma cystogram involves instillation of at least 300 cc of contrast with multiple projections and complete drainage films. The cystogram on CT scan has not been shown to be a reliable alternative to the trauma cystogram.

Posterior urethral distraction injuries occur almost exclusively with pelvic fracture, with 5%–10% of pelvic fractures resulting in posterior urethral distraction injuries. In pelvic fracture, the bladder and prostate tend to travel with the bones as they are displaced, whereas the anterior urethra remains relatively fixed, distracting the relatively weak membranous urethra. Long term sequelae of pelvic fracture and posterior urethral distraction are impotence and, in some patients, incontinence. Signs associated with posterior urethral distraction include the presence of blood at the urethral meatus and an impalpable or ''high-riding'' prostate on rectal examination.

The treatment of posterior urethral distraction injury typically consists of placement of suprapubic urinary diversion. In addition, with the advent of flexible endoscopic techniques, the placement of an aligning catheter is much easier and has proven beneficial. Neither an aligning catheter nor a suprapubic diversion prevent obliteration of the urethra. However, in many patients, distraction injury does not completely disrupt the continuity of the urethra, and in those patients, an aligning catheter can make the difference between a stricture that is readily manageable by conservative techniques and one that needs complex open reconstruction.

Anterior urethral injuries can be classified as either contusions or disruptions. The location depends on the angle of the patient as the perineum impacts an immovable object. The immovable object acts as a hammer and the pubis acts as an anvil, resulting in injury to the tissues that lie in between. Patients who have sustained straddle perineal trauma should be evaluated with retrograde urethrography just as in the case of suspected posterior urethral distraction. Many of these injuries can be managed initially with placement of an indwelling urethral catheter. In most cases, anterior urethral injuries resulting from penetrating trauma mandate exploration, debridement, and immediate reconstruction.

Trauma to the external genitalia has been classified by Culp as either non-penetrating, penetrating, avulsion, burns, or radiation injuries. The most common non-penetrating injuries are penile or scrotal contusion. Testicular fracture occurs from non-penetrating trauma, and scrotal ultrasound differentiates a scrotal contusion from a fractured testicle.

A unique non-penetrating injury in the male is the corporal or penile fracture. This occurs with buckling of the penis during intercourse. When the injury disrupts the tunica albuginea of the corpora along with Buck's fascia, findings of immediate detumescence associated with ecchymosis and a hematoma collection in the penis are noted. Many patients either disrupt only one layer of the tunica albuginea or both layers of the tunica without disrupting Buck's fascia. Although these patients do not have the dramatic findings of the classic patient with penile fracture, the sequelae of indentation and curvature of the penis can be seen. Because urethral injury can be associated with injury to the corpora cavernosa, this possibility should be evaluated.

Penetrating injuries to the external genitalia can range from simple injuries to amputation of the penis and/or scrotum and testicles. In simpler penetrating injuries, debridement and anatomic reconstruction are the preferred treatment approach. Microsurgical replantation is the treatment of choice for amputation injuries.

Avulsion injuries can be dramatic in appearance. Unique to the male genitalia, the tissues of the scrotum, penis, and underlying elastic fascial structures are integral to this injury. Avulsion injuries occur when these tissues become entangled, usually in clothing, and are torn off with the clothing, leaving behind the deep structures of the penis and often the denuded testicles. After an avulsion injury, there should be a period of observation to clarify the extent of the injury. Urethral and rectal examination should be accomplished. Reconstruction can be undertaken approximately 12–24 hours after presentation.

Burn injuries to the genitalia are treated the same as burn injuries to the rest of the body. Debridement of the penis should be executed carefully. Aggressive debridement of the penis usually is not needed due to the unique vascular characteristics of the penis. Urethral injuries must be dealt with later after healing of the burn. Diversion of urine during the acute phase may be indicated. A suprapubic tube can be placed through burned tissue without concern.

Fortunately, as enthusiasm for treatment of genital neoplasm with radiation has waned, direct radiation injuries to the genitalia are no longer seen. However, the genitalia can be involved with ''malignant'' edema associated with radiotherapy of the pelvis. These patients' injuries are reconstructible with excision of the edematous tissues and with grafting to the deep structures of the penis and testicles with a split thickness skin graft. The use of local flaps and/or full thickness skin are associated with significant reaccumulation of edema in these tissues. Because split thickness skin grafts will not become edematous, they are the graft of choice for reconstruction of radiation edema.

Bent Penis

Congenital

Curvature of the penis can be either congenital or acquired. The most frequent cause of congenital curvature of the penis is hypospadias. The constellation of congenital curvatures associated with hyperdistensibility of the corporal bodies is the second most frequent cause of congenital curvature of the penis. These curvatures can be either ventral, lateral (left), dorsal, or complex. The least common congenital curvature of the penis is the dorsal curvature associated with epispadias/exstrophy.

The curvature of hypospadias is believed to be caused by the presence of dysgenic tethering tissue on the ventrum of the penis and/or dissymmetric development of the ventral and dorsal surfaces. Correction of curvature of the penis caused by hypospadias involves resection of the dysgenetic tissue. If resection proves inadequate, shortening of the opposite dorsal side allows for straightening.

In congenital curvatures of the penis associated with hyperdistensibility of the corpora, the flaccid penis is of average size, but the erect penis becomes impressively large. Curvature results in this congenital defect if dyssymmetry exists in the expansion of one aspect of the corpora compared to another. Techniques to lengthen the short side of the penis have involved grafting of a corporotomy defect, which potentially has ill effects on the erectile mechanism. Therefore, because length of penis is usually not a problem with these patients, techniques to shorten the longer, opposite, side are favored over techniques that lengthen the shorter side.

Length is a common complaint of patients with dorsal curvature caused by exstrophy/epispadias complex. For these patients, the curvature is treated by excision of the dysgenetic dorsal tissues, and lengthening of the dorsal aspect with the creation of a corporotomy defect and grafting. These curvatures can also be corrected by rolling the corpora laterally, resulting in cancellation of the curvature and relative straightening of the penis.

Acquired

Acquired curvature of the penis is usually a result of buckling trauma. In the young individual, buckling trauma leads either to true or subclinical fracture of the corporal body. In the bilaminar tunica albuginea, there is an inner circular and an outer longitudinal layer of fibers. With buckling, the outer layer can be disrupted, while the blood tight integrity of the corpus is maintained by the intact, inner, circular layer. These patients do not experience the classic symptoms of pain, snapping, and immediate detumescence with hematoma. However, within days to weeks, they notice a bend and indentation at the site of the trauma.

With true fracture of the corpus, both layers of the tunica, and often Buck's fascia, are disrupted. These patients also notice curvature with indentation at the site of trauma within days to weeks. Pre-existing lateral curvature of the penis is thought to be a predisposing cause of fracture or subclinical fracture of the penis. Although the injury actually serves to straighten the penis in these patients, the indentation at the site of injury may be disabling in that it leads to easy buckling of the penis with intercourse.

In the older man, buckling trauma leads to Peyronie's disease. In these men, buckling trauma tends to occur in a dorsal, ventral direction as opposed to a lateral one. This places stress at the site of the implantation of the septal fibers, leading to disruption of the fibers as they interweave with the tunica albuginea, and/or a delamination injury at the site of the dorsal or ventral interweaving of the septal fibers of the inner lamina of the tunica albuginea. In the predisposed individual, the inflammatory phase that follows leads to scarring and functional tethering of the involved aspect of the penis.

Acute treatment for acquired curvatures involves reassurance and medical therapy. Although a number of oral agents have been used, none have been demonstrated to be effective via good double-blind drug studies. The most frequently used oral agents are vitamin E, Potaba, antihistamines, nonsteroidal inflammatory agents, and colchicine. A number of intralesional injection protocols have been used, including: injection of steroid, injection of collagenase, and injection of calcium channel blockers. The injection of steroids is ineffective. The effects of intralesional injection with collagenase and calcium channel blockers are currently the topic of study protocols. Ultrasound therapy with steroids (iontophoresis) has enjoyed some enthusiasm, but its efficacy has also not been proven in well-designed clinical trials.

Radiotherapy has been used at some centers during the inflammatory phase of the acquired curvatures of the penis. Used as a means of delivering anti-inflammatory therapy, it may be effective in shortening the painful stage of acquired curvature, but it has no effect on the curvature itself.

The surgical management of acquired curvatures involves either shortening the long side or lengthening the short side of the penis. Synthetic graft materials have also been used to fill the corporotomy defect, but their use is discouraged without concomitant use of a prosthesis. However, if erectile dysfunction coincides with a disabling curvature, it is acceptable to place a prosthesis, incising the area of scar, and filling the defect with either autologous or synthetic graft material. In some cases, when a prosthesis is to be placed (with Peyronie's disease in particular), the penis can be straightened by a technique termed "corporal remodeling." Corporal remodeling involves cracking or stretching of the scarred area after the prosthesis is placed, with the inherent straightening characteristics of the prosthesis then serving to splint the straightened penis.

Evaluation and Management of Benign Prostatic Disease

Benign prostatic hypertrophy (BPH), or proliferation of the epithelium and stromal components of the prostate, afflicts the majority of men after the age of 50 years. Although histologic evidence of BPH is found in 90% of men over the age of 50, the clinical manifestations are found in only 50%.

Although approximately 5% of men receive some form of intervention for the symptoms of prostatism, with the development of medical therapy for these symptoms, the incidence of surgical intervention has decreased. However, the number of patients treated overall will most likely continue to increase because of the availability of less invasive means to get symptomatic relief.

Prostatism is believed to be secondary to two factors: one static and the other dynamic. The dynamic factor has been recognized more recently; it is descriptive of increased tone at the area of the bladder neck and base, which leads to obstructive symptoms. There is a predominance of alpha receptors at the bladder base and neck, and an increase in either the number or sensitivity of these receptors leads to an increase in the resistance to urinary flow. One of the current therapies for prostatism is the administration of alpha blockers. Alpha blockers, developed as antihypertensive medications, are clinically useful for bladder neck relaxation.

The static component of prostatism results from epithelial and stromal hypertrophy, causing an increase in the volume of the prostate that impinges on the prostatic urethral lumen, producing mechanical obstruction. Although epithelial and stromal hypertrophy that occurs with aging are undoubtedly related to an alteration in the hormonal milieu, the precise alteration and its relative effects have not been defined. Five-alpha reductase is an enzyme that converts testosterone to dihydrotestosterone. Dihydrotestosterone is fifty times more potent than testosterone and is the dominant hormone in prostatic development. Males who are 5-alpha reductase

deficient, a genetic defect recognized in families in the Dominican Republic, do not develop prostatic enlargement with aging, and blockade of the conversion of testosterone to dihydrotestosterone is believed to reverse the process of prostatic hypertrophy in some individuals without adverse effects. Randomized trials are now in progress with finasteride, a 5-alpha reductase inhibitor, for the pharmacologic treatment of the static component of prostatism.

Mandatory indications for treatment of prostatism and prostatic hypertrophy include azotemia, recurrent urinary tract infections, recurrent hematuria, and urinary retention. However, these symptoms occur infrequently, and the indications for treatment of prostatism generally involve evaluation of the degree to which symptoms interfere with the patient's lifestyle.

Recently published guidelines for the diagnosis and treatment of BPH recommend transurethral resection. In addition, a number of less invasive procedures have recently been introduced, including: thermal therapy, laser and radial frequency ablation, transurethral incision of the prostate, balloon dilation of the prostate, insertion of implantable prostatic stents, and high intensity focused ultrasound. The place these modalities will eventually take in standard treatment guidelines is yet to be determined.

Evaluation and Treatment of Genitourinary Tumors

Adrenal Gland Carcinoma

With an incidence of one per 1.5 million, adrenocortical carcinoma is rare. These tumors can occur at any age, but they are seen most often in the fifth to seventh decade. Women are afflicted more commonly than males and the tumor is on the left more commonly than on the right. Adrenocortical tumors often reach a large size before they are diagnosed and are variably endocrinologically active. In general, endocrine activity reflects a certain degree of differentiation. If little evidence exists of endocrine activity, the tumor is more likely a poorly differentiated lesion and is associated with a poor prognosis.

Approximately 50% of patients present with symptoms of excess cortisol production, central obesity, plethora, hirsutism, and acne. At the time of diagnosis, these tumors have commonly metastasized to the retroperitoneal nodes, liver, or lungs. Increased androgen production may cause sterilization in about 15%–20% of female patients.

Computed tomography and magnetic resonance imaging procedures appear equally effective in demonstrating adrenal tumors. Laboratory evaluation usually shows increased urinary 17-hydro corticosteroids, and

17-ketosteroids are often significantly elevated in patients with carcinoma. Adrenocorticotrophic hormone (ACTH) assays are now available, and a low ACTH level with a high cortisol production is indicative of a tumor.

Surgery is the only effective therapy for localized tumors. Once metastases have occurred, although some patients may respond to mitotane ($o_1$1-DDD) therapy, the prognosis is poor.

Renal Neoplasms

Renal Cell Carcinoma

Renal cell carcinoma arises from the cells of the proximal collecting tubule. There are 27,000 of these tumors diagnosed each year in the United States, and 11,000 patients die of this cancer each year. Although its etiology is unknown, it has been linked to tobacco use, and recent studies have suggested genetic defect. The study of familial and sporadic cases of renal cell carcinoma have linked its etiology to a loss of the short arm of chromosome 3. Von Hippel-Lindau syndrome is an example of familial renal cell carcinoma, which is characterized by multiple tumors, bilateral tumors, and occurrence at a young age.

In the past, the most common presenting complex of signs and symptoms leading to an evaluation for possible renal cell carcinoma were flank pain, gross hematuria, and renal mass. This was often referred to as the "too late triad." Since the advent of computed tomography, however, an increasing number of renal cell carcinomas are found incidentally during evaluation of other symptoms. Patients whose tumors are detected incidentally typically have smaller tumors of a lower stage and a greater likelihood for surgical cure.

Renal cell carcinoma tends to invade the renal vein and can extend to the vena cava and right atrium. It may present with various manifestations of paraneoplastic syndromes, including polycythemia, anemia, hypercalcemia, and liver function abnormalities. These syndromes resolve with surgical extirpation.

The primary treatment for renal cell carcinoma is radical nephrectomy. However, because smaller tumors are now being detected by incidental CT imaging, more patients are being considered for partial nephrectomy. Unfortunately, options are limited for the treatment of metastatic renal cell carcinoma. Chemotherapy has been unsuccessful in most cases. Since renal cell carcinoma has been associated with spontaneous regression, several biologic therapies have been tested using IL-2 interferon, cellular therapy [lymphokine activated killer (LAK) cells], or tumor infiltrating infiltrates. Long term responses have been achieved in 10%–20% of patients with metastatic disease.

Angiomyolipoma

Angiomyolipoma is a relatively common, benign tumor that does not metastasize. Tuberous sclerosis is associated with bilateral or multiple angiomyolipoma. In the absence of tuberous sclerosis, the lesions are usually solitary, unilateral, and with a female preponderance. Angiomyolipoma presents clinically with hematuria and is often detected by CT scans done for other reasons. The characteristic kids of fat within the mass differentiates it from renal cell carcinoma by CT scan or ultrasound. If the tumor is less than 4 cm in size and is asymptomatic, it can be followed. Surgery is appropriate if hemorrhage is present or if the size exceeds 4 cm in diameter.

Wilms' Tumor

Wilms' tumor is a malignant renal tumor that occurs predominantly in children, although it can appear in adolescents and adults. The incidence is the same for males and females. Approximately 5% are bilateral at the time of diagnosis. An abnormality of chromosome 11 has been reported in patients with a Wilms' tumor. Histology is associated with a poor prognosis if the predominate cell type is anaplastic, rhabdoid, or of the clear cell variant.

Chemotherapy has had a dramatic impact on the survival of children with Wilms' tumors. The National Wilms' Tumor Project has systematically studied the effects of chemotherapy and radiotherapy combined with surgery. Treatment protocols have been modified to produce the least possible morbidity with the best possible cure rate.

Transitional Cell Carcinoma of the Bladder

Each year, 50,000 cases of bladder cancer are diagnosed in the United States with 10,000 deaths being attributed to this disease. Over 90% of tumors are of a transitional cell variety. The etiology of bladder cancers has been attributed to tobacco use. In countries with lax regulation on its chemical industries, chemical carcinogens are thought to be causative in a much larger number of cases. Artificial sweeteners have been implicated as an etiologic factor, but this relationship has not been confirmed. Nontransitional bladder cancer is a result of metaplastic dedifferentiation of the multipotential urothelium towards squamous and/or adenomatous histology. Squamous cell carcinoma, secondary to the irritative infestation of the bladder by a parasite (Schistosoma haematobium) is a unique form of bladder cancer found in the Nile River Delta.

The most frequent presenting symptom of bladder cancer is gross hematuria. Other important symptoms are bladder irritability and dysuria. In patients who are older than 40 years with negative urine cultures or without prior history of urinary tract infections, a detailed urologic evaluation should be given. This should include evaluation of the upper tract, urinary cytology, and cystoscopy. Microscopic hematuria should be evaluated similarly. The greatest delay in the diagnosis of bladder cancer is treatment with prolonged courses of antibiotics for presumed urinary tract infections.

The critical staging distinction for transitional cell carcinoma of the bladder is invasion of the muscular wall of the bladder. Superficial tumors involve only the mucosa and submucosa. The loss of chromosome 9-P has been found in superficial tumors, whereas tumors that invade the muscle are characterized by the additional loss of chromosome 17. These patients also have alterations in the retinoblastoma (RB) suppressor gene, loss of P-53, and mutations in epidermal growth factor receptors (EGFR). Seventy-five percent of bladder tumors are superficial on presentation. Of this group, approximately 50% recur, and approximately 20% progress to disease with muscle invasion.

Superficial tumors are managed by transurethral resection and fulguration, and by a variety of adjuvant intravesical agents directed at reducing recurrences and decreasing the possibility of the muscular invasion. Intravesical agents used in the past have included a number of chemotherapeutic agents (thiotepa, adriamycin, and mitomycin) and immunologic or biologic agents (most commonly Bacille Calmette Guérin [BCG]).

Muscle invasive transitional cell carcinoma may be treated by a variety of options. Partial cystectomy is used for tumors that are solitary and localized to a portion of the bladder that lends itself to extirpation (usually the dome). External beam radiation therapy is reserved for patients in poor health or of increased age. Radical cystectomy should be employed in most cases of invasive disease. Until recently, radical cystectomy implied the need for external urinary drainage. Over the past decade, advances in the understanding of the mechanics of reconfigured bowel have permitted reconstruction of continent urinary reservoirs and orthotopic bladders that avoid the need for external appliances. Protocols combining radiation with surgery, chemotherapy with radiation, and chemotherapy with surgery in a neoadjuvant or adjuvant fashion are under investigation.

Because patients with transitional cell carcinoma of the bladder are at increased risk for development of tumors of the renal pelvis and ureter, periodic radiologic and cytologic monitoring are mandatory.

Carcinoma of the Prostate

Over 240,000 new cases of carcinoma of the prostate and 40,500 related deaths occur yearly in the United States. Carcinoma of the prostate is now the most common cancer in men. The incidence of prostate cancer is directly proportional to age. About 30% of men in their seventh decade will have the disease. This figure increases to two-thirds of men in their eighth decade. There appears to be a genetic predisposition to development of prostate cancer. A family history of the disease in a first order relative increases the risk, particularly if the cancer was diagnosed in a relative under 65 years of age. Caucasian men in the United States have a 1:11 chance of developing the disease, whereas African-American men have a 1:9 chance. When prostate cancer occurs in African-American men, it tends to occur earlier in life and has a more aggressive course.

In addition to age and genetic predisposition, hormonal factors, diet, environment, and possibly infection may play roles in the development of prostate cancers. Prostate cancer has not been observed in eunuchs, and the presence of testosterone appears to be required for the tumor to develop. Testosterone is known to stimulate prostate cells and cause the development of prostate cancers in rats. The supposition that environment and/or diet may be causative is supported by the fact that the incidence of prostate cancer in Japan is 10% of that in the United States. Second and third generation Japanese-Americans are known to develop the disease at rates comparable to American Caucasians. Studies suggest that a high fat diet, exposure to cadmium, or infections with various viral or bacterial agents may predispose the male population to the development of prostate cancer. However, no cause and effect relationship has been demonstrated.

Prostate cancers are adenocarcinomas and arise from the acinar cells. Seventy percent of tumors arise in the peripheral zone of the prostate gland, 15%–20% arise in the central zone, and 10%–15% arise in the transition zone.

Tumor grading is an important factor in the prognosis of prostate cancer. The Gleason grading system has supplanted older systems. In this system, the pathologist assigns two grades to the cancer based on a major and minor pattern of glandular differentiation. Tumors arising in the prostate spread by local extension and lymphatic metastasis. When spreading locally, they may invade either through the capsule at the apex or base or at the seminal vesicles. Metastases tend to follow a predictable pattern, with early metastases occurring in the internal iliac and obturator nodal bed. Subsequent metastasis to bone can include the lumbar spine, pelvis, proximal femur, thoracic spine, ribs, sternum, and skull. Metastases to the liver, spleen, and brain occur rarely, and generally only in advanced disease.

Prostate specific antigen (PSA) is a glycoprotein produced by the acinar cells of the prostate whose function is liquefaction of semen. The older marker, prostatic acid phosphatase, has now been supplanted largely by PSA. PSA is not specific for carcinoma. Elevations have been observed in prostatitis and prostatic infarction. However, PSA is helpful in diagnosis and is indispensable for the follow-up of patients who have undergone definitive treatment for prostate cancer. Normal values range from 0 to 4.0 ng/dl, although age-specific ranges have also been suggested.

In select patients, CT scans of the pelvis may demonstrate nodal metastasis. After staging, localized disease may be treated by external beam radiotherapy, interstitial implantation with radioactive iodine or palladium, or radical surgery via the retropubic or perineal route. In elderly patients with concomitant medical problems and an expected life span of less than 10 years, no treatment may be recommended. Patients with symptomatic metastatic disease should be treated with hormonal therapy, most often luteinizing hormone-releasing hormone (LH-RH) agonist, with or without concomitant antiandrogens. Spot radiotherapy to localized symptomatic lesions or SR89, a radioisotope, may be helpful in managing late stage disease.

Primary Urethral Cancer

Primary urethral cancer is extremely rare. Tumors occur more often in whites than in non-whites, and they present most commonly between the ages of 50 and 70 years.

In men, the majority of tumors are squamous cell carcinoma, with transitional cell carcinoma and adenocarcinoma appearing less frequently. The tumor site generally reflects the site of origin (for example, transitional cell carcinoma is predominant in the prostatic urethra). In women, squamous cell carcinoma is also the most commonly encountered, with transitional cell, adenocarcinoma, and melanoma next in frequency.

The staging system most commonly used for these tumors is the AJC TNM (American Joint Committee, Tumors, Nodes, Metastases) system. The survival of both male and female patients with tumors in the distal urethra is significantly better than those with more proximal urethral lesions. In both men and women, tumors presenting in the distal urethra tend to be of a lower grade and stage than more proximal lesions.

For small superficial lesions, treatment includes excision, laser therapy, and radiotherapy. For larger lesions, partial or total penectomy or anterior exenteration may be required. Large tumors are unresponsive to radiation, and nodal involvement implies a poor prognosis. Chemotherapy and immunotherapy have been largely ineffective for primary urethral cancer.

Malignant Tumors of the Testis

Malignant tumors of the testis are rare, with only two to three cases per 100,000 men reported each year. They occur most often in young men between the ages of 17 and 30. The etiology of testis tumors is unknown, but a close association exists with cryptorchidism. In the patient with the cryptorchidic testicle in the abdomen, the relative risk of developing a neoplasm is 1:20, whereas if the cryptorchidic testicle is in the inguinal canal, the relative risk is 1:80. Orchidopexy is not thought to alter the risk of neoplasm.

Approximately 95% of testis tumors arise in the germ cells, and the remainder are nongerminal (Sertoli cell, Leydig cell, or gonadoblastoma). There are five types of germinal tumors: seminoma, teratoma, teratocarcinoma, embryonal cell carcinoma, and choriocarcinoma. Because cell type is an important consideration in treatment, tumors are classified as either seminomas or non-seminomatous germ cell tumors.

Seminomatous Germ Cell Tumors

Seminoma is the most common tumor type, comprising 35% of all testis tumors. Syncytiotrophoblastic elements are seen in 10%–15% of classical seminomas, corresponding to the incidence of beta human chorionic gonadotropin (hCG) production in these tumors. Approximately 5%–10% of seminomas are classified as anaplastic. These tumors tend to present with a higher stage than classic seminomas, but they have a similar stage for stage prognosis. Another 5%–10% of seminomas are classified as spermatocytic. These tumors occur more commonly in patients older than 50 years of age.

Nonseminomatous Germ Cell Tumors

Embryonal cell carcinoma constitutes 20% of all germinal cell tumors. Two sub-types are seen: adult, and the juvenile embryonal cell tumor or yolk sac tumor. Teratomas contain more than one germ cell layer in various stages of maturation. Teratocarcinoma is actually a mixed cell tumor, composed of teratoma and embryonal cell carcinoma. Seminoma may also comprise part of a mixed germ cell tumor. Mixed tumors constitute 35%–40% of all testis tumors, and treatment is based on the most malignant component.

Testicular ultrasound is helpful in determining the nature of scrotal masses. Beta hCG, elaborated by the syncytiotrophoblastic cells, is commonly elevated in non-seminomatous tumors. It is also elevated in a small percentage of seminomas. Alpha feta protein is elaborated by juvenile embryonal tissues and is never present in seminoma. LDH, particularly LDH isoenzyme-1, may reflect tumor burden in some non-seminomatous germ cell tumors. After histologic diagnosis has been established by orchiectomy, careful staging with chest radiograph and CT scan in combination with markers should be done. A number of staging systems have been proposed. The tumor staging system used at Memorial Sloan-Kettering Cancer Center has been applied most widely, whereas the UICC/A.C. TNM system has not been as clinically useful.

Testicular tumors tend to metastasize to the retroperitoneal lymph nodes around the renal hilum. The exception is choriocarcinoma, which often spreads by hematogenous routes. Initial treatment is inguinal orchiectomy for all stages. Treatment of low stage seminomas is with radiation therapy. Non-seminomatous germ cell tumors and bulky metastatic seminomas are treated with retroperitoneal lymph node dissection, with or without adjuvant multi-drug chemotherapy.

The choice of therapy depends on the pathology and extent of disease.

Cancer of the Penis

Cancer of the penis presents in the sixth decade and is usually associated with poor hygiene. The disease is almost unheard of in cultures where infant circumcision is practiced. It is rare in the United States, but in parts of Africa and South American it comprises up to 20% of male genital tumors.

Most penile cancers are squamous cell tumors that first appear as raised ulcers with an indurated base. Verrucous carcinomas are a variant of squamous cell carcinoma, seen in 10%–15% of patients. These lesions predominate on the glans and may be ulcerative or papillary. Carcinoma-in-situ, known as erythroplasia of Queyrat, may present on the glans or prepuce.

Treatment of the primary lesion is surgical. This usually involves local excision, laser therapy, and/or penile amputation. Enlarged inguinal nodes should be treated with a 6-week course of antibiotic therapy and then reassessed. If they resolve, careful follow-up is indicated. If the enlarged nodes persist, inguinal and pelvic node dissection may be curative.

Tumor spread occurs via the superficial and deep inguinal nodes and subsequently the pelvic nodes. Involvement of the pelvic nodes generally implies a worse prognosis. Distant metastases are unusual, and death is usually caused by infection and hemorrhage resulting from groin involvement. Distant metastatic disease generally has a poor response to chemotherapy, and the prognosis is poor.

Summary

A brief compendium of urology and the urinary system were presented in this chapter. Complex imaging and endourologic techniques have been available to the urologic surgeon for a number of years. Therefore, it is unusual for genitourinary surgery to be exploratory in nature. The genitourinary surgeon generally has an excellent appreciation of the type and extent of the disease process before approaching the operating table and an excellent idea of the prognosis early in the course of treatment.

SUGGESTED READINGS

Bosniak MA. The small (<3.0 cm) renal parenchyma tumor: Detection, diagnosis and controversies. Radiology 1991;179:307–317.

Bosnik MA, Retik AB, guest ed. Pediatric urinary tact obstruction. Urol Clin North Am 1990;17(2):247–447.

Horstman WG, Meadleton WD, Nelson GL, et al. Color doppler ultrasound of the scrotum. Radiographics 1991;11:941–959.

Howards S. Treatment of male infertility. New Engl J Med 1995;332(5): 312–317.

Kelalis PP, King LR, Belman AB, eds. Clinical pediatric urology. Vol. 1, 2. Philadelphia: W.B. Saunders, 1985.

King LR. Pediatric urologic surgery, section XI. In Walsh PC, Retik AB, Stamey TA, et al. Campbell's urology. 6th ed. Philadelphia: WB Saunders Company, 1992:1687–2002.

King LR, ed. Urologic surgery in neonates and young infants. Philadelphia: WB Saunders Company, 1988.

Lipschultz L, Howards S, eds. Infertility in the male. 2nd ed. St. Louis: Mosby Year Book, 1990.

Mitchell DG, Crovello M, Matteuui T. Benign adrenal cortical masses: Diagnosis with chemical shift imaging. Radiology 1992;185:339–340.

Sigman M. Assisted reproductive techniques and male infertility. Urol Clin North Am, 1994;21(3):505–515.

24 Anesthesia

Mack A. Thomas / *James M. Riopelle*

Anesthesia is the loss of sensation in a part of the body or in the entire body, generally induced by the administration of a drug. The choice of anesthetic technique is usually referred to by the terms *general* and *conductive* anesthesia. General anesthesia is associated with the loss of consciousness. Conductive anesthesia refers to the administration of an agent in an anatomically appropriate site so that painful sensation is interrupted. An adequate anesthetic state is characterized by minimal response to painful stimuli and is indicated by stability of the cardiovascular and respiratory systems. Adequate reflex blockade prevents troublesome cardiovascular, respiratory, and gastrointestinal responses. Because of the nature of this chapter, the basic pathophysiologic discussions will be tied closely with clinical applications in the anesthetized patient.

Theories of General Anesthesia

How general anesthetics produce their effect is the subject of much discussion. The elements of general anesthesia frequently described include amnesia, analgesia, inhibition of noxious reflexes, and skeletal muscle relaxation. A single theory explaining these various effects will be fraught with varying deficiencies.

Volatile agents are believed to produce general anesthesia by modulating synaptic function from within cell membranes. Volatile anesthetics depress excitatory transmission regardless of the specific neurotransmitter. Sodium and chloride channels may be affected by volatile agents. Few data exist to support the theory that volatile anesthetics affect synthesis, release, or binding of neurotransmitters. No particular region of the brain is solely responsible for the pharmacologic control of consciousness or all of the central nervous system elements of general anesthesia.

All discussions of anesthetic mechanisms acknowledge the observations of the Meyer-Overton lipid solubility theory. Lipid solubility correlates directly with potency of anesthetic drugs. It is believed that the primary actions of anesthetics occur in the lipid portion of all membranes.

Drug receptor interactions have been described for most of the intravenous drugs used in anesthesia. Opioids work by occupying opiate receptors in the brain and spinal cord. Analgesia results from the modulation of peptide functions (endorphins and enkephalins) that are endogenous ligands for opiate receptors.

Neurotransmitters may have either inhibitory or excitatory properties. τ-aminobutyric acid (GABA) is the major inhibitory neurotransmitter in the brain, and glycine is the major inhibitory neurotransmitter in the spinal cord. Glutamate is the major excitatory neurotransmitter in the brain. Data have accumulated supporting the concept that several aspects of anesthesia may result from modulation of GABA function (1). Benzodiazepines, barbiturates, and other intravenous drugs have been shown to enhance inhibitory tone mediated by GABA. When benzodiazepines bind to specific receptors that are contingent to the GABA receptor, inhibitory tone is enhanced. Similar barbiturate receptors are adjacent to GABA receptors, and the barbiturate receptor occupied is thought to enhance the inhibitory tone of GABA. This is believed to account for the sedative and anticonvulsant effects of these drugs.

Pharmacology

To appreciate basic concepts, several principles of pharmacology must be reviewed. Pharmacokinetics describe how a drug is absorbed, distributed, and eliminated from the body. Pharmacodynamics refer to the relative potency of a drug and are often related to a blood or tissue concentration necessary to evoke a given response. A receptor is the component of a cell or organ that interacts with the drug leading to the pharmacologic effect. Receptors determine selectivity and the quantitative relationship between dose and effect. An agonist regulates the function of the receptor molecule as a direct result of the drug binding to it. An antagonist binds to the receptor without directly altering the receptor function and prevents an agonist from stimulating the receptor to function. Two types of antagonism are identified. Competitive antagonism occurs when increasing concentrations of the antagonist progressively inhibit the response to a fixed concentration of agonist. Noncompetitive antagonism occurs when, after administration of an antagonist, increasing concentration of agonists cannot overcome antagonism.

Tissue Uptake

The capacity of tissue uptake of drugs is governed by organ blood flow, concentration gradient, and physicochemical properties of the drug. Approximately 70% of cardiac output is directed to the brain, kidney, liver, lung, and heart, which are termed the vessel-rich group. These highly perfused tissues receive a high concentration of the total dose of drug administered. As the plasma concentration decreases, drugs leave these tissues to be delivered to less perfused sites, which will initiate termination of the clinical effects of the drug. The rapid entry and rapid egress of such drugs are related to their lipid solubility and are termed redistribution. Redistribution accounts for the rapid onset and short duration of action of hypnotic drugs.

Cell membranes are lipid structures, and the lipid solubility is an important factor in the ability of a drug to diffuse across cell membranes. Most drugs are weak bases or weak acids and present as ionized and nonionized molecules in solutions. Nonionized drug is usually lipid soluble and is the active portion pharmacologically. The degree of ionization of a given drug is a function of its dissociation constant (K_a) and the pH of surrounding fluid. If the K_a and pH are identical, then 50% of the drug exists in the ionized form. Relatively small pH changes may cause significant changes in ionization. Acid drugs such as barbiturates tend to be highly ionized at an alkaline pH, as opposed to basic drugs such as local anesthetics and opioids that are highly ionized at an acid pH.

Protein binding has a significant effect on drug action because only free or unbound drug can cross cell membranes. Drug clearance is influenced by protein because it is the unbound portion that is accessible to hepatic metabolism and renal excretion. Acidic drugs tend to bind to albumin, whereas basic drugs bind with α_1-acid glycoprotein. Protein binding generally parallels lipid solubility.

Drug Distribution

The volume of distribution (V_d) is the parameter that governs the extent of drug distribution. Physiologically, the factor that governs the extent of drug distribution is the tissue capacity for a drug versus the capacity of blood for that drug. Tissue capacity is a function of the total tissue volume into which a drug distributes. The following equation presents an arithmetic approach: V_d = total amount of drug/concentration (2). If a drug is distributed extensively, then the concentration is lower, meaning it has a larger volume of distribution. Clinically, this means if a drug has a large volume of distribution, then a larger loading dose is required to achieve the same concentration as another drug with a small volume of distribution.

Drug Clearance

Drug clearance primarily depends on hepatic metabolism, renal elimination, or both. Most drugs given in therapeutic dose ranges are cleared from plasma at a rate proportional to the amount of drug present. If a constant plasma concentration of drug is desired, they must be administered at a rate equal to the clearance.

Drug Response

Drug response is affected not only by hepatic and renal function but also by cardiac function, age, enzyme activity, and genetic differences. Reduction in cardiac output will decrease renal and hepatic blood flow, causing delays in clearance. Lidocaine used to suppress cardiac dysrhythmias may reach toxic levels in patients with cardiac failure if doses are not reduced. Immaturity of the renal and hepatic systems in the newborn may result in toxic levels if conventional doses are administered. Geriatric patients may exhibit decreased renal function, decreased cardiac output, reduced protein binding, and an enlarged fat compartment. Decreased delivery of drug to liver and kidney may prolong the action of drugs dependent on these organs for excretion.

Autonomic Nervous System

The portion of the central and peripheral nervous system concerned with the involuntary regulation of cardiac muscle, smooth muscle, glandular, and visceral function throughout the body is known as the autonomic nervous system (ANS). The system is exquisitely responsive to changes in somatic motor and sensory activities of the body. Inasmuch as neither somatic nor ANS activity occurs in isolation, the ANS is not as distinct as the term suggests.

Traditionally, the ANS has been viewed as a peripheral efferent system. It is now recognized that most ANS efferent fibers are accompanied by sensory fibers now commonly thought of as components of the system. The afferent fibers cannot be divided as distinctively as can the efferent fibers.

In 1921, Langley divided this system into two parts, retaining the term *sympathetic* for one part and introducing the term *parasympathetic* for the second part (3).

Anatomy

Central autonomic organization is principally located in the hypothalamus, with integration occurring at all levels of the cerebrospinal axis. Sympathetic functions are controlled by nuclei in the posterolateral hypothalamus. The medulla and pons are centers of acute ANS organization and together integrate momentary hemodynamic adjustments. Maintenance of tonicity is second-by-second activity controlled by the ANS. Regulation of peripheral vascular resistance is a dynamic example of this tonic activity.

Physiologic anatomy consists of the aforementioned central area and peripheral system consisting of the sympathetic nervous system (SNS) and parasympathetic nervous system (PNS) divisions. Most organs receive fibers from both divisions. The anatomy of ANS and the sensory pathways are essentially identical, but motor pathways are different. The somatic motor efferent fibers are composed of a single neuron with its cell body in the spinal cord ventral gray matter. Its axon extends directly to the striated muscle unit. In contrast, the efferent ANS is a two-neuron (bipolar) chain from the central nervous system to the effector organ. It then relays the impulse to a second station known as the autonomic ganglion, which contains the cell body of the second (postganglionic) neuron. Its axon contacts the effector organ. Preganglionic fibers of both divisions are myelinated and postganglionic fibers are unmyelinated.

Sympathetic Nervous System

The preganglionic fibers of the SNS originate in the intermediolateral gray columns of the 12 thoracic and the first 3 lumbar segments of the spinal cord. These myelinated axons leave the spinal cord with motor fibers to form the white myelinated communicating rami. Rami enter the paired 22 sympathetic ganglia at their respective levels. After entry into the paravertebral ganglia, the preganglionic fibers may synapse with postganglionic fibers at the same level, course upward or downward in the trunk of the SNS to synapse in ganglia at different levels, or exit without synapsing to terminate in an outlying collateral ganglion. The exception is the adrenal gland, in which preganglionic fibers pass directly into the adrenal medulla without synapsing in a ganglion. Neuronal cells of the adrenal medulla are analogous to postganglionic neurons.

Activation of the SNS produces a mass reflex response. A single preganglionic fiber influences a large number of postganglionic fibers, which are dispersed to many organs. In addition, release of catecholamines from the adrenal medulla augments the response.

Parasympathetic Nervous System

The PNS has both preganglionic and postganglionic neurons, sometimes called the craniosacral outflow because preganglionic cell bodies originate in the brainstem and sacral segments of the spinal cord. Preganglionic fibers are found in cranial nerves III, VII, IX, and X. Sacral outflow originates in the intermediolateral gray horns of the second, third, and fourth sacral nerves. The vagus (cranial nerve X) accounts for more than 75% of PNS activity. In contrast to the sympathetic side of the system, parasympathetic preganglionic fibers pass directly to the organ that is innervated. Postganglionic cells are situated within or near the innervated viscera. Postganglionic fibers do not have an extensive secondary distribution from a single preganglionic fiber as does the SNS. This is consistent with the discrete effect of the PNS. For example, vagal bradycardia may occur without concomitant change in intestinal motility or salivation.

Pharmacology of the ANS

Transmission of excitation in the ANS occurs through the mediation of liberated chemicals. Pharmacologic terminology designates the SNS and PNS as adrenergic and cholinergic, respectively. PNS postganglionic fibers release acetylcholine (ACh). Norepinephrine (NE) is the neurotransmitter at postganglionic sympathetic terminals, with the exception of sweat glands. Preganglionic fibers of both systems secret ACh.

The entire system is modulated via a system of receptors, which appears to be protein macromolecules located in the cellular plasma membrane. Several thousand receptors have been demonstrated in the membrane of a single cell. Cholinergic receptors found in the ANS may be subdivided into muscarinic and nicotinic because muscarine and nicotine stimulate them selectively. Both respond to ACh stimulation. Muscarinic receptors may be blocked by atropine without effect on nicotinic receptors. Muscarinic receptors are found at PNS junctions of cardiac and smooth muscle. They are also known to exist at other than PNS postganglionic junctions. They are found on the presynaptic membranes of sympathetic nerve terminals in the myocardium, coronary vessels, and peripheral circulation. These have been referred to as adrenergic muscarinic receptors because of their location. Stimulation of these receptors inhibits release of NE.

Nicotinic receptors are found at synaptic junctions of both SNS and PNS ganglia. Inasmuch as both junctions are cholinergic, ACh or ACh-like substances will excite postganglionic fibers of both systems. Especially important in clinical anesthesia are nicotinic receptors found at the neuromuscular junction because pharmacologic blockade of these receptors produces muscular paralysis.

Adrenergic receptors typically are divided into α and β types, and each type can be divided further (α_1, α_2, and β_1, β_2). In addition, dopaminergic (DA) receptors have been identified. The receptors are located in the CNS, renal, mesenteric, and coronary vessels. Their physiologic importance is a matter of some controversy. These receptors may explain the action of dopamine (dopaminergic receptor effect) on renal and mesenteric vasculature.

α-receptors are subdivided into two sets: α_1 and α_2. The α_1-receptors are postsynaptic in location and are found in smooth muscle cells of the peripheral vasculature of the coronary arteries, skin, uterus, intestinal mucosa, and splanchnic beds. Activation results in either decreased or increased tone, depending on the effector organ. Stimulation of α_1-receptor in resistance and capacitance vessels produces vasoconstriction. Stimulation of presynaptic α_2-receptors mediates inhibition of NE release, resulting in a negative-feedback mechanism. Blockade of presynaptic α_2-receptors abates normal inhibition of NE release, causing vasoconstriction. Distinction between the two is based on the difference in order of potency for a series of agonists and antagonists.

β-adrenergic receptors also are subdivided into two subsets. Receptors of the β_1-type predominate in the myocardium and SH node. Similarly, β_2-receptors are located in smooth muscle of blood vessels in the skin, muscle, mesentery, and bronchial musculature. The β_2-receptors are more sensitive to epinephrine than norepinephrine.

Recent investigations have complicated the receptor locations, as α_2-receptors have been found not only at postsynaptic locations but also at extra synaptic sites. α_1-receptors have been located in human platelets, caudate nucleus of human brain, and rat lung. Many other different isoreceptors may be found in mammalian tissue.

Autonomic reflexes are frequently seen in clinical practice. These are mediated via baroreceptors. Such reflexes are operative in the moment-to-moment control of cardiac output, blood pressure, and heart rate. Pressor receptors located in the carotid sinus and the aortic arch respond to alterations in pressure. Increased blood pressure creates stretch of the receptors, causing an increase in impulses to the central vasomotor center, which produces an increase in vagal tone and a decrease in sympathetic firing. This results in vasodilation. Venous baroreceptors also exist in the right atrium and great veins. A reduction in venous tone produces an increase in heart rate. The integration of the autonomic system as a coordinated unit is of critical importance in the mechanics of autoregulation of organ perfusion.

General Anesthesia

The type of general anesthesia may be characterized by the route of administration. The most common routes use inhalation or intravenous techniques. A combination of inhalation and intravenous drugs is referred to as balanced anesthesia. Characteristics of general anesthesia include unconsciousness, amnesia, and sedation. The need for a quiet surgical field dictates the need for motor blockade; therefore, drugs that produce muscular paralysis are commonly used.

Inhalation Anesthesia

Inhalation agents may be of several chemical classes, but those clinically useful are halogenated ethers and hydrocarbons. Active research is continuing in an effort to develop the ideal agent.

Uptake and Distribution

Inhaled anesthetics are administered as gases and enter the body via ventilation. Many factors are involved in the uptake and distribution of inhalation agents.

Inspired Concentration. The rate of rise of alveolar concentration bears a direct relationship to the concentration inspired. The higher the inspired concentration, the more rapid the rise in alveolar concentration. Alveolar tension results from a balance between the delivery of the anesthesia to the lung and rate of uptake of the anesthetic from the lung by blood and tissues. Administration of high concentrations of one gas (e.g., N_2O) will facilitate the increase in alveolar concentration of another gas (e.g., halothane); a phenomenon known as the second gas effect.

Alveolar Ventilation. The greater the minute ventilation, the more rapidly alveolar gas tension will approach inspired concentrations. Lung volume is the only limiting factor, i.e., the larger the functional residual capacity (FRC), the slower the wash-in of new gas.

Anesthetic Uptake. Anesthetic uptake from the lung depends on solubility of the agent in blood, cardiac output, and the pulmonary venous blood to alveolar gas tension difference. Increasing any factor will increase anesthetic uptake, thereby decreasing the concentration in the alveolus.

Solubility. Solubility refers to the extent to which an anesthetic agent dissolves in blood and tissues. Equilibrium exists when the partial pressure of an anesthetic agent in the two phases is equal. If other factors remain stable, the greater the blood/gas solubility coefficient, the greater the uptake of agent and the slower the increase in alveolar concentration. If an anesthetic is totally insoluble (blood/gas coefficient = 0), then none will be taken into the circulation. At a fixed concentration of inspired anesthetic agent, alveolar concentration will rise at a rate determined solely by ventilation and FRC and will soon equal the inspired concentration. Conversely, if an agent has a low blood solubility, then only small quantities can be removed, allowing alveolar concentration and tension to rise rapidly. Tension in arterial blood will rise rapidly even though only a small amount is present in the circulation. As distribution to various tissues is accomplished, the anesthetic agent is given up so that venous blood returning to the lung has a reduced tension, creating a gradient. Translated into clinical practice, the following may be stated: If the anesthetic vapor has a high solubility, then large amounts can be absorbed, as if blood were like a sponge that would not allow a rapid rise in alveolar concentration. Low alveolar concentration means low blood tension, so anesthetic induction is slow.

Output. Cardiac output carries anesthetic away from the lungs. High cardiac output carries the anesthetic agent away from the lungs, resulting in a slow rate of rise in the alveolar concentration. The magnitude of this effect is related to solubility. The most soluble agents are affected more than the least soluble agents. Cardiac output will have no effect on completely insoluble agents and, therefore, will have no effect on alveolar concentration. Inhalation induction in patients with a high cardiac output (i.e., thyrotoxicosis) will be prolonged with a soluble agent. Low cardiac output states lead to rapid rate of induction.

Venous/Alveolar Difference. Mixed venous to alveolar difference is determined by the amount taken up by tissues. During induction, tissues remove nearly all of the anesthetic delivered to them. The result is a large alveolar-to-venous gradient that causes maximum anesthetic agent uptake. As tissues become saturated, a rise in venous partial pressure occurs, narrowing the venoalveolar gradient, thereby reducing uptake.

Tissues. Anesthetic delivery to tissues depends primarily on blood flow and volume. Tissue-blood partition coefficients vary far less than blood/gas solubility coefficients. Organs that are highly perfused include brain, heart, kidney, splanchnic bed, and endocrine glands. These organs make up only about 10% of body mass, but they receive 70% of the cardiac output. The high flow rates result in rapid equilibration to arterial anesthetic partial pressures. Equilibrium is usually established within 5 to 10 minutes of induction.

Recovery

Recovery from inhalation anesthesia is governed by the same factors that affect induction. Pulmonary venti-

lation will lower alveolar concentration but will be opposed by an increase in cardiac output, venous-to-alveolar anesthetic gradient, and solubility of agents in blood.

Potency

The potency of anesthetic agents is commonly referred to as minimum alveolar concentration (MAC) of the agent. It is the alveolar concentration of anesthesia at 1 atm that prevents a response, in 50% of subjects, to a painful stimulus. Many factors, both physiologic and pharmacologic, may influence MAC. Examples of agents that may increase MAC when given concomitantly are chronic ethanol abuse, hyperthermia, and drugs that cause increased central neurotransmitter levels (cocaine, ephedrine, monamine oxidase inhibitors). Examples of factors that may decrease MAC are hypothermia, metabolic acidosis, hypoxia, induced hypotension, acute ethanol administration, and drugs that cause decreased central neurotransmitter levels (α-methyldopa, reserpine). Addition of other drugs, such as nitrous oxide, barbiturates, benzodiazepines, and opioids, will lower MAC requirements.

Intravenous Agents

The intravenous anesthetics may be classified as hypnotics, dissociative, benzodiazepines, and opioids. These drugs are used as induction agents, maintenance agents, and primary anesthetics as well as sedatives to augment regional or general anesthesia.

The goal of anesthetic induction is to provide a physiologically and psychologically stress-free state. Anesthesia management thereby encompasses the proper pharmacologic recipe, which is tailored to the patient's physiologic state and the anticipated surgical procedure. Induction is accomplished most commonly by the inhalation or intravenous route. Induction agents are typically drugs with a rapid onset and short duration of action.

Muscle Relaxants

The use of a drug to produce neuromuscular blockade is a part of the anesthetic plan in the daily administration of general anesthesia. Use of muscle relaxants allows the patient to be maintained at lighter levels of general anesthesia, which translates to patient safety. The use of muscle relaxants has become more prominent as halogenated inhalation agents have replaced ether compounds in the practice of anesthesiology.

Neuromuscular Function

A motor unit consists of a single nerve fiber, with its branches innervating many muscle fibers so that muscular contraction occurs in an organized fashion. Electrochemical balance in the resting state is such that a high concentration of extracellular Na^+ and intercellular K^+ exists. Balance is maintained through the Na^+/K^+ pump, so that the resting membrane potential is about -90 mV. When stimulation takes place, Na^+ channels open, causing the nerve membrane to become selectively permeable to Na^+. Reversal in polarity of the action potential occurs when Na^+ channels close and K^+ channels open, returning the transmembrane potential to its resting level. During this period, the nerve membrane is refractory to additional excitation.

There is a junctional gap between motor nerve endings and muscle motor endplates of about 50 nm. When an action potential reaches a nerve ending, a neurotransmitter is released from vesicles into the junctional gap, carrying the electrical stimulation to nicotinic cholinergic receptors on the motor endplate. Muscle contraction is thus produced. Acetylcholine is synthesized from choline and acetylcoenzyme A (acetyl-CoA) in the axoplasm of the nerve terminal, with choline acetylase catalyzing the reaction. Under normal conditions, the amount of ACh released is about five times that required to induce muscular contraction.

Ca^{2+} must be present to aid in the release of ACh and receptor activation. Cyclic AMP serves as a cofactor in the synthesis and storage of ACh in nerve terminals and may play a role in ACh release.

The inactivation of ACh occurs in the junctional cleft between nerve and muscle. Acetylcholinesterase (AChE) inactivates ACh by hydrolyzing it to choline and acetate. Choline is then captured by the nerve terminal for synthesis of new ACh.

Muscle contraction occurs when its nerve is stimulated, allowing movement of Na^+ into the cell. This causes depolarization of the membrane (creating a less negative intracellular atmosphere) and generates the action potential. The action potential is propagated along the muscle membrane, initiating Ca^{2+} release from sarcoplasmic reticulum into the sarcoplasm where myosin ATPase activation leads to excitation contraction coupling of the myofilaments. Potency of the muscular contraction depends on successive, summated, and fused muscular contractions rather than the amplitude of individual action potentials (4).

Pharmacology

Neuromuscular-blocking drugs are classified as either depolarizing or nondepolarizing, depending on the effect at the motor endplates. The clinical effect of these drugs is to produce muscular weakness, which has allowed the term *muscle relaxants* to be used synonymously in anesthesia.

Blockade of muscles occurs so that the muscles of ventilation are the last to be paralyzed but also the first to recover. Small facial and hand muscles, trunk, and extremities are blocked before the ventilatory musculature. This is a relevant clinical observation when recovery from neuromuscular blockade is assessed.

Depolarizing Muscle Relaxants

Depolarizing muscle relaxants possess chemical structures similar to ACh, but they are resistant to hydrolysis by AChE. The motor endplates remain in a state of persistent depolarization. Repolarization does not occur and clinical weakness of the muscle results.

Hyperkalemia

Hyperkalemia may result after administration of depolarizing muscle relaxants under certain circumstances. In normal individuals, depolarization results in an elevation of serum K^+, averaging 0.5 to 1.0 mEq/liter. Traumatized or denervated muscle may extrude sufficient K^+ to result in cardiac arrest after injection. Similar rises in serum K^+ have been observed in patients who have sustained large burn injuries. Explanation of the mechanism involved may be the loss of cellular membrane integrity that might interfere with the return of potassium into its intracellular position.

Denervation type injuries such as quadriplegia or paraplegia are said to result in a proliferation of extra junctional cholinergic receptors in response to lack of neural stimulation. Administration of depolarizing muscle relaxants under these conditions results in a large efflux of potassium, which may prove lethal. Patients suffering upper motor neuron lesions, recent cerebrovascular accidents, or severe Parkinson's disease also must be considered at risk as long as the nerve dysfunction remains unresolved.

Nondepolarizing Muscle Relaxants

Nondepolarizing muscle relaxants act by competitive inhibition of the neuromuscular junction. They work by binding to the postsynaptic cholinergic receptor. This action prevents ACh from activating Na^+ channels so that initiation of an action potential is inhibited. Blockade of Na^+ channels at presynaptic sites may also occur, resulting in impairment of ACh mobilization from synthesis sites to release sites.

The nondepolarizing neuromuscular blocking agents include two groups, which can be divided according to their duration of action. In the moderately long duration of action group are *d*-tubocurarine (*d*Tc), metocurine, pancuronium, and gallamine. Vecuronium and atracurium have an intermediate duration of action.

Conduction Anesthesia

Pharmacodynamics

Communication along human peripheral nerves is encoded digitally as a temporal series of transient, localized membrane polarity reversals (depolarizations). These depolarizations are propagated along axonal membranes at speeds of between 0.5 and 130 m/sec. Impulses travel inward from the periphery along sensory nerve axons and outward from the cord along neuroeffector (including motor) axons. At the molecular level, membrane depolarization is lined to the movement of ions, especially sodium, across the nerve membrane through specialized pores, or channels. Local anesthetic drugs block these pores and, when present in sufficient concentration, prevent both propagation of electrical nerve impulses and the messages (including pain) they encode. Catastrophic complications from local anesthetic drug administration result when these drugs exert their membrane-stabilizing effects on the wrong excitable tissues, vis-à-vis the brain, heart, and cervical spinal cord.

Chemistry

Organic compounds with many different chemical structures exert local anesthetic activity in vitro and in vivo. Only a few are sufficiently safe and effective to be clinically useful. The chemical structure of most commercially available local anesthetic drugs includes one hydrophilic terminal (usually a tertiary amine) and one hydrophobic terminal (usually a substituted benzene ring); these are linked by an ester or amide group (Fig. 24.1). Procaine, chloroprocaine, and tetracaine contain ester linkages. Lidocaine, mepivacaine, bupivacaine, and etidocaine are amides. The chemical structures of dyclonine and benzocaine are atypical. Dyclonine's hydrophilic and hydrophobic terminals are linked by a ketone group. Benzocaine has an ester linkage but no hydrophilic terminal.

Pharmacokinetics

Local Diffusion

Some local anesthetic solutions are effective when applied topically; others must be injected. After administration by either route, drug diffusion occurs, facilitated by local and lymphatic circulation. Only a fraction of the local anesthetic molecules reach their specific targets—the sodium channels within the membranes of the nerves innervating the surgical field. Speed of action and extent of drug spread depend on tissue variables,

such as vascularity, pH, P_{CO2}, and the natures of any anatomic (e.g., fascial) barriers. Additional variables are the diffusivity of the particular local anesthetic and volume and concentration of the agent. The clinical effects of local anesthetics are apparent within seconds after topical or intradermal injection.

Termination of drug action results from redistribution away from the relevant nerve membranes. The following classification of the commonly used agents is based on duration of action: short acting (procaine, chloroprocaine); intermediate acting (lidocaine, mepivacaine); and long acting (bupivacaine, etidocaine, tetracaine).

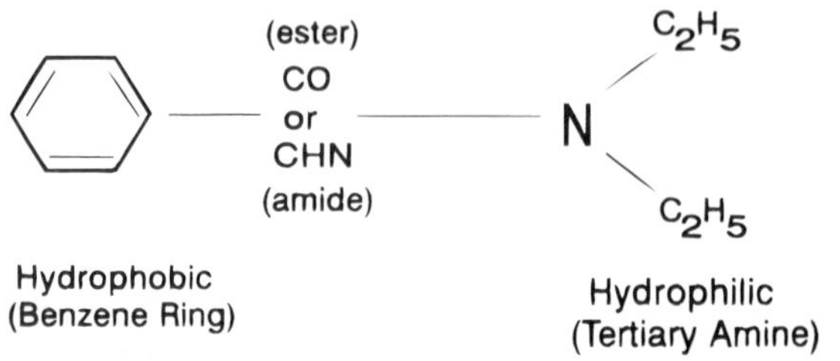

Systemic Absorption and Metabolism

The molecules of all administered local anesthetics (with the possible exception of benzocaine, which is absorbed poorly) eventually reach the systemic circulation. The time interval between local anesthetic administration and peak blood level is highly variable and depends on the anatomic site of application.

Metabolism of commercially available ester-linked anesthetics occurs predominantly within the bloodstream by plasma cholinesterases. Amide-linked anesthetics are metabolized primarily in the liver. Large or repeated doses of these drugs must be given with great caution to patients with reduced hepatic function.

Hazards of Local Anesthetic Administration

Local anesthesia is occasionally misperceived as being uniformly safer than general anesthesia. Catastrophic complications of regional anesthesia are generally the result of one of the following events: elevation of blood concentrations (secondarily brain and heart); anesthetic levels above the toxic threshold; injection of a large amount of anesthetic into the CSF, producing total spinal anesthesia; and needle-induced tissue or blood vessel injury. Clinically significant methemoglobinemia has been reported after administration of benzocaine, especially in children. Rarely, life-threatening allergic reactions to local anesthetics occur. These are thought to be especially infrequent after administration of amide-linked compounds.

Recognition and Treatment of Systemic Toxicity

Dangerously elevated concentrations in blood can occur after inadvertent intravascular injection of local anesthetics. Toxic blood levels can also arise from absolute drug overdose even when proper injection techniques are used. In the former case, symptoms and signs of toxicity occur immediately. In the latter case, symptoms and signs of toxicity may be delayed for 45 minutes.

A grand mal seizure, coma, apnea, or cardiovascular collapse may be the initial manifestation of systemic tox-

Figure 24.1. Chemical structure of local anesthetic.

icity. Often a patient first complains of sudden wooziness or drowsiness, sometimes accompanied by tinnitus, auditory distortions, or a metallic taste. Objectively, the patient may become disoriented or start to twitch. These ominous symptoms and signs should never be discounted. Their presence should result in the immediate discontinuation of drug administration until the presence of systemic toxic reaction can be excluded conclusively. Support of ventilation and the cardiovascular system are required frequently. Even when drug doses are weighted for intrinsic potency, the longer-acting agents appear to be more cardiotoxic than either intermediate- or short-acting agents.

Prevention of systemic toxicity depends on avoiding unintentional intravascular injection and keeping total drug dosages within recommended guidelines. A strategy to prevent systemic toxicity is to monitor patient pulse and use epinephrine-containing solutions with temporal fractionation: an increase in heart rate of 20/min or more within 30 to 60 seconds after injection of 3 to 4 mL local anesthetic with 5 μg/mL epinephrine (1:200,000) strongly suggests the occurrence of intravascular injection. Patients with heart disease, with implanted cardiac pacemakers, or taking β-agonists may not demonstrate heart rate increase.

Neuro Axial Blockade (Spinal and Epidural)

Spinal blockade may be produced by epidural or subarachnoid injection of local anesthetics. Nerve fibers are classified on the basis of size and degree of myelination. Larger fibers (α) are associated with motor and proprioceptive function. Small fibers transmit sharp pain, temperature, and sympathetic tone. Blockade may vary, but ultimately all pathways are partially or completely interrupted.

Physiologic Effects

Pain and motor blockade are the sought-after results of Neuro axial block. Sympathetic fibers are blocked most easily. Sympathetic blockade may extend two to four segments farther than sensory blockade, which may result in a decrease in systemic vascular resistance and increased venous capacitance. Translated into clinical terms, this results in a decrease in venous return and a decrease in cardiac output. The most common side effect of Neuro axial blockade is hypotension. Uncorrected hypovolemic patients are not considered good candidates for Neuro axial blockade. If the sensory level rises to the thoracic dermatomes, cardiac accelerator fibers may be interrupted, producing a refractory bradycardia that further compromises the hypotensive patient.

Ventilatory effects may be those related to hypoperfu-sion of the medullary respiratory area and cervical blockade of the phrenic nerve. Abdominal and intercostal blockade also effects ventilation. This is of significant concern in patients using accessory muscles of ventilation.

Regional blood flow depends on the level of blockade and presence of hypotension. Little effect on cerebral, cardiac, renal, or hepatic perfusion is found when sensory levels of blockade do not exceed the T-10 dermatome. At higher levels, decreases in blood flow to these organs may occur. A marked increase in blood flow in the lower extremities occurs with spinal and epidural anesthesia. Myocardial oxygen demand is decreased because of afterload reduction (arterial vasodilation), preload reduction (decreased venous return), and decreased heart rate (block of cardiac accelerator fibers). Myocardial oxygen supply is decreased less than myocardial oxygen demand.

Effects of Anesthesia on Organs and Systems

Central Nervous Systems

Inhaled anesthetics produce significant change in mental function, cerebral oxygen requirements, cerebral blood flow, cerebrospinal fluid (CSF) dynamics, and electrophysiology.

The obvious effect is an unconscious state with lack of response to painful stimuli. Some studies have alluded to decrease in intellectual function, psychomotor skills, and driving skills. Other studies have failed to confirm these impairments. It is reasonably safe to assume that concentrations of anesthetics in the brain several hours after termination are too low to impair most tests of mental function.

All of the potent inhalation agents decrease cerebral metabolic rate (CMR_{O2}) with isoflurane > enflurane > halothane. A decrease in CMR_{O2} is linked closely to cerebral electrical activity. This effect offers some cerebral protection if electrical activity has not been abolished by oxygen deprivation itself.

Cerebral vasodilation is produced by all inhalation agents, including nitrous oxide. The order of potency for this effect is halothane > enflurane > isoflurane. This cerebral vasodilation will cause an increase in cerebral blood flow (CB) and cerebral blood volume. Increases in CB tend to attenuate with time. In humans, the blood flow at which EEG evidence of cerebral ischemia occurs is significantly lower with isoflurane than with halothane (approximately 10 mL/100 g/min and 18 to 20 mL/100 g/min, respectively). Many of these effects may be blunted with moderate hypocarbia (25 to 30 mm Hg). CSF production or reabsorption is essentially unchanged with isoflurane. Halothane decreases the rate of

CSF production but decreases reabsorption. Enflurane increases CSF production and decreases reabsorption. All evidence indicates that enflurane is the least favorable drug regarding control of CSF pressure.

EEG patterns with all inhalation agents are similar in that with increasing concentrations, EEG wave frequency is decreased and voltage is increased. Electrical silence may be produced at high concentrations. Enflurane may produce high-voltage spiking patterns that may be abolished by decreasing the concentration of drug. Patients with epileptic loci are not believed to be at risk from seizures with enflurane administration.

Sensory evoked potential response may be changed in inhaled anesthetics. Cortical responses are more affected than subcortical responses.

Neuromuscular System

Potent inhaled anesthetics have inherent muscle relaxant properties. Neuromuscular blockade by inhalation agents may be the result of central upper motor neuron depression or an effect at the myoneural junction. These agents may potentiate the action of neuromuscular-blocking agents.

Endocrine System

Islet Cell Function and Glucose Metabolism

During anesthesia, blood glucose is usually elevated. The plasma insulin response to glucose administration is blunted. Peripheral use of glucose is reduced as is insulin release from pancreatic islet cells.

The metabolic response to stress is characterized by a number of autonomic and neuroendocrine responses. Increased catecholamine and cortisol levels suppress pancreatic insulin release. Glucagon release is stimulated, resulting in glycogenolysis, gluconeogenesis, and hyperglycemia. Release of glycerol and amino acids, which are used by the liver during gluconeogenesis, contributes to the hyperglycemia.

Antidiuretic Hormone

Inhalation agents and opioid analgesics are believed to affect antidiuretic hormone (ADH) release. This augments the massive release of ADH caused by surgical stress. Free water clearance is decreased and urinary osmolarity increases.

Stress Response

Stress response is the combined result of surgical stimulation and the administration of anesthesia. Induction and inhalatory agents are greater stimuli than intravenous induction. A general discharge of catecholamines has been quantitatively noted with norepinephrine levels elevated within the first 15 minutes. These return to normal within the first hour. An increase in adrenal cortical discharge, renin levels, and aldosterone is found with surgical stimulation. One of the goals of anesthesia, especially in patients with cardiac disease, is to limit the stress response.

Renal System

Generally, all inhalation anesthetics cause a decrease in urine formation. A decrease in glomerular filtration rate is seen with virtually all anesthetic techniques. This may be caused by direct effects on renal blood flow and changes in renovascular autoregulation. Some effects seen are undoubtedly due to the effects on the cardiovascular system; however, others are secondary to the stress responses of surgical stimulation and ADH secretion.

Hepatic System

The subject of anesthesia and liver function has been the basis for much controversy and confusion. Different anesthetics affect liver function in various ways. Perioperative hepatic dysfunction may be caused directly by the anesthetic agent or decreased oxygen and blood supply. More complex mechanisms, such as the development of antibodies and involvement of the immune mechanisms, may contribute to hepatic dysfunction. All inhalation agents are metabolized by the liver to some degree (halothane, 18% to 20% > enflurane, 2% > isoflurane, 0.5%).

Blood flow to the liver is normally about 25% of the cardiac output. Anesthetic agents may affect hepatic blood flow by changes in cardiac output or via direct effects on hepatic vasculature. Events occurring during the surgical procedure may be stressful enough to cause the release of catecholamines, thereby reducing hepatic blood flow.

Halothane is the anesthetic studied most regarding possible hepatotoxicity. When the liver is exposed to halothane, histologically a number of changes occur (rounding up of the mitochondria, increased granularity of the rough endoplasmic reticulum, etc.), indicating increased metabolic activity. Strong evidence in the literature indicates certain factors may enhance the risk of halothane hepatotoxicity. They include multiple exposures to halothane, obesity, gender (females > males), middle age, and ethnic origins (Mexican-Americans seem to be more susceptible than others). Mechanisms proposed for halothane hepatotoxicity are direct hepatotoxic effects of intermediaries of halothane metabolism, hepatic oxygen deprivation secondary to halothane-induced circulatory changes, and immunologically mediated hepatic necrosis.

The frequency of halothane-induced liver necrosis varies from 1 in 6,000 to 1 in 20,000 administrations. The U.S. National Halothane Study analyzed 850,000 anesthetics with 250,000 instances of halothane administration. The incidence in the study was 1:35,000 (5).

The incidence of hepatic injury after enflurane and isoflurane is extremely low, thus an actual estimation of the incidence is impossible.

Cardiovascular System

Inhalation anesthetics, when studied in vitro (isolated papillary muscle preparations), produce a dose-dependent depression of contractility. Papillary muscles taken from animals with congestive heart failure are depressed to a greater extent than muscles from normal animals. Patients with impaired contractility as a result of congestive heart failure are known to be particularly sensitive to the direct myocardial depressant effects of inhaled anesthetics. In vivo, cardiac depression is not observed consistently, probably because of compensatory hemostatic mechanisms.

Effects on the conduction system have been noted with all potent inhalation agents. All exert a direct negative chronotropic effect at the sinoatrial node. Atrioventricular junctional rhythms are common with all anesthetics. Heart rate changes least with halothane and increases most with isoflurane. Inhalatory agents decrease cardiac output and systemic arterial pressure; therefore, myocardial work is decreased.

Physiology

Cardiac performance is determined by the following physiologic parameters: preload; afterload; contractility; rate; and rhythm. The objective of invasive monitoring is to assess each parameter and the interplay among the parameters. Cardiac output (CO) equals stroke volume (SV) times heart rate (HR):

$$CO = SV \times HR$$

Preload. Physiologists define preload as actual fiber length at end diastole. Preload from a clinical perspective may be defined as the amount of blood returning to the atria for delivery into the ventricles. Clinically, it is assessed indirectly via right atrial measurement (CVP) for the right ventricle and left atrial pressure (PCWP) for the left ventricle. It must be appreciated that these are mean values and represent estimates of ventricular diastolic pressures. Adequate preload depends on venous return because the heart cannot pump more than it receives. Because 60% to 70% of vascular volume is contained in the venous system, it is important to have a clear understanding of venous return. The arterial system is relatively fixed in its ability to alter volume compared with the venous system. For adequate venous return, a pressure gradient must be created between the peripheral veins and the atrium.

Venous tone is defined as the state of contraction of smooth muscles within venous walls. This is controlled primarily by sympathetic activity and local factors. When venotone increases, venous capacitance decreases, creating a real decrease in pressure. This is associated with fluid depletion. Atrial filling decreases with a resultant decrease in preload. With maximal venotone, which may occur as a compensatory mechanism in hypovolemia, venous capacitance may be decreased. This may lead to improper interpretation of data.

Increasing driving pressure (venoconstriction) is the common response in the stressed state. Improving conductance (fluid administration) is the most common mechanism used in supportive care. To summarize, optimizing the vascular space in regard to intravascular volume is the primary means to optimize preload.

Afterload. Afterload is the force opposing ventricular fiber shortening during ejection. Size, shape, radius, and wall thickness are all factors affecting afterload. The principal factors are radius (related to preload) and aortic or pulmonic impedance. Aortic impedance is dominated by systemic vascular resistance (SVR) and arterial compliance. Pulmonic impedance is affected by pulmonary vascular resistance (PVR) and compliance. Clinically, SVR is used frequently as an estimate of afterload, but it reflects arteriolar tone and not ventricular systolic wall tension. Accurate measurement requires intraventricular measurements combined with echocardiographic studies. Reduction of afterload allows the ventricle to shorten more rapidly and more completely. Increases in afterload decrease the extent and velocity of shortening.

Contractility is the inherent strength of ventricular muscle when preload and afterload are constant. Quantitation remains an illusive entity in the intact system. Such terms as *stroke work indices* and *force velocity measurements* have been used to describe contractility. Certain ions, such as calcium, potassium, sodium, and magnesium, affect contractile power.

Heart rate becomes a critical factor in patients with impairment of coronary blood flow. As rate increases, coronary perfusion is compromised because diastole is shortened to a greater degree than systole and coronary perfusion occurs only in diastole. It is not surprising that many ischemic episodes occur during periods of tachycardia.

All of these cardiac factors are interrelated. Alteration of one factor may affect another determinant, and one must be aware of all these changes to interpret data properly. An example would be vasodilator therapy that may result in a decrease in BP (afterload), venous pooling (preload), and a reflex tachycardia.

Respiratory System

Effects of general anesthesia on respiratory function produce central effects and changes in lung mechanics.

Central Effect

All inhaled agents cause a decrease in ventilatory drive in a dose-related fashion. Narcotics are well-known to decrease respiratory rate as well. Inhaled agents produce a decrease in tidal volume with an initial increase in ventilatory rate. As the concentration of inhaled agents increases, a decrease in rate occurs. Narcotic anesthesia with increasing dosage leads to apnea. The responsiveness of the respiratory center to Pa_{CO2} becomes depressed.

Response to hypoxia, even with subanesthetic doses of inhalation agents, is significantly depressed. Augmentation of ventilation produced by hypercarbia or hypoxia in the awake state is not observed during anesthesia.

Approximately 60% of normal tidal breathing is contributed by the diaphragm and 40% by intercostal activity. Depressed intercostal function prohibits stabilization of the rib cage. Diaphragmatic function is also depressed, but phrenic nerve activity is more resistant to the depressive effects of anesthetic agents.

The effect of inhalation agents on hypoxic pulmonary vasoconstriction is controversial. In animal studies, there is general agreement that the response is depressed in a dose-related manner. This factor is important, but it does not preclude the use of inhalation agents. The disease status of the lung and the effects of anesthetic agents are of relatively greater importance in the selection of agents to be used in the clinical setting.

Lung Mechanics and Anesthesia

Pulmonary complications undoubtedly constitute a major source of morbidity and mortality in the postoperative patient. Reported incidences of pulmonary problems vary from 3% to 70%. This discrepancy stems in part from differences in definitions of complications, types of surgery, and patient population. Physicians should have a reasonable grasp of the effects of surgery and anesthesia as they relate to lung function.

Upper Airway. Stiff hairs in the anterior nasal fossa and the spongy mucous membrane act as important bacterial defense mechanisms. Humidification and warming of inspired gas are probably the most important functions of the nose. The great vascularity of the mucosa helps maintain a constant temperature. Despite wide variations in external temperature, inspired air is warmed to 36° to 37°C by the time it reaches the midtracheal area. The daily production of about 1 liter of nasal secretions is used in saturating inspired gas. Bronchi and alveoli require 95% humidity for adequate function.

Artificial airway placement bypasses these mechanisms, allowing relatively dry gases to reach the tracheobronchial tree. The mucosa in this area is then compelled to perform the duties of the nasal mucosa.

Administration of dry gases leads to cessation of ciliary activity. Cellular degeneration accompanied by mild tracheitis is common after the administration of an endotracheal anesthesia.

The continuous activity of the mucociliary escalator apparatus is probably the most important factor in the

prevention of the accumulation of secretions. The coordinated movement of these fine hair-like projections act to move secretions toward the larynx and pharynx. Decrease in temperature, mucus production, and changes in pH decrease ciliary activity. Volatile anesthetics in high concentrations and opiates have a depressant effect on ciliary functions.

These functions of the upper airway are adversely affected by the administration of narcotic premedicants and by dry volatile anesthetic gases. The loss of the ability to mobilize secretions produces a viable setting for derangement of pulmonary protective mechanics.

Lung Volumes. Lung volumes commonly used in respiratory physiology generally refer to expired measurements (Fig. 24.2). The amount exhaled during quiet breathing is known as the tidal volume (TV). Maximal inhalation followed by maximal exhalation is known as the vital capacity (VC). Some gas remains in the lung after a maximal exhalation and is known as the residual volume (RV). The combination of the vital capacity and residual volume is the total lung capacity (TLC). The volume of gas in the lung after a normal expiration is the functional residual capacity (FRC). It is this particular lung capacity that is of critical importance in the surgical patient.

Inspiration is usually accomplished in less than 1 second. During the greater portion of minute ventilation, fresh gas enters the lung for only 10 to 20 seconds. If one were to monitor arterial oxygen tensions constantly, these values would vary minimally on a minute-to-minute basis, although fresh gas only enters the lung during inspiration. Oxygenation is maintained by gas exchanges occurring in the FRC. Any decrease in the FRC would, therefore, lead to less volume available and hence oxygenation problems. Because anesthesia and surgery produce restrictive deficits in lung volumes (decreased lung volume), the goal should be to protect and maintain FRC.

Several important factors must be considered during the perioperative period. To appreciate these, several other definitions of lung mechanics must be understood. Lung compliance is defined as the volume change per unit of pressure change. In the normal range, the lung

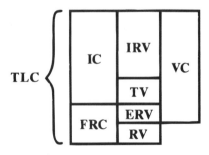

Figure 24.2. Lung volumes as a portion of total lung capacity. *IC*, inspiratory capacity; *IRV*, inspiratory reserve volume; *ERV*, expiratory reserve volume.

is remarkably distensible, or very compliant. Measurement of compliance in normal human lungs is about 150 to 200 mL/cm H_2O. At higher volumes, the lung is stiffer and compliance is reduced. Compliance is also reduced at lower lung volumes. This may be of critical importance in maintaining FRC. Engorgement of the lung with blood, increased pulmonary venous pressure, increased unventilated areas of the lung, and interstitial fibrosis may all lead to a decrease in lung compliance. Emphysema, with loss of elastic recoil fibers, leads to easier distensibility and causes an increase in lung compliance.

Surfactant produced by alveolar type II cells is a surface tension-reducing agent that allows the distending pressures in the alveoli to be less than would be necessary if surfactant were not present. As long as intra-alveolar pressure is greater than pressures in the interstitium of the lung, patency is maintained. The pressure necessary to maintain patent alveoli is, therefore, decreased by the presence of surfactant. Almost all anesthetic techniques using positive pressure ventilation decrease or inhibit surfactant production. This produces a tendency for airway closure to occur at lower lung volumes.

Ventilatory Mechanics. Normal spontaneous ventilation occurs because there is a pressure difference between the mouth and the alveolus. The subatmospheric pressure within the pleural cavity is created by the elastic force of the lung and chest wall. A gradient of pleural pressures exists in the upright lungs at end expiration varying from 0 to 10 cm of water. Inasmuch as alveoli at the apex of the upright lung are distended to a greater degree because of greater subatmospheric pressure, airflow tends to be distributed to a greater number of alveoli in the lower half of the lung. Gravitational effects and weight of the lung distribute blood to this same area. Hence, during spontaneous ventilation, gas exchange is relatively well-matched.

Airflow occurs into the lungs due to a pressure gradient that must be developed to overcome the nonelastic or dynamic resistance of the lungs. Orifice size and pattern of airflow affect resistance. Laminar flow occurs down parallel sided tubes at less than a certain critical velocity. When flow exceeds the critical velocity it becomes turbulent. Orifice flow occurs at a constriction such as the larynx.

Total cross-sectional area of the airways increases as branching occurs, thereby decreasing the velocity of airflow. Laminar flow is chiefly confined to airways below the main bronchi, orifice flow occurs at the larynx, and turbulent flow occurs in the trachea during most of the respiratory cycle.

Effects of Surgery. Position during surgery causes definite decreases in lung volumes. In changing from the upright to the supine position, FRC decreases by 0.5 to 1.0 liter with similar decreases in VC. Changes in diaphragmatic function with position have been shown to be of great importance with regard to lung volumes. Excursion of the diaphragm varies from 1 to 2 cm during quiet tidal breathing to as much as 5 to 6 cm during rigorous ventilation. Diaphragmatic motion is restricted in the supine position because of compression by the liver and gravitational changes. Paralysis is accomplished with the use of muscle relaxants and produces a flaccid diaphragm that tends to remain in the end-expiratory state. This position leads to compression of lung volumes.

Location of the surgical procedure produces a predictable quantitative change in lung volumes. Bedside measurement of vital capacity offers a serial measurement of changes in lung mechanics. With upper abdominal procedures, vital capacity may decrease by 60% to 70%, whereas procedures in the lower abdomen are associated with decreases of 40% to 50%. Chest surgical procedures have not been as well-studied because most data represent extrapolations from abdominal surgery. Limitation of excursion of the diaphragm, inability to inspire deeply, and lack of an effective cough have been attributed to postoperative pain in the surgical patient. All respiratory care maneuvers in the postoperative patient are aimed at improving inspiration and mobilization of secretions.

Direct Anesthetic Effects. Anesthesia vapors produce a paralysis of mucociliary function and depress surfactant production. Coupled with the use of positive-pressure ventilation and position problems, it is not difficult to understand why the patient has a decrease in lung compliance and loss of lung volume during anesthesia.

The direct effect on airway caliber of all potent inhalation agents is to decrease airway resistance by producing bronchodilation. Antigens and histamines produce bronchoconstriction that is blocked by potent inhalation agents. If the patient is breathing spontaneously and extubated, at the end of the operation, all effects caused by the administration of anesthesia should disappear within 4 to 6 hours.

Most volatile anesthetics are said to decrease or abolish hypoxic pulmonary vasoconstriction. If the anesthetized patient has normal lungs and a nonthoracic procedure, this is probably of little consequence. In the thoracic surgical patient or in the patient with lung disease, the abolition of this reflex may be an important cause of intrapulmonary shunting.

All of the aforementioned factors lead to an intrapulmonary shunt of 10% to 15% in the anesthetized surgical patient with no previous cardiopulmonary disease. Any decrease in ventricular function, excessive fluid administration, or sepsis may cause a decrease in lung compliance and further add to the loss of lung volumes. These problems are additive as far as decreasing FRC.

Carbon Dioxide

CO_2 production in the unstressed patient is in the range of 3 cc/kg body weight. Anesthetic techniques generally decrease CO_2 production due to a decrease in metabolic activity in the anesthetized state.

Exhaled CO_2 is an excellent measurement of alveolar ventilation, and assuming reasonable cardiac and normal lung function, values obtained approach arterial CO_2 findings.

Capnography

Systems are available that allow graphic display of the capnogram during anesthesia. A normal capnogram consists of five basic components as illustrated in Figure 24.3. The waveform can be analyzed for frequency, rhythm, baseline, shape, and height.

Frequency and rhythm depend on the state of the patient's respiratory center and ventilatory function. Height is a quantitative measure of expired CO_2. Shape depends on expiratory gas flow. A summary of the changes in expired CO_2 and the possible mechanisms is given in Table 24.1.

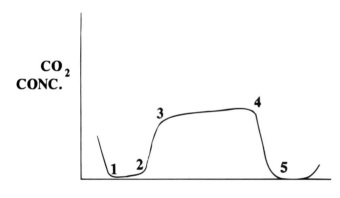

CO₂ CONC.

Time

1-2 - Anatomic dead space
2-3 - Alveolar gas & mixed dead space.
4-3 - Alveolar gas
4-5 - Last portion of alveolar gas.

Figure 24.3. Normal capnogram. The line represents CO_2 concentration in expired gas through a respiratory cycle.

Table 24.1.
Table for Capnography

Expired CO_2	Etiology
Rapid decrease to zero	Airway obstruction (kinked ETT)
	Circuit disconnection
	Defective ventilator
	Technical error (sampling line blocked)
Slower decrease (1–3 min)	Decreased cardiac output
	Pulmonary embolism, air embolism
	Hypotension
	Hyperventilation
Increase	Hypoventilation
	Rapid increase in body temperature
	Absorption from external source as CO_2 during laparoscopic surgery
	Increased pulmonary blood flow
	Release of vascular clamps
	Defective CO_2 absorption

Oxygenation and Oxygen Delivery

Oxygen is the energy source for mammalian cellular metabolism. Organ function represents the unified activity of cells. Any derangement in cellular function results in organ dysfunction. The inability to maintain O_2 delivery is, therefore, the most appropriate definition of circulatory failure. Most information gained in the clinical setting involves use of the senses and invasive and noninvasive techniques. Basic concepts concerning O_2 delivery need to be understood so that clinical observations and interventions are appropriate.

Oxygen delivery may be defined as the amount of oxygen available to tissues each minute. It is a combination of cardiac output and oxygen content. One must be familiar with hemoglobin physiology to gain a clear understanding of oxygen delivery. Hemoglobin combines reversibly with oxygen to form oxyhemoglobin. Oxyhemoglobin is intimately related to arterial oxygen tension but does not exert a partial pressure because it is in the chemically bound state. The bulk of oxygen is bound to hemoglobin, thus the pressure gradient created by dissolved oxygen is important because diffusion from plasma to cells is a pressure-related process. Therefore, almost all oxygen must first break the bond with hemoglobin so it becomes available to the cells.

The strength with which hemoglobin binds oxygen is referred to as oxygen-hemoglobin affinity. An increased affinity will allow fewer molecules to be transferred per unit time, whereas a decreased affinity will result in greater transfer.

Each hemoglobin molecule has four O_2 binding sites. Normal O_2 demand is met by release from one binding site, leaving three sites occupied. Therefore, normal mixed venous saturation (Pv_{O_2}) is 75%. Venous oxygen tension represents the lowest oxygen tension in that particular capillary bed. At an arterial O_2 tension of 26 mm, Hg hemoglobin saturation is 50%. If one applies these concepts, the oxygen-hemoglobin dissociation curve can be recalled easily.

Oxygen content defines the amount of oxygen available in blood. Because hemoglobin is expressed in volume percent (vol %), content values are expressed in terms of O_2/100 mL blood. Oxygen exists as oxyhemoglobin and is dissolved in plasma. When hemoglobin is fully saturated, it will combine with 1.34 mL of oxygen. The amount dissolved can be converted by multiplying the P_{O_2} times 0.0031 (solubility coefficient).

If one now examines oxygen availability based on the preceding facts, one sees by examining the oxygen-hemoglobin dissociation curve that a change in P_{O_2} from 95 to 65 mm Hg (33% decrease) results in a decrease in saturation from 97% to 92%. Thus, one sees a considerable protection during changes in arterial oxygen tension. As one approaches the venous portion of the curve (Pv_{O_2} 40 mm Hg/75%), small changes in P_{O_2} affect greater changes in saturation. Changes in venous P_{O_2} have important implications with respect to oxygen unloading at the tissue level.

The preceding points may be summarized as follows: (a) 98% of oxygen is combined with hemoglobin and less than 2% is dissolved; and (b) Pa_{O2} is a major determinant of hemoglobin saturation.

Oxygen transport represents the amount of oxygen delivered by the cardiovascular system per unit of time. Cardiac function now becomes a major determinant of oxygen delivery. Oxygen transport may be calculated by multiplying cardiac output (liter/min) times arterial O_2 content (mL/100 mL blood) times 10 to convert to liters per minute. If arterial oxygen content is 20 mL/100 mL blood and cardiac output is 5 liters/min, then 1000 mL of O_2 is delivered to tissues each minute.

Once oxygen is delivered, tissues use a certain amount, and the term *oxygen consumption* is introduced. If the quantity delivered is known and the amount returning via the venous system is calculated, the difference is the amount consumed. In the clinical setting, oxygen content from the arterial and mixed venous samples are collected. Cardiac output is available via thermodilution techniques, and O_2 consumption may be calculated as follows: arterial O_2 content = 20.4 mL; mixed venous O_2 content = 15.4 mL/5 mL/100 blood consumed; cardiac output = 5 liters/min × 10 = 50; therefore, O_2 consumed = 50 × 5 = 250 mL. With an arterial O_2 content of 20.4 mL/100 mL blood and a cardiac output of 5 liters, the total oxygen available is 1000 mL; a reserve or safety factor is built into the system.

What factors in the clinical setting may threaten the homeostasis? The major factors are (a) decrease in cardiac output; (b) decreased hemoglobin; and (c) decrease in arterial P_{O2}. One also must be aware of the compensatory mechanism that may be used under stress. Two fundamental steps are to increase cardiac output and to increase extraction from capillary blood, producing a decrease in venous saturation. Most normal individuals can triple cardiac output and also increase extraction by a factor of three. These mechanisms are seen in the anemic patient.

The common denominator in the shock syndrome (whether it is cardiogenic, hemorrhagic, or septic) is the development of lactic acidosis. Regardless of the etiology of the problem, an elevated blood lactate is associated with an ominous prognosis. The anemic patient who is able to compensate will not develop lactic acidosis in the unstressed state. Patients may compensate to a hemoglobin of 1.6 g/100 mL by tripling cardiac output and A–V extraction.

Decreases in arterial saturation with concomitant increases in cardiac output and maximal extraction will not result in lactic acidosis. Arterial hypoxemia without other complications will not lead to lactic acidosis unless other problems ensue. The chronic lung disease patient exemplifies this axiom.

The final factor regarding oxygen availability is cardiac output. A fall in cardiac output is qualitatively a much greater threat to oxygen consumption. A lessened cardiac output not only threatens the homeostasis in the same way that anemia and arterial desaturation do, but it removes one of the major compensatory mechanisms. Instead of a ninefold increase in the safety factor, there is only a threefold margin. The only mechanism that remains is for the body to extract more oxygen, thereby decreasing venous saturation. Failure of perfusion represents the most common cause of lactic acidosis.

Oxygenation is a complex process. From the clinical viewpoint, by assessment of hemoglobin levels, saturation, and cardiovascular function, an attempt is made to define the defect by using concepts of tissue oxygenation in the context of hemodynamic monitoring.

Temperature

Hypothermia

Hypothermia is the most common temperature disorder resulting from anesthesia and surgery. Anesthetized patients are poikilothermic. At least 70% of patients have temperatures of less than 36°C on admission to the postanesthesia care unit (PACU). Important factors contributing to heat loss are (a) cold operating room (temperature <21°C); (b) administration of nonwarmed intravenous fluids; (c) nonwarmed, unhumidified anesthetic gases; (d) use of cold irrigating solutions; (e) interference with thermoregulatory mechanism by anesthetic agent(s); (f) reduction of metabolic rate by the anesthetic agent(s) anesthesia; and (g) vasodilatation induced by the anesthetic agent(s). Heat loss occurs by the following mechanisms: radiation (60%); conduction (5%); convection (10%); and evaporation (25%).

Infants produce heat differently from adults through the mechanism of nonshivering thermogenesis. Brown fat located between the scapulae and around blood vessels becomes metabolically active in response to sympathetic discharge. Cardiac output is diverted to brown fat so that heat is distributed to the rest of the body.

Physiologic consequences resulting from hypothermia include prolonged drug metabolism, increased blood viscosity, and decreased perfusion. Upon emergence, shivering to increase body temperature may increase oxygen consumption by as much as 400% to 500%. Such an increase in oxygen demand causes an increase in cardiac output and minute ventilation. If a patient does not possess the cardiopulmonary reserves to meet the increase in oxygen demand, the result may be organ dysfunction. Ischemic myocardium damage may result.

Hyperthermia

Hyperthermia intraoperatively may be the result of infection, hyperthyroidism, excessive external warming, and malignant hyperthermia.

Malignant Hyperthermia. A genetically transmitted syndrome, malignant hyperthermia (MH) is estimated to occur in 1 in 50,000 anesthetized adults and 1 in 15,000 anesthetized children. The pathophysiology of MH remains unclear, but grossly elevated Ca^{2+} levels in the muscle myoplasm have been found in laboratory studies. This process is initiated by drugs that are referred to as "triggering agents." Triggering agents are believed to release large amounts of Ca^{2+} from the sarcoplasmic reticulum. Triggering agents include all inhalation agents (except N_2O), depolarizing muscle relaxants (SCh), and potassium salts. Classic signs of MH are tachypnea (usually not seen in the anesthetized, paralyzed patient), tachycardia, and hypercarbia. If expired CO_2 is measured, hypercarbia will be the first sign noted. Muscle rigidity, temperature elevation (1° to 2°C increases every 3 to 4 minutes), hypertension, acidosis, hypoxemia, hyperkalemia, and cardiac dysrhythmias may all be seen. Management includes discontinuance of all inhaled agents and SCh, hyperventilation with 100% oxygen, administration of dantrolene (2.5 mg/kg intravenous), cooling techniques, and $NaHCO_3$ administration. Other supportive measures include fluid administration and monitoring of urine output.

Dantrolene is a muscle relaxant that will completely reverse all of the clinical signs of malignant hyperthermia. It is unique because it operates within the muscle cell by reducing intracellular calcium levels. This may be the result of reduced sarcoplasmic reticulum calcium release with inhibition of excitation contracture coupling.

Pain Management

Pain management in the surgical patient is one of the most important tasks a physician accomplishes, yet patients often recall periods of inadequate postoperative pain relief. This scenario occurs because very little medical education is devoted to teaching physicians how to treat pain effectively.

Anatomical and Physical Basis of Pain

Under normal circumstances, pain results from activation of nociceptors in the periphery. Pain perception can be divided into the sensory discriminative aspect, which describes the location and quality of the stimulus, and the motivational-afferent portion, which leads to the aversion of pain.

Nociceptors are unencapsulated nerve endings that discharge when noxious stimuli threaten or produce injury. Information is transmitted to the spinal cord. These small primary afferents enter the spinal cord primarily in the lateral portion of the dorsal root, then bifurcate into rostral and caudal branches. The nociceptor signal is then relayed to projection cells for transmission to the brain. Individual pathways in the anterolateral cord presumed to be responsible for pain transmission are the spinothalamic, spino reticular, and spino mesencephalic tracts.

Pain can be alleviated by blockade of receptors at the spinal cord level. When stimulated, these small primary afferent fibers release neurotransmitters. Inhibition of release of these neurotransmitters or blockade of the nociceptor information within the dorsal horn are mechanisms that may play a role in pain modulation.

Opiates are morphine-like analgesics with spinal and central sites of action. They interact at specific opioid receptors where their properties are similar to endogenous peptides (enkephalins, endorphins, and dynorphins). Four distinct opioid receptors have been identified: (*a*) μ-receptor mediates analgesia, miosis, respiratory depression, and opioid withdrawal syndrome; (*b*) κ-receptor mediates spinal analgesia but not opioid withdrawal; (*c*) σ-receptor mediates pupillary dilatation, tachypnea, and dysphoria; and (*d*) δ-receptor-modulates effects of the μ-response. Studies have suggested that visceral pain may be more responsive to κ-receptor agonists, whereas cutaneous (somatic) pain responds best to μ- and δ-agonists.

Techniques

Intravenous Narcotics

Small intravenous doses of narcotics have been shown to provide satisfactory pain relief as opposed to the traditional intramuscular injection. Intravenous administration may be by continuous infusion or self-administered via mechanisms controlled by the patient. This latter system allows patients to administer small calculated doses of analgesics with a lockout interval that limits overdosing.

Intrathecal and Epidural Narcotics

The highly specific opioid receptors (μ, κ) are located in high concentrations in the lamina I and II of the substantia gelatinosa. These areas coincide with termination areas for nociceptive fibers. Most opioids act at these receptor sites to inhibit release of substance P, a neurotransmitter of nociceptive stimuli. Numerous studies have demonstrated the efficacy of both epidural and intrathecal narcotics in the control of pain.

Intrathecal analgesia may be accomplished by a variety of drugs, but single-dose morphine is used most commonly. Epidural analgesia may be produced by similar drugs as those used intrathecally. Epidural administration permits more precise control and is more amenable to continuous or long-term therapy.

Side effects of both methods include pruritus, nausea and vomiting, urinary retention, and respiratory depression. Small doses of naloxone will control these problems without disturbance in pain relief. Motor sensory and sympathetic function is not disturbed by epidural or intrathecal narcotics.

Others

Other methods of pain relief include intercostal nerve block, intrapleural instillation of local anesthetics, and catheters placed via the interscalen or axillary approach for upper extremity analgesia. Recent work on transdermal opioids using fentanyl has shown promise, providing serum drug levels similar to continuous intravenous infusion.

GLOSSARY

Shunt—passage of blood from pulmonary artery to pulmonary vein without gas exchange.

Venus admixture—Shunting caused by perfusion in excess of ventilation, uneven distribution of ventilation, VA:Q inequality; shunt effect.
(a) **VA**—alveolar ventilation.
(b) **Q**—blood flow.

Dead space ventilation—Ventilation without gas exchange.
(a) **Anatomic dead space**—conducting air space (trachea, bronchi).
(b) Alveolar dead space is alveolar air that does not exchange with blood.

Restrictive lung disease—pulmonary dysfunction with an overall decrease in lung volume.

Obstructive lung disease—pulmonary dysfunction with an overall increase in lung volume.

REFERENCES

1. Richter JJ. Mechanisms of general anesthesia. In: Barash PG, Cullen BF, Stoelting RK, eds. Clinical anesthesia. Philadelphia: JB Lippincott, 1989:282.
2. Hudson RJ. Basic principles of pharmacology. In: Barash PG, Cullen BF, Stoelting RK, eds. Clinical anesthesia. Philadelphia: JB Lippincott, 1989:152.
3. Durett LR, Lawson NW. Autonomic nervous system physiology and pharmacology. In: Barash PG, Cullen BF, Stoelting RK, eds. Clinical anesthesia. Philadelphia: JB Lippincott, 1989:1966.
4. Lebowitz PW, Ramsey FM. Muscle relaxants. In: Barash PG, Cullen BF, Stoelting RK, eds. Clinical anesthesia. Philadelphia: JB Lippincott, 1989:362.
5. Subcommittee on the National Halothane Study of the Committee on Anesthesia. National Academy of Sciences-National Research Council. Summary of the National Halothane Study. Possible association between halothane anesthesia and postoperative necrosis. JAMA 1966;197:775.
6. Tuman KJ, McCarthy RS, Spiess BD, et al. Does choice of anesthetic agent significantly affect outcome after coronary artery surgery? Anesthesiology 1989;70:189.
7. American Society of Anesthesiologists. New classification of physical status. Anesthesiology 1963;24:111.
8. Steen PA, Tinker JH, Tarhan S. Myocardial reinfarction after anesthesia and surgery. JAMA 1978;239:2655.
9. Barash, PG. Preoperative evaluation of the cardiac patient for noncardiac surgery. In: Kaplan JA, ed. Cardiothoracic and vascular anesthesia update. Vol. 2. Philadelphia: JB Lippincott Co., 1991:1–10.

SUGGESTED READINGS

Barash PG, Cullen BF, Stoelting RK, eds. Clinical anesthesia. Philadelphia: JB Lippincott, 1989.
Birmingham, PK, Cheney FW, Ward RW. Esophageal intubation: a review of detection techniques. Anesth Analg 1986;65:886.
Blitt CD, ed. Monitoring in anesthesia and critical care medicine. New York: Churchill Livingstone, 1985.
Carpenter RL, Eger EI II, Johnson BH, et al. The extent of metabolism of inhaled anesthetics in humans. Anesthesiology 1986;65:201.
Cousins MJ, Bridenbaugh PO. Neural blockade in clinical anesthesia and management of pain. 2nd ed. Philadelphia: JB Lippincott, 1988.
Eger EI II, ed. Anesthetic uptake and action. Baltimore: Williams & Wilkins, 1974.
Finck AD. Opiate receptors and endorphins: significance for anesthesiology. In: Hershey SG, ed. Refresher courses in anesthesiology. Vol 7. Philadelphia: JB Lippincott, 1979.
Miller RD, ed. Anesthesia. 2nd ed. New York: Churchill Livingstone, 1981.
Oden RV, ed. Management of postoperative pain. Vol 7. No 1. Anesthesiology clinics of North America. Philadelphia: WB Saunders, 1989.
Shapiro BA, Harrison RA, Cane RD, et al. Clinical application of blood gases. 4th ed. Chicago: Year Book Medical, 1982.
Stoelting RK, ed. Pharmacology and physiology in anesthesia practice. Philadelphia: JB Lippincott, 1987.
Stout DM, Bishop MJ. Perioperative laryngeal and tracheal complications of intubation. In: Bishop MJ, ed. Problems in anesthesia, Vol 2. No 2. Philadelphia: JB Lippincott, 1988:225–233.
Wylie WD, Churchill-Davidson HC, eds. A practice of anesthesia. 4th ed. Philadelphia: WB Saunders, 1978.

25 Selected Technologies and General Surgery

Randolph B. Reinhold / Frederick J. Doherty / Frank M. Mele / Devika N. Jajoo

The goal of this chapter is to understand the basic principles behind selected diagnostic and therapeutic technology commonly used in general surgery. Modern diagnostic advances primarily center on the concept of sector and tomographic imaging as typified by ultrasound, computed tomography (CT) and magnetic resonance imaging (MRI). Nuclear medicine adds the functional dimension as it depends on biochemical uptake and biologic activity for the imaging process.

Application of technology for general surgical therapy is focused primarily on the electrocautery, laser, and ultrasonic scalpel. When viewed as a continuum, these applied energy sources have surprisingly similar tissue responses. Technical variations dictate the best situation in which each can be used. Diagnostic ultrasound depends heavily on clinical information, and in good hands, it can provide a wealth of details. In a clinical vacuum, it can be useless and at times nonspecific.

Selected Diagnostic Technologies

Ultrasound

Modern diagnostic ultrasound has evolved over the past three decades from a rather crude imaging device to a sophisticated high-resolution real-time imager with broad applications. The unique ability to obtain 2-D images with ultrasound waves has always required specialized technical and artistic skills by the operator, and operator dependence continues to the present time. As the operator becomes more experienced and the equipment more advanced, more detailed information is available.

The Sonar Connection

Imaging with ultrasound is a direct spin off from the navy's efforts with sonar (sound navigation and ranging) in World War II. Fish and bats navigate with sound waves. It is known that sound travels better in water than in air, and the navy was able to use the elastic properties of sound in water to detect objects in the sea. Sonar was able to determine how far away these objects were and in what direction they were located. Sonar was developed to plot the terrain of the invisible ocean floor and to search under the sea's surface for submarines.

A sonar transducer is a piezoelectric crystal that both transmits sound waves in the ocean and receives echoes returning from objects under water. Time equals distance when sound is at a constant velocity. The distance to an object from the transducer can be calculated because the velocity of sound in water is known. The farther away an object is, the longer it will take for an echo to return to the transducer. Knowing the position of the transducer and the direction of the transmitted sound wave localizes the direction of the object. Modern ultrasound scanners behave like sonar. Their images depend on the transmission of sound waves into body tissues of water density, the reception of echoes reflected from tissue interfaces, and machine knowledge of the position of the transducer on the body surface (Fig. 25.1).

Modern Ultrasound Scanning

A modern ultrasound machine is a portable, real-time 2-D imager equipped with numerous probes for different specific applications. A hand-held probe contains the ultrasound transducer and is connected to the scanner by a flexible cable. The probe is placed on the skin of the patient, and a relatively small planar area deep to the probe is imaged. The probe can be oriented in any of an infinite variety of scanning planes. The image is updated so rapidly that it appears to be in real time. Motion is observed directly. The probe is not like a flashlight, magic wand, or divining rod. Only a small planar area under an available skin window is imaged.

Modern scanners are equipped with needle guides for direct visualization of targets during percutaneous interventional procedures. Inasmuch as these scanners are portable, the probes can be wrapped with sterile covers for use in a sterile field in the operating room. They

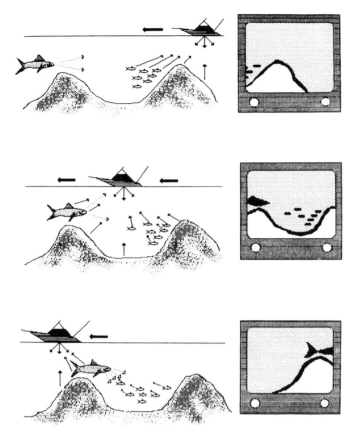

Figure 25.1. The principle of sonar is shown. A fishing boat moving along the ocean's surface is scanning the water underneath with a sonic transducer. As the boat moves along, the changing profile of the ocean floor as well as any fish swimming below the boat are plotted on a videoscope, as they reflect echoes back to the transducer. The image on the scope is updated as the boat travels along the ocean surface. The y-axis of the image on the scope is the depth below the boat. The x-axis is motion of the boat along the sea surface. Diagnostic ultrasound imaging is similar to this process. Note that the large shark also is using sonar to find a meal and to watch the boat.

are also equipped with Doppler packages, which allow direct visualization of blood flowing in vessels as well as spectral analysis of the dynamic wave forms of flowing blood. A complement of different probes is available for various applications so that the best imaging for a specific situation can be accomplished. There are probes for all-purpose scanning, for obese patients, for thin patients, and for superficial scanning. Endoluminal probes are used in the vagina and rectum for high-resolution scanning of adjacent organs. Transesophageal and intravascular probes are also currently in use.

The Production of an Ultrasound Image. An ultrasound system is made up of a series of several in-line components, consisting basically of a probe, a scanner, and an image recorder. A hand-held probe houses the transducer and is connected to the basic scanning machine. The probe's job is the transmission, reception, and aim of the sound waves.

The sound waves used medically are high frequency ones in the 1 to 10 MHZ range. These are far above

audible sound, which ranges in frequency from 16 to 16,000 cycles per second (cps); 1 MHZ is equal to 1 million cps. Higher frequency sound waves have smaller wavelengths than lower frequency ones. In other words, the distance from one cycle to the next gets longer as the frequency decreases. There are less cps with a lower frequency wave front.

The scanner is a "black box" housing all the electrical components of the system. Its job is the control of the signals sent out to the probe and the processing of signals received from it. The received analogue signals are converted to digital format, processed, analyzed, and stored in digital memory. The digital information is assigned to pixels and is displayed on a video monitor. The acquisition and display of signals is done rapidly so that the image displayed is updated continually at many frames a second, and the resulting video display is in a real-time format. The real-time image can be frozen to produce a static image. Once an image is produced on a video monitor, it is recorded for further analysis, review, and storage. Various recording devices are available, such as video recorders, multi format cameras, color paper printers, laser printers, and 35-mm cameras.

For Doppler ultrasound, audio speakers are used for the operator to hear the sounds of blood flowing. Doppler ultrasound is described later in this section.

The Ultrasound Transducer. The critical first element in a scanning system is the transducer, which is housed in the probe. The transducer is a ceramic crystal that has a piezoelectric quality that allows electricity to be converted to sound and sound to be converted back to electricity. The piezoelectric effect results in a change in the shape of the crystal when an electrical current is applied. The transducer has two important actions. It serves both as a transmitter of ultrasound waves and as a receiver of sound waves (reflected echoes).

The transducer does not transmit sound continuously. It requires temporal resolution. It must first be pulsed with a current to send out a sound wave. Then it must listen for a period of time to collect all the reflected echoes from that transmitted sound wave before it sends out its next sound wave. In effect, the transducer is listening more than 99% of the time between pulses. In this listening stage, each returning echo will produce a voltage that will be processed by the scanner. The axial resolution of an ultrasound system is its most discriminating. This is the transducer's ability to detect structures at different depths along the sound beam path. It relates to the temporal resolution of the system and is effectively in the order of about 1 mm (Fig. 25.2).

The 2-D Image. The probe housing the transducer is placed on the surface of the body and sound waves are sent deeper into the body along a thin path. This path provides the y-axis of a 2-D image—a collection of reflected echoes are displayed as dots along a thin path. Motion of the probe along the surface of the body to

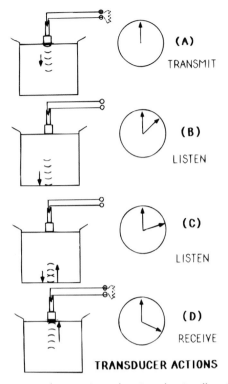

Figure 25.2. Transducer actions; the piezoelectric effect is demonstrated. **A,** At time = 0, a transducer in a beaker is pulsed with a short current of electricity. The resulting vibration propagates a short sound wave deep into the beaker. Current stops flowing as the sound goes into the water. **B,** The transducer listens, as time marches on, although the sound wave goes deeper, hitting the bottom of the beaker. No electrical current is flowing. **C,** The sound wave is reflected off the beaker's bottom as an echo returning to the transducer, which is still listening as the clock ticks. There is still no current in the transducer. **D,** The reflected echo strikes the transducer, causing it to change shape and emit a voltage in the transducer. The time from transmit to receive can be measured, and the distance to the beaker calculated, as the electrical impulse is processed in the scanner.

different scanning positions in a straight line provides the x-axis of the image. The image is made up of multiple dots of different shades of gray, depending on the strengths of the reflected echoes. It is similar to an electronic sketch made of echoes drawn on a background. The customary display is against a black background (nighttime scanning) although a white background can also be used (daytime scanning).

The transducer in the probe is moved along the surface of the body in an automated way. The practical effect is a series of thin scan lines, each representing a transmitted sound wave path. This is done generally in either linear or sector format. In linear format, numerous parallel scan lines are produced, originating perpendicularly from the surface of a probe that is several centimeters in length. In sector format, the probe has a much smaller footprint and produces diverging scan lines in a windshield-wiper fashion, scanning back and forth from a central point at the probe surface. Sector probes have fields of view that become wider with increasing depth. The very near field, in the tight apex of the sector,

has little information. Linear probes have more near field information, but the field does not enlarge with increasing depth (Fig. 25.3).

Image Display.   When any probe is used, its transducer operates at a single given frequency. The echoes that return to the transducer will return at the same frequency, although they may have different amplitudes. The amplitude of the echo refers to its strength, and it is independent of the frequency. A good strong echo will have a high amplitude, and a weak echo will have a low amplitude that is barely off the baseline when displayed in graphic format. When echoes are displayed in dot format, the highest amplitude echoes will be seen as white dots on a black background, and low amplitude weak echoes will be dark gray (almost black) and barely visible. Echoes of amplitudes between the strongest and weakest will be displayed in a gray scale fashion from white to almost black (Fig. 25.4).

Although sector or linear formats are generally used for image display, newer scanners have subtle modifications of these shapes. Sector images can be displayed in a trapezoidal format, when some type of standoff is used and a few centimeters of skin surface are displayed in the apex of the sector, as opposed to the image originating at a point on the skin surface. Curved linear probes produce an image with a good near field and less divergence of the scan lines with increasing depth. Curved linear probes are a good compromise between sectors and linears. Some endoluminal probes rotate to produce a circular image, with the probe site in the center (Fig. 25.5).

Physical Properties of Diagnostic Ultrasound

In the previous section, the basic concepts of obtaining an image were described. However, certain physical characteristics of ultrasound are factors in everyday imaging, and an awareness of these properties is necessary to understand the modality. In the following sections, some of the eccentric properties of ultrasound will be discussed in light of their influences in routine scanning.

Water Density Medium Necessary.   The best ultrasound transmission is in water, which has the proper elastic properties for the efficient propagation of a sound wave front. Different body tissues of water type-density have slight differences in their speed of sound transmission when they are compared with one another. These differences in sound transmission between two tissues is a property referred to as the acoustic impedance of the tissue, which allows the reflection of echoes from the different interfaces as sound is transmitted deeply into the body. The difference between the speed of transmission of sound in water versus air or bone is great. Bone is too hard and inelastic for transmission, and it serves as too strong a reflector of sound, allowing no transmission deeper into the body. This results in an area in back of bone with no echoes. This is called an

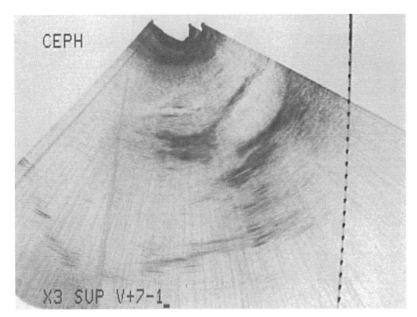

Figure 25.3. Scan lines. This is an antique static "B" scan image of a liver, which shows the scan lines composing the image. The lines are seen clearly in the deeper portions (*bottom*) of the image as they diverge, and are identified less clearly in the more superficial area closer to the skin (*top*).

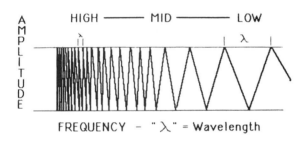

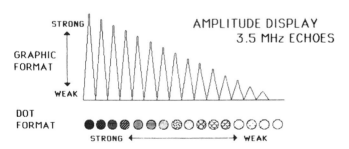

Figure 25.4. Amplitude, frequency, and gray scale. **Top,** Sound waves of changing frequencies are shown with equal amplitude (strength). Note how the wavelength of a high-frequency sound wave is much smaller than that of a low-frequency wave. **Bottom,** Echoes of a single frequency but of diminishing amplitude are shown in graphic format; the height of an echo relates to its strength. Just below the graphic picture of amplitude changes, the same information is displayed in dot format; high-amplitude echoes are shown as dark bright dots, and weak ones are shown as weak dots almost equal to the background. This is the principle of "B" scanning and gray scale.

acoustic shadow. Calcifications also behave like bones. However, gas or air have molecules too far apart for effective transmission of a wave front, which also will result in shadowing deep to that area. In other words, ultrasound cannot be transmitted through bones, stones, air, or gas, and imaging of structures deep to such areas is impossible. A water density window is needed for sound transmission.

The liver and spleen are seen easily against the body wall without any interposing air or gas. Acoustic windows are available in the lower intercostal surfaces. The liver and spleen are good windows for imaging the kidneys. A full urinary bladder lifts small bowel loops out of the pelvis, which allows imaging of the female organs. Neonates have open fontanelles with no bone to allow intracranial imaging.

With all ultrasound scanning, a thick, watery gel is used as an acoustic coupler on the body to eliminate the air at the transducer/skin interface. Bandages, ostomies, and open wounds will all trap air and hence interfere with the transmission of diagnostic ultrasound waves.

As with air and bone, fat is also the enemy. These macroscopic cells have numerous angled interfaces that scatter the sound beam. Fat effectively works as a filter. It scatters the sound being transmitted as well as the echoes returning to the probe. The more adipose tissue that exists between the transducer and at the region of interest, the less information there is that is available.

Bones, air, gas, and fat all cause severe limitations to ultrasound. They may not be absolute limitations, but it should be recognized that the confidence levels of these scans are severely reduced, and often only the grossest information is obtainable. Looking for an abdominal abscess in an obese postoperative patient with an ileus is generally fruitless.

Attenuation. In life it is necessary to pay a price for everything, and unfortunately the power of an ultra-

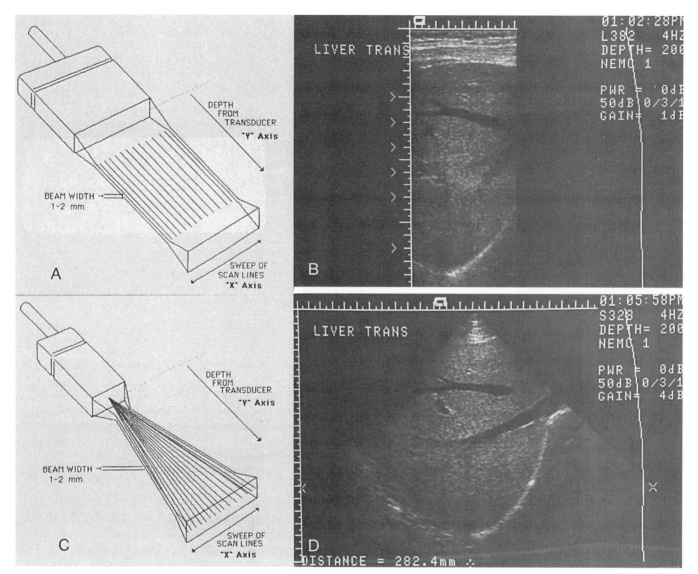

Figure 25.5. Linear and sector probes. The difference between a linear transducer probe and a sector probe are shown here. **A,** The linear transducer images by scanning with parallel lines (y-axis) originating along its surface in perpendicular fashion (x-axis). The beam width is also shown here. Note that it is narrowest in its focal zone and wider in the near and far fields. **B,** A liver imaged with a linear probe. The skin surface and abdominal wall are shown, as is a large branching hepatic vein. The depth of the image is 20 cm, and its width remains at 8 cm throughout.

C, The sector probe produces diverging scan lines from a small probe, with the image originating at a point in the center of the probe. This probe has a beam width profile similar to the linear one. **D,** The same liver as in **B.** Again the depth is 20 cm but the width covered is 28 cm in the far field. The near field has less information than the linear probe, and the resolution in the far field is somewhat less than the linear probe because of the diverging scan lines. This probe is an excellent tool for surveying large areas.

sound beam is rather limited. As sound is sent into the body and echoes are reflected, the sound beam is attenuated. Each returning echo strips off a little energy from the transmitted wave. As the sound goes deeper into the body, and more echoes are returned, the sound beam becomes progressively weaker, until it no longer can reflect any echoes back to the transducer. The energy lost by attenuation comes off as heat, but at diagnostic power levels, there appears to be no actual tissue damage (Fig. 25.6).

Controls on the scanner are used to counteract the process of attenuation. Both the transmit power and the

receiver gain can be adjusted, and the time gain compensation (TGC) control is used. The gain is similar to the volume on a stereo. The longer an echo takes to return to the transducer (the deeper it is), the more it can be amplified (Fig. 25.7). Constant adjustment of these controls by the operator is necessary when scanning.

Scatter. The strongest echoes that are reflected back to the transducer come from structures oriented in a plane perpendicular to the direction of the sound beam. As reflective structures become oriented in a direction more parallel to the beam, the returning echoes become increasingly scattered, similar to the effect of skipping a stone on the surface of a lake. Scattered echoes do not return to the transducer. When a reflector is at a critical angle somewhat more than 50° off the perpendicular plane, the sound beam will be scattered and lost, and the area deep to this point will be shadowed. This phenomenon is seen at the edges of cysts or rounded organs such as the aorta, kidney, and gallbladder. Fibrous structures, such as Cooper's ligaments in the breast, behave in a similar fashion. Usually, there is no problem identifying this process during real-time scanning (Fig. 25.8).

Tissue Characteristics. As mentioned earlier, tissues are displayed with varying types of echogenicity. Cysts are fluid-filled structures with no internal components to reflect echoes; therefore, they are anechoic. Calcified structures as well as pockets of air or gas produce strong echoes at the first soft tissue/calcified object interface or soft tissue/air interface, with acoustic shadowing of all structures deep to these areas. Soft tissue structures are displayed with gradually changing echogenicities along the gray scale from a hypoechoic to a hyperechoic presentation. Soft tissue structures also have different abilities to transmit sound. Often they transmit sound well, with good visualization of deeper areas, or they can attenuate the sound beam somewhat, resulting in some type of partial shadowing of deeper

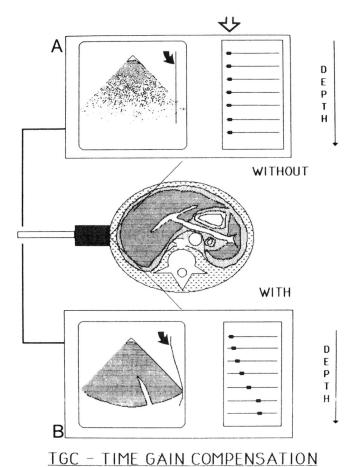

TGC — TIME GAIN COMPENSATION

Figure 25.7. Time gain compensation. The TGC control is shown. A liver is being scanned from a lateral approach. **A,** The video monitor on the scanner is shown, and the TGC control is to its right. A *solid curved arrow* points to the TGC curve on the image. It is a straight line, corresponding to the settings of the slide pods on the TGC control (*open arrow*). Note how there is no information in the image of the liver. It vanishes with increasing depth because of attenuation. **B,** By smoothly and progressively adjusting the slide pods to the right with increasing depth, deeper areas of the liver are increasingly amplified to counteract the effects of attenuation. The TGC curve is no longer flat (*solid curved arrow*) and the liver is adequately imaged. Note the appearance of the image on the monitor, with the apex at the top of the screen, and how it relates to the position of the sector originating at the probe's surface on the patient's right side.

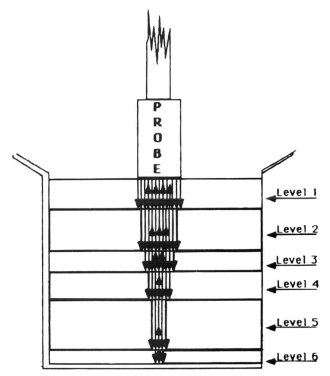

Figure 25.6. Attenuation with depth; attenuation is demonstrated. This is a diagram of a phantom with different horizontal levels. The probe is aimed toward the bottom. The sound is loudest and strongest as it leaves the probe. Echoes are reflected off each deeper layer. As echoes are returned to the transducer off each layer, the sound wave going deeper becomes weaker at each level, until it has little power remaining as it approaches the bottom of the beaker. Each reflected echo strips away some of the power of the sound wave as it is attenuated progressively with increasing depth.

areas. Fibroid tumors of the uterus often display relative attenuation of the sound beam (Fig. 25.9, A–D).

Beam Thickness. In addition to the number of scan lines in the image, the width of the sound beam also affects the lateral resolution of an ultrasound scan. Although the ideal ultrasound beam would be infinitely thin, it unfortunately has an actual thickness roughly in the range of 1 to 2 mm. Beam thickness may result in partial imaging of small cysts, which can appear to have internal echoes, or lack of shadowing deep to small stones. For a stone to shadow, it must be larger than the beam width to block the sound transmission. If it is smaller, then sound can pass on either side of the stone and there will be no shadow.

PHANTOMS   US IMAGES

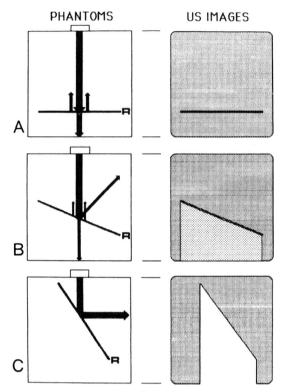

Figure 25.8.   Reflection and scatter. **A,** A bright horizontal reflector (*R*) in a phantom is imaged. Echoes are reflected strongly, although the sound is transmitted deeper. **B,** As the reflector is elevated to 30°, some of the sound waves are scattered out of the field. The resultant image shows slightly less information deep to the reflector, which also is imaged with echoes of slightly less amplitude. **C,** The reflector has been elevated to 60° off horizontal, resulting in complete scattering of the sound waves out of the field. The corresponding image shows a weaker presentation of the reflector itself in addition to complete shadowing in back of it. The sound waves scattered off the reflector are lost, never to return to the transducer.

Cysts

One of the original and important diagnostic uses of ultrasound is its ability to differentiate cysts and other fluid-filled structures from solid tissue. Although cysts are generally rounded in shape, they often exhibit irregular shapes, with wrinkles in their walls or lobulated appearances. Blood vessels or ligaments can tether the walls of cysts. These will exert an influence on them, resulting in changes in shape secondary to the external pressure on them. Nevertheless, the appearance of sharp near and deep walls still is seen, and a clearly defined strong back wall remains a hallmark of a cyst.

With modern scanners, cysts are often filled with internal echoes that represent particles or debris. These particles can be seen more clearly when the gain is increased, and they can also be observed to move during real-time scanning. When fine internal echoes are seen in a cyst, they are hypoechoic and homogeneous. Inasmuch as a cyst may no longer appear as strictly anechoic, it will usually be represented with the most hypoechoic appearance of any structure in the image. It is helpful

to compare a cyst with other known fluid structures in the image, such as the urinary bladder, the gallbladder, or a blood vessel that is seen clearly. Hydroceles, spermatoceles, and endometriomas frequently show internal echoes. Even blood vessels will show moving internal echoes when imaged optimally with modern scanning.

Hemangiomas of the liver and a thick secretory endometrium almost always show increased through transmission. It is a nice feature if seen, but by itself it is somewhat of an antique sign. However, although a cyst may not necessarily show posterior acoustic enhancement, it will never attenuate the sound (Fig. 25.10).

Resolution and Penetration

The resolution of an ultrasound transducer is directly related to its frequency. As the frequency of sound increases, its wavelength decreases. A smaller wavelength is capable of discriminating between smaller objects. A larger wavelength sound beam may detect two small objects as only a single larger object. Hence, to increase the resolution of an ultrasound system, higher frequency transducers are used. Unfortunately, a price is paid in penetration. Higher frequency sound waves reflect more echoes more frequently from smaller structures, and they are attenuated more easily than lower frequency transducers. When a lower frequency ultrasound probe is used, more penetration into the body can be achieved, but there will be less resolution. With a higher frequency transducer, increased resolution of smaller structures can be achieved, but there will be less penetration. Higher frequency transducers offer superb resolution but are limited to superficial parts scanning. The situation here is similar to playing a stereo system in an apartment building. The music sounds fine in the room where the speakers are and where all the instruments are heard. In the adjacent apartments, the music will be muffled with loss of the high-frequency instruments such as violins, and only the annoying booming of low-frequency sounds such as bass drums will be heard through the walls.

The frequencies of diagnostic ultrasound transducers vary from approximately 2 MHZ up to about 10 MHZ. The low-frequency probes (2 MHZ) are used for imaging large body areas such as the right upper quadrant in an obese person. Midrange probes (3–5 MHZ) are used for all-purpose imaging in normal to thin individuals. High-frequency probes (7–10 MHZ) are used for superficial parts scanning.

Recently, endoluminal probes have been introduced in which high-frequency transducers are used on long probes inserted into body openings. This allows superficial parts-type imaging of the rectum, prostate, and the female pelvic organs with a clarity previously unknown. Transesophageal probes are used in cardiac evaluation and intravascular probes also are currently available (Fig. 25.11).

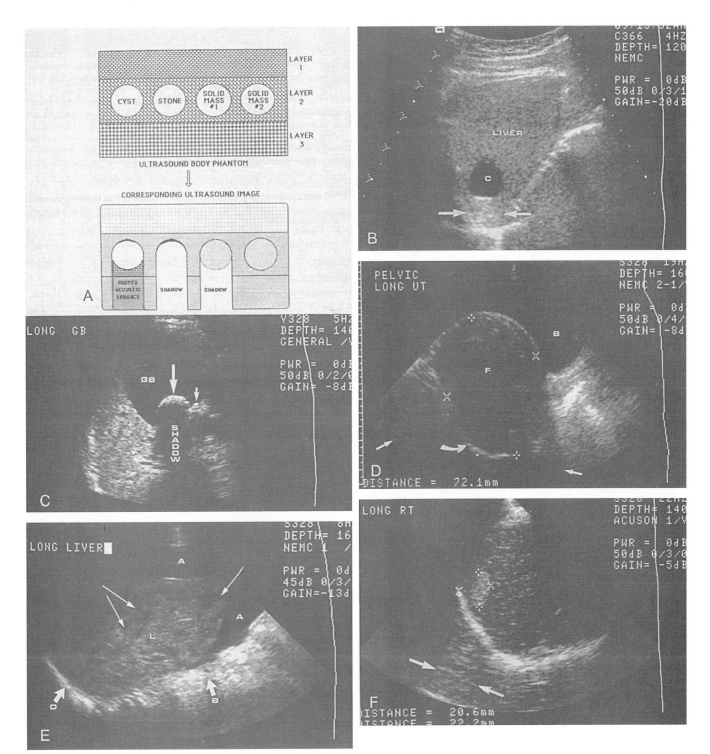

Figure 25.9. Sonographic tissue characteristics. **A,** This is a diagram of a phantom with several objects inside as well as their corresponding images. A fluid-filled cyst is depicted as an anechoic structure with sharp near and far walls along with posterior acoustic enhancement or increased through transmission. A stone is shown with a bright echo from its leading edge and an acoustic shadow deep to this edge. Solid mass #1 is imaged as a hypoechoic structure. Its back wall is seen, but it attenuates the sound somewhat and causes a shadow deep to the back wall. Solid mass #2 has a similar appearance as #1, but the sound is not attenuated and deeper tissue is seen. **B,** An anechoic *cyst (c)* in the liver is shown. *Arrows* point to the edge of the area of posterior acoustic enhancement deep to the cyst. This image was taken with a curvilinear transducer. **C,** A large *arrow* points to the leading edge of a large gallstone in the gallbladder (*GB*). Note the strong shadow deep to the stone. A *small arrow* points to a second tiny gallstone. This has no shadow because it is too small to block the sound beam, which has a width greater than the stone. **D,** A huge fibroid (*F*) of the uterus is shown deep to the filled urinary bladder (*B*). Calipers measure the fibroid at 10 × 7 cm. A *curved arrow* points to the back wall of the fibroid. Smaller *straight arrows* point to the edges of the shadow in back of the fibroid caused by its attenuating effect. Note how much brighter the echoes are deep to the bladder in contrast to the area deep to the fibroid. **E,** *Long thin arrows* point to a few of the multiple hypoechoic metastases in this liver (*L*) surrounded by anechoic ascites (*A*). *Short broad arrows* point to the hyperechoic diaphragm (*D*) and posterior body wall (*B*). **F,** Calipers measure a 2-cm hyperechoic hemangioma in the liver adjacent to the diaphragm. *Arrows* point to the edges of a path of increased through transmission deep to the hemangioma; a quality that is not limited to cysts.

625

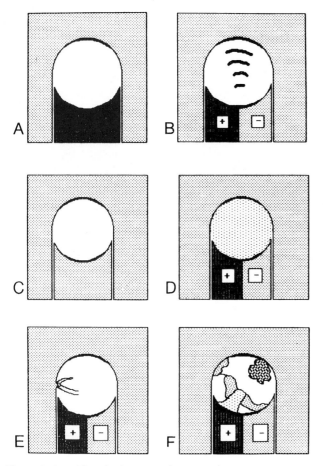

Figure 25.10. The classic cyst with its nonclassic appearances are shown. **A,** A perfectly rounded anechoic cyst with strong near and deep walls, lateral edge shadows (from tangential scatter) and increased through transmission. **B,** The same cyst qualities without any posterior acoustic enhancement. This is a common cyst presentation when scanned off its center. More than 50% of cysts can produce such an image. **C,** A cyst with a blood vessel running around its surface is depicted. The vessel causes a wall irregularity, which can be recognized at real-time scanning as a peripheral tubular curvilinear defect that can be recognized easily as a surface vessel. This appearance is seen commonly in the liver, kidney, and breast. The positive and negative appearances in back of the cyst refer to the inconsistent presence or absence of increased through transmission, depending on the position of the scan plane. **D,** These are reverberation artifacts that produce internal echoes within the cyst. These have been described in a previous section and are obvious at real-time scanning. **E,** This cyst is filled with homogenous internal echoes—either secondary to beam width artifact or representing actual debris within the cyst. The echoes from debris in a cyst can often be seen moving at real-time scanning. **F,** A complex mass—a cyst with solid internal components. These masses have a wide differential from benign hemorrhagic events to abscesses and cystic neoplasms. Change on a repeat scan can be diagnostic.

Motion

The beauty of real-time scanning lies in its ability to detect motion, and the resultant static images that are usually available fail to show this feature. Fetal behavior can be assessed because body motion, breathing, and heart rate changes can be observed. Particles can be observed moving in cyst fluid, and blood flowing through vessels can be seen. Stones in the gallbladder will move to a dependent position when the patient's position on the table is changed. Polyps in the gallbladder will not move into a dependent position. Masses often can be palpated and imaged simultaneously for diagnostic purposes. A palpable lump in the breast could be a tumor, a cyst, or a ridge of normal tissue. This is shown clearly at real-time scanning.

Needle Guides

Many modern probes are available with needle guides for direct image-guided interventional purposes. If a deep target can be seen from the skin, it can usually be punctured percutaneously from the same window. Brackets are attached to the probe where the needle is held in a fairly rigid fashion along a path at an angle to the sound beam and in the plane of the image. Software in the scanner places a target pathway on the image. The target is lined up in the path, and the needle is watched as it enters the target. This has multiple applications, among which are the aspiration of abscesses or small fluid collections, biopsy of nonpalpable masses, endovaginal oocyte retrieval from ovarian follicles for in vitro fertilization procedures, and transrectal biopsy of prostate nodules (Fig. 25.12).

Doppler Ultrasound

Doppler ultrasound has evolved into a sophisticated tool with ever-increasing applications for evaluating the dynamics of blood flow. Current scanners using color Doppler have remarkable sensitivity and resolution, by which slow flow can be detected easily in small blood vessels throughout the body. Graphic displays of vascular flow patterns are now obtained easily and confidently using color Doppler for guidance.

Doppler ultrasound is basically an extension of imaging—extracting information that is available in the echoes reflected back to the ultrasound transducer. Modern Doppler ultrasound usually refers to image-guided pulsed Doppler evaluation of blood vessels, by which the flow dynamics in a selected site in an imaged vessel are displayed in graphic format. This is known as duplex scanning. Color Doppler is another way of displaying the same information in a direct visual manner, without using a graphic format.

The Doppler effect is the change in the perceived frequency of sound when there is relative motion between the source of the sound and the detector. The classic example of the Doppler effect is the change heard in the pitch of a train whistle as the train approaches and then passes by an observer standing on the side of the tracks. The engineer on the moving train only hears a whistle of unchanging frequency, because he or she also is moving along with the train. An observer on the ground first hears the pitch of the whistle increase as the train approaches because the sound wave essentially is chasing itself. Its wavelength effectively shortens as the wave

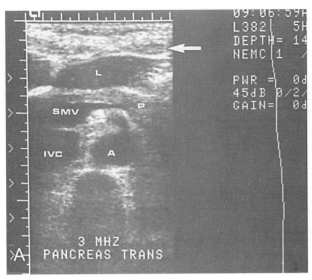

Figure 25.11. Resolution. **A,** Transverse image of the mid-abdomen taken with a 3-MHZ probe. An *arrow* points to one of the anterior abdominal wall muscles, where the detail is suboptimal. Nevertheless, the depth of the entire image is 14 cm. The liver (*L*), pancreas (*P*), superior mesenteric vein (*SMV*), abdominal aorta (*A*), and inferior vena cava (*IVC*) are labeled. **B,** This image is taken with a 7-MHZ probe, and its depth here is only to 4 cm. Both the right (*RRAM*) and left (*LRAM*) rectus abdominis muscles are shown as they contact each other in the midline. The skin is next to the probe. The subcutaneous tissue (*SQ*) is imaged, as is the first 1.5 cm of the liver.

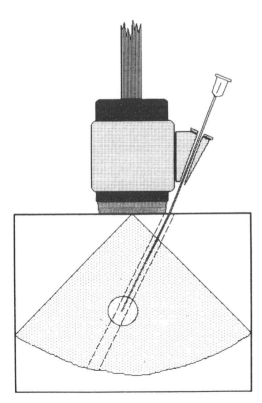

Figure 25.12. Needle guidance. The concept of needle guidance is shown. A probe is fitted with a needle guide, and software in the scanner places a target path in the image. The target to be punctured percutaneously is lined up in the needle path during real-time scanning. The needle is introduced into a fairly rigid system that positions the needle into the plane of the image for direct real-time visualization of the needle placement.

front becomes compressed. When the train passes the observer on the tracks, the frequency of the whistle then decreases as the wave front stretches out because the sound now is running away from itself (Fig. 25.13).

When ultrasound waves are used in the body, the echoes reflected are the same frequency as those transmitted if there is no motion: MHZ waves will be transmitted, and 3-MHZ echoes will be received. If something is moving in the body (e.g., red blood cells), echoes reflected from these structures will return at different frequencies than what was transmitted. Doppler scanners are able to detect and analyze these frequency changes. Thus, an echo from a red cell in a vessel in which blood is flowing toward the transducer will return at a slightly higher frequency than what was transmitted and would be assigned a positive frequency shift. Conversely, blood cells flowing away from the transducer will produce a negative frequency shift. The changes in frequency of reflected echoes can be detected in any pixel in the image. The frequency shifts above or below the baseline (the frequency of the transmitted sound) are displayed in graphic format. This allows the concept of duplex scanning. An image is produced by pulsing the transducer and collecting the echoes returning from the pulse. Those returning echoes have Doppler information, and this is referred to as pulsed Doppler. Using a real-time image to select the sampling site for simultaneous pulsed Doppler analysis is known as duplex scanning (Fig. 25.14).

Color Doppler is another way of displaying pulsed Doppler information. Rather than choosing a specific site for Doppler analysis, the entire image is analyzed pixel by pixel, and the average frequency shift in each pixel is determined. Instead of using a separate graphic format for Doppler display, the positive and negative shifts are generally displayed in two different colors that are superimposed on the appropriate pixels in the 2-D black-and-white image. If there is no flow, no color will appear in the image. Flow toward the probe will be shown in one of the two colors, although flow away from the probe will be displayed in the opposite color. Within each color there is also a color scale. Slow flow (low-frequency shifts) will be assigned a deeper color, and higher velocities (high-frequency shifts) will be displayed with brighter intensities of that color (Fig. 25.15).

The colors that are used are arbitrary and can be changed with a switch on the scanner. Several different color scales are usually available for different purposes. It must be emphasized that arteries are not necessarily red and veins blue. Only the relative direction of the blood flow in relation to the transducer is shown. A single tortuous vessel changing course up and down relative to the probe will be displayed in two different colors.

Although the best echoes in an image come from structures that are oriented at 90° to the direction of the sound beam, the best Doppler information is obtained

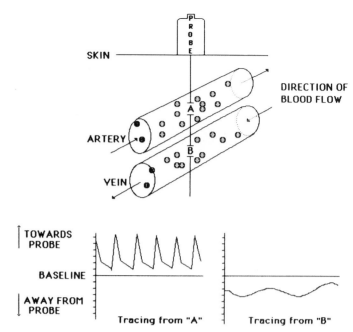

Figure 25.14. Duplex scanning–image-guided pulsed Doppler. **Top,** An artery and a vein are imaged. Two different sites are separately selected for pulsed Doppler analysis (*A* and *B*). **Bottom,** The graphic format of the pulsed Doppler sampling of these two vessels. The pattern from site *A* in the artery shows systolic peaks with a positive deflection from the baseline. At the end of the systolic peak, the flow velocity decreases in diastole, but it never reaches the baseline (no flow) until the next systole. This is typical of a blood-hungry organ with low peripheral vascular resistance, always receiving flow throughout the entire cardiac cycle. The tracing from the accompanying vein at site *B* shows a variable but constant flow, representative of the changes in intrathoracic pressure with respirations.

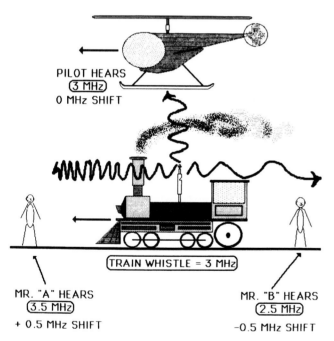

Figure 25.13. The Doppler effect. The classic example of the Doppler effect is demonstrated. A train blowing a whistle at a constant frequency is shown as it moves along its track. A helicopter travels above and along with the train at the same speed as the train. The pilot hears the whistle at the same frequency as the engineer because there is no relative motion between these two people. An observer in front of the train (*Mr. "A"*) hears the whistle increasing in pitch as the train approaches him because the sound wave is being compressed as the train chases its whistle. Another observer of the train (*Mr. "B"*) hears the whistle decreasing in pitch as the source of the sound runs away from itself, stretching out the sound wave. Mr. "A" hears a positive frequency shift (higher frequency/shorter wavelength) and Mr. "B" hears a negative frequency shift (lower frequency/longer wavelength).

along the path of the sound wave at 0°. Doppler information is often available even when imaging is suboptimal. It is frequently difficult to aim the probe down the barrel of a blood vessel, but good Doppler requires at least a 45° to 60° angle off the vessel. Color Doppler is used to identify the vessels and to assess rapidly their dynamics as well as to develop a good scanning site for the best Doppler angle. Then, pulsed Doppler is used at a specific site selected by its color appearance to obtain a graphic analysis of the flow dynamics at this site. Pulsed Doppler allows accurate quantitative measurements of velocities, the amounts of systolic and diastolic flow, resistive indices, pulsatility indices, and comparisons.

Continuous wave Doppler is used in high-velocity situations. These situations normally do not exist outside of the heart. Continuous wave Doppler is not image guided. A continuous wave Doppler probe has two transducers: one that is constantly transmitting and one that is constantly receiving. High velocities, such as those through a tight aortic stenosis, can be measured accurately in this way.

Conclusion

This section explained the basic concepts of ultrasound imaging while avoiding excess detail. However,

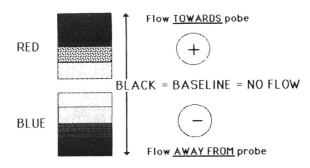

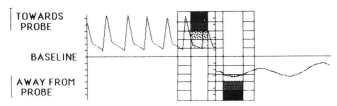

Figure 25.15. Color Doppler. The same graphic format of the pulsed Doppler tracing in Figure 25.14 is shown as it is translated into a color format. The baseline, where no detectable flow exists, is depicted as black. The deflections above and below the baseline are assigned different colors. The degree of deflection off the baseline is displayed with varying intensities of each color from dark to bright. These colors and their variable intensities are then superimposed on the real-time black-and-white 2-D image. The normally black blood vessel lumens will be filled with colors, representing the direction and velocity of the blood flowing within them.

it must be stressed that the physics of ultrasound are far more complicated than this simplistic presentation.

Operator and machine dependency are critical factors in diagnostic ultrasound imaging, and those clinicians not involved regularly with this modality are urged to use caution in self-interpretation. Frequently, the diagnosis is obvious, but subtleties and artifacts can often confuse the picture.

The field is changing constantly, and users are always adapting to these changes. Equipment currently in use is of various ages. Generally, newer equipment is better. Modern scanners have become expensive, and the use of a scanner is committed to whatever is available from that specific manufacturer for that specific machine (1–6).

CT

CT is a technique that allows cross-sectional or tomographic images of the body through the use of a narrow beam of radiographs. The patient is placed on a mobile tabletop that slides into and out of the gantry. The gantry is a circular structure containing both the radiograph tube and the detectors necessary to detect the amount of radiation that passes through the patient (i.e., is transmitted).

Evaluation of the transmitted radiographs is then done by computer, and an image is generated. The principle is illustrated in Figure 25.16. Assume you have nine boxes (in jargon, "pixels" or individual picture elements in a 2-dimensional image) arranged in a grid pattern. Each box is arbitrarily assigned a different fixed numeric value. Assume the numeric values themselves are unknown. To determine an unknown numeric box/pixel value requires knowing the values of the sums of the pixels from each different projection. This is analogous to the process of acquiring a CT image. A known quantity of radiation is passed through the patient from a series of different projections (horizontal, vertical, and diagonal in the above analogy). The sum of the radiographs can be determined by the surrounding radiograph detectors. The number of radiographs attenuated by tissue is the difference between the original number of radiographs and those transmitted. Working backward it is possible to determine the number of radiographs attenuated in each pixel so that the sum of radiographs transmitted equals the same number that the detectors have sensed.

The final CT image is constructed by simultaneously displaying the total number of pixels assigned to the vertical and horizontal dimensions. The number of pixels in each dimension (i.e., the matrix size) is typically fixed at 512 pixels by 512 pixels for a standard CT image. The pixel size, however, is variable, because it depends on the diameter of the field of view (FOV) being imaged. Pixel size is calculated simply by dividing the FOV by the matrix size. Each pixel is thus assigned a numeric value known as a Hounsfield Number (HN) or Hounsfield Unit. This value reflects the ability of the tissues within the pixel to attenuate the radiograph beam.

By convention, water has a HN of 0, air has a HN of −1000, and cortical bone has a measurement of +1000. Fat is typically −80 to −100 HN. However, the obtained HN values depend on the kVp (120 to 140) and filtration used for the exam and are thus approximate values.

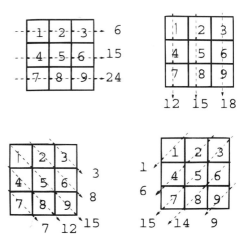

Figure 25.16. Determination of HU value per pixel is performed before an image is generated (see text for details).

Figure 25.17. Window widths describe the number of HU over which the shades of gray are distributed. **A,** Wide window (2000 HU). **B,** Narrow window (100 HU).

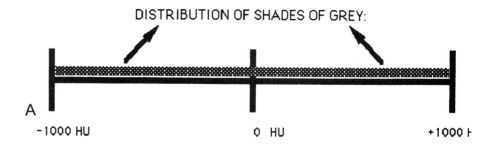

DISTRIBUTION OF SHADES OF GREY:

A

-1000 HU   0 HU   +1000 H

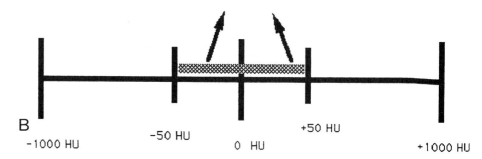

DISTRIBUTION OF SHADES OF GREY:

B

-1000 HU   -50 HU   0 HU   +50 HU   +1000 HU

Therefore, rather than relying on absolute HN, characterization of tissues is often best accomplished by using known structures within the body as internal standards (e.g., a patient's subcutaneous fat as lipid density and muscles as soft tissue density). Using filtered back projection image reconstruction algorithms, a black-and-white image is then constructed based on each pixel's HN. A high negative value (i.e., air) will appear black, and a high positive HN (i.e., cortical bone) will appear white. Values in between are assigned varying shades of gray. Each machine has 20 available shades of gray.

To optimize visualization of specific structures of interest (e.g., bones in trauma patient), the acquired image data can be manipulated by altering the window width and center. The window width determines the number of attenuation values (HN) chosen to represent these shades of gray. The width may be wide, such as 2000 HN (range from 1000 to +1000 HN) (Fig. 25.17A). Alternatively, a narrow width, such as 100 HN (range from −50 to +50 HN), may be selected (Fig. 25.17B). In the last instance, all CT values of −50 or less will be displayed as black and all values of +50 or more will be displayed as white. Values in between are assigned the 20 shades of gray. The narrow window width maximizes contrast and is therefore particularly useful when searching for subtle attenuation differences between tissues (Fig. 25.18). The window center is that HN about which the shades of gray are distributed. The average HN value of the tissue of interest is selected as the window center.

In the above examples, a center of 0 was chosen. However, one could just as easily choose a center of +100. If a window width of 1000 were chosen, the shades of gray would then range from 500 units above (+600 HN)

to 500 units below (−400 HN) the center of 100. Manipulation of both the window width and the center are thus used to idealize the visualization of various structures and pathologic anatomy (Fig. 25.19). Most routine CTs are done at a 5- to 10-mm slice thickness and thus can cover a large area. However, if one is interested in evaluating small structures, such as the adrenal gland, larynx, or distal pulmonary airways, thin slices are performed (typically in the 1- to 4-mm range).

The maximum radiation dose imparted to the patient in a single CT slice is estimated at 40 mGy (4 rads) for a head CT and 20 mGy (2 rads) for a body CT. The total radiation dose thus depends on the number of acquired slices. Other factors, such as slice thickness, scan time, and scan parameters of voltage and current, also affect patient dose. When imaging the body, the dose to the skin may be twice the dose to the center of the patient. When imaging the head, the skin to center dose ratio is virtually equal. Of note, even tissue not directly imaged but adjacent to the imaged region receives radiation exposure caused by the presence of scatter radiation.

Artifacts

CT images occasionally contain some rather typical artifacts that degrade the images. As in standard photography, any motion that takes place during the acquisition of the image will limit its definition. Thus, motion artifacts are frequently seen secondary to bowel peristalsis, respiration, or cardiac pulsation. Rapid acquisition of image data (1 to 3 sec/image) helps to reduce motion artifact. A second type of artifact is produced by metal joint prostheses, surgical clips, electronic pacing devices, and other high-density structures. In this case, any high-

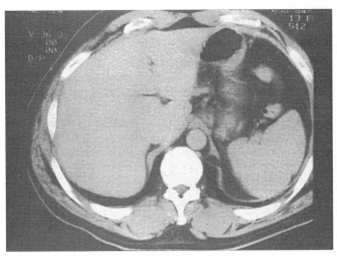

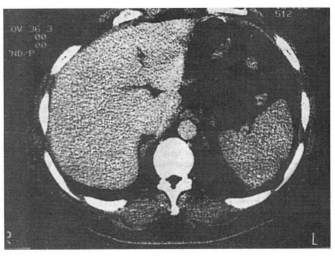

Figure 25.18. **Left,** Soft tissue window distributes the shades of gray over a relatively wide window. **Right,** Liver window distributes shades of gray over a relatively narrow window. Subtle attenuation differences between adjacent tissues are detected more easily.

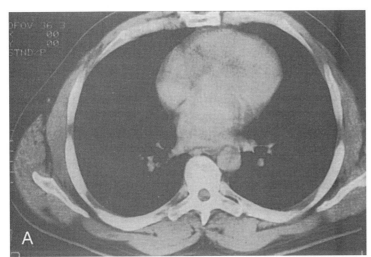

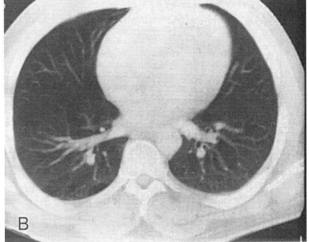

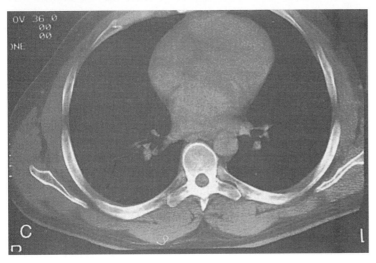

Figure 25.19. **A,** Mediastinal windows allow detail of the soft tissues. Notice the entire lung parenchyma is black, and no evaluation of this area is possible. **B,** Lung windows allow visualization of the parenchyma and vasculature within the lung. Note that the detail of the mediastinum and subcutaneous tissues is no longer evident. **C,** Bone windows (wide window width) allow evaluation of bony trabeculae and cortex, but contrast within the soft tissues has diminished relative to the mediastinal windows. The lung parenchyma is again black, and vessels are not visible.

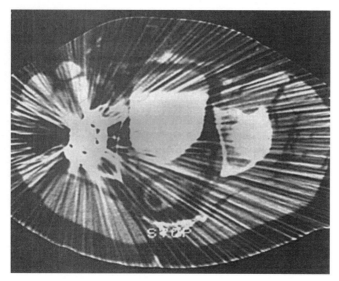

Figure 25.20. Metal joint prosthesis causes attenuation of x-rays and loss of detail adjacent to the structure.

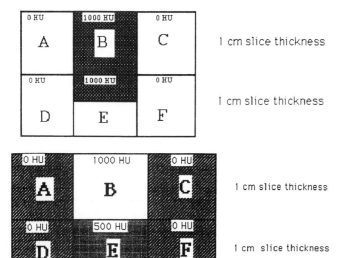

Figure 25.21. **A,** Partial volume artifact (see text for details). **B,** Partial volume artifact: image display. Box E now contains an artifactual intermediate density of 500 HU (see text for details).

density material acts to stop or attenuate many of the radiographs such that image quality is reduced and information adjacent to the devices is lost (Fig. 25.20). A third common artifact in CT is known as partial volume artifact. Here, the partial inclusion of a structure in an axial slice leads to false attenuation values and thus alters the final image. Assume pixel B (Fig. 25.21, **top**) is filled with a "mass" having a HN value of +1000; this mass also fills half of pixel E. All other pixels contain water and thus have HN equal to 0. Pixel E is half-filled with the mass, and therefore, half of the pixel has a HN of 0 and half of the pixel has a HN of +1000. The computer is forced to assign the entire pixel an intermediate value of 500 HN. When the final image is displayed (Fig.

25.21, **bottom**), only pixel B will contain the mass. Pixel E will contain an artifactual intermediate value.

However, if the slice thickness were narrowed to 0.5 cm, pixel E would now be composed of pixels H and K (Fig. 25.22A). The mass would totally fill pixels B, E, and H. Pixel K would contain only water and would thus maintain a HN of 0. Now when the final image is generated, an artifactual intermediate gray structure no longer results (Fig. 25.22B). As this example illustrates, if partial volume artifact is suspected, thinner slices eliminate or reduce the artifact.

Contrast

There are two types of contrast administration important to CT images: gastrointestinal and intravenous. Gastrointestinal (oral, rectal, or both) contrast material usually consists of either a water-soluble iodine compound or a dilute barium solution. Although the barium is the same barium used in upper and lower GI studies, it is of a much lower concentration, typically 2% to 3% rather than the 55% to 85% used for the GI studies. If the higher concentration were used, it would act to attenuate a large percentage of the radiographs and give artifacts similar to those seen with metal joint prosthesis (see the previous "Artifacts"). Thus, if a patient is to undergo both a CT of the abdomen and a GI study, either do the CT first or allow all of the barium from the GI study to clear before doing the CT. Gastrointestinal contrast administration is crucial in the evaluation of the abdomen and pelvis in search of an abscess. Nonopacified loops of bowel may look identical to an abscess and differentiation between the two often relies on filling the bowel with contrast material (Fig. 22.23).

The second type of contrast important to CT images is the intravenous type, often called "dye" in lay terms. These materials are various water-soluble solutions containing iodine. Iodine acts to attenuate radiographs, and this appears as a whiter area on the CT images. The liver, spleen, kidneys, pancreas, and major vessels can be seen to enhance (brighten) after intravenous contrast administration (Fig. 25.24). Tissues such as renal cysts, various neoplasms, and infarcted areas often do not enhance to the degree of surrounding tissue and thus appear relatively dark on the CT image. Today, there are two large categories of intravenous contrast material available: the ionic and the nonionic groups. Both of these agents contain iodine, but the carrier molecule to which the iodine is bound is different, as is the osmolality and number of ions in solution. In general, there are less adverse effects with the nonionic contrast (although severe reactions are possible). However, the cost of the nonionic material ranges from 10 to 15 times that of ionic contrast. Thus, each patient must be evaluated individually to determine which type of intravenous contrast is to be used. Some common indications for nonionic contrast use are shown in Table 25.1.

RESOLUTION OF PARTIAL VOLUME ARTIFACT USING NARROW SLICE SELECTION:

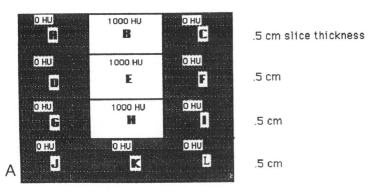

WITH THINNER SLICE THICKNESS, FINAL IMAGE DISPLAY NO LONGER INCLUDES AN ARTIFACTUAL GREY AREA.

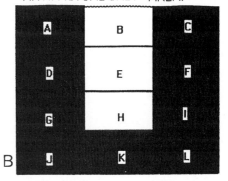

Figure 25.22. **A,** Narrow slice selection aids in eliminating partial volume artifact (see text for details). **B,** Narrow slice selection: image display (see text for details).

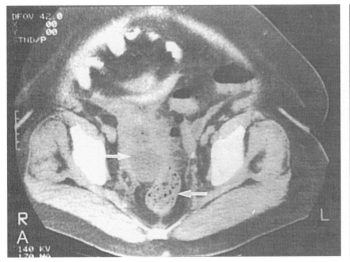

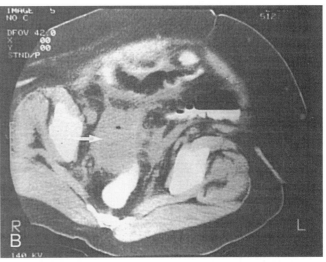

Figure 25.23. **A,** Axial image of the pelvis demonstrates several fluid- and air-filled structures in a patient in whom an abscess was suspected. **B,** After rectal contrast administration, the more posterior "collection" is seen to represent bowel. The more anterior fluid structures never opacified with contrast and were abscesses.

The degree of enhancement is a function of the concentration and amount of intravenous contrast given as well as the method in which it is administered. Typically, 100 to 180 ml of a 60% iodine solution are administered. Maximal enhancement is seen when the contrast is given quickly (1.5 to 2.5 ml/sec) and images are acquired rapidly during the inflow of contrast. Once equilibrium between the intravascular and interstitial components of tissue is reached, lesions may become isodense (indistinguishable/same HN) with the surrounding tissue. Contrast may be administered through an intravenous catheter via an electronically powered injector or manually with a syringe. The power injector allows both a steady delivery of contrast and rapid infusion and requires relatively proximal good venous access (i.e., antecubital veins).

Intravenous contrast material carries some inherent risks to the patient. Mild side effects such as sneezing, nausea, vomiting, hives, or a heat sensation are relatively common. More serious reactions, such as cardiac arrhythmia, anaphylaxis, or renal failure, occur in approximately 1/10,000 patients. The overall risk of death from ionic intravenous contrast is estimated at 1/40,000 or roughly the same risk as having a fatal reaction to penicillin. Although it is generally accepted that nonionic contrast poses less risk to the patient, it is currently less well defined which risk of adverse effects should warrant the use of nonionic material.

Caution should be exercised when contemplating intravenous contrast administration to patients with pheochromocytoma, multiple myeloma, or myasthenia gravis. A hypertensive crisis can be induced in a patient

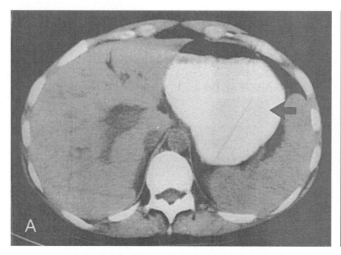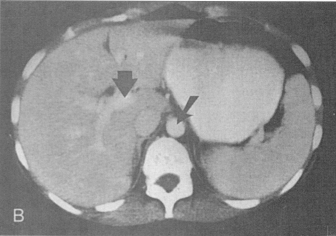

Figure 25.24. **A,** Unenhanced axial CT through the liver, spleen, and stomach. Note oral contrast in stomach. **B,** After intravenous contrast, the liver and spleen enhance. The aorta (*arrow*) and portal veins (*arrow-* *head*) are now seen as bright structures because of the iodine in the contrast.

Table 25.1.
Indications for Non-ionic Contrast

1. Children
2. Prior Contrast Reaction Requiring Treatment
3. Elderly
4. Cardiac Disease
5. Multiple Allergies/Asthma

High risk patients who have a documented need for IV contrast can be given non-ionic material and premedicated with steroids.

with a pheochromocytoma. Similarly, a myasthenia gravis crisis can rarely be induced after intravenous contrast, ultimately leading to respiratory difficulty or failure. Patients with multiple myeloma are at risk of precipitating abnormal proteins in the renal-collecting tubules and thus inducing acute renal failure. Recent reports have disputed this argument and maintain that intravenous contrast can be administered safely to multiple myeloma patients if they are well-hydrated.

Spiral/Helical Computed Tomography

Spiral/helical CT has revolutionized the field of computed tomography. Since its clinical introduction in 1989, tremendous expansion of the clinical applications of computed tomography has occurred, and the performance of existing applications has improved. The advantage of spiral CT over traditional CT is based primarily on the ability to simultaneously acquire data and advance gantry position. The radiograph tube rotates around the patient as the patient is moved along the horizontal axis, thereby circumscribing a spiral path. Projection data acquired at selected locations along this spiral path are interpolated to achieve image reconstruc-

tion. This simultaneous operation of data acquisition and patient translation is made possible by the development of slip ring technology.

In the existing third and fourth-generation scanners, gantry rotation is limited by numerous electrical cables running between the gantry and the stationary CT housing. Despite special cable wind/unwind mechanisms, these cables, essential for data acquisition from the detectors and power supply to the radiograph tubes, filters, and collimators in the gantry, restrict gantry rotation to two complete rotations, after which a reversal in rotation is required for continued scanning. Slip ring design of spiral CT eliminates these restricting cables and instead links the stationary CT housing via several electrically conductive brushes to parallel conductive rings on the gantry. The modifications in gantry along with development of high heat capacity radiograph tubes and faster computers with larger memory capacities have signficantly shortened scan time. Scan time has been reduced further by elimination of the 6 to 7 second interscan delay needed for traditional CT scanners. These innovations translate into an approximately seven-fold decrease in scan time with spiral CT. Typical spiral acquisitions of the chest, abdomen or pelvis, for example, are completed in 30 to 40 seconds, roughly a single breath hold.

Besides the obvious advantage of shortening scan time, complete imaging during a single breath hold improves detection of small lesions, previously easily missed because of respiratory variation and misregistration. Furthermore, rapid coverage of large areas allows imaging to be performed at the most optimal stage of contrast enhancement, which again improves lesion detection. Finally, small lesion conspicuity can be enhanced further by overlapping reconstruction, thus reducing partial volume effects. For example, 10 mm sections can be reconstructed at 5 mm intervals. Also, high quality coronal, sagittal or 3 D reconstruction of images can be obtained, which, unlike conventional CT, does not suffer from motion artifact, assuming the patient was able to hold still for the 30 to 40 seconds. Also, the use of non-ionic contrast material has been suggested, which is better tolerated by the patient, with less nausea and vomiting.

The total volume of contrast required for certain applications of spiral scanning can be reduced substantially. Contrast enhanced spiral scans of the chest, for example, can be performed with half the usual dose (60 ml instead of 120 ml of 60% contrast) and yet allow imaging during peak opacification of the major vascular structures. Thus, spiral CT has many advantages over conventional CT. Its improved technology can be applied to all the usual CT imaging indications, along with promising strides being made in more innovative fields, such as CT angiography of the cerebrovascular and peripheral circulations and oncologic applications.

In summary, CT uses ionizing radiation to generate its images which are predominately in the axial plane. It frequently requires administration of both oral and intravenous contrast material, either ionic or nonionic. The ionic contrast material carries more risk of adverse side effects to the patient. Manipulation of the window level and center allows the image display to vary according to the particular tissue of interest (7–10).

MRI

Magnetic resonance (MR) is a newer imaging modality that relies on strong magnetic fields to generate its images. Unlike CT, no ionizing radiation is used. Images may be acquired in virtually any plane, unlike CT, for which images are restricted to the axial plane. As in CT, the image is composed of pixels, and each pixel is assigned a numeric value. In CT, the value reflects the attenuation of radiographs by a given area of tissue. In MR, the value reflects the intensity of the MR signal arising from the tissue. The intensity is a function of the number of resonating nuclei (proton density) and two tissue parameters known as T_1 and T_2.

A nucleus that has an odd number of either protons or neutrons generates a small magnetic field or moment when it spins. Thus, when these nuclei are placed in strong magnetic fields, their magnetic moments tend to align with those of the external field. When a short burst of radio waves is applied (radio frequency, or RF, pulse), the nuclei are disturbed from their alignment with the external magnetic field. As they attempt to realign with the magnetic field, they emit a signal that can be detected and processed to generate an MR image. Because of the abundance of water within the body, hydrogen is the nucleus most often used to generate MR images. The number of available protons (proton density) in a sample of tissue is an important determinant of signal strength. Areas of high proton density such as urine are

capable of giving off strong signals. Areas of low proton density (i.e., low water content) such as cortical bone, air, and tendons typically give off weak signals and are seen as black areas in the images.

In addition to proton density, the T_1 and T_2 values of a given tissue determine final signal intensity. Both T_1 and T_2 are time constants measured in milliseconds. T_1 describes the rate at which the protons disturbed by the RF pulse will realign with the external magnetic field. T_2 relaxation refers to a process in which spinning protons no longer spin in phase with one another and, therefore, cancel each other's magnetic moments. This cancellation causes a loss of signal. T_1 and T_2 are independent of one another and are distinct for each tissue.

Every MR image is composed of T_1, T_2, proton density, and flow information. Certain parameters can be adjusted to alter the contribution from each of the previous tissue characteristics. Thus, a T_1-weighted image contains mainly information about the T_1 relaxation time, although contributions are also present from T_2, proton density, and flow information. In general, tissues with short T_1 values (e.g., fat) will be bright on a T_1-weighted image. On the contrary, tissues with long T_2 values (e.g., water) will be bright on a T_2-weighted image. Many pathologic areas have a longer T_1 and T_2 than surrounding normal tissue. The effects of flowing blood on the final images are complex and beyond the realm of this discussion. Depending on the parameters chosen, flowing blood may be black or white in the MR image.

Hazards

The strength of most clinical magnets in use today ranges from 0.5 to 1.5 Tesla (1 Tesla = 10,000 gauss). This is approximately 20,000 times the force of gravity on earth! It is precisely this intense magnetization that is the source of potential hazards. One must remember that unlike CT, for which radiographs are turned on and off, in MR *the magnet is always on!* It is costly and potentially injurious to the equipment to turn the MR "off." Thus, although one cannot see or hear it, the external magnetic field is always on. The magnetic force of the magnet can transform a normally benign object into a potentially lethal projectile. Objects such as scissors, oxygen tanks, "crash carts," intravenous poles, jewelry, and keys have been drawn into the magnet. It is crucial, therefore, that patients and physicians be screened for such objects before entering the MR area. Similarly, patients with certain types of implanted metal, surgical clips, or shrapnel are at risk if the metal is a type that is attracted to the magnetic field. Such objects may then be torqued, moved, or disabled. Not all implanted metals pose a threat to patient safety. Some are not attracted to the external magnetic field and thus do not run the risk of displacement. However, they do cause a distortion of the local magnetic field and thus image degradation. Examples would include most prosthetic joints, dental braces, and most rods, nails, and screws used in orthopedic hardware. Patients with implanted pacemakers risk pacer malfunction when exposed to high electromagnetic forces.

A less common hazard exists as a result of the heating effects of the RF energy generated by the MR systems. This energy can potentially heat the wires and gating devices attached to the patient to the point at which they burn the patient or set fire to combustible material. ECG leads, pacing leads, and electrodes should be used and placed with care. The wires should not be excessively long, coiled, or touching the sides of the magnet.

Long-term risks of MRI exposure are unknown. Most data suggest that diagnostic MRI is safe, although effects on MRI workers who are exposed daily is uncertain. Similarly, any long-term effects on pregnant women or fetuses are not known.

Uses

MRI has several advantages over other radiologic exams. Its noninvasive nature allows painless evaluation of patients. There is relatively little manipulation required, which allows patients to be scanned after an acute injury. MRI images may be obtained in virtually any plane, unlike CT for which images are usually limited to the axial (or infrequently coronal) plane.

The inherent soft tissue contrast of MRI is particularly useful in interpreting musculoskeletal abnormalities. Muscles, tendons, cartilage, and ligaments that are poorly seen on plain radiographs are seen in exquisite detail by MRI (Fig. 25.25). On the contrary, cortical bone is better evaluated by plain radiographs or CT. Bone marrow or medullary bone is well seen by MRI and a process that replaces normal marrow is readily detected (Fig. 25.26).

MRI has also been useful in the evaluation of the neurologic system. The brain and spinal cord are well-imaged without the artifact from overlying bone, which can be problematic on CT.

More recent uses of MRI include evaluation of the male and female pelvis, for which the anatomy can be well-defined, and staging of pelvic neoplasms performed (Fig. 25.27). MRI of the abdomen is often limited by motion artifact from breathing, bowel peristalsis, and pulsatile blood flow. Despite these limitations, abdominal MRI can be of use in selected cases. Detection of subtle hepatic metastasis and extent of renal cell carcinoma are two situations for which MRI may be useful (Fig. 25.28A).

Patients who cannot receive the iodinated contrast material used in CT may benefit from an MRI exam. Flowing blood provides inherent contrast in MR images, and thus adequate information can often be obtained without the use of intravenous contrast (Fig. 25.28B).

Although it can be a particularly useful examination, MRI does have several drawbacks. Patients with pace-

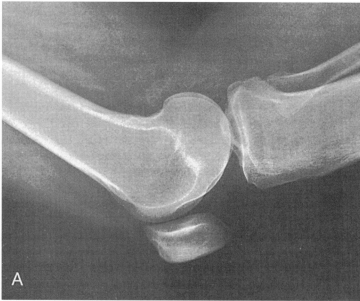
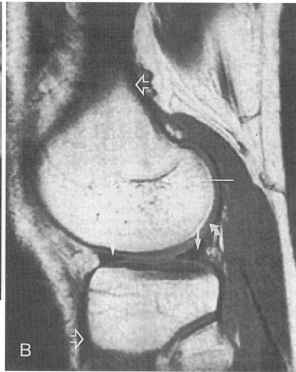

Figure 25.25. **A,** A normal lateral plain film of the knee displays the bony structures, but soft tissues such as menisci, cartilage, and muscular detail can not be visualized. **B,** A normal T$_1$-weighted sagittal view of the knee depicts the internal architecture in detail. Cortical bone (*arrowheads*) is black. Medullary bone (*straight long arrow*) appears bright. The menisci (*short straight arrows*) are low signal intensity because of their low water content. Articular cartilage (*curved arrow*) can be clearly seen. Muscle bundles can be clearly defined posterior to the femur and tibia.

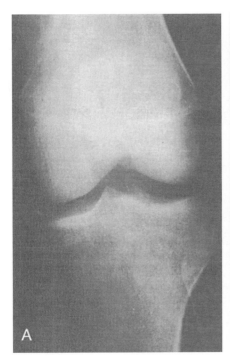
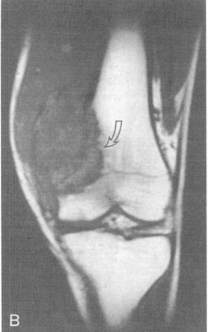
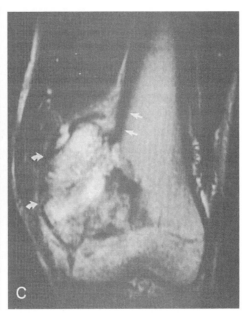

Figure 25.26. **A,** Plain film of the knee demonstrates periosteal reaction and mottled appearance to the distal femur in a patient with an osteosarcoma. **B,** A T_1-weighted MR image clearly shows involvement of the marrow of the distal femur. The tumor does not extend to the proximal tibia. **C,** A T_2 coronal image demonstrates tumor extension through the cortex into the adjacent soft tissues. Note that the lesion is low-signal intensity on T_1- and higher-signal intensity on T_2-weighted images.

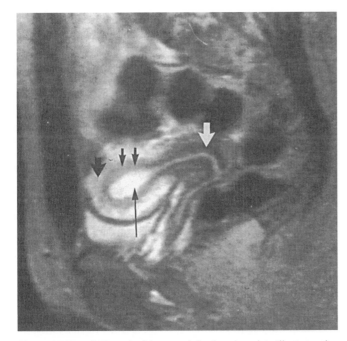

Figure 25.27. A T_2 sagittal image of the female pelvis illustrates the internal architecture of the uterus. The endometrium can be seen as a central bright area (*long arrow*). The myometrium is of intermediate signal intensity (*dark arrow*) and the junctional zone (*short arrows*) appears as a dark band. The cervix (*white arrow*) contains a significant amount of fibrous tissue and thus has a relatively lower signal intensity. The dark circular structures represent air-filled bowel.

makers, certain cardiac prosthetic valves, or any implanted ferromagnetic (attracted to the magnetic field) material should not be placed in the MRI unit. As mentioned previously, many implanted metals do not pose a hazard to the patient, but they may cause significant image degradation.

In summary, MRI is an imaging technique that uses no ionizing radiation to generate its images. The ability to depict soft tissue detail and provide inherent detection of flowing blood are among its major advantages. Unfortunately, it is currently a more costly exam that either CT or ultrasound, and the high magnetic field strengths preclude evaluation of some patients. To determine the most appropriate study to be performed, it is imperative to correlate the patient's condition with the clinical information desired (11).

Nuclear Imaging

Nuclear medicine is a dynamic specialty that uses radioactive compounds in the diagnosis and treatment of diseases. The standard cross-sectional radiologic modalities (ultrasound, CT, and MRI) use external energy sources to create detailed anatomical images. In contrast, nuclear imaging uses primarily intravenously administered radiopharmaceuticals ("tracers"). Localization of these organ-specific tracers generates unique functional images that not only reflect the underlying pathophysiology but also demonstrate important morphologic characteristics of the organ system under study.

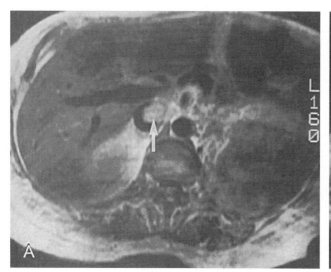
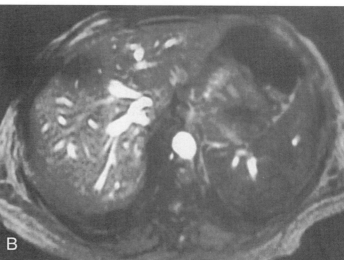

Figure 25.28. Alteration of various scan parameters allows flowing blood to be depicted clearly. The flow may be of either low- (**A**) or high- (**B**) signal intensity, depending on the parameters and pulse sequences chosen. **A,** The patient demonstrates a left renal cell carcinoma with extension of tumor thrombus into the cava (*arrow*). Flowing blood in the cava is black. **B,** Different scan parameters now cause the flowing blood in hepatic and portal veins to appear white.

A γ-camera collects photons (γ-rays) emitted from the patient's body during decay of the radioactive tracer. Routine 2-D (planar) images are obtained either directly from the γ-camera (analogue images) or via an interfaced computer system (digital images). Specialized nuclear tomographic imaging (single photon emission computed tomography, SPECT) has widespread clinical applications, e.g., brain and cardiac imaging. This technique creates higher resolution images oriented in transverse, coronal, and sagittal planes, yielding improved detection and localization of certain disease processes compared with planar imaging.

^{99m}Tc, ^{67}Ga, and ^{111}In are three of the radionuclides commonly used in the evaluation of the surgical patient. These tracers are injected either without modification (e.g., ^{67}Ga) or complexed to various carrier molecules (e.g., ^{99m}Tc sulfur colloid for liver/spleen imaging and ^{111}In-labeled white blood cells for infection imaging).

The differential diagnosis of right upper quadrant abdominal pain includes acute cholecystitis. Hepatobiliary imaging used ^{99m}Tc-labeled iminodiacetic acid (IDA) compounds that are taken up and excreted into bile by the same hepatocellular mechanism as is bilirubin. Hyperbilirubinemia, through competition with IDA agents for biliary handling, may adversely affect study outcome. Best results are achieved with bilirubin levels <10 mg/dl, although diagnostic studies may be obtained with levels exceeding 20 mg/dl. Failure to visualize the gallbladder identifies cystic duct obstruction, the hallmark of acute cholecystitis. To shorten study time from the conventional 4 hours to 90 minutes and to decrease false-positive results, pharmacologic intervention with intravenous morphine sulfate is often used. Via its physiologic action of increasing sphincter of Oddi tone, morphine promotes retrograde filling of the gallbladder

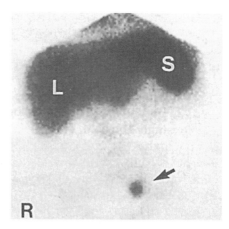

Figure 25.29. Discrete focal accumulation of ^{111}In WBC in the left lower quadrant of the abdomen (*arrow*), typical of abscess formation. *L,* liver; *S,* spleen; *R,* right.

with radioactive bile, thereby establishing cystic duct patency.

Postoperative infection is an unwelcome complication. CT or ultrasonography alone is unable to establish the physiologic significance of intra-abdominal fluid collections or soft-tissue abnormalities in the febrile postoperative patient. Both ^{67}Ga and radio-labeled autologous white blood cells (WBC) possess high sensitivity and specificity for localizing abdominal infection (Fig. 25.29). Two major limitations to the use of ^{67}Ga, which is available ready for injection, are (*a*) delay in imaging (typically 48 to 96 hours after injection) and (*b*) prominent physiologic bowel excretion that can obscure abnormal accumulation at sites of intra-abdominal infection. Labeled WBC require several hours of careful preparation to maintain cell viability and function under sterile conditions, but imaging is usually completed within 24 hours after injection. The abdomen is evaluated more readily with WBC than with ⁶⁷Ga because any radioactivity outside the liver, spleen, and bone marrow is abnormal and may represent a site of infection or inflammation. Both chronicity of infection and prior antibiotic therapy may decrease the sensitivity of WBC imaging; despite its limitations, ⁶⁷Ga may be the preferred imaging agent under these circumstances.

The site of active gastrointestinal bleeding in the small bowel or colon may be identified readily by the intraluminal extravasation of ⁹⁹ᵐTc sulfur colloid or ⁹⁹ᵐTc-labeled RBC. When intraluminal, this tracer activity moves and changes configuration over time (Fig. 25.30). The study is less sensitive for localizing gastric

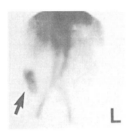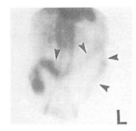

Figure 25.30. **Left,** Early anterior abdominal image showing initial site of ⁹⁹ᵐTc RBC extravasation in the region of the cecum (*arrow*) with rapid transit through the transverse and descending colon. **Right,** At 40 minutes later (*arrowheads*). Possible etiologies include arteriovenous malformation, tumor, angiodysplasia, previous biopsy sites, and diverticular disease. *L*, left.

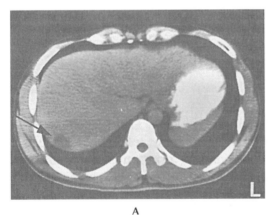

A

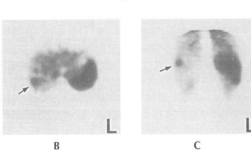

B   C

Figure 25.31. **A,** Transverse CT image showing a 2-cm lesion in the posterior superior right lobe of the liver (*arrow*). Comparable transverse (**B**) and coronal (cfbC) SPECT images demonstrate focal accumulation of ⁹⁹ᵐTc RBC (*arrows*) whose activity exceeds that of the remainder of the liver, an appearance characteristic of cavernous hemangioma. *L,* left.

and duodenal sites of bleeding. Bleeding rates as low as 0.1 ml/min can be detected; by comparison, standard angiography requires much faster bleeding rates of 0.5 to 1.0 ml/min. The nuclear bleeding scan best serves as a precursor to more definitive therapy by directing the site of surgery, colonoscopy with laser therapy, or selective angiography with intra-arterial vasopressin or embolization.

A problematic patient is one with a surgically resectable primary tumor (e.g., colon carcinoma) and an asymptomatic solitary liver mass. The differential diagnosis includes metastasis and cavernous hemangioma, a common, benign liver tumor found in up to 10% of the general population. The ⁹⁹ᵐTc RBC scan with SPECT imaging can accurately identify a hemangioma as small as 1.4 cm (Fig. 25.31), eliminating the need for more extensive evaluation.

Nuclear imaging, by providing physiologic information complementary to the more conventional anatomic radiologic modalities, has a unique role in the evaluation of the surgical patient (12,13,14).

Stereotactic Guided Core Breast Biopsy

As the public becomes increasingly aware of breast cancer detection by screening mammography, the greater number of mammograms performed has resulted in the increased discovery of non-palpable breast lesions. In the past, these lesions were excised surgically after mammographic needle localization. Subsequently, fine-needle aspiration biopsy (FNAB) techniques became popular. FNAB, however, has been somewhat limited due to often difficult cytologic evaluation, insufficient material obtained, and limited availability of competent cytopathologists. Recently, percutaneous biopsy of non-palpable breast lesions with stereotactic mammography has been successful in histopathologic diagnoses.

The candidates for stereotactic biopsy are patients in whom a non-palpable suspicious breast lesion is present, or one in whom suspicious calcifications exist. The patient lies prone with the breast exposed beneath the table. The apparatus, including imaging equipment, compression device, and the automated core biopsy device are located beneath the table, allowing easy accessibility for the physician. An initial digital image of the breast is obtained to visualize the suspect lesion. Stereo images are obtained at 15° off center to the lesion in each direction. These coordinates can then be measured in relation the film as radiographs are taken. By this mathematical relationship, the lesion position is determined by the computer with respect to X, Y, and Z coordinates. The coordinates are sent to the biopsy device, and the position is again verified before deployment with addition stereo views.

A skin incision is made with a scalpel for needle passage. A fourteen-gauge needle is advanced through the incision and deployed. After firing, post-biopsy images are obtained to verify that the needle has traversed the area of interest. Specimen radiographs are obtained to evaluate for the presence of calcification(s). Through the same skin incision, multiple passes are made to provide adequate tissue sampling. Initial sampling may be done centrally, followed by cores at 12-, 3-, 6-, and 9-o'clock positions.

Indications for using stereotactic breast biopsy for non-palpable breast lesions include suspicious masses without calcifications, suspicious masses with calcifications; and suspicious calcifications without associated mass. The method and number of samples may vary with the type of lesion. For masses with calcification and suspicious calcifications alone, a sufficient number of passes is made to adequately sample the lesion. Specimen radiographs are then performed to evaluate for the calcifications. Diagnostic yield may reach 92–99% with six or more samples. Five samples are suggested for all masses. For lesions with calcification, specimen radiographs may be taken after five cores. If no calcifications are seen, more samples should be obtained. However, with greater than ten samples, specimens tend to be composed mainly of hemorrhage. The average time for a trained physician to perform this procedure is approximately 20 minutes.

Stereotactic breast biopsy allows specific histopathologic diagnoses. With respect to benign appearing lesions mammographically, periodic surveillance by mammography is the method of choice. There are, however, two instances when a core biopsy may be useful: first, when periodic follow-up will not occur, as with poor patient compliance; second, when patient anxiety can be relieved. A benign diagnosis by core biopsy (i.e. fibroadenoma or inframammary lymph node) can be made and open biopsy can be avoided. In patients with malignant-appearing lesions, a definitive surgical procedure may be planned based on the findings at core biopsy. Stereotactic breast biopsy may thus convert a two stage procedure (surgical biopsy followed by definitive surgical procedure) into a one-stage procedure. Other advantages of stereotactic breast biopsy include: 1) ease of scheduling, 2) minimal trauma, 3) no scarring, 4) short recovery, and 5) no confusing scars for future mammographic interpretation. Potential pitfalls include: 1) fibroadenomas may be difficult to penetrate or diagnose and some calcifications may be displaced by the core needle, 2) lesions with mammographic findings suggestive of radial scar may have core findings similar to carcinoma, 3) lesions near the chest wall are not accessible, and 4) hematoma formation. In summary, stereotactic breast biopsies performed by a trained physician is a reliable method to obtain tissue for histopathologic evaluation (15–22).

Selected Therapeutic Technologies Useful in General Surgery

Electrosurgery

Most of the common technology used in clinical general surgery depends on the effect of transfer of energy to tissue. By understanding the basic principles of the most common surgical tool in use, electrosurgery, it is possible to create the framework for understanding different and newer forms of energy transfer: laser, ultrasonic aspiration, and lithotripsy. The biologic principles remain surprisingly constant.

By virtue of the high water and electrolyte concentrations, living tissue is a good conductor of electrical current. Electrical current used in clinical surgery is predominantly alternating. Standard electrical current is relatively slow oscillations (60 cps, i.e., 60 Hz) and leads to polarization/depolarization of the neuromuscular junction, manifested clinically as twitching. At 100,000 cps (100 kHz), the effect is one of tetanic contraction. At 200 kHz to 5 MHZ, the oscillations are so rapid that tetany never occurs, but rather the high-frequency molecular oscillations generate heat. At the high end of electrosurgical frequencies, e.g., 4 MHZ, the energy is similar to the electromagnetic energy of radio waves and difficult to contain within tissue (Fig. 25.32). For this

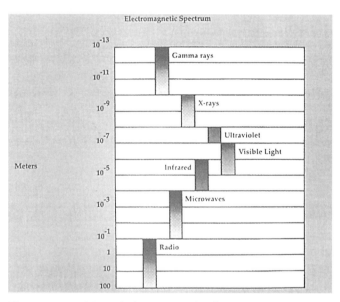

Figure 25.32. This graph demonstrates the electromagnetic spectrum. The speed of light is constant. As the wavelength shortens, the frequency increases. Notice the continuum between electrosurgical current, radio waves, microwave, visible light, and radiograph. The principles of harnessing the electromagnetic spectrum and the tissue reaction are surprisingly constant. Devices and techniques for containing the energy in a useful form is the basis for the different technologies used.

reason, most electrosurgical units function in the midrange of 500 kHz. Because the spectrum of electrical frequencies approaches those of classic radiofrequency, electrical energy is grouped with other forms of radiofrequency electromagnetic energy.

One of the unifying principles of surgical technology is the response of cellular proteins and water to electromagnetic energy. The major determinants of biologic response are (*a*) power density, (*b*) resistance/absorption, and (*c*) time of application.

Power density refers to watts of energy per square centimeter of tissue. Power or current density is inversely proportional to the cross-sectional area of the affected tissue. Therefore, the identical energy (Watts) dispersed over a broad surface has a vastly different biologic effect than pinpoint application. For example, by reducing the area of the electrode (e.g., from surgical clamp to endoscopic wire), the power density and tissue effect is magnified. The electrical current in the monopolar Bovie unit flows through the patient to the indifferent "ground" plate and back to the electrosurgical unit, completing the circuit. The ground plate is in fact active, but the dispersal of the current over a large area greatly reduces power density, resulting in the perception that the ground plate is cold (Fig. 25.33). Too small a ground plate can result in a localized skin burn by concentrating the current to a small area.

When energy is applied to biologic tissue, one of four possible phenomena may occur: (*a*) transmission; (*b*) reflection; (*c*) scatter; and (*d*) absorption. In general, transmission and reflection have minimal direct biologic effect. However, these phenomena are responsible for most secondary accidents to unexpected tissues, e.g., arcing burns with electrocautery. The tissue effect of energy on tissue relates primarily to the effect of absorption and, to a lesser extent, local scatter (diffusion). The

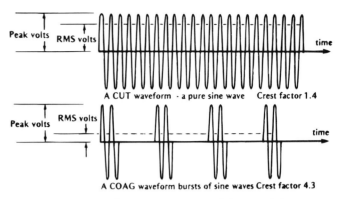

A CUT waveform - a pure sine wave   Crest factor 1.4

A COAG waveform bursts of sine waves Crest factor 4.3

Figure 25.34. Notice the intermittent nature of the coagulation waveform even at the same peak volt setting. The pulsed nature of COAG current is responsible for lower average volts delivered to the tissue, resulting in intermediate tissue heating. *RMS,* root mean square.

net results of these effects are an increase in molecular motion and heat. The power and rate (time intervals) at which the energy is applied determines the speed and magnitude of heating. The characteristics of this tissue heating relate directly to the observed surgical effects of coagulation or incision.

Time and power density are two of the prime determinants of the differential biologic effect on tissue. Intermediate tissue heating (from 37° to 60° C) results in protein denaturation and slow water evaporation. The most obvious result of this effect is tissue desiccation and blood coagulation. The coagulating current (COAG) of an electrosurgical unit produces this form of intermediary tissue heating by rapid discharge of >400 kHz energy with intermittent pause (Fig. 25.34). This pattern results in a deep, relatively even heating. COAG current uses high voltage to drive the current deeper into the tissue as the surface layer dries. Thus the current is able to burn or fulgurate the tissue even after much of the water has evaporated from the cell.

Water is the main conducting medium in cells. As heating occurs, water evaporates, the tissue begins to desiccate, and resistance increases. Increased resistance leads to decreased observed coagulation effect. If the response to increasing resistance is to increase the power, the higher current creates the potential for electrical arcing to tissues of lower, more normal, resistance and unexpected distant tissue injury. This is the probable mechanism of GI tract injury seen with electrocautery and laparoscopic cholecystectomy.

By contrast, instantaneous heating to 100° C results in evaporation, i.e., cellular vaporization at the point of contact. This instantaneous tissue lysis produces steam and cellular debris with minimal surrounding tissue damage (Fig. 25.35). Cutting current is a continuous application of low-voltage, higher frequency, 500-kHz current energy. If COAG settings are high enough, incision can be achieved but with increased local tissue damage compared with cutting current. BLEND is a combination of the two energy patterns, i.e., longer pulses resulting

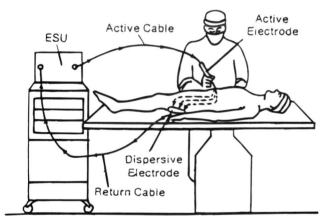

Figure 25.33. This figure shows the practical implications of power density. In an electrosurgical unit, the dispersal of the current over a wide area accounts for the relative neutrality of the cold ground plate electrode by reducing power density. The same current when concentrated within a small focused power density, i.e., scalpel electrode, will result in cutting or coagulation. Notice the similarity to the focusing and defocusing used in laser surgery.

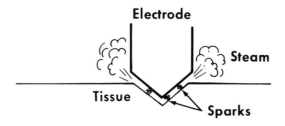

TYPICAL CURRENT=0.1 AMP RMS

Figure 25.35. The cutting current results in instantaneous heating to the boiling point of water and vaporization to steam even at low amperage. Blended current represents a combination of these two wave patterns and leads both to cutting and coagulation.

in heating and vaporization. This same phenomenon of cellular micro evaporation is seen with the application of continuous cutting laser energy as well. Defocused laser energy results in coagulation similar to the principles of coagulating electrosurgical current.

Monopolar versus Bipolar Electrosurgical Current

Electricity will only flow when the circuit is completed or grounded. In monopolar current, the active electrode is in contact with the patient's tissue; the current passes through the patient, with the ground plate completing the circuit through the electrosurgical unit. Monopolar current has the principal advantage of providing a wide spectrum of energy forms, i.e., cutting, coagulation, and blended currents. The primary disadvantage is the arcing phenomenon to nearby tissues as desiccation occurs.

In bipolar current, both electrodes are in close proximity. The circuit is completed between the local tissue only. Bipolar current requires greatly reduced power density because the conducting tissue is small. Waveforms similar to monopolar coagulating current are used in bipolar cautery. Bipolar current is typically used through endoscopes and is effective for coagulation. Recent adaptations of bipolar current are being explored in laparoscopic cholecystectomy.

Argon Beam Coagulation

The argon beam electrocoagulator is an alternative way of current delivery, not a new technology per se. In essence, the jet of argon gas replaces the 3-cm metal tip of the typical electrosurgical unit. Argon gas conducts the electrical current, completing the typical current of a coagulation unit. Because of the gas, small amounts of blood can be blown away from the area to be coagulated, leading to more efficient coagulation with no crusting of the metal tip. Penetration is minimal at usual power density. The argon beam is useful for the coagulation of surface capillaries, e.g., in liver and spleen surgery but is rarely of use in vessels more than 1 mm in size (23,24,25).

Laser

Laser is the acronym for light amplification by stimulated emission of radiation. Normal light energy is dispersed in small packets of electromagnetic waves (photons) when electrons decay from a higher energy to a more stable lower energy state. Normal light is dispersed randomly without synchronicity. Different atoms/molecules release light of different wavelengths; therefore, most natural and artificially produced light is polychromatic. By contrast, laser light is monochromatic in-phase synchronous parallel beam of light, resulting in amplification, power, and direction (Fig. 25.36).

If high-energy electrons are pumped into a given atomic compound (e.g., carbon dioxide or argon), progressively more atoms are raised to a high-energy level. When the rate of energy input exceeds spontaneous decay, a state defined as population inversion occurs, i.e., excessively high energy atoms. Photons are emitted spontaneously by these high-energy atoms. As the photons strike other nearby hyperexcited atoms, further light energy is released. This phenomenon of population inversion and subsequent stimulated emission of electromagnetic light produces a beam of pure monochromatic light unique to the atomic structure of the excited substance.

In clinical lasers, the excited atoms in their population inversion state are contained within a mirrored resonator. Initially, the photons are emitted at directions. As the photons are reflected within the mirrored chamber, the stimulated emission of photons line themselves in a coherent in-phase beam. In addition to being parallel, the waves are synchronous, i.e., positive and negative amplitudes match. This coherent beam is permitted to exit the calibrated point in their reflective chamber, producing the laser beam that is a coherent monochromatic of a single wavelength. It is the synchronicity of wavelength and phase that confers amplification, power, and direction to laser energy.

Laser energy, like other electromagnetic energy, is measured in Watts. Power density is defined as Watts per square centimeter and varies according to the excited substance and the degree of focus. Lasers that can be focused to a very narrow pinpoint, e.g., CO_2, can be used to make incisions, whereas others are useful in coagulation (see "Electrosurgery"). Laser light interaction with tissue produces four possible events: (*a*) reflection, (*b*) transmission, (*c*) scatter, and (*d*) absorption. It is the absorption of laser energy that results in the biologic effect. Reflection, transmission, and scatter are responsible for the complications of laser therapy.

The absorption of laser energy depends on the nature of the monochromatic beam. Like electrosurgery, absorption that results in gradual tissue heating produces coagulation, hemostasis, and even necrosis. Instantaneous heating higher than 100°C results in cellular vaporization and is useful as a cutting instrument. Ultra-

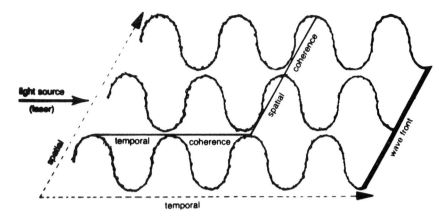

Figure 25.36. Laser light. It is the parallel synchronous nature of laser light that produces its amplification and precision. The randomness dispersion typical of normal radiofrequency energy light has been replaced by a synchronous wave front.

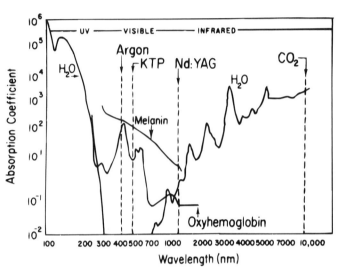

Figure 25.37. Because tissue absorption coefficients differ, the effect of the laser varies. Notice that water absorbs argon and KTP lasers poorly but has a high absorption coefficient for CO_2 laser. Thus, the focused CO_2 beam will lead to rapid heating and cutting characteristics. Argon and KTP lasers are absorbed by oxyhemoglobin because of the absorption coefficient.

sonic effects result in membrane disruption secondary to cavitation.

Clinical lasers depend on the substance exalted (e.g., CO_2, Nd-YAG, and argon) and, therefore, the monochromatic light emitted and the absorption of that specific wavelength by local tissue chromophores. The presence of melanin, hemoglobin, etc., determines which wavelength will be most useful for a given function (Fig. 25.37). Because of the focus and precision of clinical lasers, the area affected is small. In general surgery, the combination of safety precautions, especially in the retina, and small areas leads to longer operating times in most situations.

CO_2 Laser

CO_2 laser light is in the midportion of the infrared spectrum and principally absorbed by water. (Note: infrared radiation is invisible and, therefore, a guiding beam of red light is integrated with the laser only for

directional purposes.) Because of the water absorption, the accuracy of focusing determines whether coagulation is achieved (defocused beam) versus an incision (a precisely focused narrow beam leading to vaporization). Although the CO_2 laser has the advantage of broad application in terms of both cutting and coagulation, its major disadvantage is the inability to be transmitted along fiber optic bundles, i.e., endoscopes.

Nd-YAG Laser

Nd-YAG laser is based on yttrium aluminum garnet crystal doped with Nd, leading to laser light in the near infrared spectrum. Deep tissue penetration is achieved with the Nd-YAG because there is a limited chromophore absorption at this wavelength and moderate scatter. The Nd-YAG laser is most effective when high power heat coagulation is required such as for removing obstructive tumors in the bronchus.

Argon Laser

The argon laser works in the visible light spectrum at approximately 500 nm and is well-absorbed by tissue chromophores, particularly melanin and hemoglobin. For these reasons, argon is ideally suited for treating pigmented lesions of the skin and neovascularization of the retina.

Dye Laser

The dye laser group depends on the solution of organic fluorescent compounds in water or alcohol. The different dyes allow for the production of different wavelengths and, therefore, laser beams with different properties. In contrast to more classical continuous wave lasers, dye lasers are typically pulsed (shuttered) at higher peak energy for brief periods of time. By varying the medium and the exciting source, these pulse dye lasers can result in highly selective tissue damage, depending on the absorbed wavelength. The specific wavelength can be matched to the absorbed property of the tissue chromophore, maximizing laser absorption and minimizing tissue effect.

Excimer Lasers

Excited dimers (halide gases in their excited state) are the basis of the high-energy ultraviolet light excimer lasers. Depths of penetration are extremely shallow ($<100\ \mu$) and can be used for precise cuts (dominantly in ophthalmology) (26).

Ultrasonic Fragmentation

The basic principle underlying the ultrasonic aspirator is the fragmentation of cells by cavitation, i.e., the rapid formation and collapse of vapor bubbles in liquids. Sound waves produce a local change in pressure, typically depicted as a positive and negative sine wave. These waves represent regions of relative compression and rarefaction within tissue water as the wave passes through a specific point (Fig. 25.38). Frequency represents the number of peaks (or troughs) passing a particular point per second and is an inverse function of the inverse of the wavelength.

Sound waves produce local pressure variations in the surrounding cellular fluid. At supersonic speed, the sudden compression and release caused by sound waves encourages submicroscopic bubbles to grow, leading to the phenomenon of cavitation, an effect not unlike the wake seen from high-speed propellers in water. The rapidity of the collapse of the bubble is accelerated by the arrival of the next pressure wave, resulting in magnified pressure changes, molecular motion, heat, and ultimately tissue destruction. It is the cavitation effect, not the sound wave itself, that leads to tissue fragmentation with the ultrasonic scalpel (CUSA). The same cavitation is the phenomenon responsible for stone fragmentation with lithotripsy.

At the cellular level, with normal sound waves, cavitation is insignificant. The repetitive release of energy at the cavity expands and collapses at millions of cycles per second; however, it has a cumulative destructive effect. The aggregate effect of cavitation results in rupture of cells when the ultrasonically vibrating probe is brought in contact with living tissue. In addition, water under the action of cavitation decomposes partially into free radicals, producing hydroxy radicals, and causing secondary effects and local tissue death.

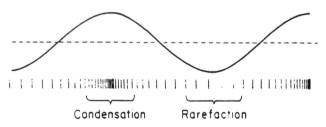

Figure 25.38. The compression and rarefaction effect of a sound wave passing to tissue is depicted diagrammatically. It is this compression and relaxation at ultra high-speed that leads to cavitation.

These two actions are responsible for the biologic usefulness of the ultrasonic aspirator. Water is injected in a spray with the CUSA to dissipate heat. Local heat production leads to coagulation of blood and cellular proteins. Suction is necessary to remove cellular debris and water.

REFERENCES

1. Sanders RC, James AE. The principles and practice of ultrasonography in obstetrics and gynecology. 2nd ed. Norwalk, CT: Appleton, Century, Crofts, 1980.
2. Kremaku FW. Diagnostic ultrasound principles, instrumentation and exercises. 2nd ed. New York: Grune & Stratton, 1984.
3. Fleischer AC, James AE. Introduction to diagnostic sonography. New York: Wiley, 1980.
4. Sarti DA. Diagnostic ultrasound text and cases. 2nd ed. Chicago: Year Book Medical, 1987.
5. Grant EG, White EM. Duplex sonography. New York: Springer-Verlag, 1988.
6. Rose JL, Golberg BB. Basic physics in diagnostic ultrasound. New York: Wiley, 1979.
7. Lee JKT, Sagel SS, Stanley RJ. Computed tomography with MRI correlation. New York: Raven, 1989.
8. Moss A. Computed tomography of the body. Philadelphia: WB Saunders, 1983.
9. Fishman EK, Jeffrey RB, Jr. Spiral CT: Principles, techniques, and clinical applications. New York: Raven, 1995.
10. Zeman RK, Brink JA, Costello P, et al. Helical/Spiral CT: a practical approach. New York: McGraw Hill, 1995.
11. Jackson HG. Fundamentals of magnetic resonance imaging. JAMA 1987;258:3417.
12. Mettler FA, Jr., Guiberteau MJ. Essentials of nuclear medicine imaging. 3rd ed. Philadelphia: WB Saunders, 1991.
13. Gottschalk A, Hoffer PB, Potchen EJ. Diagnostic nuclear medicine. 2nd ed. Baltimore: Williams & Wilkins, 1988.
14. Fogelman I, Maisey M, eds. An atlas of clinical nuclear medicine. St. Louis: CV Mosby, 1988.
15. Liebermann L, Dershaw D, Rosen P, et al. Stereotactic 14-gauge breast biopsy: how many core specimens are needed? Radiology 1994;192:793–795.
16. Parker S, Lovin J, Jobe W, et al. Stereotactic breast biopsy with a biopsy gun. Radiology 1990;176:741–747.
17. Parker S, Lovin J, Jobe W, et al. Nonpalpable breast lesions: Stereotactic large-core biopsies. Radiology 1991;180:403–407.
18. Liebermann L, Dershaw D, Rosen P, et al. Stereotactic core biopsy of breast cancer: Accuracy at predicting invasion. Radiology 1995:194:379–381.
19. Sickles E, Parker S. Appropriate role of core breast biopsy in the management of probably benign lesions. Radiology 1993;188:315.
20. Jackman R, Nowels K, Shepard M, et al. Stereotactic large-core needle biopsy of 450 non-palpable breast lesions with surgical correlation in lesions with cancer or atypical hyperplasia. Radiology 1994;193:91–95.
21. Elvecrog E, Lechner M, Nelson M. Nonpalpable breast lesions: correlation of stereotactic large-core needle biopsy and surgical biopsy results. Radiology 1993;188:453–455.
22. Sickles E. Periodic mammographic followup of probably benign lesions: results in 3,184 consecutive cases. Radiology 1991;179:463–468.
23. Papp JP. Endoscopic treatment of gastrointestinal bleeding: electrocoagulation. In: Sivak MV, ed. Gastroenterologic endoscopy. Philadelphia: WB Saunders, 1987:8:143–157.
24. Odell RC. Principles of electrosurgery. In: Sivak MV, ed. Gastroenterologic endoscopy. Vol. 7. Philadelphia: WB Saunders, 1987:128–142.
25. Hunter JG. Laser or electrocautery for laparoscopic cholecystectomy. Am J Surg 1991;161:345.
26. Absten CT, Joffee SN. Lasers in medicine: an introductory guide. Cambridge, UK: Cambridge University Press, 1985.

Subject Index

Page numbers followed by "t" denotes tables. Page numbers in italics denotes figures.